Fourth Edition
MEDICAL PHARMACOLOGY & THERAPEUTICS

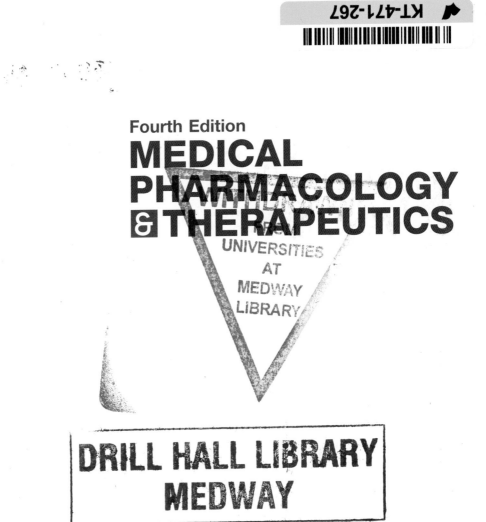

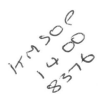

Dedication

To our families

Content Strategist: Jeremy Bowes
Content Development Specialist: Helen Leng
Project Manager: Sukanthi Sukumar
Designer: Christian Bilbow
Illustration Manager: Jennifer Rose
Illustrator: Hardlines, Oxford, Ian Ramsden, David Gardner

Fourth Edition
MEDICAL PHARMACOLOGY &THERAPEUTICS

DEREK G. WALLER BSc (HONS), DM, MBBS (HONS), FRCP

Consultant Physician and Honorary Senior Clinical Lecturer in Medicine and
Clinical Pharmacology
University Hospital Southampton NHS Foundation Trust
Southampton, UK

ANTHONY P. SAMPSON MA, PhD, FHEA, FBPharmacolS

Reader in Clinical Pharmacology
University of Southampton Faculty of Medicine
Southampton, UK

ANDREW G. RENWICK OBE, BSc, PhD, DSc

Emeritus Professor
University of Southampton Faculty of Medicine
Southampton, UK

KEITH HILLIER BSc, PhD, DSc

Former Senior Lecturer in Pharmacology
University of Southampton Faculty of Medicine
Southampton, UK

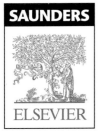

SAUNDERS

ELSEVIER

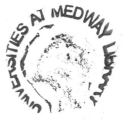

Edinburgh   London   New York   Oxford   Philadelphia   St Louis   Sydney   Toronto 2014

SAUNDERS
ELSEVIER

First edition 2001
Second edition 2005
Third edition 2010
Fourth edition 2014
  Reprinted 2014

ISBN 9780702051807

British Library Cataloguing in Publication Data
A catalogue record for this book is available from the British Library

Library of Congress Cataloging in Publication Data
A catalog record for this book is available from the Library of Congress

Notices

Knowledge and best practice in this field are constantly changing. As new research and experience broaden our understanding, changes in research methods, professional practices, or medical treatment may become necessary.

Practitioners and researchers must always rely on their own experience and knowledge in evaluating and using any information, methods, compounds, or experiments described herein. In using such information or methods they should be mindful of their own safety and the safety of others, including parties for whom they have a professional responsibility.

With respect to any drug or pharmaceutical products identified, readers are advised to check the most current information provided (i) on procedures featured or (ii) by the manufacturer of each product to be administered, to verify the recommended dose or formula, the method and duration of administration, and contraindications. It is the responsibility of practitioners, relying on their own experience and knowledge of their patients, to make diagnoses, to determine dosages and the best treatment for each individual patient, and to take all appropriate safety precautions.

To the fullest extent of the law, neither the publisher nor the authors, contributors, or editors, assume any liability for any injury and/or damage to persons or property as a matter of products liability, negligence or otherwise, or from any use or operation of any methods, products, instructions, or ideas contained in the material herein.

ELSEVIER your source for books,
journals and multimedia
in the health sciences
www.elsevierhealth.com

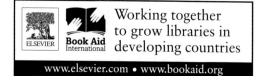

Working together to grow libraries in developing countries

ELSEVIER | Book Aid International

www.elsevier.com • www.bookaid.org

The publisher's policy is to use paper manufactured from sustainable forests

Printed in China

Last digit is the print number: 9 8 7 6 5 4 3 2

Contents

SECTION 8 THE IMMUNE SYSTEM

SECTION 9 THE ENDOCRINE SYSTEM AND METABOLISM

SECTION 10 THE SKIN AND EYES

SECTION 11 CHEMOTHERAPY

SECTION 12 GENERAL FEATURES: TOXICITY AND PRESCRIBING

Preface

The fourth edition of *Medical Pharmacology and Therapeutics* has been extensively revised and updated while preserving the popular approach of the third edition. The text is structured to reflect the ways that drugs are used in clinical practice. It provides information suitable for all healthcare professionals who require a sound knowledge of the basic science and clinical applications of drugs.

As before, a disease-based approach has been taken wherever possible with the aim of explaining clinical pharmacology and therapeutics and the principles of drug use for the management of common diseases. *Medical Pharmacology and Therapeutics* provides sound basic pharmacology background material sufficient to underpin the clinical context. New sections on headache and drug treatment in palliative care have been added and many of the diagrams are new or have been modified to further clarify complex areas of pharmacology.

Each chapter in this fourth edition has the following features.

- An updated and succinct explanation of the major pathogenic mechanisms of the disease and consequent clinical symptoms and signs, helping the reader to put into context the actions of drugs and the consequences of their therapeutic use.
- An updated comprehensive review of major drug classes relevant to the disease in question. Example drugs are used to illustrate pharmacological principles and to introduce the reader to drugs currently in widespread clinical use.
- Basic pharmacology and mechanisms of drug action, key pharmacokinetic properties and important unwanted effects associated with individual drugs and drug classes.
- A structured approach to the principles of disease management, outlining core principles of drug choice and planning a therapeutic regimen for many common diseases.
- An updated drug compendium giving details of most drugs in the classes discussed in the chapter that are available in the UK. For easy reference these tables set out key similarities and differences among drugs in each class and complement the information provided in the chapter.
- Fully revised self-assessment questions and case-based exercises to enable the reader to test their understanding of the principles covered in each chapter.

Chapters covering generic concepts of pharmacology and therapeutics have been extensively updated and include: how drugs work at a cellular level, drug development, drug metabolism and pharmacokinetics, drug toxicity and drug prescribing and genetic variations in drug handling and drug responses.

It is our intention that the fourth edition of this book will encourage readers to develop a deeper understanding of the principles of drug usage that will help them to become safe and effective prescribers and to carry out basic and clinical research and to teach. As medical science advances these principles should underpin the life-long learning essential for the maintenance of these skills.

DGW
APS

Drug dosage and nomenclature

DRUG NOMENCLATURE

In the past, the non-proprietary (generic) names of some drugs have varied from country to country, leading to potential confusion. Progressively, international agreement has been reached to rationalise these variations in names and a single recommended International Non-proprietary Name (rINN) given to all drugs.

Where the previously given British Approved Name (BAN) and the rINN have differed, the rINN is now the accepted name and is used through this book.

A source of minor irritation, however, is that in most authoritative publications issuing from the UK the internationally accepted name is still being called its BAN or new BAN, and this is likely to continue. For full information on this, the reader is referred to: ***www.mhra.gov.uk/How-weregulate/Medicines/Namingofmedicines/Changes-tomedicinesnamesBANstorINNs/CON009669***.

A special case has been made for two medicinal substances: adrenaline (rINN: epinephrine) and noradrenaline (rINN: norepinephrine). Because of the clinical importance of these substances and the widespread European use and understanding of the terms adrenaline and noradrenaline, manufacturers have been asked to continue to dual-label products adrenaline (epinephrine) and noradrenaline (norepinephrine). In this book, where the use of these agents as administered drugs is being described dual names are given. In keeping with European convention, however, adrenaline and noradrenaline alone are used when referring to the physiological effects of the naturally occurring substances.

DRUG DOSAGES

Medical knowledge is constantly changing. As new information becomes available, changes in treatment, procedures, equipment and the use of drugs become necessary. The authors and the publishers have taken care to ensure that the information given in the text is accurate and up to date. However, readers are strongly advised to confirm that the information, especially with regard to drug usage, complies with the latest legislation and standards of practice.

1

General principles

1 Principles of pharmacology and mechanisms of drug action

Much of the success of modern medicine is based on pharmacological science, and this book is confined to pharmacology as it relates to human medicine. Some of the objectives of learning about medical (or clinical) pharmacology are:

- to understand the ways that drugs work to affect biological systems, as a basis for safe and effective prescribing,
- to appreciate that pharmacology cannot be fully understood without a parallel understanding of related biological and clinical sciences, including biochemistry, physiology and pathology,
- to develop numeracy skills for calculating drug doses and dilutions, and to enable accurate comparison of the relative benefits and risks of different drugs,
- to be able to comprehend and participate in research studies advancing knowledge of better treatment of patients.

The answer to the frequently asked question 'What do I need to know?' will depend upon the individual requirements of the course you are studying, your year of study and the examinations you will be taking. The depth and type of knowledge required in different areas and topics may vary as you progress through your studies; for example, early in the course you might not be required to have detailed knowledge of drug monitoring, but you should know whether a drug has a narrow safety margin between its wanted and unwanted effects. Your personal enthusiasm for pharmacology is important and should be driven by the recognition that prescribing medicines is the commonest intervention that most doctors (and, increasingly, other health professionals) make to improve the health of their patients.

Learning about pharmacology is best approached using a variety of resources, in a range of learning scenarios and preferably in the context of clinical care, not from memorising lists of drug facts. We suggest that the following items cover the types of information that you should aim to encounter:

- the non-proprietary (*generic*) drug name (not the *proprietary* or *trade name*),
- the class to which the drug belongs,
- the way the drug works (its *mechanism of action* and its *clinical effects*) and whether these vary significantly among patients,
- the main reasons for using the drug (its *indications*),
- any reasons why the drug should not be used in a particular case (its *contra-indications*),
- whether the drug is available without prescription,
- how the drug is given (*route*, *drug monitoring*),
- the absorption, distribution, metabolism and excretion ('ADME') of the drug (its *pharmacokinetics*), particularly where these show unusual characteristics,

STUDYING PHARMACOLOGY

Pharmacology is the study of the effects of drugs on biological systems. A drug is an active substance administered in an attempt to prevent, diagnose or treat disease, to alleviate pain and suffering, or to extend life. Drugs may be chemically synthesised, or purified from natural sources with or without further modification, but their development and use are based on rational evidence of efficacy and safety derived from controlled experiments and randomised clinical trials. Drugs can be contrasted with placebos (*placebo* is Latin for 'I will please'), defined as inactive substances administered as though they are drugs, but which have no therapeutic effects other than pleasing the patient. Pharmacology evolved on the principle of studying known quantities of purified, active substances to identify their specific mechanisms of action and to quantify their effects in a reproducible manner compared to a placebo or other control.

- the drug's unwanted effects, including its propensity to cause interactions with other drugs or foods,
- whether there are non-pharmacological treatments that are effective alternatives to drug treatment or will complement the effect of the drug.

The key reference for prescribers in the UK is the *British National Formulary* (BNF), available online at www.bnf.org/bnf/index.htm, which contains monographs for nearly all drugs licensed for use in the UK. The Appendix at the end of this chapter provides a formulary of core drugs in each drug class, which gives students in the early stages of training a manageable list of the drugs they are most likely to encounter in clinical practice.

RECEPTORS AND RECEPTOR-MEDIATED MECHANISMS

Pharmacology is a materialist science in the sense that it describes how the material (physical) interaction of drug molecules with their macromolecular targets ('receptors') in the body modifies cellular processes to generate a desired effect. Drugs have been designed to interact with many different types of macromolecules, which evolved to facilitate endogenous signalling between cells, tissue and organs. The activities of most cellular processes are closely controlled to optimise homeostatic conditions in relation to physiological and metabolic requirements. Control can be divided typically into three main stages.

1. **The generation of a biological signal.** Homeostasis is maintained by communication between cells, tissues and organs to optimise bodily functions and responses to external changes. Communication is usually by signals in the form of chemical messengers, such as neurotransmitters, local mediators or endocrine hormones. The chemical signal is termed a *ligand*, because it ligates (ties) to the specialised cellular macromolecule. The cellular macromolecule is a *receptor* because it receives the ligand.
2. **Cellular recognition sites (receptors).** The signal is recognised by responding cells by interaction of the signal with a site of action, binding site or receptor, which may be in the cell membrane, the cytoplasm or the nucleus. Receptors in the cell membrane react with extracellular ligands that cannot readily cross the cell membrane (such as peptides). Receptors in the cytoplasm often react with lipid-soluble ligands that can cross the cell membrane.
3. **Cellular changes.** Interaction of the signal and its site of action in responding cells results in functional changes within the cell that give rise to an appropriate biochemical or physiological response to the original homeostatic stimulus.

Each of these three stages provides important targets for drug action and this chapter will outline the principles underlying drug action mainly in stages 2 and 3.

ACTIONS OF DRUGS AT BINDING SITES (RECEPTORS)

For very many drugs the first step in producing a biological effect is by interaction of the drug with a receptor, either on the cell membrane or inside the cell, and it is this binding that triggers the cellular response. Drugs may be designed to mimic, modify or block the actions of endogenous ligands at that receptor. The receptor table at the end of this chapter shows that cell-membrane and cytosolic receptors tend to occur in different families (receptor types), reflecting their evolution from common ancestral receptors. Within any one family of receptors, different receptor subtypes have evolved divergently to facilitate increasingly specific signalling and distinct biological effects. As might be expected, different receptor families have different characteristics, but subtypes within each family retain common family traits.

In pharmacology, the perfect drug would be one that binds only to one type or subtype of receptor and consistently produces only the desired biological effect, without the unwanted effects that can occur when drugs bind 'off target'. Although this ideal is impossible to attain, it has proved possible to develop drugs that bind avidly to their target receptor to produce their desired effect and have very much less (but not zero) ability to bind to other receptors, even ones within the same family, which might produce unwanted effects.

Where a drug binds to one type of receptor in preference to another it is said to show *selectivity of binding* or *selectivity of drug action*. Selectivity is never absolute but is high with some drugs and low with others. A drug with a high degree of selectivity is likely to show a greater difference between the dose required for its biological action and the dose that produces an unwanted or toxic action.

MAJOR TYPES OF RECEPTORS

Despite the great structural diversity of drug molecules, most act on the following major types of receptors to bring about biological change.

- **Transmembrane ion channels.** These control the passage of ions across membranes and are widely distributed.
- **Seven-transmembrane (heptahelical) receptors.** This is a large family of receptors, most of which signal via guanine nucleotide-binding proteins (G-proteins). Following activation by a ligand, second messenger substances are formed which can bring about cellular molecular changes, including the opening of transmembrane ion channels.
- **Enzyme-linked transmembrane receptors.** This is a family of transmembrane receptors with an integral or associated enzymic component, such as a kinase or phosphatase. They signal changes in cells by phosphorylating or dephosphorylating intracellular proteins, thereby altering their activity.
- **Intracellular (nuclear) receptors.** These receptors are found in the nucleus or translocate to the nucleus from the cytosol to modify gene transcription and the expression of specific cellular proteins.

It should be noted that some mechanisms, such as the opening of ion channels, can be operated by direct interactions of drugs with the channel, or by G-protein-coupled mechanisms occurring as a first step with subsequent intracellular events activating the ion channels.

Transmembrane ion channels

Transmembrane ion channels that create pores across phospholipid membranes are ubiquitous and allow the transport of ions into and out of cells. The intracellular concentrations of ions are controlled by a combination of ion pumps and transporters, which transport specific ions from one side of the membrane to the other in an energy-dependent manner, and ion channels, which open to allow the selective, passive transfer of ions down their concentration gradients. Based on concentration gradients across the cell membrane:

- both Na^+ and Ca^{2+} ions will diffuse into the cell if the channels are open, making the electrical potential of the cytosol more positive and causing depolarisation of excitable tissues,
- K^+ ions will diffuse out of the cell, making the electrical potential of the cytosol more negative and inhibiting depolarisation,
- Cl^- ions will diffuse into the cell, making the cytosol more negative and inhibiting depolarisation.

The two major families of channel are the *ligand-gated ion channels* (*LGICs*) and the *voltage-gated ion channels* (*VGICs*; also called *ionotropic receptors*). LGICs are opened by the binding of a ligand, such as acetylcholine, to an extracellular part of the channel. VGICs are opened at particular membrane potentials by voltage-sensing segments of the channel. Both channel types can be targets for drug action. Both LGICs and VGICs can control the transport of a specific ion, but a single type of ion may be transported by more than one type of channel, including both LGIC and VGIC types. The complexity that has evolved can be seen in the example of the multiple types of K^+ channel listed in Table 8.1.

LGICs include nicotinic acetylcholine receptors, γ-aminobutyric acid (GABA) receptors, glycine receptors and serotonin (5-hydroxytryptamine) 5-HT$_3$ receptors. They are typically pentamers, with each subunit comprising four transmembrane helices clustering around a central channel or pore. Each peptide subunit is orientated so that hydrophilic chains face towards the channel and hydrophobic chains towards the membrane lipid bilayer. Binding of an agonist to the receptor causes a conformational change in the protein and results in extremely fast opening of the ion channel. The nicotinic acetylcholine receptor is a good example of this type of structure (Fig. 1.1). It requires the binding of two molecules of acetylcholine for channel opening. Channel opening lasts only milliseconds because the ligand rapidly dissociates and is inactivated. Drugs may modulate LGIC activity by binding directly to the channel, or indirectly by acting on G-protein-coupled receptors (see below) with the subsequent intracellular events then affecting the status of the LGIC.

VGICs include Ca^{2+}, Na^+ and K^+ channels. The latter consist of four peptide subunits, each of which has between two and six transmembrane helices; in Ca^{2+} and Na^+ channels there are four domains, each with six transmembrane helices, in a single large protein. The pore-forming regions of the transmembrane helices are largely responsible for the selectivity of the channel for a particular ion. Both Na^+ and K^+ channels are inactivated after opening; this is produced by an intracellular loop of the channel, which blocks the

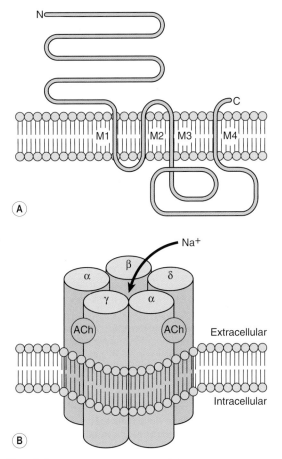

Fig. 1.1 The acetylcholine nicotinic receptor, a typical ligand-gated transmembrane ion channel.
(A) The receptor is constructed from subunits with four transmembrane regions (M1–M4). (B) Five subunits are assembled into the ion channel, which has two sites for acetylcholine binding, each formed by the extracellular domains of two adjacent subunits. On acetylcholine binding, the central pore undergoes conformational change that allows selective Na^+ ion flow down its concentration gradient into the cell. N, amino terminus; C, carboxyl terminus.

open channel from the intracellular end. The activity of VGICs may thus be modulated by drugs acting directly on the channel, such as local anaesthetics which maintain Na^+ channels in the inactivated site by binding at the intracellular site (Ch. 18). Drugs may also modulate VGICs indirectly via intracellular signals from other receptors. For example, L-type Ca^{2+} channels are inactivated directly by calcium channel blockers, but also indirectly by drugs which reduce intracellular signalling from β$_1$-adrenoceptors (see Fig. 5.5).

The ability of highly variable transmembrane subunits to assemble in a number of configurations leads to the existence of many different subtypes of channel for a single ion. For example, there are many different voltage-gated Ca^{2+} channels (L, N, P/Q, R and T types).

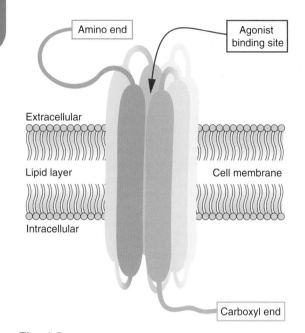

Fig. 1.2 Hypothetical seven-transmembrane (7TM) receptor. The 7TM receptor is a single polypeptide chain with its amino (N-) terminus outside the cell membrane and its carboxyl (C-) terminus inside the cell. The chain is folded such that it crosses the membrane seven times, with each hydrophobic transmembrane region shown here as a thickened segment. The hydrophilic extracellular loops create a confined three-dimensional environment in which only the appropriate ligand can bind. Other potential ligands may be too large for the site or show much weaker binding characteristics. Selective ligand binding causes conformational change in the three-dimensional form of the receptor, which activates signalling proteins and enzymes associated with the intracellular loops, such as G-proteins and nucleotide cyclases.

Seven-transmembrane receptors

Also known as 7TM receptors or the heptahelical receptor family, this is an extremely important group of receptors since the human genome has about 800 sequences for 7TM receptors and they are the targets of about 40% of modern drugs. The structure of a hypothetical 7TM receptor is shown in Figure 1.2; the N-terminal region of the polypeptide chain is on the extracellular side of the membrane and the polypeptide traverses the membrane seven times with helical regions, so that the C terminus is on the inside of the cell. The extracellular loops provide the receptor site for an appropriate agonist (a natural ligand or a drug), the binding of which alters the three-dimensional conformation of the receptor protein. The intracellular loops are involved in coupling this conformational change to the second messenger system, usually via a heterotrimeric G-protein, giving rise to the term G-protein-coupled receptor (GPCR).

The G-protein system

The heterotrimeric G-protein system (Fig. 1.3) consists of α, β and γ subunits.

- **The α-subunit.** More than 20 different types have been identified, belonging to four families (α_s, α_i, α_q and $\alpha_{12/13}$). The α-subunit is important because it binds GDP and GTP in its inactive and active states, respectively; it also has GTPase activity, which is involved in terminating its own activity. When an agonist binds to the receptor, GDP (which is normally present on the α-subunit) is replaced by GTP. The active α-subunit–GTP dissociates from the $\beta\gamma$-subunits and can activate enzymes such as adenylyl cyclase. The α-subunit–GTP complex is inactivated when the GTP is hydrolysed back to GDP by the GTPase.
- **The $\beta\gamma$-complex.** There are many different isoforms of β- and γ-subunits that can combine into dimers, the normal function of which is to inhibit the α-subunit when the receptor is unoccupied. When the receptor is occupied by a ligand, the $\beta\gamma$-complex dissociates from the α-subunit and can itself activate cellular enzymes, such as phospholipase C. The α-subunit–GDP and $\beta\gamma$-subunit then recombine with the receptor protein to give the inactive form of the receptor–G-protein complex.

Second messenger systems

Second messengers are the key distributors of an external signal, as they are released into the cytosol and are responsible for affecting a wide variety of intracellular enzymes, ion channels and transporters. There are two complementary second messenger systems (Fig. 1.4).

Cyclic nucleotide system

One system is based on cyclic nucleotides, such as:

- cyclic adenosine monophosphate (cAMP), which is synthesised from adenosine triphosphate (ATP) by adenylyl cyclase; cAMP induces numerous cellular responses by activating protein kinase A (PKA), which phosphorylates proteins, many of which are enzymes; phosphorylation can either activate or suppress cell activity;
- cyclic guanosine monophosphate (cGMP), which is synthesised from guanosine triphosphate (GTP) via guanylyl cyclase; cGMP exerts most of its actions through protein kinase G, which, when activated by cGMP, phosphorylates target proteins.

There are many isoforms of adenylyl cyclase; these show different tissue distributions and could be important sites of selective drug action in the future. The cyclic nucleotide second messenger (cAMP or cGMP) is inactivated by hydrolysis by phosphodiesterase (or PDE) isoenzymes to give AMP or GMP. There are 11 different families of phosphodiesterase isoenzymes, some of which are currently the targets of important drug groups (Table 1.1).

The phosphatidylinositol system

The other second messenger system is based on inositol 1,4,5-triphosphate (IP_3) and diacylglycerol (DAG), which are synthesised from the membrane phospholipid phosphatidylinositol 4,5-bisphosphate (PIP_2) by phospholipase C (Fig. 1.4). There are a number of isoenzymes of phospholipase C, which may be activated by the α-subunit–GTP or $\beta\gamma$-subunits of G-proteins. The main function of IP_3 is to mobilise Ca^{2+} in cells. With the increase in Ca^{2+} brought about by IP_3, DAG is able to activate protein kinase C (PKC) and

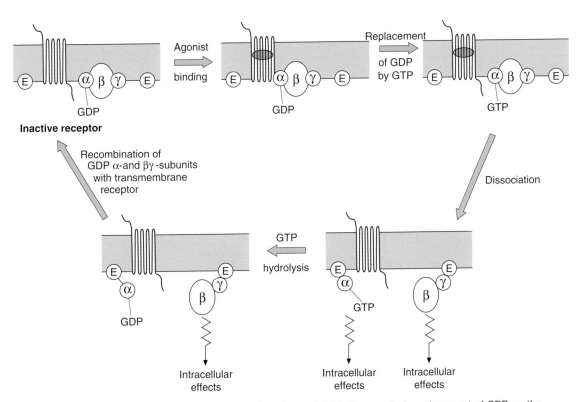

Fig. 1.3 The functioning of G-protein subunits. Ligand (agonist) binding results in replacement of GDP on the α-subunit by GTP and the dissociation of the α- and βγ-subunits, each of which can affect a range of intracellular systems (shown as E on the figure) such as second messengers (e.g. adenylyl cyclase and phospholipase C), or other enzymes and ion channels (see Figs 1.4 and 1.5). Hydrolysis of GTP to GDP inactivates the α-subunit, which then recombines with the βγ-dimer to reform the inactive receptor.

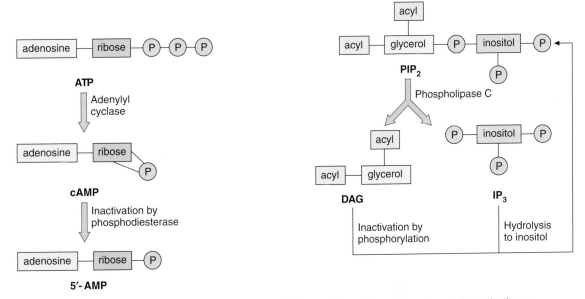

Fig. 1.4 Second messenger systems. Stimulation of GPCRs produces intracellular changes by activating or inhibiting cascades of second messengers. Examples are cyclic adenosine monophosphate (cAMP), diacylglycerol (DAG) and inositol triphosphate (IP_3) formed from phosphatidylinositol 4,5-bisphosphate (PIP_2). See also Figure 1.5.

Table 1.1 Isoenzymes of phosphodiesterase (PDE)

Enzyme	Main substrate	Main site(s)	Drug(s)	Therapeutic potential
PDE1	cAMP + cGMP	Heart, brain, lung, vascular smooth muscle	Under development (vinpocetine)	Undefined
PDE2	cAMP + cGMP	Adrenal gland, heart, lung, liver, platelets	Under development	Undefined
PDE3	cAMP + cGMP	Heart, lung, liver, platelets, adipose tissue, inflammatory cells, smooth muscle	Aminophylline Enoximone Milrinone Cilostazol	Asthma (Ch. 12) Congestive heart failure (see Ch. 7) Peripheral vascular disease (Ch. 10)
PDE4	cAMP	Sertoli cells, kidney, brain, liver, lung, inflammatory cells	Aminophylline Roflumilast	Asthma, COPD (Ch. 12) Inflammation IBD
PDE5	cGMP	Smooth muscle, endothelium, neurons, lung, platelets	Sildenafil Tadalafil Dipyridamole	Erectile dysfunction (Ch. 16) Pulmonary hypertension
PDE6	cGMP	Photoreceptors	Dipyridamole	Undefined
PDE7	cAMP	Skeletal muscle, heart, kidney, brain, pancreas, T-lymphocytes	Under development	Inflammation (combined with PDE4 inhibitor)
PDE8	cAMP	Testes, eye, liver, skeletal muscle, heart, kidney, ovary, brain, T-lymphocytes	Under development	Undefined
PDE9	cGMP	Kidney, liver, lung, brain	Under development	Undefined
PDE10	cAMP + cGMP	Testes, brain	Under development	Schizophrenia?
PDE11	cAMP + cGMP	Skeletal muscle, prostate, kidney, liver, pituitary and salivary glands, testes	Under development	Undefined

cAMP, cyclic adenosine monophosphate; cGMP, cyclic guanosine monophosphate; COPD, chronic obstructive pulmonary disease; IBD, inflammatory bowel disease.

phosphorylate target proteins. IP_3 and DAG are then inactivated and converted back to PIP_2.

Which second messenger systems are activated when a GPCR binds a selective ligand depends primarily on the nature of the $G\alpha$-subunit, as illustrated in Figure 1.5:

- G_s: stimulation of adenylyl cyclase (increases cAMP), activation of Ca^{2+} channels,
- $G_{i/o}$: inhibition of adenylyl cyclase (reduces cAMP), inhibition of Ca^{2+} channels, activation of K^+ channels,
- $G_{q/11}$: activation of phospholipase C, leading to DAG and IP_3 signalling,
- $G_{12/13}$: activation of cytoskeletal and other proteins via the Rho family of GTPases, which influence smooth muscle contraction and proliferation.

The $\beta\gamma$-complex also has signalling activity: it can activate phospholipases and modulate some types of K^+ and Ca^{2+} channels.

Activation of these second messenger systems by G-protein subunits thus affects many cellular processes such as enzyme activity (either directly or by altering gene transcription), contractile proteins, ion channels (affecting depolarisation of the cell) and cytokine production. The many different isoforms of G_α, G_β and G_γ proteins may represent important future targets for selective drugs.

It is increasingly recognised that GPCRs may assemble into dimers of identical 7TM proteins (homodimers) or into heterodimers of different receptor proteins; the functional consequences of GPCR dimerisation and its implications for drug therapy are unclear.

Protease-activated receptors

Protease-activated receptors (PARs) are GPCRs stimulated unusually by a 'tethered ligand' located within the N terminus of the receptor itself, rather than by an independent ligand. Proteolysis of the N-terminal sequence by serine proteases such as thrombin, trypsin and tryptase enables the residual tethered ligand to bind to the receptor within the second extracellular loop (Fig. 1.6). To date, four protease-activated receptors (PAR 1–4) have been identified, each with distinct N-terminal cleavage sites and different tethered ligands. The receptors appear to play roles in platelet activation and clotting (Ch. 11), and in inflammation and tissue repair. Most of the actions of PAR are mediated by G_i, G_q and $G_{12/13}$.

Enzyme-linked transmembrane receptors

Enzyme-linked receptors, most notably the receptor tyrosine kinases, are similar to the GPCRs in that they have a ligand-binding domain (or LBD) on the surface of the cell membrane, they traverse the membrane and they have an

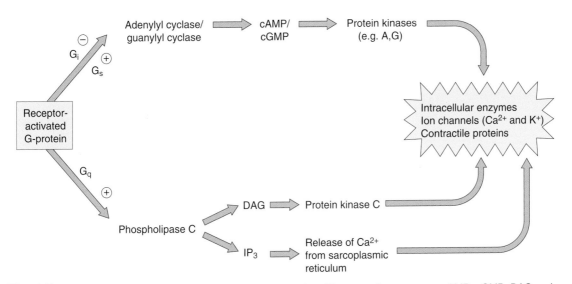

Fig. 1.5 The intracellular consequences of receptor activation. The second messengers cAMP, cGMP, DAG and IP_3 produce a number of intracellular changes, either directly, or indirectly via actions on protein kinases (which phosphorylate other proteins) or by actions on ion channels. The pathways can be activated or inhibited depending upon the type of receptor and G-protein and the particular ligand stimulating the receptor. The effect of the same second messenger can vary depending upon the biochemical functioning of cells in different tissues.

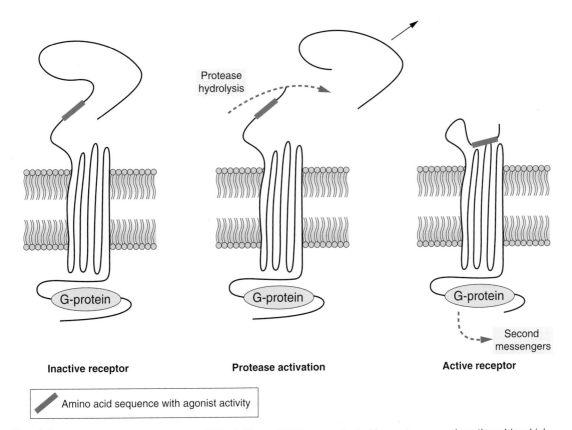

Fig. 1.6 Protease-activated receptors (PARs). These GPCRs are activated by proteases such as thrombin which hydrolyse the extracellular peptide chain to expose a segment that acts as a tethered ligand (shown in red) and activates the receptor. The receptor is inactivated by phosphorylation of the intracellular (C-terminal) part of the receptor protein.

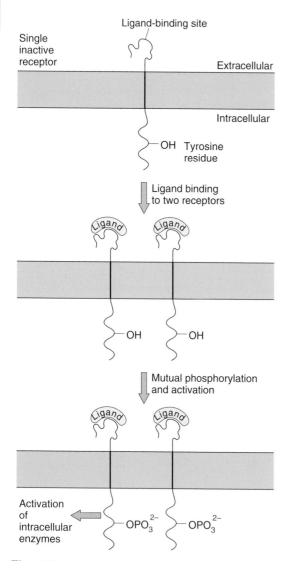

Fig. 1.7 Enzyme-linked transmembrane receptors.
This receptor tyrosine kinase has a large extracellular domain, a single transmembrane segment and an integral kinase domain. Ligand binding causes phosphorylation of tyrosine residues on the receptor and on other target proteins, leading to intracellular changes in cell behaviour. Other enzyme-linked receptors have tyrosine phosphatase, serine-threonine kinase or guanylyl cyclase enzymic activity.

intracellular effector region (Fig. 1.7). They differ from GPCRs in their extracellular ligand-binding site, which is very large to accommodate their polypeptide ligands (including hormones, growth factors and cytokines), and in having only one transmembrane helical region. Importantly, their intracellular action requires a linked enzymic domain, most commonly an integral kinase domain which activates the receptor itself or other proteins by phosphorylation. Activation of enzyme-linked receptors enables binding and activation of many intracellular signalling proteins, leading to changes in gene transcription and in many cellular

functions. There are five families of enzyme-linked transmembrane receptors.

- Receptor tyrosine kinase (RTK) family: ligand binding causes receptor dimerisation and transphosphorylation of tyrosine residues within the receptor itself and sometimes in associated cytoplasmic proteins. Up to 20 classes of RTK include receptors for growth factors, many of which signal via proteins of the mitogen-activated protein (MAP) kinase cascade, leading to effects on gene transcription, apoptosis and cell division. Constitutive over-activity of an RTK called Bcr-Abl causes leucocyte proliferation in chronic myeloid leukaemia, which is treated with imatinib, a drug that blocks the uncontrolled RTK activity.
- Tyrosine phosphatase receptor family: they dephosphorylate tyrosines on other transmembrane receptors or cytoplasmic proteins; they are particularly common in immune cells.
- Tyrosine kinase-associated receptor family (or non-receptor tyrosine kinases): these lack integral kinase activity but activate separate kinases associated with the receptor; examples include inflammatory cytokine receptors and signalling via the Jak/Stat pathways to affect inflammatory gene expression.
- Receptor serine-threonine kinase family: activation of these phosphorylates serine and threonine residues in target cytosolic proteins; everolimus is a serine-threonine kinase inhibitor used in renal and pancreatic cancer.
- Receptor guanylyl cyclase family: members of this family catalyse the formation of cGMP from GTP via a cytosolic domain.

Intracellular (nuclear) receptors

Many hormones act at intracellular receptors to produce long-term changes in cellular activity by altering the genetic expression of enzymes, cytokines or receptor proteins. Such hormones are lipophilic to facilitate their movement across the cell membrane. Examples include the thyroid hormones and the large group of steroid hormones, including glucocorticoids, mineralocorticoids and the sex steroid hormones. Their actions on DNA transcription are mediated by interactions with intracellular receptors (Table 1.2) located either in the cytoplasm (type 1) or the nucleus (type 2).

The intracellular receptor typically includes a highly conserved DNA-binding region with zinc-containing loops and a variable LBD (Table 1.3). The sequence of hormone binding and action for type 1 intracellular receptors is shown in Figure 1.8. Type 1 receptors are typically found in an inactive form in the cytoplasm linked to chaperone proteins such as heat-shock proteins (HSPs). Binding of the hormone induces conformational change in the receptor; this causes dissociation of the HSP and reveals a nuclear localisation sequence (or NLS) which enables the hormone–receptor complex to pass through nuclear membrane pores into the nucleus. Via their DNA-binding domain, the active hormone–receptor complexes can interact with hormone response elements (HRE) at numerous sites in the genome. Binding to the HRE usually activates gene transcription, but sometimes it silences gene expression and decreases mRNA synthesis.

Table 1.2 Some families of intracellular receptors

Type 1 (cytoplasmic)	
Oestrogen receptors	ER (α, β)
Progesterone receptors	PR (A, B)
Androgen receptor	AR
Glucocorticoid receptor	GR
Mineralocorticoid receptor	MR
Type 2 (nuclear)	
Thyroid hormone receptors	TR (α, β)
Vitamin D receptor	VDR
Retinoic acid receptors	RAR (α, β, γ)
Retinoid X receptors	RXR (α, β, γ)
Liver X (oxysterol) receptors	LXR (α, β)
Peroxisome proliferator-activated receptors	PPAR (α, γ, δ)

Table 1.3 The structure of steroid hormone receptor proteins

Section of protein	Domain	Role
A/B	N-terminal regulatory domain	Regulates transcriptional activity
C	DNA-binding domain	Highly conserved; binds receptor to DNA by two zinc-containing regions
D	Hinge region	Enables intracellular translocation
E	Ligand-binding domain	Enables specific ligand binding; also binds chaperone proteins and facilitates receptor dimerisation
F	C-terminal domain	Highly variable; unknown function

Translocation and binding to DNA involves a variety of different chaperone, co-activator and co-repressor proteins, and the system is considerably more complex than indicated in Figure 1.8. Co-activators are transcriptional cofactors that also bind to the receptor and increase the level of gene induction; an example is histone acetylase, which facilitates transcription by increasing the ease of unravelling of DNA from histone proteins. Co-repressors also bind to the receptor and repress gene activation; an example is histone deacetylase, which prevents further transcription by tightening histone interaction with the DNA.

Type 2 intracellular receptors, such as the thyroid hormone receptors (TR) and the peroxisome proliferator-activated receptor (PPAR) family (Table 1.2), are found within the nucleus bound to co-repressor proteins, which are liberated by ligand binding without a receptor translocation step from the cytoplasm. PPAR nuclear receptors

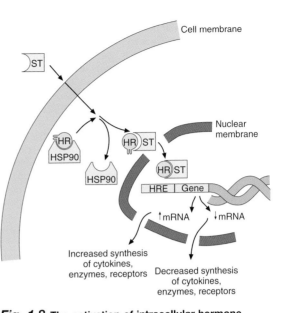

Fig. 1.8 The activation of intracellular hormone receptors. Steroid hormones (ST) are lipid-soluble compounds which readily cross cell membranes and bind to their intracellular receptors (HR). This binding displaces a chaperone protein called heat-shock protein (HSP90) and the hormone–receptor complex enters the nucleus, where it can increase or decrease gene expression by binding to hormone response elements (HRE) on DNA. Intracellular receptors for many other ligands are activated in the nucleus itself.

function as sensors for endogenous fatty acids, including eicosanoids (Ch. 29), and regulate the expression of genes that influence metabolic events.

Intracellular receptors are the molecular targets of 10–15% of marketed drugs, including steroid drugs acting at type 1 receptors and other drugs acting at type 2 receptors. Steroids show selectivity for different type 1 intracellular receptors (ER, PR, AR, GR, MR; see Table 1.2 for a list of abbreviations), which determine the spectrum of gene expression that is affected (Chs 14, 44, 45 and 46). Steroid effects are also determined by differential expression of these receptors in different tissues. Intracellular hormone–receptor complexes typically dimerise to bind to their HRE sites on DNA. Steroid receptors form homodimers (e.g. ER–ER) while most type 2 receptors form heterodimers, usually with RXR (e.g. RAR–RXR). The thiazolidinedione drugs used in diabetes mellitus (Ch. 40) and the fibrate class of lipid-lowering drugs (Ch. 48) act on specific members of the PPAR family of type 2 receptors.

OTHER SITES OF DRUG ACTION

Probably every protein in the human body has the potential to have its structure or activity altered by foreign compounds. Traditionally, all drug targets were described pharmacologically as 'receptors', although many drug targets would not be defined as receptors in biochemical terms; in addition to the receptor types discussed above, drugs may act at numerous other sites.

- **Cell-membrane ion pumps.** In contrast to passive diffusion, primary active transport of ions against their concentration gradients occurs via ATP-dependent ion pumps, which may be drug targets. For example, Na^+/K^+-ATPase in the brain is activated by the anticonvulsant drug phenytoin whereas that in cardiac tissue is inhibited by digoxin; K^+/H^+-ATPase in gastric parietal cells is inhibited by proton pump inhibitors (Ch. 33).
- **Transporter (carrier) proteins.** Secondary active transport involves carrier proteins which transport a specific ion or organic molecule across a membrane; the energy for the transport derives not from a coupled ATPase but from the co-transport of another molecule down its concentration gradient, either in the same direction (symport) or the opposite direction (antiport). Examples are:
  - Na^+/Cl^- co-transport in the renal tubule, which is blocked by thiazide diuretics (Ch. 14),
  - the reuptake of neurotransmitters into nerve terminals by a number of transporters selectively blocked by classes of antidepressant drugs (Ch. 22).
- **Enzymes.** Many drugs act on the intracellular or extracellular enzymes that synthesise or degrade the endogenous ligands for extracellular or intracellular receptors, or which are required for growth of bacterial, viral or tumour cells. Table 1.4 gives examples of drug groups that act on enzyme targets. The family of phosphodiesterase isoenzymes that regulate second messenger molecules are important drug targets and are listed in Table 1.1. As well as being sites of drug action, enzymes are involved in inactivating many drugs, while some drugs are administered as inactive precursors (prodrugs) that are enzymatically activated (Ch. 2).

- **Adhesion molecules.** These regulate the cell-surface interactions of immune cells with endothelial and other cells. Natalizumab is a monoclonal antibody directed against the α_4-integrin component of vascular cell adhesion molecule (VCAM)-1 and is used to inhibit the autoimmune activity of lymphocytes in acute relapsing multiple sclerosis. Other monoclonal antibody-based therapies are targeted at cellular and humoral proteins including cytokines and intracellular signalling proteins to suppress inflammatory cell proliferation, activity and recruitment in immune disease.
- **Organelles and structural proteins.** Examples include some antimicrobials that interfere with the functioning of ribosomal proteins in bacteria, and some types of anticancer drug that interrupt mitotic cell division by blocking microtubule formation.

The sites of action of some drugs remain unknown or poorly understood. Conversely, many orphan receptors have been discovered, the natural ligands of which are not yet recognised; these receptors may represent targets for novel drugs when their pharmacology is better understood.

PROPERTIES OF RECEPTORS

Receptor binding

The binding of a ligand to its receptor is normally reversible; consequently, the intensity and duration of the intracellular changes are dependent on repeated drug–receptor interactions that persist as long as the drug molecules remain in

Table 1.4 Examples of enzymes as drug targets

Enzyme	Drug class or use	Examples
Acetylcholinesterase (AChE)	AChE inhibitors (Ch. 27)	Neostigmine, edrophonium, organophosphates
Angiotensin-converting enzyme (ACE)	ACE inhibitors (Ch. 6)	Captopril, perindopril, ramipril
Carbonic anhydrase	Carbonic anhydrase inhibitors (Chs 14, 50)	Acetazolamide
Cyclo-oxygenase (COX)-1	Non-steroidal anti-inflammatory drugs (NSAIDs) (Ch. 29)	Aspirin, ibuprofen, indometacin, naproxen
Cyclo-oxygenase (COX)-2	Selective COX-2 inhibitors (Ch. 29)	Celecoxib, etoricoxib
Dihydrofolate reductase	Folate antagonists (Chs 51, 52)	Trimethoprim, methotrexate
DOPA decarboxylase	Peripheral decarboxylase inhibitors (PDIs) (Ch. 24)	Carbidopa, benserazide
HMG-CoA reductase	Statins (Ch. 48)	Atorvastatin, simvastatin
Monoamine oxidases (MAOs) A and B	MAO inhibitors (Chs 22, 24)	Moclobemide, selegiline
Phosphodiesterase (PDE) isoenzymes	PDE inhibitors (Chs 12, 16)	Theophylline, sildenafil (see Table 1.1)
Reverse transcriptase (RT)	Nucleoside RT inhibitors (Ch. 51)	Zidovudine
Thrombin	Direct thrombin inhibitors (Ch. 11)	Dabigatran
Viral proteases	HIV/hepatitis protease inhibitors (Ch. 51)	Saquinavir, boceprevir
Vitamin K epoxide reductase	Coumarin anticoagulants (Ch. 11)	Warfarin
Xanthine oxidase	Xanthine oxidase inhibitors (Ch. 31)	Allopurinol

the local environment of the receptors. The duration of activity of a reversible drug therefore depends mainly on its distribution and elimination from the body (pharmacokinetics), not on the duration of binding of a drug molecule to a receptor. For a reversible drug, the extent of drug binding to the receptor (receptor occupancy) is proportional to the drug concentration; the higher the concentration, the greater the occupancy. The interaction between a reversible ligand and its receptor does not involve covalent chemical bonds but weaker, reversible forces such as:

- ionic bonding between ionisable groups in the ligand (e.g. NH_3^+) and the receptor (e.g. COO^-),
- hydrogen bonding between amino-, hydroxyl-, keto- and other groups in the ligand and the receptor,
- hydrophobic interactions between lipid-soluble sites in the ligand and receptor,
- van der Waals forces, which are very weak inter-atomic attractions.

The receptor protein is not a rigid structure: binding of the ligand alters the conformation and biological properties of the protein.

Receptor selectivity

There are numerous possible extracellular and intracellular chemical signals produced in the body, which can affect many different processes. Therefore, a fundamental property of a ligand–receptor interaction is its *selectivity*; that is, the extent to which the receptor can recognise and respond to the correct signals, represented by one ligand or group of related ligands. Some receptors show high selectivity and bind a single endogenous ligand (e.g. acetylcholine is the only endogenous ligand that binds to N_1 nicotinic receptors; see Ch. 4), whereas other receptors are less selective and will bind a number of related endogenous ligands (e.g. the β_1-adrenoceptors on the heart will bind noradrenaline, adrenaline and to some extent dopamine, all of which are catecholamines).

The ability of receptors to recognise and bind the appropriate ligand depends on the intrinsic characteristics of the chemical structure of the ligand. The formulae of a few ligand families that bind to different receptors are shown in Figure 1.9; differences in structure that determine selectivity of action between receptors may be subtle, such as the differences illustrated between the structures of testosterone and progesterone, which nevertheless have markedly different hormonal effects on the body due to their receptor selectivity. Receptors are protein chains folded into tertiary and quaternary structures such that the necessary arrangement of specific bonding centres is brought together in a small volume: the receptor site (Fig. 1.10). Receptor selectivity occurs because the three-dimensional organisation of the different sites for reversible binding (such as anion and cation sites, lipid centres and hydrogen-bonding sites) corresponds better to the three-dimensional structure of the endogenous ligand than to that of other ligands.

There may be a number of subtypes of a receptor, all of which can bind the same common ligand but which differ in their ability to recognise particular variants or derivatives of that ligand. For example, α_1-, α_2-, β_1-, β_2- and β_3-adrenoceptors all bind adrenaline, but isoprenaline, a synthetic derivative of adrenaline, binds selectively to the

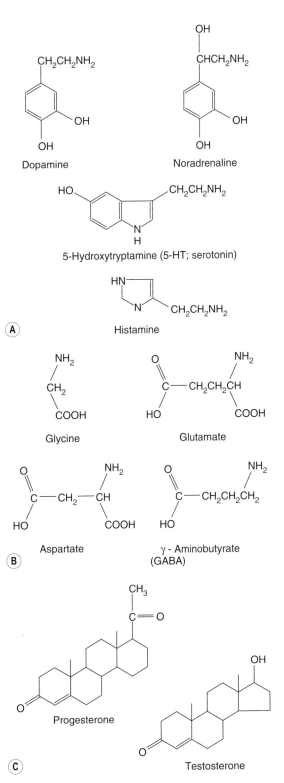

Fig. 1.9 Groups of related chemicals that show selectivity for different receptor subtypes in spite of similar structure. (A) Biogenic amines; (B) amino acids; (C) steroids.

Adrenoceptor

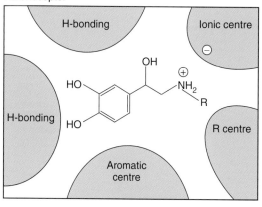

Muscarinic receptor

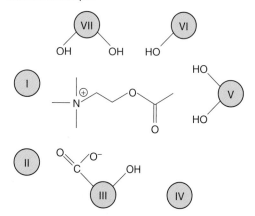

Fig. 1.10 Receptor ligand-binding sites. The coloured areas are schematic representations of the regions of the adrenoceptor (top) and muscarinic receptor (bottom) responsible for binding their respective catecholamine and acetylcholine ligands. In the muscarinic receptor, cross-sections of the seven transmembrane segments are labelled I–VII. Different segments provide different properties (hydrogen bonding, anionic site, etc.) to make up the active binding site.

Traditionally, receptor subtypes were discovered pharmacologically when a new agonist or antagonist compound was found to alter some, but not all, of the activities of a currently known receptor class. Developments in molecular biology, including the Human Genome Project, have accelerated the recognition and cloning of new receptors and receptor subtypes, including orphan receptors for which the natural ligands are unknown, and these developments are important in developing new drugs with greater selectivity and fewer unwanted effects. Based on such information it is recognised that there are multiple types of most receptors, and that there is genetic variation among individuals in the structures, properties and abundance of these receptors, which can lead to differences in drug response (pharmacogenetic variation; see end of this chapter and of Ch. 2). Greater understanding of genetic differences underlying human variability in drug responses offers the potential for individualisation of the mode of treatment and selection of the optimal drug and dosage.

Drug stereochemistry and activity

Receptors have a three-dimensional spatial organisation so the ligand has to have the correct configuration to fit the receptor, analogous to fitting a right hand into a right-handed glove. Drugs and other organic molecules show stereoisomerism when they contain four different chemical groups attached to a single carbon atom, or one or more double bonds, with the result that molecules with the same molecular formula have different three-dimensional configurations. If a drug is an equal (racemic) mixture of two stereoisomers, the stereoisomers may show different binding characteristics and biological properties. Most often, one stereoisomer is pharmacologically active while the other is inactive, but in some cases the inactive isomer may be responsible for the unwanted effects of the racemic mixture. Alternatively the two isomers may be active at different receptor subtypes and have synergistic or even opposing actions. The different isomers may also show different rates of metabolism (see Ch. 2). In consequence, there has been a trend for the development of single stereoisomers of drugs for therapeutic use; one of the earliest examples was the use of levodopa (the levo-isomer of DOPA) in Parkinson's disease (Ch. 24).

Receptor numbers

The number of receptors present in a cell is not static. There is usually a high turnover of receptors being formed and removed continuously. Cell-membrane receptor proteins are synthesised in the endoplasmic reticulum and transported to the plasma membrane; regulation of functional receptor numbers in the membrane occurs both by transport to the membrane (often as homo- or heterodimers) and by removal by internalisation. The number of receptors within the cell membrane may be altered by the drug being used for treatment, with either an increase (*upregulation*) or a decrease (*downregulation*) in receptor number and a consequent change in the ability of the drug to effect the desired theraputic response. This change may be an unwanted loss of drug activity contributing to tolerance to the effects of the drug (e.g. opioids, Ch. 19); as a result,

three β-adrenoceptor subtypes rather than the two α-adrenoceptor subtypes (Ch. 4). As the adrenoceptor subtypes occur to a different extent in different tissues, and produce different intracellular changes when stimulated or blocked, drugs can be designed with highly selective and localised actions. The cardioselective β-adrenoceptor antagonists such as atenolol are selective blockers of the β₁-adrenoceptor subtype that predominates on cardiac smooth muscle, with much less binding to the β₂-adrenoceptors that predominate on bronchial smooth muscle. The different characteristics of the receptor subtypes therefore allow a drug (or natural ligand) with a particular three-dimensional structure to show selective actions by recognising one receptor preferentially, with fewer unwanted effects from stimulation or blockade of related receptors. Although ligands may have a much higher affinity for one receptor subtype over another, this is never absolute, so the term selective is preferred to specific.

increased doses may be needed to maintain the same activity. Alternatively, the change in receptor number may be an important part of the therapeutic response itself. An example is the tricyclic antidepressants (Ch. 22); these produce an immediate increase in the availability of monoamine neurotransmitters but the therapeutic response is associated with a subsequent, adaptive downregulation in monoamine receptor numbers occurring over weeks.

PROPERTIES OF DRUG ACTION

Drug actions can show a number of important properties:

- dose–response relationship,
- selectivity,
- potency,
- efficacy.

DOSE–RESPONSE RELATIONSHIPS

Using a pure preparation of a single drug, it is possible to define accurately and reproducibly the relationship between the doses of drug administered (or concentrations applied) and the biological effects (responses) at each dose. The results for an individual drug can be displayed on a dose–response curve. In many biological systems, the typical relationship between increasing drug dose (or concentration) and the response is a hyperbola. Plotting instead the logarithm of the dose or concentration against response (on a linear scale) generates a sigmoid (S-shaped) curve. A sigmoid response curve has a number of advantages: a very wide range of doses can be accommodated easily, the maximal response plateau is illustrated clearly and the central portion of the curve (between about 15 and 85% of maximum) approximates to a straight line, allowing the collection of fewer data points to delineate the relationship accurately.

Figure 1.11 shows the log dose–response relationship between a drug and its responses at two types of adrenoceptors. In each case, the upward slope of the curve to the right reflects the Law of Mass Action, the physical principle that a greater number of reversible molecular interactions of a drug (D) with its receptor (R), due in this case to increasing drug dose, leads to more intracellular signalling by active drug–receptor complexes (DR) and hence a greater response of the cell or tissue (within biological limits). This principle is diametrically opposed to the principle of homeopathy, which argues that serially diluting a drug solution until no drug molecules remain *enhances* its activity, a belief that is not supported theoretically or experimentally.

Selectivity

As drugs may act preferentially on particular receptor types or subtypes, such as β_1- and β_2-adrenoceptors, it is important to be able to measure the degree of selectivity of a drug and to express it numerically. For example, it is important in understanding the therapeutic efficacy and unwanted effects of the bronchodilator drug salbutamol to recognise that it is approximately 10 times more effective in stimulating the β_2-adrenoceptors in the airway smooth muscle than the β_1-adrenoceptors in the heart.

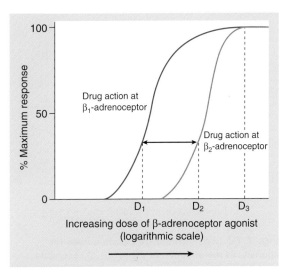

Fig. 1.11 Dose–response relationship and receptor selectivity. Each curve shows the responses (expressed as percentage of maximum on a linear vertical axis) produced by a hypothetical β-adrenoceptor agonist drug at a range of doses shown on a logarithmic horizontal axis. Plotting the logarithmic dose allows a very wide range of doses to be shown on the same axes and transforms the dose–response relationship from a hyperbolic curve to a sigmoid (S-shaped) curve, in which, conveniently, the central portion is close to a straight line. The two curves illustrate the relative selectivity of the same drug for the β_1-adrenoceptor compared to the β_2-adrenoceptor. At most doses the drug produces β_1-adrenoceptor stimulation with less effect on β_2-adrenoceptors. If dose D_1 is 10 times lower than dose D_2, the selectivity of the drug for the β_1-adrenoceptor is 10-fold higher. This selectivity diminishes at the higher end of the log dose–response curve and is completely lost at doses that produce a maximum response on both β_1- and β_2-adrenoceptors (D_3).

In pharmacological studies this type of experiment is likely to be performed by studying the effects of the drug *in vitro* on different cells or tissues, each expressing one of the receptors of interest. Comparison of the two log dose–response curves in Figure 1.11 shows that for a given response, smaller doses of the drug being tested are required to stimulate the β_1-adrenoceptor compared with those required to stimulate the β_2-adrenoceptor; the drug is therefore said to have selectivity of action at the β_1-adrenoceptor. The degree of receptor selectivity is given by the ratio of the doses of the drug required to produce a given level of response via each receptor type. It is clear from Figure 1.11 that the ratio is highly dose-dependent and disappears at very high drug doses, when a maximal response is mediated by both receptor subtypes due to the limits of the biological system being tested.

Potency

The potency of a drug *in vitro* is largely determined by the strength of its binding to the receptor, which is a reflection

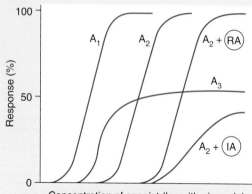

Fig. 1.12 Concentration–response curves for agonists in the absence or presence of reversible (competitive) or irreversible (non-competitive) antagonists. Responses are plotted at different concentrations of two different full agonists (A$_1$ being more potent than A$_2$) and also a partial agonist (A$_3$), which is unable to produce a maximal response even at high concentrations. Responses are also shown for the full agonist A$_2$ in the presence of a fixed concentration of a reversible antagonist (RA) or a fixed concentration of an irreversible antagonist (IA). The reversible antagonist reduces the potency of A$_2$ (the curve is shifted to the right), but A$_2$ remains able to produce a maximal response at higher concentrations. The irreversible antagonist reduces both the potency and the maximal response achievable by A$_2$.

of the receptor affinity, and the ability of the drug/receptor complex to elicit downstream signalling events. The more potent a drug, the lower will be the concentration needed to bind to the receptor and give a specified response (for an agonist) or to block a response (for an antagonist). In Figure 1.12, drug A$_1$ is more potent than drug A$_2$ because it produces a specified level of response at a lower concentration. It is important to recognise that potencies of different drugs are compared using the doses required to produce (or block) the *same response* (often chosen arbitrarily as 50% of the maximal response). The straight-line portions of *log* dose–response curves are usually parallel for drugs that share a common mechanism of action, so the potency ratio is broadly the same at most response values, for example 20, 50 or 80%, but not at 100% response. A drug concentration sufficient to produce half of the greatest response achievable by that drug is described as its EC$_{50}$ (the effective concentration for 50% of the maximal response). The EC$_{50}$ (or ED$_{50}$ if drug *dose* is considered) is a convenient way to compare the potencies of similar drugs; the lower the EC$_{50}$ (or ED$_{50}$) the more potent the drug.

In vivo, the potency of a drug, defined as the dose of the drug required to produce a desired clinical effect, depends not only on its affinity for the receptor, the receptor number and the efficiency of the stimulus-response mechanism, but also on pharmacokinetic variables that determine the delivery of the drug to its site of receptor action (Ch. 2).

Therefore, the potencies of a series of related drugs *in vivo* may not directly reflect their *in vitro* receptor-binding properties.

Efficacy

The efficacy of a drug is its ability to produce the maximal response possible for a particular biological system and relates to the extent of functional change that can be imparted to the receptor by the drug. For example, agonists are traditionally divided into two main groups (Fig. 1.12):

- full agonists (curves A$_1$ and A$_2$), which give an increase in response with an increase in concentration until the maximum possible response is obtained for that system,
- partial agonists (curve A$_3$), which also give an increase in response with increase in concentration but cannot produce the maximum possible response.

A third group, the inverse agonists, are described below. Drug efficacy is arguably of greater clinical importance than potency because a greater therapeutic benefit may be obtained with a more efficacious drug, while switching to a more potent drug may merely allow a smaller dose to be given for the same clinical benefit. In turn, efficacy and potency need to be balanced against drug toxicity to produce the best balance of benefit and risk for the patient. Drug toxicity and safety are discussed in Chs 3 and 53.

TYPES OF DRUG ACTION

Drugs can be classified by their receptor action as:

- agonists,
- antagonists,
- partial agonists,
- inverse agonists,
- allosteric modulators,
- enzyme inhibitors or activators,
- non-specific,
- physiological antagonists.

AGONISTS

An agonist, whether a therapeutic drug or an endogenous ligand, binds to the receptor or site of action and changes the conformation of the receptor to its active state, leading to signalling via its second messenger pathways. An agonist shows both *affinity* (the strength of binding for the receptor) and *intrinsic efficacy* or *activity* (the extent of functional change imparted to the receptor). Drugs may differ in their affinity and intrinsic activity at the same receptor as well as between different receptors.

Affinity and intrinsic activity

The affinity of a drug is related to the aggregate strength of the atomic interactions between the drug molecule and its receptor site of action, which determines the relative rates of drug binding and dissociation. The higher the affinity, the lower the drug concentration required to occupy a given fraction of receptors. Affinity therefore determines the drug concentration necessary to produce a certain response and is directly related to the potency of the drug. In Figure 1.12, drug A_1 is more potent than drug A_2, but both are capable of producing a maximal response (they have the same efficacy).

Intrinsic efficacy or activity describes the ability of the bound drug to induce the conformational changes in the receptor that induce receptor signalling. Although affinity is a prerequisite for binding to a receptor, a drug may bind with high affinity but have low intrinsic activity. A drug with zero intrinsic activity is an antagonist (see below).

It should be noted that the rate of binding and rate of dissociation of a reversible drug at its receptor are of negligible importance in determining its rate of onset or duration of effect *in vivo*, because these depend mainly on the rates of delivery of the drug to, and removal from, the target organ; that is, on the overall absorption or elimination rates of the drug from the body (Ch. 2).

Spare receptors

For compounds with relatively low intrinsic activity a maximal response may require all of the receptors to be occupied. However, many drugs have sufficient affinity that the maximal response can be produced even though many receptors remain unoccupied; that is, there may be *spare receptors*. The concept of spare receptors does not imply a distinct pool of permanently redundant receptors, only that a proportion of the receptor population is unoccupied at a particular point in time. Spare receptors may enhance the speed of cellular response, because an excess of available receptors reduces the time and distance that a ligand molecule needs to diffuse to find an unoccupied receptor; an example is the excess of acetylcholine nicotinic N_2 receptors that contributes to fast synaptic transmission in the neuromuscular junction (Ch. 27).

The concept of spare receptors is also helpful when considering changes in receptor numbers during chronic treatment, particularly receptor downregulation. As maximal responses are often produced at drug concentrations that do not attain 100% receptor occupancy, the same maximal response may still be produced when receptor numbers are downregulated, but only with higher percentage occupancy of the reduced number of receptors and hence with a higher drug dose or concentration. Receptor downregulation may therefore contribute to drug tolerance.

ANTAGONISTS

A competitive antagonist binds to the active site of a receptor, either alone or in competition with a drug agonist or natural ligand, but the antagonist cannot cause the conformational change that converts the receptor to its active state. In other words, it has affinity (which may be as high as that of any agonist), but it has no intrinsic activity. The antagonist will, however, reduce access of an agonist ligand to the receptor-binding site and thereby reduce receptor activation. The antagonist effect may therefore only be detectable when an agonist is present, and the extent of antagonism will depend on the relative amounts of agonist and antagonist. For example, β_1-adrenoceptor antagonists lower the heart rate markedly only when it is already elevated by endogenous agonists such as adrenaline and noradrenaline. The binding of most clinically useful competitive antagonists is reversible; in consequence, the receptor blockade can be overcome (surmounted) by an increase in the concentration of an agonist. Therefore, reversible antagonist drugs move the dose–response curve for an agonist to the right but do not alter the maximum possible response (as shown in curve $A_2 + RA$ when compared with A_2 alone in Fig. 1.12).

Like agonists, antagonists exhibit selectivity of action. For example, propranolol is a non-selective antagonist blocking β_1- and β_2-adrenoceptors equally, whereas atenolol shows selective antagonism of β_1-adrenoceptors.

Irreversible competitive antagonists bind covalently to the receptor site of action so a full response cannot be achieved even by a very large increase in agonist concentration (as shown in curve $A_2 + IA$ compared with A_2 alone in Fig. 1.12). Irreversible antagonism is therefore *insurmountable*; an example of irreversible antagonism is the action of phenoxybenzamine at α-adrenoceptors.

PARTIAL AGONISTS

An agonist that is unable to produce a maximal response is a partial agonist (e.g. drug A_3 in Fig. 1.12). Even maximal occupancy of all available receptors produces only a submaximal response due to low intrinsic activity of the partial agonist, for example because of incomplete amplification of the receptor signal via the G-proteins. Partial agonists can be considered to have both agonist and antagonist properties depending on the presence and type of other ligands. A partial agonist shows agonist activity in the absence of another ligand, and such partial agonism can be blocked by an antagonist. But, at high concentrations of a full agonist, a partial agonist will behave as an antagonist because it prevents access to the receptor of a molecule with higher intrinsic ability to initiate receptor signalling; this results in a reduced response. Partial agonism is responsible for the therapeutic efficacy of several drugs, including buspirone, buprenorphine, pindolol and salbutamol. These drugs can act as stabilisers of the variable activity of the natural ligand, as they enhance receptor activity when the endogenous ligand levels are low, but block receptor activity when endogenous ligand levels are high.

INVERSE AGONISTS

The descriptions above of agonists, partial agonists and antagonists reflect the classic model of drug–receptor interactions, in which an unoccupied receptor has no signalling activity. It is now recognised that many GPCRs show constitutive signalling independently of an agonist. Inverse agonists were first recognised when some compounds were found to show negative intrinsic efficacy: they acted alone on unoccupied receptors to produce a change opposite to that caused by an agonist. Inverse agonists shift the receptor equilibrium towards the inactive state, thereby reducing the level of spontaneous receptor activity. An inverse agonist can be distinguished from the 'neutral' antagonists discussed above, which, on their own, bind to the receptor without affecting receptor signalling. The action of a neutral antagonist depends on depriving the access of agonists to

Table 1.5 Examples of drugs with inverse agonist activity

Receptor	Drugs
α_1-Adrenoceptor	Prazosin, terazosin
β_1-Adrenoceptor	Metoprolol
Angiotensin II receptor AT_1	Losartan, candesartan, irbesartan
Cannabinoid CB1	Rimonabant
Cysteinyl-leukotriene $CysLT_1$	Montelukast, zafirlukast
Dopamine D_2	Haloperidol, clozapine, olanzapine
Histamine H_1	Cetirizine, loratadine
Histamine H_2	Cimetidine, ranitidine, famotidine
Muscarinic M_1	Pirenzepine

the receptor; a neutral antagonist can therefore block the effects of either a positive or inverse agonist at a receptor with spontaneous signalling activity.

The role of inverse agonism in the therapeutic effects of drugs remains to be fully elucidated, but a number of drugs exhibit this type of activity (Table 1.5). The same drug may even show full or partial agonism, inverse agonism or antagonism at different receptors. Some drugs, for example some β-adrenoceptor antagonists, can act as neutral antagonists at a receptor in one tissue and as inverse agonists when the same receptor is expressed in a different tissue, probably due to association of the receptor with different G-proteins.

ALLOSTERIC MODULATORS

An allosteric modulator does not compete directly with an agonist for access to receptor active site (also called the orthosteric site), but binds to a different (allosteric) site on the receptor. Binding to the allosteric site can change receptor activity by altering the conformation of the protein so as to affect the normal (orthosteric) binding site and thereby enhance or decrease the binding of the natural ligand or other drugs to the receptor. An example is the benzodiazepine anxiolytic drugs, which allosterically alter the affinity of chloride channels for the neurotransmitter ligand GABA (Ch. 20). Alternatively, allosteric modulators may change the conformation of the receptor protein so that it alters domains required for receptor signalling without affecting the orthosteric site. Allosteric modulators may be reversible or irreversible.

ENZYME INHIBITORS/ACTIVATORS

Many drugs have a site of action that is an enzyme. Drugs act reversibly or irreversibly either on the catalytic site or at an allosteric site on the enzyme to modulate its catalytic activity; most often the effect is inhibition. Important examples are shown in Table 1.4.

NON-SPECIFIC ACTIONS

A few drugs produce their desired therapeutic outcome without interaction with a specific site of action on a protein; for example, the diuretic mannitol exerts an osmotic effect in the lumen of the kidney tubule which reduces reabsorption of water into the blood (Ch. 14).

PHYSIOLOGICAL ANTAGONISTS

Physiological antagonism is said to occur when a drug has a physiological effect opposing that of an agonist but without binding to the same receptor. The increase in heart rate produced by a β_1-adrenoceptor agonist, an effect which mimics the action of the sympathetic autonomic nervous system, can be blocked *pharmacologically* with an antagonist at β_1-adrenoceptors or *physiologically* by a muscarinic receptor agonist, which mimics the opposing (parasympathetic) autonomic nervous system. The site of action of the physiological antagonist may be on a different cell, tissue or organ to that of the agonist.

TOLERANCE TO DRUG EFFECTS

Tolerance to drug effects is defined as a decrease in response with repeated doses. Tolerance may occur through pharmacokinetic changes in the concentrations of drug available at the receptor or through pharmacodynamic changes at the drug receptor. Pharmacokinetic effects are discussed in Chapter 2; some drugs stimulate their own metabolism, so they are eliminated more rapidly on repeated dosage and lower concentrations of drug are available to produce a response.

Most clinically important examples of tolerance arise from pharmacodynamic changes in receptor numbers and in concentration–response relationships. Desensitisation is used to describe both long-term and short-term changes arising from a decrease in response of the receptor. Desensitisation can occur by a number of mechanisms:

- decreased receptor numbers (downregulation),
- decreased receptor-binding affinity,
- decreased G-protein coupling,
- modulation of the downstream response to the initial signal.

GPCRs can show rapid desensitisation (within minutes) during continued activation, which occurs through three mechanisms.

- **Homologous desensitisation.** The enzymes activated following selective binding of an agonist to its receptor–G-protein complex include G-protein coupled receptor kinases (GRKs), which interact with the $\beta\gamma$-subunit of the G-protein and inactivate the occupied receptor protein by phosphorylation; a related peptide, β-arrestin, enhances the GRK-mediated desensitisation.
- **Heterologous desensitisation.** Also known as cross-desensitisation, this occurs when an agonist at one receptor causes loss of sensitivity to other agonists. The agonist increases intracellular cAMP which activates

protein kinase A or C; these phosphorylate the cross-desensitised receptors (whether occupied or not) and inactivate them by uncoupling their G-proteins. Other mechanisms of heterologous desensitisation exist.

- **Receptor internalisation.** Internalisation can occur within minutes when constant activation of a GPCR makes the receptor unavailable for further agonist action by uncoupling the G-protein from the receptor. The phosphorylated receptor protein is endocytosed and may undergo intracellular dephosphorylation prior to re-entering the cytoplasmic membrane.

Downstream modulation of the signal may also occur through feedback mechanisms or simply through depletion of some essential cofactor. An example of the latter is the depletion of the thiol (-SH; or sulphydryl) groups necessary for the generation of nitric oxide during chronic administration of organic nitrates (Ch. 5).

GENETIC VARIATION IN DRUG RESPONSES

Biological characteristics, including responses to drug administration, vary among individuals and genetic differences can contribute to these inter-individual variations. For most drugs, the nature of the response is broadly similar in different individuals, but the magnitude of the response to the same dose can differ markedly, at least partly due to genetic factors. Such variability creates the need to individualise drug dosages for different people.

Drug responses may follow a unimodal (Gaussian) distribution, reflecting the sum of many small genetic variations in receptors, enzymes or transporters that respond to or handle the drug (Fig. 1.13A). Genetic variation may also give rise to discrete subpopulations of individuals in which a drug shows distinctly different responses (Fig. 1.13B), such that some individuals may have no response to a standard dose while others show toxicity. Understanding genetic variation is of increasing importance in drug development (see Ch. 3) because it allows the possibility of genetic screening to optimise drug and dosage selection (personalised or individualised medicine).

Pharmacogenetics has been defined as the study of genetic variation that results in differing responses to drugs, including those arising due to differences in the metabolic fates of drugs in the body (Ch. 2). Pharmacogenetic research has been undertaken for many decades, largely in relation to variability *in vivo*, and has often used classic genetic techniques such as studies of patterns of inheritance in twins.

Pharmacogenomics has been defined as the investigation of variation in DNA and RNA characteristics related to drug response, and the term refers mainly to genome-wide approaches that define the presence of single-nucleotide polymorphisms (SNPs) which affect the activity of the gene product. Molecular biological techniques have predicted more than 3 million SNPs in the human genome. SNPs can be:

- in the upstream regulatory sequence of a coding gene, which can result in increased or decreased expression of the gene product; this is otherwise identical to the normal or 'wild-type' gene product,
- in the coding region of the gene resulting in a gene product with an altered amino acid sequence; this may have higher activity (although this is unlikely), similar activity, lower activity or no activity at all, compared to the wild-type protein,

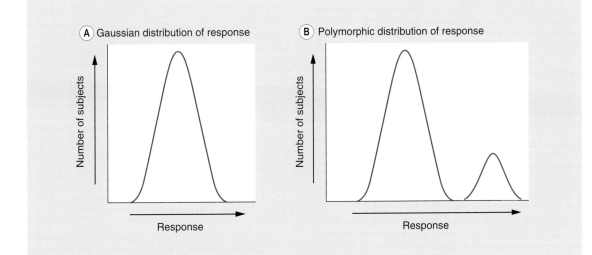

Fig. 1.13 **Inter-individual variation in response.** The graphs show the numbers of individual subjects in a population plotted against their varying levels of response to a single dose of a drug. (A) In the unimodal distribution most individuals show a middling response and the overall shape is a normal (Gaussian) distribution. Part of this variability may result from polymorphism in multiple genes encoding drug receptors and proteins involved in the drug's absorption and elimination. (B) The bimodal distribution shows discrete responder and non-responder subgroups, possibly due to a single genetic polymorphism in a drug receptor or drug-metabolising enzyme.

- inactive, because they are in non-coding or non-regulatory regions of the genome, or, if in a coding region, because the base change does not alter the amino acid encoded, due to the redundancy of the genetic code.

In consequence, a major challenge is defining the functional consequences of the large numbers of identified SNPs (functional genomics), particularly in the context of combinations of genetic variants (haplotypes). Such studies often require very large numbers of subjects to allow comparison of function in multiple, small haplotype subgroups.

Rapid advances in molecular biology have allowed analysis of inter-individual differences in the sequences of many genes encoding drug receptors and proteins involved in drug metabolism and transport. Polymorphisms in the latter are likely to have the greatest impact on dosage selection, while polymorphisms in drug targets may be more important in determining the optimal drug for a particular condition. For example, genetic variation in angiotensin AT_1 receptors, β_1-adrenoceptors and calcium ion channels may determine the relative effectiveness of angiotensin II receptor antagonists, β-adrenoceptor antagonists (β-blockers) and calcium channel blockers in the treatment of essential hypertension.

In practice, although genetic polymorphisms have been reported in many receptor types and these have been a major focus of research in relation to the aetiology of disease, relatively few studies to date have demonstrated a clear influence on drug responses. Common polymorphisms have been identified in the human β_2-adrenoceptor gene *ADRB2* and certain variants have been associated with differences in receptor downregulation and loss of theraeputic response in people with asthma while using β_2-adrenoceptor agonist inhalers (Ch. 12). The clinical response in people with asthma to treatment with leukotriene modulator drugs is influenced by genetic polymorphism in enzymes of the leukotriene (5-lipoxygenase) pathway. Variants in the epidermal growth factor receptor (EGFR), a RTK, have been reported to predict tumour response to the EGFR inhibitor gefitinib in individuals with non-small-cell lung cancer. Such examples may support genotyping to target drug treatments to those individuals most likely to respond.

Conversely, pharmacogenetic information may be used to avoid a particular treatment in people likely to experience serious adverse reactions to a specific drug. Variation in human leucocyte antigen (HLA) genes has been associated with adverse skin and liver reactions to several drugs, including abacavir, an antiretroviral drug used in HIV infection.

Compared to pharmacodynamic targets, genetic variation has been more extensively characterised in drug-metabolising enzymes, particularly in cytochrome P450 isoenzymes and others involved in glucuronidation, acetylation and methylation. Gene variations in drug-metabolising enzymes are discussed at the end of Chapter 2. Information on human genotypic variation can be found on the Online Mendelian Inheritance in Man (OMIM) database (Johns Hopkins University; www.ncbi.nlm.nih.gov/omim). Therapeutic exploitation of genotypic differences will require specific information about individuals based on detailed genetic testing. Until such genetic information is available routinely, careful monitoring of clinical response will remain the best guide to successful treatment.

CONCLUSIONS

The therapeutic benefits of drugs arise from their ability to interact selectively with target receptors, most of which are regulatory molecules involved in the control of cellular and systemic functions by endogenous ligands. Drugs may also cause unwanted effects; judging the balance of benefit and risk is at the heart of safe and effective prescribing. Increasing knowledge of the complexity of receptor pharmacology and improvements in drug selectivity offer the promise of safer drugs in the future, especially when information on genetic variation is more routinely available.

SELF-ASSESSMENT

True/false questions

1. Clinical pharmacology is the study of drugs that doctors use to treat disease.
2. Drugs act at receptors only on the external surface of the cell membrane.
3. Diluting drugs enhances their pharmacological effects.
4. Drugs produce permanent chemical changes in their receptors.
5. Plotting drug dose (or concentration) against response usually produces a sigmoid curve.
6. The EC_{50} is the concentration of drug that produces a half-maximal response.
7. On a log dose–response plot the drug with a curve to the right is more potent than a drug with its curve on the left.
8. An antagonist has zero affinity for the receptor.
9. A competitive antagonist shifts the log dose–response curve of an agonist to the right, without affecting the maximal response.
10. A partial agonist is one that, even at its highest dose, cannot achieve the same maximal response as a full agonist at the same receptor.
11. A full agonist achieves a maximal response when all its receptors are occupied.
12. Changes in receptor numbers can cause tolerance to drug effects.

True/false answers

1. **True**. Clinical pharmacology also deals with drugs used in disease prevention and diagnosis and in the alleviation of pain and suffering.
2. **False**. While many types of receptors are found on the cell membrane, including ion channels, G-protein-coupled receptors and tyrosine kinase receptors, other drug targets, including steroid receptors and many enzymes (e.g. cyclo-oxygenase, phosphodiesterase), are intracellular.

3. **False**. Drug effects depend on the number of interactions between drug molecules and their molecular targets (Law of Mass Action), so are usually greater at higher drug concentrations.

4. **False**. Molecular interactions between most drugs and their receptors are weak and transient and the conformational changes induced in the receptor are reversible; irreversible drugs may act by covalent chemical bonding.

5. **False**. Plotting drug dose or concentration against dose typically produces a hyperbola; a sigmoid (S-shaped) curve is produced by plotting the logarithm of dose or concentration against response.

6. **True**. The EC_{50} (or ED_{50}) is the concentration (or dose) effective in producing 50% of the maximal response and is a convenient way of comparing drug potencies.

7. **False.** A drug with its log dose–reponse curve to the left is the more potent as it produces the same response at lower concentrations.

8. **False**. An antagonist must have affinity to bind to its receptor, but it has zero intrinsic ability to activate the receptor.

9. **True**. A fixed dose of a competitive antagonist can be surmounted by increasing the dose of agonist, so that the same maximal response can be achieved.

10. **True**. A partial agonist has low intrinsic ability to induce conformational change in the receptor so does not elicit a maximal response even with full receptor occupancy.

11. **False**. Many full agonists are able to elicit a maximal response when less than 100% of receptors are occupied; the unoccupied receptors are termed 'spare receptors'.

12. **True**. Tolerance may be caused by downregulation or desensitisation of receptors, or by pharmacokinetic changes in drug concentrations available to interact with the receptor.

FURTHER READING

Ackerman MJ, Clapham DE (1997) Ion-channels – basic science and clinical disease. *N Engl J Med* 336, 1575–1586

Alexander SPH, Mathie A, Peters JA (2011) Guide to receptors and channels (GRAC), 5th edition. *Br J Pharmacol* 164, S1–S324

Bender AT, Beavo JA (2006) Cyclic nucleotide phosphodiesterases: molecular regulation to clinical use. *Pharmacol Rev* 58, 488–520

Berger JP, Akiyama TE, Meinke PT (2005) PPARs: therapeutic targets for metabolic disease. *Trends Pharmacol Sci* 26, 244–251

Boswell-Smith V, Spina D, Page CP (2006) Phosphodiesterase inhibitors. *Br J Pharmacol* 147, S252–S257

Costa T, Cotecchia S (2005) Historical review: negative efficacy and the constitutive activity of G-protein coupled receptors. *Trends Pharmacol Sci* 26, 618–624

Hall IP (2006) Pharmacogenetics of asthma. *Chest* 130, 1873–1878

Hirano K, Yufu T, Hirano M, Nishimura J, Kanaide H (2005) Physiology and pathophysiology of proteinase-activated receptors (PARs): regulation of the expression of PARs. *J Pharmacol Sci* 97, 31–37

Katritch V, Cherezov V, Stevens RC (2012) Diversity and modularity of G protein-coupled receptor structures. *Trends Pharmacol Sci* 33, 17–27

Kenakin T (2004) Principles: receptor theory in pharmacology. *Trends Pharmacol Sci* 25, 186–192

Kobilka BK, Deupi X (2007) Conformational complexity of G-protein-coupled receptors. *Trends Pharmacol Sci* 28, 397–406

Maxwell S, Walley T (2003) Teaching safe and effective prescribing in UK medical schools: a core curriculum for tomorrow's doctors. *Br J Clin Pharmacol* 55, 496–503

Privalsky ML (2004) The role of corepressors in transcriptional regulation by nuclear hormone receptors. *Annu Rev Physiol* 66, 315–360

Rosenbaum DM, Rasmussen SGF, Kobilka BK (2009) The structure and function of G-protein-coupled receptors. *Nature* 459, 356–363

Shi Y (2007) Orphan nuclear receptors in drug discovery. *Drug Discov Today* 12, 440–445

Strange PG (2003) Mechanisms of inverse agonism at G-protein-coupled receptors. *Trends Pharmacol Sci* 23, 89–95

Traynelis SF, Trejo J (2007) Protease-activated receptor signaling: new roles and regulatory mechanisms. *Curr Opin Hematol* 14, 230–235

Violin JD, Lefkowitz RJ (2007) β-Arrestin-biased ligands at seven-transmembrane receptors. *Trends Pharmacol Sci* 28, 416–422

Wang L, McLeod HL, Weinshilboum RM (2011) Genomics and drug response. *N Engl J Med* 364, 1144–1153

Examples of cell surface receptor families and their properties

Type	Typical location(s)	Principal transduction mechanism	Major biological actions	Agonists	Antagonists
G-protein-coupled receptors (GPCRs)					
Acetylcholine					
Muscarinic					
M_1	CNS, salivary, gastric; minor role in autonomic ganglia	G_q	Neurotransmission in CNS, gastric secretion	*Non-selective for all M receptors:* carbachol	Pirenzepine *Non-selective for all M receptors:* atropine, ipratropium, diphenhydramine, oxybutynin, tolterodine
M_2	Heart, CNS	G_i	Bradycardia, smooth muscle contraction (GI tract, airways, bladder)		
M_3	Smooth muscles, secretory glands, CNS	G_q	Contraction, secretion	I	Darifenacin, tiotropium
M_4	CNS	G_i	Unclear		
M_5	CNS	G_q	Unclear		
Adrenergic					
α-Adrenoceptors					
α_1 (α_{1A}, α_{1B}, α_{1D})	CNS; postsynaptic in sympathetic nervous system; human prostate (α_{1A})	G_q	Contraction of arterial smooth muscle, decrease in contractions of gut, contraction of prostate tissue	Phenylephrine, methoxamine, NA ≥ Adr	Prazosin, indoramin (tamsulosin α_{1A})
α_2 (α_{2A}, α_{2B}, α_{2C})	Presynaptic (in both α- and β-adrenergic neurons)	G_i	Decreased NA release	Clonidine, Adr > NA (oxymetazoline α_{2A})	Yohimbine
β-Adrenoceptors					
β_1	CNS, heart (nodes and myocardium), kidney	G_s	Increased force and rate of cardiac contraction, renin release	Dobutamine, NA > Adr	Atenolol, metoprololol
β_2	Widespread	G_s	Bronchodilation, decrease in contraction of gut, glycogenolysis	Salbutamol, salmeterol, terbutaline, Adr > NA	Butoxamine
β_3	Adipocytes, bladder	G_s	Lipolysis; bladder emptying	Adr = NA	–
Cannabinoids					
CB_1	Cortex, hippocampus, amygdala, basal ganglia, cerebellum	$G_{i/o}$	Behaviour, pain, nausea, stimulation of appetite, addiction, depression, hypotension	Tetrahydrocannabinol, anandamide, 2-arachidonylglycerol	Rimonabant (withdrawn)
CB_2	Leucocytes, osteocytes	$G_{i/o}$	Immunity, bone growth	Tetrahydrocannabinol, anandamide	

Examples of cell surface receptor families and their properties (cont'd)

Type	Typical location(s)	Principal transduction mechanism	Major biological actions	Agonists	Antagonists
Cholecystokinin					
CCK_A (CCK_1)	Primarily GI tract, some CNS	G_q/G_s	Gall bladder emptying, inhibits gut motility	CCK-4, CCK-8, CCK-33, gastrin	Proglumide
CCK_B (CCK_2)	Primarily CNS, some GI tract	G_s	CNS nociception, anxiety, appetite	CCK-4, CCK-8, CCK-33, gastrin	Proglumide
Dopamine					
D_1	CNS (N, O, P, S – see footnote for key to CNS areas), kidney, heart	G_s	Vasodilation in kidney	Fenoldepam	Chlorpromazine
D_2	CNS (C, N, O, SN), pituitary gland, chemoreceptor trigger zone gastrointestinal tract	G_i	Cognition (schizophrenia), prolactin secretion, nigrostrial control of movement, memory	Cabergoline, pramipexole, ropinirole, rotigotine	Butyrophenones, chlorpromazine domperidone, metoclopramide, sulpiride
D_3	CNS (F, Me, Mi) (limbic system)	G_i	Cognition, emotion	Cabergoline, pramipexole, ropinirole, rotigotine	Chlorpromazine, sulpiride
D_4	CNS, heart	G_i	Cognition (schizophrenia)	Cabergoline, ropinirole, rotigotine	Chlorpromazine, clozapine
D_5	CNS (Hi, Hy)	G_s	Similar to D_1		
5-Hydroxytryptamine (5-HT, serotonin)					
$5-HT_{1A}$	CNS, blood vessels	G_i	Anxiety, appetite, mood, sleep	Buspirone	
$5-HT_{1B}$	CNS, blood vessels	G_i	Vasoconstriction presynaptic inhibition	Sumatriptan, eletriptan	
$5-HT_{1D}$	CNS, blood vessels	G_i	Anxiety, vasoconstriction	Sumatriptan, eletriptan	Metergoline
$5-HT_{1E}$	CNS, blood vessels	G_i			
$5-HT_{1F}$	CNS	G_i		Sumatriptan, eletriptan	
$5-HT_{2A}$	CNS, GI tract, platelets, smooth muscle	G_q	Schizophrenia, platelet aggregation, vasodilation/vasoconstriction	LSD, psilocybin	Ketanserin
$5-HT_{2B}$	CNS, GI tract, platelets	G_q	Contraction, morphogenesis		
$5-HT_{2C}$	CNS, GI tract, platelets	G_q	Satiety		
$5-HT_4$	CNS, myenteric plexus, smooth muscle	G_s	Anxiety, memory, gut motility	Metoclopramide, renzapride	
$5-HT_5$	CNS	G_i	Anxiety, memory, mood		
$5-HT_6$	CNS	G_s	Anxiety, memory, mood		

Examples of cell surface receptor families and their properties (cont'd)

Type	Typical location(s)	Principal transduction mechanism	Major biological actions	Agonists	Antagonists
5-HT_7	CNS, GI, blood vessels	G_s	Anxiety, memory, mood	LSD	
Histamine					
H_1	CNS, endothelium, smooth muscle	G_q	Sedation, sleep, vascular permeability, inflammation		Cetirizine, desloratadine
H_2	CNS, cardiac muscle, stomach	G_s	Gastric acid secretion	Dimaprit	Cimetidine, ranitidine
H_3	CNS (presynaptic), myenteric plexus	G_i	Appetite, cognition		Thioperamide
H_4	Eosinophils, basophils, mast cells	G_i		4-Methylhistamine	
Gamma-aminobutyric acid receptor type B ($GABA_B$)					
$GABA_B$	Brain neurons, glial cells, spinal motor neurons and interneurons	G_i	Inhibition of neurotranmission in brain and spinal cord	Baclofen	
Peptides					
Angiotensin II					
AT_1	Blood vessels, adrenal cortex, brain	G_q/G_o	Vasoconstriction, salt retention, aldosterone synthesis, increased noradrenergic activity, cardiac hypertrophy		Candesartan, losartan, valsartan
AT_2	Blood vessels, endothelium, adrenal cortex, brain	$G_{i/o}$, tyrosine and ser/thr phosphatases	Weak vasodilation (endothelial nitric oxide release), fetal development, vascular growth		
Bradykinin					
B_1 (induced)	Widespread (induced by injury, cytokines)	G_q	Acute inflammation; stimulates nitric oxide synthesis	ACE inhibitors (indirect, by blocking bradykinin breakdown)	
B_2 (constitutive)		G_q	Chronic inflammation. Most kinin actions (vasodilation, pain)		Icatibant
Endothelin					
ET_A	Endothelium	G_q	Vasoconstriction, angiogenesis		Bosentan
ET_B	Endothelium	G_q, G_i	Indirect vasodilation (nitric oxide release), direct vasoconstriction, natriuresis		Bosentan

Examples of cell surface receptor families and their properties (cont'd)

Type	Typical location(s)	Principal transduction mechanism	Major biological actions	Agonists	Antagonists
Opioids					
DOP (δ), KOP (κ), MOP (μ), nociceptin	Brain, spinal cord, peripheral sensory neurons	G_i	Analgesia, sedation, respiratory depression	Endogenous opioids, opiate drugs (morphine)	Naloxone, naltrexone
Protease-activated receptors					
PAR_1, PAR_2, PAR_3, PAR_4	Platelets, endothelial cells, epithelial cells, myocytes, neurons	G_q, G_i	Activated by proteolytic cleavage	Trypsin, thrombin, tryptase	
Vasopressin and oxytocin					
Vasopressin V_{1a}	Brain, uterus, blood vessels, platelets	G_q	Vasoconstriction, platelet aggregation	Desmopressin	Conivaptan, demeclocycline
Vasopressin V_{1b}	Pituitary, brain	G_q	Modulates ACTH secretion	Desmopressin	Conivaptan, demeclocycline
Vasopressin V_2	Kidney	G_s	Antidiuretic effect on collecting duct and ascending limb of loop of Henle	Desmopressin	Conivaptan demeclocycline, tolvaptan
Oxytocin OXT	Brain, uterus	G_q, G_i	Lactation, uterine contraction, CNS actions (mood)	Oxytocin > arginine-vasopressin	Atosiban
Purinergic receptors (purinoceptors)					
Adenosine A_1	Heart, lung	G_i	Cardiac depression, vasoconstriction, bronchoconstriction		Methylxanthines
Adenosine A_{2A}	Widespread	G_s	Vasodilation, inhibition of platelet aggregation, bronchodilation	Regadenoson	Methylxanthines
Adenosine A_{2B}	Leucocytes	G_s	Bronchoconstriction		Methylxanthines
Adenosine A_3	Leucocytes	G_i	Inflammatory mediator release		Methylxanthines
Purinergic P2Y family ($P2Y_1$, $P2Y_2$, $P2Y_4$, $P2Y_6$, $P2Y_{11}$–$P2Y_{14}$)	Widespread	G_q, G_s or G_i	Depends upon G-protein coupling	ATP, ADP, UTP, UDP, UDP-glucose	$P2Y_{12}$: clopidogrel, ticlopidine
Ligand-gated ion channels (LGICs)					
Nicotinic N_1	Autonomic ganglia	Ligand-gated ion channel	Ganglionic neurotransmission	Carbachol, nicotine	Trimetaphan, mecamylamine
Nicotinic N_2	Neuromuscular junction	Ligand-gated ion channel	Skeletal muscle contraction	Nicotine, suxamethonium (depolarising)	Gallamine, vecuronium, atracurium
Serotonin $5\text{-}HT_3$	CNS (A), enteric nerves, sensory nerves	Ligand-gated Na^+/K^+ channel	Emesis		Granisetron, ondansetron, metoclopramide

Examples of cell surface receptor families and their properties (cont'd)

Type	Typical location(s)	Principal transduction mechanism	Major biological actions	Agonists	Antagonists
$GABA_A$	Brain neurons, spinal motor neurons and interneurons	Ligand-gated Cl^- channel (open)	Inhibition of neurotransmission in brain and spinal cord	Muscimol, barbiturates, benzodiazepines, zolpidem	Picrotoxin, flumazenil (benzodiazepine antagonist)
Glycine GlyR	Brain neurons, spinal motor neurons and interneurons	Ligand-gated Cl^- channel (open)	Inhibition of neurotransmission in brain and spinal cord	Intravenous anaesthetics, alanine, taurine	Strychnine, caffeine, tropisetron, endocannabinoids
Ionotropic glutamate (NMDA) receptor	CNS (B, C, sensory pathways)	Ligand-gated Ca^{2+} channel (slow)	Synaptic plasticity, excitatory transmitter release, excessive amounts may cause neuronal damage	NMDA	Ketamine, phencyclidine, memantine
Ionotropic glutamate (kainate) receptor	CNS (Hi)	Ligand-gated Ca^{2+} channel (fast)	Synaptic plasticity, transmitter release	Kainate	
Ionotropic glutamate (AMPA) receptor	CNS (similar to NMDA receptors)	Ligand-gated Ca^{2+} channel (fast)	Synaptic plasticity, transmitter release	AMPA	
Purinergic P2X family ($P2X_1$–$P2X_7$)	CNS, autonomic nervous system ($P2X_2$), smooth muscle ($P2X_1$), leucocytes	Ligand-gated ion channels (Na^+, Ca^{2+}, K^+)	Neuronal depolarisation, influx of Na^+ and Ca^{2+}, efflux of K^+	ATP	Suramin
Voltage-gated ion channels (VGICs)					
Epithelial sodium channel (ENaC)	Renal tubule, airways, colon	Na^+ channel, tonically open	Sodium reabsorption in aldosterone-sensitive distal tubule and collecting duct	Expression upregulated by aldosterone	Amiloride, triamterene
L-type calcium channels (Ca_v1.1–1.4)	Widespread	Voltage-gated Ca^{2+} channels (dihydropyridine-sensitive)	Vascular and cardiac smooth muscle contraction, prolong cardiac action potential		Nifedipine, amlodipine, diltiazem, verapamil
Ryanodine (RyR1, RyR2, RyR3)	Skeletal muscle (RyR1), heart (RyR2), widespread (RyR3)	Ca^{2+} channels	Calcium-induced Ca^{2+} release (CICR)	Cytosolic Ca^{2+}, ATP, ryanodine, caffeine	Dantrolene

This table lists some important families of G-protein-coupled receptors, ligand-gated ion channels and voltage-gated ion channels, many of which are drug targets. See Tables 1.2 and 1.4 for examples of important intracellular receptors and enzymes targeted by therapeutic drugs. For further information see Alexander et al. (2011).

Abbreviations: ACE, angiotensin-converting enzyme; ACTH, adrenocorticotropic hormone (corticotropin); Adr, adrenaline; AMPA, α-amino-3-hydroxy-5-methyl-4-isoxazole propionic acid; CNS, central nervous system; GI, gastrointestinal; LSD, lysergic acid diethylamide; NA, noradrenaline; NMDA, N-methyl D-aspartate.

Key to CNS areas: A, Area postrema; B, basal ganglia; C, caudate putamen; F, frontal cortex; Hi, hippocampus; Hy, hypothalamus; Me, medulla; Mi, midbrain: N, nucleus accumbens; O, olfactory tubercle; P, putamen; S, striatum; SN, substantia nigra.

Appendix: Student formulary

This student formulary has been derived from the formulary described by Maxwell and Walley (2003) and from the formulary of University Hospital Southampton NHS Foundation Trust. It is used in the University of Southampton Faculty of Medicine to introduce medical students to representative examples of the most commonly prescribed drugs and their major uses. It is not intended to be exhaustive.

Therapeutic problem	Core drugs
Gastrointestinal system	
Emergency treatment of poisoning	Adsorbant: activated charcoal Paracetamol antidote: acetylcysteine Acetylcholinesterase inhibitor: physostigmine Opiate antagonist: naloxone Organophosphate antidote: pralidoxime
Dyspepsia, GORD and gastric ulcer healing	Antacids, e.g. magnesium salts Compound alginates, e.g. Gaviscon Proton pump inhibitors, e.g. omeprazole, lansoprazole H_2 receptor antagonists, e.g. ranitidine, cimetidine *Helicobacter pylori* antibiotics: clarithromycin, amoxicillin, metronidazole Motility stimulants, e.g. metoclopramide Others: misoprostol, sucralfate
Inflammatory bowel disease (ulcerative colitis, Crohn's disease)	Corticosteroids, e.g. prednisolone Aminosalicylates, e.g. sulfasalazine, mesalazine Cytokine inhibitors, e.g. infliximab
Antibiotic-associated colitis	Antibiotics for *Clostridium difficile*, e.g. metronidazole, vancomycin
Diarrhoea	Oral rehydration therapy Opiate anti-motility drugs, e.g. loperamide
Constipation	Bulk-forming laxatives, e.g. ispaghula, methylcellulose Stimulant laxatives, e.g. senna, docusate Osmotic laxatives, e.g. magnesium hydroxide, lactulose
Anti-spasmodics	Anti-muscarinics, e.g. atropine, hyoscine Others: mebeverine
Cardiovascular system	
Hypertension	β-Adrenoceptor antagonists, e.g. atenolol α-Adrenoceptor antagonists, e.g. doxazosin Centrally acting drugs, e.g. clonidine Angiotensin-converting enzyme inhibitors, e.g. captopril, ramipril Angiotensin receptor antagonists, e.g. candesartan, losartan Thiazide diuretics, e.g. bendroflumethazide, metolazone Loop diuretics, e.g. furosemide Potassium-sparing diuretics, e.g. amiloride, spironolactone Compound potassium-sparing diuretic: co-amilofruse Calcium channel antagonists, e.g. amlodipine, verapamil Potassium channel openers, e.g. minoxidil, nicorandil
Heart failure	Many of the above plus the following positive inotropic drugs Cardiac glycosides, e.g. digoxin Phosphodiesterase inhibitors, e.g. milrinone β-Adrenoceptor antagonist: bisoprolol
Acute coronary syndrome (angina, myocardial infarction)	Many drugs listed under hypertension plus the following Inhibitors of platelet aggregation, e.g. low-dose aspirin, dipyridamole, clopidogrel, abciximab Thrombolytics, e.g. streptokinase, tenecteplase Heparin (unfractionated) Heparins (low molecular weight), e.g. enoxaparin Oral anticoagulants, e.g. warfarin
Hyperlipidaemia	Statins, e.g. simvastatin Fibrates, e.g. fenofibrate
Arrhythmias	Anti-arrhythmic drugs, e.g. digoxin, adenosine, amiodarone, lidocaine, β-adrenoceptor antagonists, calcium channel blockers

Appendix: Student formulary (cont'd)

Therapeutic problem	Core drugs
Respiratory system	
Asthma, COPD, respiratory failure	Oxygen β_2-Adrenoceptor agonists, e.g. salbutamol, salmeterol Anti-muscarinics, e.g. ipratropium, tiotropium Methylxanthines, e.g. theophylline, aminophylline, roflumilast Leukotriene antagonists, e.g. montelukast Anti-allergic drugs, e.g. cromoglicate Magnesium sulphate Inhaled corticosteroids, e.g. beclometasone, fluticasone Oral corticosteroid, e.g. prednisolone β_2-Agonist/steroid coformulations, e.g. Seretide
Allergy, anaphylaxis	Anti-histamines, e.g. chlorphenamine, cetirizine Adrenaline, e.g. Epipen
Cough suppression	Codeine
Central nervous system	
Insomnia, anxiety	Benzodiazepines, e.g. temazepam, diazepam Z-drugs, e.g. zopiclone Others, e.g. buspirone, propranolol
Schizophrenia, mania	Classical anti-psychotics, e.g. chlorpromazine, haloperidol, flupentixol Atypical anti-psychotics, e.g. olanzapine, risperidone, quetiapine (Depot preparations, e.g. fluphenazine decanoate) Mood stabilisers, e.g. lithium
Depression	Tricyclic anti-depressants (TCAs), e.g. amitriptyline Selective serotonin reuptake inhibitors (SSRIs), e.g. fluoxetine, citalopram Other reuptake inhibitors, e.g. venlafaxine Monoamine oxidase inhibitors (MAOIs), e.g. phenelzine
Analgesia	Non-steroidal anti-inflammatory drugs (NSAIDs): see section on Musculoskeletal disease Compound analgesics, e.g. co-codamol, co-dydramol Moderate opioids, e.g. tramadol Opioid analgesics, e.g. codeine, morphine, fentanyl
Nausea and vertigo	Dopamine antagonists, e.g. metoclopramide Serotonin receptor antagonists, e.g. ondansetron Muscarinic receptor antagonists, e.g. hyoscine Others: betahistine
Migraine	Acute: 5-HT$_1$ receptor agonists, e.g. sumatriptan Prophylaxis: 5-HT$_2$ receptor antagonists, e.g. pizotifen
Epilepsy	Anticonvulsant drugs, e.g. diazepam, phenobarbital, phenytoin, carbamazepine, valproate, gabapentin
Parkinson's disease	Levodopa/DOPA decarboxylase coformulations, e.g. co-careldopa, co-beneldopa Dopamine receptor agonists, e.g. bromocriptine, ropinirole COMT inhibitors, e.g. entacapone MAO-B inhibitor: selegiline Anti-muscarinic drugs, e.g. procyclidine
Dementia (Alzheimer's)	Anticholinesterases, e.g. donepezil NMDA receptor antagonists, e.g. memantine

Appendix: Student formulary (cont'd)

Therapeutic problem	Core drugs
Infectious diseases	
Community- and hospital-acquired infections	Penicillins, e.g. benzylpenicillin Penicillinase-resistant penicillins, e.g. flucloxacillin Broad-spectrum penicillins, e.g. amoxicillin, co-amoxiclav Cephalosporins, e.g. cefalexin, cefuroxime Tetracyclines, e.g. oxytetracycline Folate inhibitors, e.g. trimethoprim Aminoglycosides, e.g. gentamicin Vancomycin (for *C. difficile*) Macrolides, e.g. erythromycin Chloramphenicol Quinolones, e.g. ciprofloxacin Metronidazole (for anaerobes and protozoans) Antituberculosis drugs, e.g. isoniazid, rifampicin, ethambutol Antifungal drugs, e.g. amphotericin, fluconazole, nystatin Antiviral drugs, e.g. aciclovir (herpes), ganciclovir (CMV), zanamivir (influenza) Reverse transcriptase inhibitors, e.g. zidovudine, abacavir Protease inhibitors, e.g. saquinavir Antimalarial drugs, e.g. mefloquine, proguanil, malarone
Endocrine system	

Diabetes mellitus, thyroid disease and hypothalamo-pituitary hormones	Insulins (long- and short-acting)
	Secretagogues
	    Sulfonylureas, e.g. gliclazide
	    Meglitinides, e.g. repaglinide
	    GLP agonists, e.g. exenatide
	Sensitisers
	    Biguanides, e.g. metformin
	    Thiazolidinediones, e.g. pioglitazone
	Thyroid disease, e.g. levothyroxine, carbimazole
	ADH mimetics, e.g. desmopressin
	LHRH, e.g. gonadorelin
	Human growth hormone, e.g. somatropin

Osteoporosis	Calcium, vitamin D, calcitonin. Bisphosphonates, e.g. alendronic acid Selective oestrogen receptor modulators (SERMs), e.g. clomifene
Genito-urinary system	
Urinary retention	α-Adrenoceptor antagonists, e.g. doxazosin
Benign prostatic hypertrophy and prostate cancer	Anti-androgens (5α-reductase inhibitors), e.g. finasteride
Urinary frequency/incontinence	Anti-muscarinic drugs, e.g. tolterodine
Erectile dysfunction	Phosphodiesterase inhibitors, e.g. sildenafil
Obstetrics and gynaecology	
Steroidal contraception	Combined oral contraceptives Progestogen-only contraceptives Emergency contraception (progestin), e.g. Levonelle Injectable contraception, e.g. medroxyprogesterone acetate Progestogen-containing intra-uterine device
Menstrual disorders Dysmenorrhoea Menorrhagia Endometriosis	Mefenamic acid Progestogens Antifibrinolytic agent, e.g. tranexamic acid, combined oral hormonal contraceptive, danazol
Induction of labour	Oxytocics, e.g. prostaglandins, oxytocin

Appendix: Student formulary (cont'd)

Therapeutic problem	Core drugs
Myometrial relaxation and prevention of pre-term labour	Calcium channel blockers, e.g. nifedipine β-Adrenoceptor agonists, e.g. terbutaline
Induction of abortion	Oxytocics, mifepristone
Post-partum haemorrhage	Oxytocics, ergometrine
Menopause	Oestrogens (natural and synthetic), progestins

Malignant disease and immunosuppression

Cancer and immunosuppression	Alkylating agents, e.g. cyclophosphamide Cytotoxic antibiotics, e.g. doxorubicin Anti-metabolites, e.g. methotrexate, fluorouracil Vinca alkaloids, e.g. vinblastine Other cytotoxic drugs, e.g. crisantaspase, cisplatin Anti-oestrogens, e.g. tamoxifen, anastrazole, trastuzumab Immunosuppressant drugs, e.g. azathioprine, corticosteroids, cyclosporin Immunobiologicals, e.g. rituximab (anti-CD20), interferon alfa

Musculoskeletal disease

Rheumatoid arthritis	Non-steroidal anti-inflammatory drugs (NSAIDs), e.g. indometacin, diclofenac Corticosteroids, e.g. prednisolone Disease-modifiers, e.g. gold, azathioprine, sulfasalazine Anti-malarial: hydroxychloroquine Cytokine inhibitors, e.g. infliximab, etanercept
Myasthenia gravis	Anticholinesterases, e.g. pyridostigmine
Spasticity	Skeletal muscle relaxants, e.g. baclofen
Gout	Acute: colcichine; chronic: allupurinol

Ophthalmology

Glaucoma	β-Adrenoceptor antagonists, e.g. timolol Prostaglandin analogues, e.g. latanoprost Sympathomimetics, e.g. brimonidine Carbonic anhydrase inhibitors, e.g. acetazolamide Miotics, e.g. pilocarpine
Conjunctivitis	Topical antibiotics, e.g. chloramphenicol
Tear deficiency	Ocular lubricants, e.g. hypromellose
Others	Mydriatics, e.g. phenylephrine Mydriatics/cycloplegics, e.g. atropine, tropicamide Topical formulations (eye drops) of many drugs including anti-inflammatory steroids (e.g. betamethasone), antivirals and local anaesthetics (e.g. tetracaine)

Surgery, anaesthetics and intensive care

Surgery, anaesthetics and intensive care	Many drugs used are listed in other sections, including opiate analgesics, sympathomimetics and anti-emetics, plus the following. Intravenous (induction) anaesthetics, e.g. thiopental, propofol Inhalation (maintenance) anaesthetics, e.g. isoflurane Muscle relaxants, e.g. suxamethonium, atracurium Anti-muscarinics, e.g. atropine, glycopyrronium Anticholinesterases, e.g. neostigmine Local anaesthetics, e.g. lidocaine, bupivacaine

ADH, antidiuretic hormone; CMV, cytomegalovirus; COMT, catechol-O-methyltransferase; COPD, chronic obstructive pulmonary disease; GLP, glucagon-like peptide; GORD, gastro-oesophageal reflux disease; LHRH, luteinizing hormone-releasing hormone; MAO-B, monoamine oxidase B; NMDA, N-methyl D-aspartate.

2 Pharmacokinetics

PHARMACOKINETICS OF BIOLOGICAL DRUGS

The type of response experienced by an individual to a particular drug depends on the inherent pharmacological properties of the drug at its site of action. However, the speed of onset, the intensity and the duration of the response usually depend on parameters such as:

- the rate and extent of uptake of the drug from its site of administration,
- the rate and extent of distribution of the drug to different tissues, including the site of action,
- the rate of elimination of the drug from the body.

Overall, the response of an individual depends upon a combination of the effects of the drug at its site of action in the body (*pharmacodynamics*) and the way the body influences drug delivery to its site of action (*pharmacokinetics*) (Fig. 2.1). Both pharmacodynamic and pharmacokinetic aspects are subject to a number of variables, which affect the dose–response relationship. Pharmacodynamic aspects are determined by processes such as drug–receptor interaction and are specific to the class of the drug (Ch. 1). Pharmacokinetic aspects are determined by general processes, such as transfer across membranes, metabolism and renal elimination, which apply irrespective of the pharmacodynamic properties.

Pharmacokinetics may be divided into four basic processes, sometimes referred to collectively as 'ADME':

- **absorption**: the transfer of the drug from its site of administration to the general circulation,
- **distribution**: the transfer of the drug from the general circulation into the different organs of the body,
- **metabolism**: the extent to which the drug molecule is chemically modified in the body,
- **excretion**: the removal of the parent drug and any metabolites from the body; metabolism and excretion together account for drug *elimination*.

Each of these processes can be described qualitatively in biological terms, involving biochemical and physiological processes, and also in mathematical terms, which determine many of the quantitative aspects of drug prescribing.

THE BIOLOGICAL BASIS OF PHARMACOKINETICS

Most drug structures bear little resemblance to normal dietary constituents such as carbohydrates, fats and proteins, and they are handled in the body by different processes. Drugs that bind to the same receptor as an endogenous ligand rarely resemble the natural ligand

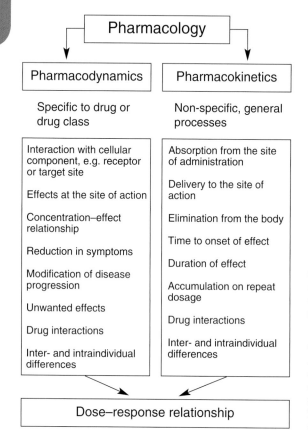

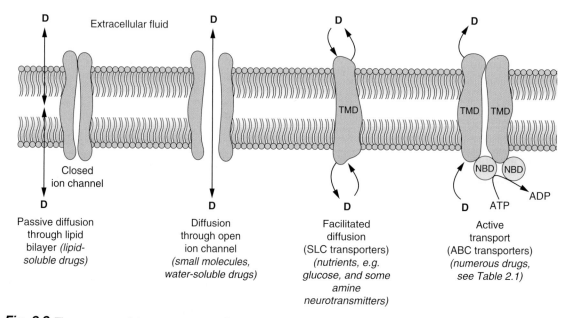

sufficiently closely in chemical structure to share the same carrier processes or metabolising enzymes. Consequently, the movement of drugs in the tissues is mostly by simple passive diffusion rather than by specific transporters, whereas metabolism is usually by enzymes of low substrate specificity that can handle a wide variety of drug substrates and other xenobiotics (foreign substances).

GENERAL CONSIDERATIONS

Passage across membranes

With the exception of intravenous or intra-arterial injections, a drug must cross at least one membrane in its movement from the site of administration into the general circulation. Drugs acting at intracellular sites must also cross the cell membrane to exert an effect. The main mechanisms by which drugs can cross membranes (Fig. 2.2) are:

- passive diffusion through the lipid layer,
- diffusion through pores or ion channels,
- carrier-mediated processes,
- pinocytosis.

Passive diffusion

All drugs can move passively down a concentration gradient. To cross the phospholipid bilayer directly (Fig. 2.2) a drug must have a degree of lipid solubility, such as ethanol or steroids. Eventually a state of equilibrium will be reached in which equal concentrations of the diffusible form of the drug are present in solution on each side of the membrane. The rate of diffusion is directly proportional to the concentration gradient across the membrane, and to the area and permeability of the membrane, but inversely proportional to

Fig. 2.1 Factors determining the response of an individual to a drug.

Fig. 2.2 The passage of drugs across membranes. Molecules can cross the membrane by simple passive diffusion through the lipid bilayer or via a channel, or by facilitated diffusion, or by ATP-dependent active transport. D, drug; TMD, transmembrane domain; NBD, nucleotide-binding domain; ABC, ATP-binding cassette superfamily of transport proteins; SLC, solute carrier superfamily of transporters (see Table 2.1).

Table 2.1 Examples of carrier molecules involved in drug transport

Transporter	Typical substrates	Sites in the body
ABC superfamily	ATP-binding cassette superfamily of transport proteins; use ATP for active transport. Although there are a number of transporters in each family, the four ABC transporters listed below can explain multidrug resistance in most cells analysed to date.	
MDR1 or P-glycoprotein (ABCB1)	Hydrophobic and cationic (basic) molecules; numerous drugs, including anti-cancer drugs	Apical surface of membranes of epithelial cells of intestine, liver, kidney, blood–brain barrier, testis, placenta and lung
MRP1 (ABCC1)	Numerous, including anti-cancer drugs, glucuronide and glutathione conjugates	Basolateral surface of membranes of most cell types with high levels in lung, testis and kidney and in blood–tissue barriers
MRP2 (ABCC2)	Numerous, including anti-cancer drugs, glucuronide and glutathione conjugates	Apical surface of membranes; mainly in liver, intestine and kidney tubules
BCRP (ABCG2) Breast cancer resistance protein	Anti-cancer, antiviral drugs, fluoroquinolones, flavonoids	Apical surface of breast ducts and lobules, small intestine, colon epithelium, liver, placenta, brain barrier and lung
SLC superfamily	Solute carrier superfamily of transporters. Comprises organic anion transporters (OATs) and organic cation transporters (OCTs)	
OAT1 (SLC22A6)	Numerous, including NSAIDs, penicillins, diuretics and phase 2 drug metabolites	Kidney (basolateral), brain, placenta, smooth muscle
OAT2 (SLC22A7)	Salicylate, acetylsalicylate, PGE_2, dicarboxylates	Kidney (basolateral), liver
OAT3 (SLC22A8)	Similar to OAT1	Kidney (basolateral), liver, brain, smooth muscle
OAT4 (SLC22A11)	Steroid sulphate conjugates	Kidney (apical), placenta
OCT1 (SLC22A1)	Serotonin, noradrenaline, histamine, agmatine, aciclovir, ganciclovir	Mainly in the liver, but also in kidney, small intestine, heart, skeletal muscle and placenta
OCT2 (SLC22A2)	Serotonin, noradrenaline, histamine, agmatine, amantadine, cimetidine	Mainly in the kidney, but is also in placenta, adrenal gland, neurons and choroid plexus
OCT3 (SLC22A3)	Serotonin, noradrenaline, histamine, agmatine	Liver, kidney, intestine, skeletal and smooth muscle, heart, lung, spleen, neurons, placenta and the choroid plexus

ABC, ATP-binding cassette; NSAIDs, non-steroidal anti-inflammatory drugs; PGE_2, prostaglandin E_2; SLC, solute carrier.

its thickness (Fick's Law). In the laboratory, transient water-filled pores can be created in the phospholipid bilayer by applying a strong external electric field, and this process (electroporation) is used to introduce large or charged molecules, such as DNA, drugs and probes into live cells in suspension.

Passage through membrane pores or ion channels

Movement through channels occurs down a concentration gradient and is restricted to extremely small water-soluble molecules (<100 Da), such as ions. This is applicable to therapeutic ions such as lithium and also to radioactive iodine. Water itself crosses membranes rapidly via a ubiquitous family of aquaporins.

Carrier-mediated processes

Two carrier-mediated processes are of widespread importance in the transport of drugs, particularly those with low lipid solubility, across membranes.

- **Active transport** utilises energy (ATP) and transports drugs into or out of cells against their concentration gradient. It is performed by a family of non-specific carriers termed the ATP-binding cassette (ABC) superfamily of membrane transporters (Fig. 2.2, Table 2.1).

- **Facilitated transport** of a molecule by a carrier aids its passive movement down a concentration gradient, or uses the electrochemical gradient of a co-transported solute to transport the molecule against its own gradient; the latter is energy-dependent but does not utilise ATP. The major examples are the solute carrier (SLC) superfamily of transporters (Fig. 2.2, Table 2.1).

In humans, the ABC active-transporter superfamily contains 49 members organised into seven subfamilies (A–G) based on their relative sequence homology. Interest in this area has expanded rapidly since the discovery of P-glycoprotein (P-gp), also known as multidrug resistance 1 (MDR1) or ABCB1 transporter. P-gp transports a wide range of drug substrates, including anti-cancer drugs, steroids and immunosuppressive agents, from the cytoplasm to the extracellular side of the cell membrane, and therefore acts as an efflux transporter. Verapamil increases the concentrations of anti-cancer drugs at their intracellular sites of action by inhibiting P-gp (Ch. 52). ABCB transporter proteins contain two hydrophobic transmembrane domains, which consist of different numbers of membrane-spanning α-helices (12 in P-gp), and two hydrophilic nucleotide (ATP)-binding domains, which bind and hydrolyse intracellular ATP. The transporter is on the apical surface and acts as an efflux pump that transports substrates from the cell into the interstitial fluid, plasma, bile, urine or gut lumen. Examples of other ABC transporters are given in Table 2.1.

The SLC superfamily comprises over 400 types of organic anion transporters (OATs) and organic cation transporters (OCTs) (Table 2.1). OAT1 to OAT4 are present in various tissues; OAT1 is the classic organic anion transporter in the kidney, which secretes urate and penicillins and is blocked by probenecid (Ch. 33). Organic cation transporters (OCT1, OCT2 and OCT3) effect facilitated diffusion and can transport cations in both directions across the membrane. Substrates common to all three OCT transporters are serotonin (5-hydroxytryptamine, 5-HT), noradrenaline, histamine and agmatine; although some drugs are substrates for the transporters (Table 2.1), many basic drugs act as inhibitors of the transporters.

Pinocytosis

This can be regarded as a form of carrier-mediated entry into the cell cytoplasm. Pinocytosis is normally concerned with the uptake of endogenous macromolecules and may be involved in the uptake of recombinant therapeutic proteins; drugs can also be incorporated into a lipid vesicle or liposome for pinocytotic uptake (e.g. amphotericin and doxorubicin; Ch. 51).

Drug ionisation and membrane diffusion

Ionisation is a fundamental property of most drugs that are either weak acids, such as aspirin, or weak bases, such as propranolol. The presence of an ionisable group(s) is essential for the mechanism of action of most drugs, because ionic forces represent a key part of ligand–receptor interactions (Ch. 1). The extent of ionisation may also influence the extent of absorption of a drug, its distribution into organs such as the brain or adipose tissue and the mechanism and route of its elimination from the body.

Drugs with ionisable groups exist in equilibrium between charged (ionised) and uncharged (un-ionised) forms (Fig. 2.3). The extent of ionisation of a drug depends on the strength of the ionisable group and the pH of the solution. The extent of ionisation is given by the acid dissociation constant, K_a.

$$K_a = \frac{[\text{conjugate base}][H^+]}{[\text{conjugate acid}]} \quad (2.1)$$

The term conjugate acid refers to a form of the drug able to *release a proton*, such as:

- an un-ionised acidic drug (Drug–COOH), or
- an ionised basic drug (Drug–NH$_3^+$).

The conjugate base is the corresponding equilibrium form of the drug that has *lost a proton*, such as:

- an ionised acidic drug (Drug–COO$^-$), or
- an un-ionised basic drug (Drug–NH$_2$).

The value of K_a is normally much less than 1, so it is easier to compare compounds using the negative logarithm of K_a, which is called pK_a. For example, a K_a of 10^{-5} becomes pK_a 5, and a K_a of 10^{-10} becomes pK_a 10. Based on the equation above, a strong acid (such as an –SO$_3$H functional group) that readily donates its H$^+$ ion will have a relatively high K_a value (e.g. 10^{-1} or 10^{-2}) and hence a low pK_a (i.e. 1 or 2), whereas weakly acidic groups, which donate their H$^+$ ion less readily, have a pK_a of 4–5. Conversely, for basic functional groups, the stronger the base, the greater will be its ability to retain the H$^+$, resulting in low K_a and high pK_a values. Thus, strongly basic groups have a pK_a of 10–11, while weakly basic groups have a pK_a of 7–8.

Drugs are 50% ionised when the pH of the solution equals the pK_a of the drug. Acidic drugs (low pK_a values) are least ionised in acidic solution (low pH) and most ionised in alkaline solutions (high pH). Basic drugs (high pK_a values) are least ionised in alkaline solutions (high pH), and most ionised in acid solutions (low pH). In either case, the ionised form of the molecule can generally be regarded as the water-soluble form and the un-ionised form as the lipid-soluble form. The ease with which a drug can diffuse across a lipid bilayer is determined by the lipid solubility of its un-ionised form (Fig. 2.4).

The pH of body fluids is controlled by the buffering capacity of the ionic groups present in endogenous molecules such as phosphate ions and proteins. When the fluids on each side of a membrane have the same pH value there will be equal concentrations of both the diffusible (un-ionised) form and the non-diffusible (ionised) form of the drug on each side of the membrane at equilibrium (Fig. 2.4).

When the fluids on each side of a membrane are at different pH values, the concentrations of the un-ionised form on each side of the membrane at equilibrium will remain equal as it can diffuse reversibly across the membrane, but the concentrations of the ionised drug will be determined by the pH of the solution. This results in pH-dependent

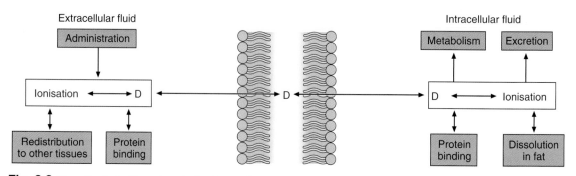

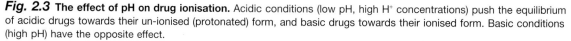

Fig. 2.3 The effect of pH on drug ionisation. Acidic conditions (low pH, high H$^+$ concentrations) push the equilibrium of acidic drugs towards their un-ionised (protonated) form, and basic drugs towards their ionised form. Basic conditions (high pH) have the opposite effect.

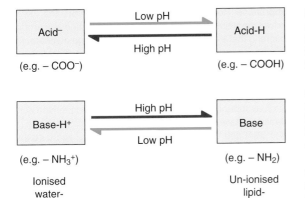

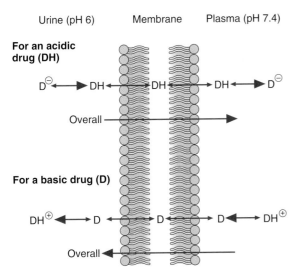

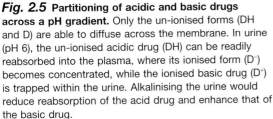

Fig. 2.4 Passive diffusion and the factors that affect drug concentrations in equilibrium between un-ionised and ionised forms. In this case, the pH is assumed to be the same on each side of the membrane; see Fig. 2.5 for drug partitioning when there is a pH gradient across the membrane.

Fig. 2.5 Partitioning of acidic and basic drugs across a pH gradient. Only the un-ionised forms (DH and D) are able to diffuse across the membrane. In urine (pH 6), the un-ionised acidic drug (DH) can be readily reabsorbed into the plasma, where its ionised form (D⁻) becomes concentrated, while the ionised basic drug (D⁺) is trapped within the urine. Alkalinising the urine would reduce reabsorption of the acid drug and enhance that of the basic drug.

differences in total drug concentration on each side of a membrane (pH trapping or partitioning), with the total drug concentration being higher on the side of the membrane on which it is most ionised. This is exemplified by the pH difference between urine (pH 5–7) and plasma (pH 7.4), which can influence renal elimination of drugs (Fig. 2.5). The relatively low pH of the urine forces an acidic drug to become predominantly un-ionised, allowing its reabsorption into the

plasma, while the higher pH in plasma (7.4) converts the drug to the ionised form, preventing it diffusing back and trapping (partitioning) it in the plasma. The opposite situation prevails with basic drugs, which are enabled to diffuse from the plasma into urine, where they become trapped.

After drug overdose, when the aim is to enhance drug elimination, alkalinisation of the urine can be used to reduce reabsorption of acidic drugs, leading to their faster elimination in the urine. Acidification of the urine can enhance ionisation and renal elimination of basic drugs, such as dexamfetamine.

The pH difference between gastric contents (pH 1–2) and plasma (pH 7.4) affects the absorption of many oral drugs. The acidity of stomach contents means that an acidic drug is present largely in its un-ionised (protonated) form, allowing it to pass into plasma where its ionised form becomes partitioned. In contrast, basic drugs are highly ionised in the stomach and absorption is negligible until the stomach empties and the drug can be absorbed from the more alkaline lumen of the duodenum (pH ~8).

Drugs that are fixed in their ionised form at all pH values, such as the quaternary amine compound suxamethonium (Ch. 27), cross cell membranes extremely slowly or not at all; they are given by injection (because of lack of absorption from the gastrointestinal tract) and have limited effects on the brain (because of lack of entry).

ABSORPTION

Absorption is the process of transfer of the drug from the site of administration into the general or systemic circulation.

ABSORPTION FROM THE GUT

The easiest and most convenient route of administration of medicines is orally by tablets, capsules or syrups. The large surface area of the small intestine combined with its high blood flow can give rapid and complete absorption of orally administered drugs. However, this route presents a number of obstacles for a drug before it reaches the systemic circulation.

Drug structure

Drug structure is a major determinant of absorption. Drugs need to be lipid-soluble to be absorbed from the gut. Highly polar acids and bases tend to be absorbed only slowly and incompletely, with much of the unabsorbed dose being voided in the faeces. High polarity may, however, be useful for delivery of the drug to a site of action in the lower bowel (see Ch. 34). The structures of some drugs can make them unstable either at the low pH of the stomach (e.g. benzylpenicillin) or in the presence of digestive enzymes (e.g. insulin). Such compounds have to be given by injection, but administration by other routes may be possible (e.g. inhalation for insulin).

Drugs that are weak acids or bases undergo pH partitioning between the gut lumen and mucosal cells. Acidic drugs will be least ionised in the stomach lumen and most absorption would be expected at this site, but absorption in the stomach is limited by its relatively low surface area (compared to the small intestine) and the presence of a zone of neutral pH on the immediate surface of the gastric mucosal cells (the mucosal bicarbonate layer; see Ch. 33). In consequence, the bulk of the absorption of drugs, even weak acids such as aspirin, occurs in the small intestine.

Drug formulation

A drug cannot be absorbed when it is taken in a tablet or capsule until the vehicle disintegrates and the drug is dissolved in the gastrointestinal contents to form a *molecular solution*. Most tablets disintegrate and dissolve quickly and completely and the whole dose rapidly becomes available for absorption. However, some formulations are designed to disintegrate slowly so that the rate of release and dissolution of drug from the formulation determines the rate of absorption. In modified-release (i.e. slow-release) formulations the drug is either incorporated into a complex matrix from which it diffuses slowly, or in a crystallised form that dissolves slowly. Dissolution of a tablet in the stomach can also be prevented by coating it in an acid-insoluble layer, producing enteric-coated formulations. This is useful for drugs such as omeprazole (Ch. 33), which is unstable in an acid environment, and allows delivery of intact drug to the duodenum.

Gastric emptying

The rate of gastric emptying determines how soon a drug taken orally is delivered to the small intestine, the major site of absorption. Delay between oral drug ingestion and the drug being detected in the circulation is usually caused by delayed gastric emptying. Drugs that slow gastric emptying, for example antimuscarinics, can delay the absorption of other drugs taken at the same time.

Food has complex effects on drug absorption; it slows gastric emptying and delays drug absorption, and it can also bind drugs and reduce the total amount of drug absorbed.

First-pass metabolism

Metabolism of drugs can occur before and during their absorption, and this can limit the amount of parent compound that reaches the general circulation. Drugs taken orally have to pass four major metabolic barriers before they reach the general circulation. If there is extensive metabolism of a drug at one or more of the sites below, only a fraction of the original oral dose reaches the general circulation as the parent compound. This process is known as first-pass metabolism because it occurs at the first passage through the organ.

Intestinal lumen

The intestinal lumen contains digestive enzymes secreted by the mucosal cells and pancreas that are able to split amide, ester and glycosidic bonds. Intestinal proteases prevent the oral administration of peptide drugs, such as insulin and other products of molecular biological

approaches to drug development. In addition, the lower bowel contains large numbers of aerobic and anaerobic bacteria that are capable of performing a range of metabolic reactions on drugs, especially hydrolysis and reduction.

Intestinal wall

The walls of the upper intestine are rich in cellular enzymes such as monoamine oxidase (MAO), aromatic L-amino acid decarboxylase, cytochrome P450 isoenzymes (e.g. CYP3A4) and the enzymes responsible for phase 2 conjugation reactions described below. In addition, the luminal membrane of the intestinal cells (enterocytes) contains efflux transporters such as P-gp (see above), which may limit the absorption of a drug by transporting it back into the intestinal lumen. Drug molecules that enter the enterocyte may thus undergo three possible fates; that is, diffusion into the hepatic portal circulation, metabolism within the cell or transport back into the gut lumen (by P-gp). The substrate specificities of CYP3A4 and P-gp overlap and for common substrates their combined actions can prevent most of the oral dose of some drugs reaching the hepatic portal circulation.

Liver

Blood from the intestine is delivered by the splanchnic circulation directly to the liver, which is the major site of drug metabolism in the body. Hepatic first-pass metabolism can be avoided by administering the drug to a region of the gut from which the blood does not drain into the hepatic portal vein, for example the buccal cavity or rectum; a good example of this is the buccal administration of glyceryl trinitrate (Ch. 5).

Lung

Cells of the lung have high affinities for many basic drugs and are the main site of metabolism for many local hormones via monoamine oxidase or peptidase activity.

ABSORPTION FROM OTHER ROUTES

Percutaneous (transcutaneous) administration

The human epidermis (especially the stratum corneum) is an effective permeability barrier to water loss and to the transfer of water-soluble compounds. Although lipid-soluble drugs are able to cross this barrier, the rate and extent of entry are very limited. In consequence, this route is only effective for use with potent, non-irritant drugs, such as glyceryl trinitrate (Ch. 5) or fentanyl (Ch. 19), or to produce a local effect. The slow and continued absorption from dermal administration (e.g. via adhesive patches) can be used to produce low, but relatively constant, blood concentrations of some drugs; for example nicotine-replacement therapy (Ch. 54).

Intradermal and subcutaneous injection

Intradermal or subcutaneous injection avoids the barrier presented by the stratum corneum and entry into the general circulation is limited mainly by the rate of blood flow to the site of injection. However, these sites only allow the administration of small volumes of drug and tend to be used mostly for local effects, such as local anaesthesia, or to deliberately limit the rate of drug absorption, for example insulin (Ch. 40).

Intramuscular injection

The rate of absorption from an intramuscular injection depends on two variables: the local blood flow and the water solubility of the drug. An increase in either of these factors enhances the rate of removal from the injection site. Absorption of drugs from the injection site can be prolonged intentionally either by incorporation of the drug into a lipophilic vehicle, such as flupentixol decanoate (Ch. 21) or by formation of a sparingly soluble salt, such as benzathine benzylpenicillin (Ch. 51), creating a depot formulation from which the drug is released over days or weeks.

Intranasal administration

The nasal mucosa provides a good surface area for absorption, combined with low levels of proteases and drug-metabolising enzymes compared with the gastrointestinal tract. In consequence, intranasal administration is used for the administration of some drugs, such as triptan drugs for migraine (Ch. 26), and desmopressin (Ch. 43), as well as for drugs designed to produce local effects, such as nasal decongestants and topical corticosteroids (Ch. 39).

Inhalation

Although the lungs possess the characteristics of a good site for drug absorption (a large surface area and extensive blood flow), inhalation is rarely used to produce systemic effects. The principal reasons for this are the difficulty of delivering non-volatile drugs to the alveoli and the potential for local toxicity to alveolar membranes. Therefore, drug administration by inhalation is largely restricted to:

- volatile compounds, such as general anaesthetics (Ch. 17),
- locally acting drugs, such as bronchodilators and corticosteroids used in the treatment of airway disease such as asthma and chronic obstructive pulmonary disease (Ch. 12).

Drugs in the latter group are not volatile and have to be given as either aerosols containing droplets of dissolved drug or fine particles of the solid drug (dry powder) (see Ch. 12). Particles greater than 10 μm in diameter settle out in the upper airways, which are poor sites for absorption, and the drug then passes back up the airways via ciliary motion and is eventually swallowed. It was estimated that only 5–10% of an inhaled dose is absorbed from the airways, although the percentage may be higher with modern inhaler devices delivering particle sizes closer to the optimum for airways deposition (2–5 μm). Particles less than 1 μm in diameter are not deposited in the airways and are exhaled.

Minor routes

Drugs may be applied to any body surface or orifice to produce a local effect. Absorption from the site of administration may be important in limiting the duration of local action and the production of unwanted systemic actions.

DISTRIBUTION

Distribution is the process by which the drug is transferred reversibly from the general circulation into the tissues as the concentrations in blood increase, and from the tissues into blood when the blood concentrations decrease. For most drugs this occurs by passive diffusion of the un-ionised form across cell membranes (Fig. 2.2) until equilibrium is reached (Fig. 2.4). At equilibrium, any process that removes the drug from one side of the membrane results in movement of drug across the membrane to re-establish the equilibrium (Fig. 2.4).

After an intravenous injection there is a high initial plasma concentration and the drug may rapidly enter well-perfused tissues such as the brain, liver and lungs (Table 2.2). This may be so rapid that these tissues may be assumed to equilibrate instantaneously with plasma and represent part of the 'central' compartment (see below). However, the drug will continue to enter poorly perfused tissues, and this will lower the plasma concentration. The high concentrations in the rapidly perfused tissues then decrease in parallel with the decreasing plasma

Table 2.2 Relative organ perfusion rates in a typical adult male at rest

Organ	Proportion of cardiac output (%)	Blood flow (mL·min⁻¹ per 100 g of tissue)
Well-perfused organs		
Lung	100	1000
Adrenals	0.5	200
Kidneys	15	350
Thyroid	1.5	500
Liver	27	110
Heart	4	100
Gastrointestinal tract	15	300
Brain	12	56
Placenta (full term)	–	10–15
Poorly perfused organs		
Skin	5	12
Skeletal muscle	12	4
Bone, connective tissue	3	3
Adipose (fat)	4	3

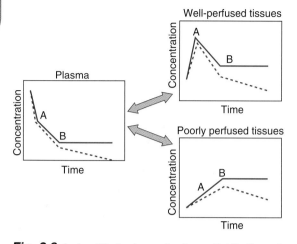

Table 2.3 Examples of drugs that undergo extensive binding to plasma protein

Bound to albumin	Bound to α₁-acid glycoprotein
Digitoxin	Chlorpromazine
Furosemide	Propranolol
Ibuprofen	Quinidine
Indometacin	Tricyclic antidepressants
Phenytoin	Lidocaine
Salicylates	
Sulphonamides	
Thiazides	
Tolbutamide	
Warfarin	

***Fig. 2.6* A simplified scheme for the redistribution of drugs between tissues.** The initial decrease in plasma concentrations results from uptake into well-perfused tissues, which essentially reaches equilibrium at point A. Between points A and B, the drug continues to enter poorly perfused tissues, resulting in a decrease in the concentrations in both plasma and well-perfused tissues. At point B all tissues are in equilibrium. The additional presence of an elimination process would produce a decrease from point B (shown as a dashed line), which would be parallel in all tissues.

concentration, resulting in a transfer of drug back into the plasma (Fig. 2.6). This redistribution is important for terminating the action of some drugs given as a rapid intravenous injection or bolus. For example, intravenous thiopental produces rapid anaesthesia, but effects in the brain are short-lived because continued uptake into muscle lowers the concentrations in the blood and therefore in the brain (Fig. 2.6; see also Fig. 17.2).

The processes of elimination (such as metabolism and excretion) are of major importance and are discussed in detail below. Elimination results in a net transfer of drug from other tissues via the circulation to the organ(s) of elimination (see dashed lines in Fig. 2.6).

REVERSIBLE PROTEIN BINDING

Many drugs show an affinity for sites on non-receptor proteins, resulting in reversible binding:

$$\text{Drug} + \text{protein} \rightleftharpoons \text{drug–protein complex}$$

Such binding occurs with plasma proteins, most commonly albumin, which binds many acidic drugs, and α₁-acid glycoprotein, which binds many basic or neutral drugs (Table 2.3). Drugs may also bind reversibly with intracellular proteins (Fig. 2.4). The drug–protein binding interaction resembles the drug–receptor interaction since it is rapid, reversible and saturable, and different ligands can compete for the same site. It does not result in a pharmacological effect but lowers the free concentration of drug available to act at receptors; the amounts of drug remaining available may be

only a minute fraction of the total body load. Proteins such as albumin can therefore act as depots, rapidly releasing the bound drug when the free drug is distributed to other compartments or eliminated.

Competition for binding to proteins in plasma or inside cells can occur between different drugs (drug interaction; see Ch. 56), and also between drugs and endogenous ligands. A highly protein-bound drug such as aspirin can displace another drug such as warfarin from its binding sites on plasma proteins; the increase in unbound drug concentration can increase the biological activity of the displaced drug. An example of interaction with an endogenous ligand is the displacement of bilirubin from albumin-binding sites by sulphanilamide drugs, causing a potentially dangerous increase in the bilirubin concentration in plasma, leading to kernicterus.

IRREVERSIBLE PROTEIN BINDING

Certain drugs, because of chemical reactivity of the parent compound or a metabolite, undergo covalent binding to plasma or tissue components such as proteins or nucleic acids. When the binding is irreversible, for example the interaction of some cytotoxic drugs with DNA, this can be considered as equivalent to elimination, because the parent drug cannot re-enter the circulation. In contrast, some covalent binding may be slowly reversible, such as the formation of disulphide bridges by captopril with its target ACE and with plasma proteins (Ch. 6); the covalently bound drug will not dissociate rapidly in response to a decrease in the concentration of unbound drug, and such binding represents a slowly equilibrating reservoir of drug.

DISTRIBUTION TO SPECIFIC ORGANS

Two systems require more detailed consideration of drug distribution: the brain, because of the difficulty of drug entry, and the fetus, because of the potential for drug toxicity.

Brain

Lipid-soluble drugs readily pass from the blood into the brain, and for such drugs the brain represents a typical well-perfused tissue (Table 2.2). In contrast, the entry of

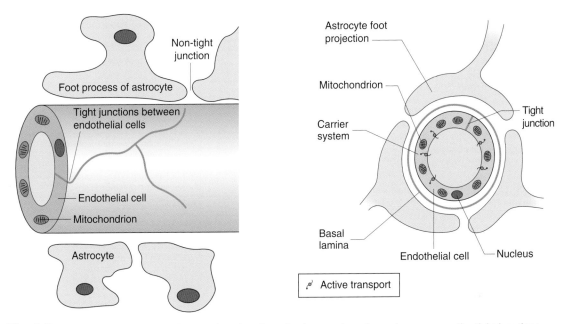

Fig. 2.7 **The blood–brain barrier.** The barrier arises from the low number of membrane pores, the tight junctions between adjacent cells and the presence of efflux transporters that remove any drug that enters the endothelial cell. The presence of astrocytes is the stimulus for these changes in endothelial structure and function. Astrocytes are one of the several types of cells found in the CNS that make up the glia; they have numerous sheet-like processes and may provide nutrients to neurons.

water-soluble drugs into the brain is much slower than into other well-perfused tissues, giving rise to the concept of a blood–brain barrier. The functional basis of the barrier to water-soluble drugs (Fig. 2.7) is reduced permeability of brain capillaries owing to:

- tight junctions between adjacent endothelial cells (capillaries are composed of an endothelial layer a single cell thick, with no smooth muscle),
- smaller size and lower number of pores in the endothelial cell membranes,
- the presence of a surrounding layer of astrocytes.

In addition, efflux transporters in the endothelial cells are an important part of the blood–brain barrier and return drug molecules back into the circulation, thereby preventing their entry into the brain and reducing effects in the central nervous system.

Water-soluble endogenous compounds needed for normal brain functioning, such as carbohydrates and amino acids, enter the brain via specific uptake transporters of the SLC superfamily (Table 2.1). Some drugs, for example levodopa, may enter the brain using these transport processes, and in such cases the rate of transport of the drug will be influenced by the concentrations of competitive endogenous substrates.

There is limited drug-metabolising ability in the brain and drugs leave by diffusion back into plasma, by active transport processes in the choroid plexus or by elimination in the cerebrospinal fluid. Organic acid transporters of the SLC superfamily (Table 2.1) are important in removing polar neurotransmitter metabolites from the brain.

Fetus

Lipid-soluble drugs can readily cross the placenta and enter the fetus. The placental blood flow is low compared to that in the liver, lung and spleen (Table 2.2); consequently, the fetal drug concentrations equilibrate slowly with the maternal circulation. Highly polar and very large molecules (such as heparin; see Ch. 11) do not readily cross the placenta. The fetal liver has only low levels of drug-metabolising enzymes so it is mainly the maternal elimination that clears the fetal circulation of drugs.

After delivery, the neonate may show effects from drugs given to the mother close to delivery (such as pethidine for pain control; see Ch. 19): such effects may be prolonged because the neonate now has to rely on his/her own immature elimination processes (Ch. 56).

ELIMINATION

Elimination is the removal of drug from the body and may involve metabolism, in which the drug molecule is transformed into a different molecule, and/or excretion, in which the drug molecule is expelled in the body's liquid, solid or gaseous 'waste'.

METABOLISM

A degree of lipid solubility is a useful property of most drugs, since it allows the compound to cross lipid barriers

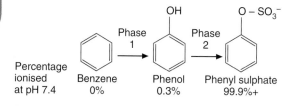

Percentage
ionised
at pH 7.4

Benzene 0% →Phase 1→ Phenol 0.3% →Phase 2→ Phenyl sulphate 99.9%+

Fig. 2.8 The two phases of drug metabolism. Phase 1 and phase 2 reactions are also called preconjugation and conjugation, respectively.

and hence to be given via the oral route. Metabolism is necessary for the elimination of lipid-soluble drugs from the body, because it converts a lipid-soluble molecule (which would otherwise be reabsorbed from urine in the kidney tubule; see below) into a water-soluble species capable of rapid elimination in the urine (often via an anion transporter).

Metabolism of the drug produces a new chemical entity, which may show different pharmacological properties from the parent compound:

- **decrease in biological activity**: the most common result of drug metabolism; arises from increased polarity which reduces receptor binding,
- **increase in activity**: the metabolite is more potent than the parent drug; a prodrug is an inactive compound that is converted by metabolism into the active molecular species,
- **change in the nature of the activity**: the metabolite shows qualitatively different pharmacological or toxicological properties.

The various steps of drug metabolism can be divided into two phases (Fig. 2.8). Although many compounds undergo both phases of metabolism, it is possible for a drug to undergo only a phase 1 or a phase 2 reaction, or for a proportion of the drug to be excreted unchanged. Phase 1 metabolism (oxidation, reduction and hydrolysis) is often described as preconjugation, because it produces a molecule that is a suitable substrate for a phase 2 or conjugation reaction. The enzymes involved in these reactions have low substrate specificities and can metabolise a wide range of drug substrates and other xenobiotics.

Phase 1

Cytochrome P450 is a superfamily of membrane-bound haemoprotein enzymes (Table 2.4). They are present in the smooth endoplasmic reticulum of cells (Fig. 2.9), particularly in the liver which is the major site of drug oxidation; the amounts in other tissues are low in comparison. The cytochrome P450 families CYP1–4 are involved in drug metabolism; the specific isoenzymes CYP2C9, CYP2D6 and CYP3A4 are involved in the phase 1 metabolism of approximately 10, 24 and 55% of drugs respectively.

Oxidation reactions (Table 2.5) are the most important of the phase 1 reactions and can occur at carbon, nitrogen or sulphur atoms within the drug structure. In most cases, an oxygen atom is retained in the metabolite, although some reactions, such as dealkylation, result in loss of the oxygen atom in a small fragment of the original molecule. Oxidation

Table 2.4 Cytochrome P450 superfamily

Isoenzyme	Comments
CYP1A	Important for methylxanthines and paracetamol; induced by smoking
CYP2A	Limited number of substrates; significant inter-individual variability
CYP2B	Limited number of substrates
CYP2C	CYP2C9 is an important isoform; CYP2C19 shows genetic polymorphism
CYP2D	Metabolises numerous drugs; CYP2D6 shows genetic polymorphism
CYP2E	Metabolises alcohol
CYP3A	Main isoform in liver and intestine; metabolises 50–60% of current drugs
CYP4	Metabolises fatty acids

Human liver contains at least 20 isoenzymes of cytochrome P450. Families CYP1–4 are involved in drug metabolism.

Table 2.5 Examples of oxidation, reduction and hydrolytic reactions

Oxidation	
Alkyl groups	$RCH_3 \rightarrow RCH_2OH \rightarrow RCHO \rightarrow RCOOH$
Deamination	$RCH_2NH_2 \rightarrow RCHO + NH_3$
Amines	$R'-N-R \rightarrow R'-N-R$ (H → OH)
Reduction	
Aldehydes	$RCHO \rightarrow RCH_2OH$
Disulphides	$R-S-S-R' \rightarrow RSH + HSR'$
Hydrolysis	
Esters	$RCO \cdot OR' \rightarrow RCOOH + HOR'$
Amides	$RCO \cdot NHR' \rightarrow RCOH + H_2NR'$

R, R', aliphatic groups

reactions are catalysed by a diverse group of enzymes, of which the cytochrome P450 system is the most important. The cytochrome P450 isoenzyme binds both the drug and molecular oxygen (Fig. 2.10), and catalyses the transfer of one oxygen atom to the substrate while the other oxygen atom is reduced to water:

$$RH + O_2 + NADPH + H^+ \rightarrow ROH + H_2O + NADP^+$$

The reaction involves initial binding of the drug substrate to the ferric (Fe^{3+}) form of cytochrome P450, followed by reduction (via a specific cytochrome P450 reductase) and then binding of molecular oxygen. Further reduction is followed by molecular rearrangement, with release of the reaction products (drug metabolite and water) and regeneration of ferric cytochrome P450.

Oxidations at nitrogen and sulphur atoms are frequently performed by a second enzyme of the endoplasmic

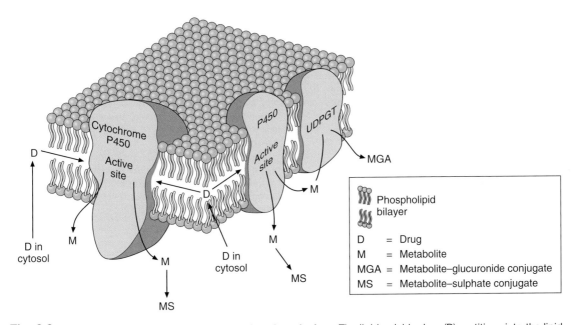

Fig. 2.9 **Drug metabolism in the smooth endoplasmic reticulum.** The lipid-soluble drug (D) partitions into the lipid bilayer of the endoplasmic reticulum. The cytochrome P450 oxidises the drug to a metabolite (M) that is more water-soluble and diffuses out of the lipid layer. The metabolite may undergo a phase 2 (conjugation) reaction catalysed by UDP-glucuronyl transferase (UDPGT) in the endoplasmic reticulum to give a glucuronide conjugate (MGA) or with sulphate in the cytosol to give a sulphate conjugate (MS).

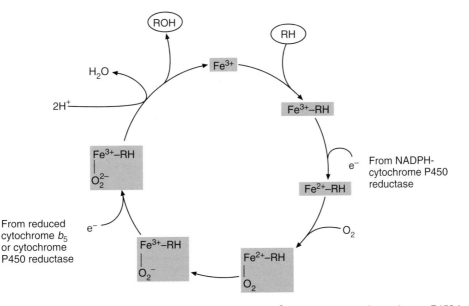

Fig. 2.10 **The oxidation of substrate (RH) by cytochrome P450.** Fe^{3+}, the active site of cytochrome P450 in its ferric state; RH, drug substrate; ROH, oxidised metabolite. Cytochrome b_5 is present in the endoplasmic reticulum and can transfer an electron to cytochrome P450 as part of its redox reactions.

reticulum, the flavin-containing mono-oxygenase, which also requires molecular oxygen and NADPH. A number of other enzymes, such as alcohol dehydrogenase, aldehyde oxidase and MAO, may be involved in the oxidation of specific functional groups.

Reduction reactions (Table 2.5) are less than common than oxidation reactions, but occur at unsaturated carbon

atoms and at nitrogen and sulphur centres by the actions of cytochrome P450 and cytochrome P450 reductase, and also by the intestinal microflora.

Hydrolysis and hydration reactions (Table 2.5) involve addition of water to the drug molecule. In hydrolysis, the molecule is then split by the addition of water. A number of ubiquitous enzymes are able to hydrolyse ester and amide bonds in drugs. The intestinal bacteria are also important for the hydrolysis of esters and amides and of drug conjugates eliminated in the bile (see below). In hydration reactions, the water molecule is retained in the drug metabolite. Hydration of an epoxide ring by epoxide hydrolase is an important reaction in the metabolism and toxicity of a number of aromatic drugs, for example carbamazepine (Ch. 23).

Phase 2

Phase 2 (conjugation) reactions involve the formation of a covalent bond between the drug, or its phase 1 metabolite, and an endogenous substrate. Table 2.6 shows the types of phase 2 reactions, the functional group necessary in the drug molecule and the activated species needed for the reaction. The products of conjugation reactions are usually highly water-soluble and lack biological activity.

The activated endogenous substrate for glucuronide synthesis is uridine-diphosphate glucuronic acid (UDPGA). UDP-glucuronyl transferases in the endoplasmic reticulum close to the cytochrome P450 system (Fig. 2.9) transfer glucuronate to the drug. Glucuronide conjugation in the gut wall and liver is important in the first-pass metabolism of substrates such as simple phenols.

Sulphate conjugation is performed by a cytosolic enzyme, which utilises high-energy sulphate (3′-phosphoadenosine-5′-phosphosulphate or PAPS) as the rate-limiting endogenous substrate. Saturation of sulphate conjugation contributes to the hepatotoxic consequences of overdose with paracetamol (acetaminophen) (see Ch. 53).

Acetylation and methylation reactions often decrease polarity because they block an ionisable functional group (Table 2.6), but they mask active groups such as amino and catechol moieties. These reactions are primarily involved in inactivation of neurotransmitters such as noradrenaline and local hormones such as histamine.

The conjugation of drug carboxylic acid groups with amino acids is unusual because the drug is converted to a high-energy form (a CoA derivative) prior to the formation of the conjugate bond by transferase enzymes. Conjugation with the tripeptide glutathione (GSH or L-α-glutamyl-L-cysteinylglycine) is catalysed by a family of transferases which covalently bind the drug to the thiol group in the cysteine (Fig. 2.11). The substrates are often reactive drugs or activated metabolites, which are inherently unstable (see Ch. 53), and the reaction can also occur non-enzymatically. The glutathione conjugate then undergoes further metabolic reactions. Glutathione conjugation is a detoxification process in which glutathione acts as a scavenging agent to protect the cell from toxic damage. Glutathione conjugates, and endogenous cysteine conjugates such as the cysteinyl-leukotriene (LT) C_4, are transported out of cells by the MRP1 transporter (Table 2.1).

The complex array of biotransformation reactions typically involved in drug metabolism is illustrated by the anxiolytic drug diazepam (Ch. 20), which is metabolised to biologically active intermediates before undergoing conjugation with glucuronide (Fig. 2.12).

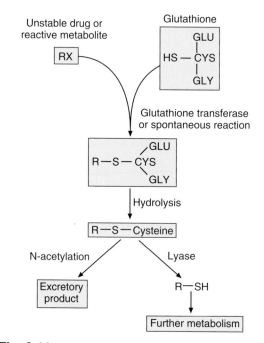

Fig. 2.11 The formation and further metabolism of glutathione conjugates.

Table 2.6 Major conjugation reactions

Reaction	Functional group	Activated species	Products
Glucuronidation	–OH –COOH –NH$_2$	Uridine-diphosphate glucuronic acid (UDPGA)	Glucuronide conjugates
Sulphation	–OH –NH$_3$	3′-Phosphoadenosine-5′-phosphosulphate (PAPS)	–O–SO$_3$H –NH–SO$_3$H
Acetylation	–NH$_2$	Acetyl-CoA	–NH–COCH$_3$
Methylation	–OH –NH$_2$ –SH	S-Adenosyl methionine	–OCH$_3$ –NHCH$_3$ –SCH$_3$
Amino acid conjugation	–COOH	Drug-CoA	CO–NH·CHR·COOH
Glutathione conjugation	Various	–	Glutathione conjugates

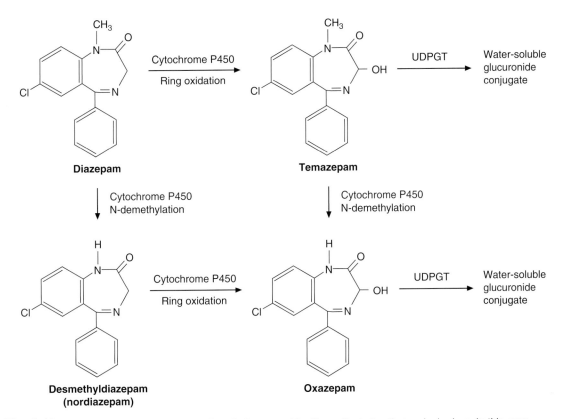

Fig. 2.12 Complex pathways of metabolism in humans. The figure illustrates that a single drug, in this case diazepam, may generate a number of active metabolites before phase 2 conjugation terminates the activity of the parent drug and metabolites.

Factors affecting drug metabolism

The liver is the main site of drug metabolism; the large surface area of the sinusoids, combined with high levels of enzyme activity in hepatocytes, can result in very rapid drug uptake and metabolism as the blood flows through the liver (see Ch. 56 for normal sinusoid architecture and the effects of liver disease on hepatic drug uptake). Environmental influences including chemical contaminants and therapeutic drugs may induce or inhibit the activity of hepatic drug-metabolising enzymes, particularly cytochrome P450 (Table 2.7). This can affect both the bioavailability and the elimination of other drugs undergoing hepatic elimination (see below).

Inducing agents increase the cellular expression of cytochrome P450 enzymes. This occurs over a period of a few days, during which the inducer interacts with nuclear receptors to increase mRNA transcription of genes coding for cytochrome P450. The increased amounts of the enzyme last for a few days after the removal of the inducing agent, and are removed by normal protein turnover. Environmental contaminants such as organochlorine compounds (e.g. dioxins) and polycyclic aromatic hydrocarbons (e.g. benzo[a]pyrene in cigarette smoke) induce CYP1A. Therapeutic drugs can induce members of the CYP2 and CYP3 families. Chronic consumption of alcohol induces CYP2E.

In contrast, inhibition of cytochrome P450 by drugs occurs by direct reversible competition for the enzyme site, not a change in enzyme expression, so the time course follows closely the absorption and elimination of the inhibitor substance. Examples of inhibitors are the histamine H_2 receptor antagonist cimetidine (Ch. 33) and components of grapefruit juice (Table 2.7).

The activity of drug-metabolising enzymes is also dependent on the delivery of their drug substrates by the circulation. Metabolism of many drugs is affected significantly by lower hepatic blood flow in the very young and in the elderly (Ch. 56). Genetic variation in drug-metabolising enzymes is discussed at the end of this chapter.

EXCRETION

Drugs and their metabolites may be eliminated from the circulation by various routes:

- **in fluids (urine, bile, sweat, tears, breast milk, etc.)**: important for low-molecular-weight polar compounds; urine is the major route; milk is important because of the potential for exposure of the breastfed infant,
- **in solids (faeces, hair, etc.)**: faecal elimination is most important for high-molecular-weight compounds excreted in bile; the sequestration of drugs into hair is not quantitatively important, but the distribution of a drug along the hair shaft can indicate the history of drug intake during the preceding weeks,
- **in gases (expired air)**: important only for volatile compounds.

Table 2.7 Common substrates, inhibitors and inducers of cytochrome P450 (CYP) isoenzymes

Isoenzyme	Substrates (examples)	Inhibitors (examples)	Inducers (examples)
CYP1A2	Caffeine, paracetamol, theophylline, verapamil	Cimetidine, clarithromycin, erythromycin, grapefruit juice, isoniazid, ketoconazole	Omeprazole, charbroiled foods, cigarette smoke, dioxins
CYP2A6	Coumarin, halothane, nicotine	Grapefruit juice, ketoconazole, tranylcypromine	Dexamethasone, phenobarbital, rifampicin
CYP2B6	Bupropion, cyclophosphamide, efavirenz, ifosfamide	Fluoxetine, orphenadrine, paroxetine	Carbamazepine, phenobarbital, phenytoin, rifampicin
CYP2C9	Diclofenac, glibenclamide, ibuprofen, losartan, tolbutamide, S-warfarin	Amiodarone, cimetidine, fluconazole, fluoxetine, ketoconazole, omeprazole, valproic acid	Carbamazepine, dexamethasone, phenobarbital, rifampicin
CYP2C19	Clopidogrel, diazepam, omeprazole	Cimetidine, fluvoxamine, moclobemide, omeprazole	Carbamazepine, rifampicin
CYP2D6	Amitriptyline, bisoprolol, codeine, desipramine, encainide, many SSRIs, metamfetamine, metoprolol, ondansetron, propranolol	Amiodarone, cimetidine, fluoxetine, haloperidol, methadone, quinidine	Carbamazepine, phenobarbital, phenytoin, rifampicin
CYP2E	Chlorzoxazone, ethanol, halothane, paracetamol	Disulfiram, isoniazid	Ethanol
CYP3A4	Numerous drugs of different classes, e.g. alfentanil, amiodarone, carbamazepine, diltiazem, erythromycin, fluconazole, lidocaine, midazolam, montelukast, nifedipine, saquinavir, tamoxifen, terfenadine	Cimetidine, clarithromycin, clotrimazole, erythromycin, fluconazole, grapefruit juice, ketoconazole, saquinavir	Carbamazepine, dexamethasone, ethosuximide, isoniazid, phenobarbital, phenytoin, rifampicin

SSRIs, selective serotonin re-uptake inhibitors.

Excretion via the urine

There are three processes involved in the handling of drugs and their metabolites in the kidney: glomerular filtration, reabsorption and tubular secretion. The total urinary excretion of a drug depends on the balance of these three processes:

Total excretion = glomerular filtration
+ tubular secretion – reabsorption

Glomerular filtration

All molecules less than about 20 kDa undergo filtration under positive hydrostatic pressure through pores of 7–8 nm diameter in the glomerular membrane. The glomerular filtrate contains about 20% of the plasma volume delivered to the glomerulus, and hence about 20% of all water-soluble, low-molecular-weight compounds free in the plasma enter the filtrate. Plasma proteins and protein-bound drugs are not filtered, so the efficiency of glomerular filtration for a drug is influenced by the extent of plasma protein binding.

Reabsorption

The glomerular filtrate contains numerous constituents that the body cannot afford to lose. There are specific tubular uptake processes for carbohydrates, amino acids, vitamins, etc., and most of the water is also reabsorbed (see Ch. 14). A few drugs pass from the tubule back into the plasma as they are substrates for these specific uptake processes. The urine is concentrated on its passage down the renal tubule; as the tubule-to-plasma concentration gradient increases, only the most polar molecules remain in the urine. Because of extensive reabsorption, lipid-soluble drugs are not eliminated via the urine, but are returned to the circulation until they are metabolised to water-soluble products, which are efficiently removed from the body. The pH of urine is usually less than that of plasma; consequently, pH partitioning between urine (pH 5–6) and plasma (pH 7.4) may increase or decrease the tendency of the compound to be reabsorbed (Fig. 2.5).

Tubular secretion

The renal tubule has secretory transporters (Table 2.1) on both the basolateral and apical membranes for compounds that are acidic (organic anion transporters, OATs) or basic (organic cation transporters, OCTs). Drugs and their metabolites, especially the glucuronic acid and sulphate conjugates, may undergo an active carrier-mediated elimination, primarily by OATs but also by multidrug-resistance-associated proteins (MRPs). Because tubular secretion rapidly lowers the plasma concentration of unbound drug there will be a rapid dissociation of any drugs bound to proteins in the plasma. As a result, even highly protein-bound drugs may be cleared almost completely from the blood in a single passage through the kidney.

Excretion via the faeces

Uptake into hepatocytes and subsequent elimination in bile is the principal route of elimination of larger molecules (molecular weight >500 Da). Conjugation with glucuronic acid increases the molecular weight of the substrate by

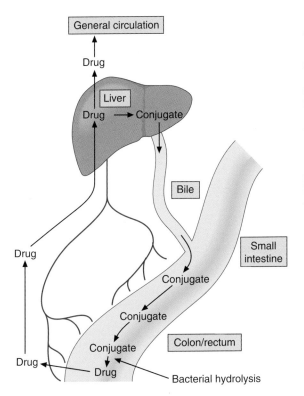

Fig. 2.13 **Enterohepatic circulation of drugs.** Drug molecules may circulate repeatedly between the bile, gut, portal circulation, liver and general circulation, particularly if the drug conjugate is hydrolysed by the gut flora.

almost 200 Da, so bile is an important route for eliminating glucuronide conjugates. Once the drug or its conjugate has entered the intestinal lumen via the bile (Fig. 2.13) it passes down the gut and may eventually be eliminated in the faeces. However, some drugs may be reabsorbed from the lumen of the gut and re-enter the hepatic portal vein. As a result, the drug is recycled between the gut lumen, hepatic portal vein, liver, bile and back to the gut lumen; this is described as *enterohepatic circulation*. Some of the reabsorbed drug may escape hepatic extraction and proceed into the hepatic vein, maintaining the drug concentrations in the general circulation.

Highly polar glucuronide conjugates of drugs or their oxidised metabolites that are excreted into the bile undergo little reabsorption in the upper intestine. However, the bacterial flora of the lower intestine may hydrolyse the conjugate, so the original, lipid-soluble drug or its metabolite may be reabsorbed and undergo enterohepatic circulation (Fig. 2.13).

THE MATHEMATICAL BASIS OF PHARMACOKINETICS

The use of mathematics to describe the fate of a drug in the body can be complex and daunting for undergraduates.

Nevertheless, a basic knowledge is essential for understanding many aspects of drug handling and the rational prescribing of drugs:

- why oral and intravenous treatments may require different doses,
- the interval between doses during chronic therapy,
- the dosage adjustment that may be necessary in hepatic and renal disease,
- the calculation of dosages for the very young and the elderly.

GENERAL CONSIDERATIONS

The processes of drug absorption, distribution, metabolism and excretion are described in mathematical terms as it is important to quantify the rate and extent to which the drug undergoes each process.

For nearly all physiological and metabolic processes the rate of reaction is not uniform but proportional to the amount of substrate (drug) available: this is described as a *first-order reaction*. Diffusion down a concentration gradient, glomerular filtration and enzymatic hydrolysis are examples of first-order reactions. At higher concentrations, more drug diffuses or is filtered or hydrolysed than at lower concentrations. Protein-mediated reactions, such as metabolism and active transport, are also first-order, because if the concentration of the substrate is doubled then the rate of formation of product is also doubled. However, as the substrate concentration increases the enzyme or transporter can become saturated with substrate and the rate of reaction cannot respond to a further increase in concentration. The process then occurs at a fixed maximum rate independent of substrate concentration, and the reaction is described as a *zero-order reaction*; examples are the metabolism of ethanol (Ch. 54) and phenytoin (Ch. 23). When the substrate concentration has decreased sufficiently for protein sites to become available again, then the reaction will revert to first-order.

Zero-order reactions

If a drug is being processed (absorbed, distributed or eliminated) according to zero-order kinetics then the change in concentration with time (dC/dt) is a fixed amount per time, independent of concentration:

$$\frac{dC}{dt} = -k \qquad (2.2)$$

The units of k (the reaction rate constant) will be an amount per unit time (e.g. $mg \cdot min^{-1}$). A graph of concentration against time will produce a straight line with a slope of $-k$ (Fig. 2.14A).

First-order reactions

In first-order reactions the change in concentration at any time (dC/dt) is proportional to the concentration present at that time:

$$\frac{dC}{dt} = -kC \qquad (2.3)$$

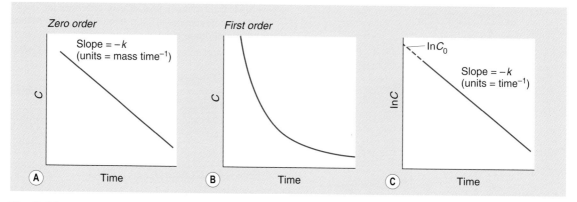

Fig. 2.14 Zero- and first-order kinetics. (A) The zero-order reaction is a uniform change in concentration C over time. (B) The first-order reaction is an exponential curve in which concentrations fall fastest when they are highest. (C) Plotting the natural logarithm of the concentration (ln C) in a first-order reaction against time generates a straight line with slope $-k$ (where k is the rate constant) and the intercept gives the concentration at time zero, C_0.

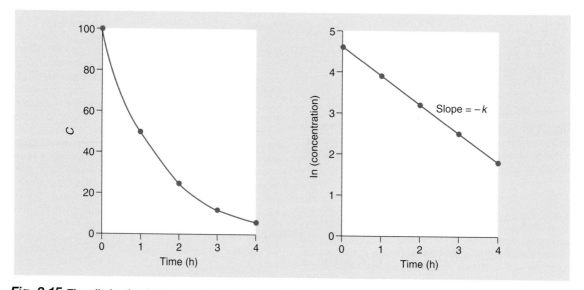

Fig. 2.15 The elimination half-life of a drug in plasma. Here the concentration C decreases by 50% every hour, i.e. the half-life is 1 h.

The rate of change will be high at high drug concentrations but low at low concentrations (Fig. 2.14B), and a graph of concentration against time will produce an exponential decrease. Such a curve can be described by an exponential equation:

$$C = C_0 e^{-kt} \qquad (2.4)$$

where C is the concentration at time t and C_0 is the initial concentration (when time = 0). This equation may be written more simply by taking natural logarithms:

$$\ln C = \ln C_0 - kt \qquad (2.5)$$

and a graph of ln$C$ against time will produce a straight line with a slope of $-k$ and an intercept of lnC_0 (Fig. 2.14C).

The units of the rate constant k (time^{-1}, e.g. h^{-1}) may be regarded as the proportional change per unit of time but are difficult to use practically, so the rate of a first-order reaction is usually described in terms of its half-life ($t_{1/2}$),

which is the time taken for a concentration to decrease by one-half. In the next half-life, the drug concentration falls again by one-half, to a quarter of the original concentration, and then to one-eighth in the next half-life, and so on. The half-life is therefore independent of concentration and is a characteristic for a particular first-order process and a particular drug. The intravenous drug shown in Figure 2.15 has a $t_{1/2}$ of 1 h.

The relationship between the half-life and the rate constant is derived by substituting $C_0 = 2$ and $C = 1$ into the above equation, when the time interval t will be one half-life ($t_{1/2}$), giving:

$$\ln 1 = \ln 2 - kt_{1/2}$$
$$0 = 0.693 - kt_{1/2} \qquad (2.6)$$
$$t_{1/2} = 0.693/k \text{ or } k = 0.693/t_{1/2}$$

(Note: 0.693 = ln2)

A half-life can be calculated for any first-order process (e.g. for absorption, distribution or elimination). In practice, the 'half-life' normally reported for a drug is the half-life for the elimination rate from plasma (the slowest, terminal phase of the plasma concentration–time curve; see below).

ABSORPTION

The mathematics of absorption apply to all non-intravenous routes (e.g. oral, inhalation, percutaneous, etc) and are illustrated by absorption from the gut lumen.

RATE OF ABSORPTION

The rate of absorption after oral administration is determined by the rate at which the drug is able to pass from the gut lumen into the systemic circulation. Following oral doses of some drugs, particularly lipid-soluble drugs with very rapid absorption, it may be possible to see three distinct phases in the plasma concentration–time curve, which reflect distinct phases of absorption, distribution and elimination (Fig. 2.16A). However, for most drugs slow absorption masks the distribution phase (Fig. 2.16B). A number of factors can influence this pattern.

- **Gastric emptying.** Basic drugs undergo negligible absorption from the stomach, so there can be a delay of up to an hour between drug administration and the detection of drug in the general circulation.
- **Food.** Food in the stomach slows drug absorption and also slows gastric emptying.
- **Decomposition or first-pass metabolism before or during absorption.** This will reduce the *amount* of drug that reaches the general circulation but will not affect the *rate* of absorption, which is usually determined by lipid solubility.
- **Modified-release formulation.** If a drug is eliminated rapidly, the plasma concentrations will show rapid fluctuations during regular oral dosing, and it may be

necessary to take the drug at very frequent intervals to maintain a therapeutic plasma concentration. The frequency with which a drug is taken can be reduced by giving a modified-release formulation that releases drug at a slower rate. The plasma concentration then becomes more dependent on the rate of absorption than the rate of elimination.

EXTENT OF ABSORPTION

Bioavailability (F) is defined as the fraction of the administered dose that reaches the systemic circulation as the parent drug (not as metabolites). For oral administration, incomplete bioavailability ($F < 1$) may result from:

- **incomplete absorption and loss in the faeces**, because either the molecule is too polar to be absorbed or the tablet did not release all of its contents,
- **first-pass metabolism** in the gut lumen, during passage across the gut wall or by the liver before the drug reaches the systemic circulation.

The bioavailability of a drug has important therapeutic implications, because it is the major factor determining the drug dosage for different routes of administration. For example, if a drug has an oral bioavailability of 0.1, the oral dose needed for therapeutic effectiveness will need to be 10 times higher than the corresponding intravenous dose.

The bioavailability is a characteristic of the drug and independent of dose, providing that absorption and elimination are not saturated. Bioavailability is normally determined by comparison of plasma concentration data obtained after oral administration (when the fraction F of the parent drug enters the general circulation) with data following intravenous administration (when, by definition, $F = 1$, as 100% of the parent drug enters the general circulation). The amount in the circulation cannot be compared at a single time point, because intravenous and oral dosing show different concentration–time profiles, so instead the total area under the plasma concentration–time curve (AUC) from $t = 0$ to $t =$ infinity is used, as this reflects the total

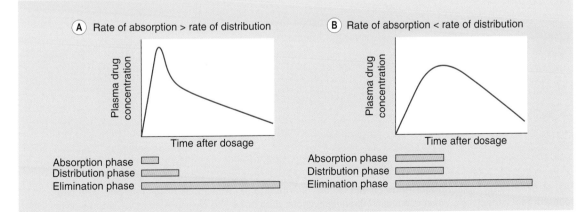

Fig. 2.16 **Plasma concentration–time profiles after oral administration of drugs with different rates of absorption.** The processes of distribution and elimination start as soon as some of the drug has entered the general circulation. (A) A clear distribution phase is seen if the rate of absorption is so rapid as to be essentially complete before distribution is finished. (B) For most drugs, the rate of absorption is slower and masks the distribution phase.

amount of drug that has entered the general circulation. If the oral and intravenous (iv) doses administered are equal:

$$F = \frac{AUC_{oral}}{AUC_{iv}} \qquad (2.7)$$

or if different doses are used:

$$F = \frac{AUC_{oral} \times Dose_{iv}}{AUC_{iv} \times Dose_{oral}} \qquad (2.8)$$

This calculation assumes that the elimination is first-order.

An alternative method to calculate F is to measure the total urinary excretion of the parent drug (Aex) following oral and intravenous administration of identical doses:

$$F = \frac{Aex_{oral}}{Aex_{iv}} \qquad (2.9)$$

DISTRIBUTION

Distribution concerns the rate and extent of movement of the parent drug from the blood into the tissues after administration and its return from the tissues into the blood during elimination.

RATE OF DISTRIBUTION

Because a distinct distribution phase is not usually seen when a drug is taken orally (Fig. 2.16B), the rate of distribution is normally measured following an intravenous bolus dose. Some intravenous drugs reach equilibrium between blood and tissues very rapidly and a distinct distribution phase is not apparent. In Figure 2.17A the slope of plasma concentration against time therefore mainly reflects elimination of the drug; this is described as a *one-compartment model*.

Most intravenous drugs, however, take a finite time to distribute into the tissues; the initial distribution out of the plasma, combined with underlying elimination, produces a steep initial slope (slope A–B in Fig. 2.17B), followed by a slower terminal phase (B–C) in which distribution has been largely completed and elimination predominates. Back-extrapolation of this terminal phase to time zero gives an initial value D, which is the theoretical concentration that would have been obtained if distribution had been instantaneous. The actual rate of distribution can therefore be estimated by the difference between the rapid initial fall in concentration (distribution plus elimination, A–B) and the underlying rate of elimination alone (D–B). In practice,

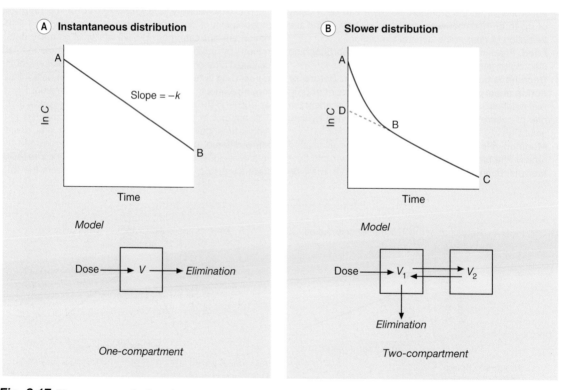

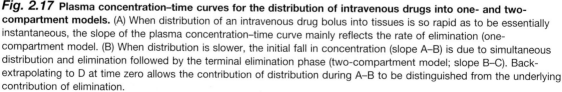

Fig. 2.17 **Plasma concentration–time curves for the distribution of intravenous drugs into one- and two-compartment models.** (A) When distribution of an intravenous drug bolus into tissues is so rapid as to be essentially instantaneous, the slope of the plasma concentration–time curve mainly reflects the rate of elimination (one-compartment model). (B) When distribution is slower, the initial fall in concentration (slope A–B) is due to simultaneous distribution and elimination followed by the terminal elimination phase (two-compartment model; slope B–C). Back-extrapolating to D at time zero allows the contribution of distribution during A–B to be distinguished from the underlying contribution of elimination.

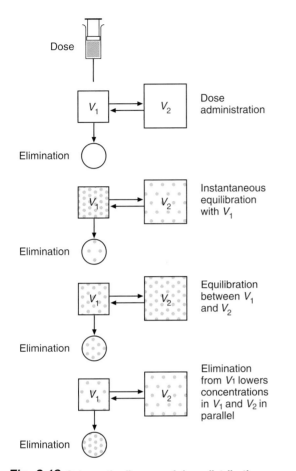

Fig. 2.18 **Schematic diagram of drug distribution.**
Distribution from the circulation into tissues is reversed as the drug in the circulation is gradually eliminated. At equilibrium, the free drug concentrations are transiently the same in volumes V_1 and V_2; the total drug concentrations may nevertheless be different due to drug binding to proteins in the plasma or accumulation in tissue fat.

knowing the rate of drug distribution is rarely of clinical importance.

Such a two-compartment model in which the drug in one compartment (e.g. blood) equilibrates more slowly with a second compartment (e.g. poorly perfused tissues; or a fetus) is also shown in Figure 2.18. The rate of distribution into the second compartment is dependent on the solubility of the drug:

- for *water-soluble drugs*, the rate of distribution depends on the rate of passage across membranes, i.e. the diffusion characteristics of the drug,
- for *lipid-soluble drugs*, the rate of distribution depends on the rate of delivery (the blood flow) to those tissues, such as adipose tissue, that accumulate the drug.

The plasma concentration–time curves of some drugs show three distinct phases; such *three-compartment models* are of limited practical value.

EXTENT OF DISTRIBUTION

The *extent* of distribution of a drug from plasma into tissues is more important clinically than the rate because it determines the total amount of a drug that has to be administered to produce a particular plasma concentration (and therapeutic effect). In humans only the concentration in blood or plasma can be measured easily, so the extent of distribution has to be estimated from the amount remaining in blood, or more usually plasma, after completion of distribution.

The parameter that describes the extent of distribution is the *apparent volume of distribution* (V_d). In general terms, the concentration of a drug solution is the amount (or dose) of drug dissolved in a volume; rearranging this gives:

$$V_d = \frac{\text{Total amount (dose) of drug in the body}}{\text{Plasma concentration}} \quad (2.10)$$

If an intravenous dose of 50 mg of a particular drug is injected, and, after an appropriate interval to allow time for distribution to reach equilibrium, the total concentration of the drug in plasma is found to be 1 mg·L^{-1}, then the apparent volume of distribution (V_d) is:

$$V_d = \frac{\text{Total amount (dose)}}{\text{Plasma concentration}} = \frac{50\,\text{mg}}{1\,\text{mg} \cdot \text{L}^{-1}}$$
$$= 50\,\text{L}$$

In other words, after giving the dose, it appears that the drug has been dissolved in 50 L of plasma. However, the plasma volume in adult humans is only about 3 L, so much of the drug must have left the plasma and entered tissues in order to give the low concentration remaining in the plasma (1 mg·L^{-1}).

V_d is a characteristic of a particular drug and is independent of dose; its clinical usefulness becomes apparent when a physician needs to calculate how much of the drug should be given to a patient to produce a desired plasma concentration. If an initial plasma concentration of 2.5 mg·L^{-1} of the drug is needed for a clinical effect, this could be produced by giving an intravenous dose of (the known V_d × the desired plasma concentration) or (50 L × 2.5 mg·L^{-1}); that is, a dose of 125 mg.

In practice, in measuring the V_d value of a drug it has to be remembered that distribution usually takes time to reach equilibrium, and also that during this time elimination is steadily reducing the total amount of drug in the body. In calculating V_d, therefore, it is usual to extrapolate the plasma-concentration curve back to time zero (as illustrated in Fig. 2.17b) to find the theoretical concentration as if the drug has distributed instantaneously and significant elimination has not yet occurred:

$$V_d = \frac{\text{Total amount (dose)}}{\text{Extrapolated plasma concentration at time zero}} \quad (2.11)$$

It is important to recognise that V_d may not be a true physiological volume. If the V_d calculated for a drug is 2.5–3 L, this might indicate that it has been confined within the circulatory volume, while a V_d value of about 40 L might mean it has been able to pass into tissues and is distributed uniformly into the total volume of body water, which is about 40 L in adults. However, V_d is only a theoretical measure based on how much the concentration of drug remaining in the plasma has been diluted by its distribution in the body. While a large V_d may indeed occur when the drug is distributed at uniform concentrations into a large body compartment (such as total body water), the same high V_d may also occur if the drug has been highly bound or sequestered by a tissue component within one or more smaller compartments. For example, binding tightly to tissue proteins in a single organ, or sequestration of a lipophilic drug at high concentrations into adipose (fat) cells, may reduce the plasma drug concentration to the same extent (and produce the same large V_d). Identifying such effects can be achieved only by measuring drug concentrations in tissues, which is rarely practicable in humans.

The V_d of a drug is nevertheless an important concept. It indicates the theoretical volume that has to be cleared of the drug by the organs of elimination, such as the liver and kidneys, which extract the drug from the plasma for metabolism and excretion. Together with clearance (the volume of plasma from which the drug can be cleared in a certain time), it determines the overall rate of elimination and therefore the half-life of the drug. In turn, the half-life determines the duration of action of a single dose and hence the optimal interval between repeated doses of the drug (see below).

Table 2.8 Pharmacokinetic parameters of selected drugs (in a 70 kg adult male)

Drug	Clearance (CL), mL·min^{-1}	Apparent volume of distribution (V_d), L	Half-life ($t_{1/2}$), h
Warfarin	3	8	37
Digitoxin	4	38	161
Diazepam	27	77	43
Valproic acid	76	27	5.6
Digoxin	130	640	39
Ampicillin	270	20	1.3
Amlodipine	333	1470	36
Nifedipine	500	80	1.8
Lidocaine	640	77	1.8
Propranolol	840	270	3.9
Imipramine	1050	1600	18

Half-life ($t_{1/2}$) = $0.693 V_d$/CL. A long half-life may result from a high apparent volume of distribution (e.g. amlodipine), a low clearance (e.g. digitoxin), or both.

ELIMINATION

The rate at which the drug is eliminated is important because it usually determines the duration of response, the time interval between doses and the time to reach equilibrium during repeated dosing.

RATE OF ELIMINATION

The rate of elimination of a drug from the circulation (and its associated plasma half-life) is usually indicated by the terminal slope of the plasma concentration–time curve (slope B–C in Fig. 2.17B). The elimination half-lives of drugs range from a few minutes to many days (and, in rare cases, weeks).

The activity of the organ of elimination

The main organs of elimination (the liver and kidneys) can only remove drug delivered to them via the blood. The first key concept in understanding drug elimination is that as long as the elimination process is not saturated, a constant *proportion* (not a constant amount) of the drug carried in the blood will be removed on each passage through the organ of elimination, whatever the drug concentration in the blood. In effect, this is equivalent to saying that a constant proportion of the blood flow to the organ is cleared of drug. For example, if 10% of the drug carried to the liver by the plasma (at a flow rate of 1000 mL·min^{-1}) is cleared by uptake and metabolism, this is equivalent to a clearance of 10% of the plasma flow (100 mL·min^{-1}); if the drug is metabolised more efficiently such that 20% of the drug is cleared, this gives a clearance of 200 mL·min^{-1}.

Clearance is therefore the volume of blood cleared of drug per unit time, not the amount of drug cleared in that time, which will vary depending on the drug concentration in the blood. If the drug concentration in the blood is high there will be a greater amount of the drug in the volume that is cleared per unit time, resulting in a greater rate of elimination; if the drug concentration is low the same clearance will eliminate a smaller amount of the drug per unit time. Overall, the rate of drug elimination from the body is therefore the product of plasma concentration of the drug and its plasma clearance (CL), a relationship which can be rearranged to:

$$CL = \frac{\text{Rate of elimination from the body}}{\text{Drug concentration in plasma}} \quad (2.12)$$

$$\text{For example } \frac{\mu g \cdot min^{-1}}{\mu g \cdot mL^{-1}} = mL \cdot min^{-1}$$

The plasma clearance is a characteristic value for a particular drug (see Table 2.8); it is a constant for first-order reactions and is independent of dose or concentration.

Reversible passage of drug from the blood into tissues

The organs of elimination can only act on drug that is delivered to them via the blood supply, and the amount of drug eliminated depends on its concentration within the volume of plasma being cleared per unit time. By definition, a drug that is distributed at equilibrium into a large apparent volume of distribution has a low plasma concentration; hence the rate of elimination is inversely proportional to apparent V_d:

$$\text{Elimination} \propto \frac{1}{V_d} \qquad (2.13)$$

The overall rate constant of elimination (k) can therefore be related directly to the volume of plasma cleared per minute (CL) and inversely to the total apparent volume of plasma that has to be cleared (V_d):

$$k = \frac{CL}{V_d} \qquad (2.14)$$

Since also (equation 2.6):

$$k = \frac{0.693}{t_{1/2}}$$

Therefore:

$$t_{1/2} = \frac{0.693 V_d}{CL}$$

The relationship between elimination, volume of distribution and clearance is illustrated in Figure 2.19. The elimination rate constant (k) or half-life ($t_{1/2}$) are the best indicators of a fall in drug concentration with time, and for most drugs this will be accompanied by a decrease in therapeutic activity.

Clearance is the best measurement of the ability of the organs of elimination to remove the drug and determines the average plasma concentrations (and therefore therapeutic activity) at steady-state (see below). Clearance is

usually determined using the area under the plasma concentration–time curve (AUC) extrapolated to infinity after an intravenous dose. Clearance and the AUC of a given dose of drug are inversely related; if clearance was zero, the drug would not be eliminated and its plasma concentration would remain at equilibrium indefinitely (the AUC would be infinitely large). Conversely, if the clearance was infinite, the AUC would be zero, as the drug would be eliminated instantly. The ratio of an intravenous drug dose to the area under its plasma concentration–time curve (note: not the logarithm of plasma concentration) is therefore a measure of clearance:

$$CL = \frac{\text{Dose}}{\text{AUC}} \qquad (2.15)$$

If an oral drug is used instead, the dose in this equation would be corrected by its bioavailability (i.e. $F \times$ Dose).

The two equations for clearance (2.14 and 2.15) can be combined to derive equation 2.16, which is used to calculate V_d more reliably than the extrapolation method given in equation 2.11 and Figure 2.17b:

$$CL = \frac{\text{Dose}}{\text{AUC}} = k \cdot V_d$$
$$V_d = \frac{\text{Dose}}{\text{AUC} \times k} \qquad (2.16)$$

The plasma clearance of a drug is the sum of all possible clearance processes (metabolism + renal excretion + biliary excretion + exhalation + etc.). Measurement of its component processes is only really possible for renal clearance, performed by relating the rate of urinary excretion to the mid-point plasma concentration. Subtracting renal clearance from the total plasma clearance gives a reasonable estimate of metabolic (mainly hepatic) clearance, which cannot be measured directly. Being able to estimate both renal and hepatic clearance values can be useful in predicting the impact of renal or liver disease.

EXTENT OF ELIMINATION

The extent of elimination is of limited value because eventually all the drug will be removed from the body. Measurement of the parent drug and its metabolites in urine and faeces can give useful insights into the extent of renal and biliary elimination.

CHRONIC ADMINISTRATION

Repeated drug doses are used to maintain a constant concentration of the drug in the blood and at the site of action for a persistent therapeutic effect. In practice, a perfectly stable concentration can only be achieved by maintaining a constant intravenous infusion that has reached a steady-state balance between drug input and drug elimination (Fig. 2.20).

TIME TO REACH STEADY-STATE

During constant infusion, the time to reach steady-state is dependent on the elimination half-life; as a rule of thumb,

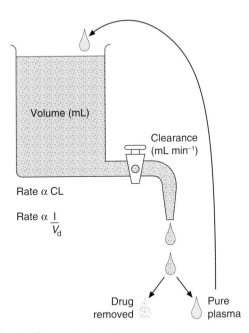

Volume (mL)

Clearance (mL min⁻¹)

Rate α CL

Rate $\alpha \dfrac{1}{V_d}$

Drug removed

Pure plasma

Fig. 2.19 The relationship between clearance, apparent volume of distribution and overall elimination rate. The drug is eliminated by the clearance process, which removes whatever amount of the drug is present in a fixed volume of plasma, per unit time. The drug is then separated and the pure plasma added back to the reservoir to maintain a constant volume (the apparent volume of distribution, V_d). The fluid, therefore, continuously recycles via the clearance process and the concentration of drug decreases exponentially.

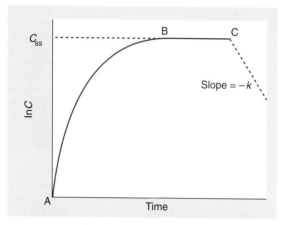

Fig. 2.20 Constant intravenous infusion (between points A and C). A steady-state concentration (C_{ss}) is reached at point B and can be used to calculate clearance (CL = rate of infusion/C_{ss}). Clearance can also be calculated from the total dose infused between A and C and the area under the total curve (AUC). The negative slope after ending the infusion gives the terminal elimination phase (k). The rate of elimination determines the time taken to reach C_{ss}, approximately four to five half-lives.

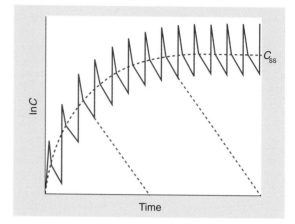

Fig. 2.21 Chronic oral therapy (solid line) compared with intravenous infusion (dashed red line) at the same dosage rate. Each oral dose shows rapid absorption and distribution to reach a peak, followed by a slower elimination phase in which concentrations fall to a trough. Successive peaks (or successive troughs) align with the dose interval. Cessation of therapy after any dose would produce the lines shown in blue.

steady-state is approached after four or five times the elimination half-life. A drug with slow elimination takes a long time to reach its steady-state as it will accumulate to high plasma concentrations before its elimination rate rises to match the rate of drug infusion (because the elimination rate depends on plasma concentration) (equation 2.12). Since the elimination half-life is also dependent on volume of distribution (equation 2.14), a high V_d can also contribute to delay in achieving steady-state. It is easy to envisage the slow 'filling' of such a high volume of distribution during regular administration.

PLASMA CONCENTRATION AT STEADY-STATE

Once steady-state has been reached, the plasma and tissues are in equilibrium, and the distribution rate and V_d will no longer affect the plasma concentration. The key insight is that a steady-state concentration (C_{ss}) is achieved when the rate of elimination equals the rate of infusion. From equation 2.12 the rate of elimination equals CL × C_{ss}, so at steady-state the rate of infusion also equals CL × C_{ss}, or:

$$C_{ss} = \frac{\text{Rate of infusion}}{\text{CL}} \qquad (2.17)$$

Alternatively, the rate of an intravenous infusion and the C_{ss} achieved can be used to calculate plasma clearance:

$$CL = \frac{\text{Rate of infusion}}{C_{ss}} \qquad (2.18)$$

Clearance and volume of distribution can also be calculated using the AUC between zero and infinity and the terminal slope after cessation of the infusion (see Fig. 2.20).

ORAL ADMINISTRATION

Most chronic administration of drugs is by the oral route, and the rate and extent of absorption affect the shape of the plasma concentration–time curves. Because oral therapy is by intermittent doses there will be a series of peaks and troughs matching the intervals between repeated doses (Fig. 2.21). The rate of absorption will influence the profile, since very rapid absorption will exaggerate fluctuations, while slow absorption will dampen down the peaks. As not all the administered dose (D) will be absorbed, the rate of dosage during chronic oral therapy is corrected for bioavailability (F):

$$\frac{D \times F}{t} \qquad (2.19)$$

where t is the *interval* between doses. When steady-state is achieved, the rate of input is equal to the rate of elimination, which is the clearance (CL) multiplied by the drug concentration averaged between the peaks and troughs (C_{ss}), so:

$$\frac{D \times F}{t} = CL \times C_{ss} \qquad (2.20)$$

Therefore:

$$C_{ss} = \frac{D \times F}{t \times CL} \qquad (2.21)$$

This important equation means it is possible to alter plasma C_{ss} by altering either the dose (D) or the dose interval (t). The bioavailability (F) depends largely on the drug formulation and clearance (CL) is usually constant unless there is a change in hepatic or renal function.

LOADING DOSE

A problem may arise when a rapid onset of effect is required for a drug that has a very long half-life; for example, if the half-life of the drug is 24 h, the steady-state conditions will not be reached until 4–5 days, and if the half-life is 1 week, reaching a steady-state will take over 4 or 5 weeks. Increasing the dose rate (by increasing the dose or shortening the dose interval) would accelerate the rise in plasma concentrations, but, if the higher dose-rate were sustained it would lead to a higher steady-state concentration being achieved than desired.

Delay between starting treatment and reaching the steady-state therapeutic concentration can be avoided by administering a *loading dose*. This is a high initial dose that 'loads up' the body to shorten the time to steady-state. The key principle is that the loading dose is the single dose required to produce the desired steady-state concentration in the apparent volume of distribution (i.e. C_{ss} = loading dose/V_d; see equation 2.10), so:

$$\text{Loading dose} = C_{ss} \times V_d \qquad (2.22)$$

The loading dose is equivalent to the total body load of drug that would be achieved more slowly by the chronic dosage regimen (equation 2.21).

In cases where C_{ss} or V are not known, the loading dose can be calculated based on the parameters of the proposed maintenance regimen by replacing C_{ss} with equation 2.21 and V_d by equation 2.14:

$$
\begin{aligned}
\text{Loading dose} &= \frac{D \times F}{t \times CL} \times \frac{CL}{k} \\
&= \frac{D \times F}{t \times k} \qquad (2.23)\\
&= \frac{D \times F \times 1.44 \times t_{1/2}}{t}
\end{aligned}
$$

It is clear from this last equation that the magnitude of any loading dose compared with the maintenance dose is proportional to the half-life.

If a drug has a very long half-life such that a very large loading dose is required, it may be given in divided doses over 24–36 h, as local variations in the rate of distribution to different tissues may otherwise cause high localised concentrations and hence toxicity.

Following the loading dose, the steady-state plasma concentration can be sustained indefinitely by the *maintenance* dosage regimen given by equation 2.21.

PHARMACOKINETICS OF BIOLOGICAL DRUGS

The first recombinant protein drug was human insulin, marketed in 1982, and there are now over 100 biological drugs available, including monoclonal antibodies, cytokines, growth factors and blood products. Such biopharmaceuticals can create special pharmacokinetic problems, mainly due to their protein structures, as follows.

- **Absorption**: pH-dependent and enzymatic breakdown of proteins in the gastrointestinal tract (>99%) precludes oral administration; administration of biopharmaecuticals is by parenteral routes (intravenous, subcutaneous, intramuscular), including – occasionally – intranasal and inhaled routes. Bioavailability of protein drugs may be low due to local proteolysis, such as at subcutaneous or intramuscular injection sites. Larger molecules (>30 kDa) cross the capillary endothelium poorly and may enter the systemic circulation by the lymphatic system.
- **Distribution**: biological drug distribution may be confined to the blood and extracellular tissues. Protein drugs may bind extensively to albumin and other plasma proteins, affecting their distribution and rate of metabolism.
- **Elimination**: biological drugs are not excreted unchanged but undergo extensive proteolysis in the blood, liver, kidneys and other tissues to small peptides and amino acids, which enter the general pool of amino acids used in endogenous protein synthesis. Degradation depends on molecular weight, charge and the extent of glycosylation; recombinant drug molecules may be designed to lack common sites of proteolytic cleavage, or coated with polyethylene glycol (pegylation) to improve solubility and resistance to proteolysis. The elimination kinetics of biopharmaceuticals can be variable and complex; concentrations of monoclonal antibodies in plasma fall initially as they bind tightly to their targets, but their terminal elimination half-life may be as slow as that of endogenous immunoglobulins (14–28 days), enabling long dosing intervals.
- **Toxicity and clinical use**: biopharmaceuticals are often highly species-specific and their toxicity is usually receptor-dependent or immunogenic in origin. Immunogenicity is reduced in drugs based on human protein sequences, but these are more difficult to develop as they may lack efficacy in animal models. The complex tertiary structure of recombinant proteins makes them more vulnerable to degradation by heat, pH effects and shear forces during manufacture, storage and handling.

GENETIC VARIATION AND DRUG KINETICS

The earliest studies on pharmacogenetics were on enzymes involved in drug metabolism. N-Acetyltransferase (NAT) was one of the first drug metabolism pathways found to show a genetic polymorphism that influenced both the plasma concentrations of a drug (isoniazid) and its therapeutic response. Individuals with low enzyme activity, so-called slow acetylators, had higher blood concentrations and a better response to isoniazid but a greater risk of toxicity than did 'fast acetylators'.

Because N-acetylation is a minor pathway of drug metabolism, pharmacogenetics remained of largely academic interest until the late 1970s, when it was found that the cytochrome P450 isoenzyme CYP2D6, which is involved in the phase 1 metabolism of 20–25% of all drugs, showed functionally important genetic polymorphisms. Developments in genotyping have allowed the identification of many polymorphisms in a number of cytochrome P450 isoenzymes with consequences for the phase 1 metabolism and elimination of many drugs; examples are listed in Table 2.9.

Table 2.9 Pharmacogenetic differences in drug-metabolising enzymes

Enzyme	Incidence of deficiency or slow-metaboliser phenotype in white people	Typical substrates	Consequences of deficiency or slow-metaboliser status
Phase 1 reactions			
Pseudocholinesterase (butyrylcholinesterase, plasma cholinesterase)	1 in 3000	Suxamethonium (succinylcholine)	Prolonged paralysis and apnoea for up to 3 h after a dose
Alcohol dehydrogenase, acetaldehyde dehydrogenase	5–10% (>50% in Asians)	Ethanol and acetaldehyde	Profound vasodilation on ingestion of alcohol
CYP1A1	10%?	Polycyclic aromatic hydrocarbons	Increased risk of low birth weight in smokers
CYP2A6	15%	Nicotine, coumarin	Reduced nicotine metabolism
CYP2B6	3–4%	Ifosfamide, efavirenz	Numerous SNPs identified; significance unclear; reduced bioactivation of cyclophosphamide
CYP2C9	About 10% in white and 3% in black subjects	Tolbutamide, diazepam, warfarin	Increased response if parent drug is active, e.g. increased risk of haemorrhage with warfarin
CYP2C19	5% (about 20% in Asians)	Omeprazole	Increased response if parent drug is active
CYP2D6	5–10%	Codeine, nortriptyline, tamoxifen	Increased response if parent drug is active, but reduced response if oxidation produces the active form, e.g. codeine
Dihydropyrimidine dehydrogenase (DPD)	1% are heterozygous	Fluorouracil	Enhanced drug response
Phase 2 reactions			
N-Acetyltransferase	50% (10–20% in Asians)	Isoniazid, hydralazine, procainamide	Enhanced drug response in slow acetylators
UDP glucuronyl transferase (UGT1A1)	10% (1–4% Asians)	Irinotecan (bilirubin)	Enhanced effect (Gilbert's syndrome; increased bilirubin)
Glutathione transferase family		Reactive compounds or metabolites	Increased risk of cancer from environmental carcinogens; therapeutic implications unclear
Thiopurine-S-methyl transferase (TPMT)	0.3%	Mercaptopurine, azathioprine	Increased risk of toxicity (because the doses normally used are close to toxic)
Catechol-O-methyltransferase	25%	Levodopa	Slightly enhanced drug effect
Transporters			
ABCB1 (P-gp)	A number of SNPs have been identified (incidences vary with ethnic origin)	Digoxin, anti-cancer drugs, dihydropyridine calcium channel blockers	Possibly higher drug levels with some SNPs, but lower drug levels due to increased activity with other SNPs

P-gp, P-glycoprotein; SNP, single-nucleotide polymorphism.

Polymorphisms have also been identified in a number of phase 2 metabolic enzymes; notable is the *28 variant in UDP glucuronyl transferase (UGT1A1*28), which results in impaired metabolism of the topoisomerase inhibitor irinotecan and greater adverse effects when the drug is used for treatment of colon cancer.

The prevalence of such gene variants may differ between ethnic groups; people from the Indian subcontinent have a lower systemic clearance of nifedipine (a CYP3A4 substrate) compared with white people, and intolerance to alcohol ingestion associated with polymorphisms in alcohol dehydrogenase (ADH) and acetaldehyde dehydrogenase (ALD) is common in people of Chinese and Japanese origin.

Polymorphisms that alter the elimination pathways of drugs may influence their efficacy and safety by altering plasma concentrations of the active drug, or by modifying the amounts of active or toxic metabolites. They may also alter the enzymatic conversion of prodrugs into their active metabolites, or change the distribution of drugs by altering their transport across membranes. There are functional polymorphisms in some ABC transporter proteins, including the *MDR1* gene which codes for P-gp, and in OATs in the kidney, although the consequences of these for drug transport are unclear. Genetic polymorphisms are likely to be of greatest clinical significance when the polymorphic protein is in the main pathway affecting bioavailability and/or elimination and when the drug has a narrow therapeutic index (Ch. 53).

The influence of genetic variation must be set against environmental factors, including age, pregnancy, interactions with other drugs (including alcohol and tobacco) and concurrent conditions including impairment of renal or hepatic function, which may be of greater importance in predicting drug efficacy and unwanted effects (Ch. 56). A number of commercial tests have been marketed for specific gene polymorphisms in drug-metabolising enzymes, including some of those listed in Table 2.9. There are nevertheless formidable obstacles to widespread use of genetic testing, including issues of cost and privacy. In most cases, individual gene polymorphisms have limited predictive value, and testing for haplotypes of multiple polymorphisms in the same gene or in other genes within the same metabolic pathways may be more predictive, but also more costly and difficult to interpret. A major hurdle to genetic testing at present is that reliable clinical trial data are not usually available in people with diverse genotypes to guide prescribers in making appropriate alterations in drug regimens.

SELF-ASSESSMENT

True/false questions

Are these statements true or false?

1. Un-ionised molecules cross phospholipid membranes more readily than their ionised forms.
2. Weak acidic drugs are mostly ionised in acid solutions.
3. Weak acidic drugs, such as aspirin, are mostly absorbed in the stomach.
4. Basic drugs may bind reversibly to α_1-acid glycoprotein in the plasma.
5. The plasma clearance of a drug usually decreases with increases in the dose prescribed.
6. First-pass metabolism may limit the bioavailability of orally administered drugs.
7. Drugs that show high first-pass metabolism in the liver also have a high systemic clearance.
8. The half-life of many drugs is longer in babies than in children or adults.
9. A decrease in renal function affects oral bioavailability.
10. Depot injections of drugs have a prolonged half-life because their renal clearance is reduced.
11. Nifedipine is eliminated more rapidly in cigarette smokers.
12. Chronic treatment with phenobarbital can increase the systemic clearance of co-administered drugs.

13. A loading dose is not necessary for drugs that have short half-lives.
14. An obese person is likely to show an increased volume of distribution of lipid-soluble drugs and would require higher dosage than a non-obese subject during chronic therapy.
15. Alcohol intolerance due to genetic polymorphism is common in some ethnic groups.

One-best-answer (OBA) questions

1. Which of the following statements about cytochrome P450 (CYP) isoenzymes is the *least* accurate?
   A. CYP enzymes catalyse drug conjugation reactions.
   B. CYP isoenzyme activity can be influenced by diet.
   C. The major site of CYP-mediated drug metabolism is the liver.
   D. The activity of CYP enzymes varies among individuals.
   E. CYP enzymes may be induced by their substrates.
2. Which of the following statements regarding apparent volume of distribution (V_d) is the *least* accurate?

   A. The V_d will be low if the drug is highly bound to plasma proteins.
   B. The V_d is the dose of intravenous drug divided by the plasma concentration extrapolated back to time zero.
   C. The V_d depends on the dose of drug administered.
   D. The elimination half-life of a drug depends on the V_d and on clearance (CL).
   E. The V_d is used to calculate the loading doses of drugs.

Descriptive question

Figure 2.22 shows the changes in plasma levels of two drugs, A and B, each given as 10 mg doses by both the oral and intravenous routes to an adult man. From the plasma concentration–time curves, describe how the drugs compare for the following properties.

A. Absorption from the gut.
B. Oral bioavailability.
C. Distribution to tissues.
D. Elimination half-life.
E. Extent of accumulation with once-daily administration of each drug.

Case-based questions

Case 1

Treatment with oral theophylline is started in a 7-year-old girl (weighing 31 kg) admitted to the accident and emergency department with asthma. The desired steady-state plasma concentration is 15 $\mu g \cdot mL^{-1}$. The apparent volume of distribution (V_d) of theophylline is 0.5 $L \cdot kg^{-1}$ and its oral bioavailability is 60% ($F = 0.6$). Which of the following would be the most appropriate loading dose?

A. 139 mg
B. 232 mg

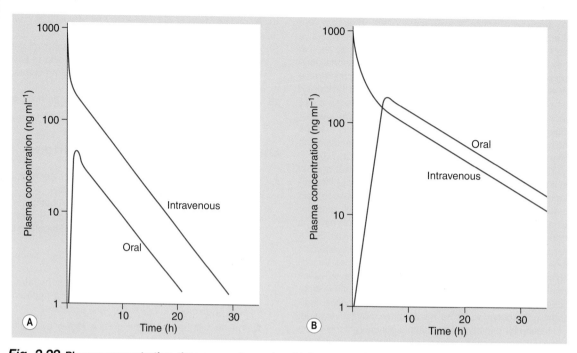

Fig. 2.22 Plasma concentration–time curves for oral and intravenous doses of drugs A and B.

C. 387 mg
D. 644 mg
E. 696 mg

Case 2

A man weighing 70 kg was admitted to hospital with a serious infection and was treated with two antibacterials. Gentamicin is given by intravenous administration, and cefalexin is given orally with bioavailability of 90% ($F = 0.9$).

	Gentamicin	Cefalexin
Volume of distribution (V_d) (L)	18	18
Clearance (CL) (L·h^{-1})	5.4	18
Half-life (h)	2–3	0.9

Gentamicin is very toxic and its therapeutic plasma concentrations should not exceed 5 mg·L^{-1}, since higher concentrations can lead to ototoxicity and nephrotoxicity.

A. You have calculated that you will give him 900 mg of gentamicin by injection as a bolus (single) dose. Is this a safe dose?
B. Because of the short half-life of gentamicin you then decide that it will be best to give him a continuous intravenous infusion to maintain a steady-state plasma concentration of 2.5 mg/L. What rate of infusion should be given?
C. What maximum plasma concentration would be obtained if a single oral loading dose of 500 mg cefalexin was given?

Case 3

Mrs J (body weight 70 kg) was diagnosed with congestive heart failure and atrial fibrillation. Treatment was started with digoxin, which has an apparent volume of distribution (V_d) of 9 L·kg^{-1} and a half-life ($t_{1/2}$) of 42 h. The plasma concentrations for therapeutic effectiveness are 0.8–2 ng·mL^{-1}, and toxic effects occur above 2 ng·mL^{-1}.

A. Approximately how long would it take to reach a steady-state concentration in plasma?
B. What dose should be given as a loading dose to achieve a plasma level of 0.8 ng mL^{-1}?

True/false answers

1. **True.** Ionisation reduces lipid solubility and improves solubility in water.
2. **False.** Weak acids are least ionised in acid solutions and most ionised in basic solutions.
3. **False.** Although low pH in the stomach renders aspirin into its un-ionised, lipid-soluble form, the low surface area of the stomach wall limits the extent of drug absorption; the bulk of most oral drugs is absorbed across the much larger surface area of the small intestine.
4. **True.** Basic (or neutral) drugs may bind reversibly to α_1-acid glycoprotein, while many acidic drugs bind to albumin.
5. **False.** Provided the elimination processes are not saturated, clearance (like bioavailability and apparent volume of distribution) is independent of dose and is a characteristic of the drug. The increase in plasma concentration following an increase in drug dose causes an increase in the *amount* of drug eliminated per unit time, but the *volume* of plasma cleared of drug per unit time (clearance) is unaltered.
6. **True.** This statement is true for all 'pre-systemic' sites of metabolism of the oral dose, e.g. gut lumen, intestinal

wall and liver. Low bioavailability may also arise from poor absorption.

7. **True.** If the liver is able to clear a high proportion of the drug as it is absorbed from the gastrointestinal tract (on first pass), then the drug fraction that survives to enter the general circulation will experience further rapid clearance on subsequent passes through the liver.

8. **True.** Infants under 12 months have relatively low hepatic metabolism and renal excretion, so many drugs are cleared more slowly and have longer half-lives than in older children and adults.

9. **False.** A decrease in renal function could affect systemic clearance, but bioavailability is simply the fraction of the oral dose that reaches the general circulation, and the kidneys are not part of the route between gut lumen and general circulation.

10. **False.** Using a depot injection of a drug prolongs its apparent elimination half-life due to slower, sustained release from the site of injection. Once absorbed into the blood, the circulating drug is handled by the kidneys as normal; the volume of plasma cleared of the drug per unit time is unaltered.

11. **False.** From Table 2.7, nifedipine is metabolised by CYP3A4, while smoking induces CYP1A2, so no interaction is likely to occur.

12. **False.** Phenobarbital is a potent inducer of several cytochrome P450 isoenzymes and this can increase the ability of the liver to metabolise many co-administered drugs.

13. **True.** Drugs with short elimination half-lives do not accumulate significantly so there is relatively little delay before the drug reaches therapeutic concentrations and a loading dose is unnecessary.

14. **False.** A lipid-soluble drug would have an increased apparent V_d in an obese person so its half-life would be longer (due to slower elimination). However, clearance (the volume of plasma cleared of drug per unit time) is unaffected, so C_{ss} is also unaffected as it depends on CL but not on V_d (see equation 2.21). There would consequently be no need to modify chronic drug dosage because of an increase in V_d in an obese person. It would, however, take longer to achieve the steady-state plasma concentration (C_{ss}), and the total body load of drug at steady-state ($C_{ss} \times V_d$) would be higher.

15. **True.** Genetic polymorphisms that alter the activity of alcohol dehydrogenase and acetaldehyde dehydrogenase underlie the alcohol intolerance (facial flushing, etc.) experienced by many people of Chinese and Japanese ancestry.

OBA answers

1. **Answer A** is the least accurate.
   A. **False**. CYP enzymes are involved in many types of oxidation, reduction, hydrolysis and hydration reactions during phase 1 drug metabolism, but phase 2 (conjugation) reactions are catalysed by other enzymes (such as UDPGT and glutathione transferases).
   B. True. CYP isoenzymes can be inhibited or induced by dietary items such as grapefruit juice and charred meat.
   C. True. The liver has higher levels of CYP isoenzymes than other tissues.
   D. True. Pharmacogenetic variation is particularly marked for CYP2C19 and CYP2D9.
   E. True. For example, ethanol induces CYP2E and is also a substrate for this isoenzyme

2. **Answer C** is the least accurate.
   A. True. Drugs confined within the circulation (e.g. by plasma protein binding) have a low apparent V_d. (The total drug concentration in plasma, both free and bound, is used when calculating V_d. Extensive binding of the drug to proteins in tissues *outside* the circulation could inflate the apparent V_d.)
   B. True. Extrapolation of the plasma concentration to time zero estimates the apparent V_d before elimination reduces the total amount of drug in the body.
   C. **False.** Apparent V_d is a characteristic of a particular drug, but is independent of dose.
   D. True. The half-life is proportional to V_d and inversely proportional to clearance.
   E. True. The loading dose is $C_{ss} \times V_d$.

Descriptive answers

A. The rate of absorption is determined by the rate of increase after oral dosing. Drug A is absorbed rapidly, while drug B takes about 6 h to reach a peak concentration.

B. Bioavailability (*F*) is determined by the ratio of the area under the oral and intravenous curves (AUC_{oral}/AUC_{iv}). For drug A, bioavailability (*F*) is visibly much less than 1, while for drug B the AUC_{oral} approximately equals the AUC_{iv}, so *F* is approximately 1.

C. The rates of distribution are given by the slopes of the *intravenous* drug curves from time zero to the establishment of the terminal elimination phase, which is at about 1 h for drug A and at 4 h for drug B, so drug A distributes more rapidly. Extrapolating the slope of the terminal phase back to time zero gives similar intercepts (apparent V_d), indicating the drugs have a similar extent of distribution.

D. The slope of the elimination phase (*k*) is greater for drug A than for B, so its elimination is faster and half-life is shorter ($t_{1/2} = 0.693/k$). This must be due to a lower clearance (CL) of drug B, since it was shown above that the volume of distribution is similar for both drugs. This is also apparent from the greater AUC for intravenous drug B, as the doses were the same (10 mg).

E. The potential for accumulation depends on the difference between half-life and dose interval (once-daily = 24 h). It is clear that after 24 h nearly all of drug A has been removed from the plasma but considerable amounts of B remain, so drug B would show significant accumulation.

Case-based answers

Case 1

Answer C is correct. Note that the apparent V_d is given as 0.5 L per kilogram of the child's bodyweight (31 kg), and also that the plasma concentration (15 $\mu g \cdot mL^{-1}$) should be converted to 15 $mg \cdot L^{-1}$. Loading dose is given by $C_{ss} \times V_d$, so:

Loading dose = 15 $mg \cdot L^{-1} \times$ (0.5 $L \cdot kg^{-1} \times$ 31 kg) = 232 mg

However, 232 mg is the dose required to be *absorbed*; as the bioavailability (*F*) of theophylline is only 0.6, the *administered* dose needs to be 232/0.6 = 387 mg (Answer C).

Case 2

A. The maximal recommended dose is given by maximal plasma concentration (C_{ss}) × volume of distribution (V_d) so 5 $mg \cdot L^{-1} \times$ 18 L = 90 mg. Your calculation of a bolus dose of 900 mg is therefore not safe, as it would give a plasma concentration 10 times higher than recommended.

B. At steady-state, the rate of infusion = the rate of elimination = CL (clearance) × C_{ss} (equation 2.17), so for a plasma concentration of 2.5 $mg \cdot L^{-1}$ you will need to give an infusion rate of 5.4 $L \cdot h^{-1} \times$ 2.5 $mg \cdot L^{-1}$ = 13.5 $mg \cdot h^{-1}$.

C. For a single oral dose the peak concentration is approximately equal to the *absorbed* dose divided by the apparent volume of distribution (V_d) (equation 2.10). Including a correction for the bioavailability (*F* = 0.9) of the oral dose (*D* = 500 mg), the concentration is:
$C = (D \times F)/V_d = $ (500 mg × 0.9) /18 L = 25 mg L^{-1}
Due to some elimination occurring before the peak concentration is reached, the peak concentration achieved would be lower than 25 $mg \cdot L^{-1}$, but this could be ignored in clinical practice.

Case 3

A. Drugs take about four to five times their elimination half-life to reach a steady-state. For digoxin ($t_{1/2}$ = 42 h) this is 168–210 h, or about 7–9 days, hence the need for a loading dose.

B. Using equation 2.22, and correcting V_d (9 $L \cdot kg^{-1}$) for the patient's body weight (70 kg) gives:
Loading dose = $C_{ss} \times V_d$ = 0.8 $\mu g \cdot L^{-1} \times$ (9 $L \cdot kg^{-1} \times$ 70 kg) = 504 μg

FURTHER READING

Baumann A (2006) Early development of therapeutic biologics – pharmacokinetics. *Curr Drug Metab* 7, 15–21

Choudhuri S, Klaassen CD (2006) Structure, function, expression, genomic organization, and single nucleotide polymorphisms of human ABCB1 (MDR1), ABCC (MRP), and ABCG2 (BCRP) efflux transporters. *Int J Toxicol* 25, 231–259

Cole SPC, Deeley RG (2006) Transport of glutathione and glutathione conjugates by MRP1. *Trends Pharmacol Sci* 27, 438–446

Daly AK (2010) Pharmacogenetics and human genetic polymorphisms. *Biochem J* 429, 435–449

De Boer AG, van der Sandt ICJ, Gaillard PJ (2003) The role of drug transporters at the blood–brain barrier. *Annu Rev Pharmacol Toxicol* 43, 629–656

Evans WE, McLeod HL (2003) Pharmacogenomics – drug disposition, drug targets, and side effects. *N Engl J Med* 348, 538–549

Feero WG, Guttmacher AE, Collins FS (2010) Genomic medicine — an updated primer. *N Engl J Med* 362, 2001–2011

Fromm MF (2004) Importance of P-glycoprotein at blood–tissue barriers. *Trends Pharmacol Sci* 25, 423–429

Gabrielsson J, Green AR (2009) Quantitative pharmacology or pharmacokinetic-pharmacodynamic integration should be a vital component in integrative pharmacology. *J Pharmacol Exp Ther* 331, 767–774

Handschin C, Meyer UA (2003) Induction of drug metabolism: the role of nuclear receptors. *Pharmacol Rev* 55, 649–673

Kirchheiner J, Seeringer A (2007) Clinical implications of pharmacogenetics of cytochrome P450 drug metabolizing enzymes. *Biochim Biophys Acta* 1770, 489–494

Koepsell H (2004) Polyspecific organic cation transporters: their functions and interactions with drugs. *Trends Pharmacol Sci* 25, 375–381

Lee G, Dallas S, Hong M, Bendayan R (2001) Drug transporters in the central nervous system: brain barriers and brain parenchyma considerations. *Pharmacol Rev* 53, 569–596

Lee W, Kim RB (2004) Transporters and renal drug elimination. *Annu Rev Pharmacol Toxicol* 44, 137–166

Miyazaki H, Sekine T, Endou H (2004) The multispecific organic anion transporter family: properties and pharmacological significance. *Trends Pharmacol Sci* 25, 654–662

Nebert DW, Vesell ES (2007) Can personalised drug therapy be achieved? A closer look at pharmaco-metabonomics. *Trends Pharmacol Sci* 27, 581–586

Pelkonen O, Turpeinen M, Hakkola J, Honkakoski P, Hukkanen J, Raunio H (2008) Inhibition and induction of human cytochrome P450 enzymes: current status. *Arch Toxicol* 82, 667–715

Pirmohamed M (2011) Pharmacogenetics: past, present and future. *Drug Discov Today* 16, 852–861

Rees DC, Johnson E, Lewinson O (2009) ABC transporters: the power to change. *Nat Rev Mol Cell Biol* 10, 218–227

Szakacs G, Varadi A, Ozvegy-Laczka C, Sarkadi B (2008) The role of ABC transporters in drug absorption, distribution, metabolism, excretion and toxicity (ADME-Tox). *Drug Discov Today* 13, 379–393

Tukey RH, Strassburg CP (2000) Human UDP-glucuronosyltransferases: metabolism, expression, and disease. *Annu Rev Pharmacol Toxicol* 40, 581–616

Verkmann AS (2009) Aquaporins: translating bench research to human disease. *J Exp Biol* 212, 1707–1715

Wang L, McLeod HL, Weinshilboum RM (2011) Genomics and drug response. *N Engl J Med* 364, 1144–1153

Weinshilboum RM, Wang L (2006) Pharmacogenetics and pharmacogenomics: development, science, and translation. *Annu Rev Genom Hum Gen* 7, 223–245

Xie H-G, Kim RB, Wood AJJ, Stein MC (2001) Molecular basis of ethnic differences in drug disposition and response. *Annu Rev Pharmacol Toxicol* 41, 815–850

3 Drug discovery, safety and efficacy

Historically, most medicines were of botanical or zoological origin and most had dubious therapeutic value. During the 20th century there were major advances in chemistry allowing the synthesis and purification of huge arrays of small organic molecules to be screened for pharmacological activity. Advances in drug development for the treatment of disease are illustrated most dramatically with antimicrobial chemotherapy, which revolutionised the chances of people surviving severe infections such as lobar pneumonia, the mortality from which was 27% in the pre-antimicrobial era but fell to 8% (and subsequently lower) following the introduction of sulphonamides and then penicillins. Latterly, advances in molecular biology have enabled the development of a number of 'biologic' drugs based on the structures of antibodies, receptors and other human proteins. Meanwhile, the Human Genome Project, and the growth of technologies that allow systematic study ('omics') of the entire range of cellular RNAs, proteins and small molecules, known as transcriptomics, proteomics and metabolonomics, respectively, have expanded knowledge of the range of gene products and processes that might present targets for novel drugs.

Early medicines consisting of crude extracts of plants or animal tissues usually contained a mixture of many organic compounds, of which one, more than one or none may have had useful biological activity. The active constituents of some plant-derived preparations are bitter-tasting organic molecules known as alkaloids. For example, opium from the opium poppy contains high concentrations of the alkaloid morphine, and various preparations of opium have been used more or less successfully for the treatment of pain and diarrhoea (e.g. dysentery) for thousands of years. Promising therapeutic approaches also included the use of foxglove extracts (which contain cardiac glycosides) for the treatment of 'dropsy' (fluid retention); however, there was also considerable toxicity, because the plant preparations contained variable amounts of the active glycoside and other compounds which have a narrow therapeutic index (Ch. 7). Similarly, for centuries, extracts of white willow bark have been used to ease joint pain and reduce fever, although their active ingredient, salicylic acid, also carries substantial toxicity.

A major advance in the safety of plant-derived medicines was the isolation, purification and chemical characterisation of the active component. This had three main advantages, as follows.

- The administration of controlled amounts of the purified active compound removed biological variability in the potency of the crude plant preparation.
- The administration of the active component removed the unwanted and potentially toxic effects of contaminating substances in the crude preparations.
- The identification and isolation of the active component allowed the mechanism of action to be defined, leading to the synthesis and development of chemically related compounds based on the structure of the active component but with greater potency, higher selectivity, fewer unwanted effects, altered duration of action and better bioavailability. For example, chemical modification of salicylic acid by acetylation produced acetylsalicylic acid, or aspirin, first marketed in 1899, with greater analgesic and antipyretic activity and lower toxicity than the parent compound.

Thus, although drug therapy has natural and humble origins, it is the application of scientific principles, particularly the use of controlled experiments and clinical trials to generate reliable knowledge of drug actions, which has given rise to the clinical safety and efficacy of modern medicines. In the age of 'scientific reason' it is surprising that so many people believe that 'natural' medicinal products offer equivalent therapeutic effectiveness with fewer unwanted effects.

A major advantage of modern drugs is their ability to act selectively; that is, to affect only certain body systems or processes. For example, a drug that both lowers blood glucose and reduces blood pressure may not be suitable for the treatment of someone with diabetes mellitus (because of unwanted hypotensive effects) or a person with hypertension (because of unwanted hypoglycaemic effects), or even of those with both conditions (because different doses may be needed for each effect).

DRUG DISCOVERY

The discovery of a new drug can be achieved in several different ways (Fig. 3.1). The simplest method is to subject new chemical entities (novel chemicals not previously

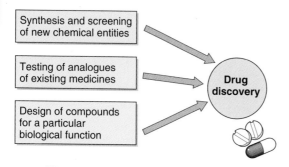

Fig. 3.1 Approaches to drug discovery.

synthesised) to a battery of screening tests that are designed to detect different types of biological activity. These include *in vitro* studies on isolated tissues, as well as *in vivo* studies of complex and integrated systems, such as animal behaviour. Novel chemicals for screening may be produced by direct chemical synthesis or isolated from biological sources, such as plants, and then purified and characterised. This approach has been revolutionised in recent years by developments in high-throughput screening (or HTS), which takes advantage of laboratory robotics for liquid handling combined with *in vitro* cell lines expressing cloned target proteins in tiny reaction volumes in microplates containing hundreds or thousands of reaction wells. Active compounds, which may be small-molecule libraries derived from bacterial or fungal sources, or proteins derived from solid-phase peptide synthesis, can then be selected based on interactions with cells that express a range of possible sites of action, such as G-protein-coupled or nuclear receptors or enzymes important in drug metabolism. Such methods allow the screening of many hundreds of compounds each day and the selection of suitable 'lead compounds', which are then subjected to more labour-intensive and detailed tests.

A second approach involves the synthesis and testing of chemical analogues and modifications of existing medicines; generally, the products of this approach show incremental advances in potency, selectivity and bioavailability (structure–activity relationships). However, additional or even new properties may become evident when the compound is tried in animals or humans; for example, minor modifications of the sulphanilamide antimicrobial molecule gave rise to the thiazide diuretics and the sulfonylurea hypoglycaemics.

More recently, attempts have been made to design substances to fulfil a particular biological role, which may entail the synthesis of a naturally occurring substance (or a structural analogue), its precursor or an antagonist. Good examples include levodopa, used in the treatment of Parkinson's disease, the histamine H_2 receptor antagonists and omeprazole, the first proton pump inhibitor. Logical drug development of this type depends on a detailed understanding of human physiology both in health and disease. High-throughput screening is particularly useful in such a focused approach. *In silico* (computer-based) approaches to the modelling of receptor binding sites have facilitated the development of ligands with high binding affinities and, often, high selectivity.

The recent phenomenal advances in molecular biology have led to the increasing use of genomic techniques, both to identify genes associated with pathological conditions and subsequently to develop compounds that can either mimic or interfere with the activity of the gene product. Such compounds are often proteins, which gives rise to problems of drug delivery to the relevant tissue and to the site of action, which may be intracellular, and also raises issues related to safety testing (see below). A good example of the potential of genomic research is the drug imatinib (Ch. 52), which was developed to inhibit the Bcr-Abl receptor tyrosine kinase, which was implicated in chronic myeloid leukaemia cells by molecular biological methods; imatinib is a non-protein organic molecule with a high oral bioavailability.

Irrespective of the approach, drug development is a long and costly process, with estimates of approximately 14 years and over GB£500 million to bring one new drug to market. Much of this cost lies in gaining the preclinical and clinical evidence required for approval of a new drug by regulatory bodies.

DRUG APPROVAL

Each year, many thousands of new chemical entities and also compounds purified from plant and microbial sources are screened for useful and novel pharmacological activities. Potentially valuable compounds are then subjected to a sequence of *in vitro* and *in vivo* animal studies and clinical trials in humans, which provide essential information on safety and therapeutic benefit (Fig. 3.2).

All drugs and formulations licensed for sale in the UK have to pass a rigorous evaluation of:

- safety,
- quality,
- efficacy.

In the European Union (EU), new drugs are approved under a harmonised procedure of drug regulation. The European Medicines Agency (EMA; www.ema.europa.eu/ema) is a decentralised body of the EU with headquarters in London and is responsible for the regulation of medicines within the EU. It is broadly comparable to the Food and Drug Administration (FDA; www.fda.gov) in the USA. The EMA receives advice from the Committee for Medicinal Products for Human Use (CHMP), which is a body of international experts who evaluate data on the safety, quality and efficacy of medicines. Other EMA committees are involved in evaluating paediatric medicines, herbal medicines and advanced therapies such as gene therapy. Under the current EU system, new drugs are evaluated by the CHMP and national advisory bodies have an opportunity to assess the data before a final CHMP conclusion is reached.

The UK Commission on Human Medicines (CHM) was established in 2005 to replace both the Medicines Commission (MC) and the Committee on Safety of Medicines (CSM), which previously had evaluated medicines regulated in the UK under the Medicines Act (1968). The CHM is one of a number of committees established under the Medicines and Healthcare products Regulatory Agency (MHRA; www.mhra.gov.uk). The MHRA provides advice to the Secretary of State for Health.

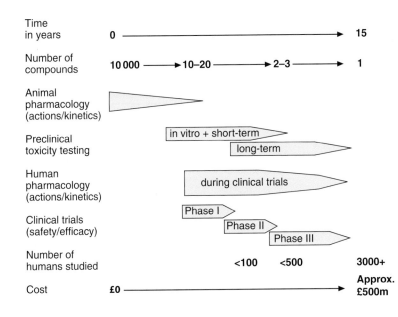

Fig. 3.2 The development of a new drug to the point at which a licence is approved. Post-marketing surveillance will continue to add data on safety and efficacy.

SAFETY

Historically, the introduction of new drugs has been bought at a price of significant toxicity, and regulatory systems have arisen as much to protect patients from drug toxicity as to ensure benefit. In the USA, the FDA was established in 1937, following a dramatic incident in which 76 people died of renal failure after taking an elixir of sulphanilamide which contained the solvent diethylene glycol. Similarly, some 30 years later, the occurrence of limb malformations (phocomelia) and cardiac defects in infants born to mothers who had taken thalidomide for the treatment of nausea in the first trimester of pregnancy led to the establishment of the precursor of the CSM in the UK.

Today, major tragedies are avoided by a combination of *in vitro* studies and animal toxicity tests (preclinical testing) and by careful observation during clinical studies on new drugs (see below). The development and continuing refinement of preclinical toxicity testing has increased the likelihood of identifying chemicals with direct organ toxicity. During clinical trials, immunologically mediated effects are likely to be seen at the lower end of the dose ranges that are used in such trials (see Ch. 53).

QUALITY

An important function of regulatory bodies is to ensure the consistency of prescribed medicines and their manufacturing processes. Drugs have to comply with defined criteria for purity and limits are set on the content of any potentially toxic impurities. The stability and, if necessary, sterility of the drug also have to be established. Similarly, licensed formulations must contain a defined and approved amount of the active drug, released at a specified rate. There have been a number of cases in the past in which a simple change to the manufactured formulation affected tablet disintegration, the release of drug and the therapeutic response. The quality of drugs for human use is defined by the specifications in the European Pharmacopoeia (Ph.Eur.) and the British Pharmacopoeia (BP).

EFFICACY

All medicines, apart from homeopathic products, must have evidence of efficacy for their licensed indications. Efficacy, i.e. the ability to produce a predefined level of clinical response, can be established only by trials in people with the disease, for whom the medicine is intended, and therefore the demonstration of efficacy is a major aim of the later phases of clinical research (Fig. 3.2).

ESTABLISHING SAFETY AND EFFICACY

Regulatory bodies such as the CHMP and CHM require supporting data from *in vitro* studies, animal studies and clinical investigations before a new drug is approved. Although there is some overlap, the basic aims and goals are:

- **preclinical studies**: to establish the basic pharmacology, pharmacokinetics and toxicological profile of the drug and its metabolites, using animals and *in vitro* systems,
- **phase I clinical studies**: to establish the human pharmacology and pharmacokinetics, together with a simple safety profile,
- **phase II clinical studies**: to establish the dose–response relationship and to develop the dosage protocol for clinical use, together with more extensive safety data,
- **phase III clinical studies**: to establish the efficacy and safety profile of the drug in people with the proposed disease for which the drug will be indicated,
- **pharmacovigilance**: to monitor adverse events following approval and marketing of the drug.

PRECLINICAL STUDIES

Preclinical studies must be carried out before a compound can be administered to humans. These studies investigate three areas:

- **pharmacological effects**: *in vitro* effects using isolated cells, tissues or organs; receptor-binding characteristics; *in vivo* effects in animals and/or animal models of human diseases; prediction of potential therapeutic use,
- **pharmacokinetics**: identification of metabolites (since these may be the active form of the compound); evidence of bioavailability (to assist with the design of both clinical trials and *in vivo* animal toxicity studies); establishment of principal route and rate of elimination,
- **toxicological effects**: a battery of *in vitro* and *in vivo* studies undertaken with the aim of identifying toxicity as early as possible, and before there is extensive *in vivo* exposure of animals or, subsequently, humans.

TOXICITY TESTING

Toxicity testing has two primary goals: identification of hazards and prediction of the likely risk of that hazard occurring in humans receiving therapeutic doses of the new medicine. A wide range of doses is studied; high doses are required to increase the ability to detect hazards and lower doses are needed to analyse dose–response relationships to predict the risk at doses producing the anticipated therapeutic effect. Toxicity tests include the following (see also www.emea.europa.eu/htms/human/humanguidelines/nonclinical.htm).

- **Mutagenicity**: a variety of *in vitro* tests using bacterial cells (such as the Ames test) and in cell lines from rodents are employed at an early stage to define any damage to DNA or chromosomal structures that may be linked to carcinogenicity or teratogenicity; *in vivo* studies may be undertaken to investigate the mechanism of genotoxicity.
- **Acute toxicity**: a single dose is given to animals by the route proposed for human use; this may reveal a likely site for toxicity and is essential in defining the initial dose for human studies. Acute toxicity data, including information on the doses causing lethality, are essential for safe manufacture; the LD_{50} (a precise estimate of the dose required to kill 50% of an animal population) has been replaced by simpler and more humane methods that define the dose range associated with acute toxicity.
- **Subacute toxicity**: repeated doses are given to animals for 14 or 28 days; this will usually reveal the target for toxic effects, and comparison with single-dose data may indicate the potential for accumulation.
- **Chronic toxicity**: repeated doses are given to animals for up to 6 months; this reveals the target for toxicity (except cancer). The aim is to define dose regimens associated with adverse effects and a 'no observed adverse effect level' (NOAEL; the 'safe' dose).
- **Carcinogenicity**: repeated doses are given throughout the lifetime of the animal (usually 2 years in a rodent).
- **Reproductive toxicity**: repeated doses are given to animals from before mating and throughout gestation to assess any effect on fertility, implantation, fetal growth, the production of fetal abnormalities (teratogenicity) or neonatal growth.

Table 3.1 EMA guidelines for the length of animal toxicity studies necessary to support phase I and phase II studies in humans

Duration of proposed phase I or II clinical trials	Minimum recommended duration of repeat-dose animal toxicity studies	
	Rodents	*Non-rodents*
Single dose	2–4 weeks	2 weeks
Up to 2 weeks	2–4 weeks	2 weeks
Up to 1 month	1 month	1 month
Up to 3 months	3 months	3 months
More than 3 months	6 months	9 months

Support of phase III clinical studies may require longer animal toxicity studies than shown here.

The extent of animal toxicity testing required prior to the first administration to humans is related to the proposed duration of human exposure and the population to be treated. All drugs are subjected to an initial *in vitro* screen for mutagenic potential: if satisfactory, this is followed by acute and subacute studies for up to 14 days of administration to two animal species. Doses studied are usually a low dose sufficient to cause the pharmacological/therapeutic effect, a high dose sufficient to cause target organ toxicity and an intermediate dose, together with a control group of untreated animals. Teratogenicity and reproductive toxicity studies are required if the drug is to be given to women of childbearing age; since the thalidomide tragedy, rabbits have been used for teratogenicity studies because, unlike rodents, they show fetal abnormalities when treated with thalidomide. Carcinogenicity testing is necessary for drugs that may be used for long periods, for example over 1 year.

An international review of the extent of *in vivo* animal testing necessary prior to phase I and phase II clinical trials concluded that the duration of animal toxicity tests should be the same as proposed human exposure (Table 3.1). In Japan and the USA, the same advice applies for phase III studies, but the EU recommends more extensive animal toxicity studies to support phase III trials. Dogs are the 'non-rodent species' usually studied.

The use of animals for the establishment of chemical safety is an emotive issue, and there is extensive current research to replace *in vivo* animal studies with *in vitro* tests based on known mechanisms of toxicity. However, toxicology as a predictive science is still in its infancy and at present it is impossible to replicate the complexity of mammalian physiology and biochemistry by *in vitro* systems. *In vivo* studies remain essential to investigate interference with either integrative functions or complex homeostatic mechanisms. Carefully controlled safety studies in animals are an essential part of the current procedures adopted to prevent extensive human toxicity, which would inevitably result from the use of untested compounds. Although toxicology has failed in the past to prevent some tragedies (see above), these have led to improvements in methods and current tests provide an effective predictive screen. Nevertheless, there have been examples of approved drugs being withdrawn because of reactions that were not detected in preclinical studies; for example, the high rate of rhabdomyolysis produced by cerivastatin, which was withdrawn worldwide in 2001. This may be increasingly important in the future because drugs developed using molecular biological methods to act specifically at human proteins may show limited or no activity at the analogous rodent receptors; however, animal studies will still provide a useful screen for non-specific, non-receptor-mediated effects.

Students should recognise that not all hazards detected at high doses in experimental animals are of relevance to human health. An important function of expert advisory bodies such as the CHMP is to assess the relevance to human health of effects detected in experimental animals at doses that may be two orders of magnitude (or more) above human exposures. Many drug 'scare stories' in the media are based on a hazard detected at experimental doses in animals much higher than the relevant doses for humans.

CLINICAL TRIALS: PHASES I–III

The purposes of pre-marketing clinical studies are:

- to establish that the drug has a useful action in humans,
- to define any toxicity at therapeutic doses in humans,
- to establish the nature of common (type A) unwanted effects (see Ch. 53).

Subjects in clinical studies give informed consent to participate and the trials are approved by ethical committees and regulatory agencies. Traditionally, pre-marketing clinical studies have been subdivided into three phases. Although the distinction between these is blurred, the following classification system provides a useful framework

Phase I studies

Phase I is the term used to describe the first trials of a new drug in humans, with typically between 20 and 100 volunteers. A principal aim of these studies is to define basic properties, such as route of administration, pharmacokinetics and tolerability. The studies are usually carried out by the pharmaceutical company, often using a specialised contract research organisation. Subjects taking part in phase I studies are often healthy volunteers recruited by open advertisement, especially when the compound is of low predicted toxicity and has wide potential use; for example, an antihistamine. In some cases, people suffering from the condition in which the drug will be used may be studied, such as cytotoxic agents used for cancer chemotherapy.

The first few administrations are usually in a very small number of subjects ($n < 10$) who receive an oral dose that may be as low as one-fiftieth or one-hundredth of the minimum required to produce a pharmacological effect in animals (after scaling for differences in body weight). Such a 'microdose' study may be termed a phase 0 trial. The dose may be then built up incrementally in larger subject groups until a pharmacological effect is observed or an unwanted action occurs. During these studies toxic effects are sought by routine haematology and biochemical investigations of liver and renal function; other tests, including an electrocardiogram, will be performed as appropriate.

It is also usual to study the disposition, metabolism and main pathways of elimination of the proposed new drug in humans at this stage. Such studies help to identify the most suitable dose and route of administration for future clinical studies. Investigations of drug metabolism and pharmacokinetics often necessitate the use of radioactively labelled compounds containing carbon-14 or tritium (^3H) as part of the drug molecule.

Peptide drugs have to be given intravenously in clinical trials to mimic the route of proposed clinical use. Very low doses are studied in the first instance, especially with peptides that are designed to interact specifically with human homeostatic or signalling systems, because studies in animals may not reveal the full biological activities. Despite these safeguards, TGN 1412, a monoclonal antibody directed against CD28, a co-stimulatory molecule for T-cell receptors, caused multiple organ dysfunction in its first phase I trial in six human volunteers in March 2006. The severe toxicity occurred at a dose 500 times lower than the dose found to be safe in animals, including non-human primates.

Phase II studies

During phase II studies, the detailed clinical pharmacology of the new compound is determined, typically in groups of 100–300 individuals with the intended clinical condition. A principal aim of these studies is to define the relationship between dose and pharmacological/therapeutic response in humans. Evidence of a beneficial effect may emerge during phase II studies, although a placebo control is not always used. Additional studies may be undertaken at this stage in special groups such as elderly people, if it is intended that the drug will be used in that population. Other studies may investigate the mechanism of action, or test for interactions with other drugs. Phase II studies normally define the optimum dosage regimen, and this is then used in large clinical trials to demonstrate the efficacy and safety of the drug.

Phase III studies

Phase III studies are the main clinical trials, usually performed in 300–3000 people with the condition that the drug is intended to treat, in multiple centres, in comparison with a placebo that looks (and tastes) the same as the active compound. Allocation to active compound or placebo requires randomisation, which reduces selection bias in the assignment of treatments and facilitates the blinding (masking) of the identity of treatments from the investigators. The advantages and disadvantages of the new compound may also be compared with the best available treatment or the leading drug in the class. It may be difficult to justify the use of a placebo if an effective form of treatment has been established for the condition being studied, as substituting the novel drug for the established treatment in the trial could result in significant risk to those participating. The drug under evaluation may therefore be used in addition to the established treatment and compared with the established treatment plus a placebo.

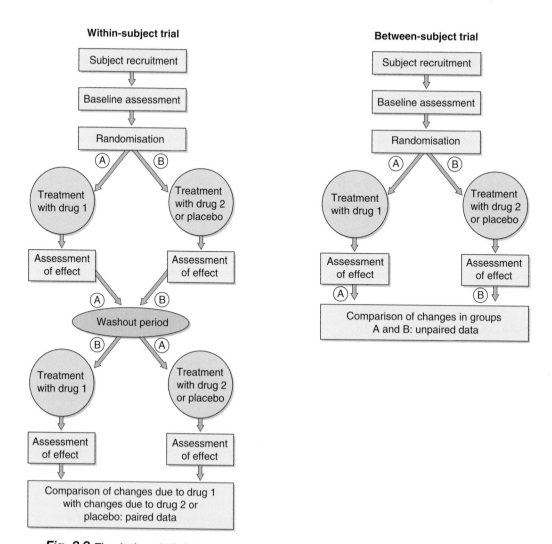

Fig. 3.3 The design of clinical trials. Subjects are randomly allocated to group A or group B.

Clinical trials are of two main types: within-subject and between-subject comparisons (Fig. 3.3). In within-subject trials, an individual is randomly allocated to commence treatment either with the new compound or with a placebo (or comparator drug) before 'crossing over' to the alternative therapy, usually with a washout period in between. In contrast, between-subject comparisons involve randomisation of subjects to receive only one of two (or more) treatments for the duration of the study.

Within-subject comparisons (also called crossover trials) can usually be performed on a smaller number of subjects, since the individuals act as their own controls and most non-treatment-related variables are eliminated. However, such studies often require a longer involvement of each individual. Also, there may be carry-over effects from one treatment that affect the apparent efficacy of the second treatment, although statistical analysis should be able to deal with this problem. Studies of this type may be difficult to interpret when there is a pronounced seasonal variation in the severity of a condition, such as Raynaud's

phenomenon or hay fever. Crossover studies (Fig. 3.3) cannot be used if the treatment is curative; for example, an antimicrobial for treating acute infections.

Between-subject comparisons (also called parallel-group studies) require roughly twice as many participants as within-subject trials but have the advantages that each subject will usually be studied for a shorter period and carry-over effects are avoided. Although it is not possible to provide a perfect match between subjects entering the two (or more) different treatment groups, this approach to the evaluation of new drugs is preferred by many drug regulatory authorities.

Whichever form of comparison is made, measurements of benefit (and adverse effects) are made at regular intervals using a combination of objective and subjective techniques (Table 3.2). Throughout these studies, careful attention is paid to detecting and reporting both unwanted effects (type A reactions) and unpredictable (type B) reactions (Ch. 53). Rare type B reactions are not usually seen prior to the marketing of a new drug, because they may occur only

Table 3.2 Examples of response measurements during clinical trials

New drug type	Measurement techniques	
	Objective	Subjective[a]
Anti-anginal	Exercise tolerance Blood pressure Heart rate Glyceryl trinitrate use	Fatigue Frequency of anginal attacks Pain intensity
Anti-arthritic	Grip strength	Duration of morning stiffness
	Joint size Paracetamol use	Pain intensity

[a]Subjective effects are often scored on a numerical scale, e.g. 0 = no pain at all, 10 = the worst imaginable pain.

once in every 1000–10 000 or more individuals treated with the drug. It is salutary to note that by the time a new medicine is marketed only 2000–3000 people may have taken the drug, often for relatively short periods such as 6 months, amounting to only a few hundred patient-years of drug exposure.

POST-MARKETING SURVEILLANCE: PHASE IV (PHARMACOVIGILANCE)

The full spectrum of benefits and risks of medicines may not become clear until after they are marketed. Reasons for this include the low frequency of certain adverse drug reactions, and the tendency to avoid the inclusion of children, the elderly and women of childbearing age in pre-marketing clinical trials. Another factor is the widespread use of other medicines in normal clinical practice, which could produce an unexpected interaction with the new drug. Phase IV studies involve post-marketing surveillance of efficacy and adverse reactions, sometimes in clinical indications additional to those licensed. Pharmacovigilance is the identification of risk/benefit issues for authorised medicines arising from their use in clinical practice, and includes the effective dissemination of information to optimise the safe and effective use of medicines.

Pharmacovigilance reports across the EU are coordinated by the EudraVigilance network (http://eudravigilance.ema.europa.eu/human/). Within the UK, a number of systems of post-marketing surveillance are in use. The most important is known as the Yellow Card system; it depends on doctors reporting suspected serious adverse reactions to the MHRA, either online (see MHRA website, www.mhra.gov.uk) or using postage-prepaid cards included in the *British National Formulary* (BNF) and the *Monthly Index of Medical Specialties* (MIMS). In addition to reporting suspected serious adverse effects of established drugs, doctors are asked to supply information about all unwanted effects of medicines that have been marketed recently. Each year the MHRA receives some 20 000 yellow cards/slips. In return, doctors are supplied regularly with information about current drug-related problems.

A second form of pharmacovigilance involves systematic post-marketing surveillance of recently marketed medicines. This may be organised by the pharmaceutical company responsible for the manufacture of the new drug (companies also receive information via their representatives). The MHRA administers the Clinical Practice Research Datalink (CRPD; www.cprd.eu), formed in 2012 from the General Practice Research Database, which collects the anonymised, longitudinal patient records from participating UK general practices. It is used in conjunction with the Yellow Card scheme to provide a warning system for approved medicines.

Prescription event monitoring (PEM) provides a further method for detailed study of possible associations provided by pharmacovigilance programmes. This involves:

- identification of a possible health problem associated with an approved medicine,
- identification by the UK Prescription Pricing Authority of individuals who have been prescribed a drug of interest,
- the subsequent distribution of 'green cards' to those individuals' GPs, with a request that they complete all details about the person and events that occurred.

The cards are returned to the Drug Safety Research Unit (DSRU) in Southampton (www.dsru.org), which collates and analyses the data. PEM has the advantage that it does not require doctors to make a judgement concerning a possible link between the prescription of a drug and any medical event that occurs while the person is taking the drug. At first sight, a broken leg may be thought an unlikely drug-related adverse effect, but it could be the result of drug-induced hypotension, ataxia or metabolic bone disease.

Finally, detailed monitoring of adverse reactions to drug therapy takes place in some hospitals. These data contribute further to our overall knowledge.

When assessing efficacy and associated toxicity, combining the data from a number of clinical trials (meta-analysis) can provide an overview of the validity and reproducibility of clinical findings. Meta-analysis is complex and only well-designed trials should be combined. The Cochrane Library (www.thecochranelibrary.com) provides a regularly updated collection of evidence-based meta-analyses.

The UK National Institute for Clinical Excellence (NICE) was established in 1999 and became the National Institute for Health and Care Excellence (still known as NICE) in 2005 following its merger with the Health Development Agency. NICE is responsible for providing national guidance on treatments and care for people using the NHS in England and Wales. It provides advice on the clinical value and cost-effectiveness of new treatments, but also on existing treatments if there is uncertainty about their use. NICE produces guidance on:

- the use of new and existing medicines and treatments in the NHS in England and Wales (technology appraisals),
- the appropriate treatment and care of people with specific diseases and conditions in the NHS in England and Wales (clinical guidelines),
- whether interventional procedures used for diagnosis or treatment are safe and work well enough for routine use (interventional procedures).

SELF-ASSESSMENT

One-best-answer (OBA) questions

1. In which phase of drug development is a placebo most likely to be used?
   A. Phase 0
   B. Phase I
   C. Phase II
   D. Phase III
   E. Phase IV

2. Which of the following statements best describes a phase III crossover trial?
   A. Randomisation is not required in a crossover trial.
   B. People with the most severe disease are allocated to receive the active drug first.
   C. The second treatment period starts as soon as the first treatment period ends.
   D. Crossover trials are preferred for trials of curative drugs.
   E. Participants receive two or more treatments in a random sequence.

OBA answers

1. **Answer D** is correct. A drug is most likely to be compared with a placebo in large-scale (phase III) trials, although a placebo may also be used in phase II trials. The drug (and placebo) may be added to the existing best treatment, or compared with a leading drug for the same condition.

2. **Answer E** is correct. Randomisation is designed to produce treatment groups that match in all important characteristics, including disease severity. In a within-subject (or crossover) trial, randomisation of the sequence of treatments that each subject receives reduces the probability of confounding by an effect of one treatment persisting into the second treatment period; an interval between treatments (washout) helps to ensure this. Crossover trials are generally not used to test curative drugs for acute conditions (e.g. antimicrobials) as the condition may not persist through both treatment periods.

FURTHER READING

Adams CP, Brantner VV (2006) Estimating the cost of new drug development: is it really $802 million? *Health Affairs* 25, 420–428

Austin CP (2004) The impact of the completed human genome sequence on the development of novel therapeutics for human disease. *Annu Rev Med* 55, 1–13

Dollery C (2003) The clinical pharmacologist's view; drug discovery and early development. In: Wilkins MR (ed.), Experimental Therapeutics. London: Martin Dunitz, Taylor and Francis; pp 3–24

Kerwin R (2004) The National Institute for Clinical Excellence and its relevance to pharmacology. *Trends Pharmacol Sci* 25, 346–348

Layton D, Hazell L, Shakir SA (2011) Modified prescription-event monitoring studies: a tool for pharmacovigilance and risk management. *Drug Safety* 34(12), e1–e9

Lynch A, Connelly J (2003) The toxicologist's view: non-clinical safety assessment. In: Wilkins MR (ed.), Experimental

Therapeutics. London: Martin Dunitz, Taylor and Francis; pp 25–50

Marchetti S, Schellens JH (2007) The impact of FDA and EMEA guidelines on drug development in relation to Phase 0 trials. *Br J Cancer* 97, 577–581

Persidis A (1998) High-throughput screening. Advances in robotics and miniaturization continue to accelerate drug lead identification. *Nat Biotechnol* 16, 488–489

Schneider G, Fechner U (2005) Computer-based *de novo* design of drug-like molecules. *Nat Rev Drug Discov* 4, 649–663

Shah RR, Branch SK, Steele C (2003) The regulator's view; regulatory requirements for marketing authorizations for new medicinal products in the European Union. In: Wilkins MR (ed.), Experimental Therapeutics. London: Martin Dunitz, Taylor and Francis; pp 51–75

Walker DK (2004) The use of pharmacokinetic and pharmacodynamic data in the assessment of drug safety in early drug development. *Br J Clin Pharmacol* 58, 601–608

4 Neurotransmission and the peripheral autonomic nervous system

• •

This chapter deals predominantly with details of the peripheral autonomic nervous system; the general principles relating to the central nervous system and the somatic nervous system are similar, but specific details are dealt with in Section 5 and Chapter 27, respectively.

ARRANGEMENT OF THE CENTRAL AND PERIPHERAL NERVOUS SYSTEMS

There are two principal neuronal control systems in the body. Functionally they are highly integrated and should be considered holistically, but for educational clarity they are introduced separately.

■ The *central nervous system* (CNS) comprises neuronal networks of the brain, brainstem and spinal cord (Section 5).
■ The *peripheral nervous systems*, which interconnect the CNS to the organs of the body, include:
  ■ the *autonomic* (automatic or involuntary) nervous system, which comprises sympathetic and parasympathetic nervous systems and also includes the enteric nervous system of the gut,
  ■ the *somatic* (voluntary) nervous system, which innervates skeletal muscle (Ch. 27).

The CNS integrates, processes and responds to sensory messages.

■ It receives sensory information from all parts of the body, including visceral sensory afferent nerves (e.g. from viscera, smooth muscle and cardiac muscle) and somatic sensory afferents (e.g. from skeletal muscle).
■ It responds by sending instructions via the autonomic efferent nerves of the sympathetic and parasympathetic systems (e.g. to glands, smooth muscle and cardiac muscle) and via somatic motor efferents to skeletal muscle.

PRINCIPLES OF NEUROTRANSMISSION

Action potentials (APs) passing along axons provide instructions to other neurons or non-neuronal cells (e.g. smooth muscle cells). Instructions are transferred by the release of chemical neurotransmitters from the presynaptic endings of the neuron, which then diffuse through a small physical space, called the synaptic cleft, and stimulate the receiving (postsynaptic) cells via recognition proteins (receptors) (Fig. 4.1). The transmitters may instruct the receiving cells to increase (excite) or reduce (inhibit) their activity.

Neurotransmitters can be either synthesised within the presynaptic region (e.g. noradrenaline) or transported from the cell body to the synaptic region (e.g. peptides). The neurotransmitter is taken up from the cytosol using specific vesicular transporters within the nerve ending and stored within membrane vesicles. The transmitter in the vesicle may form a complex; for example, noradrenaline forms a complex with adenosine triphosphate (ATP), which reduces the free concentration of noradrenaline within the vesicle.

The release of the neurotransmitter can be 'fine-tuned' by axo-axonic connections and by presynaptic receptors

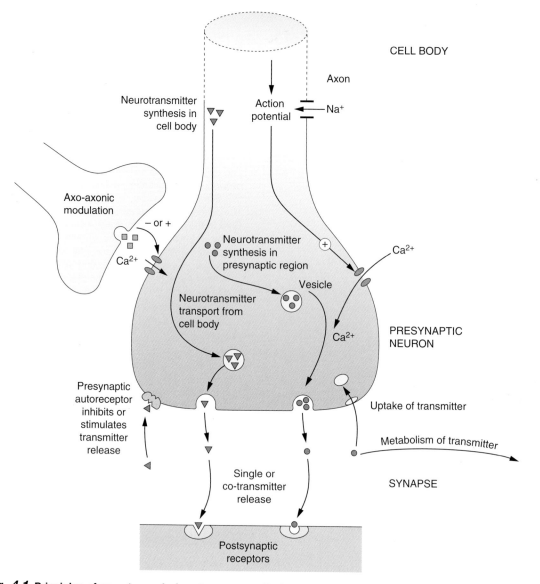

Fig. 4.1 **Principles of neurotransmission at a synapse.** Basic pathways of synthesis, storage, release, action and inactivation of a typical neurotransmitter are shown, as described in the text. At many synapses co-transmission of different neurotransmitters occurs.

(which are discussed below). A generalised scheme for neurotransmission is as follows (Fig. 4.1):

a. The cell body (or soma) responds to an appropriate stimulus by generating an AP.

b. The AP is conducted along the axon by the opening of voltage-gated Na^+ channels and the influx of Na^+; when the AP reaches the presynaptic nerve terminal it results in an influx of Ca^{2+} through voltage-dependent channels.

c. Ca^{2+}-dependent processes result in fusion of neurotransmitter-containing vesicles with the presynaptic membrane and the release of stored neurotransmitter into the synaptic space.

d. The released neurotransmitter binds to and stimulates the appropriate receptors in the postsynaptic

membranes and generates biochemical changes in the recipient cells; these may be functional changes in cells (e.g. smooth muscle contraction) or excitation or inhibition of another neuron (e.g. transmission of the AP to postsynaptic nerve fibres).

e. The released neurotransmitter may also stimulate autoreceptors in the presynaptic membranes, and thereby modulate the further release of the neurotransmitter.

f. The transmitter is degraded by enzymes or taken back into the presynaptic neuron for re-use.

Neurons may release a single transmitter, but often more than one transmitter is released; there are many examples of *co-transmission*, which are described later in this book.

Table 4.1 The control of transmitter release by presynaptic receptor mechanisms

Neurotransmitter	Presynaptic receptors inhibiting release	Presynaptic receptors facilitating release
Acetylcholine (ACh)	M_2, α_2, D_2/D_3, 5-HT_3	N_1, NMDA
Dopamine	D_2/D_3, M_2	N_1, NMDA
γ-Aminobutyric acid (GABA)	$GABA_B$	–
Histamine	H_3	–
Serotonin (5-hydroxytryptamine, 5-HT)	5-HT_{1D}, α_2	5-HT_3
Noradrenaline	α_2, H_3, M_2, D_2, opioid	β_2, N_1, angiotensin II

NMDA, *N*-methyl-D-aspartate.

PRESYNAPTIC RECEPTORS AND MODULATION OF TRANSMITTER RELEASE

An important characteristic of neurons is the presence of presynaptic receptors (Fig. 4.1 and Table 4.1). Presynaptic receptors may increase or decrease the release of the neurotransmitter and are described as facilitatory and inhibitory, respectively. There are two main sources of ligands for presynaptic receptors:

- neurotransmitter released from the vesicles that can act presynaptically (autoreceptors),
- neurotransmitter released from other neurons, usually by axo-axonal synapses (Fig. 4.1), involving a different neurotransmitter to that released by the neuron itself (heteroreceptors).

Inhibition of transmitter release is usually achieved by limiting Ca^{2+} entry through voltage-gated ion channels into the neuron.

The first recognition of a clinically important presynaptic receptor came with the discovery that the antihypertensive agent clonidine lowers blood pressure via stimulation of presynaptic α_2-adrenoceptors, with subsequent inhibition of the release of vasoconstricting noradrenaline. Presynaptic receptors (Table 4.1) are increasingly recognised to have important roles in the clinical effects produced by many drugs.

THE PERIPHERAL AUTONOMIC NERVOUS SYSTEM

The peripheral autonomic nervous system (ANS) is an important site for drug action because:

- the ANS either controls or contributes to the control of the functioning of nearly all of the major organ systems of the body,
- ANS dysfunction is present in many diseases,
- ANS dysfunction can occur as an unwanted effect of drug treatment,
- the ANS utilises two major different neurotransmitters and a number of receptor subtypes; these provide a variety of sites for drug action (Box 4.1), which allows modification of particular body functions with some degree of selectivity.

Box 4.1   Targets for drug action within the ANS

- Muscarinic receptors at postganglionic nerve endings in the parasympathetic nervous system (muscarinic receptor subtypes)
- Adrenergic receptors for noradrenaline and adrenaline in the sympathetic nervous system (α- and β-adrenoceptor subtypes)
- Presynaptic receptors in the parasympathetic and sympathetic nervous systems
- Modification of synthesis, storage, release and inactivation of ACh
- Modification of synthesis, storage, release and inactivation of noradrenaline

The peripheral ANS is subdivided into two main branches (Fig. 4.2, Box 4.2):

- *parasympathetic nervous system*, which utilises acetylcholine (ACh) as the final transmitter at muscarinic receptors on the cells that are being stimulated (called the innervated or effector cells or organs),
- *sympathetic nervous system*, which utilises noradrenaline as the transmitter at adrenoceptors on most, but not all, effector organs; the release of adrenaline and noradrenaline from the adrenal medulla during sympathetic nervous system stimulation is also an important and integral part of the sympathetic nervous system response.

Anatomically, in both branches of the ANS, the efferent neurons innervating effector organs are linked to neurons in the CNS via ganglia. The distribution and neuronal interconnections differ between the two branches (Fig. 4.2).

- The parasympathetic efferents give more discrete innervation of organs; the ganglia are close to the innervated organs and they therefore have long preganglionic fibres; there are few or no interconnections between ganglia, so that innervated organs can be affected independently.
- The sympathetic efferents are classically described as being involved in the flight-or-fight response and affect many body systems simultaneously. Many of the ganglia are close to the spinal column in the paravertebral sympathetic ganglion chain that lies along each side of the spinal column, so these nerves have long postganglionic fibres to effector organs. All neurons in the sympathetic system can be activated simultaneously because of numerous neuronal interconnections within

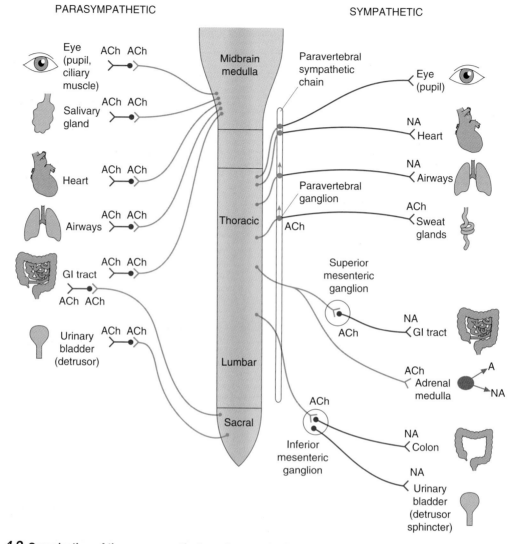

Fig. 4.2 Organisation of the parasympathetic and sympathetic autonomic nervous systems. Activation of the sympathetic nervous system leads to widespread neuronal release of noradrenaline supplemented by release into the circulation of adrenaline (and noradrenaline) from the adrenal medulla; these act at α- and β-adrenoceptors (see Table 4.2). Stimulation of the parasympathetic nervous system is more localised to particular organs, mediated by acetylcholine acting at muscarinic receptors (see Table 4.3). Some tissues, such as airways, have sparse sympathetic innervation and sympathetic effects are mainly a result of circulating adrenaline. Sympathetic innervation of sweat glands is mediated, unusually, by acetylcholine. The ganglia innervating some organs are not part of the paravertebral chain but grouped together to form the coeliac, superior mesenteric or inferior mesenteric ganglia; the transmitter at all ganglia is acetylcholine acting at nicotinic type 1 receptors. ACh, acetylcholine; NA, noradrenaline; A, adrenaline; GI, gastrointestinal.

the paravertebral chain; also, axons passing through the chain without synapsing can interconnect with ganglia such as the inferior mesenteric ganglion and can then diversify to innervate several organs (Fig. 4.2).

Many organs are innervated by both the parasympathetic and sympathetic nervous systems, which act in concert and may have opposite effects on the organ function. Physiological functions therefore often require inverse coordination of sympathetic and parasympathetic activities; for example, urination is brought about by a decreased

sympathetic activity on the sphincter muscle and increased parasympathetic activity on the detrusor muscle (see urinary bladder, Tables 4.2 and 4.3, and Ch. 15).

The concept of opposing actions, although imperfect, can be useful in remembering the effects that each part of the nervous system has on tissue function. Tables 4.2 and 4.3 show the effects that stimulation of the sympathetic or parasympathetic nervous systems have on major tissues and the primary receptors that are involved. Under resting conditions, the predominant drive to many organs is from the parasympathetic nervous system.

Box 4.2   **Organisation of the ANS**

- Parasympathetic and sympathetic efferent nerves from the spinal cord synapse at intermediate ganglia before synapsing with the effector cells at their postganglionic nerve endings
- ACh and noradrenaline are the principal neurotransmitters in the ANS but other transmitters also have neurotransmitter roles.
- Stimulation of the sympathetic nervous system has a widespread effect in the body because of interconnections between efferent fibres, whereas the parasympathetic nervous system is more organ-specific (Fig. 4.2).
- The neurotransmitters are synthesised in the presynaptic neuron, stored and released into the synapse in response to depolarization and Ca^{2+} influx caused by an AP.
- At all ganglia, the neurotransmitter is ACh, acting on nicotinic N_1 receptors, which then elicits an AP in the postganglionic nerve.
- Parasympathetic efferents have muscarinic receptors at neuroeffector synapses.
- Most sympathetic efferents have noradrenergic receptors at neuroeffector synapses.
- Adrenaline and noradrenaline are synthesised and released in the adrenal medulla in response to sympathetic stimulation and enhance the effects of local noradrenaline release.

Table 4.2 Effects of sympathetic nervous system activity via adrenoceptor subtypes in major tissues

Tissue	Effect	Main receptor type
Heart rate	Increase	β_1 (β_2 in heart disease)
Contractility	Increase	β_1 (β_2 in heart disease)
Atrioventricular conduction	Increase	β_1
Blood vessels in skin/gut	Constriction	α_1
Blood vessels in skeletal muscle	Dilation[a]	β_2
Bronchial smooth muscle	Dilation[a]	β_2
Gastrointestinal motility	Relaxation	α_1, β_2
Gastrointestinal sphincter tone	Contraction	α_1
Uterine smooth muscle	Contraction Relaxation	α_1, β_2
Bladder detrusor	Relaxation	β_2, β_3
Bladder sphincter	Constriction	α_1
Penis	Ejaculation	α_1
Pilomotor muscles	Constriction	α_1
Sweat glands	Secretion	Muscarinic
Pupil (radial muscle)	Contraction dilates pupil	α_1
Hepatic glycogenolysis	Increase	β_2, α
Skeletal muscle glycogenolysis	Increase[a]	β_2
Fat cell lipolysis	Increase[a]	β_1, α, β_3
Pancreas insulin secretion	Decrease	α_2
Platelets	Aggregation	α_2
Presynaptic nerve terminal (noradrenergic)	Inhibition of NA release Increased NA release	α_2 β_2
Presynaptic nerve terminal (muscarinic)	Inhibition of ACh release	α_2
Kidney (juxtaglomerular) renin release	Increase	β_1

[a]Respond to circulating adrenaline; little noradrenergic innervation.

Table 4.3 Effect of stimulation of parasympathetic nerves (via muscarinic M receptor subtypes) in major tissues

Tissue	Effect	Main receptor type
Heart rate	Decrease	M_2
Contractility of atria	Decrease	M_2
Atrioventricular conduction velocity	Decrease	M_2
Vascular endothelium	Dilates blood vessel: NO release	M_1, M_3
Bronchial smooth muscle	Constriction	M_2, M_3
Gut motility	Contraction, relaxation	M_2, M_3
Gut sphincter tone	Increased	M_3
Gut secretions	Increased	M_3
Bladder detrusor	Contraction	M_3
Bladder sphincter	Relaxation	M_3
Penis	Erection	M_3
Eye pupil circular muscle	Contraction (miosis)	M_3
Ciliary muscle	Contraction (accommodates for near vision)	M_3
Pancreatic insulin secretion	Increased	M_1, M_3
Salivary glands	Secretion	M_1, M_3
Emesis	Increased	M_3

THE SYMPATHETIC NERVOUS SYSTEM AND NORADRENERGIC TRANSMISSION

Noradrenaline and adrenaline are members of a group of amine transmitters called catecholamines (a catechol is a benzene ring with two adjacent hydroxyl groups; Fig. 4.3A). Both the catechol and amino groups are important for receptor binding. The receptors that noradrenaline and adrenaline stimulate are described as adrenoceptors and the effects of noradrenaline and adrenaline at these receptors are described as noradrenergic and adrenergic effects.

The approved European names of noradrenaline and adrenaline when they are formulated and used therapeutically as medicines are *norepinephrine* and *epinephrine*, respectively; however, when their physiological actions are being described, the terms noradrenaline and adrenaline are retained. Most preparations of adrenaline and noradrenaline in Europe are dual-labelled with both terms. In the USA, the terms epinephrine and norepinephrine are used for both therapeutic and physiological descriptions.

SYNTHESIS AND STORAGE OF CATECHOLAMINES: NORADRENALINE, ADRENALINE AND DOPAMINE

Catecholamine neurotransmitters are synthesised from inactive precursors (Fig. 4.3B). The basic carbon skeleton of catecholamines is derived from phenylalanine or tyrosine, which are aromatic amino acids used predominantly in protein synthesis. The sequence of synthesis of adrenaline (via dopamine and noradrenaline) is shown in Figure 4.3B. The oxidation of tyrosine to levodopa by tyrosine hydroxylase, which occurs within the neuron, commits the molecule to become a neurotransmitter. This step is subject to negative feedback by the catecholamines that are subsequently produced, thereby regulating supply. Conversion of levodopa to dopamine is catalysed by a cytosolic enzyme, aromatic L-amino acid decarboxylase (also known as dopa decarboxylase). The amine product, dopamine, is taken up by vesicles via a specific transporter termed the vesicular monoamine transporter 2 (VMAT2). In neurons that use dopamine as their primary transmitter this is the end of the synthetic pathway. Dopamine is a vital neurotransmitter in some parts of the peripheral nervous system and also widely in the CNS (Chs 7, 21 and 24).

The vesicles present in noradrenergic neurons contain dopamine-β-hydroxylase. This enzyme is largely present in the membranes of the vesicles, but on exocytosis some is lost into the synapse, after which it diffuses into the bloodstream and is slowly cleared; its levels in the blood can therefore be used as a marker of peripheral noradrenaline release. In noradrenergic neurons this is the end of the synthetic pathway. Noradrenaline and its precursor dopamine are stored in the vesicles complexed with ATP and proteoglycans.

The chromaffin cells of the adrenal medulla contain an additional cytosolic enzyme (phenylethanolamine-N-methyl transferase), which converts noradrenaline to adrenaline by the addition of a methyl group (Fig. 4.3B). Adrenaline is then transferred into chromaffin cell granules by vesicular monoamine transporter 1 (VMAT1), where it is stored ready for release.

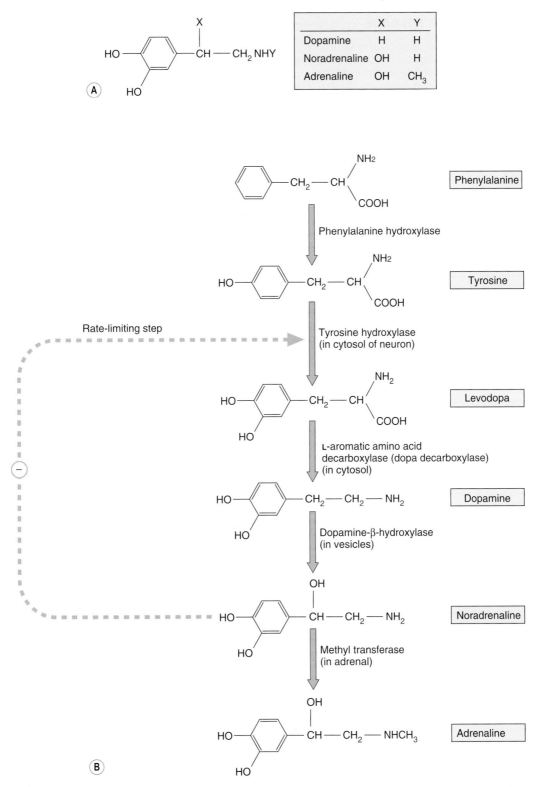

Fig. 4.3 The structure of the main physiological catecholamines (A) and their synthesis from amino acid precursors (B). The catecholamine synthetic pathway is described in the text.

NORADRENALINE RELEASE

Release in response to a nerve impulse occurs following Ca^{2+} influx and Ca^{2+}-mediated fusion of the noradrenaline-containing vesicle with the cytoplasmic membrane.

Noradrenaline in the presynaptic neuron may also be released by so-called indirectly acting sympathomimetic amines, which are low-molecular-weight basic compounds; for example, food constituents (such as tyramine), therapeutic drugs (such as ephedrine) and some drugs of abuse (such as amfetamine and metamfetamine). These compounds are taken into the presynaptic cytosol and into the vesicles, from which they displace noradrenaline. Increased noradrenaline release into the synapse is responsible for the biological effects produced by ingestion of compounds like tyramine, ephedrine and amfetamine.

UPTAKE AND METABOLISM OF RELEASED NORADRENALINE

The principal mechanism for the removal of noradrenaline from the synapse is uptake (approximately 70–90%) into the presynaptic neuron via a specific high-affinity carrier called uptake 1 (or the norepinephrine transporter, NET); it also takes up dopamine but not adrenaline (Fig. 4.4). Both noradrenaline and dopamine can then be transferred from the cytosol into the vesicles by VMAT2. Some of the noradrenaline remaining in the synapse is taken up into

non-neuronal tissues by a low-affinity carrier called uptake 2, which can also transport adrenaline; some of the remaining noradrenaline and the majority of any adrenaline released into the circulation as a co-transmitter is metabolised. Separate transporters exist for reuptake of serotonin (5-hydroxytryptamine, 5-HT) and dopamine from their respective neurons, termed the serotonin transporter (SERT) and dopamine transporter (DAT), respectively. Therapeutic agents that block NET or SERT increase the amount of neurotransmitter in the synaptic cleft and are used in treating depression (Ch. 22). The uptake of noradrenaline by NET is also blocked by cocaine and amfetamine.

There are two main enzymes involved in the initial steps in the catabolism of noradrenaline: monoamine oxidase (MAO) and catechol-O-methyltransferase (COMT).

Monoamine oxidase

MAO is present on the surface of the mitochondria of the presynaptic neuron, where it oxidises free cytoplasmic noradrenaline. It is also present in many other sites such as the gastrointestinal epithelium and liver. Oxidative removal of the amino group on noradrenaline via MAO is the major pathway of catabolism of noradrenaline and other aminergic neurotransmitters. Loss of the amino group prevents binding to the postsynaptic receptor, and therefore is an inactivation process. In the periphery, metabolism results in the formation of vanillylmandelic acid, which is the main

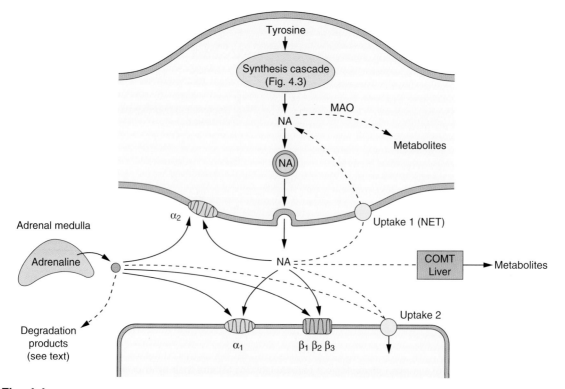

Fig. 4.4 A noradrenergic nerve terminal (varicosity) showing the synthesis and sites of action of noradrenaline and adrenaline. Dashed lines show the ways that the actions of the catecholamines are curtailed. COMT, catechol-O-methyltransferase; MAO, monoamine oxidase; NA, noradrenaline; NET, norepinephrine transporter (uptake 1).

Table 4.4 Monoamine oxidase (MAO) and its inhibitors

Isoenzyme	Location in human tissues	Main substrates	Examples of inhibitors	
			Irreversible	*Reversible*
MAO-A	Gastrointestinal tract, placenta	Serotonin, noradrenaline		Moclobemide
MAO-B	Brain[a], liver[a], platelets	Phenylethylamine, tyramine	Selegiline, rasagiline	
MAO-A or MAO-B		Tyramine, dopamine, adrenaline	Isocarboxazid, phenelzine, tranylcypromine	

[a]Both isoenzymes are present, but in humans the amount of MAO-B exceeds that of MAO-A.

urinary metabolite. In the CNS, the metabolites are conjugated with sulphate before being excreted in the urine. There are two main MAO isoenzymes, MAO-A and MAO-B, which differ in their organ distribution and substrate affinities (Table 4.4). The use of inhibitors of MAO-A and/or MAO-B isoenzymes in depression and Parkinson's disease is discussed in Chapters 22 and 24.

Catechol-O-methyltransferase

COMT occurs only at low levels in noradrenergic neurons, but is present in many other tissues, including the adrenal gland and liver. The enzyme catalyses the transfer of a methyl group onto the aromatic ring; this removes the catechol centre and prevents binding to the postsynaptic receptor. COMT is a minor route of inactivation of both dopamine and noradrenaline. Inhibitors of COMT are used as an adjunct to levodopa therapy for Parkinson's disease (Ch. 24).

SYMPATHETIC NERVOUS SYSTEM RECEPTORS

All ganglia utilise ACh as a neurotransmitter, acting predominantly on nicotinic type 1 (N_1) receptors to elicit an AP in the postganglionic axon. The receptor type at most postganglionic nerve endings in the sympathetic nervous system are adrenergic receptors (adrenoceptors).

Based on the effects of a number of agonists and antagonists, the adrenoceptors are divided into two types, α and β, and further into α-subtypes (α_1 and α_2) and β-subtypes (β_1, β_2 and β_3) (see Table 4.2 and the drug receptor table at the end of Ch. 1). It is now understood that there are multiple forms of some of these subtypes (i.e. α_{1A}, α_{1B} and α_{1D}, and α_{2A}, α_{2B} and α_{2C}) and these are discussed in later chapters where clinically relevant. The receptor subtypes show different affinities for the endogenous catecholamines, noradrenaline and adrenaline:

α_1: noradrenaline $\geq$ adrenaline
α_2: adrenaline > noradrenaline
β_1: noradrenaline $\geq$ adrenaline
β_2: adrenaline > noradrenaline
β_3: noradrenaline = adrenaline

Selective stimulation or blockade of individual adrenoceptor subtypes forms the basis of significant areas of pharmacology and therapeutics and is dealt with in relevant chapters.

THE PARASYMPATHETIC NERVOUS SYSTEM AND CHOLINERGIC TRANSMISSION

SYNTHESIS OF ACETYLCHOLINE

ACh is synthesised within the cytosol of the cholinergic neuron from choline and acetyl-CoA (Fig. 4.5). Choline is a highly polar, quaternary amino compound that is also present in phosphatidylcholine; it is obtained largely from the diet. Because of its fixed positive charge it does not readily cross cell membranes and there are specific transporters to allow uptake into the presynaptic neuron (Fig. 4.5) and from the gastrointestinal tract and across the blood–brain barrier (Ch. 2). Acetylation of choline to form ACh is catalysed by choline acetyltransferase. The rate of synthesis of ACh is closely controlled and related to ACh turnover, so that rapid release of ACh stores is associated with enhanced synthesis.

STORAGE OF ACETYLCHOLINE

Cytosolic ACh is taken up into membrane vesicles by a specific transmembrane transporter (the vesicular ACh transporter, VAChT) and is stored in the vesicles in association with ATP and acidic proteoglycans (which are also released on exocytosis of the vesicles). Each vesicle contains 1000–50 000 ACh molecules, and neuromuscular junctions (Ch. 27) contain about 300 000 vesicles.

RELEASE OF ACETYLCHOLINE

Release occurs by Ca^{2+}-mediated fusion of the vesicle membrane with the cytoplasmic membrane and exocytosis (Fig. 4.5). This process can be inhibited by botulinum toxin from *Clostridium botulinum* bacteria and stimulated by latrotoxin from the black widow spider (*Latrodectus* spp.). The number of vesicles released depends on the site of the synapse, with between 30 and 300 vesicles undergoing exocytosis, releasing from 30 000 to over 3 million ACh molecules into the synaptic cleft. Neurons within the CNS are more sensitive to ACh release and require fewer ACh molecules to be released to stimulate a recipient axon compared with the neuromuscular junction, which requires millions of ACh molecules for skeletal muscle contractility to occur.

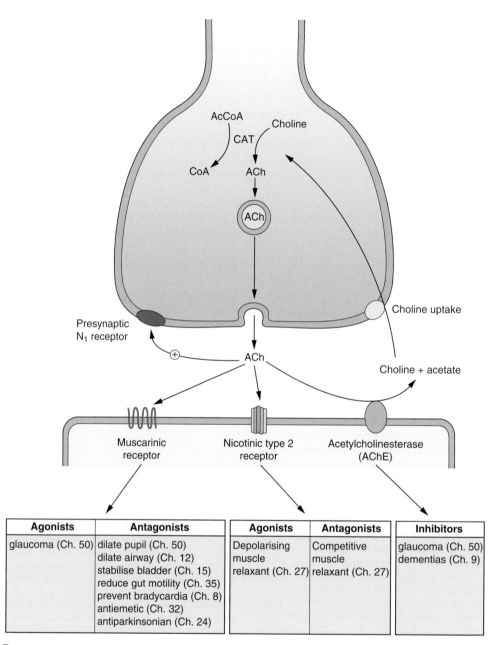

Fig. 4.5 **The mechanisms involved in the synthesis, release and inactivation of acetylcholine.** The actions of agonists and antagonists of muscarinic (M) and nicotinic receptors and acetylcholinesterase are shown with the relevant chapters dealing with their pharmacology. ACh, acetylcholine; AcCoA, acetyl-CoA; CAT, choline acetyltransferase.

METABOLISM AND INACTIVATION OF RELEASED ACETYLCHOLINE

Both presynaptic and postsynaptic membranes are rich in acetylcholinesterase (AChE); hence the released ACh is hydrolysed very rapidly (in usually <1 ms) to give choline and acetate. This rapid hydrolysis, and the rapid equilibration between ACh bound to the receptor and free in the synapse, mean that the 'receptor phase' of the transmission process only lasts for 1–2 ms (the postsynaptic changes may be more prolonged; see below).

AChE is an important target for drug action and for the toxic effects of some chemicals; the active site of the esterase has two critical features involved in the metabolism of ACh (Fig. 4.6):

- an anionic site, which forms an ionic bond with the quaternary nitrogen of the choline part of ACh,
- a hydrolytic site, which contains a serine moiety; the hydroxyl group of the serine accepts the acetyl group from ACh and very rapidly transfers it to water to complete the hydrolysis reaction.

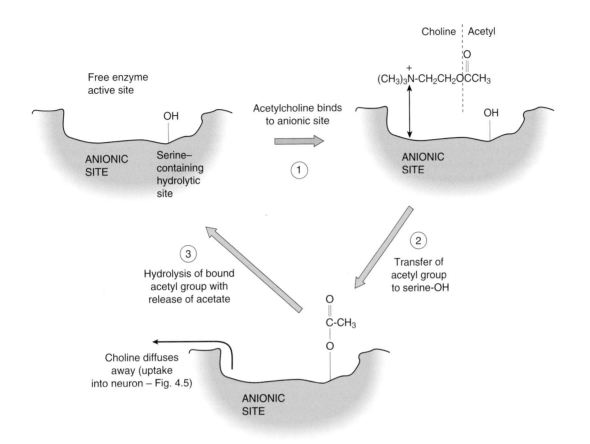

Fig. 4.6 The mechanism of hydrolysis of acetylcholine by acetylcholinesterase. The choline moiety of acetylcholine binds to the anionic site of the acetylcholinesterase active site, allowing hydrolysis of the acetyl group, with subsequent release of choline and acetate.

Inhibition of AChE will prevent the breakdown of ACh and lead to prolonged receptor occupancy, the consequences of which depend on the nature of the receptor and the innervated cell/tissue.

AChE inhibitors can be divided into three types.

- **AChE inhibitors that bind to the anionic site.** The enzyme can be inhibited by an agent binding reversibly to the anionic site, for example edrophonium (Ch. 28).
- **AChE inhibitors that carbamylate the serine group.** Some inhibitors bind to the anionic site and transfer a carbamoyl group instead of an acetyl group from the drug to the serine hydroxyl group. The carbamoyl group is hydrolysed more slowly from the serine than is an acetyl group and, as a result, prolonged and profound (but reversible) inhibition of the enzyme occurs; examples include neostigmine and pyridostigmine, which are used for reversing neuromuscular block produced by competitive neuromuscular junction blockers (Ch. 27) and in treatment of myasthenia gravis (Ch. 28). Reversible AChE inhibitors such as donepezil and rivastigmine are used in treatment of Alzheimer's disease (Ch. 9).
- **AChE inhibitors that phosphorylate the serine group.** Some inhibitors such as the organophosphates react with the serine hydroxyl group (with or without binding to the anionic site) to produce a phosphorylated enzyme. The phosphorylated enzyme is resistant to hydrolysis

and, therefore, these inhibitors cause inhibition which is irreversible (or very slowly and partially reversible). Such permanent changes in enzyme activity are of limited clinical use. The drug ecothiopate acts via phosphorylation of AChE and has a limited clinical use in ophthalmology. Compounds in this group may also be encountered clinically in people suffering accidental or intentional poisoning with organophosphate pesticides, and there has been concern in recent years over low-level exposure of agricultural workers to such compounds, for example in sheep dips. Organophosphates have also been developed as nerve gases for chemical warfare (e.g. sarin). The active serine hydroxyl group may be regenerated soon after exposure by administration of the drug pralidoxime (2-PAM), which is an antidote to organophosphate poisoning, although its efficacy is contentious. A few hours after exposure the phosphorylated enzyme undergoes changes, known as ageing, and pralidoxime cannot reactivate the enzyme after ageing has occurred.

Unlike many other neurotransmitters, ACh is not inactivated by a specific reuptake process, but because choline is a limited resource there is a specific reuptake mechanism to allow choline to re-enter the presynaptic neuron for re-use, rather than simply diffuse away. No such process occurs for acetate because it is readily available from intermediary metabolism. Presynaptic uptake of choline can be inhibited by structural analogues, such as hemicholinium, but such drugs are not useful clinically because of the widespread and non-specific consequences of impairment of ACh uptake, synthesis and release.

CHOLINERGIC RECEPTORS

The cholinergic receptors can be divided into nicotinic and muscarinic types. Two nicotinic and five muscarinic subtypes have been characterised (see drug receptor table at the end of Ch. 1). The receptors were originally named after nitrogen-containing basic compounds (alkaloids) present in plants (*nicotine*) or fungi (*muscarine*). Figure 4.5 gives information about the general effects of stimulants and inhibitors of muscarinic and nicotinic type 1 receptors and AChE inhibitors and identifies the chapter(s) describing the clinical relevance of these actions.

Nicotinic (N$_1$) receptors

These occur within the CNS and on the postsynaptic membranes of all ganglia of both the sympathetic and parasympathetic branches of the ANS.

Nicotinic (N$_2$) receptors

These occur at the junction between the somatic motor nerves and skeletal muscles (the neuromuscular junction; see Ch. 27).

The nicotinic receptor is a ligand-gated ion channel of five subunits (see Fig. 1.1), with disulphide cross-linking between adjacent subunits; there are different types of subunit (α, β, γ and δ), and different combinations give rise to neuronal N$_1$ receptors and neuromuscular junction N$_2$ receptors. The differences between N$_1$ and N$_2$ receptors in their agonist/antagonist binding characteristics are clinically very important, because they allow neuromuscular blockade (paralysis) without major effects on the ANS.

Muscarinic (M) receptors

These are G-protein-coupled receptors (GPCRs) widely distributed in the CNS and in pre- and postganglionic fibre/effector organ junctions of the parasympathetic branch of the ANS. They are also present on most sweat glands (other than the palms of the hands), which are, however, innervated by the *sympathetic* branch of the ANS. Table 4.3 shows the effect of stimulation of the muscarinic receptors in major tissues and the principal muscarinic receptor subtype that is involved. Application of molecular biology has identified five subtypes of muscarinic receptor (M$_1$–M$_5$; see drug receptor table at the end of Ch. 1). The distribution and functions of M$_1$, M$_2$ and M$_3$ receptors have been well characterised (Table 4.3).

In addition to occurring on postsynaptic sites, N$_1$ and M receptors are also found presynaptically; recent data suggest that the main role of N$_1$ receptors in the CNS may be as a presynaptic neuromodulator.

It should be appreciated that AChE inhibitors increase the concentrations of ACh at all nicotinic and muscarinic receptor sites, and therefore produce a diverse array of effects. For example, when an AChE inhibitor is used to overcome reversible neuromuscular blockade (see Ch. 27) it increases ACh-mediated effects produced via the parasympathetic nervous system, such as on the gastrointestinal tract and heart. These unwanted effects of ACh can be blocked by co-administration of an antimuscarinic agent (see drug receptor table at the end of Ch. 1).

The distribution of key neurotransmitters and receptors of the somatic and autonomic nervous systems is summarised in Figure 4.7. Students should familiarise themselves with Figure 4.7 and with the possible sites of drug action (Tables 4.2 and 4.3). Such knowledge is fundamental to understanding both the principal mechanisms of action for many drugs and the source of unwanted effects for others.

OTHER TRANSMITTERS IN THE PERIPHERAL NERVOUS SYSTEM

In addition to ACh and noradrenaline, there are other transmitters with roles in neurotransmission and function in the peripheral nervous system. Many of these are also of considerable importance in the CNS. The different transmitters are dealt with in the chapters that describe their clinical importance, and include:

- amines, e.g. dopamine, histamine, serotonin,
- amino acids, e.g. glutamate, glycine, γ-aminobutyric acid (GABA), agmatine,
- peptides, e.g. opioids, substance P,
- purines, e.g. adenosine, ATP.

Nitric oxide, calcitonin gene-related peptide, vasoactive intestinal peptide (VIP), neuropeptide Y, ghrelin and others are described later in the book.

AMINES

Dopamine

Dopamine is an important neurotransmitter in both the CNS and the periphery, and subsequent chapters cover its actions (Chs 7, 21, 24 and 32).

Synthesis and storage of dopamine

Synthesis and storage of dopamine have been described above under noradrenaline.

Release of dopamine

Nerve stimulation causes release of dopamine present in vesicles (see noradrenaline). Dopaminergic neurons are not important in the clinical responses to indirectly acting sympathomimetics, although certain behavioural responses to amfetamines are linked to dopamine D$_2$ receptor activity. The antiviral drug amantadine, which is of some value in Parkinson's disease, causes release of dopamine (Ch. 24).

Removal of activity of released dopamine

Dopamine is removed by similar mechanisms to those described above for noradrenaline, with reuptake by the dopamine transporter (DAT) representing the major pathway.

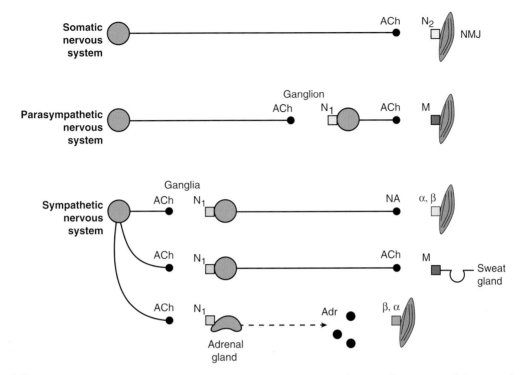

Fig. 4.7 Schematic diagram of the distribution of the main neurotransmitters and receptors of the somatic, parasympathetic and sympathetic nervous systems. α, β, adrenoceptors; ACh, acetylcholine; Adr, adrenaline; M, muscarinic receptor; N_1, N_2, nicotinic receptors; NA, noradrenaline; NMJ, neuromuscular junction.

Dopamine receptors

There are a number of types of dopamine receptors, and relatively selective therapeutic agents are available for some of these (see drug receptor table at the end of Ch. 1). Dopamine receptors are classified into those that increase cAMP (D_1 and D_5) and those that decrease cAMP (D_2, D_3 and D_4). The D_4 receptor shows polymorphic expression; subtypes D_2 and D_4 are associated with schizophrenia and relatively selective antagonists of each are valuable antipsychotic drugs and have some different biological properties (Ch. 21).

Serotonin (5-hydroxytryptamine)

Serotonin (or 5-HT; Fig. 4.8A) is a neurotransmitter in the CNS and periphery that has properties similar to the catecholamines.

Synthesis of serotonin

Serotonin is synthesised from the amino acid tryptophan by two reactions that are similar to those involved in the conversion of tyrosine to dopamine. The first reaction is oxidation of the benzene ring to form 5-hydroxytryptophan, catalysed by tryptophan hydroxylase, which is the rate-limiting step and only found in serotonin-producing cells. Conversion to serotonin is catalysed by aromatic L-amino acid decarboxylase (see noradrenaline synthesis).

Serotonin is present in the diet but undergoes essentially complete first-pass metabolism by MAO-A in the gut wall and liver. Serotonin is not synthesised by blood platelets, but they accumulate high concentrations of serotonin from the circulation which can be released when platelets aggregate and during migraine episodes.

Storage of serotonin

The major site of serotonin storage in the body (>90%) is the enterochromaffin cells of the gastrointestinal tract. Platelets accumulate serotonin and neurons utilizing serotonin are widely distributed in the brain. In presynaptic neurons serotonin is stored in vesicles as a complex with ATP, and there is an active uptake process which transfers cytoplasmic serotonin into the storage vesicle.

Release of serotonin

The release of serotonin vesicles is by Ca^{2+}-mediated exocytosis. A rise in intraluminal pressure in the gastrointestinal tract stimulates the release of serotonin from the chromaffin cells. Release of serotonin from chromaffin cells contributes to nausea following cancer chemotherapy with cytotoxic drugs by stimulation of the chemoreceptor trigger zone (Ch. 32) and of sensory receptors within the gastrointestinal tract. There is a significant release of platelet serotonin in migraine (Ch. 26).

Metabolism and removal of serotonin activity

The principal mechanism of inactivation of released serotonin is via its reuptake into the presynaptic nerve by the serotonin transporter (SERT), which shows a high affinity for serotonin and is distinct from the noradrenaline transporter (NET). Dual inhibitors of serotonin and noradrenaline

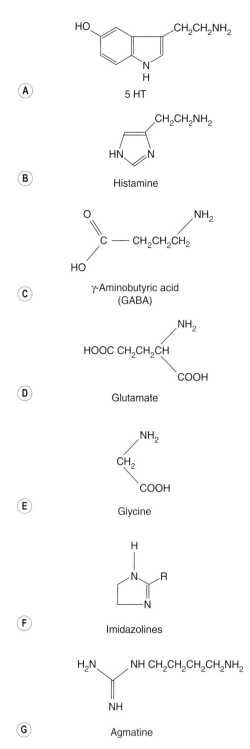

Fig. 4.8 Diverse structures of important amine and amino acid neurotransmitters.

reuptake (SNRIs) and selective serotonin reuptake inhibitors (SSRIs) are useful antidepressants (Ch. 22). Serotonin reuptake is also carried out by a low-affinity plasma membrane monoamine transporter (PMAT), which is insensitive to SSRIs.

Metabolism within the neuron is by MAO, which generates the excretory product 5-hydroxyindoleacetic acid (5-HIAA). There is a considerable turnover of serotonin in the chromaffin and nerve cells, and 5-HIAA is a normal constituent of human urine.

Serotonin receptors

There is a family of serotonin receptors, which has allowed the development of selective drugs (see drug receptor table at the end of Ch. 1). Thus far, the different serotonin receptors comprise 13 different G-protein-coupled 7TM receptors and one ligand-gated ion channel, which are divided into seven classes ($5\text{-}HT_1$ to $5\text{-}HT_7$) on the basis of their structural and functional characteristics. Not all of the subtypes of receptors have recognised physiological roles. Receptors in the $5\text{-}HT_1$ group are mostly presynaptic and inhibit adenylyl cyclase, whereas those in the $5\text{-}HT_2$ group are mostly postsynaptic in the periphery and activate phospholipase C. Identification of receptor subtype functions and selective inhibitors or stimulants has facilitated progress in the treatment of diseases including depression (Ch. 22) and migraine (Ch. 26).

Histamine

Histamine (Fig. 4.8B) is an important transmitter both in the CNS and in the periphery, as well as being an allergic mediator released from mast cells and basophils.

Synthesis of histamine

The amino acid histidine is decarboxylated to histamine by histidine decarboxylase. In addition to the synthesis and storage of histamine by mast cells and basophils there is continual synthesis, release and metabolic inactivation by growing tissues and in wound healing.

Storage of histamine

Most attention has focused on the storage of histamine in mediator-releasing cells such as mast cells and basophils (Ch. 12). In these cells it is present in granules associated with heparin. The presence of histidine decarboxylase and the synthesis of histamine in neurons in the CNS, although less well explored, appear to be associated mainly with the hypothalamus, from where projections run to many parts of the brain. Histamine plays a role in wakefulness, memory, appetite and many other functions.

Release of histamine

The release of histamine from mast cells and basophils has been studied extensively in relation to allergic reactions (Chs 12 and 39). In chromaffin cells in the gut and enterochromaffin-like (ECL) cells in the gastric mucosa, histamine is synthesised rapidly when required (Ch. 33). The release of histamine from neurons may be similar to the release of other amine neurotransmitters, but this has not been demonstrated unequivocally.

Removal of histamine activity

Histamine is rapidly inactivated by oxidation to imidazole acetic acid. Histamine is not a substrate for MAO and the oxidation is catalysed by diamine oxidase (or histaminase).

A second, minor route of metabolism is methylation by histamine-N-methyltransferase, and the product is then a substrate for MAO. Histamine is also eliminated as an N-acetyl conjugate.

Histamine receptors

There are four receptors for histamine (see drug receptor table at the end of Ch. 1). H_1 receptors have been studied extensively in relation to inflammation and allergy (Chs 12 and 39). Histamine-containing neurons are found in the brain, particularly in the brainstem, with pathways projecting into the cerebral cortex. H_1 receptors are probably important in these pathways, because sedation is a serious problem with H_1 receptor antagonists that are able to cross the blood–brain barrier (Ch. 2). The second generation of H_1 antihistamines produce less sedation. H_1 receptors are also involved in emesis (Ch. 32).

The discovery of H_2 receptors affecting the release of gastric acid led to the development of important H_2-selective antihistamines that reduce acid secretion and contribute to the treatment of dyspepsia and to ulcer healing (Ch. 33). H_2 receptors are also present in the brain and are probably responsible for the confusional state associated with the use of the H_2 receptor antagonist cimetidine. H_3 receptors are found in the CNS and other sites and H_4 receptors are localised mainly to leucocytes, but their functions are poorly understood.

AMINO ACIDS

Gamma-aminobutyric acid

GABA is an important inhibitory neurotransmitter responsible for about 40% of all inhibitory activity in the CNS (Fig. 4.8C).

Synthesis and storage of GABA

GABA is formed by the decarboxylation of glutamate by glutamate decarboxylase in GABAergic neurons. GABA is stored in membrane vesicles in the brain and in interneurons in the spinal cord (particularly laminae II and III).

Release of GABA

GABA is released by Ca^{2+}-mediated exocytosis. Co-transmitters such as glycine, metenkephalin and neuropeptide Y are stored in GABA vesicles and released with GABA.

Removal of GABA activity

Uptake by the GAT family of transporters is the principal mechanism for the removal of GABA from the synaptic cleft. The antiepileptic drug tiagabine may act as an inhibitor of GABA uptake by GAT-1 (Ch. 23).

GABA is metabolised by transamination with α-ketoglutarate, which forms the corresponding aldehyde (succinic semialdehyde) and amino acid (glutamic acid). The antiepileptic drug vigabatrin inhibits GABA transamination.

GABA receptors

There are two main types of GABA receptor, with different mechanisms of action (see drug receptor table at the end of Ch. 1). Stimulation of both receptors produces hyperpolarisation of the cell membrane, with $GABA_A$ causing rapid inhibition and $GABA_B$ producing a slower and more prolonged response. The $GABA_A$ receptor comprises a number of subunits. There are multiple forms of each subunit and numerous possible combinations (see Fig. 20.1); consequently, the $GABA_A$ receptor should be regarded as a family of receptors. Hyperpolarisation following $GABA_A$ receptor stimulation results from the opening of Cl^- channels and influx of Cl^-. $GABA_B$ receptors are G-protein-linked receptors that hyperpolarise the cell indirectly by closing Ca^{2+} channels and opening K^+ channels. A subtype of $GABA_A$ receptor ($GABA_A$-ρ) is found in the retina, where its significance remains unclear. Both $GABA_A$ and $GABA_B$ receptors are found presynaptically and inhibit neurotransmitter release by hyperpolarising the cell (by opening Cl^- or K^+ channels) and reducing release of the vesicles of the innervating cell (by closing Ca^{2+} channels). Many important drugs act by altering GABA breakdown or by enhancing GABA activity at its receptor (Chs 20 and 23).

Glutamate

Glutamate (Fig. 4.8D) is an important excitatory amino acid neurotransmitter with wide-reaching actions in physiological and pathological conditions. The functions of glutamate are described in later chapters. Aspartate (which is similar to glutamate but has only one CH_2 group) acts at the same receptors. Administration of glutamate or aspartate causes CNS excitation, tachycardia, nausea and headache, and convulsions at very high doses. Hyperactivity at glutamate receptors has been proposed as a factor in the generation of epilepsy (Ch. 23).

Synthesis and storage of glutamate

Glutamate (glutamic acid) is an amino acid that is found in most cells and is widely distributed within the CNS. Glutamate is stored in presynaptic vesicles in the neurons.

Release of glutamate

Exocytosis of vesicles is mediated via the influx of Ca^{2+} into the presynaptic nerve terminal, as occurs for other neurotransmitters. Some antiepileptic drugs, for example lamotrigine and valproate (Ch. 23), inhibit glutamate release.

Removal of glutamate activity

The action of glutamate in the synapse is terminated by excitatory amino acid transporters (EAATs), which take up glutamate (and aspartate) into the neuron and surrounding glial cells.

Glutamate receptors

There are two major types of glutamate receptor, the ionotropic family (AMPA (α-amino-3-hydroxy-5-methyl-4-isoxazole propionic acid)/kainate/NMDA (N-methyl-D-aspartate)) and the metabotropic family (metabotropic glutamate receptors, or mGluRs), which have a range of biological actions (see drug receptor table at the end of Ch. 1). The NMDA antagonist memantine is used in treating Alzheimer's disease (Ch. 9).

Glycine

Glycine (Fig. 4.8E) is a widely available amino acid that acts as an inhibitory neurotransmitter. It is released in response to nerve stimulation and acts in the spine, lower brainstem and retina.

Synthesis and storage of glycine

Glycine is present in all cells and is accumulated by neurons. It is stored within neurons in vesicles.

Release of glycine

Vesicle release accompanies an AP, as described above for other neurotransmitters. Tetanus toxin prevents glycine release, and the decrease in glycine-mediated inhibition results in reflex hyperexcitability.

Removal of glycine activity

Released glycine undergoes cellular uptake via the high-affinity transporters GLYT-1 and GLYT-2 in glial and neuronal cells.

Glycine receptors

Glycine receptors (GlyRs) are ligand-gated Cl⁻ channels similar in structure to GABA$_A$ channels: they are present mainly on interneurons in the spinal cord. Strychnine produces convulsions through the blockade of glycine receptors. Glycine is important for the activity of NMDA receptors (see drug receptor table at the end of Ch. 1).

Imidazoline receptor ligands

Studies of the centrally acting α_2-adrenoceptor agonists clonidine, moxonidine and rilmenidine showed their antihypertensive effects could be not be interpreted wholly by actions on the α_2-adrenoceptor. These imidazoline compounds (Fig. 4.8F) are thought to act at least partly at imidazoline (I)-binding sites, of which there are three main types. The I_1 receptor mediates the sympatho-inhibitory actions on blood pressure in the brainstem, the I_2 receptor is an allosteric binding site on monoamine oxidase and the I_3 receptor regulates insulin secretion from pancreatic β cells. The putative natural ligand for I receptors, agmatine (Fig. 4.8G), is a decarboxylated derivative of the amino acid arginine; it also binds to α_2-adrenoceptors and activates nitric oxide synthase, but its role in disease is unclear.

PEPTIDES

The importance of peptides as neurotransmitters has been appreciated in recent years, largely because of the development of highly specific and sensitive probes, combined with histochemical techniques, which has allowed their detection and measurement. Unlike other classes of neurotransmitter, peptides are synthesised in the cell body as precursors, which are transported down the axon to the site of storage. There are specific receptors for different peptides (see drug receptor table at the end of Ch. 1). An AP causes the release of the peptide from its precursor; inactivation is probably via hydrolysis by a local peptidase.

Peptide neurotransmitters are often found stored in the same nerve endings as other transmitters (described above) and undergo simultaneous release (co-transmission).

Peptides do not cross the blood–brain barrier readily. A major problem for exploiting our increasing knowledge of the importance of peptides is devising ways to deliver the novel products derived from molecular biology to the sites within the brain where they can have an effect.

Substance P is released from C-fibres (Ch. 19) by a Ca²⁺-linked mechanism and is an important neurotransmitter for sensory afferents in the dorsal horn. It is also present in the substantia nigra, associated with dopaminergic neurons, and may be involved in the control of movement.

Opioid peptides are a range of endogenous peptides that are the natural ligands for opioid receptors; opioid receptors were recognised in the brain and gastrointestinal tract for many years before the natural ligands were identified. These are discussed in Chapter 19.

A number of other peptides are detectable in the CNS particularly in the hypothalamus and/or pituitary gland (e.g. neurotensin, oxytocin, somatostatin, vasopressin; see Chs 43 and 45) or in the gastrointestinal tract (e.g. cholecystokinin and vasoactive intestinal peptide).

PURINES

Adenosine and guanosine are endogenous purines and exist in the body in the free form, attached to ribose or deoxyribose (as nucleosides), and as mono-, bi- or triphosphorylated nucleotides. Purines within cells are usually incorporated into nucleotides, which are involved in the energetics of biochemical processes (e.g. ATP), act as intracellular signals (e.g. cAMP and cGMP; see Ch. 1) and are involved in the synthesis of RNA and DNA. ATP is present in the presynaptic vesicles of some other neurotransmitters and is released along with the primary neurotransmitter, following which it may act on postsynaptic receptors (co-transmission). Extracellular ATP is rapidly hydrolysed via adenosine diphosphate (ADP) to adenosine. Adenosine itself is very rapidly metabolised and inactivated.

There is a family of purine receptors that show individual selectivity for different purines and give different responses (see drug receptor table at the end of Ch. 1). G-protein-coupled purinergic receptors (P2Y) are specific for the adenosine and uridine phosphates, and ADP causes platelet aggregation via P2Y$_{12}$-type receptors. This effect of ADP can be inhibited with clopidogrel and ticagrelor, which have important anti-aggregatory actions (Ch. 11). Ligand-gated P2X receptors for ATP are widely distributed in the brain. The adenosine receptors A$_1$–A$_3$, formerly called P1 receptors, show very high selectivity for adenosine itself. Adenosine is used therapeutically to terminate supraventricular tachycardia.

SELF-ASSESSMENT

True/false questions

1. The sympathetic division of the ANS utilises adrenaline as its primary transmitter substance.

2. The parasympathetic and sympathetic nervous systems have opposite effects in every organ.
3. Sympathetic nervous stimulation to the gut inhibits gut motility and sphincter tone.
4. Acetylcholine is metabolised by plasma cholinesterase in the synaptic cleft.
5. Dopamine and noradrenaline are synthesised from levodopa.
6. Dopamine is a transmitter in the peripheral autonomic nervous system.
7. Tyramine is metabolised by both isoenzymes of monoamine oxidase (MAO-A and MAO-B).
8. Both α_1- and α_2-adrenoceptor antagonists can be used to lower blood pressure.
9. Botulism is caused by poisoning with a bacterial toxin.
10. Botulinum toxin enhances acetylcholine release from all cholinergic neurons.
11. There are two subtypes of β-adrenoceptor.
12. Blockade of presynaptic adrenoceptors by propranolol increases noradrenaline release.
13. The actions of synaptic serotonin and noradrenaline are curtailed mainly by metabolism by MAO and COMT.
14. The synaptic uptake of noradrenaline and serotonin can be inhibited selectively.
15. The vagal cranial nerve to the eye decreases pupil size.
16. Blockade of H_1 histamine receptors reduces gastric acid secretion.
17. Glutamate and glycine are inhibitory amino acid transmitters.
18. Substance P is a transmitter in the dorsal horn of the spinal cord

One-best-answer (OBA) question

Which of the following is the *most accurate* statement about neurotransmission?

A. Neurotransmitters are synthesised in the presynaptic nerve terminal.
B. Neurotransmitters are taken up into the presynaptic neuron by passive diffusion.
C. Acetylcholine release is modified by receptors on the presynaptic membrane.
D. Each postganglionic sympathetic neuron releases a single neurotransmitter.
E. Fusion of vesicles with the presynaptic membrane is facilitated by K^+ influx triggered by the AP.

True/false answers

1. **False.** Noradrenaline is the main transmitter substance at the sympathetic postganglionic nerve endings. Adrenaline is released only from the adrenal medulla and acetylcholine is the transmitter only in sweat glands and hair follicles.
2. **False.** While the two autonomic systems have broadly opposing actions on many organs, other organs may be controlled by only one system (e.g. the lens of the eye).
3. **False.** Sympathetic nervous stimulation releases noradrenaline and inhibits motility but increases the tone of the sphincters.

4. **False.** Within the synaptic cleft acetylcholine is broken down rapidly by acetylcholinesterase.
5. **True.** Levodopa is converted into dopamine by DOPA decarboxylase and then to noradrenaline by dopamine-β-hydroxylase.
6. **True.** Dopamine is predominantly an important transmitter in the CNS but also in some peripheral sites, for example the renal vascular smooth muscle.
7. **True.** This is important, as selective inhibitors of MAO-A used in the treatment of depression leave MAO-B unaffected so this is available to metabolise tyramine in food, thereby avoiding the 'cheese reaction' (see Ch. 22).
8. **False.** Antagonism of α_1-adrenoceptors on peripheral resistance vessels causes relaxation and lowers blood pressure, but presynaptic α_2-adrenoceptors reduce noradrenaline release so blockade of these receptors would increase noradrenaline release and raise blood pressure.
9. **True.** Botulinum toxin from the anaerobic bacterium *Clostridium botulinum* can cause fatal poisoning.
10. **False.** Botulinum toxin inhibits acetylcholine release and causes skeletal muscle paralysis; it can be used locally where there is muscle spasm or excessive sweating.
11. **False.** A third type, the β_3-adrenoceptor, is found in adipocytes, the heart, colon, bladder and some other tissues, but is less widespread than the β_1- and β_2-adrenoceptors.
12. **True.** Propranolol is a non-selective antagonist of β-adrenoceptors, and the role of the presynaptic β_2-adrenoceptor is to increase noradrenaline release. (Noradrenaline release is decreased by presynaptic α_2-adrenoceptors.)
13. **False.** The actions of serotonin and noradrenaline are curtailed mainly by reuptake into the presynaptic neuron by their respective transporters, SERT and NET.
14. **True.** The SERT and NET uptake transporters can be inhibited by SSRIs and other selective antidepressant drugs.
15. **True.** Vagal (parasympathetic) stimulation causes miosis of the pupil and also accommodates the lens for near vision.
16. **False.** Gastric acid secretion is promoted by histamine released from enterochromaffin-like (ECL) cells acting at H_2 receptors, and is reduced by H_2 antihistamines such as ranitidine.
17. **False.** Glycine is an inhibitory transmitter but glutamate is excitatory.
18. **True.** Substance P in the dorsal horn is an important transmitter in sensory afferents.

OBA answer

Answer C is correct.

A. Incorrect. Peptides are synthesised in the cell body and transported to the postganglionic nerve ending.
B. Incorrect. Active transporters transfer neurotransmitters back into the presynaptic neuron.
C. **Correct.** On parasympathetic nerve endings, stimulation of presynaptic N_1 receptors increases acetylcholine release whereas stimulation of presynaptic M_2 receptors decreases acetylcholine release.

D. Incorrect. Co-transmission is common, such as noradrenaline and vasoactive intestinal polypeptide released from sympathetic nerve endings to the gut.

E. Incorrect. An influx of Ca^{2+} is associated with transmitter release.

FURTHER READING

Abrams P, Andersson K-E, Buccafusco J et al. (2006) Muscarinic receptors: their distribution and function in body systems, and the implications for treating overactive bladder. *Br J Pharmacol* 148, 565–578

Berger M, Gray J, Roth BL (2009) The expanded biology of serotonin. *Annu Rev Med* 60, 355–366

Bowery NG, Bettler B, Froestl W et al. (2002) International Union of Pharmacology. XXXIII. Mammalian gamma-aminobutyric acid (B) receptors: structure and function. *Pharmacol Rev* 54, 247–264

Burnstock G (2006) Purinergic signalling. *Br J Pharmacol* 147 (Suppl. 1), S172–S181

Dajas-Bailador F, Wonnacott S (2004) Nicotinic acetylcholine receptors and the regulation of neuronal signalling. *Trends Pharmacol Sci* 25, 317–324

Dani JA, Bertrand D (2007) Nicotinic acetylcholine receptors and nicotinic cholinergic mechanisms of the central nervous system. *Ann Rev Pharmacol Toxicol* 47, 699–729

Eglen RM, Choppin A, Dillon MP, Hegde S (1999) Muscarinic receptor ligands and their therapeutic potential. *Curr Opin Chem Biol* 3, 426–432

Filip M, Bader M (2009) Overview on 5-HT receptors and their role in physiology and pathology of the central nervous system. *Pharmacol Rep* 61, 761–777

Foster AC, Kemp JA (2006) Glutamate- and GABA-based CNS therapeutics. *Curr Opin Pharmacol* 6, 7–17

Frishman WH, Kotob F (1999) Alpha-adrenergic blocking drugs in clinical medicine. *J Clin Pharmacol* 39, 7–16

Gether U, Andersen PH, Larsson OM, Schousboe A (2006) Neurotransmitter transporters: molecular function of important drug targets. *Trends Pharmacol Sci* 27, 375–383

Grace AA, Gerfen CR, Aston-Jones G (1998) Catecholamines in the central nervous system. Overview. *Adv Pharmacol* 42, 655–670

Haas HL, Sergeeva OA, Selbach O (2008) Histamine in the nervous system. *Physiol Rev* 88, 1183–1241

Head GA, Mayorov DN (2006) Imidazoline receptors, novel agents and therapeutic potential. *Cardiovasc Hematol Agents Med Chem* 4, 17–32

Hieble JP (2000) Adrenoceptor subclassification: an approach to improved cardiovascular therapeutics. *Pharm Acta Helv* 74, 163–171

Insel PA (1996) Adrenoceptors – evolving concepts and clinical implications. *N Engl J Med* 334, 580–585

Kirstein SL, Insel PA (2004) Autonomic nervous system pharmacogenomics: a progress report. *Pharmacol Rev* 56, 31–52

Ogden KK, Traynelis SF (2011) New advances in NMDA receptor pharmacology. *Trends Pharmacol Sci* 32, 726–733

Olsen RW, Sieghart W (2008) $GABA_A$ receptors: subtypes provide diversity of function and pharmacology. *Neuropharmacology* 56, 141–148

Piascik MT, Perez DM (2001) Alpha-1 adrenergic receptors: new insights and directions. *J Pharmacol Exp Ther* 298, 403–410

Romanelli MN, Gualtieri F (2003) Cholinergic nicotinic receptors: competitive ligands, allosteric modulators, and their potential applications. *Med Res Rev* 23, 393–426

Salio C, Lossi L, Ferrini F, Merighi A (2006) Neuropeptides as synaptic transmitters. *Cell Tissue Res* 326, 583–598

Simons FE (2004) Advances in antihistamines. *N Engl J Med* 351, 2203–2217

Small KM, McGraw DW, Liggett SB (2003) Pharmacology and physiology of human adrenergic receptor polymorphisms. *Annu Rev Pharmacol Toxicol* 43, 381–411

Thurmond RL, Gelfand EW, Dunford PJ (2008) The role of histamine H_1 and H_4 receptors in allergic inflammation: the search for new antihistamines. *Nat Rev Drug Discov* 7, 41–53

Wallukat G (2002) The beta-adrenergic receptors. *Herz* 27, 683–690

Youdim MBH, Edmondson D, Tipton K (2006) The therapeutic potential of monoamine oxidase inhibitors. *Nat Rev Neurosci* 7, 295–309

2

The cardiovascular system

5 Ischaemic heart disease

• •

The heart receives about 5% of the cardiac output at rest via the coronary arteries, and extracts about 75% of the oxygen from the perfusing blood. When the metabolic demand from the myocardium becomes greater (for example with exercise) there is little increase in the percentage of oxygen extracted from the blood passing through the myocardium and coronary artery blood flow increases by up to three- to fourfold to supply the necessary oxygen. Myocardial perfusion occurs largely during diastole, when the muscle of the heart is relaxed and not compressing the intramyocardial vessels. Therefore, unlike for other organs, myocardial perfusion is reliant on the diastolic blood pressure.

Ischaemic heart disease most frequently arises as a result of restriction of blood flow to cardiac muscle by development of atheromatous plaques in the large epicardial coronary arteries (Fig. 5.1). Myocardial ischaemia can sometimes occur in the presence of structurally normal epicardial coronary arteries. In this situation it arises either from abnormal regulation of the microvascular circulation within the myocardium, or from intense vasoconstriction of an epicardial artery (coronary vasospasm).

Atheromatous plaques tend to form in areas of flow disturbance, such as bends in the vessels or near branching vessels. The major risk factors for atheromatous coronary artery disease (in common with atheroma in other parts of the vascular tree) are male sex, smoking, hypertension, hypercholesterolaemia and diabetes mellitus. The effects of these risk factors are additive, and when several are present coronary atheroma occurs more extensively and at a younger age.

Early atheromatous plaques enlarge by stretching the medial smooth muscle (remodelling) and do not narrow the lumen of the vessel until 40–50% of the cross-sectional area of the vessel is diseased. Even when luminal narrowing occurs, symptoms only arise when 75% of the cross-sectional area of the vessel lumen is occluded.

Although atheroma can diffusely involve a long segment of the vessel, plaques are often confined to a small segment of the coronary artery. Localised plaques frequently involve only part of the circumference of the arterial wall, leaving the rest free of significant disease and still able to respond to vasoconstrictor and vasodilator influences. At the site of an atheromatous plaque there is turbulent blood flow. The consequent changes in shear stress at the endothelial surface impair endothelial function and reduce local generation of vasodilator substances such as nitric oxide (see organic nitrates below). Therefore, diseased segments of an artery are particularly prone to vasospasm, which produces dynamic flow limitation superimposed on the fixed atheromatous narrowing. If the coronary artery disease is long-standing, then collateral vessels can develop around the atheromatous narrowing and improve perfusion distal to the diseased segment of the artery.

There are two morphological types of atheromatous plaque. Some have a lipid-rich core, with a substantial infiltration of inflammatory cells and a thin fibrous cap. Such plaques are relatively unstable ('vulnerable' plaques) and are more prone to plaque disruption by ulceration or rupture of the cap, leading to thrombus formation (see below). Other plaques have a fibrotic core, with a thick fibrous cap, and are more stable. The reasons why both stable and unstable plaques can coexist in the coronary circulation is not well understood.

Reversible myocardial ischaemia is the consequence of an imbalance between oxygen supply and oxygen demand in a part of the myocardium (Fig. 5.2) due to an inability to increase coronary blood flow sufficiently to meet the metabolic demands of the heart. Rupture of an atheromatous plaque is responsible for most acute ischaemic cardiac events (presenting as an acute coronary syndrome).

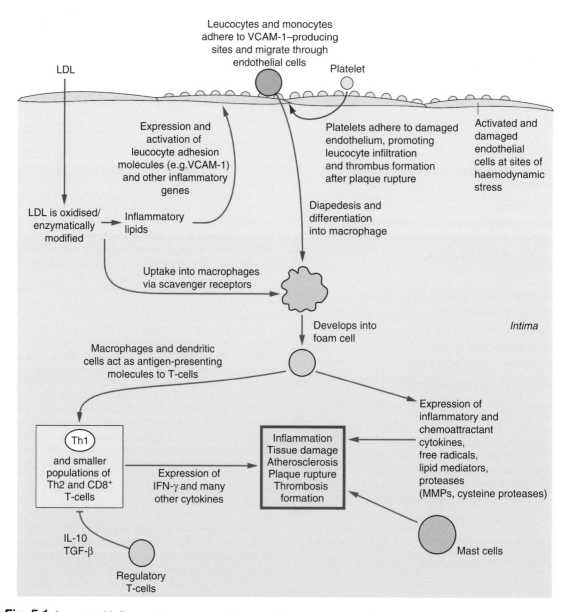

Fig. 5.1 **Aspects of inflammatory processes that contribute to coronary heart disease.** Multifactorial processes contribute to coronary heart disease; endothelium is damaged and activated; platelets adhere and promote leucocyte infiltration and thrombus formation; low-density lipoprotein (LDL) is oxidised and taken up via scavenger receptors into monocyte-macrophages, subsequently forming foam cells. Dysfunctional expression of a host of cytokines, lipid mediators, free radicals and proteases exacerbates inflammation, endothelial damage, atheroma formation, plaque rupture and thrombus formation. These processes are influenced by risk factors such as smoking, heredity, hypercholesterolaemia, hypertension, obesity, diabetes, age and gender. IFN-γ, interferon-γ; IL-10, interleukin-10; MMPs, matrix metalloproteases; TGF-β, tumour growth factor β; Th, T-helper cell; VCAM-1, vascular cell adhesion molecule 1.

CLINICAL MANIFESTATIONS OF MYOCARDIAL ISCHAEMIA

STABLE ANGINA

Angina pectoris is pain arising from heart muscle after it switches to anaerobic metabolism, and is a symptom of reversible myocardial ischaemia. Ischaemia occurs once the coronary artery lumen is narrowed sufficiently to restrict maximal blood flow to a level that cannot deliver adequate oxygen to meet the metabolic needs of the myocardium. Stable angina is relatively predictable ischaemic chest pain that is most frequently experienced as chest pain on exertion or with emotional stress and is rapidly relieved by rest. Reversible myocardial ischaemia can also present with shortness of breath (due to diastolic stiffening of the left

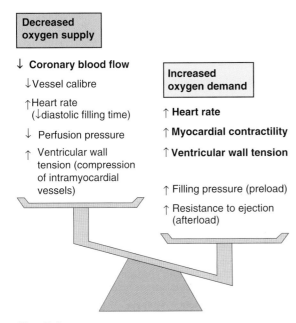

Decreased oxygen supply

↓ **Coronary blood flow**

↓Vessel calibre

↑Heart rate
(↓diastolic filling time)

↓ Perfusion pressure

↑ Ventricular wall tension (compression of intramyocardial vessels)

Increased oxygen demand

↑ **Heart rate**

↑ **Myocardial contractility**

↑ **Ventricular wall tension**

↑ Filling pressure (preload)

↑ Resistance to ejection (afterload)

***Fig. 5.2* Factors increasing myocardial oxygen demand and decreasing myocardial oxygen supply in angina.** Anti-anginal drugs act at many different sites to reduce oxygen demand and increase oxygen supply.

ventricle when a reduced cellular energy supply impairs the uptake of Ca^{2+} by the sarcoplasmic reticulum; see also heart failure with preserved ejection fraction, Ch. 7), or it can occur without symptoms (silent ischaemia). Vasospasm at the site of an atheromatous plaque accentuates the reduction in flow produced by a fixed atheromatous obstruction, and when it is present angina occurs at a lower workload.

People with stable angina have an increased risk of subsequent myocardial infarction or sudden cardiac death, due to rupture of an unstable atheromatous plaque (see below). On average the annual rate of such events is about 2%.

ACUTE CORONARY SYNDROMES (UNSTABLE ANGINA, MYOCARDIAL INFARCTION AND SUDDEN DEATH)

Acute coronary syndromes have a common pathophysiological origin, arising from disruption of an unstable atheromatous plaque (vulnerable plaque) in a coronary artery. Plaque disruption can be precipitated by sudden stresses on the cap produced by pulsatile blood flow across the plaque, by elastic recoil of the vessel in diastole or by vasospasm. As a consequence of these stresses the thin cap over the plaque fissures or ulcerates, leading to plaque rupture and exposure of the core of the plaque to circulating blood. Plaque rupture initiates platelet adhesion and then aggregation (Ch. 11), followed by thrombus formation and local vasospasm. These processes lead to a sudden reduction in blood flow. Platelet–thrombin microemboli can break off from the thrombus and become lodged in small distal vessels downstream from the thrombus, contributing to ischaemia.

Unstable angina

Unstable angina occurs if there is incomplete occlusion of the coronary artery following plaque rupture, but with critical reduction in blood flow so that oxygen supply is inadequate at rest or on minimal stress. Angina may then occur at rest or with very little exertion. Unstable angina is distinguished pathologically from other acute coronary syndromes because perfusion of the ischaemic tissue remains sufficient to prevent necrosis of myocytes. Unlike myocardial infarction, symptoms of unstable angina are usually relieved by glyceryl trinitrate (see below), or resolve spontaneously within 30 min.

Following an episode of unstable angina the thrombus may become incorporated into the plaque so that after healing the plaque is substantially larger, leading to greater long-term luminal narrowing.

Myocardial infarction and sudden cardiac death

Myocardial infarction most commonly arises from complete coronary artery occlusion following disruption of an unstable atheromatous plaque. Occlusion often occurs at the site of an atheromatous lesion that previously was only producing minor or moderate stenosis of the artery and may not have caused symptoms prior to disruption. Muscle necrosis begins when the occlusion lasts for longer than 20–30 min.

Myocardial infarction is usually associated with intense, prolonged chest pain and sympathetic nervous stimulation which increases cardiac work. However, about 15% of infarctions do not present with pain, and may go unrecognised (silent infarction). The diagnosis of acute myocardial infarction requires a rise in the plasma concentrations of sensitive biochemical markers, such as cardiac-specific myoglobin or troponin, which are released from necrotic myocytes. Cell death begins in the subendocardial muscle which is furthest from the epicardial blood supply (the endocardium receives its oxygen from the ventricular cavity), and, unless perfusion is restored, it progressively extends across the full thickness of the myocardium (transmurally) over the next few hours. Activation of endogenous fibrinolysis (Ch. 11) and the presence of a good collateral circulation are factors that favour reperfusion of the ischaemic area and naturally limit the size of the infarct. If very early reperfusion occurs the damage is usually confined to the subendocardial myocardium.

A full-thickness (or transmural) myocardial infarction often produces characteristic changes on the electrocardiograph (ECG), with early ST-segment elevation and eventually pathological Q waves. The resulting infarction is referred to as an ST-elevation myocardial infarction (STEMI). A subendocardial infarction often presents without diagnostic ECG changes. In these cases the ECG may show ST-segment depression or T-wave inversion (consistent with myocardial ischaemia), or even be normal. The resulting infarction is classified as a non-ST-elevation myocardial infarction (NSTEMI), because of the absence of the characteristic ST-segment changes usually found with more extensive myocardial damage.

Myocardial infarction principally affects left ventricular muscle, and the amount of muscle lost correlates well with both early and late survival. Infarction of the anterior muscle of the left ventricle (usually resulting from an occlusion in the left coronary artery system) causes greater myocardial loss than does inferior infarction of the ventricle (usually from right coronary artery occlusion). The amount of muscle loss also determines the extent of left ventricular remodelling (a geometrical change in the left ventricle that begins with healing of the infarct), which determines the risk of subsequent heart failure.

Sudden cardiac death results when fatal ventricular arrhythmias arise from ischaemic tissue, or from ventricular rupture.

DRUG TREATMENT OF ANGINA

Drug treatment for angina is directed either:

- to reduce oxygen demand by decreasing cardiac work, and/or
- to increase oxygen supply by improving coronary blood flow.

Drugs can be taken to relieve the ischaemia rapidly during an acute attack or as regular prophylaxis to reduce the risk of subsequent episodes. Several classes of drug are used to treat angina.

ORGANIC NITRATES

 xamples

glyceryl trinitrate, isosorbide mononitrate

Mechanism of action and effects

The organic nitrates are vasodilators that relax vascular smooth muscle by mimicking the effects of endogenous nitric oxide (NO). Enzymatic degradation of the nitrate releases NO, which combines with thiol groups in vascular endothelium to form nitrosothiols. Nitrosothiols activate guanylyl cyclase, which generates the second messenger cyclic guanosine monophosphate (cGMP; Fig. 5.3). cGMP activates protein kinase G, which reduces the availability of intracellular Ca^{2+} to the contractile mechanism of vascular smooth muscle, causing relaxation and vasodilation. Vasodilation is produced in three main vascular beds.

- **Venous capacitance vessels**, leading to peripheral pooling of blood and reduced venous return to the heart. This lowers left ventricular filling pressure (preload), decreases ventricular wall tension and therefore reduces myocardial oxygen demand. Venous dilation is produced at moderate plasma nitrate concentrations, and

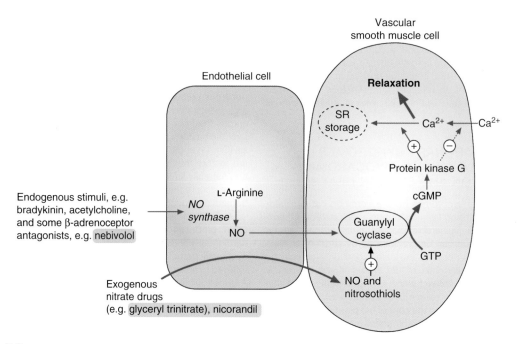

Fig. 5.3 **Actions of endogenous nitric oxide (NO) and exogenous nitrates.** Endogenous NO from endothelial cells relaxes vascular smooth muscle by activating guanylyl cyclase with subsequent formation of cGMP. This activates protein kinase G, which decreases Ca^{2+} influx into the cell, increases Ca^{2+} storage in the sarcoplasmic reticulum (SR) and increases myosin light-chain dephosphorylation. Exogenous agents such as organic nitrates and nicorandil react with tissue thiols, generating NO or nitrosothiols, which then activate guanylyl cyclase and increase cGMP.

tolerance to this action occurs rapidly during continued treatment.

- **Arterial resistance vessels**, leading to reduced resistance to left ventricular emptying (afterload). This lowers blood pressure, decreases cardiac work and contributes to a reduced myocardial oxygen demand. Arterial dilation occurs at higher plasma nitrate concentrations than venodilation, but tolerance arises less readily during long-term treatment.
- **Coronary arteries.** Nitrates have little effect on total coronary blood flow in angina; indeed, flow may be reduced because of a decrease in perfusion pressure. However, blood flow through collateral vessels may be improved, and nitrates also relieve coronary artery vasospasm. The net effect is increased blood supply to ischaemic areas of the myocardium. Coronary artery dilation occurs at low plasma nitrate concentrations, and tolerance is slow to develop.

Pharmacokinetics

Glyceryl trinitrate (GTN) is the most widely used organic nitrate. It is well absorbed from the gut but undergoes extensive first-pass metabolism in the liver to inactive metabolites. To increase its bioavailability, GTN is given by one of four routes that avoid first-pass metabolism.

- **Sublingual**: the tablet is placed under the tongue and is absorbed rapidly across the buccal mucosa. The very short half-life of GTN (less than 5 min) limits the duration of action to approximately 30 min. Tablets lose their potency with prolonged storage, and a metered-dose aerosol spray is a more stable delivery method.
- **Buccal**: a tablet containing GTN in an inert polymer matrix is held between the upper lip and gum, which permits slow release of drug to prolong the duration of action.
- **Transdermal**: GTN is absorbed well through the skin and can be delivered from an adhesive patch via a rate-limiting membrane or matrix. Steady release of the drug maintains a stable blood concentration for at least 24 h after application of the patch.
- **Intravenous**: the short duration of action of GTN is an advantage for intravenous dose titration.

Isosorbide 5-mononitrate is well absorbed from the gut and does not undergo first-pass metabolism. It has a half-life of 3–7 h so modified-release formulations are often used to prolong the duration of action.

Unwanted effects

- Venodilation can produce postural hypotension, dizziness, syncope and reflex tachycardia. Tachycardia can be reduced by concurrent use of a β-adrenoceptor antagonist.
- Arterial dilation causes throbbing headaches and flushing, but tolerance to these effects is common during treatment with long-acting nitrates.
- Tolerance to the therapeutic effects of nitrates develops rapidly if there is a sustained high plasma nitrate concentration. Tolerance is therefore a particular problem with delivery of GTN via transdermal patches or with long-acting nitrates. The cause is incompletely understood, but an important mechanism may be increased degradation of NO by oxygen free radicals (e.g. superoxides). There is limited evidence that co-administration of an angiotensin-converting enzyme (ACE) inhibitor, angiotensin receptor antagonist or hydralazine (Ch. 6) may reduce nitrate tolerance by impairing superoxide formation. Reflex activation of the sympathetic nervous system and the renin–angiotensin system in response to hypotension may also counteract the vasodilator actions of the nitrates. Tolerance can be avoided by a 'nitrate-low' period of several hours in each 24 h. This is preferable to a 'nitrate-free' period, which carries a risk of rebound angina. A nitrate-low period is achieved by asymmetric dosing with conventional formulations of isosorbide mononitrate (e.g. twice daily, at 8 a.m. and 1 p.m.) or by using a once-daily formulation that allows plasma nitrate concentrations to fall overnight. Transdermal GTN patches must be removed for part of each 24 h (e.g. overnight) to prevent tolerance.
- Drug interactions are most troublesome with phosphodiesterase inhibitors, such as sildenafil, used in the treatment of erectile dysfunction. These inhibit cGMP metabolism (Ch. 16) and co-administration can result in marked hypotension.

BETA-ADRENOCEPTOR ANTAGONISTS (β-BLOCKERS)

Examples

atenolol, bisoprolol, carvedilol, labetalol, metoprolol, nebivolol, propranolol

Mechanism of action and effects in angina

All β-adrenoceptor antagonists (often simply referred to as β-blockers) act as competitive antagonists of catecholamines at β-adrenoceptors. They achieve their therapeutic effect in angina by blockade of the cardiac β_1-adrenoceptor with reduced generation of intracellular cAMP. As a result they:

- decrease heart rate (by inhibition of the cardiac I_f pacemaker current in the sinoatrial node; see Ch. 8); this is most marked during exercise, when the rate of rise in heart rate is blunted,
- reduce the force of cardiac contraction (see Ch. 7),
- lower blood pressure by reducing cardiac output (a consequence of both the decreased heart rate and force of myocardial contraction).

The overall effect is to reduce myocardial oxygen demand. The slower heart rate also lengthens diastole and gives more time for coronary perfusion, which effectively improves myocardial oxygen supply.

Certain β-adrenoceptor antagonists have additional properties, which might reduce the incidence of unwanted effects or enhance their blood pressure-lowering actions (see below and also Chs 6 and 8), as follows.

- **Cardioselectivity.** Some β-adrenoceptor antagonists, for example atenolol, bisoprolol and metoprolol, are selective antagonists at the β$_1$-adrenoceptor. They are usually called cardioselective drugs since the most important site of action on β$_1$-adrenoceptors is the heart. Other β-adrenoceptor antagonists, for example propranolol, have equal or greater antagonist activity at β$_2$-adrenoceptors; these drugs are referred to as 'non-selective' β-adrenoceptor antagonists. The cardioselectivity of all β-adrenoceptor antagonists is dose-related, with progressively more β$_2$-adrenoceptor blockade at higher doses.
- **Partial agonist activity (PAA) or intrinsic sympathomimetic activity (ISA).** Certain β$_1$-adrenoceptor antagonists also act as partial agonists at either β$_1$- or β$_2$-adrenoceptors. For example, pindolol is a β$_1$-adrenoceptor antagonist that also has weak agonist activity at β$_2$-adrenoceptors, and as such it will produce vasodilation in some vascular beds (see Fig. 6.6). Drugs with PAA at the β$_1$-adrenoceptor have less inhibitory effect on heart rate and force of contraction and may be less effective than full antagonists in the treatment of severe angina, but their PAA means they are less likely to cause a resting bradycardia. Beta-adrenoceptor antagonists with PAA are not widely used.
- **Vasodilator activity.** Pure β$_1$-adrenoceptor antagonists do not cause vasodilation. Indeed, the reflex response to β$_1$-adrenoceptor blockade is vasoconstriction, mediated in part by the reflex sympathetic nervous system stimulation of α$_1$-adrenoceptors in response to the fall in cardiac output. However, some β-adrenoceptor antagonists have additional properties that produce arterial vasodilation. Mechanisms of vasodilation include β$_2$-adrenoceptor partial agonist activity (e.g. pindolol; see above), α$_1$-adrenoceptor blockade (e.g. carvedilol, labetalol) or an increase in endothelial NO synthesis (e.g. nebivolol) (see Fig. 6.6). Vasodilation does not have any proven advantage for the treatment of angina, but may be useful when β-adrenoceptor antagonists are given for the treatment of hypertension (Ch. 6).

Pharmacokinetics

Highly lipophilic β-adrenoceptor antagonists, such as propranolol and metoprolol, are well absorbed from the gut but undergo extensive first-pass metabolism in the liver, with considerable variability among individuals. Reduction in heart rate during exercise is closely related to the plasma concentration of the drug, so dose titration of lipophilic β-adrenoceptor antagonists is usually necessary to achieve an optimal clinical response. Most lipophilic β-adrenoceptor antagonists have short half-lives (see Compendium of drugs used to treat ischaemic heart disease at the end of this chapter), and are often available in modified-release formulations to prolong their duration of action.

Hydrophilic β-adrenoceptor antagonists, such as atenolol, are incompletely absorbed from the gut, and are eliminated unchanged in the urine. The dose range to maintain effective plasma concentrations is narrower than for those drugs that undergo metabolism. The half-lives of hydrophilic β-adrenoceptor antagonists are usually longer than those of lipophilic drugs (see Compendium at the end of this chapter).

Unwanted effects

- **Blockade of β$_1$-adrenoceptors.** A large dose of a β-adrenoceptor antagonist can precipitate acute pulmonary oedema if there is pre-existing poor left ventricular function, when high sympathetic nervous activity is necessary to maintain cardiac output. However, there is a paradox that when used at low doses with gradual-dose titration a β-adrenoceptor antagonist is part of the core therapy of heart failure (Ch. 7). A reduction in cardiac output can also impair blood supply to peripheral tissues, which can be detrimental in critical leg ischaemia (Ch. 10) or can provoke Raynaud's phenomenon (Ch. 10). Excessive bradycardia occasionally occurs, and β-adrenoceptor antagonists should be used with caution or avoided in the presence of advanced atrioventricular conduction defect (heart block). Drugs with partial agonist activity produce less bradycardia or reduction of cardiac output.
- **Blockade of β$_2$-adrenoceptors.**
  - *Bronchospasm* can be precipitated in people with asthma (including those with chronic obstructive pulmonary disease and some bronchodilator reversibility). People who are susceptible to this problem can experience bronchospasm even with cardioselective drugs.
  - *Hypoglycaemia* may be prolonged by non-selective β-adrenoceptor antagonists, which may be a problem in people with diabetes mellitus who are treated with insulin (Ch. 40). Gluconeogenesis, a component of the metabolic response to hypoglycaemia, is dependent upon β$_2$-adrenoceptor stimulation in the liver. Beta-adrenoceptor antagonists also blunt the autonomic response that alerts the person to the onset of hypoglycaemia.
- **Central nervous system effects.** These include sleep disturbance, vivid dreams and hallucinations, and are more common with lipophilic drugs, which readily cross the blood–brain barrier. Other consequences of CNS action include fatigue and subtle psychomotor effects, for example lack of concentration and sexual dysfunction.
- **Effects on blood lipid levels.** Most β-adrenoceptor antagonists raise the plasma concentration of triglycerides and lower the concentration of high-density lipoprotein (HDL) cholesterol (Ch. 48). These changes are modest but potentially atherogenic. They are most marked with non-selective β-adrenoceptor antagonists, and least if the drug has partial agonist activity.
- **Sudden withdrawal syndrome.** Upregulation of β-adrenoceptors (Ch. 1) during long-term treatment makes the heart more sensitive to catecholamines. Palpitation due to a greater awareness of the heart is common on withdrawal. Beta-adrenoceptor antagonists should be stopped gradually in people with ischaemic heart disease, to avoid precipitating unstable angina or myocardial infarction.
- **Drug interactions.** The calcium channel blocker verapamil and, to a lesser extent, diltiazem (see below) have potentially hazardous additive effects with β-adrenoceptor antagonists, since both reduce the force of cardiac contraction and slow heart rate.

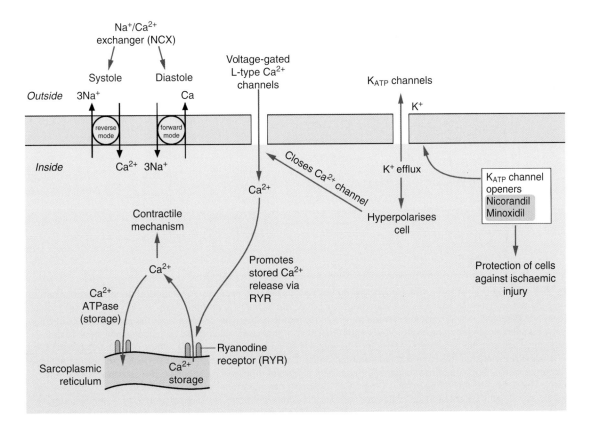

Fig. 5.4 **The control of calcium regulation and actions of potassium channel openers in cardiac myocytes and blood vessels.** Calcium concentrations in cardiac cells and in vascular smooth muscle are under the control of a number of different mechanisms. Calcium entry through voltage-gated L-type Ca^{2+} channels stimulates ryanodine receptors (RYR) in the sarcoplasmic reticulum, releasing stored Ca^{2+} (known as Ca^{2+}-induced calcium release, CICR). Intracellular Ca^{2+} is also regulated by exchange with Na^+ via the Na^+/Ca^{2+} exchangers (NCX) in the cell membrane. Vascular smooth muscle cells have ATP-sensitive inward rectifier K^+ channels (K_{IR}) which combine with sulfonylurea receptors to form ATP-sensitive K^+ channels (K_{ATP}). Hyperpolarisation of the cell by drugs which open K_{ATP} channels, such as nicorandil, closes voltage-gated L-type Ca^{2+} channels and causes relaxation.

CALCIUM CHANNEL BLOCKERS

Examples

dihydropyridines: amlodipine, nifedipine
non-dihydropyridines: diltiazem, verapamil

Mechanism of action and effects

Calcium is essential for excitation/contraction coupling in muscle cells. The following mechanisms of regulating intracellular free Ca^{2+} concentration are important pharmacologically (Figs 5.4 and 5.5).

■ Ca^{2+} can enter cells through transmembrane voltage-gated and ligand-gated channels in smooth muscle and cardiac muscle cells (Figs 5.4 and 5.5).
■ A rise in intracellular free Ca^{2+} promotes release of Ca^{2+} from the sarcoplasmic reticulum in striated and cardiac muscle cells through actions at ryanodine receptors (Figs 5.4 and 5.5).

■ Ligand-gated channels linked to G-protein-coupled receptors release Ca^{2+} from intracellular stores in the sarcoplasmic reticulum.
■ Ca^{2+} can exit cells in exchange for Na^+ via the Na^+/Ca^{2+} exchanger (Fig. 5.4).

Therefore, in striated muscle, free Ca^{2+} in the cytosol comes from the sarcoplasmic reticulum, while in smooth muscle it enters the cell through transmembrane Ca^{2+} channels. Cardiac muscle uses both mechanisms. There are at least five different types of transmembrane Ca^{2+} channel, two of which are found in cardiovascular tissues. These are listed here.

■ **Voltage-gated L-type Ca^{2+} channels** (long-acting, high-threshold-activated, slowly inactivated): these are important therapeutically and are found in the cell membranes of a large number of excitable cells, including cardiac and vascular smooth muscle. Ca^{2+} enters the cell through these channels when the cell membrane is depolarised. The cardiac and vascular L-type Ca^{2+} channels have different subunit structures.
■ **Voltage-gated T-type Ca^{2+} channels** (transient, low-threshold-activated, fast inactivated): these are found in

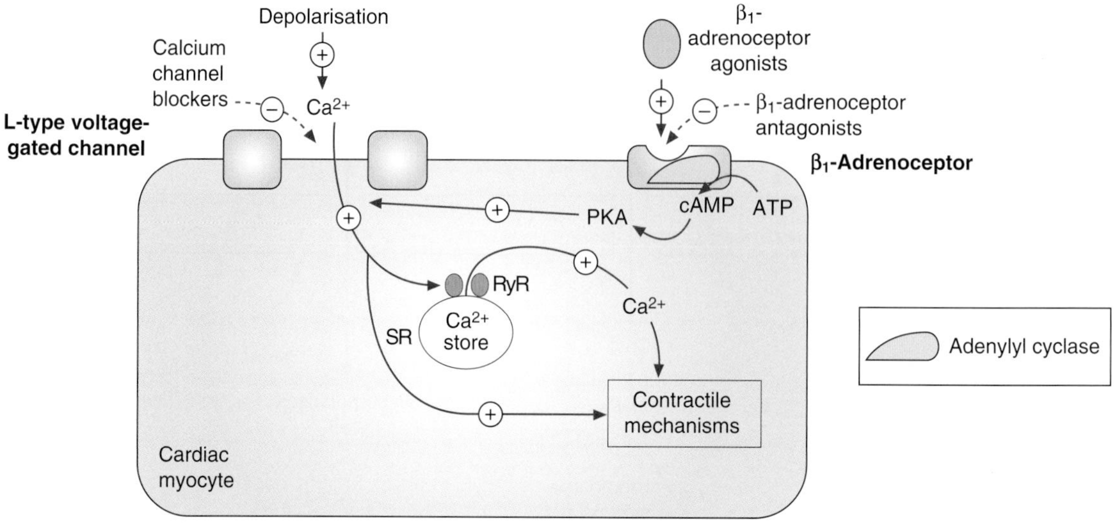

Fig. 5.5 **Contraction of the cardiac myocyte by voltage-gated and receptor-operated channels.** Depolarisation during the action potential activates the voltage-gated L-type Ca^{2+} channels and the influx of Ca^{2+} into the cell results in myosin phosphorylation and muscle contraction. It also promotes further Ca^{2+} release from the sarcoplasmic reticulum (SR) by stimulation of ryanodine receptors (RyR). Stimulation of the β_1-adrenoceptors by catecholamines activates adenylyl cyclase and the generated cAMP binds to subunits of protein kinase A (PKA), which phosphorylates the L-type Ca^{2+} channels, increasing their opening time and facilitating Ca^{2+} entry. The L-type Ca^{2+} channels can also be activated by other pathways, such as phospholipase C-dependent signalling triggered by agonism of α_1-adrenoceptors (not shown). The activity of the voltage-gated L-type Ca^{2+} channels can therefore be reduced directly by calcium channel blockers or indirectly by antagonists of β_1-adrenoceptors or other receptors. +, Stimulates activity; –, inhibits activity.

pacemaker cells of the sinoatrial and atrioventricular nodes, and are also present in vascular smooth muscle.

Calcium channel blockers (sometimes referred to inaccurately as calcium antagonists) have widely different chemical structures, but their common action is to reduce Ca^{2+} influx through voltage-gated L-type Ca^{2+} channels in smooth and cardiac muscle. None of the currently available calcium channel blockers affect T-type channels to any important extent, or influence ligand-gated Ca^{2+} channels (which are involved in neurotransmitter release and respond to endogenous agonists such as noradrenaline; Fig. 5.5).

There are clinically important differences among the calcium channel blockers, which bind to discrete receptors on the L-type Ca^{2+} channel. The receptor for verapamil is intracellular, while diltiazem and the dihydropyridines (e.g. nifedipine, amlodipine) have extracellular binding sites; however, the receptor domains for verapamil and diltiazem overlap. Verapamil and diltiazem exhibit frequency-dependent receptor binding and gain access to the Ca^{2+} channel when it is in the open state; in contrast, the dihydropyridines preferentially bind to the channel in its inactivated state. As more Ca^{2+} channels are in the inactive state in relaxed vascular smooth muscle than in cardiac muscle, dihydropyridines selectively bind to Ca^{2+} channels in vascular smooth muscle. These receptor binding characteristics account for the relative vascular selectivity of the dihydropyridines and for the anti-arrhythmic properties of verapamil and diltiazem (Ch. 8).

Calcium channel blockers produce a number of effects that are important in the treatment of angina.

- **Arteriolar dilation.** Although all calcium channel blockers are vasodilators, dihydropyridine derivatives such as nifedipine and amlodipine are the most potent and show the greatest vascular selectivity. Arterial dilation reduces peripheral resistance and lowers the blood pressure. This reduces the work of the left ventricle, and therefore reduces myocardial oxygen demand. Most dihydropyridines have a rapid onset of action and produce rapid vasodilation and reduction in blood pressure. This leads to reflex sympathetic nervous system activation and tachycardia (Fig. 5.6). Amlodipine or modified-release formulations of short-acting dihydropyridines are more slowly absorbed and gradually reduce blood pressure with little reflex tachycardia.
- **Coronary artery dilation.** Prevention or relief of coronary vasospasm improves myocardial blood flow.
- **Negative chronotropic effect.** Verapamil and diltiazem (but not the dihydropyridines) slow the rate of firing of the sinoatrial node and slow conduction of the electrical impulse through the atrioventricular node (see also Ch. 8). Thus, reflex tachycardia is not seen with these drugs and they also slow the rate of rise in heart rate during exercise.
- **Reduced cardiac contractility.** Most calcium channel blockers (but particularly verapamil) have some negative inotropic effect. Amlodipine does not impair myocardial contractility.

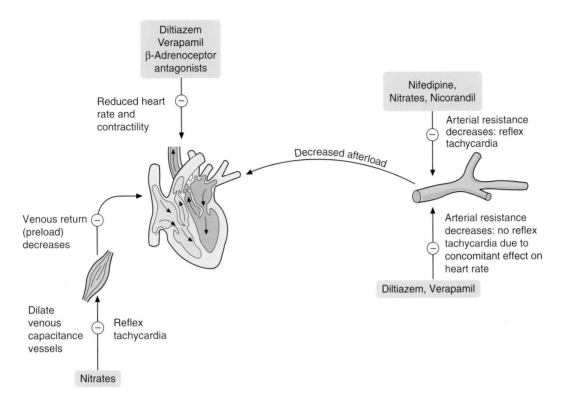

Fig. 5.6 **The major sites of action of anti-anginal drugs.** Reflex tachycardia results from the actions of dihydropyridine calcium channel blocker nifedipine and the potassium channel opener nicorandil. Nifedipine causes a rapid fall in blood pressure, triggering the reflex. This is not a problem with the non-dihydropyridines diltiazem and verapamil, which concomitantly slow the heart rate. Reflex tachycardia to nifedipine can be minimised with a modified-release formulation, or a more slowly acting dihydropyridine compound such as amlodipine can be used.

Pharmacokinetics

Most calcium channel blockers are lipophilic compounds with similar pharmacokinetic properties. They are almost completely absorbed from the gut lumen, and variable first-pass metabolism can limit bioavailability. Their half-lives are mostly in the range of 2 to 12 h, and modified-release formulations are widely used to prolong their duration of action. However, amlodipine is slowly absorbed and does not undergo first-pass metabolism. It has a high volume of distribution, due to extensive membrane partitioning in cells, and slower metabolism by the liver, which together result in a very long half-life of about 1–2 days. Verapamil can be given intravenously, a route that is usually reserved for the treatment of supraventricular arrhythmias (Ch. 8).

Unwanted effects

- Arterial dilation can produce headache, flushing and dizziness, although tolerance often occurs with continued use. Ankle oedema, which is frequently resistant to diuretics, probably arises from increased transcapillary hydrostatic pressure. Tolerance to oedema does not occur. All these unwanted effects are most common with the dihydropyridines.
- Reduced cardiac contractility can precipitate heart failure in people with pre-existing poor left ventricular

function, particularly with verapamil. Amlodipine does not depress cardiac contractility.
- Tachycardia and palpitations can arise with dihydropyridines, especially with rapid-release formulations.
- Bradycardia and heart block with verapamil and diltiazem.
- Altered gut motility: constipation is most common with verapamil, less so with diltiazem. Amlodipine and other dihydropyridines can cause nausea and heartburn.
- Gum hyperplasia.
- Drug interactions: verapamil and diltiazem can slow the heart rate excessively if they are used in combination with other drugs that have similar effects on atrioventricular nodal conduction; for example, digoxin (Ch. 8) or β-adrenoceptor antagonists. Metabolism of many calcium channel blockers can be inhibited or accelerated by drugs that affect the liver P450 cytochrome enzymes.

POTASSIUM CHANNEL OPENERS

nicorandil

Mechanism of action

There are many different K^+ channels in cell membranes (Ch. 8, Table 8.1). Of these, the ATP-inhibited K_{ATP} channels are the target for nicorandil (Fig. 5.4). K_{ATP} channels are found in many tissues, but have a variety of tissue-specific subunit configurations making targeted drug action on the channels possible. Nicorandil opens vascular smooth muscle K_{ATP} channels, so that K^+ leaves the cell and the efflux of positive ions hyperpolarises the cell. Hyperpolarisation means that the cell will be more difficult to depolarise and the membrane voltage-gated L-type Ca^{2+} channels are less likely to open (see calcium channel blockers, above). The consequence is that less Ca^{2+} is available to the muscle contractile mechanism, leading to vasodilation in systemic and coronary arteries (Fig. 5.4). Prevention of coronary vasospasm improves myocardial perfusion and blood pressure will fall, which reduces myocardial oxygen demand. In addition, enhanced K_{ATP} channel activity may protect myocardial cells against ischaemic injury.

Nicorandil also carries a nitrate moiety, and part of its vasodilator action is via generation of NO in vascular smooth muscle (see organic nitrates, above). This may account for the venodilation produced by the drug, which reduces venous return and further reduces myocardial oxygen demand.

Pharmacokinetics

Nicorandil is rapidly and almost completely absorbed from the gut. It is eliminated by hepatic metabolism and has a short half-life of 1 h. However, the tissue effects correlate poorly with the plasma concentration and the biological effect lasts up to 12 h.

Unwanted effects

- Arterial dilation causes headache in 25–50% of people, but tolerance usually occurs with continued use. Palpitation (caused by reflex activation of the sympathetic nervous system in response to a fall in blood pressure) and flushing are less common than headache.
- Dizziness.
- Nausea, vomiting.

SPECIFIC SINUS NODE INHIBITORS

ivabradine

Mechanism of action

In cardiac pacemaker cells (especially the sinoatrial node) the pacemaker I_f current is responsible for spontaneous depolarisation (Ch. 8). This is an inward current of positive ions through f-channels that carry both Na^+ and K^+, that are activated by the negative intracellular potential in diastole or by cyclic nucleotides. Ivabradine is a specific inhibitor of the I_f current, and its major effect is to slow sinus heart rate. The degree of channel inhibition is use-dependent, since ivabradine binds to the open channel from the internal side of the cell membrane. As a result, the efficacy of ivabradine increases with the frequency of channel opening and is greatest at higher heart rates. Unlike β-adrenoceptor antagonists, ivabradine has no effect on myocardial contractility.

Pharmacokinetics

Ivabradine is well absorbed from the gut and undergoes extensive first-pass metabolism in the gut wall and liver to an active metabolite. It has a half-life of 2 h.

Unwanted effects

- Bradycardia, first-degree heart block. It is recommended that the resting heart rate should not be allowed to fall below 50 beats/min.
- Ventricular ectopics.
- Headache, dizziness.
- Dose-related ocular symptoms, including phosphenes (flashes of light), stroboscopic effects and blurred vision from inhibition of the I_f in the eye.

LATE SODIUM CURRENT INHIBITORS

Example

ranolazine

Mechanism of action

Transmembrane Na^+ channels are activated during the initial electrical excitation of myocardial cells, and are mainly inactivated during the plateau phase of the action potential. However, a small proportion of the Na^+ channels remain open, giving rise to the late Na^+ current. In hypoxic tissues this current is increased and the consequent rise in intracellular Na^+ concentration activates the reverse mode of the Na^+/Ca^{2+} exchanger in the cell membrane, leading to removal of Na^+ from the cell, intracellular Ca^{2+} accumulation and increased diastolic myocardial tension (Fig. 5.4). Ranolazine attenuates the late transcellular Na^+ current in ischaemic myocardial cells, and reduces Ca^{2+} accumulation. There are two potentially beneficial consequences of this effect: the lower wall tension in the ventricles should reduce myocardial oxygen demand, and it will also reduce compression of small intramyocardial coronary vessels, thus improving myocardial perfusion.

Pharmacokinetics

Ranolazine is partially absorbed from the gut and extensively metabolised in the liver. It has a short elimination half-life of about 2 h and a modified-release formulation is used.

Unwanted effects

- Nausea, dyspepsia, constipation.
- Headache, dizziness, lethargy.
- Prolongation of the QT interval on the ECG (Ch. 8), with the potential to provoke cardiac arrhythmias if used with other drugs that have the same effect.

MANAGEMENT OF STABLE ANGINA

The principal aims of treatment for stable angina are to relieve symptoms and to improve prognosis. Angina has a pronounced circadian rhythm and occurs most frequently in the hours after waking, so a drug given for prevention of symptoms should ideally be effective at this time. There is no evidence that control of symptoms will affect either survival or the risk of a subsequent myocardial infarction. Improvement in prognosis is achieved mainly by using drugs that do not directly affect symptoms.

There are several important principles of management.

- Lifestyle changes: stopping smoking reduces the progression of coronary atheroma. It also reduces coronary vasospasm, and may improve symptoms, but importantly reduces the risk of developing an acute coronary syndrome by up to 50%. Symptoms may be improved by weight loss in people who are obese by reducing cardiac work. Regular exercise will improve fitness and attenuate the rise in heart rate on exercise, which will increase exercise duration before the onset of angina.
- Reduction of high blood pressure and control of diabetes will reduce progression of atheroma.
- Treatment of provoking or exacerbating factors for angina, such as anaemia, arrhythmias or thyrotoxicosis.
- Sublingual GTN remains the treatment of choice for an acute anginal attack. It relieves symptoms within minutes, but gives only short-lived protection (20–30 min). GTN can also be taken before an activity that is likely to produce angina.
- If anginal attacks are frequent, a prophylactic antianginal drug should be used. A rise in heart rate is one of the main precipitating factors for angina, and a drug that lowers heart rate, such as a β-adrenoceptor antagonist or a rate-limiting calcium channel blocker like verapamil or diltiazem, is first-line treatment. Ivabradine can be used if other heart-rate limiting drugs are not tolerated. Nitrates are less suitable as first-line prophylactic agents because of the risk of tolerance. If symptoms are not controlled by optimal doses of a single drug then a combination of a β-adrenoceptor antagonist with a calcium channel blocker (not verapamil) can be used. Alternatively, a β-adrenoceptor antagonist or calcium channel blocker can be combined with a long-acting nitrate. If two drugs do not control symptoms, then coronary angiography should be considered with a view to revascularisation. 'Triple therapy' (e.g. β-adrenoceptor antagonist, calcium channel blocker and a long-acting nitrate) has not been shown convincingly to be better than two agents, but such combinations may give further symptomatic benefit if coronary revascularisation is not being considered or while awaiting coronary angiography. Nicorandil is generally used in combination therapy. Ranolazine may be helpful when symptomatic hypotension precludes the use of other drugs.
- Low-dose aspirin reduces the risk of subsequent myocardial infarction by about 35%. Clopidogrel is an alternative if aspirin is not tolerated, but the combination has not been shown to have any additive benefit in stable coronary artery disease (see Ch. 11).
- Lowering the total plasma cholesterol to <4.0 mmol·L^{-1} by diet and a statin (Ch. 48) reduces the risk of subsequent non-fatal myocardial infarction, cardiac death and the need for a coronary artery revascularisation procedure by more than 30%.
- ACE inhibitors (Ch. 6) have no anti-anginal action, but reduce the risk of subsequent myocardial infarction and death by about 15%, especially in people at high risk of an event.
- Percutaneous coronary intervention (PCI) consists of angioplasty and usually insertion of a stent to maintain vessel patency. PCI improves symptoms, but only reduces cardiovascular death or myocardial infarction if there is a large area of ischaemic myocardium. Insertion of a coronary artery stent is followed by combination antiplatelet therapy with aspirin and clopidogrel (Ch. 11) for up to a year to minimise stent thrombosis which carries a high risk of myocardial infarction or death. Short-term use of a glycoprotein IIb/IIIa antagonist such as abciximab (Ch. 11) at the time of angioplasty further improves outcome for high-risk procedures. Re-stenosis after angioplasty is due to intimal hyperplasia and smooth muscle proliferation encroaching on the lumen of the vessel, and usually occurs within 6 months of the procedure. Angioplasty alone is followed by a re-stenosis rate of about 40% at 6 months, which can be reduced to about 20% by the use of a bare-metal stent. The most recent development is drug-eluting stents, which are coated with a polymer matrix containing an antiproliferative drug such as sirolimus or tacrolimus (Ch. 38). Drug-eluting stents reduce the risk of re-stenosis at 6 months to about 6%.
- Coronary artery bypass grafting (CABG) improves long-term prognosis compared with medical treatment in people with a left mainstem coronary artery stenosis, and in those with 'triple vessel disease' (significant stenoses of the left anterior descending, left circumflex and right coronary arteries) who have impaired left ventricular function. In less severe disease it is used for symptom relief.

Symptoms, and their response to treatment, are a poor guide to the severity of coronary artery disease, and quantifying the amount of ischaemic myocardium with non-invasive myocardial perfusion imaging is a more accurate predictor. A large area of ischaemic myocardium, or failure to respond to two prophylactic drugs in adequate dosages, should lead to consideration of coronary angiography, with a view to CABG or PCI.

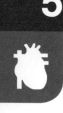

MANAGEMENT OF ACUTE CORONARY SYNDROMES

MANAGEMENT OF ACUTE CORONARY SYNDROMES WITHOUT ST-SEGMENT ELEVATION

Acute coronary syndromes require urgent treatment even if there is no ECG evidence of myocardial infarction at presentation. Unstable angina, if left untreated, progresses in about 10% of cases to myocardial infarction or death. The management of an acute coronary syndrome is initially determined by the ECG. In the absence of ST-segment elevation on the ECG, management is based on the assumption that a myocardial infarction has occurred until a sensitive marker of myocardial damage such as plasma troponin I or T is obtained about 10–12 h after the onset of pain. A rise in one of these markers will differentiate NSTEMI from unstable angina. If there is no evidence of myocardial damage and the ECG does not show ischaemic changes, then the risk of subsequent myocardial infarction or sudden death is low and treatment can then be less intensive.

- Initial treatment is with sublingual or intravenous GTN which may reduce pain by relief of coronary artery vasospasm at the site of the arterial occlusion and increase coronary blood flow. Analgesia with an intravenous opioid such as morphine (Ch. 19), together with an antiemetic, is used for pain that does not settle with a nitrate. Intramuscular injection of morphine should be avoided, since a low cardiac output and poor tissue perfusion often delay absorption. Supplementary oxygen may be required if the arterial oxygen saturation is below 94% with the aim of maintaining it between 94 and 98%, unless there is a risk of type 2 respiratory failure. Oxygen should be avoided if there is no hypoxaemia since it may increase myocardial damage.
- A loading dose of aspirin and clopidogrel (Ch. 11) should be given. If myocardial infarction is confirmed, then dual platelet inhibition with clopidogrel and low-dose aspirin is continued for up to 1 year. This reduces the risk of subsequent myocardial infarction by a further 20% compared to aspirin alone. After a year, the clopidogrel is stopped, but aspirin is continued indefinitely. Low-dose aspirin is used alone after an episode of unstable angina, when dual therapy has no advantage.
- Full anticoagulation with fondaparinux (Ch. 11) is initially used together with dual antiplatelet therapy. Fondaparinux has largely replaced low-molecular-weight heparin (which carries a higher risk of bleeding) unless coronary angiography is planned within 24 h of admission. The risk of further myocardial infarction or death within 14 days is reduced by about 60% using combined treatment with antiplatelet therapy and an anticoagulant. If PCI is carried out the direct thrombin inhibitor bivalirudin (Ch. 11) is used in combination with clopidogrel and aspirin to reduce the risk of ischaemic events during and after the procedure. Heparin combined with a glycoprotein IIb/IIIa antagonist such as tirofiban (Ch. 11) can be used instead of bivalirudin, but there is a higher risk of bleeding.

- A β-adrenoceptor antagonist is the first-choice anti-anginal treatment, and can reduce subsequent ischaemic events after presentation with unstable angina. A heart rate-limiting calcium channel blocker, such as verapamil or diltiazem, can be used if a β-adrenoceptor antagonist is contraindicated or not tolerated. If further treatment is needed, then a dihydropyridine calcium channel blocker such as nifedipine, or nicorandil or a nitrate via a buccal tablet or by intravenous infusion can be used with a β-adrenoceptor antagonist. Apart from β-adrenoceptor antagonists, anti-anginal drugs do not improve prognosis in unstable angina.
- In the acute phase of an acute coronary syndrome, angiography (followed when appropriate by CABG or PCI) is carried out for the 10% of people whose pain is refractory to full medical treatment. If the symptoms settle, those who had evidence of myocardial damage during the acute episode (an increase in the plasma concentration of troponin I or troponin T), and therefore had an NSTEMI, or those who have ongoing evidence of reversible myocardial ischaemia, should also be investigated by angiography.

MANAGEMENT OF ST-SEGMENT ELEVATION MYOCARDIAL INFARCTION

The presence of ST-segment elevation on the ECG usually heralds a more extensive myocardial infarction (STEMI) and, in contrast to NSTEMI, assisted early opening of the occluded artery to reperfuse the myocardium limits the extent of myocardial damage and improves long-term outcomes. Reperfusion should be considered if there is characteristic ST-segment elevation in two or more contiguous leads or left bundle branch block on the ECG and a good history of acute myocardial infarction. In the latter situation, an acute myocardial infarction cannot be easily diagnosed from the ECG but mortality is high. The greatest reduction in mortality is achieved in people at highest risk of death (i.e. anterior infarcts rather than inferior), older people (>65 years of age) and those with a presenting systolic blood pressure below 100 mmHg. Reperfusion therapy significantly reduces mortality if given within 12 h of the onset of pain, but the survival advantage is greater the earlier treatment is given.

- Analgesia and oxygen may be given as described above for unstable angina/NSTEMI. An intravenous β-adrenoceptor antagonist can be given to reduce cardiac work, especially if there is hypertension, but should be avoided if there are signs of heart failure.
- 'Primary' PCI (coronary angioplasty, usually with insertion of a stent) is the treatment of choice for reperfusion in STEMI if it can be started within 120 min of presentation. There is a greater reduction in mortality than using thrombolytic therapy. 'Rescue' PCI can be considered if thrombolysis has failed to reperfuse the infarct-related vessel. Anticoagulation with bivalirudin or a combination of heparin and a glycoprotein IIb/IIIa antiplatelet drug (Ch. 11) is essential at the time of primary PCI, in addition to dual oral antiplatelet therapy. A combination of aspirin with an oral ADP receptor antagonist (either prasugrel, ticagrelor or clopidogrel; see Ch. 11) is continued for at least 12

Box 5.1 Complications after myocardial infarction

Heart failure
Cardiogenic shock
Cardiac rupture
    Free wall rupture
    Ventricular septal defect
Arrhythmias
    Ventricular fibrillation
    Ventricular tachycardia
    Supraventricular tachycardias
    Sinus bradycardia and heart block
Pericarditis
Intracardiac thrombus

months after primary PCI, especially if a drug-eluting stent has been inserted.

- Natural fibrinolysis can be enhanced by intravenous fibrinolytic therapy (Ch. 11) to rapidly reperfuse the occluded artery and limit the size of the infarct. Treatment with thrombolytic therapy is now limited mainly to people who cannot be rapidly transferred to a centre that carries out primary PCI. The preferred agents are alteplase (recombinant tissue plasminogen activator, rt-PA) or a synthetic rt-PA analogue such as tenecteplase. Alteplase and related compounds are relatively short-acting, and subsequent anticoagulation reduces reocclusion of the artery. Fondaparinux (Ch. 11) for 8 days after thrombolysis reduces mortality and reinfarction by up to 25% more than heparin. Streptokinase is rarely used now, since it has a lower success rate for opening occluded arteries and produces symptomatic hypotension during about 10% of administrations.

In addition to the management discussed above, complications of myocardial infarction may need specific treatment (Box 5.1).

SECONDARY PROPHYLAXIS AFTER MYOCARDIAL INFARCTION

Secondary prophylaxis to reduce late mortality after myocardial infarction requires a broad-based approach. These interventions are additive and not mutually exclusive.

- Stopping smoking is of major benefit, and reduces mortality after a myocardial infarction by up to 50%.
- Rehabilitation programmes which include exercise reduce mortality by up to 25% and improve psychological recovery.
- Low-dose aspirin combined with clopidogrel (Ch. 11) inhibit platelet aggregation and reduce mortality in the first few weeks when started within 24 h of the onset of pain. Overall mortality is reduced by at least 25%. The combination is effective following both STEMI and NSTEMI.
- Beta-adrenoceptor antagonists, started orally soon after the infarct, reduce both death and reinfarction by about 25%. The mechanism is unknown. Greatest benefit is seen in those at highest risk, for example following anterior infarction and in those who have had serious post-infarct arrhythmias, post-infarct angina or heart failure.

Heart failure should be controlled before a β-adrenoceptor antagonist is given (Ch. 7).

- An ACE inhibitor (Ch. 6) is of greatest benefit if there is clinical or radiological evidence of heart failure after myocardial infarction, with a reduction in mortality of about 25% over the subsequent year. There is a smaller survival advantage if there is significant left ventricular dysfunction after the infarction (an ejection fraction of 40% or less) without clinical evidence of heart failure, with a 20% reduction in mortality over 3–5 years. This is accompanied by a significant reduction in non-fatal reinfarction, the mechanism of which is unknown. ACE inhibitors also reduce both non-fatal reinfarction and death when there is well-preserved left ventricular function, although the absolute benefits are smaller. The effects of an ACE inhibitor are greatest with high doses. An angiotensin receptor antagonist (Ch. 6) has similar efficacy following myocardial infarction, and should be considered if an ACE inhibitor is poorly tolerated.
- Verapamil and diltiazem produce a small reduction in reinfarction, but do not reduce mortality. They may be detrimental if there have been symptoms or signs of heart failure. These drugs should be considered as an option only for those at high risk who cannot tolerate a β-adrenoceptor antagonist and who do not have significant left ventricular dysfunction. Dihydropyridine calcium channel blockers have no effect on prognosis after myocardial infarction.
- Long-term anticoagulation with warfarin (Ch. 11) reduces mortality and reinfarction to a similar extent to low-dose aspirin. In combination with aspirin, warfarin produces an additional reduction in both fatal and non-fatal events but with an increased risk of bleeding.
- Plasma cholesterol should be reduced to <4.0 mmol·L^{-1} by diet and a statin (Ch. 48). Statins reduce reinfarction and cardiac death by 25–30%. Fibrates are less effective, but may be useful if the total cholesterol is not greatly raised but the high-density lipoprotein cholesterol is low.
- A Mediterranean diet reduces mortality after myocardial infarction. A further reduction in mortality can be achieved with supplementary omega-3 fatty acids. An anti-arrhythmic effect may be responsible for these benefits (Ch. 48).

SELF-ASSESSMENT

True/false questions

1. The increased oxygen demand produced by a rise in cardiac workload is met by an increase in coronary blood flow.
2. Nitric oxide (NO) causes vasodilation by increasing cAMP in vascular smooth muscle cells.
3. In angina, glyceryl trinitrate (GTN) increases total coronary blood flow.
4. Topical absorption of GTN from a transdermal patch avoids first-pass metabolism.
5. GTN can be taken safely with a β-adrenoceptor antagonist.

6. All β-adrenoceptor antagonists have vasodilator activity.
7. Resting bradycardia is less likely with a β-adrenoceptor antagonist with intrinsic sympathomimetic activity.
8. The anti-anginal action of amlodipine arises from its negative chronotropic and inotropic effects on the heart.
9. Enhancing the efflux of K^+ ions hyperpolarises vascular smooth muscle cells.
10. Ivabradine slows the heart rate and reduces myocardial contractility.
11. Percutaneous coronary intervention (PCI) reduces mortality after a ST-elevation myocardial infarction (STEMI) more than thrombolytic therapy.
12. Drug-eluting stents reduce the risk of re-stenosis after angioplasty.

One-best-answer (OBA) questions

1. Which statement about angina and myocardial infarction is *incorrect*?
   A. Isosorbide mononitrate does not undergo first-pass metabolism.
   B. Verapamil can reduce arterial blood pressure without causing reflex tachycardia.
   C. Antiplatelet drugs such as tirofiban can reduce the risk of myocardial infarction in high-risk individuals with unstable angina.
   D. Cholesterol reduction is of little benefit in reducing the risk of recurrence of myocardial infarction.
   E. Nifedipine does not improve prognosis after myocardial infarction.
2. Which change to the treatment regimen would is *most likely* to reduce the risk of tolerance developing to isosorbide mononitrate?
   A. Switch to its longer-acting precursor, isosorbide dinitrate.
   B. Give GTN in addition by the buccal route when necessary.
   C. Switch to a continuously applied transdermal GTN patch.
   D. Schedule doses so that there is a period of low plasma concentration of isosorbide mononitrate each day.
   E. Administer isosorbide mononitrate together with a β-adrenoceptor antagonist
3. Which drug combination is *most likely* to have an adverse effect on cardiac function in a person suffering from angina?

   A. GTN with atenolol
   B. Verapamil with atenolol
   C. Amlodipine with atenolol
   D. GTN with nicorandil
   E. GTN with low-dose aspirin

Case-based questions

Mr TK, a 65-year-old man who works as a landscape gardener, has been having episodes of chest pain that he likened to indigestion. They were brought on by moderately strenuous exercise and relieved by rest but not by antacids.

The symptoms had been present for approximately 1 year, but recently the frequency and intensity of the pains had become worse and were now occurring several times a week. He is hypertensive and his serum cholesterol is 6.6 mmol·L^{-1}. He smokes 40 cigarettes per day and is overweight. He drinks about 10 units of alcohol a week. He had a good exercise tolerance during a diagnostic exercise test but his ECG showed anterolateral ST-segment depression at peak exercise. There is no evidence of heart failure. A diagnosis of angina is made, and medical treatment started.

Six months later, despite continuing medication, Mr TK awoke with severe chest pains and dyspnoea that was not relieved by GTN. An ECG showed an acute STEMI.

A. How could his acute attacks of angina be treated?
B. The frequency of his attacks requires prophylactic treatment. What options are available to reduce the frequency of anginal attacks?
C. What other drugs could be useful to improve his prognosis?
D. Would lifestyle changes help Mr TK?
E. In unstable angina, which drug treatments would be likely to reduce the progression of the episodes to myocardial infarction or sudden death?
F. What is the likely cause of the myocardial infarction?
G. Why is it important to give fibrinolytic therapy as quickly as possible?
H. Mr TK is given the fibrinolytic agent altepase (recombinant tissue plasminogen activator, rt-PA) because of fears that he would get an allergic response to streptokinase. Is this justified?
I. He is given 150 mg aspirin orally, after an initial loading dose. Would this have any added benefit if fibrinolytic therapy is also given?
J. The normal therapeutic dose of aspirin for headache is about 650 mg. Why is the dose given to Mr TK so small?
K. Consideration is given to giving fondaparinux to Mr TK, but this is considered unnecessary because he had been given rt-PA. Is this decision correct?
L. Following his myocardial infarction, long-term prophylactic treatment of his condition was considered. Which of the following drugs would have been likely to be of benefit: an ACE inhibitor, low-dose aspirin, a β-adrenoceptor antagonist, diltiazem, verapamil or warfarin?

True/false answers

1. **True.** Increased coronary blood flow meets the increased myocardial oxygen demand, as the proportion of oxygen removed from the coronary artery blood is high (75%) even at rest.
2. **False.** Nitric oxide vasodilates by increasing synthesis of cGMP, which reduces intracellular Ca^{2+}. Organic nitrates act by the same pathway.
3. **False.** Although GTN can reduce coronary vasospasm or dilate collateral blood vessels, it does not increase total coronary blood flow. Its main actions are peripheral venodilation, which reduces venous return (preload), and reduced peripheral resistance (afterload), both of which reduce cardiac work and oxygen demand.

4. **True.** GTN taken orally undergoes extensive first-pass metabolism due to delivery to the liver in the hepatic portal circulation; this is avoided by transdermal or sublingual administration, from which the drug gains direct access to the systemic circulation.

5. **True.** The main anti-anginal action of β-adrenoceptor antagonists is to reduce myocardial oxygen demand by reducing heart rate and contractility. They thus reduce the reflex tachycardia that may occur with GTN and other nitrates.

6. **False.** βlockade of β_1-adrenoceptors produces reflex vasoconstriction, but some β-adrenoceptor antagonists produce peripheral vasodilation by partial agonism at β_2-adrenoceptors (e.g. pindolol), by α_1-adrenoceptor blockade (e.g. carvedilol) or by activation of NO synthesis (nebivolol).

7. **True.** Drugs with intrinsic sympathomimetic (partial agonist) activity at β_1-adrenoceptors produce less bradycardia at rest, but may be less effective than full antagonists in reducing heart rate on exertion.

8. **False.** Dihydropyridine calcium channel blockers mainly reduce myocardial oxygen demand by reducing peripheral arterial resistance and venous return; they do not reduce heart rate and amlodipine does not reduce myocardial contractility.

9. **True.** Potassium channel openers such as nicorandil hyperpolarise vascular myocytes by enhancing K^+ efflux; this closes voltage-gated L-type Ca^{2+} channels, leading to smooth muscle relaxation.

10. **False.** Ivabradine slows the heart by a direct action at the sinoatrial node without effect on myocardial contractility, unlike β-adrenoceptor antagonists.

11. **True.** PCI with stent insertion within 120 min of a STEMI is preferred to thrombolytic therapy and can also be used when thrombolysis has failed.

12. **True.** Stents coated with polymers that elute an antiproliferative drug (e.g. tacrolimus) can reduce restenosis compared to bare-metal stents.

OBA answers

1. **Answer D is incorrect.**
   A. Correct. Isosorbide mononitrate can therefore give a more predictable response of greater duration than the dinitrate.
   B. Correct. Unlike the dihydropyridines, verapamil also acts on the heart and reflex tachycardia does not occur.
   C. Correct. Platelet inhibition with tirofiban, an intravenous glycoprotein IIb/IIIa antagonist, reduces the risk of MI or death in those at high risk (see also Ch. 11). These agents are most effective after a non-ST-elevation myocardial infarction.
   D. **Incorrect**. Cholesterol reduction to <4.0 mmol·L^{-1} should be attempted and statins reduce reinfarction and cardiac death by 25–30% (Ch. 48).
   E. Correct. Dihydropyridine calcium channel antagonists do not improve prognosis after myocardial infarction. Verapamil and diltiazem produce a small reduction in reinfarction, but do not reduce mortality and may be detrimental if there are signs of heart failure.

2. **Answer D is correct.**

   The only way to reduce tolerance is to allow daily periods with low plasma concentrations of organic nitrate. Tolerance will develop to all the organic nitrates independent of the route given if plasma concentrations remain high continuously. A β-adrenoceptor antagonist will reduce reflex tachycardia but not the development of tolerance.

3. **Answer B is correct.**
   A. Unlikely. Atenolol prevents reflex tachycardia caused by the nitrate.
   B. **Most likely**. Verapamil and atenolol both have a negative inotropic effect and this could be a problem, particularly if there are signs of heart failure. They also have a negative chronotropic effect and the combination can cause severe bradycardia and heart block.
   C. Unlikely, although amlodipine and atenolol might cause excessive hypotension.
   D. Unlikely. Nicorandil does not have a direct effect on the heart.
   E. Unlikely. Aspirin will reduce the likelihood of development of myocardial infarction.

Case-based answers

A. Sublingual GTN is the first-choice drug for rapid relief of Mr TK's acute anginal attacks, although protection is only short-lived.

B. For prophylaxis, a β-adrenoceptor antagonist is often the treatment of first choice, or a calcium channel blocker if a β-adrenoceptor antagonist is contraindicated. If symptoms are not well controlled with either agent alone, a combination of both drugs, or the addition of a long-acting nitrate could be used, but the benefit of triple therapy is not convincing. Dual therapy with atenolol and diltiazem could significantly decrease the number of anginal attacks compared with either drug alone, and will also lower blood pressure and heart rate, which are precipitating factors for angina. The combination should be carefully monitored, however, because of the risk of compounding bradycardia or heart failure.

C. Additional therapy to improve prognosis includes low-dose aspirin or a statin drug to lower plasma cholesterol, both of which have been shown to reduce the risk of subsequent myocardial infarction.

D. Smoking, lack of exercise and obesity are all risk factors for coronary heart disease. TK is exposed to these increased risks and should address them by lifestyle changes.

E. The most consistent evidence is for combined use of aspirin with a β-adrenoceptor antagonist.

F. Coronary artery occlusion at the site of a ruptured atheromatous plaque, causing myocardial necrosis.

G. The benefit of fibrinolytic therapy is strongly dependent upon the delay between symptoms and administration. The benefit is particularly great if fibrinolytic therapy can be administered within 6 h from the onset of pain, but there is good evidence for benefit until at least 12 h.

H. Allergic reactions to streptokinase are extremely rare. Mr TK had not had a previous myocardial infarction and had not previously been given streptokinase, so would be unlikely to have high titres of streptokinase-neutralising antibodies. It would, therefore, be safe to give him streptokinase unless he had severe symptomatic hypotension. However, alteplase or an rt-PA derivative is usually preferred.

I. Aspirin and fibrinolytic therapy have additive benefit for treating acute myocardial infarction, reducing subsequent reinfarction or death.

J. Low doses of aspirin selectively reduce production of the platelet-aggregating agent thromboxane A_2 by platelets, while having less effect on the production of the platelet-disaggregating agent prostacyclin (prostaglandin I_2, PGI_2) from endothelial cells. Large doses of aspirin do not produce additional benefit, and the risk of gastric irritation or ulceration is increased.

K. The decision is incorrect. Giving fondaparinux or heparin is necessary to improve the long-term patency of the artery as rt-PA is short-acting; it would not be necessary with streptokinase, which has a longer duration of action than rt-PA.

L. ACE inhibitors, low-dose aspirin and β-adrenoceptor antagonists all reduce mortality and the risk of reinfarction. The β-adrenoceptor antagonist will need to be given under close observation, since it carries a risk of worsening heart failure. Verapamil and diltiazem may also be detrimental in people who have signs of heart failure. Warfarin reduces mortality and reinfarction to a similar extent as low-dose aspirin but with a greater risk of bleeding, so is not required unless aspirin is poorly tolerated.

FURTHER READING

General

Hansson GK (2005) Inflammation, atherosclerosis and coronary heart disease. *N Engl J Med* 352, 1685–1695

Tamargo J, Caballero R, Gomez R et al. (2004) Pharmacology of cardiac potassium channels. *Cardiovasc Res* 62, 9–33

Stable angina

Abrams J (2005) Chronic stable angina. *N Engl J Med* 352, 2524–2533

Deedwania PC, Carbajal EV (2011) Medical therapy versus myocardial revascularization in chronic coronary syndrome and stable angina. *Am J Med* 124, 681–688

Ben-Dor I, Battler A (2007) Treatment of stable angina. *Heart* 93, 868–874

Fayers KE, Cummings MH, Shaw KM et al. (2003) Nitrate tolerance and the links with endothelial dysfunction and oxidative stress. *Br J Clin Pharmacol* 56, 620–628

Feher MD (2003) Lipid lowering to delay the progression of coronary artery disease. *Heart* 89, 451–458

Heidenreich PA, McDonald KM, Haslie T et al. (1999) Meta-analysis of trials comparing β-blockers, calcium antagonists and nitrates for stable angina. *JAMA* 281, 1927–1936

Knight CJ (2003) Antiplatelet treatment in stable coronary artery disease. *Heart* 89, 1273–1278

Ko DT, Hebert PR, Coffey CS et al. (2002) β-blocker therapy and symptoms of depression, fatigue, and sexual dysfunction. *JAMA* 288, 351–357

Nash DT, Nash SD (2008) Ranolazine for chronic stable angina. *Lancet* 372, 1335–1341

Ong HT (2007) β blockers in hypertension and cardiovascular disease. *BMJ* 334, 946–949

Opie LH, Commerford PJ, Gersh BJ (2007) Controversies in stable coronary heart disease. *Lancet* 367, 69–78

Pfisterer ME, Zellweger MJ, Gersh BJ (2010) Management of stable coronary artery disease. *Lancet* 375, 763–772

Toda N (2003) Vasodilating β-adrenoceptor blockers as cardiovascular therapeutics. *Pharmacol Ther* 100, 215–234

Wei J, Wu T, Yang Q et al. (2011) Nitrates for stable angina: A systematic review and meta-analysis of randomized clinical trials. *Int J Cardiol* 146, 4–12

Unstable angina and NSTEMI

Aronow WS (2010) Office management of myocardial infarction. *Am J Med* 1213, 593–595

Chan MY, Becker RC, Harrington RA et al. (2008) Noninvasive, medical management for non-ST-elevation acute coronary syndromes. *Am Heart J* 155, 397–407

Peters RJG, Mehta S, Yusuf S (2007) Acute coronary syndromes without ST segment elevation. *BMJ* 334, 1256–1259

Rothberg MB, Celestin C, Fiore LD et al. (2005) Warfarin plus aspirin after myocardial infarction or acute coronary syndrome: meta-analysis with estimates of risk and benefit. *Ann Intern Med* 143, 241–250

STEMI

Brouwer MA, Clappers N, Verheugt FWA (2004) Adjunctive treatment in patients treated with thrombolytic therapy. *Heart* 90, 581–588

Dalal H, Evans PH, Campbell JL (2004) Recent developments in secondary prevention and cardiac rehabilitation after acute myocardial infarction. *BMJ* 328, 693–697

Keeley EC, Hillis LD (2007) Primary PCI for myocardial infarction with ST-segment elevation. *N Engl J Med* 356, 47–54

Lee VC, Rhew DC, Dylan M et al. (2004) Meta-analysis: angiotensin-receptor blockers in chronic heart failure and high-risk acute myocardial infarction. *Ann Intern Med* 41, 693–704

White HD, Chew DP (2008) Acute myocardial infarction. *Lancet* 372, 570–584

Compendium: drugs used to treat ischaemic heart disease

Drug	Kinetics (half-life)	Comments
Beta-adrenoceptor antagonists		
Beta-adrenoceptor antagonists are used in a wide variety of indications in addition to ischaemic heart disease, including hypertension and arrhythmias. All are given orally unless otherwise indicated. For completeness, all oral or parenteral β-adrenoceptor antagonists are listed in this compendium, irrespective of their licensed clinical uses.		
Acebutolol	Oral bioavailability 50–70%; active metabolite (7 h)	$β_1$-Adrenoceptor-selective (10% partial agonism); drug-induced lupus reported
Atenolol	Hydrophilic drug, eliminated by glomerular filtration (7 h)	$β_1$-Adrenoceptor-selective; given orally, or by injection or intravenous infusion
Betaxolol	Oral bioavailability 80–90%; hepatic metabolism and renal elimination (13–24 h)	$β_1$-Adrenoceptor-selective; used topically for glaucoma (Ch. 50)
Bisoprolol	High oral bioavailability 90%; hepatic metabolism and renal elimination (11 h)	$β_1$-Adrenoceptor-selective (but cardioselectivity less than atenolol)
Carvedilol	Oral bioavailability 20–30% due to first-pass metabolism; biliary and urinary elimination (6 h)	Non-selective; vasodilator action from $α_1$-adrenoceptor antagonism
Celiprolol	Poor absorption, bioavailability 30–50%; renal elimination (5 h)	$β_1$-Adrenoceptor-selective; vasodilator action due to partial $β_2$-adrenoceptor agonism
Esmolol	Rapidly hydrolysed in erythrocytes (9 min)	$β_1$-Adrenoceptor-selective; given only by intravenous infusion for termination of supraventriculoar arrhythmias
Labetalol	Oral bioavailability variable (10–90%) due to first-pass metabolism; hepatic metabolism (3 h)	$β_1$-Adrenoceptor-selective; vasodilator action through $α_1$-adrenoceptor antagonism; given orally, or by intravenous injection or infusion
Metoprolol	Oral bioavailability about 50%; wide variability in hepatic metabolism (3–10 h)	$β_1$-Adrenoceptor-selective (cardioselectivity less than atenolol); given orally, or by injection or intravenous infusion
Nadolol	Poor absorption (30%); renal and biliary elimination (17–24 h)	Non-selective
Nebivolol	Hepatic metabolism (10 h)	$β_1$-Adrenoceptor-selective (D-isomer); vasodilator from generation of NO (by D- and L-isomers)
Oxprenolol	Variable oral bioavailability (20–80%) due to first-pass metabolism; hepatic metabolism (2 h); active metabolite	Non-selective; 18% non-selective partial agonist activity
Pindolol	High oral bioavailability (> 90%); hepatic metabolism and urinary elimination (4 h)	Non-selective; vasodilator due to 35% partial $β_2$-adrenoceptor agonist activity
Propranolol	Oral bioavailability 10–50% due to first-pass metabolism; hepatic metabolism (4 h)	Non-selective; given orally or by intravenous injection
Sotalol	Renal elimination (7–18 h)	Non-selective β-adrenoceptor and K^+ channel antagonist; used mainly in arrhythmias; see under class III drugs (Ch. 8)
Timolol	Oral bioavailability 30–50%; hepatic metabolism and renal excretion (2–5 h)	Non-selective; also used topically for glaucoma (Ch. 50)
Calcium channel blockers		
Indications include angina, hypertension, Raynaud's phenomenon, arrhythmias and subarachnoid haemorrhage (see Chs 6, 8, 9, 10). All are given orally unless stated otherwise.		
Dihydropyridines		
Didhydropyridines have less effect on the myocardium than verapamil and have little or no detrimental effect in heart failure. They have no anti-arrhythmic activity. Modified-release formulations reduce fluctuations in blood pressure and reflex tachycardia and are preferred for the treatment of angina and hypertension.		
Amlodipine	Oral bioavailability 60–80%; hepatic metabolism (30–60 h)	Used once daily; no negative inotropic action
Felodipine	Oral bioavailability about 15% due to first-pass metabolism; hepatic metabolism (12–25 h)	Used once daily

Compendium: drugs used to treat ischaemic heart disease—cont'd

Drug	Kinetics (half-life)	Comments
Isradipine	Oral bioavailability 20% due to first-pass metabolism; hepatic metabolism (2–6 h)	
Lacidipine	Variable oral bioavailability (4–52%) due to first-pass metabolism in gut wall and liver; hepatic metabolism (7–8 h)	
Lercanidipine	Oral bioavailability (44%) increased by a fatty meal; hepatic metabolism (3–5 h)	Long duration of action (24 h) by an undefined mechanism; used once daily
Nicardipine	Oral bioavailability is dose-dependent (5–10% at low doses and 30–45% at high doses); hepatic metabolism (1–12 h)	Similar to nifedipine; modified-release formulation available
Nifedipine	Oral bioavailability about 40% due to first-pass metabolism in gut wall and liver; hepatic metabolism (2–4 h)	Modified-release formulations available; liquid capsule has rapid onset of action
Nimodipine	Oral bioavailability 5–10%; hepatic metabolism (8–9 h)	Selective for cerebral arteries; used in ischaemic neurological deficits following subarachnoid haemorrhage; given orally or by intravenous infusion

Non-dihydropyridines

In contrast to dihydropyridines, these drugs are also used for treatment and prevention of supraventricular arrhythmias, but are less effective for Raynaud's phenomenon. Modified-release formulations are available.

Diltiazem	Oral bioavailability about 50% due to first-pass metabolism; hepatic metabolism (2–5 h)	Reduces heart rate and some negative inotropic effect; should be avoided in heart failure
Verapamil	Oral bioavailability about 20% due to first-pass metabolism; hepatic metabolism; half-life (2–5 h) is longer after chronic dosing (5–12 h)	Reduces heart rate; marked negative inotropic effect and should be avoided in heart failure; given orally or by slow intravenous injection

Nitrates

Used for treatment of angina and in the management of heart failure; modified-release formulations are available.

Glyceryl trinitrate	Essentially complete first-pass metabolism if swallowed (1–3 min); the dinitrate metabolites are less active but have longer half-lives (40 min)	Given sublingually, buccally, topically or as an intravenous infusion
Isosorbide dinitrate	Low bioavailability from sublingual (30–60%) and topical (10–30%) administration; high first-pass metabolism to the active mononitrate (0.5–2 h)	Precursor of isosorbide mononitrate; given sublingually, orally (as normal or modified-release tablets), topically or by intravenous infusion
Isosorbide mononitrate	Complete oral bioavailability; low first-pass metabolism (3–7 h)	Given orally

Potassium channel activators

Nicorandil	Complete oral bioavailability; hepatic metabolism; biological effect much longer than predicted by half-life of 1 h	Used for angina; given orally

Specific sinus node inhibitor

Ivabradine	Metabolism and renal elimination (2 h); active metabolite	Used for angina; given orally

Late sodium current inhibitor

Ranolazine	Oral bioavailability about 35–50%; hepatic metabolism (1.5–2 h)	Used as adjunctive treatment for patients inadequately controlled by, or intolerant to, other anti-anginal agents

6 Systemic and pulmonary hypertension

SYSTEMIC HYPERTENSION

The cause of systemic hypertension in the majority of people is unknown (essential hypertension), with a complex interplay between genetic and environmental influences. Abnormal regulation of the physiological mechanisms that normally control arterial blood pressure may be an important factor. A small number of people with hypertension have an identifiable underlying cause (secondary hypertension).

CIRCULATORY REFLEXES AND THE CONTROL OF SYSTEMIC BLOOD PRESSURE

Systemic blood pressure (BP) is determined by the cardiac output (CO) and total peripheral resistance (TPR).

$$BP = CO \times TPR$$

Blood pressure is maintained within fairly narrow limits due to modulation by a series of physiological reflexes that are triggered by both acute and chronic changes in blood pressure. There are both short-term and long-term control mechanisms. Important regulatory systems are:

- the autonomic nervous system,
- the renin–angiotensin–aldosterone system,
- local chemical mediators at the vascular endothelium.

The autonomic nervous system regulates arterial blood pressure in several ways.

- **In the heart**, the sympathetic nervous system acts mainly through β_1-adrenoceptors to increase myocardial contractility and heart rate, generating a greater cardiac output and increasing blood pressure (Ch. 4). An increase in parasympathetic nervous system tone reduces heart rate and therefore cardiac output and blood pressure
- **In arterial resistance vessels**, sympathetic nervous stimulation produces arteriolar vasoconstriction through stimulation of postsynaptic α_1-adrenoceptors. Arterial vasoconstriction raises blood pressure, but also increases the afterload on the heart. In the healthy heart, cardiac output is maintained by an increase in cardiac contractility via β_1-adrenoceptors.
- **In venous capacitance vessels**, sympathetic stimulation of postsynaptic α_1-adrenoceptors produces venous constriction. This increases venous return to the heart (preload), raises cardiac output and increases blood pressure (Ch. 7).

The autonomic nervous system is normally responsible for immediate regulation of blood pressure. Change in systemic blood pressure is detected by baroreceptors (stretch receptors) in the aorta and carotid arteries. When blood pressure rises, stretch of the baroreceptors increases afferent nerve impulses to a coordinating area in the medulla which controls the autonomic outflow to the cardiovascular system. The increase in afferent impulses inhibits sympathetic nervous system output and increases parasympathetic nervous system outflow, returning the blood pressure to normal. The opposite occurs when blood pressure falls (Fig. 6.1).

A slower compensatory mechanism for a reduction in blood pressure is initiated by the release of renin from the juxtaglomerular apparatus of the kidney (Fig. 6.2). The major stimuli leading to renin release are reduced renal blood flow (often as a result of a decrease in blood pressure), decreased Na^+ in the renal distal tubule and direct sympathetic stimulation via β_1-adrenoceptors. Renin is a protease that acts on circulating renin substrate (angiotensinogen) to release the decapeptide angiotensin I. This is further cleaved by angiotensin-converting enzyme the octapeptide angiotensin II. There are several additional enzymatic pathways for generating angiotensin II that do not involve ACE (see Fig. 6.8). Angiotensin II acts on various tissues via specific angiotensin AT_1 and AT_2 receptors (Fig. 6.2). Its action at the AT_1 receptor produces potent direct vasoconstriction, and also enhances sympathetic nervous tone by facilitating presynaptic neuronal release of noradrenaline and through stimulation of central sympathetic outflow. Angiotensin II has a number of additional properties which promote salt and water retention (Fig. 6.3), one of the most powerful being the release of aldosterone from the adrenal cortex. Aldosterone acts at the distal renal tubule to conserve salt and water at the expense of K^+ loss (Ch. 14). Therefore, angiotensin II and aldosterone raise blood pressure by vasoconstriction and by increasing circulating blood volume. Some of the effects of angiotensin at the AT_1 receptor do not raise blood pressure; in the endothelium,

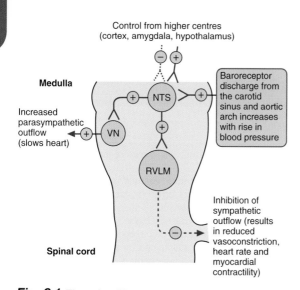

Fig. 6.1 **The role of baroreceptors.** Increased blood pressure increases neural discharge from the baroreceptors (stretch receptors) in the carotid sinus and aortic arch, resulting in a compensatory inhibition in sympathetic outflow from the rostral ventrolateral medulla (RVLM) and an increase in the parasympathetic outflow from the cardioinhibitory vagal nucleus (VN). Both effects act to lower blood pressure, which is also influenced by control from higher centres acting at the nucleus of the tractus solitarius (NTS). See Fig. 6.7 for sites of action of centrally acting antihypertensive drugs. +, stimulation; –, inhibition.

AT_1 receptor stimulation enhances nitric oxide production, resulting in vasodilation and dampening the pressor effects of angiotensin II. Angiotensin II has additional actions at the AT_2 receptor that appear to oppose some of those at the AT_1 receptor (Fig. 6.2).

The integration of the fast-responding sympathetic nervous system and the slower-responding renin–angiotensin–aldosterone system in response to a fall in blood pressure is shown in Figure 6.3. These mechanisms prevent hypotension due to peripheral pooling of blood on standing and during exercise.

Additional mechanisms involved in controlling vascular tone and blood volume include circulating or local endothelial hormones and metabolites, such as natriuretic peptides, antidiuretic hoemone, prostaglandins, bradykinin, nitric oxide, endothelin and adenosine. Their relative importance may differ in health and disease states.

AETIOLOGY AND PATHOGENESIS OF SYSTEMIC HYPERTENSION

There is no absolute cut-off between normal and high blood pressure. Blood pressure in all populations is normally distributed with a slight skew because of a small number of individuals with very high blood pressures. The risk of complications is also a continuous variable, increasing as blood pressure rises. Defining a point at which blood pressure is 'high' is therefore somewhat arbitrary but it is usually set at values greater than 140/90 mmHg. Using this definition, hypertension is a common condition found in 20–30% of the population of the developed world, with the prevalence increasing with age.

Hypertension does not usually cause symptoms but produces progressive structural changes in the heart and circulation. These include formation of atheroma, microaneurysms on intracerebral blood vessels and remodelling of the muscle in the left ventricle and arterial resistance vessels.

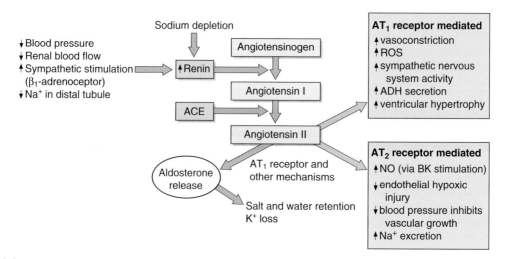

Fig. 6.2 **Formation and actions of angiotensin II.** Angiotensin II acts on type 1 (AT_1) and type 2 (AT_2) receptors. Current therapeutic drugs act predominantly to block AT_1 receptors. The number of AT_2 receptors is low relative to that of AT_1 receptors but increases in pathological conditions. ACE, angiotensin-converting enzyme; ADH, antidiuretic hormone; BK, bradykinin, NO, nitric oxide; ROS, reactive oxygen species.

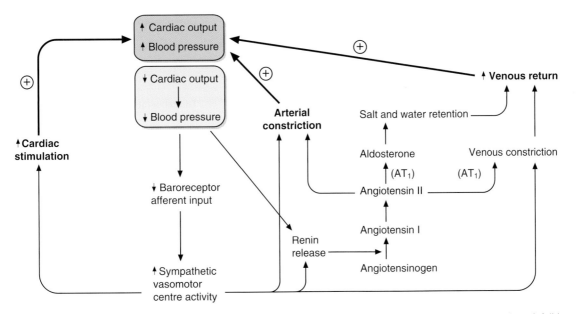

Fig. 6.3 **The control of blood pressure via the sympathetic and renin–angiotensin–aldosterone systems.** A fall in cardiac output or blood pressure (yellow box) produces relatively rapid responses mediated by increased sympathetic activity and slower responses mediated by renin–angiotensin–aldosterone mechanisms. The outcomes are increased cardiac stimulation, increased arterial constriction and increased venous return, restoring blood pressure. AT_1, angiotensin II type 1 receptor.

These changes predispose to clinical complications that are often referred to as 'target organ damage'. The principal complications of hypertension are ischaemic heart disease (especially in middle-aged Europeans and Americans), and cerebrovascular disease (especially in Asians and older people) which usually presents as thromboembolic stroke or, less commonly, as cerebral haemorrhage (Ch. 9). Ischaemic complications of hypertension are more likely to occur if it is accompanied by hypercholesterolaemia, diabetes mellitus and smoking. The underlying vascular lesions that occur in hypertension and their resulting complications are shown in Figure 6.4.

Sustained hypertension predisposes to left ventricular muscle hypertrophy (LVH). LVH is an independent risk factor for the complications of hypertension, particularly ischaemic heart disease (since the muscle outgrows its blood supply), heart failure with preserved ejection fraction (Ch. 7) and arrhythmias leading to sudden death (Ch. 8).

If target organ damage or diabetes is present, treatment reduces complications when introduced at blood pressures above 140/90 mmHg. However, if there is no target organ damage treatment may not alter outcome until the systolic pressure is sustained above 160 mmHg, or the diastolic blood pressure is sustained above 100 mmHg.

Hypertension should ideally be confirmed by ambulatory 24 h blood pressure monitoring, unless target organ damage gives a clear indication treatment is necessary. Sometimes, the blood pressure is raised only when the measurement is taken by a doctor or, to a lesser extent, by a nurse. This phenomenon is termed 'white coat' or 'office' hypertension and appears to carry little risk of complications over the subsequent few years but can eventually lead to sustained hypertension. It can be detected by ambulatory 24 h blood pressure monitoring. White coat

hypertension often persists despite drug treatment, which can then result in quite troublesome *hypotension* away from the surgery or clinic. There is also a phenomenon of 'masked' hypertension, when blood pressure is normal in the clinic but high at home. This appears to carry a similar risk of complications as sustained hypertension.

Malignant or accelerated hypertension is an infrequently encountered condition, produced by very high blood pressure or a rapid rise in blood pressure. It is characterised pathologically by arterial fibrinoid necrosis, and identified clinically by the presence of flame-shaped haemorrhages, hard exudates and 'cotton wool' spots in the retina or by papilloedema, which can lead to visual disturbance. If untreated, accelerated hypertension usually leads to death from renal failure, heart failure or stroke within 5 years.

Hypertension is usually characterised by increased peripheral arterial resistance, which arises from arteriolar smooth muscle constriction and hypertrophy leaving a smaller vessel lumen and an increase in the wall-to-lumen ratio (vascular remodelling). Cardiac output is often normal in younger people with hypertension, but is usually reduced in the elderly. The cause of the inappropriately raised peripheral resistance is unknown in the majority of people with hypertension, who are said to have 'essential hypertension'. Essential hypertension probably has a polygenic inheritance, leading to several clinical subtypes with different underlying pathogenic mechanisms. Environmental influences and factors such as diet, level of exercise, obesity and alcohol intake all interact with the genetic programming to determine the final level of blood pressure. There is evidence that reduced renal Na^+ excretion plays a central role in the pathogenesis of essential hypertension, and the kidney requires a higher-than-normal blood pressure to maintain a normal extracellular fluid volume.

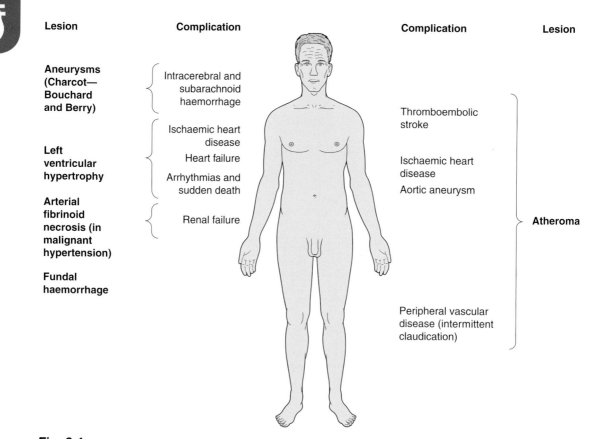

| Lesion | Complication | | Complication | Lesion |

Aneurysms (Charcot—Bouchard and Berry) — Intracerebral and subarachnoid haemorrhage

Left ventricular hypertrophy — Ischaemic heart disease / Heart failure / Arrhythmias and sudden death

Arterial fibrinoid necrosis (in malignant hypertension) — Renal failure

Fundal haemorrhage

Thromboembolic stroke

Ischaemic heart disease

Aortic aneurysm

Atheroma

Peripheral vascular disease (intermittent claudication)

Fig. 6.4 **Complications of hypertension.** Hypertension causes vascular lesions and damage throughout the body.

However, the disturbance in essential hypertension is much more widespread than the kidney, with cell membrane abnormalities found in many organs.

Isolated systolic hypertension, usually found in older people, is the consequence of stiffening of large 'conductance' arteries. These vessels normally expand to accommodate the blood expelled from the heart in systole, which slows the pulse wave and increases the time taken for it to reach the peripheral resistance vessels. The pulse wave is normally reflected back from the peripheral vessels in diastole, and supports the diastolic blood pressure and therefore coronary artery perfusion. If the compliance of the large arteries is reduced, then the pulse wave reaches the peripheral vessels early and is reflected back in systole. This increases systolic blood pressure and reduces diastolic pressure. In isolated systolic hypertension, coronary artery perfusion can be impaired, while cardiac work is increased.

A secondary underlying cause of high blood pressure, which often has a renal or endocrine origin, can be identified in about 5% of people with hypertension (Table 6.1).

Not surprisingly, since the cause of hypertension is unclear, treatment cannot be directed precisely at the underlying mechanism(s). Most antihypertensive drugs are vasodilators, and they often modulate the natural hormonal or neuronal mechanisms responsible for blood pressure regulation. Less commonly, a hypotensive action is partially achieved by reducing cardiac output. The principal classes of antihypertensive drugs and their sites of action are shown in Table 6.2 and Figure 6.5.

Table 6.1 Principal causes of secondary hypertension

	Causes
Renal	Renal artery stenosis, glomerulonephritis, interstitial nephritis, arteritis, polycystic disease, chronic pyelonephritis
Endocrine	Conn's syndrome (aldosterone excess), Cushing's syndrome (glucocorticoid excess), phaeochromocytoma (catecholamine excess), acromegaly
Pregnancy	Pre-eclampsia and eclampsia
Drugs	Oestrogen, corticosteroids, non-steroidal anti-inflammatory drugs (NSAIDs), ciclosporin

ANTIHYPERTENSIVE DRUGS

Drugs acting on the sympathetic nervous system

Beta-adrenoceptor antagonists (β-blockers)

Examples

atenolol, nebivolol, propranolol

Table 6.2 Principal classes of antihypertensive drugs and their sites of action

Sites of action	Drugs
Sympathetic nervous system	β-Adrenoceptor antagonists
	α_1-Adrenoceptor antagonists
	Selective imidazoline receptor agonists
	Centrally acting α_2-adrenoceptor agonists
	Adrenergic neuron blockers
Hormonal control (renin–angiotensin system)	Angiotensin-converting enzyme (ACE) inhibitors
	Angiotensin II receptor antagonists
	Direct renin inhibitors
Vasodilation by other mechanisms	Diuretics
	Calcium channel blockers
	Potassium channel openers
	Nitrovasodilators
	Endothelin-1 receptor antagonists

Mechanism of action in hypertension

Beta-adrenoceptor antagonists reduce blood pressure in several ways (Fig. 6.6). Selective β_1-adrenoceptor antagonists are as effective as non-selective drugs, indicating that β_2-adrenoceptor blockade makes little contribution. The more important actions are probably:

- reduction of heart rate and myocardial contractility, which decreases cardiac output,
- blockade of renal juxtaglomerular β_1-adrenoceptors, which reduces renin secretion and therefore generation of angiotensin II and aldosterone. This produces vasodilation and reduces plasma volume,
- peripheral arterial vasodilation is not a direct effect of pure β-adrenoceptor antagonists, but is an additional property of some compounds that have a hybrid action (such as nebivolol). These produce vasodilation by mechanisms other than β_1-adrenoceptor antagonism (Fig. 6.6C and see especially Ch. 5),
- blockade of presynaptic β-adrenoceptors in sympathetic neurons supplying arteriolar resistance vessels. This may reduce the release of noradrenaline and thus attenuate reflex arterial vasoconstriction, but the clinical importance of this effect is uncertain.

For further details about β-adrenoceptor antagonists and their many uses, see Chapters 5 and 8, and Box 6.1.

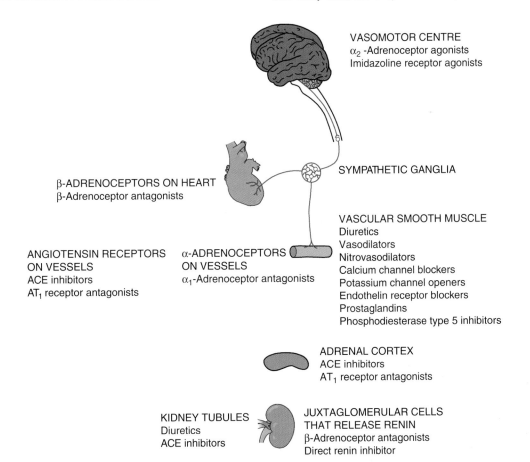

Fig. 6.5 **The main classes of antihypertensive drugs and their sites of action.** ACE, angiotensin-converting enzyme; AT_1, angiotensin II type 1 receptor.

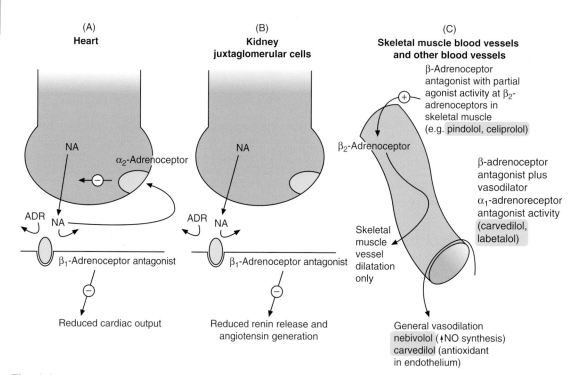

Fig. 6.6 Sites of action of the β-adrenoceptor antagonists relevant to their use as antihypertensive agents. (A) In the heart, the β₁-adrenoceptor antagonist drugs reduce stimulation of the β₁-adrenoceptors by noradrenaline (NA) and circulating adrenaline (ADR). Presynaptic stimulation of α₂-adrenoceptors, which inhibits noradrenaline release, still functions normally. (B) In the kidney, β₁-adrenoceptor blockade reduces the activity of the renin–angiotensin system. (C) Some selective β₁-adrenoceptor antagonists have hybrid activity: pindolol and celiprolol have intrinsic sympathomimetic activity, acting as partial agonists at β₂-adrenoceptors in skeletal muscle blood vessels, leading to vasodilation and reduced peripheral resistance. As partial agonists these drugs reduce heart rate and cardiac output less than full antagonists. Nebivolol may dilate blood vessels more generally by releasing nitric oxide (NO). Carvedilol and labetalol also have α₁-adrenoceptor antagonist activity, reducing peripheral resistance.

> **Box 6.1** **Clinical uses of β-adrenoceptor antagonists**
>
> Treatment of hypertension (this chapter)
> Prophylaxis of angina (Ch. 5)
> Secondary prevention after myocardial infarction
>   (Ch. 5)
> Treatment of heart failure (Ch. 7)
> Prevention and treatment of arrhythmias (Ch. 8)
> Control of symptoms in thyrotoxicosis (Ch. 41)
> Alleviation of symptoms in anxiety (Ch. 20)
> Prophylaxis of migraine (Ch. 26)
> Topical treatment of glaucoma (Ch. 50)

Alpha-adrenoceptor antagonists (α-blockers)

Examples

α₁-adrenoceptor-selective antagonists: doxazosin, prazosin
non-selective antagonists: phenoxybenzamine (irreversible), phentolamine (reversible)

Mechanisms of action

Alpha-adrenoceptor antagonists (often referred to as α-blockers) lower blood pressure by blockade of postsynaptic α₁-adrenoceptors, leading to:

- dilation of arteriolar resistance vessels, which lowers peripheral resistance,
- dilation of venous capacitance vessels, which reduces venous return and therefore cardiac output.

When blood pressure falls as a result of using an α-adrenoceptor antagonist, this is detected by arterial baroreceptors. The baroreceptors initiate an increase in sympathetic discharge from the medulla, causing a reflex tachycardia (Figs 6.1 and 6.3). However, because noradrenaline released from cardiac sympathetic nerve terminals also stimulates inhibitory α₂-adrenoceptors on the presynaptic sympathetic neuron, the degree of sympathetic stimulation and reflex tachycardia is attenuated (Fig. 6.6A). Selective α₁-adrenoceptor antagonists do not block the presynaptic α₂-adrenoceptors on sympathetic nerve terminals, and therefore reflex tachycardia is unusual with these compounds.

By contrast, non-selective α-adrenoceptor antagonists block both postsynaptic α₁-adrenoceptors and presynaptic α₂-adrenoceptors, and their use is accompanied by a marked reflex tachycardia. Non-selective agents now have little place in clinical practice except for the perioperative management of phaeochromocytoma.

Alpha-adrenoceptor antagonists produce a potentially beneficial effect on plasma lipids by increasing high-density lipoprotein (HDL) cholesterol and reducing triglycerides (Ch. 48). Whether this has any relevance for the prevention of atheroma in individuals with hypertension is uncertain. Selective α_1-adrenoceptor antagonists are also used to treat the symptoms of bladder outlet obstruction (Ch. 15).

Pharmacokinetics

Selective α_1-adrenoceptor antagonists are well absorbed from the gut and undergo extensive first-pass metabolism and subsequent elimination by the liver. The compounds differ principally in their half-lives and, therefore, duration of action; for example, prazosin has a half-life of 3 h whereas doxazosin has a half-life of 9–12 h.

Unwanted effects

- Postural hypotension caused by venous pooling; this can be particularly troublesome following the first dose.
- Lethargy, headache, dizziness.
- Nausea.
- Rhinitis.
- Urinary frequency or incontinence.
- Palpitation from reflex cardiac stimulation with non-selective drugs.

Centrally acting antihypertensive drugs

Selective imidazoline receptor agonists

moxonidine

Mechanism of action

Imidazoline I_1 receptors are important for the regulation of sympathetic drive (Figs 6.1 and 6.7). They are concentrated in the rostral ventrolateral medulla, a part of the brainstem involved in control of blood pressure. Increased neuronal activity in this area, either through baroreceptor stimulation or by direct stimulation of I_1 receptors by moxonidine, will decrease sympathetic outflow, which results in a fall in blood pressure with no reflex tachycardia. Unlike other centrally acting drugs (clonidine and methyldopa), moxonidine has a low affinity for presynaptic α_2-adrenoceptors.

Pharmacokinetics

Moxonidine is well absorbed from the gut, and its principal route of elimination is the kidney. It has a short half-life (2–3 h) but a prolonged duration of action, which may reflect its high affinity for I_1 receptors.

Unwanted effects

- Dry mouth.
- Nausea.
- Fatigue, headache, dizziness.

Centrally acting α_2-adrenoceptor agonists

clonidine, methyldopa

Unwanted effects limit the use of the centrally acting α_2-adrenoceptor agonists, although methyldopa is a drug of choice in the treatment of hypertension in pregnancy (see below).

Mechanisms of action

The α_2-adrenoceptor agonists act at presynaptic autoreceptors in the central nervous system (CNS) to reduce sympathetic nervous outflow and increase vagal outflow from the medulla (Fig. 6.7). This reduces both peripheral arterial and venous tone.

Methyldopa is a prodrug that is metabolised in the nerve terminal as a 'false substrate' in the biosynthetic pathway for noradrenaline, to produce α-methylnoradrenaline, a potent α_2-adrenoceptor agonist. Clonidine is a direct-acting α_2-adrenoceptor agonist that is also an agonist at imidazoline I_1 receptors (see above). Clonidine has some peripheral postsynaptic α_1-adrenoceptor agonist activity, which produces direct peripheral vasoconstriction; this initially offsets some of the central blood pressure-lowering effect.

Pharmacokinetics

Methyldopa is incompletely absorbed from the gut and undergoes dose-dependent first-pass metabolism, with an elimination half-life of 1–2 h. Clonidine is completely absorbed from the gut and has a half-life of about 24 h.

Unwanted effects

- Sympathetic blockade: failure of ejaculation, and postural or exertional hypotension (unusual with clonidine, owing to its direct peripheral action).
- Unopposed parasympathetic action: diarrhoea.
- Dry mouth.
- CNS effects: sedation and drowsiness occur in up to 50% of people who take methyldopa; depression is occasionally seen.
- Fluid retention with peripheral oedema.
- Methyldopa induces a reversible positive Coombs' test in 20% of people, resulting from production of IgG to red cell membrane constituents; however, haemolytic anaemia is rare.
- Sudden withdrawal of clonidine can produce severe rebound hypertension with tachycardia, sweating and anxiety.

Drugs affecting the renin–angiotensin system

Angiotensin-converting enzyme inhibitors

captopril, enalapril, lisinopril, ramipril

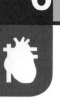

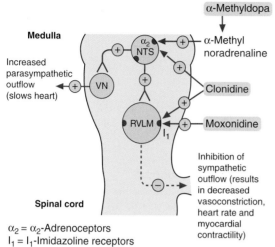

$\alpha_2 = \alpha_2$-Adrenoceptors
$I_1 = I_1$-Imidazoline receptors

Fig. 6.7 Mechanisms of centrally acting antihypertensive drugs. These drugs act on the same medullary centres that respond to raised blood pressure (Fig. 6.1). Methylnoradrenaline and clonidine stimulate α_2-adrenoceptors in the nucleus of the tractus solitarius (NTS). Moxonidine, and possibly also clonidine, act on imidazoline I_1 receptors in the rostral ventrolateral medulla (RVLM). VN, vagal nucleus (cardioinhibitory centre).

Mechanisms of action

The ACE inhibitors lower blood pressure by several mechanisms (see Figs 6.2, 6.5 and 6.8).

- Competitive inhibition of plasma ACE reduces generation of circulating angiotensin II and consequently reduces the release of aldosterone (Fig. 6.8).
- Inhibition of tissue ACE in the vascular wall is central to the hypotensive effect of these drugs (Fig. 6.8). Reduced tissue concentrations of angiotensin II lead to arterial dilation and, to a lesser extent, venous dilation. Angiotensin II production is not completely inhibited owing to alternative pathways for its generation by proteases including chymase and chymotrypsin-like angiotensin-II-generating enzyme (CAGE). The activity in these pathways is enhanced due to stimulation of renin release by the fall in blood pressure after ACE inhibition.
- Competitive inhibition of plasma ACE reduces generation of circulating angiotensin II and consequently reduces the release of aldosterone (Fig. 6.8).
- Reduction in angiotensin II-mediated potentiation of the sympathetic nervous system (Figs 6.2 and 6.3) prevents reflex tachycardia.
- Angiotensin II is implicated in the development of arterial remodelling and LVH in hypertension. ACE inhibitors are more effective in regressing LVH than diuretics or β-adrenoceptor antagonists.

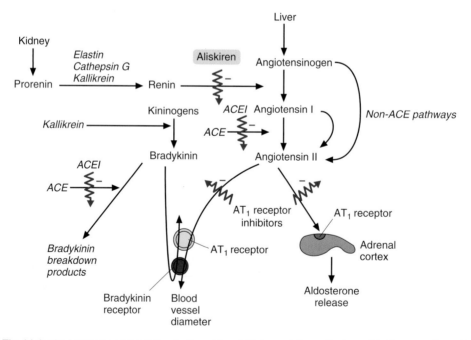

Fig. 6.8 The biological actions of angiotensin II and bradykinin and drugs that modify these actions. Angiotensin II causes vasoconstriction by stimulating AT_1 receptors in the blood vessels and causes Na^+ retention by stimulating AT_1 receptors in the adrenal cortex, which results in aldosterone release. Bradykinin causes vasodilation by acting on vascular smooth muscle cells and on endothelial cells. Angiotensin-converting enzyme inhibitors (ACEI) block angiotensin II formation from angiotensin I (although alternative, non-ACE-dependent protease pathways remain that can result in some angiotensin II formation from angiotensinogen or angiotensin I). ACE inhibitors also reduce the breakdown of bradykinin, contributing to their vasodilator effects. Angiotensin II receptor antagonists block AT_1 receptors in blood vessels and the adrenal cortex. Aliskiren directly inhibits the actions of renin on angiotensinogen.

> **Box 6.2** **Clinical uses of ACE inhibitors and angiotensin II receptor blockers**
>
> Treatment of hypertension (this chapter)
> Treatment of heart failure (Ch. 7)
> Secondary prevention after myocardial infarction (Ch. 5)
> Diabetic nephropathy (Ch. 40 and this chapter)

- ACE also degrades other peptides including bradykinin (Fig. 6.8). Increased bradykinin in the vascular wall may contribute to the hypotensive actions of ACE inhibitors.

There are many clinical uses of ACE inhibitors other than hypertension; these are listed in Box 6.2.

Pharmacokinetics

Many ACE inhibitors are given orally as prodrugs, because the active forms are polar and poorly absorbed from the gut. The prodrugs are converted in the liver to the active agent; for example, ramipril is converted to the active compound ramiprilat. In contrast, captopril and lisinopril are absorbed adequately as an active molecule. Most ACE inhibitors are excreted in the active form by the kidney. The half-lives range from about 2 h (for example, captopril and ramiprilat) to about 30–35 h (for example, enalaprilat).

Unwanted effects

- Persistent dry cough that is not dose-related and may be caused by accumulation of kinins in the lung. This occurs in 10–30% of people who take ACE inhibitors, is more common in women and can develop after many months of treatment.
- Postural hypotension, which is rare unless there is salt and water depletion, for example as a result of therapy with diuretics. Profound hypotension can occur in such individuals, particularly after the first dose. This is rarely a problem in the treatment of hypertension, but can be in the treatment of severe heart failure (Ch. 7).
- Renal impairment, especially in those with severe bilateral renal artery stenosis who rely on angiotensin-mediated efferent glomerular arterial vasoconstriction to maintain glomerular perfusion pressure.
- Disturbance of taste (which may be permanent), nausea, vomiting, dyspepsia or bowel disturbance.
- Rashes.
- Angioedema, which is more frequent in people of Afro-Caribbean origin.

Angiotensin II receptor antagonists

candesartan, losartan, valsartan

Mechanism of action

The angiotensin II receptor antagonists are selective for the AT_1 receptor subtype, which is found in the heart, blood vessels, kidney, adrenal cortex, lung and brain, and have less effect at the AT_2 receptor subtype (Fig. 6.2). Actions of angiotensin II via the AT_1 receptor include vasoconstriction, cell growth and proliferation, aldosterone release, sympathetic stimulation, salt and water retention, inhibition of renin release and an increase in reactive oxygen species. In contrast to the use of ACE inhibitors, kinin degradation is unaffected by angiotensin II receptor antagonists and inhibition of the effects of angiotensin II is more complete (Fig. 6.8). There are many clinical uses of angiotensin II receptor antagonists other than hypertension; these are listed in Box 6.2.

Pharmacokinetics

Losartan is well absorbed from the gut and partially converted to an active metabolite, which is responsible for most of the pharmacological effects and has a longer half-life (6 h) than the parent drug (2 h). Candesartan and valsartan are given as prodrugs. Most angiotensin II receptor antagonists are given once daily.

Unwanted effects

Drugs in this class are usually well tolerated. Their major advantages over ACE inhibitors are the low incidence of cough, and that angioedema is rare. Unwanted effects include:

- headache, dizziness,
- arthralgia or myalgia,
- fatigue.

Direct renin inhibitors

aliskiren

Mechanism of action

Aliskiren is a selective renin inhibitor with low affinity for other proteases. It binds competitively to the active site of the enzyme and inhibits the generation of angiotensin I (Fig. 6.8). Vasodilation is achieved by reduced angiotensin II synthesis, without the compensatory increase in plasma renin activity that occurs with an ACE inhibitor or angiotensin II receptor antagonist. The place of aliskiren in the treatment of hypertension remains to be established.

Pharmacokinetics

Aliskiren is poorly absorbed from the gut and has a very long half-life (40 h).

Unwanted effects

- Diarrhoea.
- Cough.
- Renal function may deteriorate when aliskiren is combined with an ACE inhibitor or an angiotensin II receptor antagonist.

Vasodilators

Diuretics

thiazide and thiazide-type diuretics: bendroflumethiazide, chlortalidone, hydrochlorothiazide, indapamide
loop diuretics: furosemide
potassium-sparing diuretics: spironolactone

Thiazide or thiazide-type diuretics are most frequently used to lower blood pressure, but loop and potassium-sparing diuretics are used in some situations.

Mechanism of action in hypertension

Full details of the sites and mechanisms of action of diuretics on the kidney and their unwanted effects are considered in Chapter 14. Actions involved in lowering blood pressure include the following.

- An initial hypotensive effect is produced by intravascular salt and water depletion. However, compensatory mechanisms such as activation of the renin–angiotensin–aldosterone system largely restore plasma and extracellular fluid volumes (see Fig. 6.3) (unless salt and water retention was a major component of the initial hypertension, e.g. in advanced renal failure or as a consequence of other antihypertensive treatment).
- Direct arterial dilation is responsible for the longer-term reduction in blood pressure. The mechanism of vasodilation is not well understood, but may result from reduced Ca^{2+} entry into the smooth muscle of the arteriolar resistance vessel walls (perhaps as a consequence of intracellular Na^+ depletion).

Thiazide and thiazide-type diuretics

These produce their maximum blood pressure-lowering effect at doses lower than those required for significant diuretic activity. This is an advantage, since most unwanted effects are dose-related.

Loop diuretics

Loop diuretics are usually less effective than thiazides in the treatment of essential hypertension. Despite having a more powerful diuretic action, their duration of action is too short. However, hypertension with advanced renal impairment or hypertension resistant to multiple drug treatment is more likely to be associated with fluid retention and often responds better to a loop diuretic than to a thiazide.

Potassium-sparing diuretics

Spironolactone, a specific aldosterone antagonist, is particularly effective for hypertension caused by primary hyperaldosteronism (Conn's syndrome). However, it can also be useful to treat resistant hypertension. Amiloride and triamterene (Ch. 14) are less effective than thiazides in essential hypertension.

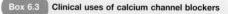

Box 6.3   **Clinical uses of calcium channel blockers**

Treatment of hypertension (this chapter)
Prophylaxis of angina (Ch. 5)
Treatment of Raynaud's phenomenon (Ch. 10)
Prevention and treatment of supraventricular arrhythmias (Ch. 8)
Subarachnoid haemorrhage (Ch. 9)

Calcium channel blockers

amlodipine, diltiazem, nifedipine, verapamil

The calcium channel blockers lower blood pressure principally by arterial vasodilation. For clinical uses, see Box 6.3. For further details, see Chapter 5.

Potassium channel openers

amlodipine, diltiazem, nifedipine, verapamil

minoxidil

Mechanism of action

Vascular smooth muscle possesses ATP-sensitive K^+ channels (K_{ATP}) that are responsible for repolarisation of the cell (see also Ch. 8). Minoxidil opens K_{ATP} channels, causing an efflux of K^+ which hyperpolarises the cell and leads to closure of voltage-gated Ca^{2+} channels and muscle relaxation (see also potassium channel openers, Ch. 5). Minoxidil is one of the most powerful peripheral arterial dilators.

Pharmacokinetics

Minoxidil is well absorbed from the gut and mainly metabolised in the liver. It has a short half-life (3–4 h).

Unwanted effects

- Arterial vasodilation produces flushing and headache.
- The reflex sympathetic nervous system response to vasodilation causes tachycardia and palpitation (which can be blunted by concurrent use of a β-adrenoceptor antagonist, ACE inhibitor or angiotensin II receptor antagonist).
- Salt and water retention occur through stimulation of the renin–angiotensin–aldosterone system (Fig. 6.2). This, along with increased transcapillary pressure from vasodilation, can produce peripheral oedema, which can be reduced by the concurrent use of diuretics.
- Hirsutism; therefore rarely used for treatment of women.

Hydralazine

Hydralazine is rarely used for long-term treatment of hypertension, but is an important treatment for hypertension in late pregnacy (pre-eclampsia), since it maintains uterine blood flow.

Mechanism of action

The mechanism of action of hydralazine is uncertain, but it may activate guanylyl cyclase, leading to the intracellular production of cGMP, and act as a nitric oxide donor. This will produce smooth muscle relaxation by mechanisms similar to those of organic nitrates (see Fig. 5.3).

Pharmacokinetics

Hydralazine undergoes extensive first-pass metabolism in the gut wall and liver, principally by N-acetylation. Some individuals, who are genetically determined slow acetylators (Ch. 2), require lower doses of hydralazine to achieve a clinical effect but are more susceptible to some of the unwanted effects.

Unwanted effects

- Arterial vasodilation with reflex sympathetic activation produces tachycardia, flushing, hypotension and fluid retention.
- Headache, dizziness.
- A systemic lupus erythematosus (SLE)-like syndrome, which usually occurs after several months of treatment, is dose-related and is more common in slow acetylators. It resembles the naturally occurring disease but does not produce renal or cerebral damage and is slowly reversed if treatment is stopped. A positive antinuclear antibody is found in many individuals who do not develop the syndrome.

Nitrovasodilators

sodium nitroprusside

Because it must be given intravenously, the use of nitroprusside is limited to the emergency management of hypertensive crises.

Mechanism of action

Nitroprusside is a nitrovasodilator with a mechanism of action similar to that of organic nitrates (Ch. 5). It produces dilation of arterioles and veins, reducing both peripheral resistance and venous return.

Pharmacokinetics

Nitroprusside is given by intravenous infusion and its duration of action is less than 5 min. Metabolism to cyanide within red blood cells (by electron transfer from haemoglobin iron) terminates its effect. The cyanide is partly bound in the erythrocyte and partly liberated, when it is taken up by cells and inhibits intracellular cytochrome oxidase. Free cyanide is converted in the liver to less toxic thiocyanate but thiocyanate accumulates with prolonged infusion. Therefore, treatment with nitroprusside is usually limited to a maximum of 3 days.

Unwanted effects

- Headache, dizziness.
- Nausea, retching, abdominal pain.

- Thiocyanate accumulation causes tachycardia, sweating, hyperventilation, arrhythmias and metabolic acidosis from inhibition of aerobic metabolism in cells.

TREATMENT OF SYSTEMIC HYPERTENSION

Morbidity and premature deaths associated with untreated hypertension are considerable (Fig. 6.4) and increase with advancing age. Therefore, treatment of older people with hypertension prevents more events in the short term than treating a similar number of younger people. However, early treatment will prevent vascular damage occurring in the younger individuals with hypertension – an important consideration since the vascular changes are not completely reversible once established.

The optimal target blood pressure in uncomplicated hypertension is a systolic blood pressure below 140 mmHg and a diastolic pressure (phase V Korotkoff sound) below 90 mmHg. When there is target organ damage or diabetes, a lower target of 130/80 mmHg is recommended, to minimise the risk of progressive vascular disease. There is no lower limit for blood pressure reduction, except in people with significant coronary artery disease. In this situation, lowering the diastolic blood pressure much below 70 mmHg may reduce coronary artery perfusion and increase the risk of myocardial infarction. Even if the target pressures cannot be achieved, any blood pressure reduction in severe hypertension will reduce the risk of complications. Treating isolated systolic hypertension (systolic >160 mmHg, diastolic <90 mmHg) in the elderly gives similar benefits to the treatment of diastolic hypertension in this age group.

It is rarely possible to correct the underlying cause of hypertension. Lifestyle modifications such as weight loss, restriction of alcohol and salt intake, and increasing exercise may be enough to lower the blood pressure satisfactorily in some individuals with mild hypertension. In people with more severe hypertension these measures can produce a substantial reduction in blood pressure but rarely restore it to normal values. It is important to advise all those with hypertension not to smoke, because smoking doubles the risk of cardiac and cerebrovascular events at any level of blood pressure.

The decision to treat hypertension with drugs should be determined largely by an assessment of the overall risk of complications in that individual. Drug treatment is usually started if blood pressure remains higher than the levels discussed above despite non-pharmacological approaches.

Drug regimens in hypertension

Lowering blood pressure by a very modest amount with drugs (even if the target levels described above are not achieved) produces a substantial ($\approx$40%) reduction in the risk of stroke, as well as reducing the risk of heart failure by 50% and reducing the incidence of renal failure. Drug treatment also reduces the risk of coronary artery disease in the elderly by about 25%; evidence for a similar reduction in the young is less convincing, but this may reflect the short duration of the trials (up to 5 years). In people with evidence of LVH, regression of left ventricular mass during treatment of hypertension will reduce cardiovascular events by 60%

compared to those in whom left ventricular mass is unchanged. ACE inhibitors, angiotensin II receptor antagonists and calcium channel blockers may be most effective in this regard.

Treatment regimens that are based on diuretics, calcium channel blockers, ACE inhibitors or angiotensin II receptor antagonists have generally shown equal efficacy in reducing vascular events. In contrast, β-adrenoceptor antagonists are less effective at preventing the complications of hypertension and are no longer recommended as first-line therapy. Treatment of hypertension should follow a 'stepped care' approach (Fig. 6.9). A single drug will achieve good blood pressure control in about one-third of people with hypertension. If the initial choice of drug fails to produce a sufficient reduction in blood pressure, then the first drug should be continued and a second drug should be added.

The British Hypertension Society has endorsed a protocol for combining blood pressure-lowering drugs, which is based on their mode of action (Fig. 6.9). The underlying principle is that younger people with hypertension are more likely to have high plasma renin concentrations, and therefore a drug that suppresses the renin–angiotensin–aldosterone system is most likely to be effective. An ACE inhibitor is usually the drug of choice, or an angiotensin II receptor antagonist if an ACE inhibitor is not tolerated. Conversely, elderly people with hypertension are more likely to have 'low renin' hypertension and a calcium channel blocker or thiazide diuretic is more likely to produce a substantial reduction in blood pressure. Use of a drug that suppresses the renin–angiotensin system creates the equivalent of a low-renin state, whereas calcium channel blockers and diuretics increase plasma renin. This provides the rationale for combination therapy with drugs from complementary

classes. The recommendations are based on the probability of achieving optimal blood pressure control and the evidence that the achieved blood pressure, rather than the means by which it was achieved, is important for improving outcome. However, the combination of an ACE inhibitor with a calcium channel blocker may be more effective at preventing cardiovascular disease than an ACE inhibitor with a thiazide diuretic. Consequently, a calcium channel blocker is preferred as the first-line treatment of older people with hypertension.

Optimal third-step therapy is an ACE inhibitor, calcium channel blocker and a thiazide or thiazide-like diuretic. Beta-adrenoceptor antagonists are only recommended as fourth-line treatment for uncomplicated hypertension. Several studies have shown that atenolol is less effective at preventing complications of hypertension than are other classes of drugs, and there is little information on outcome with other β-adrenoceptor antagonists.

Both thiazide diuretics and β-adrenoceptor antagonists increase the risk of developing new-onset diabetes, particularly when used together. This combination is not recommended for those who are at increased risk of glucose intolerance, such as people who are obese, those with a strong family history of type 2 diabetes or people of South Asian or Afro-Caribbean origin who have a higher risk of developing diabetes. In contrast, both ACE inhibitors and angiotensin II receptor antagonists reduce the risk of developing diabetes.

Resistant hypertension

If three drugs with complementary actions, taken in adequate dosage, are insufficient to control the blood pressure,

Choosing drugs for patients newly diagnosed with hypertension

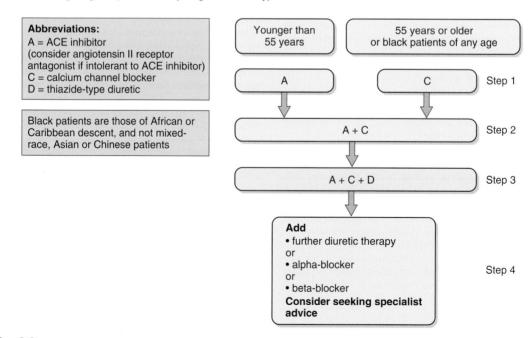

Fig. 6.9 **The British Hypertension Society recommendations for combining blood pressure-lowering drugs.** Steps 1–4 reflect hypertension severity and risk, and initial treatment is influenced by patient age and ethnic origin.

then the person is said to have 'resistant' hypertension. There are several possible causes of apparently resistant hypertension. These include:

- poor adherence to prescribed therapy (see Ch. 55),
- 'white coat' hypertension, which responds poorly to drug treatment,
- secondary hypertension, most often caused by renal artery stenosis or Conn's syndrome,
- concurrent drug use, such as a non-steroidal anti-inflammatory drug or a glucocorticoid, or excessive alcohol consumption,
- obstructive sleep apnoea,
- intravascular volume expansion, due to antihypertensive drug therapy or renal failure.

Some people with resistant hypertension benefit from treatment with a loop diuretic rather than a thiazide, which will help if expansion of the plasma volume is contributing to drug resistance. Spironolactone can be effective when added to a thiazide diuretic, especially if there is evidence of increased production of aldosterone. An α-adrenoceptor antagonist or β-adrenoceptor antagonist are further options as the fourth drug for resistant hypertension. In men, minoxidil is a particularly powerful hypotensive agent, but excess hair growth limits its use for women. In a few individuals, treatment with five or more drugs may be necessary.

Additional treatment to reduce risk of vascular complications

Hypertension should be treated as part of a strategy to tackle all factors that increase the risk of cardiovascular disease. Advice on stopping smoking is important. A statin is recommended for primary prevention of cardiovascular disease in people with hypertension and a predicted risk of cardiovascular disease greater than 20% in the subsequent 10 years, or in those with diabetes mellitus (Ch. 48).

Hypertension in special groups

There may be reasons for selecting particular classes of drugs, particularly if there are other comorbid conditions that need treatment (Table 6.3). Ethnic differences may also be important: for example, people of Afro-Caribbean origin respond less well to ACE inhibitors or angiotensin II receptor antagonists as first-line therapy than do Caucasians, since at all ages they are more likely to have low-renin hypertension.

Malignant or accelerated hypertension

Immediate treatment is important for people with hypertension who have retinal haemorrhages and exudates or papilloedema. Rapid blood pressure reduction is potentially dangerous, since autoregulation of cerebral blood flow is reset at a higher level than normal. A sudden fall in perfusion pressure can lead to a profound drop in cerebral blood flow and ischaemic cerebral damage. Intravenous drugs should usually be avoided, and oral amlodipine is the most widely recommended treatment, which gradually reduces the blood pressure over 24 h or more.

Renal artery stenosis

ACE inhibitors or angiotensin II receptor antagonists usually produce an excellent reduction in blood pressure if hypertension is caused by renal artery stenosis, but they can lead to deterioration in renal function, especially if there are bilateral stenoses. Renal artery angioplasty with insertion of a stent is not currently recommended for either preservation of renal function or blood pressure control unless the stenosis is caused by fibromuscular dysplasia. In atherosclerotic disease, embolisation of small distal arteries in the kidney during angioplasty may cause worsening of renal function.

Diabetic nephropathy

ACE inhibitors and angiotensin II receptor antagonists appear to protect the kidney more than other classes of antihypertensive drug in diabetic nephropathy. In particular, they reduce progression from microalbuminuria to overt nephropathy, and can be more effective when combined than using either drug alone. The benefit from these classes of antihypertensive drugs is probably not simply due to

Table 6.3 Selection of antihypertensive drugs for coexisting conditions

	Diuretic	β-Adrenoceptor antagonist	ACE inhibitor	Calcium channel blocker	α₁-Adrenoceptor antagonist
Angina	+/–	+	+/–	+	+/–
After myocardial infarction	+/–	+	+	–	+/–
Congestive heart failure	+	+	+	–	+/–
Diabetes mellitus (with or without nephropathy)	+/–	+/–	+	+/–	+/–
Raynaud's phenomenon	+/–	–	+	+	+
Gout	–	+/–	+/–	+/–	+/–
Prostatism	–	+/–	+/–	+/–	+
Supraventricular arrhythmias	+/–	+	+/–	+ (diltiazem or verapamil only)	+/–
Migraine	+/–	+	+/–	+/–	+/–

+, Treatment of choice; +/–, no obvious advantage/not preferred; –, usually contraindicated.

blood pressure reduction. They produce afferent glomerular artery vasodilation by inhibiting the generation or action of angiotensin II, and therefore reduce glomerular perfusion pressure. Other complications of hypertension in people with diabetes are prevented equally well by other antihypertensive drugs.

Phaeochromocytoma

Phaeochromocytoma is a catecholamine-secreting tumour, often arising from the adrenal gland. Noradrenaline-secreting tumours most often lead to sustained hypertension, through vasoconstriction mediated by α_1-adrenoceptor stimulation. Treatment should be started with an α-adrenoceptor antagonist (usually phenoxybenzamine) to prevent excessive vasoconstriction, followed by a β-adrenoceptor antagonist to block the arrhythmogenic effects of the catecholamines on the heart. Definitive treatment, whenever possible, is by surgical removal of the tumour.

Primary hyperaldosteronism

This can be caused by bilateral adrenal hyperplasia or, less commonly, by an adrenal adenoma (Conn's syndrome). The drug treatment of choice is spironolactone, to directly block the effects of aldosterone at its renal tubular receptor. If there is a tumour, surgical excision should be considered.

Pregnancy

There are two issues peculiar to pregnancy.

- **Pre-existing chronic hypertension.** The risk of hypertension to mother and fetus is probably not great until the systolic blood pressure reaches 150 mmHg, or the diastolic blood pressure reaches 95 mmHg. Treatment of blood pressure at lower levels carries a risk of impairment of fetal growth. Many antihypertensive drugs should be avoided if possible in early pregnancy because they are teratogenic, or their potential for teratogenicity is not known (Ch. 56). The drugs with the best safety record for pre-existing hypertension in women who wish to become pregnant are methyldopa, nifedipine and labetalol. In the second trimester, the risk of fetal malformations is lower, but thiazide diuretics and pure β-adrenoceptor antagonists are usually avoided because they may retard fetal growth by reducing placental blood flow. ACE inhibitors or angiotensin II receptor antagonists may cause oligohydramnios (reduced amniotic fluid production), renal failure and hypotension in the fetus, or intra-uterine death, and should be avoided at all stages of pregnancy.
- **Pre-eclampsia.** This usually occurs after 20 weeks of gestation. It presents as hypertension with oedema and proteinuria or hyperuricaemia in women whose blood pressure had previously been normal. If this condition is untreated there is a risk to the mother of convulsions, cerebral haemorrhage, abruptio placentae, pulmonary oedema and renal failure, and a risk to the fetus of severe growth retardation or even death. Once the diagnosis is established, bed rest is supplemented by antihypertensive drugs as described above for pre-existing hypertension in pregnancy. Labetalol given by intravenous infusion is favoured in severe pre-eclampsia.

PULMONARY HYPERTENSION

Pulmonary hypertension is most commonly found in people with chronic obstructive lung disease and some other lung disorders, where it arises as a result of destructive changes affecting the structure of the vascular bed. It also occurs with multiple small pulmonary emboli which silt up the peripheral pulmonary arteries and increase vascular resistance. However, some people develop increased pulmonary vascular resistance for unknown reasons (primary pulmonary hypertension, PPH), which has distinctive pathological findings of either the formation of plexiform vascular lesions or thrombotic arteriopathy. The most common presenting complaint in PPH is shortness of breath, although fatigue, chest pain, syncope, peripheral oedema and palpitation also frequently occur. The sustained increase in pulmonary vascular resistance leads to progressive right heart failure.

DRUGS FOR TREATING PULMONARY HYPERTENSION

Endothelin receptor antagonists

Example

ambrisentan, bosentan

Mechanism of action

In PPH the expression of endothelin is increased in the pulmonary vasculature. Endothelin-1 is a powerful vasoconstrictor and smooth muscle mitogen which exerts its effects via two receptors, ET_A and ET_B. ET_A receptors on vascular smooth muscle cells primarily mediate vasoconstriction and cell proliferation, while a smaller population of ET_B receptors on endothelial cells mediate vasodilation via nitric oxide release; they are also responsible for clearance of endothelin from the circulation. Bosentan is an antagonist at both endothelin ET_A and ET_B receptors, while ambrisentan is selective for ET_A receptors.

Pharmacokinetics

Ambrisentan and bosentan are metabolised in the liver.

Unwanted effects

- Gastrointestinal disturbances, including diarrhoea and gastro-oesophageal reflux.
- Vasodilator effects, including flushing, hypotension, palpitation, oedema and syncope.
- Headache.
- Drug interactions: bosentan inhibits the metabolism of warfarin by CYP2C9 with the risk of excessive anticoagulation.

Prostaglandins

Examples

epoprostenol, iloprost

Epoprostenol is naturally occurring prostacyclin (prostaglandin I_2, PGI_2) and iloprost is a synthetic PGI_2 analogue. Prostacyclin is a vasodilator that also inhibits platelet aggregation (Ch. 11), and both effects may be useful in the management of PPH. Iloprost is given by inhalation, but its short duration of action requires use every 2–3 h and it has a high incidence of flushing, headache, jaw pain and cough. Epoprostenol must be given by continuous intravenous infusion, so is only used when other treatments are ineffective.

Phosphodiesterase inhibitors

sildenafil, tadalafil

cGMP production in the pulmonary vasculature may be a protective mechanism against PPH. Oral phosphodiesterase type 5 inhibitors that inhibit breakdown of cGMP, such as sildenafil and tadalafil (Ch. 16), reduce pulmonary artery pressure, and the effects are additive to those of inhaled iloprost.

MANAGEMENT OF PULMONARY HYPERTENSION

Secondary pulmonary hypertension in chronic lung disease is most effectively managed by alleviating hypoxaemia when possible, using bronchodilators or long-term domiciliary oxygen therapy. There is no specific drug therapy. Chronic pulmonary embolic disease is treated by life-long anticoagulation, usually with warfarin.

PPH can be treated with drugs that reduce pulmonary vascular resistance. About 25% of people with PPH maintain a vasoactive pulmonary vascular bed (defined as a 20% decrease in pulmonary vascular resistance on acute challenge with a vasodilator). In this situation, treatment with a calcium channel blocker such as nifedipine will improve both symptoms and survival. However, most people with PPH show little evidence of vascular reactivity, and conventional vasodilators tend to produce excessive systemic hypotension before useful pulmonary vasodilation is achieved. For such individuals, treatment is considered with an endothelin antagonist, inhaled prostacyclin or a phosphodiesterase V inhibitor. All these drugs can improve symptoms and quality of life but have not been shown to improve survival. The role of combination therapy is under investigation.

SELF-ASSESSMENT

True/false questions

1. Stretch of baroreceptors increases the afferent impulses to the vasomotor centre, resulting in a rise in blood pressure.
2. Nifedipine lowers blood pressure principally by arterial vasodilation.
3. Moxonidine stimulates imidazoline receptors in the medulla.
4. Propranolol lowers blood pressure by peripheral vasodilation.
5. Thiazide diuretics reduce sodium and water reabsorption in the distal convoluted tubule.
6. Thiazide diuretics reduce blood pressure in the long term at doses that do not cause diuresis.
7. Thiazide diuretics are the drugs of choice for treating pregnancy-related hypertension.
8. The potassium-sparing diuretics amiloride and spironolactone have the same mechanism of action in the distal tubule and early collecting duct.
9. Selective blockade of α_1-adrenoceptors by prazosin increases noradrenaline release.
10. ACE inhibitors prevent the conversion of angiotensinogen to angiotensin I.
11. ACE inhibitors prevent the breakdown of bradykinin.
12. Minoxidil blocks K^+ channels in smooth muscle cell membranes.
13. Nitroprusside can be given for up to 3 months.
14. Phosphodiesterase type 5 inhibitors are used in primary pulmonary hypertension (PPH).
15. Ambrisentan selectively blocks pulmonary vasoconstriction mediated by endothelin ET_A receptors.

One-best-answer (OBA) question

Which of the following statements about antihypertensive drugs is the *least accurate*?

A. Thiazide diuretics increase the risk of diabetes mellitus.
B. β-Adrenoceptor antagonists are first-line therapy for hypertension.
C. Blood pressure is not always lowered adequately by a single drug.
D. Angiotensin II receptor antagonists selectively block angiotensin AT_1 receptors.
E. Nifedipine is more likely to cause reflex tachycardia than verapamil.

Extended-matching-item question

1. Choose which of the following drug classes A–D would be *good* choices for initial treatment of the people newly diagnosed with hypertension in the scenarios 1.1–1.3 below. Each drug may be selected once, more than once or never.
   A. An ACE inhibitor or angiotensin II receptor antagonist
   B. A non-selective β-adrenoceptor antagonist
   C. A calcium channel blocker
   D. A thiazide diuretic
   1.1. A black, clinically obese male aged 75 years with a blood pressure of 150/100 mmHg and no other pathology
   1.2. A white female aged 40 years with type 1 diabetes mellitus and a blood pressure of 150/100 mmHg
   1.3. A woman 24 weeks pregnant with pre-existing chronic hypertension and a blood pressure of 150/100 mmHg

Case-based question

Mr AT, a 60-year-old man with type 2 diabetes mellitus, smoked 20 cigarettes a day. His plasma lipid levels were normal and there was no proteinuria. His ECG was normal. His height was 1.70 m and his weight 95.5 kg. He had no evidence of fluid retention or heart failure. Following treatment with a calcium channel blocker, his blood pressure was reduced from 175/110 mmHg but he remained hypertensive (155/95 mmHg) and he then had a small myocardial infarction. What changes in his therapy would you consider?

True/false answers

1. **False.** Baroreceptor impulses to the vasomotor centre reduce sympathetic outflow, enhance vagal outflow and lower blood pressure.
2. **True.** Calcium channel blockers act by opening L-type voltage-gated Ca^{2+} channels, and nifedipine, a dihydropyridine, is relatively selective for these channels in arterial smooth muscle. The non-dihydropyridines verapamil and diltiazem have additional cardiodepressant properties.
3. **True.** Moxonidine selectively stimulates imidazoline I_1 receptors in the ventrolateral medulla; this decreases sympathetic outflow and increases vagal outflow, hence reducing blood pressure.
4. **False.** Propranolol lowers blood pressure by reducing cardiac output and by reducing renin production, but only β_1-adrenoceptor antagonists with partial agonist activity at β_2-adrenoceptors (such as pindolol) or those drugs with other hybrid properties (such as nebivolol) produce peripheral vasodilation.
5. **True.** All diuretics reduce sodium and water reabsorption in the renal tubule; thiazides act at the Na^+/Cl^- co-transporter (NCC) in the distal convoluted tubule.
6. **True.** The initial blood-lowering effect of thiazides is due to diuresis, but in the longer term they cause vasodilation by an unknown mechanism even at low doses.
7. **False.** Thiazide diuretics cause fetal growth retardation by reducing plasma volume and placental blood flow; methyldopa, nifedipine and labetalol are most often used in pregnancy.
8. **False.** Spironolactone competes with aldosterone for the mineralocorticoid receptor (MR), blocking its stimulation of the Na^+/K^+-ATPase pump and increased expression of the epithelial Na^+ channel (ENaC); this reduces uptake of Na^+ and loss of K^+ from the tubule. Amiloride, however, directly blocks ENaC (see Ch. 14).
9. **False.** Prazosin dilates blood vessels by its selective blockade of α_1-adrenoceptors; it does not block the presynaptic α_2-adrenoceptors, and stimulation of these receptors to limit further noradrenaline release can still take place.
10. **False.** Angiotensinogen is converted to angiotensin I by renin. ACE effects the subsequent conversion of angiotensin I to angiotensin II.
11. **True.** ACE inhibitors reduce the breakdown of bradykinin, a potent vasodilator, and this action may contribute to their antihypertensive effects.
12. **False.** Minoxidil is a potassium channel (K_{ATP}) opener; it causes an efflux of K^+ ions resulting in hyperpolarisation of arterial smooth muscle cells and vasodilation.
13. **False.** Nitroprusside is converted to cyanide and then to thiocyanate. The toxicity of these limits its use to 3 days for emergency management of some hypertensive states.
14. **True.** PPH is often associated with poor vascular reactivity, but vasodilation can be achieved by endothelin antagonists, phosphodiesterase type 5 inhibitors or prostacyclin.
15. **True.** Ambrisentan selectively blocks vasoconstriction mediated by ET_A receptors; endothelial ET_B receptors which mediate vasodilation via nitric oxide are unaffected.

OBA answer

Answer B is the least accurate.

A. True. Thiazides increase the risk of new-onset diabetes, particularly when combined with β-adrenoceptor antagonists.
B. **False.** β-Adrenoceptor antagonists are now fourth-line therapy in the British Hypertension Society guidelines, as they are less effective in reducing the risk of myocardial infarction and stroke than the other antihypertensive drugs.
C. True. Satisfactory lowering of blood pressure is achieved with a single drug in only 30–40% of people with hypertension.
D. True. Angiotensin II receptor antagonists block the vasoconstrictor and aldosterone secretory actions of angiotensin II at AT_1 receptors; AT_2 receptors are involved in vascular growth and are less affected by these drugs.
E. True. Nifedipine selective dilates arterioles and may cause reflex tachycardia; this is unlikely with verapamil, which has negative chronotropic activity.

Extended-matching-item answers

1.1. **Answer C** (a calcium channel blocker) would be a good choice in this 75-year-old black male. The elderly and black people usually have low plasma renin concentrations, so an ACE inhibitor or angiotensin II receptor antagonist would be less effective. A thiazide diuretic or a β-adrenoceptor antagonist might increase the risk of diabetes in this obese man.
1.2. **Answer A** (an ACE inhibitor or, if poorly tolerated, an angiotensin II receptor antagonist) would be a good choice in a 40-year-old white female. A thiazide diuretic or a β-adrenoceptor antagonist may exacerbate the diabetes.
1.3. **Answer C** (a calcium channel blocker) would be an appropriate first choice in a pregnant woman with pre-existing hypertension. All the other drugs can cause unwanted effects on the fetus.

Case-based answer

Mr AT's blood pressure has not reached the target level (140/90 mmHg) and he has had a myocardial infarction. His blood pressure may be reduced further by introducing an ACE inhibitor. ACE inhibitors improve survival after a myocardial infarction, especially when there is left ventricular impairment. ACE inhibitors also protect the kidney in diabetic nephropathy and could be considered in this situation. The addition of a β-adrenoceptor antagonist could also be considered for additional long-term prognostic benefit, particularly if there is left ventricular impairment.

FURTHER READING

Systemic hypertension

August P (2003) Initial treatment of hypertension. *N Engl J Med* 348, 610–617

Blood Pressure Lowering Treatment Trialists' Collaboration (2003) Effects of different blood pressure lowering regimens on major cardiovascular events: second cycle of prospectively designed overviews. *Lancet* 362, 1527–1535

Blood Pressure Lowering Treatment Trialists' Collaboration (2008) Effects of different regimens to lower blood pressure on major cardiovascular events in older and younger people: meta-analysis of randomised trials. *BMJ* 336, 1121–1123

Chiong JR, Aronow WS, Khan IA et al. (2008) Secondary hypertension: current diagnosis and treatment. *Int J Cardiol* 124, 6–21

Ernst ME, Moser M (2009) Use of diuretics in patients with hypertension. *N Engl J Med* 361, 2153–2164

Ferrario C, Levy P (2002) Sexual dysfunction in patients with hypertension: implications for therapy. *J Clin Hypertens* 4, 424–432

Grossman E, Messerli FH (2011) Drug-induced hypertension: an uanappreciated cause of secondary hypertension. *Am J Med* 125, 14–22

Kaplan N, Opie LH (2006) Controversies in hypertension. *Lancet* 367, 168–176

Moser M, Setaro JF (2006) Resistant or difficult-to-control hypertension. *N Engl J Med* 355, 385–392

Moser M, Feig PU (2009) Fifty years of thiazide diuretic therapy for hypertension. *Arch Intern Med* 169, 1851–1856

Ong HT (2007) β blockers in hypertension and cardiovascular disease. *BMJ* 334, 946–949

Oparil S, Zaman A, Calhoun DA (2003) Pathogenesis of hypertension. *Ann Intern Med* 139, 761–776

Shah SJ (2012) Pulmonary hypertension. *JAMA* 308, 1366–1374

Snow V, Weiss KB, Mottur-Pilson C et al. (2004) The evidence base for tight blood pressure control in the management of type 2 diabetic mellitus. *Ann Intern Med* 138, 587–592

Sowers JR (2004) Treatment of hypertension in patients with diabetes. *Arch Intern Med* 164, 1850–1857

Staessen JA, Wang J, Bianchi G et al. (2003) Essential hypertension. *Lancet* 361, 1629–1641

Vijan S, Hayward RA (2003) Treatment of hypertension in type 2 diabetes mellitus: blood pressure goals, choice of agents, and setting priorities in diabetes. *Ann Intern Med* 138, 593–602

Williams B (2005) Recent hypertension trials: implications and controversies. *J Am Coll Cardiol* 45, 813–827

Yoder SR, Thomberg LL, Bisognano JD (2009) Hypertension in pregnancy and women of childbearing age. *Am J Med* 122, 890–895

Pulmonary hypertension

Agarwal R, Gomberg-Maitland M (2011) Current therapeutics and practical management strategies for pulmonary arterial hypertension. *Am J Med* 162, 201–213

Archer SL, Michelakis ED (2009) Phosphodiesterase type 5 inhibitors for pulmonary arterial hypertension. *N Engl J Med* 361, 1864–1871

Badesh DB, Abman SH, Simmonneau G et al. (2007) Medical therapy for pulmonary arterial hypertension. *Chest* 131, 1917–1928

Macchia A, Marchioli R, Marfisi RM et al. (2007) A meta-analysis of pulmonary hypertension: a clinical condition looking for drugs and research methodology. *Am Heart J* 153, 1037–1047

McLaughlin VV, McGoon MD (2006) Pulmonary arterial hypertension. *Circulation* 114, 1417–1431

Rich S (2006) The current treatment of pulmonary arterial hypertension: time to redefine success. *Chest* 130, 1198–1202

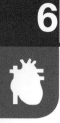

Compendium: drugs used to treat hypertension

Drug	Kinetics (half-life)	Comments
β-Adrenoceptor antagonists		
All β-adrenoceptor antagonists (except esmolol and sotalol) are used for hypertension; see Ch. 5 for individual drugs.		
Calcium channel blockers		
All calcium channel blockers (except nimodipine) are used for treatment of hypertension; see Ch. 5 for individual drugs.		
Diuretics		
Diuretics can be used to lower blood pressure; see Ch. 14 for individual drugs.		
α_1-Selective adrenoceptor antagonists		
All drugs are given orally		
Doxazosin	Oral bioavailability 65% due to incomplete absorption; hepatic metabolism (9–12 h)	Used for hypertension and benign prostatic hyperplasia
Indoramin	Oral bioavailability 10–25%; hepatic metabolism (5 h)	Used for hypertension and benign prostatic hyperplasia
Prazosin	Oral bioavailability 60% due to first-pass metabolism; hepatic metabolism (2–3 h)	Used for hypertension, congestive heart failure, Raynaud's phenomenon and benign prostatic hyperplasia
Terazosin	Oral bioavailability >90%; mainly eliminated by hepatic metabolism (12 h)	Used for hypertension and benign prostatic hyperplasia
Non-selective α-adrenoceptor antagonists		
Used in phaeochromocytoma only.		
Phenoxybenzamine	Low oral bioavailability (20–30%); hepatic metabolism (24 h)	Used for hypertensive episodes associated with phaeochromocytoma; given orally or by intravenous infusion
Phentolamine	Eliminated by metabolism and renal excretion (1.5 h)	Used for diagnosis and hypertensive episodes in phaeochromocytoma; given by intravenous injection
Angiotensin-converting enzyme (ACE) inhibitors		
These drugs are used for hypertension, heart failure, prophylaxis of ischaemic heart disease and diabetic nephropathy. All are given orally; many are prodrugs that undergo bioactivation by hepatic metabolism.		
Captopril	Good absorption (70–80%) with limited first-pass metabolism (10%); renal elimination (2 h)	Parent drug is active
Cilazapril	Prodrug is well absorbed (60%) and converted in liver to cilazaprilat, which is eliminated by the kidney (30 h)	
Enalapril	Prodrug is well absorbed (60%) and converted in liver to enalaprilat, which is eliminated by the kidney (35 h)	
Fosinopril	Poorly absorbed prodrug of which about 30% is converted in the intestine and liver to fosinoprilat; which is eliminated by the kidney and in faeces (12 h)	
Imidapril	Prodrug is well absorbed and rapidly hydrolysed to imidaprilat, which is eliminated by the kidney (8 h)	
Lisinopril	Incompletely absorbed from gut; renal elimination and in faeces (12 h)	Parent drug is active
Moexipril	Poorly absorbed prodrug converted in liver to moexiprilat; 50% excreted in faeces (10 h)	
Perindopril	Well-absorbed prodrug; about 20% is converted in liver to perindoprilat, which is eliminated by the kidney (29 h)	

Compendium: drugs used to treat hypertension—cont'd

Drug	Kinetics (half-life)	Comments
Quinapril	Well-absorbed prodrug converted in liver to quinaprilat, which is eliminated by renal tubular secretion (2 h)	
Ramipril	Well-absorbed prodrug converted in liver to ramiprilat, which is eliminated by the kidney (1–5 h)	
Trandolapril	Well-absorbed prodrug converted in liver to trandolaprilat and inactive metabolites; eliminated by the kidney and by hepatic metabolism (16–24 h)	

Angiotensin II receptor (AT$_1$) antagonists

Used for hypertension, heart failure, prophylaxis after myocardial infarction and diabetic nephropathy. All drugs are given orally.

Drug	Kinetics (half-life)	Comments
Candesartan	Given as prodrug (candesartan cilexetil) and rapidly hydrolysed during absorption to active candesartan; renal elimination and in faeces (9–12 h)	Highly selective blockade of AT$_1$ receptors
Eprosartan	Rapidly absorbed but with a low bioavailability (13%); renal elimination (5–9 h)	
Irbesartan	Oral bioavailability 60–80%; parent drug and hepatic metabolites eliminated by the kidney and in bile (11–15 h)	Highly selective blockade at AT$_1$ receptors
Losartan	Extensive (50%) first-pass metabolism to inactive products plus an active metabolite (6 h)	Highly selective competitive AT$_1$ receptor antagonist; active metabolite is non-competitive AT$_1$ antagonist
Olmesartan	Prodrug (olmesartan medoxomil) rapidly converted to olmesartan in gastrointestinal tract; renal elimination and in bile (13 h)	
Telmisartan	Good oral bioavailability (50%); eliminated in faeces (16–23 h)	Highly selective blockade at AT$_1$ receptors
Valsartan	Oral bioavailability 25%; eliminated by hepatic metabolism (5–7 h)	Highly selective blockade at AT$_1$ receptors

Direct renin inhibitors

Drug	Kinetics (half-life)	Comments
Aliskiren	Oral bioavailability only 3%; faecal elimination (40 h)	Non-peptide inhibitor; given orally

Endothelin receptor antagonists

Used for pulmonary arterial hypertension.

Drug	Kinetics (half-life)	Comments
Ambrisentan	Extensive hepatic metabolism and biliary excretion (13–16 h)	Selective antagonist of endothelin ET$_A$ receptors; given orally
Bosentan	Bioavailability 50%; induces its own metabolism by hepatic CYP2C9 and CYP3A4; biliary elimination (5 h)	Endothelin ET$_A$ and ET$_B$ receptor antagonist; given orally

Potassium channel openers

Drug	Kinetics (half-life)	Comments
Minoxidil	Complete oral bioavailability; mainly hepatic metabolism and eliminated as glucuronide conjugate (3–4 h)	Used for severe hypertension; given orally

Vasodilators

Drugs used under special circumstances.

Drug	Kinetics (half-life)	Comments
Diazoxide	Eliminated largely by the kidney; long half-life due to high protein binding (28 h)	Given in hypertensive emergencies by intravenous bolus injection

Compendium: drugs used to treat hypertension—cont'd

Drug	Kinetics (half-life)	Comments
Hydralazine	Undergoes first-pass metabolism by N-acetylation with a bioavailability of 10–15% in fast acetylators and 30–35% in slow acetylators (2–4 h)	Used as an adjunct for moderate or severe hypertension, for heart failure and for hypertensive crisis; given orally, by slow intravenous injection or by intravenous infusion
Iloprost	Eliminated by hepatic metabolism (20–30 min)	Prostacyclin analogue used for pulmonary arterial hypertension; given by nebuliser; see also epoprostenol, Ch. 11
Sodium nitroprusside	Decomposes in seconds to active NO and to cyanide, which is eliminated largely in the urine as thiocyanate	Short-lived clinical response; used for hypertensive crisis, for controlled hypotension in anaesthesia and for acute heart failure

Centrally acting antihypertensive drugs

Drug	Kinetics (half-life)	Comments
Clonidine	Oral bioavailability >70%; renal elimination (20–25 h)	Selective α_2-adrenoceptor agonist; used for hypertension, migraine and menopausal flushing; given orally or by slow intravenous injection; sudden withdrawal may give hypertensive crisis
Methyldopa	Variable oral bioavailability (10–60%) due to sulphate conjugation in the intestinal wall; eliminated by hepatic metabolism and by the kidney (1–2 h)	Selective α_2-adrenoceptor agonist; used particularly for hypertension in pregnancy; given orally
Moxonidine	Oral bioavailability about 90%; renal elimination (2–3 h)	Selective imidazoline I_1 receptor agonist; given orally
Guanethidine	Eliminated largely by the kidney (2 days)	Adrenergic neuron blocker; used only for hypertensive crisis; given by intramuscular injection

7 Heart failure

There is no universally accepted definition of heart failure. The heart failure syndrome is usually said to exist when there is inadequate oxygen delivery to peripheral tissues, either at rest or during exercise, due to dysfunction of the heart or when adequate oxygen delivery can only be maintained with an elevated left ventricular filling pressure.

MAINTENANCE OF CARDIAC OUTPUT

There are four major determinants of cardiac output:

- **preload**: this is governed by the ventricular end-diastolic volume, which in turn is related to ventricular filling pressure and therefore to venous return of blood to the heart,
- **heart rate**,
- **myocardial contractility**,
- **afterload**: the systolic wall tension in the ventricle; this reflects the resistance to ventricular emptying within both the heart (during isovolumic contraction) and the peripheral circulation.

The output from both right and left sides of the heart is normally balanced. In the healthy heart, cardiac output is regulated mainly by changes in heart rate and preload.

Heart rate is modulated by the autonomic nervous system, with sympathetic nervous stimulation increasing heart rate and parasympathetic stimulation via the vagus nerve slowing the rate.

The relationship between preload and stroke volume (the amount of blood ejected from the ventricle during systole with each contraction) is shown in Figure 7.1. The degree of stretch of the ventricular muscle (preload) determines the force of cardiac contraction (the Frank–Starling phenomenon). The curve describing this relationship is governed by intrinsic myocardial contractility: thus, the curve is shifted upwards and to the left when contractility is augmented, for example by sympathetic nervous stimulation. In a healthy heart with normal myocardial contractility, the left ventricular filling pressure lies on the steep part of the curve, making stroke volume very sensitive to small changes in preload.

The relationship between afterload and stroke volume is shown in Figure 7.2. Afterload is determined largely by peripheral resistance but also by the size of the ventricle. Enlargement of the left ventricular cavity (e.g. as a result of increased venous return or preload) increases wall tension, and the heart must generate greater pressure both to initiate and to maintain contraction. Preload and afterload are therefore interrelated. In the healthy ventricle a rise in afterload will cause a fall in stroke volume, but the consequent sympathetic stimulation will increase myocardial contractility and maintain stroke volume.

PATHOPHYSIOLOGY OF HEART FAILURE

Heart failure is a syndrome that has several underlying causes (Box 7.1). Occasionally it arises suddenly such as after acute myocardial infarction or acute mitral regurgitation from rupture of the chordae tendineae. More commonly the onset is gradual from progressive loss of myocardial function or slow degenerative change in valve function.

The underlying problem in heart failure is reduced cardiac output and therefore low blood pressure, but the syndrome of heart failure arises largely from neurohumoral counter-regulation in response to low blood pressure and reduced renal perfusion. This is principally due to the sympathetic nervous system and the renin–angiotensin–aldosterone system (Fig. 7.3). The consequences of these compensatory mechanisms are vasoconstriction of both arteries and veins and excessive salt and water retention by the kidneys. Although these are the normal physiological responses to reduced blood pressure, in the setting of a failing heart they can create additional problems.

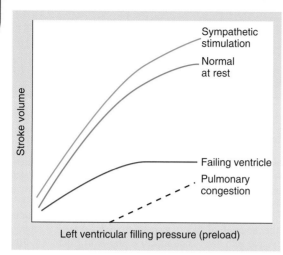

Fig. 7.1 The Frank–Starling relationship between preload (left ventricular filling pressure) and stroke volume in healthy and failing hearts. In the severely failing heart, increases in filling pressure and heart rate are insufficient to restore cardiac output, and pulmonary congestion will occur.

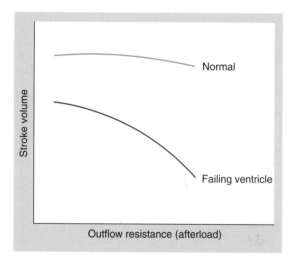

Fig. 7.2 The relationship between afterload (outflow resistance) and stroke volume in the presence of normal and reduced myocardial contractility. Sympathetic stimulation maintains the stroke volume of the normal heart against an increasing afterload, but not in the failing heart.

In the failing ventricle, the Frank–Starling curve is shifted downwards and to the right (failing-ventricle curve, Fig. 7.1) and the maximum achievable stroke volume is reduced. The curve is also flatter, indicating that stroke volume has become less responsive to changes in preload. As a result of activation of the compensatory mechanisms, salt and water retention expands plasma volume and venoconstriction enhances venous return to the heart. These factors increase the filling pressure of the left ventricle in an attempt to restore the resting stroke volume. Heart rate will also increase, which will raise cardiac output despite a lower

| Box 7.1 | Causes of heart failure |

Coronary artery disease
Hypertension
Myocardial disease: cardiomyopathies, myocarditis
Valvular heart disease
Constrictive pericarditis
Congenital: atrial septal defect, ventricular septal defect, aortic coarctation
Infiltrative: amyloid, sarcoid, iron
Iatrogenic: β-adrenoceptor antagonists (high doses), anti-arrhythmics, calcium channel blockers, cytotoxics, alcohol, irradiation
Arrhythmias, especially incessant tachyarrhythmias

stroke volume. If these responses are successful in restoring a normal resting cardiac output the heart failure is said to be *compensated.* However, the cardiac output may be unable to rise to meet the needs of the body during exertion.

Decompensation occurs when the combination of the increases in preload and heart rate fail to restore a normal resting cardiac output (Fig. 7.3). A persistent high level of symapathetic tone results in downregulation of β_1-adrenoceptors and therefore less ability to maintain cardiac output. In most cases of heart failure, the impairment of function initially affects the left ventricle. As the central blood volume continues to increase in an attempt to raise the stroke volume, the hydrostatic pressure in the pulmonary veins will rise. When the hydrostatic pressure in the pulmonary circulation exceeds the plasma colloid osmotic (oncotic) pressure that holds fluid in the blood vessel, fluid leaves the capillaries into the interstitium of the alveoli and then into the alveolar spaces, producing pulmonary oedema (Fig. 7.2). Eventually, the raised pulmonary vascular pressure leads to right heart failure (producing biventricular failure, or congestive cardiac failure), and oedema develops in the peripheral and splanchnic tissues.

Peripheral arterial resistance (afterload) will also rise as a result of the compensatory mechanisms (Fig. 7.2). The failing ventricle cannot meet this with an increase in myocardial contractility so stroke volume will fall (Fig. 7.2) with further cardiac decompensation.

Heart failure arising from myocyte loss (such as occurs with myocardial infarction or cardiomyopathies) leads to adaptive changes in the surviving cells and extracellular matrix, known as remodelling. Remodelling is driven by several factors including local effects of catecholamines, angiotensin II, aldosterone and pro-inflammatory cytokines. This eventually produces a more globular, dysfunctional left ventricle. This type of heart failure is characterized by a reduced ejection fraction (heart failure with reduced ejection fraction or systolic heart failure).

In aortic or mitral valve regurgitation, heart failure arises because the left ventricle must accommodate the normal forward stroke volume and also the regurgitant volume (the volume leaking back into the left ventricle or left atrium respectively). Eventually, the left ventricle cannot enlarge sufficiently to maintain an effective stroke volume.

Heart failure can also arise from impaired diastolic relaxation even when contractile function in systole is normal. Stroke volume is reduced, but ejection fraction is normal. This is known as heart failure with preserved ejection

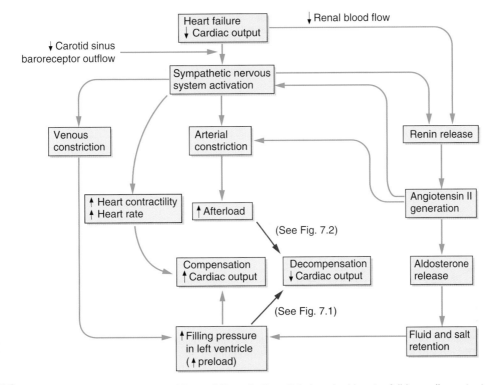

Fig. 7.3 Neurohumoral consequences of heart failure. In the mildly impaired heart a fall in cardiac output results in a cascade of compensatory events (green arrows), including sympathetic stimulation of heart rate and contractility, constriction of arteries and veins, and activation of the renin–angiotensin–aldosterone system; overall these compensatory mechanisms restore cardiac output. If cardiac function is significantly impaired (red arrows), an increased preload cannot restore an adequate stroke volume (decompensation) (see Fig. 7.1) and the increased afterload will put additional strain on the failing heart and further decrease cardiac output (see Fig. 7.2). In chronic heart failure these effects are compounded by cardiac remodelling and downregulation of cardiac β_1-adrenoceptors.

fraction or diastolic heart failure. If the left ventricle fails to relax adequately, it will not accommodate the venous return, leading to pulmonary venous congestion and a low cardiac output, activating the same compensatory neurohumoral responses. Heart failure with preserved ejection fraction characteristically occurs in older people in association with left ventricular hypertrophy, but it also contributes to heart failure in ischaemic left ventricular dysfunction (see Ch. 5).

Symptoms in heart failure are caused by a reduced cardiac output ('forward failure') or venous congestion ('backward failure'). The most common complaints are breathlessness from increased pulmonary venous pressure, and fatigue resulting from the reduced cardiac output and impaired skeletal muscle perfusion. In response to the reduced perfusion, biochemical changes also occur in skeletal muscle, making it less efficient. Other symptoms, such as the discomfort of peripheral oedema and anorexia due to bowel congestion, are attributable to a high systemic venous pressure. Increased stimulation of β-adrenoceptors in the heart can lead to life-threatening ventricular arrhythmias.

ACUTE LEFT VENTRICULAR FAILURE

Acute left ventricular failure usually results from a sudden inability of the heart to maintain an adequate cardiac output

and blood pressure. It can follow acute myocardial infarction, acute mitral or aortic valvular regurgitation, or arise from the onset of a brady- or tachyarrhythmia if there is pre-existing poor left ventricular function. The sudden fall in cardiac output leads to reflex arterial and venous constriction (Fig. 7.3). There is a rapid rise in filling pressure of the left ventricle as a result of increased venous return. If the heart is unable to expel the extra blood, the hydrostatic pressure in the pulmonary veins rises until it exceeds the plasma oncotic pressure and produces acute pulmonary oedema. The principal symptom is breathlessness, usually at rest with orthopnoea.

CARDIOGENIC SHOCK

The syndrome of cardiogenic shock arises when the systolic function of the left ventricle is suddenly impaired to such a degree that there is insufficient blood flow to meet resting metabolic requirements of the tissues. This definition excludes shock caused by hypovolaemia. The clinical hallmarks are a low systolic blood pressure (usually <90 mmHg), with a reduced cardiac output and an elevated left ventricular filling pressure. Cardiogenic shock can follow acute myocardial infarction, and in this situation usually indicates loss of at least 40% of the left ventricular myocardium. Other mechanical disturbances, such as

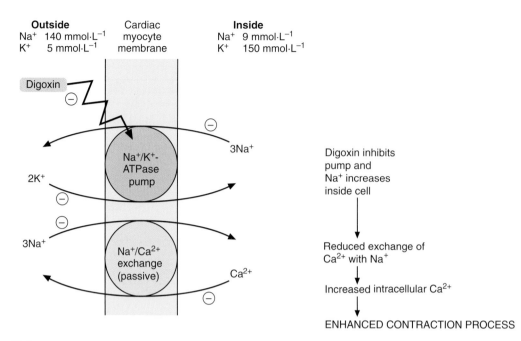

Outside
Na⁺ 140 mmol·L⁻¹
K⁺ 5 mmol·L⁻¹

Cardiac
myocyte
membrane

Inside
Na⁺ 9 mmol·L⁻¹
K⁺ 150 mmol·L⁻¹

Digoxin

Na⁺/K⁺-
ATPase
pump

3Na⁺

2K⁺

3Na⁺

Na⁺/Ca²⁺
exchange
(passive)

Ca²⁺

Digoxin inhibits
pump and
Na⁺ increases
inside cell

↓

Reduced exchange of
Ca²⁺ with Na⁺

↓

Increased intracellular Ca²⁺

↓

ENHANCED CONTRACTION PROCESS

Fig. 7.4 The action of digoxin on the cardiac myocyte. Digoxin increases intracellular Na⁺ by inhibiting the Na⁺/ K⁺-ATPase. This reduces the Na⁺ gradient for the passive export of Ca²⁺, resulting in increased intracellular Ca²⁺ and enhanced contractile responses.

acute mitral regurgitation or ventricular septal rupture, can produce cardiogenic shock in association with a lesser degree of myocardial damage. Less commonly, the syndrome is associated with right ventricular infarction. The mortality of cardiogenic shock, even with intensive treatment, is in excess of 70%.

CHRONIC HEART FAILURE

Myocardial damage from ischaemic heart disease is the most common cause of chronic heart failure, but potentially correctable causes such as valvular lesions, as well as treatable exacerbating factors such as anaemia or arrhythmias, may be identified. In most people with heart failure there are signs of both right and left ventricular failure (biventricular or congestive heart failure). Chronic heart failure is not a trivial complaint. People with left ventricular systolic dysfunction who have symptoms only on exertion have a 2-year mortality risk of about 20%, whereas the 1-year mortality is 80% if there are symptoms at rest. In heart failure with reduced ejection fraction the degree of left ventricular dysfunction is a guide to prognosis. Death is from either progressive heart failure or ventricular arrhythmias.

POSITIVE INOTROPIC DRUGS IN THE TREATMENT OF HEART FAILURE

Myocardial contractility can be improved by increasing the availability of free intracellular Ca²⁺ to interact with contractile proteins, or by increasing the sensitivity of the myofibrils

to Ca²⁺. Only drugs that increase myocardial intracellular Ca²⁺ are established in clinical use; they work by one of two distinct mechanisms:

■ an action on the cell membrane Na⁺/K⁺-ATPase pump (e.g. digitalis glycosides),
■ by increasing intracellular cAMP (e.g. sympathomimetic inotropes, phosphodiesterase inhibitors).

An additional advantage of the positive inotropic drugs that increase myocardial cAMP is their ability to enhance the reuptake of Ca²⁺ by the sarcoplasmic reticulum in diastole. This improves diastolic relaxation in addition to augmenting systolic contractility.

DIGITALIS GLYCOSIDES

Example

digoxin

Mechanism of action and effects

Effect on myocardial contractility

Digitalis glycosides are compounds with a steroid nucleus that were originally isolated from a species of foxglove (*Digitalis purpura*). Digoxin is the drug that is most widely used in clinical practice. Digoxin binds to the energy-dependent Na⁺ pump (Na⁺/K⁺-ATPase) in the myocyte membrane. This pump establishes and maintains the Na⁺ and K⁺ gradients across the cell (Fig. 7.4), producing low intracellular Na⁺ and high intracellular K⁺ concentrations. A separate passive transmembrane exchange of Na⁺ and Ca²⁺

occurs down their concentration gradients, with Na^+ entering the cell while Ca^{2+} is translocated out. The rate of this exchange is dependent on the intracellular Na^+ concentration. Digoxin partially inhibits the Na^+/K^+-ATPase, which increases the intracellular Na^+ concentration. This lowers the concentration gradient for Na^+ across the cell membrane, which in turn reduces the Na^+/Ca^{2+} exchange so that Ca^{2+} is retained in the cell. The excess intracellular Ca^{2+} is stored in the sarcoplasmic reticulum during diastole and released during cell membrane excitation, leading to enhanced myocardial contraction.

Effects on cardiac action potential and intracardiac conduction

Digoxin can be arrhythmogenic, but also has actions that are useful for treating certain arrhythmias.

Direct actions of digoxin on the heart can provoke arrhythmias by increasing myocardial cell excitability (Ch. 8), as follows.

- **Reduction of the resting membrane potential.** The cell membrane Na^+/K^+-ATPase pump extrudes three Na^+ out of the cell for every two K^+ that enter, which increases the negative intracellular electrical potential and hyperpolarises the cell, making it less excitable (see Ch. 8). Inhibition of this membrane pump by digoxin leads to the cell membrane potential becoming less negative and closer to the threshold potential for depolarisation. Arrhythmias are therefore more readily initiated.
- **Triggering of spontaneous release of Ca^{2+} from the sarcoplasmic reticulum.** This leads to transient depolarisation of the cell immediately following an action potential ('after-potentials'), which can initiate arrhythmias (Ch. 8).

Digoxin also has useful indirect actions on the heart that arise from stimulation of the central vagal nucleus and enable it to be used for treating arrhythmias (Ch. 8). The vagal effects on the heart are:

- **decreased automaticity of the sinoatrial node** which slightly slows heart rate in sinus rhythm,
- **increased refractory period of the atrioventricular node**, which slows impulse transmission to the ventricles and is useful in the management of the fast ventricular rates that result from atrial flutter and fibrillation (Ch. 8).

Pharmacokinetics

Digoxin is well absorbed from the gut and the kidney is the main route of elimination, by filtration at the glomerulus and by active tubular secretion. The half-life of digoxin is very long (about 1.5 days) and is increased if renal function is impaired. The dose must be reduced in the presence of renal impairment to avoid toxicity (see below). If an early onset of action is required, loading doses should be given over the first 24 or 36 h (Ch. 2). If a rapid response is essential, digoxin can be given by slow intravenous injection.

Unwanted effects

Digitalis glycosides have a narrow therapeutic index, and toxicity is mostly dose-related.

- **Gastrointestinal disturbances**: anorexia, nausea and vomiting (largely a central effect at the chemoreceptor trigger zone; Ch. 32), and diarrhoea.
- **Neurological disturbances**: fatigue, malaise, confusion, vertigo, coloured vision (especially yellow halos around lights, possibly from inhibition of Na^+/K^+-ATPase in the cones of the retina).
- **Distinctive changes on the ECG**: this includes non-specific T-wave changes and sagging of the S–T segment with an upright T-wave ('reverse tick') often referred to as 'digoxin effect'. These ECG effects do not indicate toxicity, but can be mistaken for myocardial ischaemia.
- **Consequences of intracellular Ca^{2+} overload**: increased excitability of the atrioventricular node and Purkinje fibres produces atrial or nodal ectopic beats, atrial or nodal tachycardia, ventricular ectopic beats or (less commonly) ventricular tachycardia.
- **Consequences of increased vagal activity**: excessive atrioventricular nodal block ('heart block') can occur. When associated with increased atrial excitability, this produces atrial tachycardia with atrioventricular nodal block, a rhythm characteristic of digitalis toxicity.
- **Gynaecomastia**: during long-term treatment the steroid structure allows digitalis glycosides to bind to, and stimulate oestrogen receptors in breast tissue.

Exacerbating factors for digitalis glycoside toxicity

- **Hypokalaemia**: reduced extracellular K^+ concentration increases the effects of digitalis glycosides on the Na^+/K^+-ATPase pump. Care must be taken if potassium-losing diuretics, such as furosemide (Ch. 14), are used with digitalis glycosides.
- **Renal impairment**: reduces the excretion of digoxin.
- **Hypoxaemia**: this sensitises the heart to digitalis glycoside-induced arrhythmias.
- **Hypothyroidism**: the renal elimination of digoxin is decreased because of a reduced glomerular filtration rate.
- **Drugs that displace digoxin from tissue binding sites and interfere with its renal excretion**: these include verapamil (Ch. 5) and quinidine (Ch. 8), which can double the plasma concentration of digoxin. Amiodarone (Ch. 8) produces a less marked effect.

Treatment of digitalis toxicity

Digitalis glycoside toxicity can be treated by:

- withholding further doses of digitalis glycoside,
- using K^+ supplementation (Ch. 14) for hypokalaemia. This is usually given orally, but should be given by slow intravenous infusion if there are dangerous arrhythmias,
- using atropine (Ch. 8) for sinus bradycardia or atrioventricular block. Temporary transvenous pacing is used for marked bradycardia unresponsive to atropine,
- digoxin-specific antibody fragments for serious digoxin toxicity (Ch. 53).

SYMPATHOMIMETIC INOTROPES

Examples

selective β$_1$-adrenoceptor agonist: dobutamine
selective β$_2$-adrenoceptor agonist and dopamine receptor
   agonist: dopexamine
non-selective β-adrenoceptor, α-adrenoceptor and
   dopamine receptor agonist: dopamine

Mechanisms of action and effects

The mechanisms of action of the inotropic sympathomimetic drugs are also considered in Chapter 4. Noradrenaline and adrenaline are not used for their inotropic action because they produce marked vasoconstriction through effects on α-adrenoceptors.

Isoprenaline is a non-selective β-adrenoceptor agonist that is now only available in the UK on special order. It is sometimes used to increase heart rate in the emergency treatment of bradycardias through its action on both β$_1$- and β$_2$-adrenoceptors (Ch. 8). *Dobutamine*, a synthetic dopamine analogue, is a selective β$_1$-adrenoceptor agonist that produces a powerful inotropic response, with relatively less increase in heart rate than isoprenaline and little direct effect on vascular tone, even at high concentrations. *Dopexamine* acts on β$_2$-adrenoceptors to increase heart rate and to vasodilate, and, to a lesser extent, on β$_1$-adrenoceptors, giving a weak direct positive inotropic effect. It also acts on peripheral dopamine receptors and produces some increase in renal blood flow, but, unlike dopamine, it does not cause peripheral vasoconstriction with high doses.

Dopamine has dose-related actions at several receptors.

- At low doses, it selectively stimulates peripheral dopamine receptors, which are structurally distinct from those in the central nervous system. This produces renal arterial vasodilation and diuresis (D$_1$ receptors) and peripheral arterial vasodilation (D$_2$ presynaptic receptors, which inhibit noradrenaline release from sympathetic nerves).

- At moderate doses, non-selective β-adrenoceptor stimulation produces a positive inotropic response (Fig. 7.5). Tachycardia is more marked than with dobutamine, because of stimulation of both cardiac β$_1$- and β$_2$-adrenoceptors and the reflex response to β$_2$-adrenoceptor-mediated peripheral arterial dilation.

- At high doses, α$_1$-adrenoceptor stimulation produces peripheral vasoconstriction, which also affects the renal arteries and overcomes D$_1$-receptor-mediated renal vasodilation.

The doses of dopamine that produce these different effects differ widely among individuals. Unfortunately there is no dose that can be relied upon to act selectively at dopamine receptors without stimulating adrenoceptors.

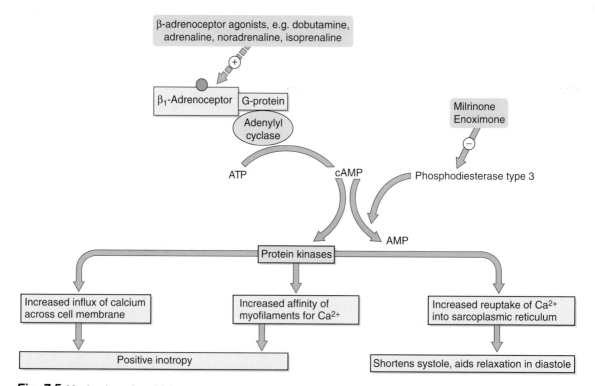

Fig. 7.5 Mechanisms by which sympathomimetics and phosphodiesterase inhibitors exert their positive inotropic effects.

Pharmacokinetics

All sympathomimetic inotropes are administered by intravenous infusion because of their very short half-lives (<12 min). Metabolic inactivation is by the same monoamine oxidase (MAO) and catechol-O-methyltransferase (COMT) pathways as for noradrenaline (Ch. 4). Desensitisation and downregulation of β-adrenoceptors (Ch. 1) rapidly reduce the response to sustained infusions over 48–72 h. Because of its unpredictable vasoconstrictor actions, dopamine is usually given into a large central vein.

Unwanted effects

- Excessive cardiac stimulation, with tachycardia, palpitations and arrhythmias.
- Nausea, vomiting.
- Chest pain, dyspnoea.
- Headache.

PHOSPHODIESTERASE INHIBITORS

Examples

enoximone, milrinone

Mechanism of action and effects

Milrinone and enoximone are specific inhibitors of the isoenzyme of phosphodiesterase (type 3) found in cardiac and smooth muscle. Their inotropic action on the heart results from an increase in intracellular cAMP with increased mobilisation of intracellular Ca^{2+} (Fig. 7.5). Unlike β-adrenoceptor agonists, the activity of phosphodiesterase inhibitors is not limited by desensitisation of cell surface receptors, because they act at a site beyond the receptor. Since they have complementary sites of action, phosphodiesterase inhibitors and β-adrenoceptor agonists will have additive effects on the heart. Phosphodiesterase type 3 inhibition in vascular smooth muscle produces peripheral arterial vasodilation.

Pharmacokinetics

Phosphodiesterase inhibitors are only given for short-term treatment by intravenous infusion. Milrinone is eliminated by the kidney and enoximone by hepatic metabolism. They have elimination half-lives of about 1 h.

Unwanted effects

- These are mainly a consequence of excessive cardiac stimulation, and include ectopic beats and both ventricular and supraventricular arrhythmias.
- Nausea, vomiting, diarrhoea (milrinone).
- Headache.
- Long-term oral use increases mortality in heart failure. Oral use has therefore been abandoned.

MANAGEMENT OF HEART FAILURE

ACUTE LEFT VENTRICULAR FAILURE

The immediate aim of pharmacological treatment in acute left ventricular failure is to reduce the excessive venous return to the heart. Treatment includes:

- oxygen in high concentration via a facemask,
- intravenous opioid analgesic such as morphine (Ch. 19), often given to relieve both distress and breathlessness,
- intravenous injection of a loop diuretic such as furosemide (Ch. 14). This initially produces venodilation, which increases peripheral venous pooling. Symptoms are therefore improved even before the onset of a diuresis that reduces plasma volume and further decreases preload,
- sublingual glyceryl trinitrate (GTN; Ch. 5). This dilates venous capacitance vessels and is a useful alternative or additional emergency treatment to diuretics.

Whenever possible, a precipitating or exacerbating cause should be treated; for example, arrhythmias, anaemia, thyrotoxicosis, acute mitral regurgitation or critical aortic stenosis. However, if the primary cause is impairment of left ventricular systolic function, then management as for chronic heart failure is subsequently necessary.

CARDIOGENIC SHOCK

The immediate aim of treatment is resuscitation, while looking for a remediable cause. If appropriate, early coronary revascularisation is crucial to increase the probability of survival. Supportive measures include the following:

- Give oxygen in high concentration via a facemask.
- Correct any acid–base imbalance (especially acidosis) and electrolyte abnormalities (particularly hypokalaemia).
- Relieve pain, usually with an intravenous opioid analgesic such as morphine (Ch. 19).
- Correct any cardiac rhythm disturbance (Ch. 8).
- Ensure an adequate left ventricular filling pressure. This can be low after right ventricular infarction, despite a high central venous pressure (right ventricular filling pressure). If intravenous volume is adequate but tissue perfusion remains impaired, dobutamine is the inotropic drug of choice. Dobutamine is often given in combination with low-dose dopamine, with the intention that the dopamine will improve renal perfusion; however, there is little evidence that the addition of dopamine is beneficial.
- Phosphodiesterase inhibitors are sometimes given to improve myocardial contractility and to produce peripheral vasodilation. They are usually reserved for those who fail to improve with maximum tolerated doses of dobutamine.
- When there is profound hypotension, noradrenaline (norepinephrine) (Ch. 4) can be infused intravenously to produce α_1-adrenoceptor-mediated peripheral vasoconstriction and maintain vital organ perfusion. The potential

disadvantage is that the increase in peripheral resistance will further impair cardiac output. Vasopressin (Ch. 43) is sometimes given to raise blood pressure, as vascular sensitivity to noradrenaline is impaired in shock. Vasopressin is a vasoconstrictor that also increases vascular sensitivity to noradrenaline.

- Vasodilators can be given to 'offload' the heart once an adequate blood pressure has been established. This strategy is particularly helpful if there is significant mitral regurgitation, since reduced resistance to left ventricular emptying will diminish the regurgitant volume. Either glyceryl trinitrate (Ch. 5) or nitroprusside (Ch. 6) is used.

CHRONIC HEART FAILURE WITH REDUCED EJECTION FRACTION

Much of the treatment of chronic heart failure is directed towards counteracting the compensatory mechanisms for the reduced cardiac output and low blood pressure generated by a failing heart; that is, arterial and venous vasoconstriction and fluid retention. When there is a reduced ejection fraction, a further desirable action is to reduce or reverse the shape change (remodelling) that occurs in the failing ventricle and makes contraction less efficient. Overall, treatment of heart failure with reduced ejection fraction has two main aims: symptom relief and improved prognosis.

Non-pharmacological treatment

A number of lifestyle changes can be helpful.

- Weight reduction should be encouraged for an obese person; this improves exercise tolerance.
- Bed rest may be appropriate to rest the heart during acute episodes of fluid retention.
- Modest salt restriction is desirable (severe salt restriction is unpleasant and unnecessary).
- Fluid restriction is rarely required unless profound hyponatraemia accompanies severe oedema. In this situation, diuretics may be ineffective until the plasma Na^+ concentration is corrected.
- If possible, drugs that exacerbate heart failure by producing myocardial depression (e.g. most calcium channel blockers) or by promoting fluid retention (e.g. non-steroidal anti-inflammatory drugs) should be withdrawn. Beta-adrenoceptor antagonists can cause myocardial depression, but should not be stopped, although a high dose may need to be reduced. Alcohol intake should be moderate at most, since alcohol depresses myocardial contractility and can be arrhythmogenic.
- A graded exercise programme for people with stable heart failure can improve symptoms.

Diuretics

Diuretics remain the mainstay of treatment for chronic heart failure with fluid retention, and are very effective for relief of symptoms (Ch. 14). A loop diuretic (usually furosemide) is typically used, taken once daily in the morning. There is no evidence that the use of a loop or thiazide diuretic alters prognosis in heart failure. Hypokalaemia is unusual when loop diuretics are used in chronic heart failure, especially as an angiotensin-converting enzyme (ACE) inhibitor or angiotensin II receptor antagonist is usually taken concurrently (see below). Nevertheless, the use of a potassium-sparing diuretic is advisable if the plasma K^+ falls below $3.5\ mmol\cdot L^{-1}$, especially if digoxin or anti-arrhythmic therapy is given concurrently (because of an increased risk of generating cardiac rhythm disturbances). Spironolactone is preferred in this situation since it improves symptoms and prognosis (at least in severe heart failure) if a low dose is added to maximal therapy with other drugs. In more severe heart failure the fluid retention may not respond to usual doses of a loop diuretic. Strategies for the management of diuretic-resistant fluid retention are considered in Chapter 14.

Angiotensin-converting enzyme inhibitors and angiotensin receptor antagonists

An ACE inhibitor (Ch. 6) is now considered to be essential in the treatment of heart failure with reduced ejection fraction, and is usually started at the same time as a diuretic. By reducing angiotensin II synthesis, ACE inhibitors produce arterial and venous dilation, which improves cardiac function by decreasing ventricular end-diastolic volume and increasing cardiac output (Figs 7.1 and 7.2). ACE inhibitors usually improve breathlessness and fatigue, and exercise tolerance increases. The full symptomatic response is often delayed for 4–6 weeks after the start of treatment, despite early haemodynamic changes. A further benefit of ACE inhibitors is improved survival, which may be due to a reversal of the remodelling of the left ventricle. High doses of an ACE inhibitor are more effective than low doses, and reduce mortality by 20–25% in heart failure with reduced ejection fraction.

There is a small risk of symptomatic hypotension after administration of the first dose of an ACE inhibitor, but the use of a small initial dose reduces the duration of any hypotension. ACE inhibitors promote K^+ retention by the kidney; the combination of an ACE inhibitor with spironolactone is used to improve prognosis in severe heart failure, but carries a small additive risk of hyperkalaemia.

If an ACE inhibitor is not tolerated, usually because of cough, an angiotensin II receptor antagonist (Ch. 6) can be substituted. These agents have similar efficacy to ACE inhibitors.

Beta-adrenoceptor antagonists

Beta-adrenoceptor antagonists (Ch. 5) are highly effective for the treatment of heart failure with reduced ejection fraction, usually after stabilising the condition with an ACE inhibitor (or an angiotensin II receptor antagonist) and a diuretic. Beta-adrenoceptor antagonists were once considered to be contraindicated in heart failure because of their negative inotropic properties. However, if introduced very gradually, and starting with a low dose, they improve both symptoms and survival. The survival advantage is additive to that produced by an ACE inhibitor, with a further reduction of 30–35% in mortality at all classes of severity of

---

Box 7.2   **Possible beneficial effects of ß-adrenoceptor antagonists in heart failure**

Reduced workload of ischaemic myocardium
Restoration of cardiac excitation–contraction coupling and improved intracellular Ca^{2+} handling
Reduced cardiac hypertrophy and fibrosis
Reduced myocyte apoptosis
Anti-arrhythmic effects

---

heart failure. Possible explanations for the benefit of β-adrenoceptor antagonists are numerous (Box 7.2), but a reduction in cardiac remodelling is probably important. Unless there are contraindications, all people who have heart failure with reduced ejection fraction should be treated with a β-adrenoceptor antagonist once they are clinically stable. The only compounds licensed for this use in the UK are bisoprolol, carvedilol and nebivolol, although there are also data to show the efficacy of a modified-release formulation of metoprolol.

Digoxin

Digoxin is widely used to control heart rate when heart failure is associated with atrial fibrillation and a rapid ventricular rate. The use of digoxin for heart failure associated with sinus rhythm has been more controversial, but there is now conclusive evidence that its positive inotropic effect can be useful as a supplement to diuretic and ACE inhibitor therapy when there is severe left ventricular systolic dysfunction and persisting symptoms. Digoxin improves symptoms and the need for hospitalisation, and survival may be improved if the serum digoxin concentration is kept low. Importantly, the effective dose of digoxin for those in heart failure who are in sinus rhythm is smaller than the dose required for control of atrial fibrillation.

Other vasodilators

Treatment with a combination of hydralazine (Ch. 6) and isosorbide dinitrate or mononitrate (Ch. 5), in addition to a diuretic and digoxin, provides balanced arterial and venous dilation. This combination improves exercise tolerance in heart failure but produces only a modest reduction in mortality, although there may be greater benefits in people of Afro-Caribbean origin. The combination can be tried for people who cannot tolerate an ACE inhibitor or angiotensin II receptor antagonist (Ch. 6).

Cardiac pacing and defibrillation

Cardiac resynchronisation therapy (CRT; biventricular electrical pacing) is helpful in severe heart failure when the ECG shows left bundle branch block and the ventricles display marked dyssynchronous contraction on echocardiography. Pacing both ventricles simultaneously restores synchronous contraction and improves cardiac output.

About half of all people with heart failure die suddenly of ventricular arrhythmias, and an implantable cardioverter ventricular defibrillator (ICD) can improve prognosis when there is severe left ventricular impairment and a propensity to ventricular arrhythmias. Combined cardiac resynchronisation–defibrillator devices (CRT-Ds) are also available.

Anti-arrhythmic drugs do not improve survival in heart failure.

HEART FAILURE WITH PRESERVED EJECTION FRACTION

The optimal management of heart failure with preserved ejection fraction is not well established. Most of the interventions that improve prognosis in heart failure with reduced ejection fraction have shown little impact on survival when ejection fraction is preserved, and therefore treatment is mainly directed at symptom relief using the drugs discussed above (with the exception of positive inotropic agents such as digoxin).

SELF-ASSESSMENT

True/false questions

1. When blood pressure falls, sympathetic outflow increases because of an increase in the sensory input from the baroreceptors in the carotid sinus.
2. In the healthy heart, a rise in afterload increases myocardial contractility.
3. Breathlessness and fatigue are common symptoms of heart failure.
4. Pulmonary oedema occurs when the hydrostatic pressure in the pulmonary veins is less than the plasma osmotic pressure.
5. In severe heart failure the attempts of the body to compensate for the cardiac dysfunction are detrimental.
6. Digoxin is the mainstay of the treatment of heart failure.
7. Digoxin inhibits the Na^+/K^+-ATPase pump on the cardiac myocyte membrane.
8. Hypokalaemia reduces the action of digoxin on the Na^+/K^+-ATPase pump.
9. Digoxin inhibits the vagus, decreasing the refractory period of the atrioventricular node.
10. Dobutamine produces peripheral vasodilation by its effect on β_2-adrenoceptors.
11. Sustained infusion of dobutamine desensitises the receptor response.
12. Milrinone is given intravenously to improve tissue perfusion in cardiogenic shock.
13. Angiotensin-converting enzyme (ACE) inhibitors should not be given together with K^+-sparing diuretics.
14. ACE inhibitors may cause cough by reducing the synthesis of bradykinin.
15. β-Adrenoceptor antagonists improve survival in chronic heart failure.
16. Hydralazine is a vasodilator with a predominant action on arteries.

One-best-answer (OBA) question

Which of the following is the *least accurate* statement about dopamine?

A. At low doses dopamine produces diuresis.
B. Effects of dopamine vary widely among individuals.
C. At moderate doses dopamine produces marked tachycardia.
D. At moderate doses dopamine is a selective β_1-adrenoceptor agonist.
E. At high doses dopamine produces renal arterial vasoconstriction.

Case-based questions

Mr DY is 78 years of age and had a large anterior myocardial infarction 3 years ago. Echocardiography revealed significant left ventricular systolic dysfunction with an ejection fraction of 30%. He presented with several symptoms, including fatigue, decreased exercise ability, shortness of breath and peripheral oedema. Examination demonstrated cardiomegaly, a raised jugular venous pressure and crackles in the lungs. An ECG showed that he is in sinus rhythm.

A. What are the choices of diuretic open to you in treating Mr DY?
B. Potassium loss produced by diuretics may lead to hypokalaemia. What is an effective way of reducing urinary K^+ loss?
C. Mr DY was then started on an ACE inhibitor. What precautionary measures should be taken in starting this new medication?
D. Could long-term oral digoxin be used as part of the treatment for Mr DY?
E. Could the use of a β-adrenoceptor antagonist make Mr DY's condition worse?

True/false answers

1. **False.** A falling blood pressure reduces the baroreceptor reflex input to the vasomotor centre, resulting in increased sympathetic outflow.
2. **True.** A rise in afterload decreases stroke volume initially but the consequent sympathetic stimulation increases contractility in the healthy heart and restores the stroke volume. In the failing heart, contractility increases less readily and stroke volume falls.
3. **True.** The breathlessness is caused by increased pulmonary venous pressure leading to pulmonary oedema; fatigue is caused by reduced cardiac output and impaired perfusion of skeletal muscle.
4. **False.** Oedema occurs when the net hydrostatic pressure, which moves fluid out of the vessel, is greater than the the plasma osmotic pressure, which moves interstitial fluid into the vessel.
5. **True.** The fall in cardiac output activates the sympathetic nervous system and the renin–angiotensin-aldosterone system; these changes are appropriate to restore blood pressure in the event of haemorrhage, but are unhelpful in severe heart failure as they increase preload, afterload and heart rate, hence increasing the workload of the failing heart.

6. **False.** Digoxin may be of benefit but the mainstay of treatment is a diuretic such as furosemide and an ACE inhibitor (or angiotensin II receptor antagonist). If diuretics are given concurrently with digoxin, a K^+-sparing diuretic such as spironolactone may also be required to prevent hypokalaemia; hypokalaemia increases the risk of digoxin-induced rhythm disturbances.
7. **True.** By blocking the Na^+/K^+-ATPase pump, cellular export of Na^+ is reduced and intracellular Na^+ concentrations rise. The reduced Na^+ concentration gradient across the cell membrane reduces the linked export of Ca^{2+} ions. Increased intracellular Ca^{2+} concentrations enhance contractility.
8. **False.** Potassium ions and digoxin compete for the pump, so hypokalaemia can increase the activity and pro-arrhythmic risk of digoxin.
9. **False.** As well as its direct effects on the heart, digoxin increases vagal outflow from the vasomotor centre. This increases the refractory period of the atrioventricular node and is the reason why digoxin is useful in some arrhythmias, such as atrial fibrillation.
10. **False.** Dobutamine is a selective β_1-adrenoceptor agonist and does not produce peripheral vasodilation.
11. **True.** Stimulation of β_1-adrenoceptors by dobutamine results in cAMP synthesis and increased cardiac contractility. Prolonged stimulation (48–72 h) desensitises the receptors; this does not occur with phosphodiesterase type 3 inhibitors, such as milrinone, which bypass the receptor and raise levels of cAMP by blocking its breakdown.
12. **True.** Milrinone inhibits the breakdown of intracellular cAMP by phosphodiesterase type 3 in cardiac and vascular smooth muscle, resulting in an inotropic effect and peripheral vasodilation; it is used in patients with cardiogenic shock not responding to full doses of dobutamine.
13. **False.** The combination of an ACE inhibitor and spironolactone provides additive clinical benefit but care must be taken to avoid dangerous hyperkalaemia, with regular monitoring of the plasma K^+ concentration. This is because ACE inhibitors reduce aldosterone-dependent reabsorption of Na^+ in the collecting duct. As Na^+ reabsorption at this site occurs in exchange for K^+ efflux, ACE inhibitors may increase K^+ retention, particularly in combination with potassium-sparing diuretics.
14. **False.** ACE inhibitors reduce the breakdown of bradykinin by ACE (also known as kininase II); increased bradykinin levels in the lungs are thought to be responsible for the cough seen in some patients receiving ACE inhibitors. An alternative strategy is to use an angiotensin II receptor antagonist.
15. **True.** Beta-adrenoceptor antagonists, ACE inhibitors and spironolactone improve survival in chronic heart failure, possibly by reducing the cardiac remodelling effects of catecholamines, angiotensin II and aldosterone respectively.
16. **True.** Hydralazine is predominantly an arterial vasodilator, while isosorbide mononitrate mainly acts as a venodilator; their combined use may be effective in chronic heart failure in people intolerant to ACE inhibitors or angiotensin II receptor antagonists.

OBA answer

Answer D is the least accurate statement as dopamine is a *non*-selective β-adrenoceptor agonist at moderate doses, resulting in a positive inotropic effect. Its action on β_2-adrenoceptors causes peripheral vasodilation leading to marked tachycardia (answer C). At low doses, dopamine causes renal arterial vasodilation via D_1 receptors, leading to diuresis (answer A), but at high doses this is counteracted by renal arterial vasoconstriction mediated by α_1-adrenoceptors (answer E). Interindividual variation in the response to dopamine is high (answer B).

Case-based answers

A. The treatment of first choice for fluid retention in chronic heart failure is a diuretic. For mild symptoms, a thiazide diuretic may be adequate, but in most people a loop diuretic such as furosemide is used. The loss of renal function in the elderly and renal underperfusion in heart failure means that thiazide diuretics are less effective in older people with this condition, such as Mr DY.

B. Hypokalaemia is arrhythmogenic and should be avoided in people with heart failure, particularly those taking digoxin. Urinary K^+ loss caused by a loop diuretic or thiazide can be reduced by combination with a K^+-sparing diuretic such as amiloride or spironolactone. Amiloride directly blocks epithelial Na^+/K^+ exchange in the collecting duct. In severe heart failure, spironolactone, which competes with aldosterone for the mineralocorticoid receptor, also improves prognosis, possibly by blocking aldosterone-dependent cardiac remodelling.

C. ACE inhibitors reduce preload and afterload by reducing the production of angiotensin II, a powerful vasoconstrictor, and by reducing blood volume (via reduced aldosterone production). They also slow the progression of heart failure and improve survival. There is a small risk of severe hypotension following the first dose, and omission of the diuretic immediately prior to this may be helpful.

D. The place of digoxin is well established in heart failure associated with atrial fibrillation and a rapid ventricular rate, but the benefit of a low dose of digoxin is now established in heart failure with severe left ventricular systolic dysfunction and sinus rhythm, when combined with a diuretic and an ACE inhibitor.

E. β-Adrenoceptor antagonists used injudiciously may worsen heart failure by reducing cardiac output, but low doses are beneficial (see Box 7.2), provided the patient's condition has been stabilised with diuretics and an ACE inhibitor.

FURTHER READING

Ahmed A, Rich MW, Love TE et al. (2006) Digoxin and reduction in mortality and hospitalization in heart failure: a comprehensive *post hoc* analysis of the DIG trial. *Eur Heart J* 27, 178–186

Amabile CM, Spencer AP (2004) Keeping your patient with heart failure safe. A review of potentially dangerous medications. *Arch Intern Med* 164, 709–720

Arroll B, Doughty R, Andersen V (2008) Investigation and management of congestive heart failure. *BM J* 341, c3657

Bangash MN, Kong M-L, Pearse RM (2011) Use of inotropes and vasopressor agents in critically ill patients. *Br J Pharmacol* 165, 2015–2033

Cleland JGF, Coletta A, Witte K (2006) Practical applications of intravenous diuretic therapy in decompensated heart failure. *Am J Med* 119 (12A), S26–S36

Eichhorn EJ, Gheorghiade M (2002) Digoxin. *Prog Cardiovasc Dis* 44, 251–266

Friedrich JO, Adhikari N, Herridge MS et al. (2005) Meta-analysis: low-dose dopamine increases urine output but does not prevent renal dysfunction or death. *Ann Intern Med* 142, 510–521

Gowda RM, Fox JT, Khan IA (2008) Cardiogenic shock: basics and clinical considerations. *Int J Cardiol* 123, 221–228

Krum H, Teerlink JR (2011) Medical therapy for chronic heart failure. *Lancet* 378, 713–721

McAlister FA, Wiebe N, Ezekovitz JA et al. (2009) β-Blocker dose, heart rate reduction, and death in patients with heart failure. *Ann Intern Med* 150, 784–794

McMurray JJV (2010) Systolic heart failure. *N Engl J Med* 362, 228–238

Metra M, Felker GM, Zaca V et al. (2010) Acute heart failure: multiple clinical profiles and mechanisms require tailored therapy. *Int J Cardiol* 144, 175–179

Molenaar P, Parsonage WA (2005) Fundamental considerations of β-adrenoceptor subtypes in human heart failure. *Trends Pharmacol Sci* 26, 368–374

Rajagopolan S, Arora A, Shafiq N et al. (2011) Pharmacotherapy of heart failure with normal ejection fraction (HFNEF) – a systematic review. *Br J Clin Pharmacol* 72, 369–380

Rathore SS, Curtis JP, Jeptha P et al. (2003) Association of serum digoxin concentration and outcomes in patients with heart failure. *JAMA* 289, 871–878

Shah AM, Mann DL (2011) In search of new therapeutic targets and strategies for heart failure: recent advances in basic science. *Lancet* 378, 704–712

Struthers AD (2006) Angiotensin blockade or aldosterone blockade as the third neuroendocrine-blocking drug in mild but symptomatic heart failure. *Heart* 92, 1728–1731

Waller JR, Waller DG (2011) Beta-blockers for heart failure with reduced ejection fraction. *BMJ* 343, c5603

Yang EH, Shah S, Criley JM (2012) Digoxin toxicity: a fading but crucial complication to recognize. *Am J Med* 125, 337–343

Compendium: drugs used to treat heart failure

Drug	Kinetics (half-life)	Comments
Digitalis glycoside		
Used in heart failure and for supraventricular arrhythmias (particularly atrial fibrillation, Ch. 8).		
Digoxin	Eliminated by glomerular filtration (20–50 h); increased half-life in renal impairment	Given once daily orally; a loading dose may be given orally in divided doses over 24 h, or by intravenous infusion in an emergency; digoxin-specific antibody is used for treatment of severe digoxin overdose
Phosphodiesterase inhibitors		
Given intravenously.		
Enoximone	Hepatic metabolism to a sulphoxide, renal elimination (4–10 h)	Used for congestive heart failure where cardiac output is reduced and filling pressure increased; given by intravenous infusion
Milrinone	Short half-life (0.8–0.9 h) due to rapid renal tubular secretion	Used for short-term treatment of severe congestive heart failure, and acute heart failure; given by intravenous injection followed by infusion for up to 12 h
Sympathomimetic inotropes		
Rapidly metabolised by the same local enzymatic pathways as noradrenaline (Ch. 4), giving very short half-lives and negligible oral bioavailability; all given by intravenous infusion.		
Dobutamine	Metabolised by MAO and COMT (2 min)	Selective β_1-adrenoceptor agonist has inotropic action with little effect on heart rate or vascular tone; used after myocardial infarction, cardiac surgery, cardiomyopathies, septic shock and cardiogenic shock
Dopamine	Metabolised by MAO and COMT (7–12 min)	Non-selective β-adrenoceptor agonist increases cardiac contractility and heart rate; agonism of peripheral dopamine receptors increases renal perfusion, offset by α_1-adrenoceptor-mediated vasoconstriction at high doses; used for cardiogenic shock in exacerbations of chronic heart failure and in heart failure associated with cardiac surgery
Dopexamine	Metabolised by MAO and COMT (7 min)	Selective β_2-adrenoceptor agonist increases cardiac contractility and rate; agonism of renal dopamine receptors increases renal perfusion; used for inotropic effect after myocardial infarction, cardiac surgery, cardiomyopathies, septic shock and cardiogenic shock

COMT, catechol-O-methyltransferase; MAO, monoamine oxidase.

8

Cardiac arrhythmias

BASIC CARDIAC ELECTROPHYSIOLOGY

Action potentials in myocardial cells and the resultant highly regulated cardiac contractions are a product of transmembrane ion currents generated by the movement of ions through membrane channels (Ch. 1). A variety of specific channels exist for transmembrane Na^+, Ca^{2+} and K^+ transport in the myocardium (Figs 8.1 and 8.2). These channels cycle through three states: resting, open or closed (inactive and refractory). Whether the ion channels are open to allow ion flow or are closed is determined by the electrical potential across the cell membrane. Therefore they are called voltage-gated ion channels. The direction in which ions move is dependent upon the type of channel, the concentration gradient of the ions and the transmembrane electrical potential (Figs 8.1 and 8.2). As a result of activity in these ion channels, the resting potential inside a cardiac cell is approximately −70 to −80 mV compared with the extracellular environment, although this varies among different types of cells in the heart.

When activated, depolarisation of these cells generates an action potential. The sinoatrial (SA) node, atrioventricular (AV) node, bundle of His and Purkinje system are part of the *specialised conducting system* of the heart that ensures the depolarizing impulse is conducted rapidly and synchronously through ventricular myocardium. In addition, the AV node slows impulse conduction to allow time for completion of mechanical events in the atrium and for ventricular filling to be completed. Once the impulse is passed to myocytes, depolarisation initiates contraction and also triggers depolarisation in adjacent myocytes. This ensures conduction of the impulse progressively through the myocardium.

The action potentials in cells of the sinoatrial (SA) and atrioventricular (AV) nodes, Purkinje fibres and ventricular muscle vary substantially in their characteristics (Figs 8.1, 8.2 and see Fig. 8.5). Action potentials in cardiac cells can be divided into four phases (Figs 8.1A and 8.2), although phases 1 and 2 are not clearly evident in the SA and AV nodes because of the different ion channels that are activated (Fig. 8.1A).

CELLS WITH PACEMAKER ACTIVITY

The myocardial cells of the specialised conducting system (SA node, AV node, bundle of His and Purkinje system) are distinguished electrophysiologically from cardiac myocytes by their intrinsic ability to depolarise spontaneously in phase 4, and independently generate an action potential. These cells are said to possess *automaticity* and are termed *pacemaker cells*. Cardiac myocytes have a stable resting potential and do not show phase 4 spontaneous depolarisation (compare Fig. 8.1A and 8.1C).

The primary pacemaker that drives normal repetitive cardiac contractions is the SA node (producing a normal sinus rhythm of 60–100 impulses per minute at rest). These secondary pacemaker, the AV node, depolarises more slowly and can generate 40–60 impulses per minute, while the tertiary pacemakers (the bundle of His, its branches and the Purkinje fibres) can fire 20–40 times per minute. The secondary and tertiary pacemakers will only be utilised if there is a failure of pacemakers that have a faster rate of spontaneous depolarisation.

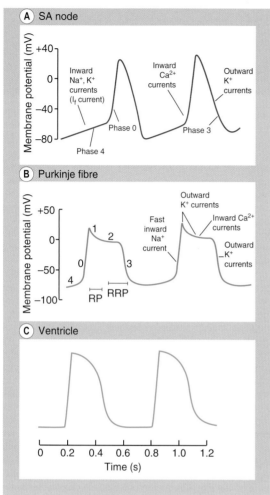

Ⓐ **SA node**

Ⓑ **Purkinje fibre**

Ⓒ **Ventricle**

Fig. 8.1 Action potentials show variations in patterns among different populations of myocytes in different regions of the heart. The patterns are determined by the opening and closing of selective gates for Na^+, Ca^{2+} and K^+, and this figure should be studied in conjunction with Figure 8.2. The overall stability of the resting transmembrane ionic balance is controlled by active pumps, such as the Na^+/K^+-ATPase pump, which maintain the Na^+ concentration gradient of 140 mM outside the cell versus 10–15 mM inside, and the K^+ concentration gradient of 140 mM inside and 4 mM outside the cell. This results in an electrical potential at rest of approximately −70 to −80 mV inside the cell relative to 0 mV outside the cell. Large ion fluxes at rest are prevented by specific pumps and closure of voltage-gated gates. Action potentials in the atrioventricular (AV) node, bundle of His and ventricle are controlled by the sinoatrial (SA) node when the heart is in sinus rhythm. The rate of spontaneous depolarisation of the SA node determines its primacy as a pacemaker in the healthy heart. Phase 0 (B, C) occurs when the membrane potential reaches a defined threshold potential and an 'all-or-none' influx of Na^+ through voltage-dependent fast Na^+ channels occurs; this is transient and the gates close after a few milliseconds. Phase 0 is much slower in the SA and AV nodes than in ventricular cells, and depends mainly upon Ca^{2+} influx (A). This causes the conduction velocity in the SA node to be considerably less than that in the Purkinje fibres, and the refractory period is longer in proportion to the total duration of the action potential. Phase 1, called the early repolarisation and notch, results from K^+ efflux (the transient outward (I_{to}) current) and reduced Na^+ influx (Fig. 8.2). The phase 2 plateau is primarily a result of Ca^{2+} influx (slow inward, or SI, current) which is balanced by K^+ efflux over a slow time course. Phase 3 repolarisation results from inactivation of Ca^{2+} influx and increasing K^+ efflux via a number of currents (see text, Table 8.1 and Fig. 8.2). Part of the overall importance of the K^+ currents is to maintain a stable resting membrane potential. Phase 4 (A, B) is termed the diastolic or pacemaker depolarisation generated on hyperpolarisation. The phase 4 inward 'funny' current (I_f) involves Na^+ and K^+ and is gated both by changes in voltage and by cAMP. I_f controls the rate of spontaneous beating of the heart and is regulated by the sympathetic and parasympathetic nervous systems. Ca^{2+} currents may also be involved in pacemaker activity in Phase 4. RP, absolute refractory period; RRP, relative refractory period.

CONTROL OF CELL DEPOLARISATION IN PACEMAKER AND NON-PACEMAKER CELLS

Slow spontaneous depolarisation in phase 4 in all pacemaker cells results from influx of positive ions (Na^+ and K^+) into the cell through f-channels that generate the strangely termed cardiac pacemaker 'funny' current (I_f) (Figs 8.1A and 8.2). The I_f is unusual in being generated by mixed-ion transport through a single channel, in being activated by the negative intracellular potential in diastole and in having slow activation and deactivation rates. Non-pacemaker cells have a minimal or no funny current.

The intrinsic rate of firing of a pacemaker cell depends on four factors:

- the resting intracellular potential,
- the resting potential at which the I_f is activated,
- the rate of spontaneous depolarisation,
- the threshold potential for initiating an impulse.

Activation of the I_f in the SA node is modulated by the autonomic nervous system via intracellular cAMP. Stimulation of β_1-adrenoceptors generates cAMP and shifts activation of the channel to a less negative intracellular voltage, while vagal stimulation via muscarinic M_2 receptors inhibits cAMP production and then activation of the channel requires a more negative intracellular voltage.

Full depolarisation of pacemaker cells occurs when, as a result of the I_f, the internal membrane potential reaches a threshold potential that opens voltage-gated L-type Ca^{2+} channels so that Ca^{2+} influx into the cell occurs (phase 0) (Fig. 8.1A; I_{CaL} in Fig. 8.2). The SA node is the dominant pacemaker because activation of the I_f current in the SA node occurs at a less negative intracellular potential and has a faster intrinsic activation rate than in the AV node or

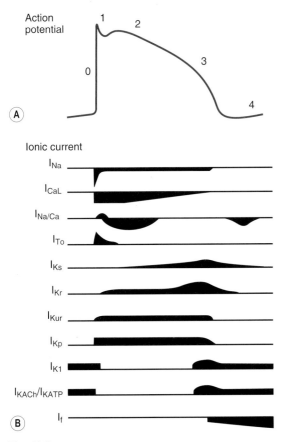

Action potential

1
2
0
3
4

(A)

Ionic current

I_{Na}

I_{CaL}

$I_{Na/Ca}$

I_{To}

I_{Ks}

I_{Kr}

I_{Kur}

I_{Kp}

I_{K1}

I_{KACh}/I_{KATP}

I_f

(B)

Fig. 8.2 A schematic representation of the influx and efflux of Na^+, Ca^{2+} and K^+ in Purkinje fibres. This figure should be examined in conjunction with Table 8.1, with other explanations given in the text. A downward inflection represents influx of the ion, and upward represents efflux. (Modified and reproduced with permission from Tamargo et al. 2004.)

Purkinje fibres. Therefore, spontaneous diastolic depolarisation in the SA node is initiated earlier and the threshold potential for full depolarisation is reached sooner.

Slow influx of Ca^{2+} in phase 0 is also the reason for slow conduction of the impulse through the AV node. In contrast, phase 0 of the action potential in Purkinje fibres and in atrial and ventricular myocytes is initiated by a rapid influx of Na^+ through voltage-gated Na^+ ion channels (fast Na^+ channels) (Fig. 8.1B; I_{Na} in Fig. 8.2).

At the end of phase 0, the intracellular voltage potential briefly becomes positive, at which point a voltage-triggered 'gate' closes and inactivates the Na^+ or Ca^{2+} channels and prevents further depolarisation (Fig. 8.1a,b).

CONTROL OF CELL REPOLARISATION IN PACEMAKER AND NON-PACEMAKER CELLS

Once depolarised, cardiac cells then undergo a process of repolarisation to return the membrane potential to its resting level. This creates the conditions for the next action

potential to be initiated (Figs 8.1 and 8.2). In both pacemaker and non-pacemaker cells, repolarisation (phase 3) is achieved by the opening of cell membrane K^+ channels known as rectifiers (see Table 8.1 for explanation). In the Purkinje system and non-pacemaker cardiac cells, repolarisation is delayed by influx of Ca^{2+} through L-type channels (phase 2, the plateau phase, I_{CaL} in Fig. 8.2), which balances K^+ efflux (Fig. 8.1B, phase 2). Eventually in these cells the K^+ current dominates and the cell returns to a negative intracellular resting potential.

In the resting phase between action potentials, Na^+ and K^+ transmembrane concentration gradients are restored by a separate exchange pump (Na^+/K^+-ATPase; see Fig. 7.4), and intracellular Ca^{2+} concentration is restored by a Na^+/Ca^{2+} exchange pump. The negative internal resting membrane potential is maintained by high K^+ permeability of resting cell membranes through inward rectifying voltage- and ligand-gated K^+ channels which close when the cell depolarises (see also Ch. 1).

During the period between phase 0 and the end of phase 2 of the action potential the myocardial cell is refractory to further depolarisation (the *absolute refractory period*, RP). This is because the depolarising channels are inactivated until a sufficiently negative potential is restored inside the cell. During phase 3, a large depolarising stimulus can open sufficient Na^+ or Ca^{2+} channels (many of which will have recovered to the resting state) to overcome the K^+ efflux and initiate a further action potential. This part of the action potential is the *relative refractory period* (RRP; Fig. 8.1B).

The sum of the individual electrical currents that pass from one cell to another through the heart can be recorded as the surface electrocardiogram (ECG) (Fig. 8.3).

MECHANISMS OF ARRHYTHMOGENESIS

Arrhythmias are disorders of rate and rhythm of the heart, which can arise as the result of either abnormal impulse generation or abnormal impulse conduction. There are three principal mechanisms of arrhythmogenesis.

■ **Increased automaticity.** Dominant ectopic pacemakers (pacemakers other than the SA node) can arise when pacemaker cells in the specialised conducting tissue develop a more rapid phase 4 depolarisation than the SA node. Ectopic pacemakers can also arise when rapid spontaneous phase 4 depolarisation develops in myocytes that usually have a stable phase 4. Ischaemia, or other changes in the microcellular environment, can create conditions that allow a non-specialised myocardial cell to express f-channels and become a pacemaker.

■ **Re-entry.** This is the cause of most clinically important arrhythmias. It is initiated when a depolarising impulse (often a premature ectopic beat from elsewhere in the heart) arrives at a part of the myocardium that is still in its refractory period. This is usually a fast conducting pathway with slow recovery from depolarisation. The impulse will bypass the refractory tissue. If this impulse is conducted through an adjacent part of the myocardium with slower conduction but fast recovery, then the impulse may subsequently arrive at the distal part of the

Table 8.1 Selected examples of K⁺ channels and associated currents

Type of gating	Examples of distribution	Comment
K$_V$ voltage-gated channel family		
K$_V$ channels carrying delayed inward rectifying currents	Widely distributed, including brain, heart, pancreas	Multiple subtypes of K⁺ channels are involved in delayed inward rectification and are responsible for slow (I$_{Ks}$), rapid (I$_{Kr}$) and ultrarapid (I$_{Kur}$) K⁺ currents involved in repolarisation in phases 2 and 3 in the heart. Inhibited by some class I and class III antiarrhythmics, e.g. amiodarone and sotalol
K$_V$ channel carrying transient outward rectifying (I$_{KTO}$) current		A genetically distinct member of the K$_V$ family of channels. Responsible for the I$_{TO}$ transient current in phase 1. Activated by adenosine; inhibited by quinidine, amiodarone
K$_{ir}$ family		
Inward rectifying	Heart, muscle, brain, pancreas	Inward rectifying, rapidly inactivates cardiac Na⁺ channels; sets resting membrane potential (I$_{K1}$, I$_{Kr}$). Inhibited by amiodarone
Ligand-gated channels		
ATP-sensitive channels (K$_{ATP}$)	Heart, muscle, pancreas, mitochondria	Comprised of coexpressed K$_{ir}$ and sulfonylurea subunits with varied configurations in different tissues. Provide a weak inward rectifying current. Opened by ischaemia, minoxidil and nicorandil; inhibited by ATP and sulfonylureas
Acetylcholine-sensitive channel (K$_{ACh}$)	SA node, AV node and atria	This is G-protein-linked in the SA node, atria and AV node and is a member of the K$_{ir}$ family resulting in an inward rectifying (K$_{ir}$) current. Opened by adenosine; inhibited by atropine and disopyramide
Two-pore channel (K$_{2P}$)	Heart, brain, pancreas	Opened by arachidonic acid; weak inward rectifying current; modulates resting membrane potential
Calcium-activated (K$_{Ca}$ family)		Members of K$_{ir}$ family of channels
Large conductance channel (B$_{KCa}$)	Heart, brain, pancreas	Being investigated for roles in neuroprotection, erectile dysfunction and other disorders
Intermediate conductance channel (I$_{KCa}$)	T-lymphocytes, smooth muscle, brain, heart	Opened by hydralazine

This table should be studied in conjunction with Fig. 8.2.

Potassium channels are diverse in structure and behaviour. Each channel consists of four membrane-spanning subunits, with each subunit consisting of two to six linked membrane segments which make up the water-filled pore. This allows many different configurations of K⁺ channels, many of which have particular physiological roles. Channels with subunit variations are associated with different types of current which are involved in repolarisation at different phases of the cardiac action potential. The channels can be open or closed depending upon the voltage across the cell or the presence of a selective ligand.

Rectifying current: an inward rectifying current means that under conditions of equivalent but opposing electrochemical potentials these channels pass more current inwards than outwards. An outward rectifying current is similar but in an outward direction.

refractory tissue when this tissue has had sufficient time to repolarise. The impulse will then be conducted retrogradely through this previously refractory tissue (Fig. 8.4C). If there has been sufficient time for the fast recovery myocardium proximal to the block to repolarise, a self-perpetuating circuit of electrical activity will be initiated (a re-entry circuit). The re-entry circuit acts as a pacemaker that initiates impulses that are then propagated through the heart. Such functional re-entry circuits can be localised within a small area of myocardium that has been damaged by fibrosis or ischaemia (micro re-entry). Micro re-entry circuits may arise in the atria, within the AV node or in the ventricles. The myocardium can also support large anatomical re-entry circuits (macro re-entry). These circuits arise when there is a congenital accessory pathway that bypasses the AV node, and conducts electrical activity between the atria and ventricles. The re-entry circuit between the atria and

ventricles includes both the accessory pathway and the AV node (such as occurs in the Wolff–Parkinson–White syndrome).

■ **Triggered activity.** A cell can develop transient depolarisations during or following repolarisation ('afterdepolarisations'), which will initiate an action potential if they reach the threshold potential of the cell. Afterdepolarisations are said to be 'early' if they occur during repolarisation (relative refractory period in Fig. 8.1B), or 'delayed' if they occur in phase 4. Early afterdepolarisations are due to opening of L-type Ca²⁺ channels or fast Na⁺ channels. Delayed afterdepolarisations are due to intracellular Ca²⁺ overload and follow spontaneous Ca²⁺ release from the sarcoplasmic reticulum during prolonged repolarisation. This activates the 3Na⁺/Ca²⁺ exchange transporter and produces a net depolarising current. Triggered activity is an uncommon mechanism of arrhythmogenesis but may be responsible for the proarrhythmic

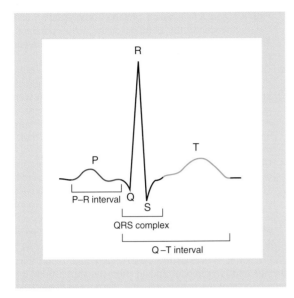

Fig. 8.3 The waveform for cardiac events seen on a surface electrocardiogram. The P wave represents the spread of depolarisation through the atria, and the QRS complex is the spread through the ventricles. The T wave represents repolarisation of the ventricle. The P–R interval is the time of conductance from atrium to ventricles, and the QRS time is the time the ventricles are activated. The duration of the ventricle action potential is given by the Q–T interval.

activity of class Ia and III antiarrhythmic agents (early afterdepolarisations) and digitalis glycosides (delayed afterdepolarisations) (see below).

CLASSIFICATION OF ANTIARRHYTHMIC DRUGS

A widely used classification of antiarrhythmic drugs (the Vaughan Williams classification) is based on their effects on the action potential (Fig. 8.5). This classification has many flaws and does not take account of the multiple actions possessed by some drugs, or the fact that the effects of drugs on diseased myocardium may be different from that on healthy myocardium. However, there is no widely accepted alternative classification.

VAUGHAN WILLIAMS CLASSIFICATION

The Vaughan Williams classification recognises four classes of drug (Table 8.2).

Class I

All class I drugs inhibit fast Na$^+$ channels and slow the rate of rise of phase 0, and therefore reduce the excitability of the myocardial cell. They are often called membrane stabilisers. They readily penetrate the phospholipid bilayers of the cell membrane, where they concentrate in the hydrophobic core and bind to hydrophobic amino acids in the

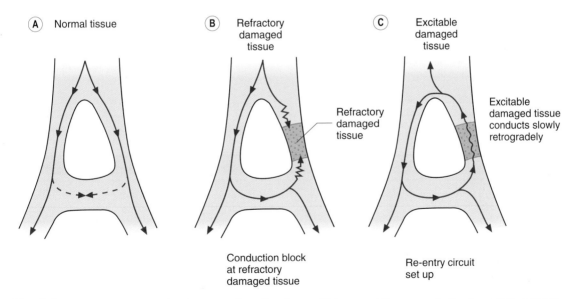

Fig. 8.4 Conduction in normal and damaged cardiac tissue. (A) In normal tissue, conduction is carefully ordered. When an action potential has been generated, the cells cannot be immediately reactivated because of refractoriness of the myocardial cells. If conducted impulses meet, they die out. (B) If an area of damage or dysfunction is present, impulses are conducted abnormally. If an action potential arrives at the area of damaged tissue and it is fully refractory, the impulse is blocked and an arrhythmia will not develop. (C) If an action potential arrives at a damaged area and it is capable of being excited and conducting in a retrograde direction, a perpetuating abnormal re-entry circuit may be set up.

Na$^+$ channel. Class I drugs are subdivided according to their effects on the duration of the action potential.

- **Class Ia drugs**, such as disopyramide, slow impulse conduction by producing moderate Na$^+$ channel blockade. In addition, they block some K$^+$ channels (Table 8.1, Figs 8.1 and 8.5A), which prolongs repolarisation and therefore extends the duration of the action potential. *They are effective for the treatment of both supraventricular and ventricular arrhythmias* (Table 8.2).

- **Class Ib drugs**, such as lidocaine, slow impulse conduction by producing weak Na$^+$ channel blockade in abnormal tissue (such as ischaemic myocardium) with no effect in healthy tissue. They do not block K$^+$ channels and have either no effect on repolarisation or may shorten it (Fig. 8.5B). *They are only effective for the treatment of ventricular arrhythmias.*

- **Class Ic drugs**, such as flecainide, slow impulse conduction by producing marked Na$^+$ channel blockade. They produce weak blockade of some K$^+$ channels (Table 8.1), and also block inward Ca^{2+} channels. There is minimal effect on repolarisation (Fig. 8.5C). *They are effective for the treatment of both atrial and ventricular arrhythmias.*

The different effects of the class I subgroups result from their diverse ion-channel binding characteristics. During the time course of the action potential, the access of the drug to its binding site is intermittent and dependent on the state of the channel. Class Ib drugs (such as lidocaine) show marked use-dependency; that is, the action increases with the frequency of opening of the channel. They associate more rapidly with Na$^+$ channels during depolarisation and they rapidly dissociate from the channel when it returns to the resting state. Therefore they are more effective when there are repetitive depolarisations, and they will effectively block premature impulses. Cells in ischaemic myocardium are more likely to be depolarised, which explains the selectivity of class Ib drugs for ventricular arrhythmias in ischaemic heart disease (ischaemia mainly affects the ventricles). Class Ic drugs (such as flecainide) also show use-dependent binding, but dissociate slowly from their binding sites in the Na$^+$ channel and therefore produce prolonged blockade. This results in a widespread reduction in cellular excitability. Class Ia drugs (such as disopyramide) have binding characteristics between those of the other two subgroups.

Class II

The class II drugs are the β-adrenoceptor antagonists (β-blockers) which block the actions of catecholamines on the heart. They reduce the rate of spontaneous depolarisation of SA and AV nodal tissue and reduce conduction through the AV node through their action on adrenoceptor-sensitive f-channels (Fig. 8.5D). They can also inhibit ectopic pacemakers that have developed

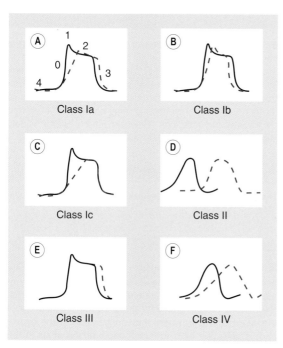

Fig. 8.5 Effects of different classes of antiarrhythmic drug on the cardiac action potential. (A, B, C, E) Drug effects on ventricular cells; (D, F) effects on the AV node. (A) Class Ia drugs. Block fast Na$^+$ channels in phase 0 with moderate potency, and some K$^+$ channels. Repolarisation is prolonged. (B) Class Ib drugs. Weakly block fast Na$^+$ channels in phase 0 only in abnormal tissue; little effect on K$^+$ channels. (C) Class Ic drugs. Potently block fast Na$^+$ channels and weakly block Ca^{2+} channels and some K$^+$ channels. (D) Class II drugs. Reduce phase 4 and phase 0 depolarisation in AV and SA nodes. Repolarisation in the AV node is prolonged. (E) Class III drugs. Block some K$^+$ channels, inhibiting repolarisation and prolonging the action potential. (F) Class IV drugs. Block L-type Ca^{2+} channels, slowing phase 0 and phase 4 depolarisation, particularly in the AV node, with less effect in the SA node. Repolarisation is prolonged.

Table 8.2 Principal indications for antiarrhythmic drugs

Class	Examples	Supraventricular arrhythmias	Ventricular arrhythmias
Ia	Disopyramide (procainamide)	+	+
Ib	Lidocaine	−	+ (especially after myocardial infarction)
Ic	Flecainide, propafenone	+	+
II	β-Adrenoceptor antagonists	+	+ (especially after myocardial infarction)
III	Amiodarone, sotalol	+	+
IV	Calcium channel blockers	+	−

automaticity. *Beta-adrenoceptor antagonists are effective for the treatment of both supraventricular and ventricular arrhythmias, particularly if these are catecholamine-dependent.*

Class III

Class III drugs such as amiodarone prolong the duration of the action potential by inhibiting some K^+ channels involved in repolarisation, thus increasing the absolute refractory period (Table 8.1, Fig. 8.5E). *They are effective for the treatment of both supraventricular and ventricular arrhythmias.*

Class IV

There are two types of Ca^{2+} channel in the heart but the class IV drugs are calcium channel blockers that selectively block the L-type Ca^{2+} channel. They slow conduction of the action potential particularly in the AV node. They have a lesser effect on the rate of depolarisation at the SA node (Fig. 8.5F). *They are only effective for the treatment of supraventricular arrhythmias.*

Unclassified drugs

Four drugs used in the treatment of rhythm disturbances do not fit into the Vaughan Williams classification: digitalis glycosides, adenosine, magnesium sulphate and atropine.

PROARRHYTHMIC ACTIVITY OF ANTIARRHYTHMIC DRUGS

Many antiarrhythmic drugs have the potential to precipitate serious arrhythmias, such as incessant ventricular tachycardia. Several of them (particularly class Ia agents and sotalol) prolong the Q–T interval on the ECG (Fig. 8.3). This predisposes to a polymorphic ventricular tachycardia known as torsade de pointes, which has a characteristic twisting QRS axis on the ECG and can degenerate into ventricular fibrillation. Drug-induced ventricular rhythm disturbances are particularly refractory to treatment.

There are probably multiple mechanisms of drug-induced arrhythmogenesis. Several risk factors have been identified, including the following.

- **Excessive slowing of cardiac impulse conduction**, such as occurs with marked blockade of Na^+ channels.
- **Excessive prolongation of the action potential**, especially if this is due to blockade of the I_{Kr} repolarising current (Table 8.1, Fig. 8.2). Prolonged repolarisation may cause early afterdepolarisations (see above), or a selective effect of the drugs on some cells in the myocardium can lead to differential rates of repolarisation that predisposes to re-entry circuits.
- **Mutations in genes** coding for channels that regulate Na^+, K^+ and Ca^{2+} transmembrane ion flows exist in 5–10% of people, and are probably subclinical variants of the congenital long QT syndrome. These individuals are more susceptible to torsade de pointes when exposed to a drug that prolongs the Q–T interval.

- **Structural heart disease**, especially ischaemic heart disease, with greater slowing of conduction in diseased myocardium.
- **Hypokalaemia**.
- **Female sex**: about 70% of those who develop torsade de pointes are women.

CLASS IA DRUGS

Disopyramide

Disopyramide is no longer widely used in the UK because of its unwanted effects.

Pharmacokinetics

Oral absorption of disopyramide is almost complete. Metabolism in the liver generates a compound with less antiarrhythmic activity but with greater antimuscarinic activity.

Unwanted effects

- Gastrointestinal disturbances.
- Powerful negative inotropic effect; disopyramide should be avoided in people with left ventricular dysfunction.
- Proarrhythmic effects (see above).
- Antimuscarinic effects (see Ch. 4), especially urinary retention, dry mouth and blurred vision.

CLASS IB DRUGS

Lidocaine

Pharmacokinetics

Extensive first-pass metabolism to a potentially toxic metabolite means that oral administration of lidocaine is not practicable. It is given intravenously, initially as a loading dose by bolus injection followed by an infusion. Lidocaine is extensively metabolised in the liver to compounds with little antiarrhythmic activity, although one can cause seizures. The half-life of lidocaine is 2 h.

Unwanted effects

- Central nervous system (CNS) toxicity: muscle twitching, seizures, respiratory depression, dizziness, drowsiness, parasthesia.
- Negative inotropic effect.
- Bradycardia.

CLASS IC DRUGS

Flecainide

Pharmacokinetics

Oral absorption of flecainide is complete. An intravenous formulation is also available for rapid onset of action. Flecainide is eliminated both by the kidneys and by hepatic metabolism, and the half-life is long (14 h).

Unwanted effects

- Oedema.
- Fever.
- Dyspnoea.
- CNS toxicity: dizziness, fatigue, visual disturbances.
- Negative inotropic effect.
- Proarrhythmic effects, possibly more marked after recent myocardial infarction, when it may increase mortality.

Propafenone

Propafenone has weak β-adrenoceptor antagonist activity in addition to its class Ic action.

Pharmacokinetics

Oral absorption of propafenone is almost complete, but extensive first-pass metabolism by cytochrome P450-mediated oxidation is saturable so the half-life is dose-dependent. Elimination is much slower in subjects with CYP2D6 genetic polymorphism.

Unwanted effects

- Gastrointestinal disturbances: nausea, vomiting, diarrhoea, bitter taste.
- Cholestasis, hepatitis.
- CNS toxicity: dizziness, anxiety, confusion, ataxia, headache, insomnia, seizures.
- Negative inotropic effect, producing hypotension.
- Weak β-adrenoceptor antagonist activity can cause bronchoconstriction in people with asthma.
- Proarrhythmic effects.

CLASS II DRUGS

Beta-adrenoceptor antagonists (β-blockers)

The antagonist activity of β_1-adrenoceptor is responsible for the therapeutic effects of this class. The most widely used agents for treatment of rhythm disturbances are atenolol, bisoprolol and propranolol, but all drugs in this class have antiarrhythmic activity. Beta-adrenoceptor antagonists are discussed in more detail in Chapter 5.

Esmolol is an ultra-short-acting β_1-adrenoceptor-selective (cardioselective) agent that is used by bolus intravenous injection exclusively for the treatment of arrhythmias. It is most often used when arrhythmias arise during anaesthesia.

Pharmacokinetics

After bolus intravenous injection, the half-life of esmolol is very short (about 9 min). Its action is terminated by esterases after uptake by erythrocytes.

CLASS III DRUGS

Amiodarone

Amiodarone is a drug with multiple antiarrhythmic actions. It has class III actions by blocking several K$^+$ channels and shows use-dependence (see above). However, amiodarone also has a class Ib-like action on Na$^+$ channels, as well as non-competitive β-adrenoceptor antagonist (class II) activity and calcium channel-blocking (class IV) actions. The antiarrhythmic effects produced early after intravenous infusion are believed to be due to β-adrenoceptor antagonist activity, since the class III effect is delayed.

Pharmacokinetics

Amiodarone is incompletely absorbed orally and has a large volume of distribution as a result of extensive uptake into adipose tissue. An intravenous formulation is available. Both amiodarone and its major hepatic metabolite have extremely long half-lives (50–60 days), so a prolonged loading dose regimen is used for both routes of administration.

Unwanted effects

- Gastrointestinal disturbances, for example constipation and nausea, most often occur during the loading period.
- Reversible corneal microdeposits develop in almost all people, and can cause dazzling by lights when driving at night.
- Amiodarone has a high iodine content and a structural relationship to thyroid hormone. In iodine-sufficient areas (such as the UK), inhibition of intracellular thyroxine (T$_4$) transport and 5′-deiodinase by amiodarone reduces the conversion of T$_4$ to active triiodothyronine (T$_3$) (Ch. 41). This produces hypothyroidism in about 10% of those treated. Hypothyroidism can be treated by thyroxine replacement without stopping amiodarone (Ch. 41). Amiodarone can also exacerbate underlying asymptomatic autoimmune thyroid disease. By contrast, in people who are iodine-deficient amiodarone can produce a destructive thyroiditis with release of preformed thyroid hormone leading to thyrotoxicosis in up to 10% of those taking it. Amiodarone-induced thyrotoxicosis is often resistant to treatment. Thyroid function should be checked every 6 months during treatment.
- Photosensitive skin rashes are common, and use of wide-spectrum sunscreen is recommended. Slate-grey skin discoloration can also occur.
- Peripheral neuropathy or myopathy.
- Hepatitis and cirrhosis occur rarely.
- Progressive pneumonitis and lung fibrosis are rare but serious effects of long-term treatment.
- Proarrhythmic effects.
- Drug interactions: the plasma concentrations of warfarin (Ch. 11) and digoxin (Ch. 7) are increased by amiodarone, with consequent potentiation of their effects. Amiodarone inhibits the metabolism of warfarin. It displaces digoxin from tissue stores and inhibits its renal excretion, both actions which increase the risk of digoxin toxicity.

Unlike most antiarrhythmic drugs, amiodarone does not have negative inotropic effects.

Sotalol

Sotalol is a non-selective β-adrenoceptor antagonist (Ch. 5) with additional class III properties. It selectively blocks the I$_{Kr}$ K$^+$ current (which is particularly involved in phase 2 and

3 repolarisation), and shows reverse use-dependency (higher receptor binding when the channel is closed) so that sotalol is most effective at slow rates of cell depolarisation (bradycardia). Sotalol is a racemic mixture; the L-isomer has both β-adrenoceptor antagonist and class III activity, whereas the D-isomer has only class III activity. The class III activity gives sotalol a greater proarrhythmic potential than other β-adrenoceptor antagonists (see above). Sotalol is reserved for treatment of significant cardiac rhythm disturbances and is not used for the other indications for β-adrenoceptor antagonists.

Pharmacokinetics

Sotalol is almost completely absorbed from the gut and excreted unchanged in the urine. Its half-life varies between 7 and 18 h.

Unwanted effects

These are discussed in Chapter 5. Sotalol also has proarrhythmic activity (see above).

CLASS IV DRUGS

Calcium channel blockers

Verapamil and diltiazem (Ch. 5), but not the dihydropyridine derivatives such as amlodipine, have antiarrhythmic activity. Verapamil can be given intravenously for a rapid effect, but should not be given together with a β-adrenoceptor antagonist, because of summation of myocardial depression and AV nodal conduction block. Details of calcium channel blockers can be found in Chapter 5.

OTHER DRUGS FOR CARDIAC RHYTHM DISTURBANCES

Those drugs used for the management of rhythm disturbances that do not fit into the Vaughan Williams classification are considered here.

Digitalis glycosides

Digitalis glycosides (such as digoxin) are not strictly antiarrhythmic, but they are useful for controlling ventricular rate in atrial flutter and atrial fibrillation by reducing conduction through the AV node. Digitalis glycosides are discussed in Chapter 7.

Adenosine

Mechanism of action and effects

Adenosine is a purine nucleoside with electrophysiological actions mediated by the A_1 subtype of specific G-protein-coupled adenosine receptors. These receptors activate inward rectifier K_{ACh} channels which enhances the flow of K^+ out of myocardial cells and hyperpolarises the resting cell (see Table 8.1). In addition, adenosine antagonises the stimulatory effects of noradrenaline on Ca^{2+} currents. These actions combine to stabilise the myocardial cell transmembrane ion fluxes. Adenosine has potent effects on the SA node, producing sinus bradycardia. It also slows impulse conduction through the AV node, but has no effect on conduction in the ventricles. Consequently, it is useful only for the management of supraventricular arrhythmias, particularly those caused by AV nodal re-entry mechanisms.

The action of adenosine at the A_2 adenosine receptor reduces Ca^{2+} uptake in vascular smooth muscle, and produces vasodilation. In the coronary circulation, preferential dilation of healthy arteries produces coronary blood flow 'steal' that reduces flow in stenosed arteries. This receptor action enables adenosine to be used as a pharmacological stress to induce ischaemia in people with coronary artery disease, which can then be assessed by radionuclide scanning, magnetic resonance imaging or echocardiography.

Pharmacokinetics

Adenosine is given by rapid bolus intravenous injection. The effect is terminated by uptake into erythrocytes and endothelial cells, followed by metabolism to inosine and hypoxanthine. Adenosine has a half-life of less than 10 s and its duration of action is less than 1 min.

Unwanted effects

Unwanted effects are common and occur in about 25% of those given adenosine, but last less than 1 min:

- Bradycardia and AV block.
- Malaise, facial flushing, headache, chest pain or tightness, bronchospasm; adenosine should be avoided in people with asthma.
- Drug interactions: dipyridamole (Ch. 11) potentiates the effects of adenosine, while methylxanthines such as aminophylline (Ch. 12) inhibit its action.

Atropine

Atropine (see Ch. 4) is an antimuscarinic drug that is given by intravenous bolus injection and reduces the inhibitory effect of the vagus nerve on the heart. Blockade of muscarinic M_2 receptors increases the rate of firing of the SA node and increases conduction through the AV node. This is due to inhibition of inward rectifying K_{ACh} channels which prevents hyperpolarisation of the cell membrane (Table 8.1) and enhanced activation of pacemaker f-channels. Atropine is used specifically for the treatment of sinus bradycardia and AV block. It is metabolised in the liver and has a half-life of 2–5 h.

Magnesium sulphate

Intravenous magnesium sulphate is used to control the ventricular arrhythmia torsade de pointes, and digitalis-induced ventricular arrhythmias. The mechanism is not well understood, but may involve blockade of transmembrane Ca^{2+} currents. Flushing is the main unwanted effect.

DRUG TREATMENT OF ARRHYTHMIAS

Arrhythmias can be asymptomatic, or they can produce a variety of consequences that range from mild symptoms to life-threatening effects on cardiac output. The probability of developing symptoms depends on several factors, the most important of which are the rate of an abnormal rhythm and the presence of underlying heart disease. The range of consequences of rhythm disturbances includes:

- awareness of palpitation,
- dizziness,
- syncope,
- precipitation of angina or heart failure,
- sudden death.

Treatment may not be necessary for benign or self-terminating arrhythmias and reassurance may be all that is required. In some cases it may be possible to remove or treat an underlying cause.

The choice of treatment depends on the situation. With most tachyarrhythmias, sinus rhythm should be restored if possible. Direct current (DC) cardioversion is used to achieve this in severe, life-threatening or drug-resistant arrhythmias. Drug therapy is used if there is less need for an immediate effect, or to control the ventricular rate if the abnormal rhythm cannot be terminated. Radiofrequency ablation of an arrhythmogenic focus or pathway is increasingly used to prevent arrhythmia. This is carried out after intracardiac electrophysiological studies, using a cardiac catheter. Long-term drug treatment for bradyarrhythmias is not possible and an implanted pacemaker may be necessary.

SUPRAVENTRICULAR TACHYARRHYTHMIAS

Atrial premature beats

Atrial premature beats are very common and usually benign, but sometimes they are a consequence of digoxin toxicity, and frequent multifocal atrial ectopics can result from organic heart disease. Other than treatment of an underlying cause, specific drug therapy is rarely needed. Some people are disturbed by a post-ectopic pause followed by a more forceful beat when sinus rhythm recommences. If treatment is required, then a β-adrenoceptor antagonist, or a calcium channel blocker such as verapamil or diltiazem, can be used to suppress the ectopics.

Atrial tachycardia

Atrial tachycardia is an infrequent rhythm disturbance usually arising from an automatic focus that produces an atrial rate of 150–250 beats·min^{-1}. There is usually AV conduction block that results in a slower ventricular rate. Atrial tachycardia is not usually associated with significant cardiac disease, but can be a manifestation of digitalis toxicity. If drug therapy is necessary an AV nodal blocking agent such as a β-adrenoceptor antagonist or a calcium channel blocker (verapamil or diltiazem) will control the ventricular rate but rarely restores sinus rhythm. Sinus rhythm can be achieved with a class Ic antiarrhythmic agent such as flecainide, given with an AV nodal blocking drug (flecainide alone increases the risk of 1:1 AV nodal conduction if the atrial rate slows sufficiently but sinus rhythm is not restored). Sotalol or amiodarone can also be used to maintain sinus rhythm. Ablation of the initiating focus may also be considered.

A less common form of atrial tachycardia is multifocal atrial tachycardia arising from several ectopic foci, usually in people with severe pulmonary disease. Calcium channel blockers are usually used for ventricular rate control if treatment is needed.

Atrial flutter

In atrial flutter, the atrial rate is usually 250–350 beats·min^{-1} and the impulses are conducted to the ventricles with 2:1 or greater degrees of AV block. Flutter waves may be obvious on the ECG, or appear if the ventricular rate is slowed by transiently increasing the degree of AV block using vagal stimulation (such as carotid sinus massage) or the administration of adenosine. Atrial flutter usually arises from a macro re-entrant circuit in the right atrium. Underlying causes include recent cardiac surgery, cor pulmonale and congenital heart disease, but it can arise for no obvious reason. It may be paroxysmal, and it can degenerate into atrial fibrillation.

Drug therapy is relatively unsuccessful for restoring sinus rhythm, and DC cardioversion (synchronised to discharge on the R wave of the ECG) or rapid 'overdrive' electrical pacing to capture the ventricle followed by a gradual reduction in the paced rate may be required. Class Ic and III antiarrhythmic agents can prevent recurrence of paroxysmal atrial flutter. If a class Ic agent such as flecainide is used, then an AV nodal blocking drug should be given concurrently, since the atrial rate could slow with 1:1 AV conduction, causing an unacceptably high ventricular rate.

Control of the ventricular rate in atrial flutter can be achieved in a similar manner to that in atrial fibrillation (see below), but treatment is often less successful. For this reason, radiofrequency ablation of the re-entrant pathway via a cardiac catheter is becoming increasingly popular. Prophylaxis against thromboembolism should be given, similar to that for atrial fibrillation.

Atrial fibrillation

Atrial fibrillation is the most common rhythm disturbance in clinical practice (apart from ectopic beats). It has a variety of underlying causes (Box 8.1), some of which may be

---

Box 8.1   **Causes of atrial fibrillation**

Structural heart disease
Hypertension
Coronary heart disease
Valvular heart disease (especially mitral)
Cardiomyopathies
Cardiac surgery
Congenital heart disease (especially atrial septal defect)

Other causes
Major infections
Thyrotoxicosis, myxoedema
Alcohol intoxication
Systemic illness (e.g. amyloid, sarcoidosis)
Pulmonary embolism

treatable. In younger people, atrial fibrillation often occurs without any obvious underlying cause, when it is called 'lone' atrial fibrillation. The arrhythmia usually arises from multiple re-entry circuits in the atria, although a rapid ectopic focus in a pulmonary vein may be responsible for triggering paroxysmal atrial fibrillation. The ventricular rate will depend on AV nodal function, so that when the AV node conducts well, atrial fibrillation produces a rapid ventricular rate. Atrial fibrillation predisposes to left atrial thrombus formation and subsequent systemic emboli, which most commonly cause stroke. Clinically, three forms of atrial fibrillation are recognised: paroxysmal (intermittent self-limiting episodes), persistent (present for more than 7 days but less than 1 year) and permanent (present for more than 1 year after unsuccessful attempts to maintain sinus rhythm, or if a decision has been made not to attempt this). Management has four underlying aims.

■ To identify and treat the underlying cause.
■ To restore or maintain sinus rhythm in paroxysmal or persistent atrial fibrillation (Box 8.2). It is desirable to attempt to restore sinus rhythm in younger people or those who tolerate the rhythm disturbance poorly. In these individuals, symptoms and exercise tolerance are usually improved by restoring sinus rhythm, but the risk of stroke is not removed (see below). However, the case for restoring sinus rhythm is less clear-cut for older people who tolerate the rhythm well, because there is no reduction in the risk of thromboembolic events (see below), and their quality of life may not improve. Restoration of sinus rhythm is usually possible in lone atrial fibrillation or when a precipitating factor has been treated. It can be achieved with drugs (pharmacological or chemical cardioversion), especially if the rhythm disturbance is of recent onset (40–80% success rate if the arrhythmia is of less than 7 days' duration), but often requires QRS-synchronised DC cardioversion. Pharmacological cardioversion is most rapidly achieved by using a single oral dose of a class Ic drug such as flecainide or propafenone. Intravenous amiodarone is also effective, but takes longer to restore sinus rhythm. Recurrence of atrial fibrillation is most frequent during the first 3–6 months after restoration of sinus rhythm. Drugs are not always recommended for prophylaxis to maintain sinus rhythm after a first cardioversion, because of their proarrhythmic effects. However, if there is a high risk of recurrence, then sinus rhythm can be maintained with a class Ic drug, sotalol, amiodarone or dronedarone (see Compendium at end of chapter). Amiodarone is the most successful single drug for long-term prevention of recurrence; although it maintains sinus rhythm in only about 75% of people at 1 year, this is superior to the 40% maintenance of sinus rhythm with the other drugs. Digitalis glycosides are ineffective for restoring or maintaining sinus rhythm in paroxysmal atrial fibrillation and should be avoided. Radiofrequency isolation of a pulmonary vein trigger area via a cardiac catheter is becoming increasingly used for younger people with paroxysmal atrial fibrillation. Other curative procedures are infrequently used.

■ To control a rapid ventricular response in persistent or permanent atrial fibrillation. For ventricular rate control both at rest and on exercise a drug that slows AV nodal conduction, such as a β-adrenoceptor antagonist, verapamil or diltiazem, should be used. Rate control at rest can be achieved with digoxin, but a rapid heart rate often still occurs during exercise (see Ch. 7), so it is only used alone for sedentary people. A β-adrenoceptor antagonist, verapamil, diltiazem or amiodarone can be used together with digoxin if rate control is difficult to achieve. Sotalol has no additional benefit in sustained atrial fibrillation and should be avoided because of its greater proarrhythmic activity compared with that of other β-adrenoceptor antagonists. Dronedarone is not used for rate control due to evidence of increased mortality. If drug combinations do not provide satisfactory rate control, then AV nodal ablation with insertion of a pacemaker can be considered.

■ To reduce thromboembolism by long-term anticoagulation (Ch. 11). Anticoagulation, usually with warfarin, is the prophylactic of choice in atrial fibrillation associated with rheumatic heart disease or thyrotoxicosis, and for 1 month before and at least 1 month after DC cardioversion. In non-rheumatic atrial fibrillation, the risk of emboli is related to the number of associated risk factors (Table 8.3). Most people with atrial fibrillation, whether sustained or paroxysmal, should take thromboprophylaxis. Warfarin (maintaining the international normalised ratio [INR] between 2 and 3; see Ch. 11) reduces the risk of thromboembolism by about two-thirds, and low-dose aspirin reduces the risk of thromboembolism by one-quarter. There are also newer oral anticoagulants with similar efficacy to warfarin, but with a lower risk of serious bleeding and no need for monitoring, such as apixaban, dabigatran and rivaroxaban (Ch. 11). Oral anticoagulation is preferred for people at moderate or high risk of embolism, but has little advantage in those at low risk, when the increased risk of bleeding outweighs the benefit. Even after restoration of sinus rhythm in paroxysmal or persistent atrial fibrillation, people at high risk of thromboembolic events should continue to take thromboprophylaxis, since the risk of stroke does not decrease. This may reflect the high risk of recurrence (often asymptomatic) of atrial fibrillation.

Junctional (nodal) tachycardias

Junctional tachycardias usually arise from a re-entry circuit, and are often initiated by an ectopic beat. A micro re-entry circuit can form within the AV node if there are two functional intranodal pathways with different recovery times (AV nodal re-entry tachycardia; AVNRT). Such circuits account

---

Box 8.2	**Factors predicting a high probability of successful restoration of sinus rhythm in people with atrial fibrillation**

Short duration of atrial fibrillation (less than 1 year)
Younger age (< 50 years)
Absence of underlying heart disease
Normal left ventricular function
Little or no enlargement of the left atrium
Withdrawal or treatment of a precipitating factor, e.g. thyrotoxicosis, alcohol

Table 8.3 Risk of stroke in non-rheumatic atrial fibrillation

Score	Annual risk of stroke (%)	Recommended thromboprophylaxis
CHADS$_2$ score[a]		
0	1.9	Use CHA$_2$DS$_2$–Vasc score
1	2.8	Use CHA$_2$DS$_2$–Vasc score
2	4.0	Warfarin or other oral anticoagulant
3	5.9	Warfarin or other oral anticoagulant
4	8.5	Warfarin or other oral anticoagulant
5	12.5	Warfarin or other oral anticoagulant
6	18.2	Warfarin or other oral anticoagulant
CHA$_2$DS$_2$–Vasc score[b]		
0	0	None (or low-dose aspirin)
1	1.3	Low-dose aspirin (or oral anticoagulant)
2	2.2	Warfarin or other oral anticoagulant
3	3.2	Warfarin or other oral anticoagulant
4	4.0	Warfarin or other oral anticoagulant
5	6.7	Warfarin or other oral anticoagulant
6	9.8	Warfarin or other oral anticoagulant
7	9.6	Warfarin or other oral anticoagulant
8	6.7	Warfarin or other oral anticoagulant
9	15.2	Warfarin or other oral anticoagulant

Based on guidelines for the management of atrial fibrillation of the European Society of Cardiology (2010).
[a]The CHADS$_2$ score is a summation of the following component scores: **c**ongestive heart failure, 1; **h**ypertension, 1; **a**ge >75 years, 1; **d**iabetes mellitus, 1; prior **s**troke or transient ischaemic attack, 2.
[b]The CHA$_2$DS$_2$–Vasc score is a summation of the following component scores: **c**ongestive heart failure, 1; **h**ypertension, 1; **a**ge >75 years, 2; **d**iabetes mellitus, 1; prior **s**troke or transient ischaemic attack, 2; **a**ge 64–74 years, 1; **vasc**ular disease (prior myocardial infarction, peripheral arterial disease, aortic plaque), 1; Age 64–74, 1; Female sex, 1.

for 60% of supraventricular tachycardias other than atrial fibrillation/flutter, and are not usually associated with structural cardiac disease. Alternatively, a macro re-entry circuit may involve an accessory AV pathway connecting the atria and ventricles such as in Wolff–Parkinson–White syndrome (AV re-entrant tachycardia; AVRT), which accounts for 30% of supraventricular tachycardias. Termination of an acute attack of nodal tachycardia can often be achieved with vagotonic manoeuvres such as carotid sinus massage, or by adenosine. For AVNRT, β-adrenoceptor antagonists, diltiazem or verapamil can be used to treat acute episodes or for prophylaxis. However, if there is an accessory AV pathway diltiazem, verapamil and digoxin should be avoided because selective blockade of the AV node by these drugs can predispose to rapid conduction of atrial arrhythmias through the accessory pathway. Junctional tachycardias involving an accessory pathway often respond well to flecainide, sotalol or amiodarone. Radiofrequency ablation of the re-entry circuit, via a cardiac catheter, is being employed increasingly for troublesome junctional tachycardias.

Immediate management of narrow-complex tachycardia of uncertain origin

If the rhythm is regular it is often not possible to determine from the ECG whether a narrow-complex tachycardia has an atrial or nodal origin. If vagotonic manoeuvres are unsuccessful, and the person is haemodynamically stable, intravenous adenosine should be given. This often converts a junctional tachycardia to sinus rhythm or can slow the ventricular rate sufficiently to identify the origin of the rhythm on an ECG. If there is a history of severe asthma, intravenous verapamil may be preferred. DC cardioversion should be considered if there is haemodynamic instability.

VENTRICULAR TACHYARRHYTHMIAS

Ventricular ectopic beats

Ventricular ectopic beats can occur in healthy individuals or in association with a variety of cardiac disorders such as ischaemic heart disease and heart failure. Frequent ventricular ectopic beats after myocardial infarction predict a poorer long-term outcome; however, suppressing such ectopics with class I antiarrhythmic drugs increases mortality and should be avoided. In contrast, β-adrenoceptor antagonists after myocardial infarction reduce the risk of sudden death (Ch. 5). A β-adrenoceptor antagonist can also suppress ventricular ectopic beats induced by stress or anxiety. In other situations, symptomatic ventricular ectopic beats can be suppressed by a class I drug such as flecainide.

Ventricular tachycardia

Ventricular tachycardia presents with broad QRS complexes on the ECG (broad-complex tachycardia). Although broad complexes can arise with supraventricular tachycardias (when there is bundle branch block), broad-complex tachycardia is usually treated on the assumption that it is ventricular tachycardia. Ventricular tachycardia is often associated with serious underlying heart disease, such as ischaemic heart disease or heart failure, and is more common following myocardial infarction. It can be either sustained or non-sustained. Sustained ventricular tachycardia can be associated with a minimal or absent cardiac output ('pulseless' ventricular tachycardia), when it is treated in the same way as ventricular fibrillation (see below). Polymorphic or incessant ventricular tachycardias can arise as a complication of antiarrhythmic drug therapy (see above) and with other drugs that prolong the Q–T interval on the ECG.

For sustained ventricular tachycardias, drug options include class Ib antiarrhythmic agents such as lidocaine (especially after myocardial infarction), and amiodarone.

Sustained ventricular tachycardia is often associated with a poor long-term outlook in ischaemic heart disease, and coronary revascularisation or an automatic implantable cardiac defibrillator (ICD) may be beneficial. During and after the acute phase of myocardial infarction, a β-adrenoceptor antagonist is the treatment of choice to suppress non-sustained ventricular tachycardias.

Polymorphic or incessant ventricular tachycardias do not respond well to conventional treatments. Withdrawal of a precipitant drug, correction of electrolyte imbalance and intravenous magnesium sulphate are the therapies of choice. Temporary transvenous overpacing at a rate of 90–110 beats·min^{-1} may prevent recurrence. In the congenital form of long QT syndrome a β-adrenoceptor antagonist is the mainstay of treatment.

Ventricular fibrillation

Ventricular fibrillation is a potentially lethal arrhythmia that constitutes one form of 'cardiac arrest'. An algorithm for the management of cardiac arrest is regularly updated by the European Resuscitation Council and is shown in Figure 8.6. The important principles of prolonged resuscitation are the maintenance of adequate cardiac output by external chest compression, and oxygenation by artificial inflation of the lungs, while attempting to restore sinus rhythm. Ventricular fibrillation is the commonest arrhythmia in acute cardiac arrest and it should be assumed to be present unless an ECG is available to show otherwise. It should be treated with immediate DC cardioversion. Adrenaline (epinephrine; Ch. 4) may be given to vasoconstrict the peripheries and thus maintain pressure in the central arteries perfusing the heart and brain. For recurrent ventricular fibrillation, suppression can be achieved by long-term use of antiarrhythmic drugs such as sotalol or amiodarone (often combined with a β-adrenoceptor antagonist), but frequently requires an automatic ICD.

BRADYCARDIAS

Sinus bradycardia

Treatment with atropine may be necessary if sinus bradycardia is causing symptoms (e.g. after myocardial infarction or an overdose with a β-adrenoceptor antagonist). Hypotension precipitated by drugs such as streptokinase (Ch. 11) or the first dose of an angiotensin-converting enzyme (ACE) inhibitor (Ch. 6) is often associated with vagally mediated bradycardia, which will respond to atropine.

Atrioventricular block ('heart block')

AV block can be congenital or may accompany a variety of heart diseases. When occuring after myocardial infarction it is usually temporary if the infarct is inferior but is often permanent after anterior infarction. First-degree heart block (prolongation of the P–R interval on the ECG but with all P waves conducted to the ventricles) or Wenckebach (Mobitz type 1) second-degree heart block (progressive P–R prolongation until there is a non-conducted P wave) rarely require treatment, but higher degrees of block (second-degree, Mobitz type 2) and third-degree heart or complete heart block (with non-conducted P waves) should be treated. If complete AV block arises suddenly, then loss of consciousness (Stokes–Adams attack) or death can occur. If the onset is acute, atropine should be given intravenously to increase AV conduction, or an intravenous infusion of the non-selective β-adrenoceptor agonist isoprenaline can be used (Ch. 7). However, external or temporary transvenous electrical cardiac pacing is usually required in an emergency. If the AV block is permanent, the implantation of a permanent electrical cardiac pacemaker is usually necessary.

SELF-ASSESSMENT

True/false questions

1. The sinoatrial (SA) node and the atrioventricular (AV) node have pacemaker activity.
2. Pacemaker cells in the SA node discharge at a higher frequency than those in other parts of the heart.
3. Spontaneous or pacemaker depolarisation during diastole results solely from the influx of Na^+.
4. The influx of Na^+ during phase 0 lasts only for milliseconds.
5. Cells are unable to generate further action potentials during phases 0, 1 and 2 of the action potential.
6. Reducing the gradient of the slope of phase 4 will slow the normal pacemaker rate.
7. Sympathetic and vagal stimulation reduce the slope of phase 4 depolarisation and reduce pacemaker rate.
8. Healthy non-pacemaker cells remain quiescent if not excited by an impulse arising from other regions in the heart.
9. Flecainide blocks Na^+ channels.
10. Beta-adrenoceptor antagonist drugs are useful in stress-induced tachycardias.
11. The antiarrhythmic action of amiodarone depends only on blockade of K^+ channels.
12. Amiodarone reaches steady-state concentrations after several months of treatment.
13. Adenosine is effective in the treatment of ventricular arrhythmias.
14. Verapamil affects both the plateau phase 2 and phase 4 of the action potential cycle.
15. Combining verapamil and a β-adrenoceptor antagonist may cause AV nodal conduction block.

One-best-answer (OBA) question

Considering the flow of ions into cardiac myocytes (inward flow) and out of myocytes (outward flow), identify which one statement most correctly describes a situation that would prevent arrhythmias.

A. Increased inward flow of Na^+ during phase 0 of the action potential
B. Increased inflow of Ca^{2+} during phase 4 of the action potential

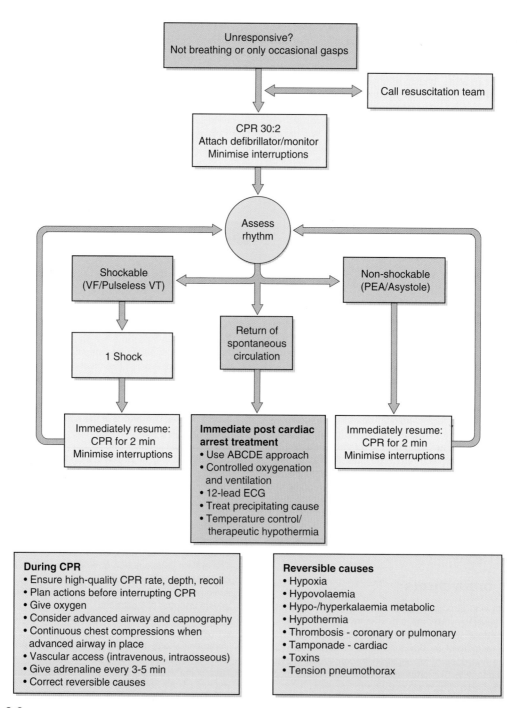

Fig. 8.6 An algorithm for the management of cardiac arrest. CPR, cardiopulmonary resuscitation; EMS, emergency medical services; PEA, pulseless electrical activity; VF, ventricular fibrillation; VT, ventricular tachycardia. Adapted from the 2010 European Resuscitation Council (ERC) Guidelines for Resuscitation (Nolan et al. 2010).

C. Decreased inflow of Na^+ during phase 0 of the action potential

D. Increased inflow of Ca^{2+} during phase 2 of the action potential

E. Decreased outflow of K^+ in phase 3 of the action potential

Case-based questions

Mr GH, aged 48 years, consulted his GP complaining of palpitations and was found to have an irregular pulse with a rate of 120 beats·min⁻¹. He had been suffering from shortness of breath and faintness for the previous 6 h. The symptoms had started after a drinking binge 36 h previously. Examination, blood tests (including thyroid function tests), ECG and chest radiograph revealed no coexisting heart disease, diabetes or hypertension. The ECG confirmed atrial fibrillation.

A. What were the options available for treating Mr GH?

Before any treatment could be instituted, Mr GH spontaneously reverted to sinus rhythm. He was well for a year but then returned to his GP with a 3-day history of palpitations, breathlessness, chest pain and dizziness. Examination and an ECG again revealed atrial fibrillation. He was referred to a cardiologist and echocardiography showed no evidence of structural cardiac disease. Electrical DC cardioversion was carried out and the rhythm reverted to sinus rhythm.

Over the next 5 years, episodes of atrial fibrillation occurred with increasing frequency, and, eventually, sinus rhythm could not be restored with a variety of antiarrhythmic drugs or by DC conversion.

B. What prophylactic treatment should be considered at the time of DC cardioversion? What drug treatments may be useful after DC cardioversion?

True/false answers

1. **True.** The SA and AV nodes, the bundle of His and the Purkinje system are pacemaker cells and form the specialised conducting system of the heart.
2. **True.** Pacemaker cells in the SA node therefore initiate cardiac rhythm.
3. **False.** Slow spontaneous depolarisation in pacemaker cells results from an inward flow of Na^+ and K^+ ions (funny current or I_f).
4. **True.** The fast Na^+ channels for influx close at the end of phase 1.
5. **True.** However, during phase 3, the cells are only relatively refractory to further depolarising stimuli and a sufficient stimulus could fire an action potential during this phase.
6. **True.** The slope in phase 4 controls the normal pacemaker rate as it determines the time taken to reach the threshold potential.
7. **False.** Vagal stimulation reduces the slope of phase 4 and slows the rate of firing, but sympathetic stimulation increases the slope and hence the firing rate.
8. **True.** However, if the intracellular Ca^{2+} concentration rises abnormally (e.g. under the influence of cardiac glycosides or catecholamines), this can exchange with Na^+ passing inwards, causing membrane depolarisations, called afterdepolarisations or 'triggered activity'.
9. **True.** All class I antiarrhythmics such as flecainide (class Ic) block fast Na^+ channels and slow the rate of rise of phase 0, therefore reducing myocardial excitability.
10. **True.** Beta-adrenoceptor antagonists reduce pacemaker depolarisation rate by inhibiting the sympathetic stimulation of the cAMP-dependent funny current (I_f) in the SA and AV nodes.
11. **False.** Like other class III agents, amiodarone blocks several types of K^+ channel, but also has a class Ib-like action on Na^+ channels, class II activity (non-competitive

β-adrenoceptor antagonism) and class IV activity (calcium channel blockade).
12. **True.** Accumulation of amiodarone to steady-state after about 6 months is due to its lipophilicity, resulting in a high apparent volume of distribution and very long half-life (50–60 days).
13. **False.** Adenosine has no beneficial effect on ventricular arrhythmias. Its main effect involves enhancing K^+ conductance and inhibiting Ca^{2+} influx, resulting in reduced AV nodal conduction and an increase in the AV nodal refractory period. Adenosine is useful in supraventricular arrhythmias, particularly when caused by AV nodal re-entry mechanisms; it has high efficacy and a very short duration of action.
14. **True.** L-type Ca^{2+} channels are involved in the phase 2 plateau while both T- and L-type channels contribute to depolarisation in phase 0 and the funny current in phase 4. Verapamil acts on both to slow the rate of the pacemaker depolarisation and to reduce the plateau phase, thus shortening the action potential. These effects make verapamil useful in supraventricular tachycardias but not in ventricular arrhythmias.
15. **True.** Verapamil is a highly negatively inotropic calcium channel blocker, reduces cardiac output, slows the heart rate, and impairs atrioventricular conduction, so it may cause AV nodal block or heart failure when used with β-adrenoceptor antagonists.

OBA answer

Answer C is correct.

A, B. Incorrect. Each of these would increase depolarisation rate in phase 4 and the rate of firing of the SA and AV nodes.
C.   Correct. This would slow the rate of depolarisation in phase 0 and is one of the mechanisms by which class I antiarrhythmics exert their therapeutic actions.
D, E. Incorrect. Each of these would shorten action potential duration, increasing the likelihood of arrhythmias.

Case-based answers

A. The aim at this stage is to restore and maintain sinus rhythm in Mr GH, who appears to have no structural heart disease. Since the arrhythmia is of short duration, pharmacological cardioversion may be successful. This could be achieved by flecainide, propafenone or amiodarone. Amiodarone is usually reserved for people with significant cardiac dysfunction or those refractory to other agents. Flecainide and propafenone should be avoided in people with significant cardiac dysfunction or concomitant ischaemic heart disease. However, they are probably suitable for this man. Digoxin, calcium channel blockers and β-adrenoceptor antagonists are ineffective for *terminating* atrial fibrillation. Synchronised DC cardioversion is successful in up to 90% of people with atrial fibrillation who have no structural heart disease or heart failure, who are aged less than 50 years and whose duration of atrial fibrillation is less

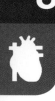

than 1 year. It could be considered if drugs are unsuccessful. About 50% of the time, recent-onset atrial fibrillation (less than 48 h duration) spontaneously converts to sinus rhythm. In Mr GH, the atrial fibrillation could have been brought on by excess alcohol (so-called 'holiday heart'). If he moderates his alcohol intake then prophylaxis would not be necessary after a single attack.

B. Anticoagulation with warfarin is essential for at least 3–4 weeks before and 4 weeks after a DC cardioversion to minimise the risk of a systemic embolus. For prophylaxis against recurrence, antifibrillatory drugs are usually given for at least 3–6 months following DC cardioversion, since this is the period of highest risk of recurrence. Digoxin, verapamil and β-adrenoceptor antagonists are not effective for prophylaxis. After 5 years of recurrence of atrial fibrillation, sinus rhythm could not be restored. Therefore, the aim in Mr GH is to control ventricular rate. Digoxin suppresses AV nodal conduction and can reduce the ventricular response rate. This is mediated through potentiation of vagal effects on the heart and is less effective during exercise; therefore, a β-adrenoceptor antagonist or calcium channel blocker (such as verapamil) is preferred. However, β-adrenoceptor antagonists (in high doses) and verapamil are negatively inotropic, and if there is significant cardiac dysfunction or heart failure they are contraindicated. The positive inotropic action of digoxin might be helpful if there is coexisting left ventricular impairment. The major long-term consequence of atrial fibrillation is the risk of thromboembolism and this is greatest in those over 75 years of age. For Mr GH, aspirin or no thromboprophylaxis is appropriate as he is at a relatively low risk of stroke because of his age and lack of any coexisting hypertension, diabetes or significant left ventricular impairment.

FURTHER READING

Calò L, Sciarra L, Lamberti F et al. (2003) Electropharmacological effects of antiarrhythmic drugs on atrial fibrillation termination. Part 1: molecular and ionic fundamentals of antiarrhythmic drug actions. *Ital Heart J* 4, 430–441

Delacrétaz E (2006) Supraventricular tachycardias. *N Engl J Med* 354, 1039–1051

Grant AO (2001) Molecular biology of sodium channels and their role in cardiac arrhythmias. *Am J Med* 110, 296–305

Gupta A, Lawrence AT, Krishnan K et al. (2007) Current concepts in the mechanisms and management of drug-induced QT prolongation and torsade de pointes. *Am Heart J* 153, 891–899

Hart RG, Pearce LA, Aguilar MI (2007) Meta-analysis: antithrombotic therapy to prevent stroke in patients who have nonvalvular atrial fibrillation. *Ann Intern Med* 146, 857–867

International Liaison Committee on Resuscitation (2005) 2005 International Consensus on Cardiopulmonary Resuscitation and Emergency Cardiovascular Care Science with Treatment Recommendations, Part 1: Introduction. *Resuscitation* 67, 181–186

Iqbal MB, Taneja AK, Lip GYH et al. (2005) Recent developments in atrial fibrillation. *BMJ* 330, 238–243

Katz AM (1998) Selectivity and toxicity of antiarrhythmic drugs: molecular interactions with ion channels. *Am J Med* 104, 179–195

Lafuente-Lafuente C, Mouly S, Longás-Tejero MA et al. (2006) Antiarrhythmic drugs for maintaining sinus rhythm after cardioversion of atrial fibrillation. *Arch Intern Med* 166, 719–728

Lau W, Newman D, Dorian P (2000) Can antiarrhythmic agents be selected based on mechanism of action? *Drugs* 60, 1315–1328

Lip GYH, Tse H-F (2007) Management of atrial fibrillation. *Lancet* 370, 604–618

Nattel S, Opie LH (2006) Controversies in atrial fibrillation. *Lancet* 367, 262–272

Nolan JP, Soar J, Zideman DA, Biarent D, Bossaert LL, Deakin C, Koster RW, Wyllie J, Böttiger B, on behalf of ERC Guidelines Writing Group (2010). European Resuscitation Council Guidelines for Resuscitation 2010 Section 1: Executive Summary. *Resuscitation* 81, 1219–1276

Page RL (2004) Newly diagnosed atrial fibrillation. *N Engl J Med* 351, 2408–2416

Reiffel JA, Reiter MJ, Blitzer M (1998) Antiarrhythmic drugs and devices for the management of ventricular tachyarrhythmias in ischemic heart disease. *Am J Cardiol* 82, 31I–40I

Reiter MJ, Reiffel JA (1998) Importance of beta blockade in the therapy of serious ventricular arrhythmias. *Am J Cardiol* 82, 9I–19I

Roden DM, Balser JR, George AL Jr, Anderson ME (2002) Cardiac ion channels. *Annu Rev Physiol* 64, 431–475

Shorofsky SR, Balke CW (2001) Calcium currents and arrhythmias: insights from molecular biology. *Am J Med* 110, 127–140

Tamargo J, Caballero, R, Gomez, R et al. (2004) Pharmacology of cardiac potassium channels. *Cardiovasc Res* 62, 9–33

Task Force on the Management of Atrial Fibrillation of the European Society of Cardiology (2010). Guidelines for the management of atrial fibrillation. *Eur Heart J* 31, 2369–2429

Compendium: Drugs used to treat cardiac arrhythmias

Drug	Kinetics (half-life)	Comments[a]
Class I drugs		
Disopyramide	Oral bioavailability 90%; main metabolite is less antiarrhythmic but more antimuscarinic (4–10 h).	Class Ia drug used for SVT, VF, VT; given orally, or by slow intravenous injection (over at least 5 min) or intravenous infusion
Flecainide	Oral bioavailability >90%; hepatic metabolism; also renal elimination (12–30 h)	Class Ic drug used for AF, SVT; given orally, or by slow intravenous injection (over 10–30 min) or intravenous infusion (for resistant ventricular tachyarrhythmias)
Lidocaine	Low oral bioavailability; hepatic metabolites retain some activity and toxicity (2 h)	Class Ib drug used for VA (especially post-myocardial infarction); given by intravenous injection or intravenous infusion
Procainamide	Metabolised by N-acetylation (3 h) to product as active as the parent drug and with longer half-life (6–9 h)	Class Ia drug used for AT, VA; given by slow intravenous injection or by intravenous infusion
Propafenone	Low oral bioavailability (10%) increased at higher doses and by food; hepatic metabolism (4h); longer half-life (17 h) in slow CYP2D6 metabolisers	Class Ic drug used for SVT, VA; also has some β-adrenoceptor antagonist activity; given orally
Class II drugs: β-adrenoceptor antagonists (β-blockers)		
Beta-adrenoceptor antagonists are used in a wide variety of indications; they are listed alphabetically in the Compendium in Ch. 5. Atenolol, bisoprolol, esmolol and propranolol are the most commonly used in arrhythmias. See also sotalol below.		
Class III drugs		
Amiodarone	Oral bioavailability 20–100%; hepatic metabolism; active metabolite has similar long half-life to parent drug (50–60 days); accumulation occurs to steady state after about 6 months	Used for all arrhythmias, with treatment usually initiated in hospital or under specialist supervision; given orally or by intravenous injection (over 3 min) for VF; significant unwanted effects – monitor thyroid function
Dronedarone	Less lipophilic than amiodarone with shorter half-life (24 h); hepatic metabolism and faecal excretion	Multichannel blocker; used for AF; given orally
Sotalol	Oral bioavailability is >90%; eliminated largely by glomerular filtration (7–18 h)	Also a class II non-selective β-adrenoceptor antagonist; used for VT (life-threatening); greater proarrhythmic risk than other β-adrenoceptor antagonists; given orally or by intravenous injection (over 10 min)
Class IV drugs: calcium channel blockers		
For calcium channel blockers, see Ch. 5. Dihydropyridine calcium channel blockers have no antiarrhythmic actvity; the non-dihydropyridine diltiazem has antiarrhythmic properties but is not licensed in the UK for this indication.		
Verapamil	Low oral bioavailability (about 20%); hepatic metabolism (2–7 h)	Used for SVT; given orally or by intravenous injection; interaction risk with β- adrenoceptor antagonists
Other drugs		
Adenosine	Cleared extremely rapidly by metabolism in erythrocytes and endothelial cells (<10 s)	Purine nucleoside; used as the treatment of choice for terminating paroxysmal SVT; given intravenously
Atropine	Liver metabolism and renal excretion (2–5 h)	Anti-muscarinic; used for bradycardia, especially if complicated by hypotension; given intravenously
Digoxin	Mainly renal excretion (20–50 h); longer half-life in renal impairment	Cardiac glycoside; used for AF; may need loading dose; oral or intravenous dosage (see Ch. 7)

[a]The types of arrhythmias commonly treated with different drugs are: AF, atrial fibrillation; AT, atrial tachycardia; SVT, supraventricular tachycardia; VA, ventricular arrhythmias; VF, ventricular fibrillation; VT, ventricular tachycardia.

9 Cerebrovascular disease and dementia

• •

STROKE

AETIOLOGY

Strokes are a major cause of morbidity and mortality, particularly in older people. They present as a transient or permanent neurological disturbance caused by ischaemic infarction or haemorrhagic disruption of neuronal pathways in the brain.

Ischaemic strokes and transient ischaemic attacks

Ischaemic strokes and transient ischaemic attacks (TIAs) account for about 85% of events. Cerebral infarction can result from intracerebral arterial thrombosis or from emboli travelling to the cerebral arteries, typically from an unstable atheromatous plaque in an internal carotid artery (see Ch. 5) or from the heart. The extent and duration of the resulting functional deficit following a stroke are very variable.

Transient (cerebral) ischaemic attacks arise from small cerebral arterial emboli that disperse rapidly. They produce short-lived neurological signs and symptoms but leave no functional deficit 24 h later. A completed stroke results from more severe cerebral ischaemia, which produces cerebral infarction. The neurological disturbance persists for more than 24 h, and frequently there is some permanent loss of function. Following a TIA there is a 5% risk of a completed stroke in the subsequent 24 h, and a 30% risk of a completed stroke in the subsequent 5 years. However, if there is a significant carotid artery stenosis at the time of the TIA the risk of completed stroke is 30% in the first month.

Haemorrhagic strokes

Primary intracerebral haemorrhage is responsible for up to 15% of strokes. It often arises from rupture of microaneurysms on intracerebral arteries, usually in association with hypertension. Haemorrhagic strokes commonly leave a permanent functional deficit.

PREVENTION AND TREATMENT

Current treatments produce only a modest limitation of the neurological deficit in acute stroke. Most management is directed to:

- primary prevention of a first event (ischaemic or haemorrhagic stroke),
- prevention of recurrence of stroke or of other cardiovascular events,
- rehabilitation after the stroke.

About one-third of strokes are recurrent. The recurrence rate for ischaemic stroke is about 3–7% per year for individuals who are in sinus rhythm and about 12% per year for those in atrial fibrillation.

Primary prevention of ischaemic stroke

- **Blood pressure reduction.** Hypertension is the single most powerful predictor of stroke. Pooled trial results indicate that a reduction in diastolic blood pressure by 5–6 mmHg reduces the risk of stroke by about 40% (Ch. 6). For isolated systolic hypertension, a similar reduction in risk has been shown after an average 11 mmHg reduction in systolic blood pressure.
- **Smoking cessation.** The risk of ischaemic stroke is reduced by up to 40% by 2–5 years after smoking cessation. This is probably due to slower progression of arterial atherothrombotic disease.
- **Reduced platelet aggregation.** Low-dose aspirin has *not* been shown to prevent a first ischaemic stroke when taken by healthy individuals who are in sinus rhythm. For people with atrial fibrillation, aspirin produces a modest reduction in the risk of a first ischaemic stroke by about one-quarter. However, aspirin is much less effective than warfarin (or other oral anticoagulants) for stroke reduction in atrial fibrillation (Ch. 8).

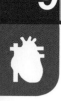

- **Inhibition of blood clotting.** Oral anticoagulation (Chs 8 and 11) in people with atrial fibrillation reduces the risk of a first ischaemic stroke by 70%. Warfarin, at a dosage giving an international normalised ratio (INR) of 2–3, or one of the newer anticoagulants such as apixaban, dabigatran or rivaroxaban, can be used. There is no advantage of warfarin over aspirin for people in sinus rhythm. Warfarin reduces the risk of stroke following myocardial infarction if there is intracardiac clot associated with an akinetic area of the left ventricular wall.
- **Cholesterol reduction.** Reduction of a raised plasma cholesterol with a statin (Ch. 48) produces a 25% reduction in the risk of a first stroke, although much of the evidence for this effect derives from trials in people who already have clinical evidence of vascular disease or who have diabetes mellitus.
- **Carotid endarterectomy or stenting.** This is sometimes recommended for asymptomatic carotid artery disease when the stenosis exceeds 60%, but the annual risk of an ischaemic stroke is low in this situation.

Primary prevention of haemorrhagic stroke

- **Blood pressure reduction.** Lowering a raised blood pressure is the only means of reducing the risk of cerebral haemorrhage.

Treatment of acute ischaemic stroke

Fibrinolytic therapy with recombinant tissue plasminogen activator (rt-PA, alteplase; Ch. 11) can reduce the long-term neurological deficit after an ischaemic stroke. If treatment is started within 3 h of the onset of symptoms, thrombolysis reduces the risk of death or dependency at 3 months, with greater benefit the earlier that treatment is given. Overall, 7% more people who are given thrombolysis after ischaemic stroke will have no or minimal disability 3 months later. However, more than half of those who are treated with

an intravenous fibrinolytic drug do not have complete or near-complete recovery. There is an increased risk of intracerebral haemorrhage after thrombolysis, particularly in those with a blood pressure above 185/110 mmHg or when treatment is delayed, which can outweigh the benefit from neuronal salvage. About 6% of people who are treated will have a symptomatic intracranial haemorrhage.

Meta-analysis of several studies shows that intravenous alteplase is moderately effective from 3 h until 4.5 h after the event. Intra-arterial alteplase is effective in large ischaemic strokes up to 6 h after the onset of symptoms.

Indications and usual contraindications for thrombolytic therapy in acute stroke are shown in Box 9.1. Anticoagulants or antiplatelet drugs should not be given for 24 h after thrombolysis.

There have been many recent advances in treatment of acute ischaemic stroke. These include the use of mechanical thrombectomy devices to reduce the size of the thrombus, and ultrasonography to improve penetration of the fibrinolytic drug into the thrombus. However, a major advance may be the use of sensitive brain imaging to identify those who have potentially recoverable neurological injury from those with irreversible infarction.

Secondary prevention of recurrent ischaemic stroke

Many treatments are similar to those used for primary prevention of ischaemic stroke (see above).

- **Blood pressure reduction.** Lowering blood pressure after a stroke will reduce the risk of recurrence by 30–40%. There is considerable reluctance to reduce blood pressure in the first few days after a stroke, because of concern that cerebral perfusion pressure may fall too much if the normal cerebral arterial autoregulation has been disturbed by the stroke. However, there is some evidence that early treatment (after the first 24 h) may be advantageous.
- **Reduced platelet aggregation.** Low-dose aspirin with dipyridamole can be used following a TIA for people who

---

Box 9.1   Usual indications and contraindications for thrombolysis in acute ischaemic stroke

Indications for thrombolysis	Potential contraindications to thrombolysis
Clinical diagnosis of ischaemic stroke causing measurable neurological deficit for at least 30 min	Severe stroke deficit on clinical assessment
	Head trauma or prior stroke in past 3 months
Onset of symptoms less than 4.5 h before beginning treatment	Any previous stroke with concomitant diabetes mellitus
	Gastrointestinal or genitourinary hemorrhage in previous 21 days
The patient and family understand the potential risks and benefits of therapy	Arterial puncture in non-compressible site during previous 7 days
	Major surgery in previous 14 days
Intracranial haemorrhage excluded by CT or MR head scan	History of previous intracranial haemorrhage
	Evidence of acute trauma or haemorrhage
	Taking an oral anticoagulant (or, if so, INR greater than 1.4 when treating in under 3 h)
	Heparin within 48 h, unless a normal activated partial thromboplastin time
	Seizure at the onset of the stroke
	Systolic blood pressure above 185 mmHg or diastolic blood pressure above 110 mmHg
	Platelet count of less than 100×10^9 L^{-1}
	Blood glucose less than 2.7 mmol·L^{-1}

are in sinus rhythm. The combination reduces the risk of a subsequent non-fatal stroke by about 35%, and is more effective than aspirin alone. This combination is recommended for up to 2 years after a TIA, when the risk of recurrent stroke is highest, after which aspirin is often used alone. Clopidogrel alone (Ch. 11) is as effective as aspirin and dipyridamole after ischaemic stroke, and is now the preferred treatment. By contrast, the combination of aspirin and clopidogrel is no more effective than aspirin alone for long-term prevention (unlike in acute coronary syndromes; see Ch. 5), and increases the risk of serious bleeds. However, there may be some benefit from the combination for short-term treatment (7–30 days) immediately after a stroke or TIA in those at high risk of recurrence. Warfarin has no role in preventing recurrent stroke in people who are in sinus rhythm.

- **Inhibition of blood clotting.** After a first stroke in people with atrial fibrillation, oral anticoagulation reduces the risk of a further stroke by two-thirds. In contrast, aspirin has no protective effect in this situation (see Ch. 11).
- **Cholesterol reduction.** Cholesterol reduction with a statin is effective in secondary prevention of ischaemic stroke, reducing recurrent stroke by 21% for every 1 mmol·L^{-1} reduction in low-density lipoprotein (LDL) cholesterol. However, the greatest advantage of cholesterol reduction in this situation is in the prevention of ischaemic cardiac events, since coronary artery disease often coexists with atheromatous cerebrovascular disease.
- **Carotid endarterectomy or stenting.** This reduces the risk of recurrent stroke if there have already been transient focal neurological symptoms in the cerebral territory served by a diseased carotid artery. If the stenosis is ≥70% of the vessel diameter (but without near total occlusion), then endarterectomy reduces the risk of recurrent stroke by about two-thirds over the subsequent 2 years (despite a perioperative risk of stroke or death of 3–5%). There is no benefit from surgery if the occlusion is less than 50%, and only marginal benefit if the occlusion is between 50 and 69%, unless the surgery is carried out soon after the event (usually within 2 weeks), when the risk of recurrence is highest.

Secondary prevention of recurrent haemorrhagic stroke

- **Blood pressure reduction.** Lowering blood pressure after a haemorrhagic stroke will reduce the risk of recurrence by up to 40%. The reduction in risk from treating hypertension is greater than for ischaemic stroke, and even lowering a 'normal' blood pressure may be effective. As for ischaemic stroke, treatment is usually delayed to allow return of autoregulation of cerebral blood flow, unless the blood pressure exceeds 185/105 mmHg.

SUBARACHNOID HAEMORRHAGE

Most subarachnoid haemorrhages are caused by rupture of a saccular (or berry) aneurysm on an intracranial artery, usually on or close to the circle of Willis. These aneurysms are acquired during life and the cause is unknown, although there is an association with hypertension and conditions that increase cerebral blood flow such as arteriovenous malformations. About 5% of all strokes are caused by subarachnoid haemorrhage. Sudden onset of severe occipital headache is the most common presenting symptom, but focal neurological signs or progressive confusion and impaired consciousness can occur. Rebleeding is a significant cause of disability and death, and early surgical intervention in survivors of the initial bleed reduces this risk. A more common cause of permanent neurological disability or later death is delayed cerebral ischaemia. This is produced by cerebral vasospasm, which develops in about 25% of cases, usually at least 3 days after the haemorrhage. The mechanism is poorly understood, but involves activation of voltage-dependent L-type Ca^{2+} channels in intracranial arteries. It presents with confusion, decreased consciousness and new focal neurological deficit.

DRUGS FOR SUBARACHNOID HAEMORRHAGE

Nimodipine

Nimodipine is a dihydropyridine L-type calcium channel blocker (for mechanism of action see Ch. 5) that is an arterial vasodilator with some selectivity for cerebral arteries. It reduces the risk of vasospasm following subarachnoid haemorrhage, but probably produces most of its benefits by protecting ischaemic neurons from Ca^{2+} overload. There is a theoretical risk that cerebral vasodilation may actually facilitate further bleeding, but this does not appear to be a problem in practice.

Pharmacokinetics

Nimodipine is well absorbed from the gut and undergoes extensive first-pass metabolism in the liver and gut wall. It has a half-life of 8–9 h, and is eliminated by metabolism in the liver.

Unwanted effects

These are mainly caused by arterial dilation:

- hypotension, which can have a detrimental effect on cerebral perfusion,
- headache, flushing.

MANAGEMENT OF SUBARACHNOID HAEMORRHAGE

Initial treatment of subarachnoid haemorrhage aims to reduce ischaemic cerebral damage. Nimodipine is usually given intravenously immediately after the event, followed by oral dosing for a total of 5–10 days. Intravenous fluids are given to avoid hypotension. The optimum blood pressure in the early period after the haemorrhage is not known, but hypotension should be avoided and blood pressure lowered modestly in those who present with significant hypertension. Dexamethasone (Ch. 44) may be used to reduce cerebral oedema.

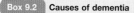

Box 9.2	Causes of dementia
Treatable causes of dementia	**Irreversible and partially treatable causes of dementia**
Hypothyroidism	Vascular dementia
Neurosyphilis	Alzheimer's disease
Vitamin B₁ deficiency	Lewy body-type dementia
Normal-pressure hydrocephalus	Parkinson's disease dementia
Frontal lobe tumours	Progressive supranuclear palsy
Cerebral vasculitis	Multiple-system atrophy
Cerebral hypoperfusion	

The definitive management of subarachnoid haemorrhage is surgical, with endovascular coil occlusion of the aneurysm or clipping of the neck of the aneurysm that produced the bleeding. In the last 20 years early surgical intervention, combined with medical therapy, has reduced mortality from 20% to about 5–10%.

DEMENTIA

Dementia usually begins with forgetfulness and is characterised by disorientation in unfamiliar surroundings, variable mood, restlessness and poor sleep. Deterioration in social behaviour with self-neglect often follows, and may be accompanied by personality change with loss of inhibition. Most dementia results from Alzheimer's disease or from cerebrovascular disease (multi-infarct dementia), but there are other causes (Box 9.2). Memory impairment in dementia tends to be associated with bilateral hippocampal damage.

ALZHEIMER'S DISEASE

Alzheimer's disease is the commonest cause of dementia in people over the age of 65 years. About 10% of people over the age of 65 and about 30% of those over the age of 85 have some signs of Alzheimer's disease. The onset of symptoms is gradual, with progressive deterioration, unlike vascular dementia. It is a neurodegenerative disorder that begins pathologically 20–30 years before the clinical onset.

The cause of Alzheimer's disease is unknown, but there are several distinct factors associated with the disease.

- **Amyloid protein**. β-Amyloid is deposited in the medial temporal lobe and cerebral cortex of people with Alzheimer's disease as senile plaques. The initiating factor in Alzheimer's disease may be an imbalance between the production and clearance of β-amyloid in the brain, leading to toxic effects on neuronal synapses. Deposition of β-amyloid may be the driver for hyperphosphorylation of tau protein (found in axons, where it promotes microtubule assembly and vesicle transport), which aggregates into neurofibrillary tangles that are characteristic of Alzheimer's disease.
- **Genetic predisposition**. This accounts for about 70% of the risk. Mutations of the apolipoprotein E ε4 allele (APOE ε4; essential for amyloid β clearance) confer a higher risk of late-onset Alzheimer's disease, while

mutations in genes coding for amyloid precursor protein and presenilin 1 and 2 explain the rare familial disease.

- **Inflammatory factors**. Activated microglia and reactive astrocytes surround the senile plaques, and there is local increase in pro-inflammatory mediators.
- **Glutamate excitotoxicity**. Amyloid deposits may promote neuronal damage by increasing neuronal release of glutamate. This acts at N-methyl-D-aspartate (NMDA) receptors to generate glutamate-induced excitotoxicity of cholinergic neurons. Hyperactivity of glutamatergic neurons is a common finding in Alzheimer's disease.
- **Oxidative stress**. There is evidence for excessive free radical production in Alzheimer's disease. Increased oxidative stress may contribute to the condition by producing vascular damage, reducing β-amyloid clearance and promoting metabolic derangement in neurons.
- **Loss of cholinergic neurotransmission**. There is a marked loss of acetylcholine neurotransmitter synthesis in the cerebral cortex and the hippocampus, particularly affecting the areas involved in cognition and in memory that are impaired in Alzheimer's disease. There is also loss of cholinergic neurons. Activity at both muscarinic and nicotinic receptors is reduced. Depletion of other neurotransmitters is a late and inconsistent finding.

DRUGS FOR ALZHEIMER'S DISEASE

Anticholinesterases

donepezil, galantamine, rivastigmine

Mechanisms of action and effects

The basis of the cholinergic hypothesis of Alzheimer's disease is that loss of cholinergic neurons in the basal forebrain nuclei results in abnormal function at cholinergic terminals in the hippocampus and neocortex, which are involved in memory and cognition. Anticholinesterases increase cholinergic transmission in the brain by inhibition of acetylcholinesterase in the synaptic cleft (Ch. 4).

- Donepezil is a reversible inhibitor of acetylcholinesterase with a high degree of selectivity for the central nervous system (CNS).
- Galantamine is a reversible competitive inhibitor of acetylcholinesterase that also has agonist activity at presynaptic nicotinic receptors by allosterically enhancing the receptor response to acetylcholine.
- Rivastigmine is a slowly reversible inhibitor of acetylcholinesterase with selectivity for the CNS, and also inhibits pseudocholinesterase (butyrylcholinesterase) present in tissues and plasma.

Pharmacokinetics

Donepezil, galantamine and rivastigmine are well absorbed from the gut. Donepezil and galantamine are metabolised in the liver, and galantamine has a half-life of 5–7 h while that of donepezil is very long, at 70–80 h. Rivastigmine is rapidly inactivated by cholinesterase-mediated hydrolysis and has a short half-life of 1–2 h.

Unwanted effects

- Anorexia, nausea, vomiting, diarrhoea, abdominal pain.
- Drowsiness, hallucination, agitation, dizziness, headache.
- Bradycardia.

NMDA receptor antagonists

memantine

Mechanism of action and effects

Memantine is a derivative of the antiviral drug amantadine (Chs 24 and 51), and is a non-competitive antagonist at glutamate NMDA receptors. This may prevent glutamate-induced excitotoxicity (by limiting long-lasting influx of Ca^{2+} into neurons), but without interfering with the actions of glutamate that are involved in memory and learning. Memantine is also a 5-HT$_3$ receptor antagonist and a non-competitive nicotinic receptor antagonist, but the significance of these actions for the treatment of dementia is unknown. It can be taken together with an anticholinesterase.

Pharmacokinetics

Memantine is well absorbed from the gut and is largely excreted unchanged by the kidneys. It has a very long half-life of 60–80 h.

Unwanted effects

- Constipation.
- Headache, dizziness, drowsiness.
- Hypertension, dyspnoea.

TREATMENT OF ALZHEIMER'S DISEASE

In the UK, drug treatment for Alzheimer's disease is started only for people who have a Mini-Mental State Examination (MMSE) score of 10–20 points (moderate dementia). The diagnosis of Alzheimer's disease should be first confirmed in a specialist memory clinic.

Cholinesterase inhibitors produce modest improvement in symptoms, and a delay in the decline of cognitive function and memory, in up to 40% of those who are treated. Efficacy should be assessed after 2–4 months of treatment at a suitable dose. Treatment should be continued only if the 'global, functional and behavioural condition remains at a level where the drug is considered to be having a worthwhile effect'. Treatment should be stopped in non-responders. The decline in mental function is delayed by about 3–6 months but not arrested. Rapid progression resumes when the drugs are stopped, but there may be limited benefit from restarting treatment more than a month after withdrawal. Anticholinesterases produce some

improvement in other functional measures and behaviour that also affect the quality of life.

Memantine produces moderate improvement in cognition and reduction in functional decline, and is usually well tolerated. However, it may be ineffective in the early stages of Alzheimer's disease. Combination of a cholinesterase inhibitor with memantine can give additive benefits.

Current treatments for Alzheimer's disease do not alter the progression of the underlying disease. New treatment strategies are being developed that are directed either at enhancing the various neurotrophic proteins which protect neuronal systems, or at altering the production or clearance of amyloid protein or tau protein found in neurofibrillary tangles. Such strategies may offer a more fundamental approach to retarding the progress of Alzheimer's disease.

Neuropsychiatric complications such as depression and severe aggression may require treatment, but the value of antidepressant therapy is uncertain and antipsychotic drugs can produce significant unwanted effects with only modest benefit.

VASCULAR DEMENTIA

Cerebrovascular disease is a particularly common cause of dementia over the age of 85 years, and overall is the second most frequent cause of dementia. The deterioration in mental function is produced by multiple cerebral infarcts (multi-infarct dementia), particularly if they affect the white matter. The risk of dementia is increased ninefold in people with stroke. In some of these, dementia may be produced by specific, strategically located infarcts, especially in the angular gyrus of the inferior parietal lobule. In contrast to Alzheimer's disease, the initial presentation is usually more acute and cognitive decline has a stepwise course arising from recurrent cerebrovascular events.

TREATMENT

- Prophylaxis against cerebral emboli with aspirin or warfarin depending on the heart rhythm (see prevention of stroke, above). However, the Cochrane database finds that there is no evidence, as yet, that aspirin is of benefit in vascular dementia.
- Control of hypertension (Ch. 6). Trials have shown that calcium channel blockers are effective for reducing the risk of vascular dementia, but it is likely to be an effect related to blood pressure reduction rather than a more specific effect of this class of drug.
- Anticholinesterases or memantine may produce some improvement in vascular dementia.
- Immunosuppressant drugs (Ch. 38) can be used in the rare cases caused by cerebral vasculitis.

SELF-ASSESSMENT

True/false questions

1. Aspirin reduces the risk of a first stroke in healthy individuals.

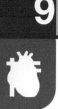

2. Aspirin cannot prevent a first stroke in people with persistent atrial fibrillation.
3. Approximately 85% of all strokes have a haemorrhagic aetiology.
4. If thrombolysis with recombinant tissue plasminogen activator (rt-PA; alteplase) is given in acute stroke, antiplatelet and anticoagulant therapies should not be given concurrently.
5. Anticoagulation with warfarin and antiplatelet therapy with aspirin are equal first-choice drugs for secondary prevention of recurrent ischaemic strokes in the presence of sinus rhythm.
6. Nimodipine reduces risk of vasospasm following subarachnoid haemorrhage.
7. Donepezil is an acetylcholinesterase inhibitor with selectivity for the CNS.
8. Cerebral ischaemia depolarises neurons and causes the release of large amounts of glutamate.
9. The NMDA receptor antagonist memantine reduces neurotoxicity caused by the excitatory transmitter glutamate.
10. Cerebral emboli arising from the heart are invariably caused by atrial fibrillation.

One-best answer (OBA) question

Choose the one *correct* statement from the following.

A. Alzheimer's disease is associated with a relative lack of cholinergic and glutamatergic neurotransmission.
B. It is recommended that rivastigmine is prescribed in Alzheimer's disease irrespective of the Mini-Mental State Examination (MMSE) score.
C. Memantine is a muscarinic receptor agonist.
D. Anticholinesterases should not be co-prescribed with memantine.
E. Unlike donepezil, rivastigmine inhibits both acetylcholinesterase and butyrylcholinesterase.

Case-based questions

A 70-year-old man had a blood pressure of 190/110 mmHg despite intensive antihypertensive drug treatment. He was admitted to hospital 6 h after the acute onset of unilateral weakness and sensory loss. At the time of admission to hospital, most of the neurological signs had resolved. He had no headache or vomiting and remained conscious. He was in sinus rhythm. Following clinical examination and a CT brain scan, this episode was diagnosed as a TIA.

A. Should thrombolysis be given?
B. What other therapies should be instituted immediately?
C. What secondary prevention strategy should be employed?

True/false answers

1. **False.** Aspirin does not reduce the risk of a first stroke in healthy individuals in sinus rhythm.
2. **False.** Aspirin reduces the risk of a first embolic stroke in atrial fibrillation by about 25%, but is less effective than warfarin.
3. **False.** About 85% of strokes have an ischaemic aetiology; up to 15% are caused by intracerebral haemorrhage.
4. **True.** The immediate risk of intracranial haemorrhage with alteplase is high and could be compounded by simultaneous administration of antiplatelet or anticoagulant agents. These should be considered later, when the effect of the thrombolytic has waned.
5. **False.** In people in sinus rhythm, aspirin alone (or together with dipyridamole) reduces the risk of stroke; warfarin is no more effective and there is a greater risk of major bleeding.
6. **True.** By blocking L-type calcium channels, nimodipine reduces vasospasm and also protects ischaemic neurons from Ca^{2+} overload.
7. **True.** Anticholinesterase drugs enhance cholinergic activity in the hippocampus and neocortex, improving memory and cognition.
8. **True.** The excitatory transmitter glutamate can cause a substantial rise in intracellular Ca^{2+}, causing Ca^{2+} overload and cell death by generation of free radicals.
9. **True.** Memantine blocks NMDA (glutamate) receptors and reduces glutamate-induced excitotoxicity of cholinergic neurons.
10. **False.** Cerebral emboli arising from the heart can also be caused by infected or damaged prosthetic valves or following damage to the myocardium

OBA answer

Answer **E is correct**.

A. Incorrect. Alzheimer's disease is associated with reduced cholinergic transmission and increased glutamatergic transmission.
B. Incorrect. In the UK, it is advised that the anticholinesterases should not be prescribed if the MMSE is below 10.
C. Incorrect. Memantine is a glutamate NMDA receptor antagonist.
D. Incorrect. Anticholinesterases and memantine can be useful co-prescribed.
E. **Correct.** But it is unclear whether additional inhibition of pseudocholinesterase (butyrylcholinesterase) by rivastigmine provides additional clinical benefit.

Case-based answers

A. Thrombolysis is inappropriate in this situation. His blood pressure is high and it is a considerable time since the onset of symptoms. Thrombolysis has been approved for use within 3 h of the onset of symptoms. The rapid resolution of signs indicates a TIA, for which thrombolysis is not given. (Although thrombolysis has been shown in some trials to be useful in the treatment of stroke, safe and effective use is determined by a rigid set of criteria as there is a significant risk of intracranial haemorrhage.)
B. His blood pressure must be brought under control. Reduction in blood pressure has a major effect on the prevention of a recurrent stroke. He should also be given low-dose aspirin and dipyridamole.

C. Antiplatelet therapy should be continued. The antiplatelet drug dipyridamole has additional benefit when given together with aspirin. Cholesterol reduction with a statin is effective in secondary prevention of ischaemic stroke. It would be worth treating this man with a statin even if his cholesterol is not raised. An important reason for cholesterol reduction is prevention of ischaemic cardiac events, since coronary artery disease often coexists with atheromatous cerebrovascular disease.

FURTHER READING

Stroke

Claiborne JS (2002) Transient ischemic attack. *N Engl J Med* 347, 1687–1692

Davis SM, Donnan GA (2012) Secondary prevention after ischaemic stroke or transient ischaemic attack. *N Engl J Med* 366, 1914–1922

Donnan GA, Fisher M, MacLeod M et al. (2008) Stroke. *Lancet* 371, 1612–1623

Feher A, Pusch G, Koltai K et al. (2011) Statin therapy in the primary and secondary prevention of ischaemic cerebrovascular disease. *Int J Cardiol* 148, 131–136

Hacke W, Donnan G, Fieschi C et al. (2004) Association of outcome with early stroke treatment: pooled analysis of ATLANTIS, ECASS, and NINDs rt-PA stroke trials. *Lancet* 363, 768–774

Lansberg MG, Bluhmki E, Thijs VN (2009) Efficacy and safety of tissue plasminogen activator 3 to 4.5 hours after acute ischemic stroke: a meta-analysis. *Stroke* 40, 2438–2441

Rashid P, Leonardi-Bee J, Bath P (2003) Blood pressure reduction and secondary prevention of stroke and other vascular events: a systematic review. *Stroke* 34, 2741–2748

Rothwell PM, Algra A, Amarenco P (2011) Medical treatment in acute and long-term secondary prevention after transient ischaemic attack and ischaemic stroke. *Lancet* 377, 1681–1692

Salman RA, Labovitz DL, Stapf C (2009) Spontaneous intracerebral haemorrhage. *BMJ* 339, b2586

Van der Worp HB, van Gijn J (2007) Acute ischemic stroke. *N Engl J Med* 357, 572–579

Wardlaw JM, Murray V, Berge E et al. (2012) Recombinant tissue plasminogen activator for ischaemic stroke: an updated systematic review and meta-analysis. *Lancet* 379, 2364–2372

Wechsler LR (2011) Intravenous thrombolytic therapy for acute ischaemic stroke. *N Engl J Med* 364, 2138–2146

Subarachnoid haemorrhage

Al-Shahi R, White PM, Davenport RJ et al. (2006) Subarachnoid haemorrhage. *BMJ* 333, 235–240

van Gijn J, Kerr RS, Rinkel GJ (2007) Subarachnoid haemorrhage. *Lancet* 369, 306–318

Dementia

Ballard C, Gauthier S, Corbett A et al. (2011) Alzheimer's disease. *Lancet* 377, 1019–1031

Farlowe MR (2006) Use of antidementia agents in vascular dementia: beyond Alzheimer disease. *Mayo Clin Proc* 81, 1350–1358

Farlowe MR, Cummings JL (2007) Effective pharmacologic management of Alzheimer's disease. *Am J Med* 120, 388–397

Mayeux R (2010) Early Alzheimer's disease. *N Engl J Med* 362, 2194–2201

O'Brien, Erkinjuntti T, Roman G et al. (2003) Vascular cognitive impairment. *Lancet Neurol* 2, 89–98

Raina P, Santaguida P, Ismalia A et al. (2008) Effectiveness of cholinesterase inhibitors and mementine for treating dementia: evidence review for a clinical practice guideline. *Ann Intern Med* 148, 379–397

Ritchie K, Lovestone S (2002) The dementias. *Lancet* 360, 1759–1766

Rodda J, Carter J (2012) Cholinesterase inhibitors and memantine for symptomatic treatment of dementia. *BMJ* 344, e2986

Salomone S, Caraci F, Leggio GM et al. (2012) New pharmacological strategies for the treatment of Alzheimer's disease: focus on disease modifying drugs. *Br J Clin Pharmacol* 73, 504–517

Compendium: drugs used to treat cerebrovascular disease and dementia

Drug	Kinetics (half-life)	Comment
Anticholinesterase drugs		
Donepezil	High oral bioavailability; metabolised in liver and excreted in urine as both parent drug and metabolites, with very long half-life (70–80 h)	Acetylcholinesterase inhibitor used for mild to moderate dementia in Alzheimer's disease; given orally once daily at night
Galantamine	Oral bioavailability >90%; metabolised in liver and excreted in urine as parent drug and metabolites (5–7 h)	Acetylcholinesterase inhibitor and nicotinic receptor agonist used for mild to moderate dementia in Alzheimer's disease; given orally
Rivastigmine	Oral bioavailability 30–70%; hydrolysed by cholinesterase activity (1–2 h); duration of effect about 10 h	Inhibitor of acetylcholinesterase and pseudocholinesterase used for mild to moderate dementia in Alzheimer's disease. Also used in Parkinson's disease; given orally or by transcutaneous patch
Other drugs		
Aspirin, clopidogrel, dipyridamole		Antiplatelet drugs (see Ch. 11)
Memantine	Oral bioavailability 100%; renal excretion (60–80 h)	Glutamate NMDA receptor antagonist; significance of additional actions at $5\text{-}HT_3$, nicotinic and dopamine D_2 receptors is unclear; used for moderate to severe dementia in Alzheimer's disease; given orally
Nimodipine	Low oral bioavailability (5–10%); liver metabolism (8–9 h)	Calcium channel blocker (Ch. 5) selective for cerebral arteries; use is confined to the prevention and treatment of ischaemic neurological deficits following aneurysmal subarachnoid haemorrhage; given orally or by intravenous infusion

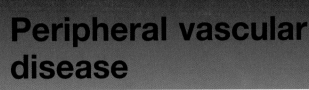

10 Peripheral vascular disease

ATHEROMATOUS PERIPHERAL VASCULAR DISEASE

Atherothrombotic disease is by far the most important cause of peripheral vascular disease. Disease in peripheral arteries principally affects the aorta and renal and lower limb arteries. The risk factors for its development are similar to those for coronary artery and cerebrovascular disease (Chs 5 and 9). The strongest associations are with increasing age, smoking and a raised systolic blood pressure, and to a lesser extent with diabetes mellitus, a raised plasma low-density lipoprotein (LDL) cholesterol and lack of exercise. Not surprisingly, symptomatic ischaemic heart disease and cerebrovascular disease coexist in up to 50% of people with peripheral vascular disease and are responsible for about 70% of their excess mortality. Only about 50% of people with peripheral vascular disease are alive 10 years after diagnosis; this is three times the mortality of people of similar age without peripheral vascular disease.

SYMPTOMS OF PERIPHERAL VASCULAR DISEASE

Peripheral vascular disease is often asymptomatic until it produces a stenosis of more than 50% of the diameter of an arterial lumen. Symptoms usually arise as a consequence of atherosclerotic stenosis of a lower limb artery, and produce intermittent claudication. This is ischaemic pain in the muscles of the lower limb that is precipitated by walking and relieved by rest. Hypoxia of skeletal muscle occurs when blood flow through the diseased artery fails to increase sufficiently to meet the increased metabolic demand of the muscle during exercise. The metabolic changes that accompany the switch to anaerobic metabolism in the muscle trigger the pain. Depending on the site of the vascular narrowing, pain can be experienced in the calf, thigh or buttock. The severity of reduction in blood flow to the limb does not correlate well with symptoms, and an important factor is ischaemia–reperfusion injury to the muscle and altered oxidative metabolism. The development of a collateral arterial circulation (see also Ch. 5) will reduce the severity of the symptoms and influence the long-term outcome. In three-quarters of those with peripheral vascular disease the symptoms stabilise within a few months of presentation. The remaining 25% experience steady progression, but only 1% of symptomatic patients per year will develop critical ischaemia which causes pain at rest, trophic changes and ultimately distal gangrene (see below).

DRUGS FOR PERIPHERAL VASCULAR DISEASE

Cilostazol

Mechanism of action

Cilostazol appears to have several actions. It is a reversible inhibitor of the enzyme phosphodiesterase type 3 (PDE3), and therefore reduces breakdown of cAMP (Table 1.1). PDE3 is present in vascular smooth muscle cells and platelets, and cilostazol causes vasodilation, inhibits platelet activation and aggregation, and prevents release of prothrombotic inflammatory substances. Cilostazol also inhibits adenosine reuptake, which promotes vasodilation, has favourable effects on plasma lipids by increasing high-density lipoprotein (HDL) cholesterol, and inhibits cell proliferation in vascular smooth muscle.

Pharmacokinetics

Cilostazol is well absorbed orally, and undergoes hepatic metabolism via cytochrome P450 to two metabolites with antiplatelet activity, one of which is more active than cilostazol. Cilostazol has a half-life of about 12 h.

Unwanted effects

- Diarrhoea.
- Headache.
- Palpitation and tachycardia.
- Other PDE3 inhibitors such as milrinone have been shown to decrease survival in people with heart failure (Ch. 7); cilostazol does not appear to increase the risk of life-threatening arrhythmias, but is contraindicated in people with heart failure, cardiac arrhythmias and ischaemic heart disease due to an increase in heart rate.
- Increased risk of bleeding when combined with aspirin and clopidogrel.

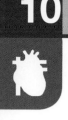

- Drug interactions: the pharmacokinetics of cilostazol will be altered by drugs that influence the liver cytochrome P450 CYP3A4 isoenzyme (Ch. 2).

Naftidrofuryl oxalate

Mechanism of action and effects

Naftidrofuryl oxalate promotes the production of high-energy phosphates (ATP) in ischaemic tissue by activating the mitochondrial enzyme succinic dehydrogenase. It is also a 5-hydroxytryptamine type 2 (5-HT$_2$) receptor antagonist, an action which leads to arterial vasodilation and reduced platelet aggregation. All these actions could improve blood flow to ischaemic tissues and tissue nutrition, but the effect on walking distance is modest.

Pharmacokinetics

Naftidrofuryl is well absorbed from the gut and metabolised in the liver. It has a half-life of 3–4 h.

Unwanted effects

- Nausea, epigastric pain.
- Rash.
- Hepatitis is a rare, but potentially serious, complication.

MANAGEMENT OF INTERMITTENT CLAUDICATION

Non-pharmacological treatment

- Stopping smoking slows the progression of peripheral atherosclerosis and may improve walking distance by improving blood oxygen transport. It will also have an impact on the risk of coronary and cerebrovascular events, and is therefore a cornerstone of long-term management.
- Regular supervised exercise, up to the point of claudication, can improve maximum walking distance by 150% over 8–12 weeks.

Pharmacological treatment

- Low-dose aspirin inhibits platelet aggregation and reduces cardiac and cerebrovascular events (Chs 11 and 29).
- Intensive management of hypertension reduces progression of atheroma. Conventional antihypertensive therapy is used (Ch. 6). Although β-adrenoceptor antagonists could theoretically exacerbate intermittent claudication by reducing cardiac output and impairing vasodilation of arteries supplying skeletal muscle (Ch. 5), there is little evidence that they are disadvantageous unless there is critical limb ischaemia.
- Lowering serum LDL cholesterol (Ch. 48) can stabilise or regress atherosclerotic plaques. It is not known whether this improves limb survival or reduces the need for subsequent surgery. A greater benefit of lowering cholesterol may be reduced morbidity and mortality from coexistent ischaemic heart disease (Ch. 5).

- Naftidrofuryl oxalate improves maximum walking distance by up to 60%. A trial of treatment may be justified for those who remain restricted by the disease after 6–12 months of conservative treatment, and for whom angioplasty is inappropriate or has failed. Withdrawal is advised after 3–6 months of treatment to assess whether spontaneous improvement has occurred.
- Cilostazol can improve maximum walking distance by up to 25% over 3–6 months of treatment, but the impact of this on quality of life is often minimal. It is not known whether cilostazol has any effect on long-term outcome or on the subsequent need for surgery.

Surgical treatment

Surgical treatment is usually considered if quality of life is significantly impaired by claudication or if tissue integrity is at risk. Percutaneous transluminal angioplasty, often with insertion of a stent, is used particularly for stenoses above the inguinal ligament, while bypass surgery is used for most other disease.

ACUTE AND CRITICAL LIMB ISCHAEMIA

An arterial embolus is the usual cause of acute limb ischaemia, and can arise from an intracardiac site, usually associated with atrial fibrillation (Ch. 8) or following a myocardial infarction (Ch. 5), or from aortic or internal iliac artery thrombus. Emboli can occlude previously healthy vessels and presents with acute onset of severe pain at rest, associated with signs of critically impaired tissue perfusion.

Critical limb ischaemia results from chronic, severe, subtotal occlusion of an artery, and may be due to partial occlusion of the vessel from thrombus on a ruptured atherosclerotic plaque. The symptoms include rest pain, often worse at night and relieved by hanging the leg out of the bed.

MANAGEMENT OF ACUTE AND CRITICAL LIMB ISCHAEMIA

Unless treatment of acute or acute-on-chronic critical limb ischaemia is rapid, the person may be left with a chronically ischaemic limb, or occasionally the limb may be lost through gangrene.

If the limb is still viable, then a peripheral arterial angiogram should be carried out. For acute embolic arterial occlusion, embolectomy is the treatment of choice. Intraarterial thrombolysis, either with streptokinase or recombinant tissue plasminogen activator (rt-PA; alteplase) (Ch. 11), is used to dissolve an acute thrombus occluding a previously diseased vessel. Alteplase produces more rapid lysis, but there is no evidence that limb salvage is any better than with streptokinase. The fibrinolytic agent can be infused via a catheter for up to 24 h or given as repeated boluses. Reperfusion takes several hours and in about 25% of acute vascular occlusions lysis is not achieved, especially if there is embolic occlusion. The risk of intracerebral haemorrhage is also a concern. A surgical bypass may be considered if there is no time for thrombolysis.

Secondary prevention measures to reduce other cardio-vascular events (see above) should also be started.

RAYNAUD'S PHENOMENON

Raynaud's phenomenon is a profound and exaggerated vasospastic response of blood vessels in the extremities on exposure to cold, change in environmental temperature or during emotional upset. This leads to episodes of ischaemia that most commonly affect the fingers (occasionally also the toes, ear lobes or the nipples). A typical attack initially produces pallor of the affected part, followed by one or both of cyanosis then erythema. Each attack can last several minutes or up to a few hours. About two-thirds of cases occur in women (typically presenting under the age of 40 years), in whom the overall prevalence is about 15%. Common symptoms include discomfort, numbness and tingling, with loss of function and pain if the condition is severe. Rarely, digital ulceration can occur.

The majority of cases of Raynaud's phenomenon are idiopathic (primary Raynaud's phenomenon; also called Raynaud's disease). The cause of the excessive vascular reactivity is unknown, although there is a genetic predispostion. Vascular function in other tissues is often abnormal in primary Raynaud's phenomenon: for example, in the cerebral vessels (giving an association with migraine), the coronary circulation (producing variant angina) or, more rarely, in the pulmonary circulation (leading to pulmonary hypertension).

In about 10% of cases, Raynaud's phenomenon is secondary to another disorder. This is most commonly scleroderma, but there are many other associated conditions (Box 10.1). Structural damage to arteries is common in secondary Raynaud's phenomenon, and digital ulceration is much more common than in the primary type.

Other disorders of the peripheral circulation should also be considered in the differential diagnosis of Raynaud's phenomenon.

- Acrocyanosis usually affects the hands and produces persistently cold, bluish fingers which are often sweaty or oedematous. The management of this condition is similar to that of Raynaud's phenomenon.
- Chilblains are an inflammatory disorder with erythematous lesions on the feet, or less commonly the hands or face, that are precipitated by cold and humidity followed by rapid rewarming. The lesions are often painful or itchy. Treatments used for Raynaud's phenomenon may help, with the addition of topical non-steroidal anti-inflammatory agents (Ch. 29).
- Erythromelalgia is a painful, burning condition often affecting the hands and feet that, unlike Raynaud's phenomenon, is usually provoked by heat. It sometimes responds to treatment with a calcium channel blocker (Ch. 5) or gabapentin (Ch. 23).
- Vibration white finger is a patchy digital vasospasm associated with prolonged use of vibrating tools. If drug treatment is necessary, it is similar to that for Raynaud's phenomenon.

Box 10.1 Conditions associated with Raynaud's phenomenon

Connective tissue disorders
Systemic sclerosis
Systemic lupus erythematosus
Rheumatoid arthritis
Dermatomyositis and polymyositis

Obstructive arterial disorders
Carpal tunnel syndrome
Thoracic outlet syndrome
Atherosclerosis
Thromboangiitis obliterans

Drugs and chemicals
Ergotamine
Beta-adrenoceptor antagonists
Bleomycin, vinblastine, cisplatin
Oral contraceptives
Vinyl chloride

Occupational
Vibrating tools
Cold environment

Blood disorders
Polycythaemia
Cold agglutinin disease
Monoclonal gammopathies
Thrombocytosis

MANAGEMENT OF RAYNAUD'S PHENOMEMON

Many people with Raynaud's phenomenon are only mildly inconvenienced by their symptoms and respond to simple measures. Drug treatment is usually reserved for those suffering from more intense vasospasm with pain, impairment of function or trophic changes. Responses to individual treatments are unpredictable, and are less satisfactory in secondary Raynaud's phenomenon because of structural changes to the vessel wall.

Non-pharmacological treatment

- Often, minimising changes in ambient temperature with insulating clothing is enough to reduce the number of attacks, although electrically heated gloves or socks may be useful for more severely affected people.
- Smoking should be strongly discouraged. Nicotine promotes vasospasm and may also reduce the threshold for other provoking factors.
- Aggravating factors should be withdrawn or corrected whenever possible (see Box 10.1). Beta-adrenoceptor antagonists (Ch. 5) produce peripheral circulatory problems sufficient to necessitate stopping treatment in about 3–5% of people with hypertension.
- Surgical sympathectomy is occasionally used for advanced disease.

Pharmacological treatment

Arterial vasodilators

- Calcium channel blockers (Ch. 5): modified-release nifedipine is the drug of first choice for Raynaud's phenomenon, and reduces the frequency, duration and intensity of vasospastic episodes. Several other dihydropyridines are probably equally effective, but diltiazem is less effective and verapamil ineffective in this condition.
- Naftidrofuryl oxalate may produce a modest reduction in the severity of attacks.
- Alpha$_1$-adrenoceptor antagonists (Ch. 6): moxisylyte is typically used and does not lower blood pressure, unlike other α-adrenoceptor antagonists.
- Angiotensin II receptor antagonists (Ch. 6)
- Sildenafil (Ch. 16) has been used successfully in secondary Raynaud's phenomenon that is resistant to other vasodilators.
- Bosentan, an endothelin receptor antagonist (Ch. 6), has shown promise in severe Raynaud's phenomenon.
- Fluoxetine (Ch. 22), a selective serotonin reuptake inhibitor (SSRI) antidepressant, is effective in some people.
- Calcitonin gene-related peptide (CGRP) is effective for prolonged periods when given by short intravenous infusions over 5 or more consecutive days. It is a neurotransmitter for vasodilator cutaneous sensorimotor nerves in the fingers and toes. CGRP is usually reserved for failure to respond to epoprostenol (see below).

Drugs acting primarily on blood components

- Prostaglandins: short intravenous infusions of epoprostenol (prostacyclin (prostaglandin I$_2$, PGI$_2$); Ch. 11) over at least 5 consecutive days produces immediate vasodilation, but long-term improvement in symptoms and healing of ulcers over a period of 10–16 weeks. These effects are believed to be caused by actions on the flow properties of blood; that is, reduced platelet aggregation, increased red cell deformability and reduced neutrophil adhesiveness. Epoprostenol is rapidly inactivated in plasma by hydrolysis, and has a very short half-life of about 3 min. Unwanted effects are due to vasodilation, and include flushing, headache and hypotension.
- Inositol nicotinate (a nicotinic acid derivative) produces a gradual onset of clinical response and only modest improvement. Its action may result more from fibrinolysis (reducing plasma viscosity) and reduction in platelet aggregation than from vasodilation.

SELF-ASSESSMENT

True/false questions

1. Diabetes mellitus, hypertension and smoking confer an additive risk of developing peripheral vascular disease.

2. People with intermittent claudication do not have an increased risk of developing coronary artery disease.
3. Statin drugs are indicated in people with symptomatic atherosclerotic peripheral vascular disease.
4. Simvastatin increases the hepatic expression of low-density lipoprotein (LDL) receptors.
5. Drugs used in migraine treatment, such as ergotamine, can precipitate Raynaud's phenomenon.
6. Verapamil is the calcium channel blocker of choice in the treatment of Raynaud's phenomenon.
7. Epoprostenol mimics the actions of thromboxane A$_2$.
8. Moxisylyte is metabolised to a compound with α_1-adrenoceptor antagonist activity.

One-best-answer (OBA) question

Choose the one *correct* statement from the following.

A. Cilostazol inhibits phosphodiesterase type 3 in vascular tissues.
B. Cilostazol is useful in the treatment of congestive heart failure.
C. Cilostazol is mainly excreted unchanged in the urine.
D. Cilostazol has little effect on platelet aggregation.
E. Cilostazol decreases plasma HDL cholesterol.

Case-based questions

Mr TH, aged 67 years, had type 1 diabetes mellitus and smoked 20 cigarettes a day. His plasma total cholesterol was raised at 7.2 mmol·L^{-1} and his blood pressure was 160/110 mmHg. After walking 50 m he developed pain in his left calf muscle, which was relieved by rest. He occasionally, but rarely, had rest pain at night. On examination, both popliteal and posterior tibial pulses were absent and femoropopliteal obstruction was diagnosed.

1. Comment on the usefulness and drawbacks of the following drugs to treat Mr TH's peripheral vascular disease.
   A. Propranolol
   B. Atenolol
   C. Nifedipine
   D. A statin
   E. Low-dose aspirin
   F. Cilostazol
2. What other therapy could be of benefit?
3. Should the use of an electric blanket be discouraged?

True/false answers

1. **True.** The risk factors for peripheral vascular disease are similar to those for coronary artery and cerebrovascular disease.
2. **False.** There is a two- to fourfold increase in risk of developing coronary disease, stroke or heart failure compared with age-matched subjects who do not have intermittent claudication.
3. **True.** Lowering serum LDL cholesterol can stabilise or regress atherosclerotic plaques.

4. **True**. By reducing cholesterol synthesis, simvastatin increases hepatic LDL receptors, which results in reduced LDL cholesterol in blood and a small accompanying increase in high-density lipoprotein (HDL) cholesterol (Ch. 48). The main potential benefit of lowered LDL cholesterol in these patients is a reduction in coronary artery disease events.

5. **True**. Ergotamine and other drugs including β-adrenoceptor antagonists can trigger Raynaud's phenomenon.

6. **False**. Verapamil is ineffective in the treatment of Raynaud's phenomenon, and the agent of choice is nifedipine.

7. **False**. Epoprostenol is prostacyclin (PGI_2), which has opposing actions on vessels and platelets to thromboxane A_2

8. **True**. The active metabolite is deacetylmoxisylyte (DAM).

OBA answer

Answer A is correct.

A. **Correct**. Cilostazol increases cAMP levels in vascular smooth muscle cells and platelets by inhibiting phosphodiesterase type 3.

B. Incorrect. Unlike other phosphodiesterase 3 inhibitors such as milrinone, cilostazol does not increase the incidence of arrhythmias. However, cilostazol is not recommended in people with congestive heart failure and cardiac arrhythmia.

C. Incorrect. Cilostazol is extensively metabolised by CYP3A4 and CYP2C19 isoenzymes in the liver.

D. Incorrect. Cilostazol inhibits platelet aggregation.

E. Incorrect. Cilostazol increases plasma HDL cholesterol.

Case-based answers

1. The usefulness and drawbacks of drugs A–F in treating Mr TH are as follows.

   A. Beta-adrenoceptor antagonists should probably be avoided in this man. They would not be the drug of choice in the initial treatment of his high blood pressure (Ch. 6), and by reducing cardiac output and inhibiting vasodilation they could further reduce blood flow in critical limb ischaemia.

   B. Cardioselective β-adrenoceptor antagonists such as atenolol do not cause deterioration in walking distance when used without a vasodilator.

   C. Vasodilators will lower blood pressure but do not improve walking distance. In some people, they may redirect blood from the maximally dilated ischaemic tissues to healthy tissues (vascular steal). This can be particularly troublesome in critical limb ischaemia, or when the cardiac output is also reduced by concurrent use of a β-adrenoceptor antagonist.

   D. Lowering LDL cholesterol can stabilise atherosclerotic plaques, perhaps reducing the consequences of coexistent heart disease; it is not known whether walking distance or limb survival are improved.

   E. Low-dose aspirin inhibits platelet aggregation and reduces future cardiac events, which are common in people with peripheral vascular disease.

   F. Cilostazol can increase walking distance by up to 25%.

2. Intensive management of blood pressure, control of diabetes and antiplatelet therapy will reduce the risk of cardiac events. An exercise programme can improve walking distance. Smoking is a major contributory factor to impaired walking distance and cardiac events.

3. An electric blanket should be discouraged as excessive warming of limbs may dilate normal arteries, 'stealing' blood from diseased arteries.

FURTHER READING

Bowling JCR, Dowd PM (2003) Raynaud's disease. *Lancet* 361, 2078–2080

Goundry B, Bell L, Langtree M et al. (2012) Diagnosis and management of Raynaud's phenomenon. *BMJ* 344, e289

Hankey GJ, Norman PE, Eikelboom JW (2006) Medical treatment of peripheral arterial disease. *JAMA* 295, 547–553

Mannava K, Money SR (2007) Current management of peripheral arterial occlusive disease: a review of pharmacologic agents and other interventions. *Am J Cardiovasc Drugs* 7, 59–66

Peach G, Griffin M, Jones KG et al. (2012) Diagnosis and management of peripheral arterial disease. *BMJ* 345, e5208

Wright C (2007) Intermittent claudication. *N Engl J Med* 356, 1241–1250

Compendium: drugs used to treat peripheral vascular disease

Drug	Kinetics (half-life)	Comments
Cilostazol	Absorption increased by food; metabolised by CYP3A4 and CYP2C19 to active metabolites (12 h)	Reversibly inhibits phosphodiesterase (PDE) type 3 and blocks adenosine reuptake in vascular smooth muscle cells, causing vasodilation; also has antiplatelet activity and increases plasma HDL cholesterol
Cinnarizine	Slow oral absorption; eliminated largely by CYP2D6 (polymorphic) hepatic metabolism (24 h)	H_1 antihistamine used primarily for vestibular disorders; at higher doses, cinnarizine has a vasodilator effect and may improve circulation in Raynaud's phenomenon and peripheral vascular disease
Epoprostenol	Must be freshly reconstituted from dry powder before intravenous infusion; eliminated very rapidly by hydrolysis (half-life <3 min)	A prostaglandin (PGI_2, prostacyclin) with vasodilator and antiplatelet activity
Inositol nicotinate	Metabolised slowly into inositol and nicotinic acid (niacin); probably eliminated by hydrolysis	Nicotinic acid (niacin) has vasodilator activity; also used for hyperlipidaemias
Moxisylyte	Good oral bioavailability; prodrug rapidly converted in plasma to its active metabolite, deacetylmoxisylyte (1 h)	An α_1-adrenoceptor antagonist used for the short-term treatment of primary Raynaud's phenomenon; formerly known as thymoxamine in UK
Naftidrofuryl oxalate	Good oral bioavailability; hepatic metabolism with some renal excretion (3–4 h)	Activates mitochondrial succinic dehydrogenase and is a 5-HT_2 receptor antagonist
Pentoxifylline	Rapidly metabolised in liver and blood (1 h)	PDE inhibitor which increases erythrocyte flexibility and decreases blood viscosity, possibly by increasing erythrocyte cAMP

All the drugs above are given orally, with the exception of epoprostenol (given intravenously).

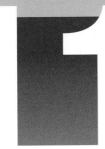

11

Haemostasis

Haemostasis is a complex process involving vasoconstriction, platelet aggregation, blood coagulation and the interactions between them. The descriptions of the processes of platelet aggregation and coagulation pathways in this chapter are restricted to essential knowledge required for understanding the actions of pharmacological agents.

PLATELETS AND PLATELET AGGREGATION

Platelets are critical components of the blood for initiating thrombus formation, and have a lifespan in the circulation of 8–10 days, with about 10–12% being replaced each day. Platelets aggregate following adhesion to an injured blood vessel and consequent activation. When the integrity of vascular endothelium is breached, subendothelial proteins such as von Willebrand factor (vWF) and collagen come into contact with blood. These proteins interact with a family of platelet-surface glycoprotein (GP) receptors (integrin receptors), particularly GPIb (vWF receptor) and GPVI (collagen receptor), resulting in platelets adhering at the site of injury and to each other (primary reversible aggregation) and the formation of a platelet plug (Fig. 11.1). Platelet adhesion then initiates a process known as platelet activation.

Extension of the platelet plug requires activation of platelets and their subsequent aggregation together (homotypic aggregation). Platelets are initially activated by exposure to soluble agonists, such as thrombin generated by local coagulation, ADP released from endothelial cells and collagen. These activators lead to an increase in intracellular Ca^{2+} and activation of (MLCK). MLCK phosphorylates myosin light chains in the platelet which interact with actin, disrupt the platelet cytoskeleton and change the shape of the platelet.

The increase in platelet intracellular Ca^{2+} activates phospholipase A_2, which liberates arachidonic acid (AA) from membrane phospholipids. AA is then converted by cyclo-oxygenase type 1 (COX-1) in the platelet to thromboxane A_2, the most potent naturally occurring pro-aggregating agent, which diffuses from the platelet. Significant disruption of the platelet cytoskeleton as the platelet changes shape also initiates a platelet release reaction, which expels mediators in platelet dense storage granules from the cell. Fusion of dense granules with the platelet cell membrane releases platelet factor 4, adrenaline, ADP and serotonin. Outside the platelet ADP, thrombin and thromboxane A_2 interact with specific platelet surface receptors and trigger intracellular pathways that express and activate GPIIb/IIIa collagen receptors on the surface of the platelets (Figs 11.1 and 11.2). Therefore, ADP released from platelets acts as a mediator for initiators of platelet activation, such as collagen and thrombin. Secondary irreversible homotypic platelet–platelet aggregation follows platelet activation when the activated GPIIb/IIIa receptors on the surface of the platelets are crosslinked by fibrinogen in the plasma.

The substances released from platelet dense granules also facilitate haemostasis by:

- reducing prostacyclin (prostaglandin I_2, PGI_2) synthesis by vascular endothelium; prostacyclin is a vasodilator and a potent inhibitor of platelet aggregation,
- inhibiting the action of heparin sulphate produced by vascular endothelium; this enhances activity of the coagulation cascade.

Expression of platelet GPIIb/IIIa surface receptors can be inhibited by an increase in the concentration of cyclic nucleotides (cAMP, cGMP) in the platelet. This is the mechanism by which prostacyclin (PGI_2) inhibits platelet aggregation (Figs 11.1 and 11.2).

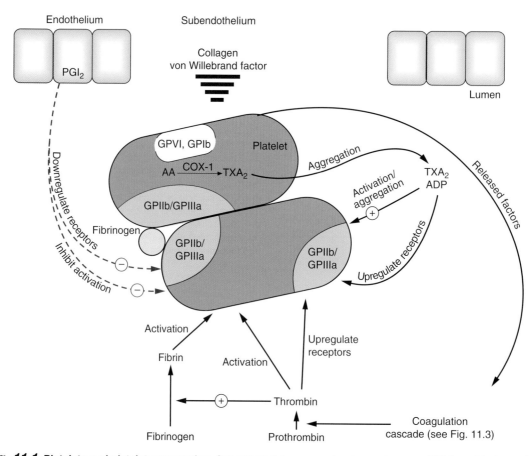

Fig. 11.1 **Platelets and platelet aggregation.** Subendothelial macromolecules such as von Willebrand factor and collagen interact with glycoprotein receptors (GPVI and GPIb) on platelets, causing activation of platelets and upregulation of GPIIb/IIIa receptors, which are crosslinked by fibrinogen, resulting in aggregation. During the initial processes of aggregation, stimulation of the synthesis and release of a number of platelet-derived substances, such as thromboxane A_2 (TXA_2) synthesised from arachidonic acid (AA) by cyclo-oxygenase-1 (COX-1), ADP, and other factors (see text) further promote aggregation by upregulation of GPIIb/IIIa receptors. Conversely, prostacyclin (PGI_2) from endothelial cells inhibits activation and upregulation of GPIIb/IIIa receptors. Thrombin is generated by the action of factor Xa on prothrombin (see Fig. 11.3).

Polyunsaturated (omega-3) fatty acids in fish oils are precursors for thromboxane A_3, which causes less platelet aggregation than thromboxane A_2; they also increase production of a modified form of prostacyclin (PGI_3) by vascular endothelium which has equal anti-aggregatory activity to PGI_2. Therefore, a high intake of fish oils creates a state in which platelets are less able to aggregate.

Heterotypic platelet aggregation can also arise when platelets aggregate with leucocytes (and particularly monocytes) in circulating blood. This process has been detected close to atherosclerotic lesions but also in a variety of inflammatory conditions, and may follow initial activation of platelets by vascular damage. Heterotypic aggregation results from expression of P-selectin on the surface of the platelet. P-selectin is one of several molecules found in platelet alpha-granules, which are released when the platelet cytoskeleton is only minimally disrupted by thrombin- or ADP-mediated activation of the cell. Heterotypic platelet aggregation is not inhibited by some antiplatelet drugs (such as aspirin) to the same extent as homotypic aggregation

BLOOD COAGULATION AND THE COAGULATION CASCADE

Both coagulant and anticoagulant factors regulate haemostasis. Activation of the coagulation cascade is divided into extrinsic and intrinsic pathways (Fig. 11.3). The factors involved in these cascades amplify the coagulation response and work together to produce a thrombus. The extrinsic pathway accounts for most of the coagulation *in vivo*, but both coagulation pathways respond to breaches in endothelial integrity much more slowly than platelet aggregation. The following description of the pathways is simplified to identify the key steps at which drugs can modulate coagulation.

The extrinsic coagulation pathway is initiated by exposure of blood to tissue factor (TF) on the surface of subendothelial cells after vascular injury, and is activated rapidly within minutes of endothelial disruption. Formation of complexes of TF with factor VIIa, and the presence of

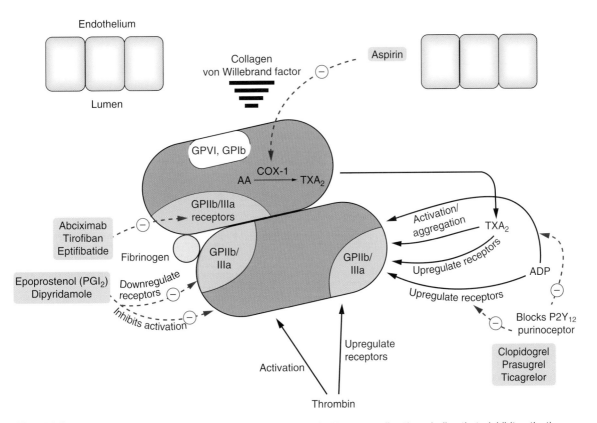

Fig. 11.2 **Sites of action of major drugs used in haemostasis.** Drugs act directly or indirectly to inhibit activation of platelets or to block or reduce upregulation of the glycoprotein GPIIb/IIIa receptors (integrin receptor family), which are necessary for aggregation of platelets. Abciximab is an antibody, tirofiban a non-peptide inhibitor and eptifibatide a peptide inhibitor of these glycoprotein receptors. Epoprostenol and dipyridamole inhibit activation of platelets and downregulate the glycoprotein receptors by increasing cAMP. Clopidogrel inhibits ADP receptors and prevents ADP-induced upregulation of the glycoprotein GPIIb/IIIa receptors and platelet aggregation. Aspirin inhibits the generation of thromboxane A_2 (TXA_2) by cyclo-oxygenase-1 (COX-1), which otherwise causes activation of platelets and upregulation of GPIIb/IIIa receptors. AA, arachidonic acid. For direct and indirect inhibitors of thrombin, see Fig. 11.3.

phospholipids and Ca^{2+}, result in the conversion of inactive factor X to active Xa.

The intrinsic pathway is triggered by contact of blood with a negatively charged surface such as subendothelial collagen, and its activation is delayed by more than 10 min after tissue disruption. The intrinsic coagulation pathway comprises a series of enzyme-mediated reactions involving activation of several clotting factors and eventually activation of factor X.

Activation of factor X, which mediates the hydrolysis of prothrombin to thrombin (factor IIa), is the point at which the two pathways of coagulation converge (Fig. 11.3). The actions of thrombin (factor IIa) and several other activated coagulation factors (Fig 11.3) are inhibited by circulating antithrombin. Antithrombin inhibits coagulation factors after forming complexes with heparin-like molecules that are produced by intact endothelial cells, and with heparin released from mast cells. Once sufficient thrombin has been produced to overcome the effect of circulating antithrombin, the soluble protein fibrinogen is converted to an insoluble fibrin

gel. Thrombin also activates factor XIII, which crosslinks the fibrin polymers and forms a fibrin mesh that traps circulating platelets, leucocytes and red blood cells.

Each activated clotting factor is inactivated extremely rapidly so that the coagulation process remains localised at the site of the initiating event. However, in some circumstances, aggregates of platelets combined with fibrin thrombi can embolise and occlude more distal parts of the circulation.

ARTERIAL AND VENOUS THROMBOSIS

There are differences in the composition of an arterial or venous thrombus. Arterial thrombosis occurs in the setting of high flow and high shear stress, and platelets play a prominent role in the initiation and growth of the thrombus. In contrast, venous thrombi form in a low-flow, low-shear stress environment. Venous thrombus usually forms initially in the valve pockets of deep veins, and consists mainly of fibrin and red cells with few platelets.

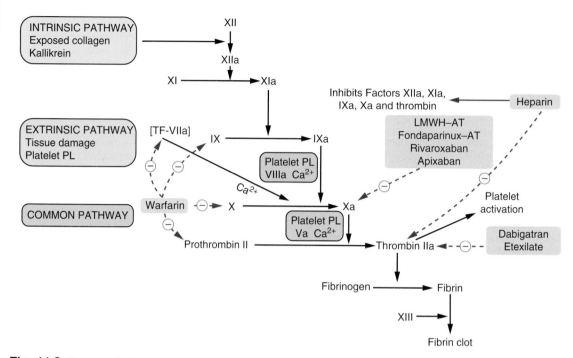

Fig. 11.3 The coagulation cascade and action of anticoagulants. The complex cascade of clotting factor synthesis is initiated extrinsically by tissue damage. Activation of the clotting factors after damage depends upon platelet factors, tissue factor, phospholipids, Ca^{2+} and vitamin K. The provision of platelet products is further enhanced by the formation of thrombin, which then activates further platelets as well as causing fibrin formation. Heparin acts at various sites in the cascade by complexing with the anticlotting factor antithrombin III (AT) and inhibiting thrombin (IIa) and the other activated clotting factors shown. Low-molecular-weight heparin (LMWH) complexes with AT but in a different manner to unfractionated heparin and inhibits only factor Xa. Bivalirudin and dabigatran etexilate inhibit thrombin (IIa) action. Warfarin inhibits the synthesis of the vitamin K-dependent clotting factors VII, IX, X and II (prothrombin). Roman numerals indicate the individual clotting factors; PL, phospholipid; TF, tissue factor.

ANTIPLATELET DRUGS

CYCLO-OXYGENASE INHIBITORS

xamples

aspirin

Mechanism of action on platelets

The highly potent platelet-aggregating agent thromboxane A_2 is formed in platelets from AA by the enzyme COX-1. After release from the platelet, thromboxane A_2 acts via TP receptors on the surface of the platelet to generate the intracellular second messengers inositol triphosphate (IP_3) and diacylglycerol (DAG). These lead to Ca^{2+} release in the cell and expression and activation of GPIIb/IIIa receptors.

Inhibition of COX-1 by aspirin reduces platelet thromboxane A_2 synthesis and inhibits platelet aggregation, but does not eliminate it completely because other pathways for platelet activation still function (Figs 11.1 and 11.2). Aspirin (acetylsalicylic acid) irreversibly inhibits COX-1 by acetylation (Ch. 29) and since platelets lack a nucleus and

cannot synthesise new enzyme, their ability to aggregate will be reduced throughout the lifespan of the platelet. The antiplatelet action of aspirin occurs at very low doses that have little analgesic or anti-inflammatory actions. At higher doses, aspirin also inhibits the production of prostacyclin by vascular endothelium which may offset some of the beneficial effects on platelets. Details of the pharmacology of aspirin can be found in Chapter 29.

PHOSPHODIESTERASE INHIBITORS

xample

dipyridamole

Mechanism of action

Dipyridamole has multiple mechanisms of action; the most important is probably inhibition of the reuptake of adenosine by cells. The increased plasma concentration of adenosine promotes vasodilation and inhibits platelet aggregation by stimulation of intracellular adenylyl cyclase and production of the intracellular cyclic nucleotides cGMP and cAMP. Dipyridamole also inhibits phosphodiesterase types 3 and 5, which degrade cyclic nucleotides. High intracellular cyclic nucleotide concentrations inhibit activation of cell surface GPIIb/IIIa receptors, leading to reduced platelet activation (Fig. 11.2). Dipyridamole has a number of other actions that are of uncertain significance, including antioxidant properties.

Pharmacokinetics

Dipyridamole is incompletely absorbed from the gut and is metabolised in the liver. It has a half-life of 12 h. A modified-release formulation is better tolerated than the standard formulation.

Unwanted effects

- Gastrointestinal effects.
- Myalgia.
- Dizziness, headache.
- Flushing, hypotension, tachycardia.
- Hypersensitivity reactions, including rash, urticaria, bronchospasm and angioedema.

ADP RECEPTOR ANTAGONISTS

clopidogrel, prasugrel, ticagrelor

Mechanism of action

ADP activates platelets via two purinergic surface receptors, P2Y$_1$ and P2Y$_{12}$. P2Y$_1$ receptors increase intracellular Ca^{2+} and initiate platelet shape change. Activation of P2Y$_{12}$ receptors inhibits adenylyl cyclase, and reduces generation of the intracellular cyclic nucleotides that inhibit activation of GPIIb/IIIa receptors.

ADP receptor antagonists inhibit platelet aggregation by binding selectively to P2Y$_{12}$ receptors (Fig. 11.2). Inhibition of P2Y$_{12}$ receptors also reduces the production of thromboxane A$_2$ by the platelet. Clopidogrel and prasugrel are irreversible receptor inhibitors, while ticagrelor binds to a different site on the receptor and produces reversible inhibition. There is considerable inter-individual variability in the degree of platelet inhibition by clopidogrel, and it has a slow onset of action (about 5 days for full effect) without a loading dose. Both prasugrel and ticagrelor are more predictable inhibitors of platelet activation than clopidogrel and have a more rapid onset of action.

Pharmacokinetics

Clopidogrel is a prodrug. It is well absorbed from the gut, and is activated by metabolism in the liver to a derivative that has a half-life of 7 h. Prasugrel is also a prodrug that is well absorbed from the gut and metabolised rapidly in the liver to an active metabolite which has a long half-life of 8 days. Ticagrelor is active as the parent drug, and also has an active metabolite. The offset of action of ticagrelor over 3 days is much slower than would be predicted from the short half-life.

Unwanted effects

- Bleeding; a greater risk with prasugrel and ticagrelor than clopidogrel.
- Gastrointestinal upset, especially dyspepsia, abdominal pain and diarrhoea with clopidogrel.
- Dyspnoea with ticagrelor.

GLYCOPROTEIN IIB/IIIA RECEPTOR ANTAGONISTS

Examples

abciximab, eptifibatide

Mechanism of action

Abciximab is a murine/human chimaeric monoclonal antibody to the GPIIb/IIIa receptors with the Fc fragment removed to prevent clearance of antibody-bound platelets from the circulation. Abciximab binds irreversibly to the GPIIb/IIIa receptors and blocks the binding of fibrinogen (Fig. 11.2). Abciximab can reduce platelet aggregation by more than 90%.

Eptifibatide is a synthetic peptide that binds reversibly to and blocks the GPIIb/IIIa receptor.

Pharmacokinetics

All GPIIb/IIIa antagonists are given intravenously, usually as an initial bolus to achieve rapid inhibition of platelets followed by continuous infusion. The duration of receptor blockade with abciximab is longer than predicted from its very short half-life of 30 min due to slow dissociation from the receptor over several hours. After stopping abciximab, platelet aggregation largely recovers by 48 h as new platelets are synthesised.

Eptifibatide has a short half-life of about 2.5 h, and is eliminated by the kidney. Platelet aggregation recovers more rapidly after treatment than with abciximab, due to rapid dissociation of the drug from the receptor after a few seconds.

Unwanted effects

- Bleeding, especially in the elderly and those of low body weight; the risk is reduced if the dose is adjusted for body weight.
- Thrombocytopenia.
- Abciximab can cause nausea, vomiting, hypotension, bradycardia, headache and, occasionally, hypersensitivity reactions.

Epoprostenol

Mechanism of action

Epoprostenol (PGI$_2$) increases platelet cAMP, which at low concentrations inhibits platelet aggregation and at higher concentrations reduces platelet adhesion. Epoprostenol is also a peripheral arterial vasodilator.

Pharmacokinetics

Epoprostenol is given by intravenous infusion. Unlike most other prostaglandins it is not significantly metabolised in the lung, as it is rapidly metabolised by hydrolysis in plasma and peripheral tissues, giving a very short half-life of about 3 min.

Unwanted effects

These can be reduced by starting the infusion with a low dose and include:

- facial flushing,
- headache,
- hypotension,
- gastrointestinal disturbances.

CLINICAL USES OF ANTIPLATELET DRUGS

Aspirin has often been used as the sole antiplatelet drug in a variety of clinical settings. However, there are some situations where clopidogrel is more effective, or where combinations of aspirin and an ADP receptor antagonist give better outcomes than aspirin alone. The suppression of thromboxane A_2 production by ADP receptor antagonists has called into question whether the concurrent use of aspirin is necessary to achieve optimal clinical outcomes, but this issue is unresolved. A combination of antiplatelet drugs inevitably carries a greater risk of bleeding than a single agent. Main uses of antiplatelet drugs are listed here.

- **Secondary prevention of embolic stroke and transient cerebral ischaemic attacks** (aspirin, clopidogrel, dipyridamole). Clopidogrel alone is more effective than aspirin alone for the secondary prevention of stroke, while the combination has no further advantage despite a higher risk of bleeding. Dipyridamole combined with aspirin is better than aspirin alone for prevention of recurrent transient ischaemic attacks, and is equally effective as clopidogrel after stroke (Ch. 9).
- **Secondary prevention after acute coronary syndrome** (aspirin, clopidogrel, prasugrel, ticagrelor, eptifibitide, tirofiban). The combination of aspirin and clopidogrel is better than aspirin alone for reducing further vascular events after myocardial infarction. Prasugrel and ticagrelor may have advantages over clopidogrel in some situations (Ch. 5).
- **Reduction of ischaemic complications produced by stent thrombosis following percutaneous coronary intervention (PCI) with stent insertion**; these complications include non-fatal myocardial infarction, death and the need for emergency surgical revascularisation. Aspirin with clopidogrel or prasugrel are given for up to a year, often with abciximab or eptifibatide added at the time of the procedure when PCI is carried out following myocardial infarction.
- **Secondary prevention of myocardial infarction in stable angina or peripheral vascular disease** (aspirin, clopidogrel): either aspirin or clopidogrel alone is

effective, and there is no evidence to support combination therapy (Chs 5 and 10).
- **Primary prevention of ischaemic heart disease** (aspirin). This is a controversial area, with the potential for serious haemorrhage offsetting much of the potential benefit. Use of aspirin should be confined to people at very high risk of developing cardiovascular disease.
- **Anticoagulation in extracorporeal circulations**; for example, cardiopulmonary bypass and renal haemodialysis (epoprostenol).
- **Symptom relief in Raynaud's phenomenon** (epoprostenol) (Ch. 10).
- **Dipyridamole is used as a pharmacological stress for the coronary circulation to detect myocardial ischaemia in people who are unable to exercise.** This is related to its ability to block the cellular uptake of adenosine. In the heart, adenosine acts on specific receptors in the small resistance coronary arteries to produce vasodilation. Dipyridamole can divert blood away from myocardium supplied by stenosed coronary arteries by preferentially dilating healthy vascular beds (vascular steal).

ANTICOAGULANT DRUGS

Anticoagulation can be achieved with either injectable or oral drug therapy. Increasingly, oral anticoagulant therapy with newer agents is likely to supersede the long-established use of heparin followed by warfarin to initiate anticoagulation.

INJECTABLE ANTICOAGULANTS

Heparins

Heparins are a family of highly sulphated acidic mucopolysaccharides (glycosaminoglycans) that are found in mast cells, basophils and endothelium. Heparins have a variable molecular weight of between 3000 and 30 000 Da according to the numbers of polysaccharide subunits.

Mechanism of action and effects

Heparin is available as an unfractionated preparation, or as low-molecular-weight heparins (LMWHs), which consist of the heparin subfractions that have molecular weights of less than 7000 Da.

Unfractionated heparin forms a complex with and alters the conformation of antithrombin III; this complex can then inactivate thrombin and factors IXa, Xa, XIa and XIIa (Fig. 11.3). LMWH interacts with antithrombin III in a different manner to unfractionated heparin, and the LMWH–antithrombin complexes have a more selective anticoagulant action, mainly inhibiting factor Xa (Fig. 11.3).

Additional actions of the heparins are as follows.

- Promotion of tissue factor pathway inhibitor (TFPI) release from the vascular wall contributes to the antithrombotic effects of heparin. TFPI inhibits formation of factor Xa.
- Inhibition of platelet aggregation through binding to platelet factor 4 (mainly unfractionated heparin).

- Activation of lipoprotein lipase, which in addition to promoting lipolysis also reduces platelet adhesiveness.

Pharmacokinetics

Heparins are inactive orally and are given intravenously or by subcutaneous injection. They have a rapid onset of action. Heparins do not cross the placenta or enter breast milk. The two principal forms of heparin have different pharmacokinetic properties.

Unfractionated heparin

This is extracted from porcine intestinal mucosa or bovine lung, and consists of a mean of 45 polysaccharide units. It has dose-dependent pharmacokinetics: the half-life is very short (about 30 min) at low doses, increasing some five-fold at higher doses. Variable binding to plasma proteins contributes to inter-individual variation in the dose required to achieve target levels of anticoagulation. Most heparin is metabolised in endothelial cells after binding to cell surface receptors. Unfractionated heparin is usually given by continuous intravenous infusion for full anticoagulation. Low-dose subcutaneous injections are used for prophylaxis against venous thrombosis, although bioavailability by this route is only about 30%.

Low-molecular-weight heparins

LMWHs have a mean of 15 polysaccharide units. They are almost completely absorbed after subcutaneous administration and only need to be given once or twice daily by subcutaneous injection for full anticoagulation. LMWHs have a low affinity for plasma protein binding sites and for endothelial cell heparin receptors. They have two routes of elimination: a rapid, saturable liver uptake and slower renal excretion. The different LMWHs have half-lives in the range 2–6 h. When the dose of a LMWH is based on body weight they produce a more predictable anticoagulant effect compared with unfractionated heparin.

Control of heparin therapy

The therapeutic index for heparin is low. The degree of anticoagulation with unfractionated heparin is usually monitored with the activated partial thromboplastin time (APTT; a global test of the intrinsic coagulation pathway), which should be prolonged by 1.5–2.0 times the control value for full anticoagulation. Monitoring is not required when unfractionated heparin is used subcutaneously for prophylaxis. The anticoagulant effect of LMWHs can be monitored by the degree of factor Xa inhibition, but this is not carried out routinely since their effect is much more predictable than that of unfractionated heparin.

Unwanted effects

- Haemorrhage is the most common problem. The risk is greater in the elderly, especially if there is a history of heavy alcohol intake. The effect of unfractionated heparin can be rapidly reversed by intravenous injection of protamine sulphate, a basic peptide which binds strongly to the acidic heparin components. Protamine binds poorly to LMWHs and only partially reverses their action.

- Osteoporosis is a rare complication which can occur when heparin is given for several weeks; heparin binds to osteoblasts, and inhibits their activity. The risk is less with LMWH.
- Heparin-induced thrombocytopenia (HIT) usually occurs 5–15 days after starting intravenous heparin in about 2% of people, and arises from the development of antibodies to the heparin–platelet factor 4 complex. This causes platelet activation, aggregation and thrombosis. LMWHs are much less likely to cause HIT, since they have much less affinity for platelet factor 4 and their lower binding to endothelium also reduces interference with platelet–vessel wall interaction. Danaparoid (see the Compendium at the end of this chapter) is often used if continued parenteral anticoagulation is necessary.
- Hyperkalaemia by inhibition of aldosterone secretion. This is most likely to occur after at least 7 days of treatment.
- Hypersensitivity reactions.

Fondaparinux

Mechanism of action

Fondaparinux is a synthetic pentasaccharide almost identical to the natural pentasaccharide sequence of heparin that binds to antithrombin. Like LMWH, it enhances the innate ability of antithrombin to inhibit factor Xa.

Pharmacokinetics

Fondaparinux is given by subcutaneous injection. It is predictably absorbed from the injection site, is eliminated unchanged by the kidney and has a long half-life (18 h).

Unwanted effects

- Haemorrhage.
- Thrombocytopenia.
- Oedema.
- Gastrointestinal upset.

ORAL ANTICOAGULANTS

Vitamin K antagonists

Examples

warfarin, acenocoumarol (especially in Europe)

Mechanism of action

These drugs inhibit hepatic vitamin K epoxide reductase, which is the enzyme that converts vitamin K to its active (hydroquinone) form. As a result, the hepatic synthesis of the vitamin K-dependent clotting factors II (prothrombin), VII, IX and X is impaired (Fig. 11.3). There is a delay in the onset of the anticoagulant effect, due to the presence of previously synthesised clotting factors, which must be cleared from the circulation.

Pharmacokinetics

Warfarin is the most widely used vitamin K antagonist. It is almost completely absorbed from the gut and is highly bound to plasma albumin. It is eliminated by cytochrome P450-mediated hepatic metabolism (CYP2C9) and has a very long half-life of 1–2 days. Functional CYP2C9 polymorphisms contribute to considerable inter-individual variability in warfarin sensitivity. The plasma concentration of warfarin does not correlate directly with the clinical effect of the drug, which is determined by the balance between the rates of synthesis and degradation of clotting factors. The maximum effect of an individual dose of warfarin is reflected in the blood coagulation time some 24–36 h later. On stopping treatment, the duration of anticoagulant action is determined largely by the time required to synthesise new clotting factors.

Control of oral anticoagulant therapy

Factor VII is the clotting factor that is most sensitive to vitamin K deficiency, since it has the shortest half-life of the vitamin K-sensitive clotting factors. Therefore, a test of the extrinsic coagulation pathway – the prothrombin time – is used as a measure of effectiveness. The degree of prolongation of the prothrombin time is standardised by comparison with control plasma from a single source, and referred to as the international normalised ratio (INR). Therapeutic INR ranges differ according to the condition being treated:

- INR 2–2.5 for prophylaxis of deep vein thrombosis (thromboprophylaxis),
- INR 2–3 for thromboprophylaxis in hip surgery and fractured femur operations, for treatment of deep vein thrombosis and pulmonary embolism, and for prevention of thromboembolism in atrial fibrillation,
- INR 3–4.5 for prevention of recurrent deep vein thrombosis and for preventing thrombosis on mechanical prosthetic heart valves.

Unwanted effects

Warfarin is an important example of a drug that has a narrow therapeutic index.

- Haemorrhage. The most effective antidote to warfarin is phytomenadione (vitamin K_1). For major bleeding, this is given intravenously and controls bleeding within 6 h. An immediate coagulant effect is achieved by also giving an intravenous injection of prothrombin complex concentrate (vitamin K-dependent clotting factors) or an infusion of fresh frozen plasma. After giving a large dose of phytomenadione, it can be difficult to restore therapeutic anticoagulation with warfarin for up to 3 weeks. If the INR is >8.0 but there is no bleeding or only minor bleeding, then a smaller dose of phytomenadione can be given intravenously or orally with less disturbance to subsequent anticoagulation.
- Alopecia, skin necrosis and hypersensitivity reactions occur rarely.
- Warfarin crosses the placenta and can have undesirable effects on the fetus. It is teratogenic and should be avoided in the first trimester of pregnancy, except when essential; furthermore, it should not be used in the last trimester, as it increases the risk of intracranial haemorrhage in the baby during delivery.

- Drug interactions are particularly important. The anticoagulant effect of warfarin can be increased by broad-spectrum antibacterial agents that suppress the production of vitamin K by gut bacteria. Drugs such as amiodarone (Ch. 8) and the histamine H_2 receptor antagonist cimetidine (Ch. 33), which inhibit CYP2C9-mediated metabolism of warfarin, enhance its effects. Drugs that induce CYP2C9 – for example, phenytoin (Ch. 23) and alcohol (Ch. 54) – reduce the effect of warfarin by increasing its elimination.

DIRECT FACTOR XA INHIBITORS

Examples

apixaban, rivaroxaban

Mechanism of action

Apixaban and rivaroxaban are orally active factor Xa inhibitors that bind reversibly to the active site of factor Xa. They inhibit both free factor Xa and that bound to the prothrombinase complex, and unlike warfarin produce a rapid onset of predictable anticoagulation.

Pharmacokinetics

Apixaban and rivaroxaban are well absorbed from the gut. They are partially metabolised in the liver and partially excreted by the kidneys. Their half-lives are around 10 h.

Unwanted effects

- Nausea, and less often other gastrointestinal upset.
- Haemorrhage. If bleeding occurs, the short half-life means that stopping treatment may be all that is required. There is no direct antidote, but serious bleeding can be reduced with intravenous prothrombin complex concentrates or activated factor X.
- Drug interactions: rivaroxaban is a substrate for P-glycoprotein (P-gp), and its excretion is reduced by drugs that inhibit P-gp, such as ketoconazole.

DIRECT THROMBIN INHIBITORS

Example

dabigatran etexilate

Mechanism of action

Dabigatran is a selective, direct competitive thrombin inhibitor that binds to and inhibits both free circulating and thrombus-bound thrombin (factor IIa). It produces a rapid onset of predictable anticoagulation.

Pharmacokinetics

Dabigatran etexilate is a prodrug that has a low oral bioavailability and undergoes first-pass metabolism to its active derivative dabigatran. The active metabolite is excreted unchanged by the kidneys, and has a short half-life of about 40 min.

Unwanted effects

- Nausea, dyspepsia, diarrhoea, abdominal pain.
- Haemorrhage, but with a lower risk than warfarin at equally effective doses. There is no direct antidote, but serious bleeding can be treated with intravenous prothrombin complex concentrates.

CLINICAL USES OF ANTICOAGULANTS

Until recently, rapid anticoagulation was usually achieved with LMWH or unfractionated heparin, and warfarin was started simultaneously for long-term anticoagulation. The heparin is stopped when the INR reaches the desired therapeutic range. The newer oral anticoagulants have a rapid onset of action (so heparin is not needed) and compared to warfarin they have fewer drug interactions and do not need monitoring of their anticoagulant effect. In most situations where warfarin is used, they have similar or greater efficacy compared to warfarin with either similar or lower risk of bleeding. Therefore, increasing use of drugs such as rivaroxaban and dabigatran in place of warfarin is likely.

VENOUS THROMBOEMBOLISM

Acute pulmonary embolism can present with a wide variety of symptoms. Massive emboli produce shock or sustained hypotension, while smaller emboli can present with chest pain, dyspnoea or haemoptysis. Pulmonary embolism is a major cause of morbidity and death. Most serious pulmonary emboli arise from deep vein thrombosis in the lower limb, particularly if the thrombus extends to the larger veins above the calf. Massive pulmonary emboli causing haemodynamic instability are fatal in about 60% of cases if untreated. Mortality is much lower in stable patients. Many episodes of deep vein thrombosis occur in hospital, particularly in people over 40 years of age following major illness, trauma or surgery. Pulmonary embolism has been estimated to be responsible for 10% of all deaths in hospital. Chronic pulmonary embolic disease can lead to pulmonary arterial hypertension with progressive dyspnoea (Ch. 6).

Factors predisposing to venous thromboembolism in hospital (Table 11.1) include prolonged immobility and a variety of coexisting medical conditions such as cancer. Spontaneous thromboembolism can occur after long journeys, such as by road or air, and in various inherited or acquired disorders of the coagulation system. Use of the combined oral contraceptive pill by older women who smoke (see Ch. 45) is also a factor.

After an initial spontaneous deep vein thrombosis, the risk of recurrence is about 25% after 4 years, but is much

Table 11.1 Risk of thromboembolism in people admitted to hospital

Risk	Procedure
Low	Minor surgery, no other risk factor Major surgery, age <40 years, no other risk factors Minor trauma or illness
Moderate	Major surgery, age ≥40 years or other risk factor Heart failure, recent myocardial infarction, malignancy, inflammatory bowel disease Major trauma or burns Minor surgery, trauma or illness in patient with previous deep vein thrombosis or pulmonary embolism
High	Fracture or major orthopaedic surgery of pelvis, hips or lower limb Major pelvic or abdominal surgery for cancer Major surgery, trauma or illness in patient with previous deep vein thrombosis or pulmonary embolism Lower limb paralysis Major lower limb amputation

lower after postoperative thrombosis. Following a deep vein thrombosis, chronic post-phlebitic syndrome can develop, with pain, swelling and ulceration of the affected leg.

Prevention of deep vein thrombosis

In hospitalised people, the most appropriate method to prevent deep vein thrombosis will depend on the degree of risk.

Mechanical methods

These are used for people in hospital who are at moderate risk of thromboembolism and include graduated elastic compression stockings and intermittent pneumatic compression devices to improve venous flow and limit stasis in venous valve pockets. They can also be used to supplement pharmacological prophylaxis in people at high risk.

Low-dose subcutaneous heparin

This is the treatment of choice for many people in hospital who are at high or moderate risk of thromboembolism. Heparin reduces both initiation and extension of fibrin-rich thrombi at doses that have little effect on other measures of blood coagulation; therefore, laboratory monitoring is unnecessary. Low-dose unfractionated heparin reduces deep venous thrombosis and fatal pulmonary emboli by about two-thirds, with minimal risk of serious bleeding, although minor bleeding is increased. LMWHs or fondaparinux are more effective than unfractionated heparin for those at highest risk.

Oral anticoagulants

Low-dose dabigatran, apixaban and rivaroxaban are at least as effective as LMWHs for thromboprophylaxis in people undergoing hip and knee orthopaedic surgery. Bleeding rates with dabigatran, apixaban and LMWH are similar, but may be higher with rivaroxaban. Prophylaxis should be started before surgery. Warfarin may be more effective than heparin for prophylaxis in people at highest risk of thromboembolism, but is not widely used. Although a meta-analysis of several studies suggests that low-dose aspirin reduces deep venous thrombosis, it is less effective than heparin.

Treatment of established venous thromboembolism

The goals of treatment for deep vein thrombosis are to prevent pulmonary emboli and to restore patency of the occluded vessel, with preservation of the function of venous valves. In about 50% of people with deep venous thrombosis, the vessel will recanalise within 3 months if appropriately treated. Use of compression stockings in the first few weeks after a deep venous thrombosis of the leg reduces the incidence of post-phlebitic syndrome.

Therapeutic anticoagulation

This is the treatment of choice for deep vein thrombosis and for most pulmonary emboli since anticoagulation substantially reduces mortality. Heparin is still the most widely used initial treatment for its rapid onset of effect. LMWH or fondaparinux given subcutaneously are preferred to unfractionated heparin, except in people with significant renal impairment. Heparin is usually given for 3–5 days, with concurrent initiation of treatment with warfarin. Heparin can be stopped once warfarin has produced adequate anticoagulation (i.e. the INR is within the therapeutic range; see above). When deep vein thrombosis occurs in someone with cancer there is a high risk of both bleeding and recurrence during treatment with warfarin. In this situation, prolonged treatment with LMWH (6 months, or lifelong if remission is not achieved) is usually advocated. The optimal duration of anticoagulant therapy is not well defined, but suggested periods are shown in Table 11.2.

Oral anticoagulants such as rivaroxaban can be used instead of sequential heparin and warfarin, and have equal efficacy. At present there is only evidence for the efficacy of dabigatran after initial treatment with LMWH.

Surgical venous thrombectomy

This may be required for massive iliofemoral thrombosis if it threatens the viability of the limb. Pulmonary embolectomy is occasionally carried out for large pulmonary emboli.

Thrombolysis and percutaneous thrombectomy

Pharmacological thrombolysis (see below) has no advantage over warfarin in uncomplicated deep venous thrombosis. However, it is used to disintegrate massive pulmonary emboli, and reduces mortality in haemodynamically unstable patients. Percutaneous mechanical thrombectomy (fragmentation and removal of the thrombus) and surgical embolectomy are occasionally used if there are contraindications to thrombolysis.

Other treatments

When pulmonary emboli recur despite adequate anticoagulation, or when anticoagulation is contraindicated, inferior vena caval plication or insertion of a 'filter' device to trap emboli in the inferior vena cava can be considered.

ARTERIAL THROMBOEMBOLISM

Warfarin is used long term for the prevention of thrombosis on prosthetic heart valves. Atrial fibrillation and mural thrombus in the left ventricle following a myocardial infarction predispose to arterial embolism and are indications for anticoagulation with warfarin. Dabigatran, apixaban and rivaroxaban are at least as effective as warfarin for prevention of thromboembolism in atrial fibrillation and may have a lower risk of haemorrhage (Ch. 8). When combined with antiplatelet therapy, apixaban reduces the composite endpoint of mortality, reinfarction and ischaemic stroke after an acute coronary syndrome (Ch. 5).

THE FIBRINOLYTIC SYSTEM

Fibrinolysis is the physiological mechanism for dissolving the fibrin meshwork in a thrombus. The process is initiated by activation of plasminogen, a circulating α_2-globulin (Fig. 11.4). Tissue plasminogen activator (t-PA) is released from damaged vessels and cleaves plasminogen to the active enzyme plasmin. In the circulation, plasminogen activator inhibitors 1 and 2 rapidly inactivate t-PA. However, t-PA binds to fibrin locally at the site of release, and converts fibrin-bound plasminogen to plasmin. Plasmin splits both fibrinogen and fibrin into degradation products, and if this occurs at the site of a thrombus it produces lysis of the clot matrix. Fibrinolytic therapy (also called thrombolytic therapy) is achieved by using a plasminogen activator in such large quantities that the inhibitory controls are overwhelmed.

FIBRINOLYTIC (THROMBOLYTIC) AGENTS

Examples

alteplase (recombinant tissue-type plasminogen activator, rt-PA), streptokinase, tenecteplase

Mechanism of action

Fibrinolytic drugs enhance fibrinolysis by substituting for the naturally occurring t-PA. They bind to and activate

Table 11.2 Suggested duration of anticoagulant therapy for venous thromboembolism

Risk of recurrence	Clinical setting	Duration
Low	Temporary risk factors for thromboembolism	3 months
Intermediate	Continuing medical risk factors for thromboembolism	3–6 months
High	Recurrent thromboembolism; inherited thrombophilic tendency	Indefinite

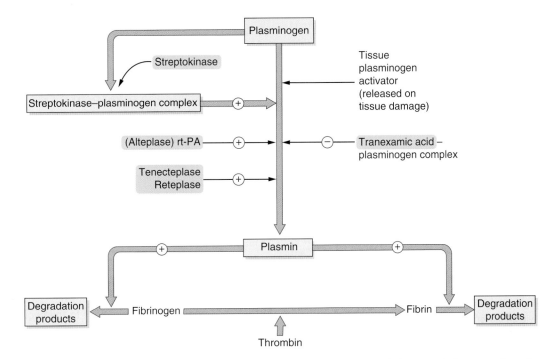

Fig. 11.4 **The fibrinolytic system.** The fibrinolytic system is linked intimately with the coagulation cascade and platelet function. When a clot is formed via the prothrombotic system, activation of plasminogen to the fibrinolytically active plasmin is initiated by several tissue plasminogen activators, thus lysing the clot. The drugs promoting this act as plasminogen activators (alteplase (recombinant tissue-type plasminogen activator, rt-PA) and derivatives) or bind to plasminogen (streptokinase), promoting plasmin activity. The antifibrinolytic drug tranexamic acid inhibits plasminogen activation.

plasminogen, which degrades fibrin thrombi. Alteplase is a genetically engineered copy of the naturally occurring t-PA that binds directly to fibrinogen and fibrin. It has a wide range of clinical uses. Tenecteplase is a genetically engineered modified form of t-PA with increased fibrin specificity, less sensitivity to plasminogen activator inhibitors and a longer duration of action than alteplase. Tenecteplase is only licensed for treatment of myocardial infarction

Streptokinase is obtained from haemolytic streptococci, and is inactive until it forms a complex with circulating plasminogen; the resultant streptokinase–plasminogen activator complex substitutes for t-PA in the fibrinolytic cascade, causing plasminogen activation. Streptokinase is now used less frequently than other fibrinolytic drugs.

The effectiveness of any fibrinolytic agent is greatest with fresh thrombus and if a large surface area of thrombus is exposed to the drug.

Pharmacokinetics

All fibrinolytic agents are given intravenously or intra-arterially. Alteplase and related compounds are metabolised in the liver. The streptokinase–plasminogen activator complex is degraded enzymatically in the circulation. Some streptokinase is cleared from the plasma before it forms an active complex, by combining with circulating neutralising antibody formed during previous exposure to streptokinase. After the use of streptokinase, or following a streptococcal infection, neutralising antibodies can persist in high titre for several years and substantially reduce the effectiveness of subsequent therapy with streptokinase. For this reason, repeat use of streptokinase is not recommended.

Alteplase and its derivatives have a more rapid onset of action than streptokinase and consequently the reperfusion of occluded vessels is faster. Infusions of alteplase are given over 1–3 h, depending on the condition being treated. Tenecteplase is given as a single bolus. Because of a short duration of action, when alteplase or its derivatives have been used to lyse coronary artery thrombus, subsequent anticoagulation with heparin for 48 h is necessary to reduce the risk of reocclusion. Streptokinase is usually given as a short (1 h) infusion for the treatment of coronary artery occlusion, although longer infusions are usual for peripheral arterial occlusions or pulmonary embolism. The long duration of action means that heparin is not necessary after streptokinase has been given.

Unwanted effects

- Nausea and vomiting.
- Haemorrhage is usually minor, but serious bleeding, for example intracerebral haemorrhage, occurs in about 1% of those treated. Bleeding can be stopped by antifibrinolytic drugs (see below) or by transfusion of fresh frozen plasma.

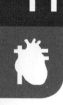

- Hypotension: this is dose-related and more common with streptokinase. It may be caused by enzymatic release of the vasodilator bradykinin from its circulating precursor. If the infusion of the fibrinolytic is stopped for a brief period, the blood pressure usually recovers rapidly and treatment can be continued.
- Allergic reactions: these are rare but can occur with streptokinase, as a consequence of its bacterial origin.

CLINICAL USES OF FIBRINOLYTIC AGENTS

Fibrinolytic agents are used to treat the following:

- acute myocardial infarction (although this use is rapidly declining with the greater availability of primary coronary angioplasty) (Ch. 5),
- ischaemic stroke (alteplase only) (Ch. 9),
- pulmonary embolism or deep venous thrombosis, in a minority of cases (see above),
- peripheral arterial thromboembolism (Ch. 10),
- central venous catheters occluded by clot (alteplase): this is particularly useful to restore patency of 'long lines' inserted for intravenous nutrition or administration of cytotoxic drugs.

ANTIFIBRINOLYTIC AND HAEMOSTATIC AGENTS

Antifibrinolytic agents

 Example

tranexamic acid

Mechanisms of action

Tranexamic acid competitively inhibits the activation of plasminogen, so fibrinolysis is inhibited. The theoretical risk of creating a thrombotic tendency does not appear to be a clinical problem.

Pharmacokinetics

Tranexamic acid is a synthetic amino acid that is incompletely absorbed from the gut and can also be given intravenously. It is excreted unchanged by the kidney and has a short half-life (1–2 h).

Unwanted effects

- Nausea, vomiting, diarrhoea.

Desmopressin

Desmopressin (Ch. 43) briefly increases the plasma concentrations of clotting factor VIII and von Willebrand factor, an adhesion protein in blood vessel walls. Factor VIII accelerates the process of fibrin formation and von Willebrand factor enhances platelet adhesion to subendothelial tissue.

CLINICAL USES OF ANTIFIBRINOLYTIC AND HAEMOSTATIC AGENTS

The use of haemostatic agents is limited, but includes the following.

- Tranexamic acid is used to prevent bleeding after surgery, for example prostatectomy or bladder surgery, or after dental extraction in individuals with haemophilia.
- Desmopressin is used in mild congenital bleeding disorders such as haemophilia A or von Willebrand's disease; it is given to reduce spontaneous or traumatic bleeding, or as a prophylactic before surgery.
- Tranexamic acid is used for the treatment of menorrhagia and epistaxis, or for bleeding following overdose of a fibrinolytic drug.
- Tranexamic acid is used for treatment of hereditary angioedema.

SELF-ASSESSMENT

True/false questions

1. Unfractionated heparin and low-molecular-weight heparin (LMWH) directly inhibit thrombin.
2. Heparin can be used to prevent clotting of blood collected in laboratory test tubes.
3. Once administered, the action of heparin cannot be reversed.
4. Fondaparinux is a pentapeptide activator of antithrombin III.
5. Warfarin readily crosses the placenta.
6. Warfarin prevents the activation of clotting factors which depend upon vitamin K for their synthesis.
7. Anticoagulant activity of warfarin is inhibited by broad-spectrum antibacterial agents.
8. Clopidogrel has its antithrombotic action by enhancing the action of ADP on platelets.
9. Abciximab is an antibody directed against the glycoprotein GPIIb/IIIa receptor on platelets.
10. Aspirin is a reversible inhibitor of cyclo-oxygenase type 1 (COX-1).
11. Aspirin inhibits platelet aggregation at doses below those needed for an anti-inflammatory effect.
12. Fibrinolytic infusions of recombinant tissue-type plasminogen activator (rt-PA; alteplase) for myocardial infarction are usually given over 1 h whereas streptokinase is given for 3–24 h.
13. Tenecteplase is a modified form of t-PA with a longer half-life than alteplase.
14. Apixaban is a direct inhibitor of factor Xa.
15. Dabigatran inhibits thrombin in the plasma and within the thrombus.
16. Tranexamic acid enhances plasminogen activation.

One-best-answer (OBA) question

Choose the one *correct* statement about anticoagulant drugs.

A. INR would need to be regularly monitored in people treated with heparin.

B. If an oral anticoagulant is required for rapid anticoagulant activity before surgery, heparin is the drug of choice.

C. Dosage adjustment of warfarin would be required if a person was prescribed concomitant treatment with the H_2 receptor antagonist cimetidine.

D. In overdose, the effects of warfarin cannot be reversed.

E. During treatment with a broad-spectrum antibacterial the anticoagulant effects of enoxaparin may be inhibited.

Case-based questions

A 51-year-old obese female was treated with oestrogen replacement therapy for 18 months because of perimenopausal symptoms. She was scheduled for a hip replacement.

1. Was anticoagulant therapy necessary for this woman?
2. Should thromboprophylaxis have been started before surgery?
3. Should heparin or warfarin have been chosen for prophylaxis and what routes of administration were appropriate?
   The hip replacement was carried out successfully and the woman was discharged from hospital after 5 days, although heparin therapy was continued for a further 5 days.
4. Why was therapy continued for this extended period and what out-of-hospital therapeutic prophylaxis could be considered?

True/false answers

1. **False.** Heparins first form a complex with antithrombin III; the complex then inactivates thrombin and other clotting factors including factors IXa, Xa and XIa. Complexes of LMWH with antithrombin have a more selective action on factor Xa.
2. **True.** The complexing of heparin with antithrombin in plasma means it can anticoagulate blood *in vitro*.
3. **False.** The action of unfractionated heparin (but not LMWH) can be reversed by the strongly basic protein protamine, which rapidly binds to it, forming an inactive complex.
4. **False.** All heparins are mucopolysaccharides. Fondaparinux is similar in structure to the pentasaccharide sequence within heparin that binds to antithrombin
5. **True.** Warfarin can cause fetal abnormalities and, unless essential, should not be given in early or late pregnancy.
6. **True.** Warfarin is a vitamin K antagonist that impairs vitamin K-dependent hepatic synthesis of factors II (prothrombin), VII, IX and X.
7. **False.** Vitamin K is produced by gut bacteria. Alteration of gut flora by broad-spectrum antibacterials will reduce vitamin K formation and hence reduce vitamin K-dependent clotting factor synthesis, enhancing the activity of warfarin.
8. **False.** Clopidogrel prevents the platelet aggregatory action of ADP by blocking purinergic ($P2Y_{12}$) receptors.

9. **True.** The increased expression of GPIIb/IIIa receptors on platelets is essential for aggregation as fibrinogen links adjacent platelets by binding to GPIIb/IIIa receptors, thereby initiating aggregation.
10. **False.** Aspirin (acetylsalicylic acid) irreversibly inhibits COX-1 by acetylating its active site.
11. **True.** Thromboxane A_2 (TXA_2) required for platelet aggregation is synthesised by COX-1, whereas prostaglandins are synthesised during inflammation predominantly by induced cyclo-oxygenase type 2 (COX-2). Aspirin is 160 times more active at inhibiting COX-1 than COX-2, so it has no anti-inflammatory effect at the low doses required to inhibit TXA_2 synthesis.
12. **False.** Streptokinase is usually infused for 1 h and alteplase for 3 h. Streptokinase has a longer half-life (1 h, alteplase 0.5 h), permitting a shorter infusion time.
13. **True.** Alteplase is identical to the naturally occurring t-PA, while tenecteplase has been modified for greater fibrin specificity and a longer duration of action.
14. **True.** The 'xabans' (apixaban, rivaroxaban) are orally active direct inhibitors of factor Xa.
15. **True.** Unlike heparin, which only inhibits plasma thrombin (via anti-thrombin III), dabigatran directly inhibits both free thrombin and thrombus-bound thrombin.
16. **False.** Tranexamic acid is an antifibrinolytic agent that inhibits plasminogen activation, reducing fibrin degradation and the risk of bleeding.

OBA answer

Answer C is correct.

A. Incorrect. Regular INR monitoring is required in people taking warfarin but not heparin, when the activated partial thromboplastin time (APTT) is used. Monitoring is not required when LMWH is used subcutaneously.

B. Incorrect. Heparin is inactive orally and must be given by intravenous or subcutaneous routes.

C. **Correct.** Warfarin is metabolised by the liver cytochrome P450 CYP2C9 and cimetidine inhibits this isoenzyme. A reduction in warfarin dose may be required or the replacement of cimetidine with another H_2 antihistamine or a proton pump inhibitor without an interaction with warfarin.

D. Incorrect. The effects of warfarin can be reversed with vitamin K_1.

E. Incorrect. Broad-spectrum antibacterials may suppress the production of vitamin K by gut bacteria and increase the activity of warfarin, but would not affect the actions of heparin.

Case-based answers

1. Anticoagulant therapy is necessary. Postoperative venous thromboembolism occurs in 40–50% of people who undergo hip replacement, and fatal pulmonary embolism in 1–5%, if prophylactic anticoagulant therapy is not given. This woman is also at increased risk because of obesity.

2. This is controversial. Initiating prophylaxis postoperatively allows more effective haemostatic control during

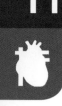

and immediately after surgery and does not reduce the effectiveness of treatment.

3. Heparins are active given intravenously or subcutaneously and their onset of action is rapid, whereas warfarin takes several days for full effectiveness but can be given orally. Heparin would therefore be chosen if started pre- or postoperatively.

4. The woman was obese, a risk factor for postoperative venous thrombosis. Daily self-administered subcutaneous prophylaxis with LMWH could be used. LMWH has a better bioavailability, a longer half-life and a lower risk of producing thrombocytopenia. Unlike unfractionated heparin, its effect is predictable.

FURTHER READING

Antiplatelet agents

Antiplatelet Trialist's Collaboration (2002) Collaborative meta-analysis of randomised trials of antiplatelet therapy for prevention of death, myocardial infarction and stroke in high risk patients. *BMJ* 324, 71–86

Cryer B (2005) Reducing the risks of gastrointestinal bleeding with antiplatelet therapies. *N Engl J Med* 352, 287–289

Gladding P, Webster M, Ormiston J et al (2008) Antiplatelet drug unresponsiveness. *Am Heart J* 155, 591–599

Gresele P, Momi S, Falcinelli E (2011) Antiplatelet therapy: phosphodiesterase inhibitors. *Br J Clin Pharmacol* 72, 634–646

Sambu N, Curzen N (2011) Monitoring the effectiveness of antiplatelet therapy: opportunities and limitations. *Br J Clin Pharmacol* 72, 683–696

Schneider DJ (2011) Antiplatelet therapy: glycoprotein IIb-IIIa antagonists. *Br J Clin Pharmacol* 72, 672–682

Wijeyeratne YD, Heppinstall S (2011) Antiplatelet therapy: ADP receptor antagonists. *Br J Clin Pharmacol* 72, 647–657

Anticoagulants

Agnelli G, Becattini C, (2010) Acute pulmonary embolism. *N Engl J Med* 363, 266–274

Blann AD, Lip YH (2006) Venous thromboembolism. *BMJ* 332, 215–219

Cayley WE (2007) Preventing deep vein thrombosis in hospital inpatients. *BMJ* 335, 147–151

DeZee KJ, Shimeall WT, Douglas et al (2006) Treatment of excessive anticoagulation with phytonadione (vitamin K). A meta-analysis. *Arch Intern Med* 166, 391–397

Ginsberg JS, Greer I, Hirsch J (2001) Use of antithrombotic agents during pregnancy. *Chest* 119, s122–s131

Kazmi RS, Lwaleed BA (2011) New anticoagulants: how to deal with treatment failure and bleeding complications. *Br J Clin Pharmacol* 72, 593–603

Kyrle PA, Eichinger S (2005) Deep vein thrombosis. *Lancet* 365, 1163–1174

Lee CJ, Ansell JE (2011) Direct thrombin inhibitors. *Br J Clin Pharmacol* 72, 581–592

Toschi V, Lettino M (2011) Inhibitors of propagation of coagulation: factors V and X. *Br J Clin Pharmacol* 72, 563–580

Fibrinolytic drugs

Khan IJ, Gowda RM (2003) Clinical perspectives and therapeutics of thrombolysis. *Int J Cardiol* 91, 115–127

Nordt TK, Bode C (2003) Thrombolysis: newer thrombolytic agents and their role in clinical medicine. *Heart* 89, 1358–1362

Haemostatic drugs

Mannucci PM, Levi M (2007) Prevention and treatment of major blood loss. *N Engl J Med* 356, 2301–2311

Wellington K, Wagstaff AJ (2003) Tranexamic acid. A review of its use in the management of menorrhagia. *Drugs* 63, 1417–1433

Compendium: drugs used to affect haemostasis

Drug	Kinetics (hallf-life)	Comments
Antiplatelet drugs		
Abciximab	Mechanism of elimination probably tissue uptake and proteolysis (0.5 h)	Antibody produces long-lasting blockade of glycoprotein IIb/IIIa receptor on platelets; specialist use only, as an adjunct to heparin and aspirin in high-risk individuals; given intravenously
Aspirin	Deacetylation (0.25–0.35 h); active salicylic acid metabolite (3–20 h)	Low dose used for the secondary prevention of thrombotic cerebrovascular or cardiovascular disease; given orally
Clopidogrel	Prodrug requiring hepatic bioactivation in two steps; acts via an unstable thiol metabolite which binds irreversibly to platelet receptors; half-life of an inactive metabolite (8 h) may not relate to the duration of clinical effect	Used for the prevention of ischaemic events in people with a history of symptomatic ischaemic disease; given orally
Dipyridamole	Metabolised largely to glucuronic acid conjugates, which are excreted in bile with some enterohepatic circulation (12 h)	Used as an adjunct to oral anticoagulants in people with prosthetic heart valves and for the secondary prevention of ischaemic stroke; given orally or by intravenous injection (for diagnostic purposes)
Epoprostenol	Eliminated very rapidly by hydrolysis (3 min)	Used intravenously in combination with heparin during renal dialysis and in combination with oral anticoagulants for primary pulmonary hypertension resistant to other treatments; potent vasodilator
Prasugrel	Prodrug activated rapidly by esterases then metabolised by several CYPs; active metabolite excreted mainly in urine (7 h)	Similar uses to clopidogrel, but has more rapid onset and inhibits platelet aggregation more completely; greater incidence of bleeding; given orally
Eptifibatide	Eliminated unchanged in urine and as a deaminated metabolite (1.5–2 h)	A cyclic hexapeptide given as an adjunct to heparin and aspirin in high-risk people with unstable angina (specialist use only); glycoprotein IIb/IIIa receptor inhibitor; given intravenously
Ticagrelor	Oral bioavailability 36%; parent drug and major metabolite are both active; hepatic metabolism and biliary excretion (7 h)	Used in combination with low-dose aspirin for the prevention of atherothrombotic events in people with acute coronary syndrome; given orally
Tirofiban	Limited metabolism; eliminated in urine and bile (2 h)	A non-peptide glycoprotein IIb/IIIa receptor inhibitor; used as an adjunct to heparin and aspirin in high-risk people with unstable angina (specialist use only); given intravenously
Anticoagulants (heparin-like)		

Heparins are polysaccharide macromolecules given by injection; they are eliminated by tissue uptake and degradation; low-molecular-weight heparins (LMWHs) are as effective as unfractionated heparin and their longer half-life allows treatment with once-daily subcutaneous injection. The LMWH half-lives below are based on anticoagulant activity not on measured drug concentrations.

Drug	Kinetics (hallf-life)	Comments
Bemiparin	Half-life 4–5 h	LMWH
Dalteparin sodium	Unlike heparin, renal elimination (2–4 h) is not dose-dependent	LMWH
Danaparoid sodium	Unlike heparin, renal elimination (17–28 h) is not dose-dependent	A heparinoid substance; useful in prophylaxis of deep vein thrombosis on a named-patient basis only
Enoxaparin	Eliminated by hepatic metabolism and limited renal excretion (3–6 h)	LMWH
Fondaparinux	Excreted in the urine unchanged (18 h)	A synthetic pentasaccharide which, like heparin, enhances the ability of antithrombin to inhibit factor Xa; used for prophylaxis in people undergoing major orthopaedic surgery of the legs
Heparin (unfractionated)	Eliminated by tissue uptake and metabolism; half-life (0.4–2.5 h) is dose-dependent	Used as the initial treatment for deep vein thrombosis and pulmonary embolism, as an intravenous loading dose followed by an intravenous infusion or intermittent subcutaneous injection; also given by subcutaneous injection for deep vein thrombosis prophylaxis in general surgery

Compendium: drugs used to affect haemostasis—cont'd

Drug	Kinetics (half-life)	Comments
Tinzaparin	Eliminated largely by renal excretion with some hepatic metabolism (3–4 h)	LMWH

Direct thrombin inhibitors

These are either peptides that are related to hirudin and are given intravenously (bivalirudin) or non-peptides that can be given orally (dabigatran etexilate).

Drug	Kinetics (half-life)	Comments
Bivalirudin	Eliminated by a combination of glomerular filtration and metabolism (peptide cleavage) (0.5 h)	Used for people undergoing percutaneous coronary intervention
Dabigatran etexilate	A prodrug; low oral bioavailability; metabolised to active derivative dabigatran which is excreted unchanged by the kidneys (40 min)	Selective, competitive thrombin inhibitor acting on both free and clot-bound thrombin (factor IIa); administered orally

Vitamin K antagonists

Warfarin is the drug of choice and the others are seldom required.

Drug	Kinetics (half-life)	Comments
Acenocoumarol	R- and S-enantiomers show different kinetics; genetic variation in hepatic metabolism of the more potent S-isomer affects drug response and risk of bleeding	Uses as for warfarin; given orally
Phenindione	Hepatic metabolism; urinary metabolites give a reddish colour to alkalinised urine (5–6 h)	Uses as for warfarin; given orally
Warfarin	Activated by oxidation; S-enantiomer more active and metabolised by CYP2C9 (18–35 h); R-enantiomer also undergoes hepatic metabolism (20–60 h)	Used for treatment of deep vein thrombosis and pulmonary embolism, and for prophylaxis of embolism in rheumatic heart disease, atrial fibrillation and after insertion of prosthetic heart valves; given orally

Thrombolytic agents (fibrinolytic agents)

Activate plasminogen to plasmin; used in the treatment of myocardial infarction; all are macromolecules given intravenously.

Drug	Kinetics (half-life)	Comments
Alteplase (recombinant tissue-type plasminogen activator,)	Hepatic uptake and degradation (0.5 h)	Tissue-type plasminogen activator; given by intravenous injection or infusion
Reteplase	Cleared by liver and kidney (0.3–0.5 h)	Given by intravenous injection over not more than 2 min
Streptokinase	Binding to plasminogen; hepatic metabolism (2 h)	Also used for life-threatening venous thrombosis and pulmonary embolism; given by intravenous infusion; rapid initial decrease in concentrations when there is a high antibody titre
Tenecteplase	Eliminated by hepatic metabolism (1.5–2 h)	A modified tissue-type plasminogen activator; higher selectivity than alteplase for fibrin; given by intravenous injection over 10 s

Antifibrinolytic drugs and haemostatic agents

Drug	Kinetics (half-life)	Comments
Etamsylate	No published kinetic data available	Reduces capillary bleeding, probably by affecting platelet adhesion; given orally
Tranexamic acid	Eliminated by glomerular filtration (1.4 h)	Used in hereditary angioedema, epistaxis and after excessive thrombolytic dosage; given orally or by slow intravenous injection

Direct factor Xa inhibitors

Drug	Kinetics (half-life)	Comments
Apixaban	Eliminated partly by metabolism and partly by urinary excretion (9–12 h)	Anticoagulant action by inhibiting factor Xa; used for prophylaxis after hip and knee replacement surgery; given orally
Rivaroxaban	Eliminated partly by metabolism and partly by urinary excretion (9–12 h)	Anticoagulant action by inhibiting factor Xa; used for prophylaxis after hip and knee replacement surgery; given orally

3

The respiratory system

12 Asthma and chronic obstructive pulmonary disease

Asthma and chronic obstructive pulmonary disease (COPD) show several similarities in their clinical features but have some distinct pathophysiological – including immunological – differences. Both are inflammatory disorders of the bronchi. Clinically, they are characterised by airflow obstruction (a forced expiratory volume in 1 second [FEV_1] below 80% of predicted and a ratio of FEV_1 to forced vital capacity of less than 70%).

ASTHMA

The characteristic feature of asthma is reversible airflow obstruction. Asthma is often associated with an atopic disposition, and exposure to allergens or other environmental air pollutants may then result in expression of the condition. However, more severe and adult-onset asthma is often non-allergic and accounts for 10–30% of cases.

The most common symptoms of asthma are chest tightness, wheeze, breathlessness and cough, although cough may be the only symptom in younger people, especially at night. Airflow obstruction in asthma typically shows marked variability over time and greater than 15% improvement in response to any inhaled bronchodilator (see below). The symptoms are due to a combination of smooth muscle constriction in the airway and bronchial inflammation.

The pathogenesis of asthma is complex, and our knowledge is incomplete (Figs 12.1 and 12.2). Immune dysfunction leads to airway inflammation in asthma and may result from impaired regulation and imbalance between different T-lymphocyte subsets and also epithelial and airway dendritic cells. Chronic inflammation of the bronchial mucosa is prominent, with infiltration of activated T-helper lymphocytes, eosinophils, mast cells, basophils and sometimes neutrophils. These inflammatory cells release several powerful chemical mediators (Figs 12.1 and 12.2). The result is hyperplasia of bronchial smooth muscle with abnormal reactivity, oedema of the bronchial wall, deposition of subepithelial collagen and increased airway secretions. Dysregulation of numerous inflammatory mediators appears to be involved in asthma, including cysteinyl-leukotrienes, histamine, proteases and a variety of cytokines and chemokines but, unlike COPD, there is relatively little evidence of an increase in reactive oxygen species.

Figure 12.1 shows how exposure of atopic individuals to a relevant allergen (such as pollen or the faeces of house-dust mite) crosslinks IgE bound to mast cell membrane receptors and causes mast cell degranulation. Degranulation and the subsequent pathological processes can also occur in hypersensitive non-atopic asthmatics with normal levels of IgE, triggered by other factors such as upper respiratory tract infections, particularly with human rhinovirus. Degranulation of mast cells produces immediate bronchoconstriction (early phase) due to the release of a number of spasmogens, of which the most potent are cysteinyl-leukotrienes (Fig. 12.1). Chemotactic mediators are also released, promoting an influx of inflammatory cells which 4–6 h later results in a delayed bronchoconstrictor response (late-phase) and the commencement of a cascade of other pathological events in the airways. The persistent release of spasmogens and inflammatory mediators by these infiltrating cells can leave the bronchi hyperreactive to various irritants for several weeks. The inflammatory mediators produce mucosal oedema, which narrows the airways, and stimulate smooth muscle contraction leading to bronchoconstriction. Excessive production of mucus can cause further airways obstruction by plugging the bronchiolar lumen.

In *mild to moderate* asthma there is an increase in the number and activation of eosinophils (accompanied by some neutrophils and macrophages) in the airway and hyperresponsiveness of the airways to irritants and spasmogens. There is a persistent and excessive T-helper cell type 2 (Th2) immune response (Fig. 12.2). All airways are involved in the inflammatory process in mild to moderate asthma, but the degree of submucosal fibrosis and mucus secretion is modest, with no parenchymal destruction.

In *severe* asthma there is evidence of additional, greater infiltration of neutrophils, tissue destruction and airways remodelling, with progressive thickening and loss of elastic recoil, especially in the peripheral airways. In addition to the changes seen in mild to moderate asthma, in severe disease there is increased expression of T-helper cell type 1 (Th1)-derived cytokines.

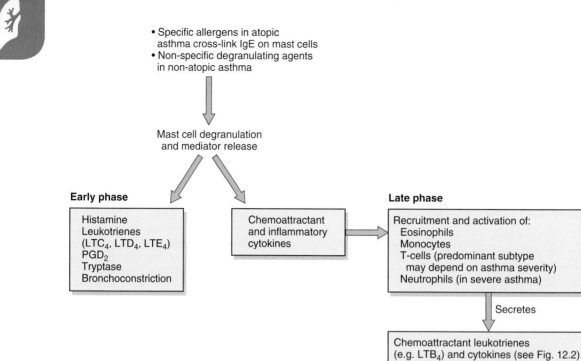

Fig. 12.1 **Some aspects of the early and late-phase responses in asthma.** Crosslinking of the over-expressed IgE on mast cells of atopic individuals, and non-immunogenic stimuli in more severe non-atopic asthma, can degranulate mast cells, resulting in secretion of mediators that contribute to the pathogenesis of asthma. These mediators directly produce bronchoconstriction, initiate the acute inflammatory response, and attract and activate cells responsible for further inflammatory mediator production and persistent chronic inflammation. LT, leukotriene; PG, prostaglandin.

CHRONIC OBSTRUCTIVE PULMONARY DISEASE

About 95% of people with COPD are, or have been, cigarette smokers. There is wide variability in the rate of decline in pulmonary function in persistent smokers, with about 10–20% showing an accelerated decline that may reflect a genetic susceptibility. Less common causes of COPD are exposure to air pollution (including biomass fuels in the developing world) and inherited α_1-antiprotease deficiency.

COPD is a symptom complex that is characterised by persistent airflow obstruction, with most people showing limited reversibility in response to a bronchodilator; however, about 10% of people with COPD do show considerable bronchodilator-induced reversibility of the airflow obstruction, and have a mixed inflammatory pattern in the airways, which probably represents an overlap between asthma and COPD (wheezy bronchitis). The airflow obstruction in COPD is usually slowly progressive and results from

a combination of decreased bronchial luminal diameter (produced by wall thickening, intraluminal mucus and changes in the fluid lining the small airways) and dynamic airways collapse due to emphysema (see below). It is often accompanied by chronic bronchitis (production of mucoid sputum for all or part of the year).

The most frequent symptoms of COPD are gradually progressive breathlessness and cough. The cough is often productive and usually worse in the morning, but its severity is unrelated to the degree of airflow obstruction. Repeated respiratory infections are common, and are often associated with exacerbations of the airflow obstruction and symptomatic deterioration.

In COPD there is an inflammatory process that particularly affects the peripheral airways. The predominant infiltrating cells are neutrophils and macrophages, but ongoing damage to the lung even after the trigger is removed is probably due to T-lymphocyte-mediated inflammation (Fig. 12.3). There is increased oxidative stress due to reactive oxygen species derived from cigarette smoke and other pollutants and released from neutrophils and inflammatory

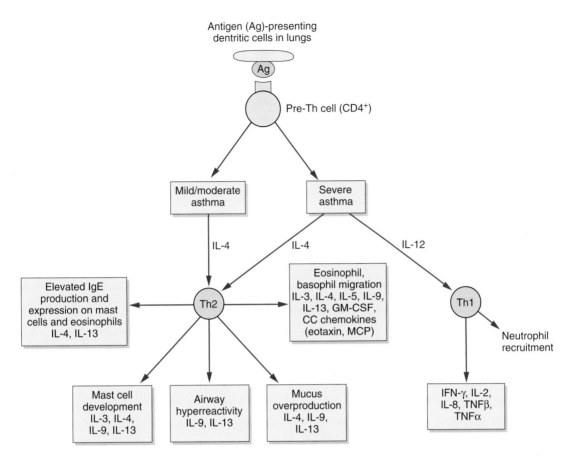

***Fig. 12.2* T-cells and asthma.** In allergic asthma there are complex and still poorly understood imbalances in the immune system. These include alterations in the functioning of several T-cell subsets and additional dysregulation in epithelial cells, fibroblasts and airway dendritic cells. In mild to moderate allergic asthma, the T-helper cell type 2 (Th2) response is amplified, and Th2 cytokines contribute to many of the pathophysiological features of asthma. In severe asthma there is an additional pathological role for T-helper type 1 (Th1) cytokines and neutrophils. IL, interleukin; GM-CSF, granulocyte–macrophage colony-stimulating factor; IFN, interferon; MCP, monocyte chemoattractant proteins, TNF, tumour necrosis factor.

macrophages. The inflammation produces a marked fibrotic reaction with parenchymal destruction and excessive bronchial mucus secretion. Corresponding histological changes include an increase in goblet cells in the bronchial mucosa and an increase in muscle mass in the bronchial wall, accompanied by interstitial fibrosis. Apoptosis of endothelial and alveolar cells reduces the ability of the lung to repair itself in response to sustained injury from the inhaled pollutants.

Emphysema is a pathological description, and is defined as enlargement of airways distal to the terminal bronchioles owing to destructive changes that may involve the entire acinus (panacinar) or the central part of the acinus (centriacinar). Lung parenchymal destruction is largely mediated by tissue proteases and cathepsins that are released by neutrophils and macrophages. Generation of excessive amounts of reactive oxygen species inhibits the antiproteases that normally protect the lung against such attack. This explains the susceptibility of people with inherited α_1-antiprotease deficiency to emphysema. Tissue destruction leads to a loss of lung recoil on expiration, which is a major

factor in generating expiratory flow. Emphysema is probably the dominant factor in severe COPD.

DRUGS FOR ASTHMA AND CHRONIC OBSTRUCTIVE PULMONARY DISEASE

DRUG DELIVERY TO THE LUNG

For the treatment of airways disease, direct delivery of drug to the lung by inhalation allows the use of smaller doses and therefore reduces the incidence of unwanted systemic effects (see Table 12.1). It also allows rapid onset of action of 'rescue' medication. The drug is usually delivered to the airways in an aerosol. The size of the aerosol particle that is inhaled is an important factor that determines whether or not it will reach the airways and where in the airways it will be deposited. The optimal particle size for treatment is 2–5 µm. Particles larger than 10 µm impact on the upper

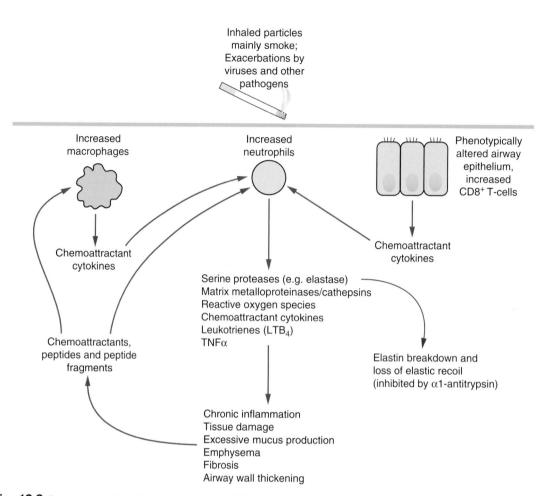

Fig. 12.3 Some pathophysiological factors in COPD. A small percentage of people who smoke are particularly susceptible to the development of COPD; susceptibility may be determined by variability in inflammatory or protective genes. Chronic alterations in the recruitment, activation and control in function of neutrophils, macrophages and subsets of T-cells results in chronic parenchymal damage, loss of elastic recoil and episodes of infection. TNF, tumour necrosis factor.

Table 12.1 Comparison of aerosol and oral therapy for asthma

	Aerosol	Oral
Ideal pharmacokinetics	Slow absorption from the lung surface and rapid systemic clearance	Good oral absorption and slow systemic clearance
Dose	Low dose delivered rapidly to target	High systemic dose necessary to achieve an appropriate concentration in the lung
Systemic drug concentration	Low	High
Incidence of unwanted effects	Low	High (but depends on drug)
Distribution in the lung	Reduced in severe disease	Unaffected by disease
Compliance	Good with bronchodilators, poor with anti-inflammatory drugs	Good
Ease of administration	Difficult for small children and infirm people[a]	Good
Effectiveness	Good in mild to moderate disease	Good even in severe disease

[a]May be improved by breath-actuated inhalers or spacing devices. Nebulisers can be used for severe exacerbations.

airways and will be swallowed. Particles smaller than 1 μm will not be deposited in the lower respiratory tract, and will either reach the alveoli and are absorbed into the blood or are exhaled. Other factors that influence aerosol deposition include the pattern of inhalation, the properties of the carrier and the type and severity of the lung disease. There are several methods for delivery of inhaled drug.

Pressurised metered-dose inhaler

This is the most common device for delivery of bronchodilator and anti-inflammatory drugs used in the treatment of asthma and COPD. The propellant in the device is a pressurised hydrofluoroalkane (HFA) (having replaced chlorofluorocarbons, or CFCs) and activation delivers a measured dose of aerosol via an atomization nozzle. Manually activated inhalers are widely used since they are convenient and inexpensive, but they require coordination of device activation and inhalation. The delivery and uptake of the drug are suboptimal if inspiratory flow is low, if inspiration is not full and is not preceded by full expiration, or if inspiration is followed by a breath hold of less than 6 s. About one-third of users find coordination difficult and, even if it is optimal, up to 70–90% of the aerosol may be deposited in the oropharynx and swallowed. The inhaler should be shaken before use.

Pressurised metered-dose inhaler with a spacer

A spacer device (a plastic reservoir) can be attached to the pressurised metered-dose inhaler to act as a chamber from which the suspended aerosol particles can be inhaled. The use of a spacer removes the need to coordinate aerosol activation and inspiration. A spacer can be large volume which retains more of the aerosol, or small volume which is more convenient but in which the aerosol impacts to a greater extent on the wall of the spacer. The spacer can be designed as a holding chamber by incorporating a one-way valve that retains the aerosol in the chamber for longer. A spacer is essential for young children, and for very young children a holding chamber can be attached to a facemask. The inhaler is activated into the spacer, and the person breathes normally through the mouthpiece. Inhalation of the contents should be completed within 10 s. The spacer allows evaporation of propellant and may create more droplets of the correct size to deposit in the airways. It also reduces drug deposition in the oropharynx, due to reduced particle velocity. Electrostatic charge on the plastic wall can attract particles and reduce drug delivery, so non-electrostatic materials are preferred. The device should be washed in mild detergent and air-dried to minimise the electrostatic charge. Addition of a spacer makes a metered-dose inhaler system less portable and may reduce adherence with treatment.

Breath-actuated metered-dose inhaler

There are several types of breath-actuated metered-dose inhaler, delivering either an aerosol or dry powder. The aerosol type is a modified metered-dose inhaler that is activated by inspiration. Actuation requires air to be drawn through the mouthpiece at a flow rate of at least 30 L·min⁻¹. People who have severe airflow obstruction cannot achieve this. Breath-actuated metered-dose inhaler devices cannot be used with a spacer.

Dry-powder inhaler

Dry-powder inhalers contain particles of drug of optimal size for deposition. Inspiration through the device generates turbulence, which disperses the particles in the inspired air. Some devices use a single dose capsule, while in others the source is a bulk powder with the device metering the dose. The delivered dose is dependent on the inspiratory effort, unless the device is power-assisted by a battery or vibrating piezoelectric crystals.

Multi-dose liquid inhaler

This novel delivery device uses a spring to force a metered dose of liquid through a narrow nozzle. It creates more fine particles and gives high drug delivery to the lungs.

Nebulisers

Nebulisers are devices that are used with a facemask or mouthpiece to deliver drug from a reservoir solution. There are two types.

- Jet nebulisers use compressed air or oxygen passing through a narrow orifice at 6–8 L·min⁻¹ to suck drug solution from a reservoir into a feed tube. There are fine ligaments in this tube, and the impact of the solution on these ligaments generates droplets (Venturi principle). Baffles trap the larger droplets.
- Ultrasonic nebulisers use a piezoelectric crystal vibrating at high frequency to create the aerosol, and do not require gas flow. The vibrations are transmitted through a buffer to the drug solution and form a fountain of liquid in the nebulisation chamber. Ultrasonic nebulisers produce a more uniform particle size than jet nebulisers, but are less widely used due to cost.

Up to 10 times the amount of drug is required in a nebuliser to produce the same degree of bronchodilation achieved by a metered-dose inhaler. Drug delivery is more efficient via a mouthpiece than via a mask from which drug can be deposited in the nasal passages.

SYMPTOM-RELIEVING DRUGS FOR AIRFLOW OBSTRUCTION (BRONCHODILATORS; 'RELIEVERS')

Beta₂-adrenoceptor agonists

Examples

short-acting: salbutamol, terbutaline
long-acting: formoterol, salmeterol
ultra long-acting: indacaterol

Mechanism of action and effects

Beta$_2$-adrenoceptors are widely distributed in the lung, and the receptor density is higher in bronchial smooth muscle than in other cell types such as epithelial and endothelial cells and mast cells. Stimulation of these receptors by an agonist stabilises the receptor in its active rather than inactive configuration. This results in increased generation of cAMP by adenylyl cyclase, and activation of protein kinase A (PKA), which phosphorylates proteins that are central to the regulation of smooth muscle tone. Major beneficial actions of a β_2-adrenoceptor agonist are:

- bronchodilation due to reduced Ca^{2+} release from intracellular stores and reduced Ca^{2+} entry into smooth muscle cells,
- inhibition of mediator release from mast cells and monocytes,
- enhanced mucociliary clearance.

However, in addition to their beneficial effects on the airway, use of a β_2-adrenoceptor agonist in asthma can enhance Th2 inflammatory pathways and also downregulate β_2-adrenoceptors. Therefore, regular use of a β_2-adrenoceptor agonist without an inhaled corticosteroid is not advised. There is evidence of synergy between inhaled corticosteroids and inhaled β_2-adrenoceptor agonists, with the latter enhancing the gene-transcription effects of corticosteroids and corticosteroids enhancing β_2-adrenoceptor gene transcription.

Some β_2-adrenoceptor agonists, such as salbutamol, terbutaline and salmeterol, have about 60% partial agonist activity at the receptor (low-efficacy agonists) compared with formoterol and indacaterol which have full agonist activity (high-efficacy agonists). The relevance of these differences to treatment outcomes and unwanted effects is unclear.

Pharmacokinetics

The selectivity of β_2-adrenoceptor agonists for the β_2-adrenoceptor subtype is dose-dependent. Inhalation of drug aids selectivity since it delivers small but effective doses to the airways and minimises systemic exposure and stimulation of β-adrenoceptors outside the lungs (Table 12.1). The dose–response relationship for bronchodilation is log-linear and a 10-fold increase in dose is required to double the effect.

Short-acting β_2-adrenoceptor agonists, such as salbutamol, have a rapid onset of action, often within 5 min, and produce bronchodilation for up to about 6 h. Their duration of action is far longer than the natural adrenoceptor agonists such as adrenaline, because they are not substrates for the uptake transporter on the presynaptic neuron or for catechol-O-methyltransferase, the enzyme that metabolises catecholamines outside adrenergic neurons (Ch. 4).

Salmeterol and formoterol have a longer duration of action (up to 12 h) because they are more lipophilic than short-acting agents and bind to the lipid of the cell membrane. Salmeterol has a slower onset of action than short-acting agents, but the onset with formoterol is rapid. Indacaterol is an ultra-long acting (up to 24 h) lipophilic, rapid-onset β_2-adrenoceptor agonist.

Salbutamol and terbutaline can also be given orally (as conventional or modified-release formulations), by subcutaneous or intramuscular injection or by intravenous infusion. Much larger doses are required to deliver an adequate amount of drug to the lungs by any of these routes compared to inhaled doses. This reduces the selectivity for β_2-adrenoceptors, and systemic unwanted effects can be troublesome.

Unwanted effects

- Fine skeletal muscle tremor from stimulation of β_2-adrenoceptors.
- Tachycardia and arrhythmias result from both β_1- and β_2-adrenoceptor stimulation in the heart when high doses of inhaled drug are used, or after oral or parenteral administration.
- Hypokalaemia with high doses, due to promotion of cellular uptake of K^+ by a cAMP-dependent action of β_2-adrenoceptor agonists on the Na^+/K^+ pump. Nebilised salbutamol is sometimes used as a treatment for hyperkalaemia. Hypomagnesaemia and hyperglycaemia can also occur. These effects do not persist during long-term use.
- Paradoxical bronchospasm has been reported with inhalation, usually when given for the first time or with a new canister.
- Headache.
- Tolerance to the bronchodilator effects with prolonged use of β_2-adrenoceptor agonists is modest, but desensitisation and downregulation of the β_2-adrenoceptor does occur. The process of receptor desensitisation appears to be more rapid for mast cells than for bronchial smooth muscle, and the prevention of exercise-induced bronchoconstriction is more affected than the symptom relief that these drugs produce. Corticosteroids reduce desensitisation by increasing β_2-adrenoceptor gene transcription and enhancing coupling of the receptor to adenylyl cyclase.

Regular use of high doses of short-acting or inhaled long-acting β_2-adrenoceptor agonists has been linked with asthma deaths. One possibility is that they precipitate serious cardiac arrhythmias during severe asthma exacerbations. It is also possible that their use might allow people to tolerate initial exposure to larger doses of allergens or irritants, which then produce an enhanced late asthmatic response. The excess mortality, although of concern, is extremely low. Recent investigation has raised the possibility that β_2-adrenoceptor polymorphism may modify the response to β_2-adrenoceptor agonists in some individuals, but it is not known whether this explains the risk of adverse events.

Antimuscarinic agents

Examples

ipratropium, tiotropium

Mechanism of action and effects

Many cell types in the respiratory system, including both neuronal and non-neuronal cells, have nicotinic and muscarinic surface receptors. These mediate a multitude of actions in response to parasympathetic nervous system stimulation. There are two main types of muscarinic receptors in the airways, as follows.

- M_3 receptors mediate direct bronchoconstriction and glandular mucus secretion and also enhance mucociliary clearance from the bronchi. M_3 receptor stimulation activates phospholipase C with subsequent formation of inositol triphosphate (IP_3) and diacylglycerol (DAG), which are key events in the signalling pathway that increases intracellular Ca^{2+} (Ch. 1, Fig. 1.5).
- M_2 receptors are more numerous and inhibit ciliary activity as well as limiting β_2-adrenoceptor-mediated bronchodilation by inhibition of adenylyl cyclase.

Therefore, blocking both M_2 and M_3 receptors could be beneficial in bronchoconstriction. However, M_2 autoreceptors are also present on presynaptic parasympathetic nerves supplying the lungs. Stimulation of these autoreceptors inhibits acetylcholine release and attenuates vagally mediated bronchoconstriction. Blocking these M_2 autoreceptors may blunt the beneficial effect of non-selective muscarinic antagonists.

Ipratropium is a non-selective muscarinic receptor antagonist, and binds to all muscarinic receptors in the lung including the presynaptic M_2 autoreceptor. Ipratropium therefore has the potential to augment vagally mediated bronchoconstriction. The recommended dose is determined by unwanted effects and is well below the dose that produces maximal bronchodilation. By contrast, tiotropium is functionally selective for the M_3 receptor. Although it has a high affinity for all muscarinic receptors, it dissociates rapidly from M_2 receptors.

The main benefit of muscarinic antagonists is in COPD; they are of less value for bronchodilation in acute mild to moderate asthma, but ipratropium has a place when added to a β_2-adrenoceptor agonist in severe exacerbations of asthma.

Pharmacokinetics

The antimuscarinic drugs used for bronchodilation are N-quaternary congeners of the tertiary-structured atropine, and are poorly absorbed orally and do not cross the blood–brain barrier. They are given exclusively by inhalation as a powder or aerosol or via a nebuliser. They have a slower onset of action (30–60 min) than salbutamol (5–10 min), probably due to slow absorption from the surface of the airways. The duration of action is related to the rate of removal locally from the airways, and not the half-life of elimination from the circulation.

Unwanted effects

Similarly to inhaled β_2-adrenoceptor agonists, direct delivery of antimuscarinic drugs to the lung is the main reason for the relative lack of unwanted systemic effects.

- Dry mouth is the most common unwanted effect.
- Nausea, constipation.
- Headache.
- Tiotropium can cause urinary retention in men with prostatism.
- Exacerbation of angle-closure glaucoma (Ch. 50).

Methylxanthines

Examples

aminophylline, theophylline

Mechanism of action and effects

Methylxanthines are a group of naturally occurring substances found in coffee, tea, chocolate and related foodstuffs. Naturally occurring theophylline (1,3-dimethylxanthine), and its ester derivative aminophylline, are the only compounds in clinical use. They are chemically similar to caffeine. Methylxanthines have vasodilatory, anti-inflammatory and immunomodulatory actions. The mechanisms of action of methylxanthines are multiple, controversial and of uncertain importance.

- Inhibition of the enzyme phosphodiesterase (PDE), which degrades cyclic nucleotide second messengers, may partly explain the actions of methylxanthines. Theophylline preferentially inhibits the isoenzymes PDE3 (which degrades cAMP and cGMP) and PDE4 (which degrades cAMP). PDE3 is found in bronchial smooth muscle and PDE4 in several inflammatory cell types, including mast cells. The rise in intracellular cAMP in bronchial smooth muscle stimulates large-conductance voltage-gated Ca^{2+}-activated K^+ channels (BK_{Ca}) in the cell membrane, leading to cell hyperpolarisation and muscle relaxation. However, theophylline only produces bronchodilation at relatively high plasma concentrations (10–20 $mg \cdot L^{-1}$) and drugs that are more effective PDE inhibitors (such as dipyridamole) do not bronchodilate. Prolonging the duration of action of cyclic nucleotides may potentiate the action of β_2-adrenoceptor agonists and produce a synergistic dilator effect on bronchial smooth muscle. PDE inhibition also stimulates ciliary beat frequency in the airways and enhances water transport across the airway epithelium, which increase mucociliary clearance. In contrast, theophylline increases the force and rate of contraction of cardiac muscle through its effect on cAMP (Ch. 7), but also causes arterial vasodilation by inhibiting the breakdown of cGMP.
- Increased diaphragmatic contractility and reduced fatigue have been reported at lower plasma theophylline concentrations than those required for bronchodilation. This may improve lung ventilation.
- Adenosine receptor antagonism may be relevant to some of the clinical effects of methylxanthines (see also adenosine; Ch. 8). Adenosine releases histamine and leukotrienes from mast cells, which results in the constriction of hyperresponsive airways in individuals with asthma. Theophylline is a potent antagonist at adenosine A_1 and A_2 receptors (Ch. 1) and may reduce bronchoconstriction by this mechanism. Adenosine receptor

antagonism is responsible for central nervous system (CNS) stimulation, which improves mental performance and alertness, and in the kidney reduces tubular Na^+ reabsorption and leads to natriuresis and diuresis.

- Activation of histone deacetylases (HDACs; see corticosteroids, below): acetylation of core histones, which form part of the structure of chromatin, activates gene transcription, while their deacetylation suppresses gene transcription, including transcription of pro-inflammatory genes. Theophylline at low concentrations activates HDAC in nuclear extracts, indicating an action independent of adenosine and other surface receptors, and also increases HDAC activity in bronchial biopsies of asthmatic patients. Anti-inflammatory effects of theophylline occur at drug plasma concentrations of $5-10$ mg·L^{-1}, similar to those that produce clinical benefit. The action of theophylline on HDAC may potentiate the anti-inflammatory effects of corticosteroids (see Ch. 44).

Pharmacokinetics

The extent of absorption of theophylline from the gut is unpredictable, with considerable inter-individual variation. This, and the short but highly variable plasma half-life, has resulted in the widespread use of modified-release formulations. Theophylline has a narrow therapeutic index, and since different formulations vary in their release characteristics they are not readily interchangeable. Theophylline is metabolised in the liver by cytochrome P450 (CYP1A2 and, to a lesser extent, by CYP3A4), giving the potential for drug interactions. Aminophylline is a more water-soluble ester prodrug, which is hydrolysed rapidly after absorption from the gut to theophylline and ethylenediamine. Aminophylline can also be given by intravenous infusion. Measurement of blood theophylline concentrations is valuable as a guide to effective dosing.

Unwanted effects

Most are dose-related and can arise within the accepted therapeutic plasma concentration range.

- Gastrointestinal upset, including nausea, vomiting (from PDE4 inhibition in the vomiting centre) and diarrhoea.
- CNS stimulation, including insomnia, irritability, headache (from PDE3 inhibition) and occasionally seizures at high plasma concentrations (from adenosine receptor antagonism).
- Hypotension from peripheral vasodilation (from PDE3 inhibition in the smooth muscle cells of many blood vessels). In contrast, cerebral arteries are constricted by methylxanthines (adenosine is a vasodilator of cranial blood vessels and methylxanthines may act as adenosine receptor antagonists in this vascular bed).
- Cardiac stimulation produces various arrhythmias.
- Hypokalaemia can occur acutely, especially after intravenous injection, which also promotes cardiac arrhythmias.
- Tolerance to the beneficial effects of methylxanthines can occur.
- Drug interactions can be troublesome, due to the narrow therapeutic index of theophylline. Hepatic CYP1A2 enzyme inhibitors such as ciprofloxacin, erythromycin, clarithromycin, fluconazole and ketoconazole (Ch. 51, Table 2.7) can precipitate theophylline toxicity.

ANTI-INFLAMMATORY DRUGS FOR AIRWAYS OBSTRUCTION ('PREVENTERS')

Corticosteroids

Examples

beclometasone dipropionate, budesonide, fluticasone propionate, hydrocortisone, prednisolone

Mechanism of action and effects

Corticosteroids with powerful glucocorticoid activity (but without significant mineralocorticoid activity) are the most effective class of drug in the treatment of chronic asthma, but are relatively ineffective in COPD. They suppress inflammation and the immune response but are not bronchodilators and are therefore of no benefit in the initial stages of an acute attack of asthma.

Intracellular events involved in the anti-inflammatory action of corticosteroids are described in Chapters 38 and 44. Inhibition of transcription of genes coding for the cytokines involved in inflammation is particularly important in asthma. Higher glucocorticoid concentrations also activate anti-inflammatory genes and genes linked to glucocorticoid unwanted effects. Following a delay of $6-12$ h, corticosteroids reduce airway responsiveness to several bronchoconstrictor mediators and, with chronic therapy, inhibit both the early and late reactions to allergen.

Anti-inflammatory effects of corticosteroids in asthma include:

- reduced airway oedema and leucocyte recruitment by induction of tight junctions in vascular endothelial cells,
- reduced inflammatory cell activation (including macrophages, T-lymphocytes, eosinophils and airway epithelial cells) with reduced inflammatory cytokine, chemokine, adhesion molecule and inflammatory enzyme expression (Ch. 38). In allergic disease, suppression of Th2 cells and their cytokines is particularly important,
- reduced inflammatory cell recruitment to the airways (eosinophils, T-lymphocytes, mast cells and dendritic cells) through reduction in chemotactic mediators and adhesion molecules, and reduced survival (enhanced apoptosis) of airway inflammatory cells,
- decreased local generation of inflammatory prostaglandins and leukotrienes by inhibition of phospholipase A_2 which reduces mucosal oedema (see also Ch. 29),
- beta$_2$-adrenoceptor upregulation and better coupling to adenylyl cyclase, which restores responsiveness to β_2-adrenoceptor agonists,
- enhanced activity of the M_2 autoreceptors on acetylcholine nerve endings inhibits acetylcholine release and relieves vagally mediated bronchoconstriction,

■ suppression of the excess epithelial cell shedding and goblet cell hyperplasia found in the bronchial epithelium in asthma.

Inhaled corticosteroids produce some improvement in asthmatic symptoms after 24 h and a maximum response after 1–2 weeks. Reduction in airway responsiveness to allergens and irritants occurs gradually over several months, but many of the chronic structural changes in the airways in asthma are not affected by corticosteroids.

Pharmacokinetics

Whenever possible, corticosteroids are given by inhalation of an aerosol or dry powder in order to minimise systemic unwanted effects, but they can be used intravenously or orally in severe asthma. Desirable properties of an inhaled corticosteroid include a low rate of absorption across mucosal surfaces (such as the lung, but also the gut for swallowed drug) and rapid inactivation once absorbed. Beclometasone dipropionate fulfils the former criterion, but it is only slowly inactivated once it reaches the systemic circulation. Inhaled budesonide (which is inactivated by extensive first-pass metabolism in the liver following oral absorption) or fluticasone (which is very poorly absorbed from the gut) may be preferred if high doses of inhaled drug are needed, or for the treatment of children, in whom the systemic effects can be more problematic.

Unwanted effects

The unwanted effects of oral and parenteral corticosteroids are described in Chapter 44. Inhaled corticosteroids only have systemic actions when given in high doses. The amount of swallowed drug can be minimised by using a large-volume spacer (see above); large aerosol particles, which would otherwise be deposited on the oropharyngeal mucosa, are trapped in the spacer and only the smaller particles are inhaled.

There are some specific problems with inhaled corticosteroids:

■ dysphonia (hoarseness), caused by deposition on vocal cords and myopathy of laryngeal muscles, occurs in up to one-third of those using inhaled corticosteroids. This may be less troublesome with breath-actuated delivery, since the method of inspiration leads to protection of the vocal cords by the false cords,
■ oral candidiasis can occur but can be prevented by using a spacer device or by gargling with water after use of the inhaler,
■ prolonged use of high doses of inhaled corticosteroid has been associated with systemic unwanted effects. These include adrenal suppression, osteoporosis and reduced growth velocity in children. In older people with COPD there is an increased risk of pneumonia.

Cromones

Examples

sodium cromoglicate, nedocromil sodium

The cromones are used to prevent asthma attacks, but they are usually less effective than inhaled corticosteroids and only about one-third of people benefit from treatment. Cromones have no bronchodilator activity and are of no use in acute attacks of asthma. The major use of cromones is as prophylactic agents in the treatment of mild to moderate antigen-, pollutant- and exercise-induced asthma. They are also used as nasal inhalants to treat seasonal allergic rhinitis (Ch. 39) and in ophthalmic solutions to treat allergic conjunctivitis (Ch. 50).

Mechanisms of action and effects

■ Mast cell stabilisation. Sodium cromoglicate was originally introduced as a mast cell stabiliser. It enhances phosphorylation of a protein that normally forms a substrate for intracellular protein kinase C, and interferes with the signal transduction for inflammatory mediator release. This action may protect against immediate bronchoconstriction induced by allergens, exercise or cold air.
■ Inhibition of sensory C-fibre neurons by antagonism of the effects of the tachykinins, substance P and neurokinin B, which are involved in generation of sensory stimuli. This is probably responsible for protection against bronchoconstriction produced by irritants such as sulphur dioxide.
■ Inhibition of accumulation of eosinophils in the lungs and reduced activation of eosinophils, neutrophils and macrophages in inflamed lung tissue. These actions may be important in preventing the 'late-phase' response to allergen and the development of bronchial hyperreactivity.
■ Inhibition of B-cell switching to IgE production probably also contributes to the long-term effects.

A single dose of either nedocromil sodium or sodium cromoglicate will prevent the early-phase bronchoconstrictor response to allergen, but treatment for 1–2 months may be necessary to block the late-phase reaction.

Pharmacokinetics

Both sodium cromoglicate and nedocromil sodium are highly ionised and poorly absorbed across biological membranes. They are therefore largely retained at the site of action on bronchial mucosa after inhalation as a powder or from a metered-dose aerosol inhaler. Swallowed drug is unabsorbed and voided in the faeces.

Unwanted effects

■ Cough, wheeze and throat irritation may be provoked transiently following inhalation.
■ Headache.
■ Nausea, vomiting, dyspepsia and abdominal pain with nedocromil sodium.

Leukotriene receptor antagonists

Examples

montelukast, zafirlukast

Mechanisms of action and effects

The leukotriene receptor antagonists are given orally and inhibit the bronchoconstriction induced by the cysteinyl-leukotrienes (LTC_4, LTD_4 and LTE_4) (Ch. 29) by blocking the $CysLT_1$ receptor on bronchial smooth muscle. Cysteinyl-leukotrienes are released from various cells, including activated mast cells and eosinophils, in response to several airway insults, and their synthesis is increased by many mediators, such as cytokines. Cysteinyl-leukotrienes can also contribute to airway oedema, enhanced secretion of mucus and airway eosinophilia (Fig. 12.1).

Leukotriene receptor antagonists reduce both the early and late bronchoconstrictor responses to inhaled allergen, and may be most useful in mild and moderate asthma, exercise-induced bronchoconstriction and asthma provoked by non-steroidal anti-inflammatory drugs (NSAIDs; Ch. 29). The effects are additive to those of inhaled corticosteroid.

Unwanted effects

- Headache.
- Gastrointestinal upset.

Phosphodiesterase type 4 inhibitors

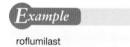

roflumilast

Mechanism of action and effects

Phosphodiesterase type 4 (PDE4) is the main isoenzyme present in cells involved in the inflammatory process in COPD. PDE4 degrades the intracellular second messenger cAMP, and inhibition of this enzyme with roflumilast has several anti-inflammatory actions:

- decreased cytokine and chemokine release from neutrophils, eosinophils, macrophages and T-lymphocytes,
- decreased expression of adhesion molecules on T-lymphocytes and other inflammatory cells. Along with the reduced chemokine release, this results in less accumulation of these cells in the airway,
- decreased apoptosis of airway cells, which may assist in sputum clearance.

Roflumilast is highly selective for PDE4, and therefore has little action in tissues that express different PDE isoenzymes. It is effective in COPD patients with chronic bronchitis (prominent cough and sputum production) who have frequent exacerbations. In these individuals, roflumilast improves lung function and reduces exacerbation frequency.

Pharmacokinetics

Roflumilast is well absorbed from the gut, and is metabolised by the liver. It has a long but variable half-life with an average of about 17 h.

Unwanted effects

PDE4 has several isoforms that are found in the gut, adipose tissue and neurons, and inhibition of these is responsible for most unwanted effects with roflumilast:

- nausea, anorexia, abdominal pain, diarrhoea,
- weight loss,
- headache, insomnia.

Magnesium sulphate

Mechanism of action and effects

Intravenous magnesium sulphate can be given for the treatment of severe asthma in adults if life-threatening features are present. Magnesium bronchodilates by blocking Ca^{2+} channels in smooth muscle cell membranes, therefore reducing Ca^{2+} influx into the cell.

Pharmacokinetics

Magnesium sulphate is given intravenously and is widely distributed. The Mg^{2+} is excreted by the kidney, with a half-life of 4 h.

Unwanted effects

- Atrioventricular block.
- Enhancement of neuromuscular blockade by neuromuscular blocking agents.
- Potentiates the hypotensive effects of calcium channel blockers.
- Diarrhoea.

Antibodies to immunoglobulin E (IgE)

Example

omalizumab

Mechanism of action

Omalizumab is a recombinant humanised IgG1k monoclonal antibody that binds selectively to IgE, to form complexes which are removed from the circulation. This leads to a reduction in IgE receptor expression and mediator release from mast cells, basophils and dendritic cells. Treatment with omalizumab gradually reduces airway inflammation in asthma, with a peak response after 12–16 weeks. Omalizumab is used for the treatment of persistent severe allergic asthma in adults and children over 12 years that cannot be controlled with high-dose inhaled corticosteroids with a long-acting β_2-adrenoceptor agonist and other standard therapies for asthma.

Pharmacokinetics

Omalizumab is given subcutaneously every 2–4 weeks in a dose that is determined by the recipient's plasma IgE concentration and body weight. It forms complexes with IgE that are removed by the reticuloendothelial system and endothelial cells. Omalizumab has a very long half-life of about 26 days.

Unwanted effects

- Anaphylaxis occurs in 1–2 of every 1000 people given omalizumab.
- Headache.
- Injection-site reactions.

MANAGEMENT OF ASTHMA

Treatment of asthma has two aims:

- relief of symptoms,
- reduction of airways inflammation.

THE ACUTE ATTACK

Mild infrequent attacks of asthma can often be controlled by occasional use of a short-acting inhaled β_2-adrenoceptor agonist. Antimuscarinic agents are less effective unless asthma coexists with chronic obstructive airways disease. More severe attacks of asthma require intensive treatment with bronchodilators and systemic corticosteroids. The signs of severe and life-threatening asthma are shown in Table 12.2.

Treatment of acute severe asthma should include:

- ensuring adequate hydration,
- high-flow oxygen via a facemask to achieve an arterial oxygen saturation of above 90%,
- inhaled short-acting β_2-adrenoceptor agonist such as salbutamol, preferably via an oxygen-driven nebuliser, or a via a metered-dose inhaler with a large-volume spacer if a nebuliser is not available,

Table 12.2 Signs of severe and life-threatening asthma

Severe asthma	Life-threatening asthma
Inability to complete a sentence	A silent chest
Pulse ≥110 beats·min^{-1}	Bradycardia or hypotension
Peak expiratory flow rate ≤50% of predicted or previous best	Peak expiratory flow rate ≤33% of predicted or previous best
	Exhaustion, confusion or coma
Arterial blood gas markers	
Normal (5–6 kPa) or high arterial carbon dioxide (P_aCO_2)	
Severe hypoxaemia (P_aO_2 <8 kPa)	
Low or high plasma pH	

- high-dose oral prednisolone or initial intravenous hydrocortisone followed by oral prednisolone.

If response to treatment is poor after 15–30 min, or if there are life-threatening features, additional treatment should be given:

- inhaled ipratropium via an oxygen-driven nebulizer.

If response is poor after a further 15–30 min, then consider:

- intravenous aminophylline,
- intravenous magnesium sulphate,
- assisted ventilation if there is not rapid clinical improvement.

After recovery from a severe asthma attack, prednisolone should be continued for at least 5 days or until there are no residual symptoms, especially at night, and the peak expiratory flow rate is at least 80% of the person's previous best. High doses of prednisolone can be stopped abruptly if used for 3 weeks or less, but should be reduced gradually if they have been used for a longer period (Ch. 44).

PROPHYLAXIS OF CHRONIC ASTHMA

An initial attempt should be made to identify and exclude precipitating factors; for example, allergens, occupational precipitants, NSAIDs (see below) and β-adrenoceptor antagonists (including eye drops) (Ch. 5). Long-term treatment is guided by a stepwise treatment plan.

Step 1. Mild intermittent asthma. Inhaled short-acting β_2-adrenoceptor agonist, such as salbutamol, taken as required. For those who are intolerant to this treatment, inhaled ipratropium and oral theophylline are alternative options but there is a higher risk of unwanted effects with the latter. Step 2 treatment should be considered if more than two doses of short-acting β_2-adrenoceptor agonist are required in a week, or if there has been an exacerbation of asthma in the previous 2 years.

Step 2. Regular inhaled preventer therapy. For adults, a regular standard-dose inhaled corticosteroid such as beclometasone is used in addition to step 1 therapy. In children under 5 years, a leukotriene receptor antagonist such as montelukast could be tried, but is generally less effective than inhaled corticosteroid.

Step 3. Inhaled corticosteroid plus long-acting inhaled β_2-adrenoceptor agonist. If symptoms in an adult are not controlled by standard doses of inhaled corticosteroid, a long-acting β_2-adrenoceptor agonist such as salmeterol is usually more effective than increasing the dose of corticosteroid. An inhaled short-acting β_2-adrenoceptor agonist can still be used as required. If there is no response to the long-acting β_2-adrenoceptor agonist, it should be stopped and the corticosteroid dose increased. The corticosteroid dose can also be increased if there was some response to a long-acting β_2-adrenoceptor agonist but the symptoms are still not controlled. For persistent poor control, sequential add-on therapy with a leukotriene receptor antagonist, a modified-release theophylline formulation or a modified-release oral β_2-adrenoceptor agonist should be tried.

For children under 5 years, a leukotriene receptor antagonist is added to regular inhaled corticosteroid with an inhaled short-acting β_2-adrenoceptor agonist as required.

Step 4. High-dose inhaled corticosteroid plus regular bronchodilators. High-dose inhaled corticosteroid with an inhaled long-acting β_2-adrenoceptor agonist plus a short-acting β_2-adrenoceptor agonist as required, and a sequential trial of one of the following:

- leukotriene receptor antagonist,
- oral modified-release theophylline formulation,
- oral modified-release β_2-adrenoceptor agonist.

Step 5. Regular oral corticosteroid. Oral prednisolone is taken in addition to high-dose inhaled corticosteroid with an inhaled long-acting β_2-adrenoceptor agonist plus a short-acting β_2-adrenoceptor agonist as required.

ASPIRIN-INTOLERANT ASTHMA

About 5–20% of people with asthma experience acute exacerbations when they take aspirin or other NSAIDs in a laboratory setting (Ch. 29). Individuals with the clinical syndrome of aspirin-intolerant asthma (or aspirin-exacerbated respiratory disease, AERD) have an eosinophilic rhinosinusitis and nasal polyposis in addition to asthma. The condition may be initiated by priming of the respiratory mucosa by an immune reaction to a viral infection or other insult which chronically upregulates the cysteinyl-leukotriene biosynthetic pathway or CysLT$_1$ receptor expression. Production of bronchoconstrictor leukotrienes nevertheless remains under partial inhibitory control of prostaglandin E$_2$ (PGE$_2$).

Aspirin is an irreversible cyclo-oxygenase type 1 (COX-1) and COX-2 inhibitor with greater effect on COX-1 inhibition. COX inhibition reduces PGE$_2$ synthesis, which removes its inhibition of leukotriene synthesis, provoking acute bronchospasm (see Fig. 29.1). Other NSAIDs that inhibit COX-1 also induce bronchoconstriction, but the selective COX-2 inhibitors do not provoke asthma. In sensitive individuals, asthma symptoms begin within 3 h of ingesting aspirin, accompanied by profuse rhinorrhoea, conjunctival injection and, sometimes, flushing or urticaria. Airways inflammation can persist for many weeks after an aspirin challenge.

Leukotriene receptor antagonists produce symptom relief in some people with aspirin-induced asthma. Treatment of acute aspirin-intolerant asthma is the same as for any other episode. Sometimes, long-term use of an oral corticosteroid is the only way to control persistent symptoms; in such cases, desensitisation to aspirin should be attempted. Nasal polypectomy may be necessary to control rhinosinusitis.

MANAGEMENT OF CHRONIC OBSTRUCTIVE PULMONARY DISEASE

There are two goals in the treatment of COPD: to minimise symptoms (including a reduction in acute exacerbations) and to preserve lung function.

- **Cessation of smoking.** Stopping smoking (see Ch. 54) is the only effective way to alter the natural history of COPD. Smoking cessation slows the rate of decline in lung function to that naturally seen with ageing, although any loss of lung function due to smoking cannot be restored. Occupational exposure to inhaled pollutants should also be minimised.
- **Pneumococcal and influenza vaccination.** These can reduce infective exacerbations in people with COPD.
- **Inhaled bronchodilators.** The principles are similar to those for asthma, although the limited reversibility of the airway obstruction means that the benefit is less marked, except during an acute exacerbation of symptoms. Some improvement in symptoms and functional capacity can occur without changes in standard lung function tests and the main benefit is improved lung emptying during expiration, with reduced hyperinflation at rest. Inhaled bronchodilators reduce the frequency of exacerbations of COPD. Short-acting β_2-adrenoceptor agonists and antimuscarinic agents are equally effective for mild symptoms. For continuing breathlessness either a long-acting β_2-adrenoceptor agonist (with a short-acting bronchodilator as required) or the long-acting antimuscarinic drug tiotropium (with a short-acting β_2-adrenoceptor agonist as required) may give better symptom relief and reduce the risk of exacerbations. Theophylline or roflumilast are usually reserved for advanced COPD when symptoms persist or there are frequent exacerbations despite use of inhaled long-acting bronchodilators and corticosteroid. Nebulised bronchodilators can be useful for severe exacerbations.
- **Corticosteroids.** Many of the chronic inflammatory changes in COPD do not respond to corticosteroids; nevertheless, an oral corticosteroid should be used for 7–14 days when treating an acute exacerbation of symptoms. Long-term use of an inhaled corticosteroid can reduce the number and severity of exacerbations, and should be considered if there are two or more exacerbations in a 12-month period. An inhaled corticosteroid can also produce some symptomatic benefit for people who remain breathless despite the use of a long-acting bronchodilator, or those with a forced expiratory volume of less than 50% of predicted. About 10% of people with COPD will have an improvement in their forced expiratory volume with an inhaled corticosteroid. However, there is an increased risk of pneumonia with inhaled corticosteroid, especially in the elderly with COPD.
- **Antibacterial drugs.** One-third of infective exacerbations are due to viral infection, but antibacterial drugs (Ch. 51) produce earlier symptomatic improvement if there is moderate-to-severe acute exacerbation of symptoms with purulent sputum.
- **Mucolytic agents.** Mecysteine hydrochloride, erdosteine or carbocisteine (Ch. 13) may reduce the frequency of exacerbations of COPD. An initial 1-month trial should be considered if COPD is accompanied by a chronic productive cough or if there are prolonged severe exacerbations. Treatment should only be continued if there is a perceived benefit.
- **Oxygen therapy.** This is extremely important to treat hypoxaemia during acute exacerbations. Care must be taken to raise the arterial oxygen saturation (if possible to ≥90%) without increasing the arterial carbon dioxide tension. To avoid suppressing hypoxic drive in type 2 respiratory failure (hypoxaemia with a raised arterial

carbon dioxide concentration), low-dose supplementary oxygen may be necessary (e.g. 24% via Venturi mask or 1–2 L·min^{-1} via nasal cannulae). Long-term domiciliary oxygen treatment, usually from an oxygen concentrator which removes nitrogen from air and delivers via nasal cannulae, improves symptoms and survival in COPD with respiratory failure (with an arterial oxygen tension less than 7.3 kPa). It should only be considered if respiratory failure persists for 3–4 weeks despite optimal drug therapy and without a clinical exacerbation. Those in the household must be warned of the fire risk if people smoke when receiving oxygen therapy. To improve survival in COPD with respiratory failure, oxygen must be used for at least 15 h per day.

- **Ventilatory support.** This may be required during exacerbations. Intubation and mechanical ventilation may be necessary, but non-invasive assisted ventilation is preferable. Nasal intermittent positive-pressure ventilation (NIPPV) is being increasingly used during exacerbations for people who fail to respond to maximal medical therapy, especially if there is carbon dioxide retention.
- **Pulmonary rehabilitation.** This improves exercise capacity and reduces the sensation of breathlessness, and can substantially improve morale.

SELF-ASSESSMENT

True/false questions

1. Asthma is defined as irreversible airflow obstruction resulting from chronic airway inflammation.
2. An influx of Th2 lymphocytes occurs in the late airway response to inhaled allergen challenge of people with asthma and atopy.
3. The β_2-adrenoceptor agonists are effective in preventing exercise-induced asthma.
4. The β_2-adrenoceptor agonists have no effect on mucus clearance.
5. Tolerance to β_2-adrenoceptor agonists can occur.
6. The mechanisms of action of theophylline are unclear.
7. The plasma concentration of theophylline is increased by simultaneous administration of erythromycin or ciprofloxacin.
8. Methylxanthines cause drowsiness.
9. An unwanted effect of theophylline is stimulation of the heart.
10. Ipratropium is more effective than salbutamol for preventing bronchospasm following challenge with an allergen.
11. Tiotropium is a selective antagonist of muscarinic M_2 receptors.
12. Ipratropium causes bradycardia.
13. Ipratropium is poorly absorbed from the bronchi into the systemic circulation.
14. Leukotriene C_4 is an important bronchodilator released from eosinophils.
15. Cysteinyl-leukotrienes are important in the precipitation of asthma in people who are intolerant to NSAIDs.
16. Montelukast inhibits 5-lipoxygenase that converts arachidonic acid to leukotrienes.

17. The leukotriene receptor antagonists (LTRA) are only given prophylactically.
18. Glucocorticoids reduce eosinophil recruitment to the bronchial mucosa.
19. Roflumilast is a selective inhibitor of phosphodiesterase (PDE) type 4.
20. Omalizumab binds to IgE receptors on mast cell membranes, preventing degranulation.

One-best-answer (OBA) questions

1. Which one of the following is the most likely unwanted effect of high-dose salbutamol?
   A. Bradycardia
   B. Hypokalaemia
   C. Hypoglycaemia
   D. Mydriasis
   E. Hypermagnesaemia
2. Which of the following is the most accurate statement about the mechanism of action of glucocorticoids in asthma therapy?

   A. They reduce airway inflammation by inhibiting eosinophil apoptosis
   B. They reduce airway narrowing by relaxing bronchial smooth muscle
   C. They reduce release of mast cell mediators by blocking allergen–IgE interaction
   D. They downregulate β_2-adrenoceptors on bronchial smooth muscle
   E. They reduce oedema by inducing endothelial tight junctions

Extended-matching-item questions

1. Match each statement below to the most appropriate option A–G.
   A. Theophylline
   B. Celecoxib
   C. Prostaglandin D_2
   D. Salbutamol
   E. Montelukast
   F. Indometacin
   G. Leukotriene B_4
      1.1. It increases the synthesis of cAMP
      1.2. It decreases the breakdown of cAMP
      1.3. It results in an increase in leukotriene synthesis in susceptible people with asthma
      1.4. It inhibits NSAID-induced bronchoconstriction
      1.5. It causes bronchoconstriction
2. Which option A–H is the most appropriate for add-on treatment to the current medication prescribed in each case scenario below?

   A. Ipratropium
   B. Ciprofloxacin
   C. Salmeterol
   D. A spacer
   E. Modified-release theophylline
   F. Intravenous magnesium sulphate
   G. Oral prednisolone
   H. Modified-release theophylline.

2.1. A 25-year-old woman was admitted to the accident and emergency department with an acute exacerbation of her asthma. Her peak expiratory flow was 150 L·min^{-1}. Her pulse rate was 145 beats·min^{-1}, her respiratory rate was 30 min^{-1}, respiration was shallow and she was confused. She was treated with 60% oxygen, nebulised salbutamol, nebulised ipratropium, intravenous aminophylline and intravenous hydrocortisone. Arterial blood gases on admission, breathing air, showed a PO_2 of 8.4 kPa, PCO_2 7.2 kPa and pH 7.29. There was little clinical improvement and she was transferred to the intensive care unit.

2.2. A 64-year-old man had mild asthma that was well controlled taking salbutamol two to three times a week and inhaled beclometasone twice daily. He complained of soreness of the mouth and hoarseness and was advised about oral hygiene.

2.3. A 67-year-old man had COPD with a chronic cough producing clear sputum. The cough and sputum production had not recently changed. He had stopped smoking 3 months previously because of his dyspnoea. Prior to that time, he had smoked 20 cigarettes a day for 50 years. He denied alcohol use. He had no other significant medical illnesses. His FEV_1 was 1.34 L (about 45% of that predicted). He was taking salbutamol four times daily. A trial of inhaled beclometasone 3 months previously had provided no benefit and had been stopped.

2.4. A 60-year-old woman attended the accident and emergency department with increasing shortness of breath, increased production of green–yellow sputum and fever over the previous 4 days. She was known to have COPD. She was taking daily salbutamol and ipratropium by breath-actuated inhalers.

2.5. A 30-year-old man had mild asthma and allergic rhinitis. He was taking inhaled salbutamol and beclometasone, both twice daily. Recently he had been waking most nights with a persistent cough. He was a non-smoker and had no other medical history.

True/false answers

1. **False.** Airflow obstruction in asthma is mostly reversible, either spontaneously or as a result of treatment.
2. **True.** Th2 lymphocytes generate cytokines that promote activation, recruitment and survival of eosinophils and other leucocytes and increase the expression of IgE receptors on mast cells and eosinophils.
3. **True.** Salbutamol is effective taken before exercise but the longer-acting β_2-adrenoceptor agonists are slower in onset. Cromoglicate taken prophylactically may also be effective.
4. **False.** Beta$_2$-adrenoceptor agonists increase ciliary action and mucus clearance.

5. **True.** Tolerance to β_2-adrenoceptor agonists may occur due to downregulation of their target receptor, an effect counteracted by administration of corticosteroids.
6. **True.** Methylxanthines may bronchodilate by inhibiting phosphodiesterases (PDEs) or blocking adenosine receptors on airway smooth muscle, while inhibition of histone deacetylase may account for reported anti-inflammatory effects at low doses.
7. **True.** Erythromycin and ciprofloxacin inhibit liver cytochrome P450 enzymes, resulting in slower metabolism of theophylline.
8. **False.** Methylxanthines present in coffee increase alertness and can cause irritability and headache.
9. **True.** All methylxanthines have positive inotropic and chronotropic activity and a narrow therapeutic index.
10. **False.** Ipratropium is less effective against allergen challenge but can be useful as an adjunct and in the management of COPD.
11. **False.** Tiotropium is a selective antagonist of M_3 receptors on airway smooth muscle, with less antagonism of inhibitory M_2 autoreceptors on parasympathetic nerves than ipratropium.
12. **False.** Ipratropium can cause a modest tachycardia owing to blockade of muscarinic receptors in the heart.
13. **True.** Ipratropium and tiotropium have quaternary structures and are therefore only poorly absorbed, minimising unwanted systemic effects.
14. **False.** Leukotriene C_4 (and its extracellular metabolite LTD_4) are potent bronchoconstrictors, and also increase mucus secretion, oedema and eosinophilia in the airway.
15. **True.** In susceptible individuals, NSAIDs that inhibit cyclo-oxygenase (COX)-1 may cause acute bronchospasm either by shunting arachidonic acid from the COX pathway to the leukotriene pathway or, more probably, by liberating the leukotriene pathway from partial inhibition by COX-derived prostaglandin E_2.
16. **False.** Montelukast and other lukast drugs are antagonists of the cysteinyl-leukotriene receptor type 1 ($CysLT_1$), not inhibitors of 5-lipoxygenase.
17. **True.** The LTRA are oral drugs taken once or twice daily for prophylaxis of asthma; they may also benefit comorbid conditions such as allergic rhinitis.
18. **True.** Glucocorticoids act at the transcriptional level to inhibit numerous steps in the inflammatory pathways involved in the pathogenesis of asthma, including the proliferation, recruitment, activation and survival of eosinophils.
19. **True.** Roflumilast is a highly selective inhibitor of PDE4, which is found in inflammatory cells.
20. **False.** Omalizumab binds to circulating and tissue IgE, leading to its clearance by endothelial cells. This results in a reduction in the numbers of IgE receptors on mast cells and other cells.

OBA answers

1. **Answer B** is correct. Salbutamol is a β_2-adrenoceptor agonist that can produce hypokalaemia by increasing cellular uptake of K$^+$. At higher doses it may cause tachycardia, hyperglycaemia and hypomagnesaemia, while mydriasis is not likely with a β-adrenoceptor agonist.

2. **Answer E** is correct. Glucocorticoids induce endothelial tight junctions, which reduces vascular permeability and leucocyte migration into tissue.

Extended-matching-item answers

1.1. Answer **D**. Salbutamol acts selectively on the β_2-adrenoceptors in airways, activating adenylyl cyclase and increasing cAMP.

1.2. Answer **A**. Theophylline inhibits the breakdown of cAMP by phosphodiesterases.

1.3. Answer **F**. Indometacin (and other NSAIDs that inhibit COX-1) can induce bronchoconstriction in aspirin-sensitive people with asthma. Celecoxib, a selective COX-2 inhibitor, is unlikely to cause this reaction, but should still be used with care.

1.4. Answer **E**. Montelukast is a selective antagonist of $CysLT_1$ receptors for the bronchoconstrictor cysteinyl-leukotrienes ($LTC_4/D_4/E_4$), synthesis of which is triggered by non-selective NSAIDs.

1.5. Answer **C**. Prostaglandin D_2 is a bronchoconstrictor released by mast cells.

2.1. Answer **F**. This woman is being treated according to the British Thoracic Society guidelines; an appropriate add-on medication for use in this life-threatening situation is intravenous magnesium sulphate.

2.2. Answer **D**. This man should additionally be advised to use a spacer with all inhaled drugs. This improves the effectiveness of the medication and will reduce deposition of corticosteroid in the mouth and oropharynx, reducing the occurrence of fungal growth and hoarseness.

2.3. Answer **A**. The antimuscarinic drug ipratropium provides equal or greater benefit to β_2-adrenoceptor agonists in COPD and will reduce the volume of sputum produced. Corticosteroids are of modest benefit in only a small percentage of people with COPD.

2.4. Answer **B**. This woman has an infection-related exacerbation of her COPD and should be treated with an appropriate antibiotic. Nebulised salbutamol and ipratropium should also be started.

2.5. Answer **C**. Approximately 80% of severe asthmatic attacks occur between midnight and 8 am. Salbutamol is a short-acting β_2-adrenoceptor agonist, providing relief for 2–6 h. A trial of salmeterol or formoterol, which provide bronchodilation for 12 h or longer, should be considered. The long-acting drugs should not be used for relief of acute asthma episodes.

FURTHER READING

Barnes PJ (2011) Glucocorticoids: current and future direction. *Br J Pharmacol* 163, 29–43

Cazzola M, Calzetta L, Matera MG (2011) β_2-Adrenoceptor agonists: current and future direction. *Br J Pharmacol* 163, 4–17

Dolovich MB, Dhand R (2011) Aerosol drug delivery: developments in device design and clinical use. *Lancet* 377, 1032–1045

Moulton BC, Fryer AD (2011) Muscarinic receptor antagonists, from folklore to pharmacology; finding drugs that actually work in asthma and COPD. *Br J Pharmacol* 163, 44–52

Asthma

Adcock IM, Caramori G, Chung KF (2008) New targets for drug development in asthma. *Lancet* 372, 1073–1087

Bush A, Saglani S (2010) Management of severe asthma in children. *Lancet* 376, 814–825

Fanta CH (2009) Drug therapy: Asthma. *N Engl J Med* 360, 1002–1014

Farooque SP, Lee TH (2009) Aspirin-sensitive respiratory disease. *Annu Rev Physiol* 71, 465–487

Holgate ST, Polosa R (2006) The mechanisms, diagnosis and management of severe asthma in adults. *Lancet* 368, 780–793

Johnson M (2006) Molecular mechanisms of β_2 adrenergic receptor function, response and regulation. *J Allergy Clin Immunol* 117, 18–24

Lazarus SC (2010) Emergency treatment of asthma. *N Engl J Med* 363, 755–764

O'Byrne PM, Parameswaran K (2006) Pharmacological management of mild or moderate persistent asthma. *Lancet* 368, 794–803

Ormiston TM, Salpeter EE (2004) Respiratory tolerance to regular β_2-agonist use in patients with asthma. *Ann Intern Med* 140, 802–814

Rees J (2006) Asthma control in adults. *BMJ* 332, 767–771

Rowe BH, Bretzlaff JA, Bourdon C, Bota GW, Camargo CA Jr (2000) Intravenous magnesium sulfate treatment for acute asthma in the emergency department: a systematic review of the literature. *Ann Emerg Med* 3, 6181–6190

Salpeter SR, Buckley NS, Ormiston TM, Salpeter EE (2006) Meta-analysis: effect of long-acting β-agonists on severe exacerbations and asthma-related deaths. *Ann Intern Med* 144, 904–912

Stevenson DD (2009). Aspirin sensitivity and desensitization for asthma and sinusitis. *Curr Allergy Asthma Rep* 9 155–163

Chronic obstructive pulmonary disease

Anzueto A (2006) Clinical course of chronic obstructive pulmonary disease: review of therapeutic interventions. *Am J Med* 119, S46–S53

Barnes PJ (2002) Theophylline. New perspectives for an old drug. *Am J Respir Crit Care Med* 167, 813–818

Barnes PJ, Ito K, Adcock IM (2004) Corticosteroid resistance in chronic obstructive pulmonary disease: inactivation of histone deacetylase. *Lancet* 363, 731–733

Brusselle GG, Joos GF, Bracke KR (2012) New insights into the immunology of chronic obstructive pulmonary disease. *Lancet*, 378, 1015–1026

Criner GJ (2007) Optimal treatment of chronic obstructive pulmonary disease: the search for the magic combination of inhaled bronchodilators and corticosteroids. *Ann Intern Med* 146, 606–608

Decramer M, Janssens W, Miravitelles M (2012) Chronic obstructive pulmonary disease. *Lancet* 379, 1341–1351

Hansel T, Barnes P (2009) New drugs for exacerbations of chronic obstructive pulmonary disease. *Lancet* 374, 744–755

Lipworth BJ (2005) Phosphodiesterase-4 inhibitors for asthma and chronic obstructive pulmonary disease. *Lancet*, 365, 167–175

Martinez FJ, Donohue JF, Rennard S (2011) The future of chronic obstructive pulmonary disease treatment – difficulties of and barriers to drug development. *Lancet* 378, 1027–1037

Niewoehner DE (2010) Outpatient management of severe COPD. *N Engl J Med* 362, 1407–1416

Plant PK, Elliot MW (2003) Chronic obstructive pulmonary disease 9: management of ventilatory failure in COPD. *Thorax* 58, 537–542

Rabe KF, Wedzicha JA (2011) Controversies in treatment of chronic obstructive pulmonary disease. *Lancet* 378, 1038–1047

Wilt J, Niewoehner D, MacDonald R et al. (2007) Management of stable chronic obstructive pulmonary disease: a systematic review for a clinical practice guideline. *Ann Intern Med* 147, 639–653

Wilt J, Weinberger S, Shekelle P et al. (2007) Diagnosis and management of stable chronic obstructive pulmonary disease: a clinical practice guideline from the American College of Physicians. *Ann Intern Med* 147, 633–638

Compendium: drugs used to treat asthma or chronic obstructive pulmonary disease

Drug	Kinetics and half-life[a] (h)	Comment
β-Adrenoceptor agonist bronchodilator drugs		
Bambuterol	Prodrug hydrolysed slowly by plasma cholinesterase to terbutaline (8–22 h)	Given orally; not recommended for children or in pregnancy
Ephedrine	High oral bioavailability; eliminated largely by renal excretion; metabolised to norephedrine, which has central stimulant effects (6 h)	Given orally; direct- and indirect-acting non-selective sympathomimetic; not recommended
Fenoterol	Eliminated by hepatic conjugation (6–7 h)	Given by inhalation in combination with ipratropium
Formoterol	Eliminated largely by hepatic conjugation (2–3 h)	Given by dry-powder inhalation; long duration of action exceeds the elimination half-life
Indacaterol	Mainly hepatic metabolism, very long half-life (40–52 h)	Ultra-long acting bronchodilator for COPD; given by dry powder inhalation
Salbutamol	Eliminated by hepatic conjugation (4–6 h)	Given by inhalation, orally, intravenously or subcutaneously; short-acting
Salmeterol	Extensively metabolised; metabolite retains some activity (3–5 h)	Given by inhalation; long-acting due to lipophilicity
Terbutaline	Eliminated by glomerular filtration and by hepatic conjugation (14–18 h)	Given by inhalation, orally, intravenously or subcutaneously; short-acting
Antimuscarinics		
Ipratropium	Little drug enters the circulation after inhalation and most is swallowed and not absorbed from the gut; the absorbed fraction is rapidly eliminated (4 h)	Short-acting; non-selective antimuscarinic; given by inhalation for short-term relief in asthma and for COPD
Tiotropium	The small amounts of drug that enter the circulation after inhalation are eliminated in the urine (5–6 days)	Long-acting, selective M_3 receptor antagonist; given by inhalation for COPD; not recommended for children
Methylxanthines		
Aminophylline	Mixture of theophylline and ethylenediamine improves solubility; very rapidly hydrolysed to its constituents (minutes)	Given orally, or by injection for acute severe asthma
Theophylline	Variable liver metabolism (1–13 h), induced by smoking and alcohol; half-life shorter in children.	Given orally, usually as a modifed release preparation, for asthma prophylaxis; narrow therapeutic index
Corticosteroids		
Given by inhalation for chronic asthma and COPD. See Ch. 44 for corticosteroids (such as prednisolone and hydrocortisone) given orally or by intravenous injection in the treatment of acute asthma; high-dose preparations are not recommended for children.		
Beclometasone dipropionate	Hydrolysed by esterases to the 17-monopropionate, which is ≈30 times more potent, or to an inactive metabolite (15 h)	Inhaled using aerosol or powder formulation; standard- and high-dose preparations available; also given in combination with formoterol
Budesonide	Low oral bioavailability (10%) reduces systemic absorption; metabolites are inactive (2 h)	Inhaled using aerosol or powder formulation; also given in combination with formoterol

Compendium: drugs used to treat asthma or chronic obstructive pulmonary disease—cont'd

Drug	Kinetics and half-life[a] (h)	Comment
Ciclesonide	Prodrug converted in lung to active product, then hepatic metabolism (7 h)	Inhaled using powder formulation
Fluticasone propionate	Hepatic metabolism to inactive metabolite, excreted in bile (3 h); any swallowed dose undergoes 100% first-pass inactivation	Inhaled using aerosol or powder formulation; commonly given in combination with salmeterol
Mometasone furoate	Hepatic metabolism; metabolites eliminated in bile (5 h)	Inhaled using powder formulation; not recommended for children
Cromones		
Nedocromil sodium	High polarity gives slow absorption from lung; negligible absorption from gut (oral half-life 23 h)	Given by inhalation for asthma prophylaxis
Sodium cromoglicate	High polarity gives slow absorption from lung; negligible absorption from gut	Given by inhalation for asthma prophylaxis
Leukotriene receptor antagonists		
Montelukast	Good oral bioavailability (about 70%); hepatic metabolism (3–5 h)	Antagonist of LTD_4 receptor ($CysLT_1$) in the human airway; given orally at bedtime for asthma prophylaxis
Zafirlukast	Believed to undergo extensive first-pass metabolism; hepatic metabolism (10 h)	Antagonist of LTD_4 receptor ($CysLT_1$) in the human airway; given orally twice daily for asthma prophylaxis; not recommended for children under 12 years
Anti-IgE antibodies		
Omalizumab	Eliminated by very slow turnover/recycling of immunoglobulins (22–28 days)	Recombinant monoclonal antibody binds to human IgE and prevents activation of IgE receptors on mast cells and other cells; given by subcutaneous injection every 2–4 weeks in severe, uncontrolled allergic asthma
Phosphodiesterase type 4 inhibitors		
Roflumilast	Good oral absorption; variable hepatic metabolism (17 h)	PDE4 inhibitor used in bronchitic exacerbations of severe COPD; given orally
Other drugs		
Magnesium sulphate	Renal excretion (4 h)	Smooth muscle relaxant; given intravenously in life-threatening acute asthma in adults

COPD, chronic obstructive pulmonary disease.
[a]The half-life refers to the systemic elimination half-life from the general circulation, which may not correlate with the duration of action following inhalation when this is dependent on very slow uptake from the airways.

13

Respiratory disorders: cough, respiratory stimulants, cystic fibrosis and neonatal respiratory distress syndrome

COUGH

Cough is a protective mechanism that removes excessive mucus, abnormal substances such as fluid or pus, or inhaled foreign material from the upper airways. A cough is initiated by a rapid inspiration followed by brief closure of the glottis. Forced expiration against the closed glottis raises intrathoracic pressure, and sudden opening of the glottis expels air together with secretions and debris. Flow rates can approach the speed of sound, producing vibration of upper airway structures and the typical sound of cough. Cough is under both voluntary and involuntary control.

The cough reflex is initiated by irritant receptors located at the epithelial surface of the airway mucosa, which can be activated by either chemical or mechanical stimuli. These receptors have been identified at and below the oropharynx in the large airways, and are probably present in the external auditory canals and tympanic membrane in the ear, as well as in other sites such as the oesophagus and stomach. Rapidly adapting receptors that respond mainly to mechanical stimuli may be of primary importance in eliciting the cough reflex. Neuropeptides produced by the mechanosensitive neurons following viral infection or allergen challenge probably sensitise the cough reflex.

Afferent fibres from the receptors in the airways travel in the vagus and superior laryngeal nerves to the medullary 'cough network' in the region of the nucleus tractus solitarius. Neuronal pathways connect this network to the respiratory pattern generator, from where efferent fibres travel in somatic nerves to respiratory muscles. Projections from the cerebral cortex to the medulla can also initiate cough or modulate the cough reflex.

Several mediators are involved in the cough reflex pathways in the medulla. One proposed model is that the afferent input to the cough centre is via glutamatergic neurons that stimulate N-methyl-D-aspartate (NMDA) receptors. These neurons can be inhibited by presynaptic serotonergic

nerve synapses via serotonin type 1 (5-hydroxytryptamine$_1$, 5-HT$_1$) receptors. Opioids facilitate the inhibitory action of the serotonergic neurons through further interneuronal connections. The complexity of these pathways is illustrated by the number of mediators and antagonists that can experimentally initiate or inhibit cough. Selective opioids such as κ- and δ-opioid receptor agonists, tachykinin receptor antagonists, bradykinin receptor antagonists and transient receptor potential vanilloid 1 (TRPV$_1$) receptor antagonists all have potential as future antitussives.

Cough has several diverse causes (Box 13.1). A cough is considered useful if it aids clearing excess secretions or inhaled foreign matter from the airway. By contrast, an unproductive cough has no useful function. An effective cough that can clear the airway depends on the ability to generate high airflow. An ineffective cough may result from respiratory muscle weakness, or when the mucus on the airway wall is thick and adhesive.

There are three clinical categories of cough: acute cough, lasting less than 3 weeks, subacute cough lasting 3–8 weeks and chronic cough. Acute cough is most often caused by acute viral upper respiratory tract infection (the common cold), and most subacute cough also results from an initial viral infection. Chronic productive cough is usually related to smoking or bronchiectasis. The most common causes of a chronic non-productive cough in non-smokers are upper airway cough syndrome (also called post-nasal drip syndrome), asthma and gastro-oesophageal reflux disease. There is also an entity called unexplained cough, predominantly affecting middle-aged women and associated with cough reflex hypersensitivity, for which investigations fail to identify a cause.

DRUGS FOR TREATMENT OF COUGH

Antitussives (cough suppressants)

Cough suppressants fall into three classes.

Centrally acting drugs (opioids)

Opioids increase the threshold for stimulation of neurons in the medullary cough centre, and probably modulate a gating mechanism in the brain analogous to that identified for pain reception. They are most effective for cough arising from the lower airways. Weak opioid analgesics (Ch. 19) are most commonly used, especially codeine and pholcodine. These are less addictive than morphine, which should be reserved for terminal conditions. Dextromethorphan is structurally related to opioids, but is a glutamate NMDA receptor antagonist with antitussive properties and no analgesic or sedative action.

Box 13.1 Common causes of cough

Acute respiratory infection

  Upper respiratory tract infection
  Pneumonia, including aspiration

Chronic respiratory infection

  Cystic fibrosis
  Bronchiectasis
  Post-nasal drip (upper airway cough syndrome)

Airway disease

  Asthma
  Chronic obstructive pulmonary disease

Parenchymal lung disease

  Interstitial fibrosis

Irritant

  Cigarette smoke
  Inhaled foreign body

Bronchopulmonary malignancy
Drug-induced

  Angiotensin-converting enzyme inhibitors
  Inhaled drugs

Peripherally acting drugs

Local anaesthetics such as lidocaine (Ch. 18) are used as an oropharyngeal spray to reduce cough during bronchoscopy. Antihistamines (Ch. 39) reduce post-nasal drip from allergic rhinitis, which can stimulate cough, but probably have little direct antitussive activity. Nevertheless, sedative antihistamines, such as diphenhydramine, are commonly used in compound cough preparations on sale direct to the public.

Locally acting drugs

Demulcents line the surface of the airway above the larynx, reducing local irritation. The syrup in simple linctus acts by this mechanism.

Expectorants and mucolytics

Expectorants such as guaifenesin and squill are often included in compound cough preparations, with the intention of improving clearance of mucus from the airways. There is no evidence that they have any clinical value.

Mucolytics such as mecysteine hydrochloride, erdosteine and carbocisteine can be given orally to reduce the viscosity of bronchial secretions by breaking disulphide crosslinking between molecules. Mucolytics can be useful in chronic obstructive pulmonary disease (Ch. 12) and bronchiectasis.

MANAGEMENT OF COUGH

An acute cough should be treated only if it is unproductive or excessive. A self-limiting non-productive acute cough,

such as that caused by a viral illness, can be suppressed by simple linctus or a weak opioid. Any cough of unknown origin that is still present after 14 days should be investigated further to identify an underlying cause.

For chronic cough, non-specific therapy has a limited role, since it should be possible to identify and treat the cause. Specific treatment for left ventricular failure, asthma, upper airway cough syndrome (with an antihistamine and a decongestant) or gastro-oesophageal reflux disease (Ch. 33) often eliminates the cough associated with those conditions.

Cough is a common unwanted effect of angiotensin-converting enzyme (ACE) inhibitors (Ch. 6) and occurs in up to 15% of people who take them. It sometimes appears hours after starting treatment, but can first arise after several months of treatment. The cough may improve with a reduction in ACE inhibitor dosage, but changing to another class of drug, such as an angiotensin II receptor antagonist, is usually necessary to eliminate the cough.

When symptomatic therapy is required for chronic cough, there are few options. Chronic non-productive cough in terminal lung cancer can be treated with a powerful opioid such as morphine. The value of mucolytics in chronic bronchitis is uncertain, but they may be useful in chronic obstructive pulmonary disease (Ch. 12). Mucolytics may make clearance of mucus easier, but are probably no more effective than hydration from inhaling steam or nebulised hypertonic saline. Mucolytics do not improve lung function in cystic fibrosis.

RESPIRATORY STIMULANTS (ANALEPTIC DRUGS)

Doxapram has a limited place in the short-term treatment of ventilatory failure, such as in hypercapnoeic respiratory failure due to chronic obstructive pulmonary disease which is causing drowsiness. It increases respiratory drive and arousal, and improves both rate and depth of ventilation. When combined with physiotherapy, doxapram may encourage coughing and clearance of excessive secretions. However, its use has largely been superseded by non-invasive ventilatory support, such as with nasal intermittent positive pressure ventilation. There is also a minor role for doxapram to reverse postoperative respiratory depression. Doxapram stimulates the medullary respiratory centre both by a direct action and by peripheral stimulation of the carotid body. Given by intravenous injection, its action is very brief, owing to rapid metabolism by the liver, and a continuous infusion is often used. Restlessness, muscle twitching and vomiting are common unwanted effects, and seizures can occur due to generalised stimulation of the central nervous system.

Acetazolamide (Ch. 14) is an inhibitor of carbonic anhydrase that stimulates the respiratory centre by creating a mild metabolic acidosis. This action may contribute to its ability to reduce the headache, nausea, vomiting and lethargy of acute altitude sickness by decreasing periodic nocturnal apnoea and maintaining arterial oxygen saturation. Use of acetazolamide is not a substitute for gradual acclimatisation to altitude.

CYSTIC FIBROSIS

Cystic fibrosis is an autosomal recessive disorder caused by a single gene mutation on the long arm of chromosome 7. This gene encodes the cystic fibrosis transmembrane conductance regulator (CFTR), a Cl^- and HCO_3^- channel in the apical membranes of many epithelial cells. The transport of negative ions is accompanied by paracellular diffusion of Na^+ and water, creating a fluid secretion from the cell. If the *CFTR* gene is faulty, then the function of the transporter is impaired or absent and Cl^- transport is defective in epithelial cells in many organs, including the respiratory, hepatobiliary, gastrointestinal and reproductive tracts and the pancreas. As a result of the defective electrolyte flows, secretions become thicker. This causes obstruction in (and destruction of) exocrine glandular ducts, and in the lungs clogs respiratory cilia with mucus. Over 1700 *CFTR* gene mutations have already been identified (although about 15 of these account for more than 75% of clinical cases), but even a single type of mutation produces different severities of disease, suggesting that there is involvement of other genes or environmental factors.

In cystic fibrosis there is a defective periciliary liquid layer of the airway suface mucus. The more viscous mucus renders the cilia ineffective and the resulting stasis creates the environment for infection. The lung becomes colonised with bacteria that are impossible to eradicate and a chronic inflammatory response is established in the airway. The consequences of infection and inflammation are bronchiectasis and chronic airflow obstruction.

The most common and disabling clinical consequences of cystic fibrosis are lung disease and pancreatic exocrine insufficiency leading to malabsorption. These problems affect about 90% of those with the gene defect. About 20% develop pancreatic endocrine insufficiency with type 1 diabetes mellitus and a smaller number develop meconium ileus in infancy or obstructive biliary tract disease. Death in 90% of people with cystic fibrosis is due to progressive lung disease, but median life expectancy is now about 37 years due to improved treatment.

DRUG TREATMENT OF CYSTIC FIBROSIS

Much of the treatment for cystic fibrosis is supportive, including physiotherapy and regular inhaled antibacterial drugs to reduce exacerbations of lung disease, and intensive antibacterial therapy to treat exacerbations of lung disease. Nebulised hypertonic saline improves mucociliary clearance, and reduces the frequency of infective exacerbations. It can sometimes produce bronchospasm, which can be prevented by prior use of an inhaled β_2-adrenoceptor agonist such as salbutamol (Ch. 12). Nutritional supplements are important because of the frequency of fat malabsorption.

Prevention of infection (and cross-infection), particularly during hospital admission, is important, and improved treatment of infection is the main reason for the prolongation of life expectancy in recent years. *Staphylococcus aureus* and *Haemophilus influenzae* are common pathogens in the very young person with cystic fibrosis, while *Burkholderia cepacia* and *Burkholderia dolosa* are particularly virulent pathogens. In the early years of life, anti-staphylococcal therapy is usually appropriate for exacerbations of lung disease (Ch. 51). By adolescence, *Pseudomonas aeruginosa* becomes the predominant pathogen, and is treated with intravenous or nebulised antibacterials. Inhalation of nebulised tobramycin or nebulised colistimethate sodium, perhaps combined with oral ciprofloxacin, is increasingly used to treat exacerbations during and after adolescence (Ch. 51). It is almost impossible to eradicate *P. aeruginosa* from sputum, but rapid and intensive treatment of clinical infection slows the decline in lung function.

Since inflammation is a major component of the airway disease, several anti-inflammatory therapies have been studied. Oral corticosteroids (Ch. 44) reduce the rate of decline in lung function and reduce the frequency of infections, but unwanted effects preclude their long-term use. Inhaled corticosteroid does not improve lung function unless there is associated airway hyperreactivity.

There are several pharmacological interventions under investigation for improving the conductance of the defective Cl^- channel in cystic fibrosis. The first of these, ivacaftor, is now available for treatment of the 5% of people with cystic fibrosis with a specific type of *CFTR* gene defect.

In addition to antibacterial treatment of respiratory infection, current therapies for respiratory and gastrointestinal symptoms of cystic fibrosis include the following.

Dornase alfa

Dornase alfa (recombinant human deoxyribonuclease I, or rhDNase I) is an enzyme that digests extracellular DNA. DNA released from dying neutrophils in the airways contributes to the increased sputum viscosity in cystic fibrosis. Dornase alfa is given by inhalation using a jet nebuliser (see Ch. 12) and is probably most effective when given on alternate days. It reduces sputum viscoelasticity, improves lung function in the short- to medium-term (although long-term benefits are much less certain) and results in fewer exacerbations of lung disease. Improved lung function should be measurable after 2 weeks in responders. Unwanted effects are rare, and include transient pharyngitis and hoarseness.

Pancreatic enzyme supplements (pancreatin)

Pancreatin consists of protease, lipase and amylase, enzymes which are inactivated by gastric acid and by heat. Supplements, therefore, must be taken with food (but not mixed with very hot food), and either with gastric acid suppression therapy (e.g. given 1 h after cimetidine; Ch. 33) or as enteric-coated formulations to protect them from gastric acid. Pancreatin preparations in clinical use are all of porcine origin. Dosage is adjusted according to the size, number and consistency of stools. Unwanted effects include irritation of the mouth and perianal skin, nausea, vomiting and abdominal discomfort. Some higher-strength formulations should be avoided in children under 15 years of age with cystic fibrosis, since they have been associated with the formation of large bowel strictures. Pancreatin is also used for pancreatic exocrine insufficiency following pancreatectomy, gastrectomy or chronic pancreatitis.

NEONATAL RESPIRATORY DISTRESS SYNDROME

Pulmonary surfactant is responsible for reducing surface tension at the air–liquid interface in the alveoli, preventing lung collapse at resting lung pressures. Surfactant is a macromolecular complex largely composed of phospholipids, mainly phosphatidylcholine (of which dipalmitoylphosphatidylcholine is the major surface-active component), neutral lipids and surfactant-specific proteins A–D. The phospholipid monolayer stabilises the lungs and prevents end-expiratory alveolar collapse by reducing the deflating force in the alveolus. Surfactant proteins B and C are hydrophobic and critical for adsorption and spreading of the surfactant layer at the air–liquid interface. The hydrophilic surfactant proteins A and D are involved in surfactant metabolism and host defence.

Surfactant is synthesised by epithelial cells lining the alveoli and is normally present in substantial amounts at full term delivery. However, preterm infants may produce too little surfactant, leading to neonatal respiratory distress syndrome.

Mortality is high in neonatal respiratory distress syndrome, but it can be reduced by administration of surfactant via an endotracheal tube into the lung. There are two natural therapeutic surfactants: beractant (bovine lung extract) and poractant alfa (porcine lung phospholipid fraction), which do not retain the surfactant proteins A and D. New synthetic compounds with peptides that mimic the natural surfactant proteins are under clinical development. The potential advantages of a synthetic compound include easier production and elimination of the infection risk associated with animal products.

The use of a surfactant in neonatal respiratory distress syndrome reduces the risk of death by 40%, whether the treatment is given prophylactically or as a rescue treatment. There is also a reduced risk of pneumothorax and of subsequent chronic lung disease. Surfactant is given as soon as possible after delivery to infants with neonatal respiratory distress syndrome, or to those considered to be at risk of developing it.

In women at risk of preterm delivery, a corticosteroid such as dexamethasone (Ch. 44) can increase the production of surfactant in the fetal lung, which may prevent neonatal respiratory distress syndrome.

SELF-ASSESSMENT

True/false questions

1. Postviral cough can last for 3–6 weeks.
2. Angiotensin II receptor antagonists frequently cause cough.
3. Many compound cough preparations sold over the counter contain sedating antihistamines.
4. Dextromethorphan is a synthetic opioid with cough suppressant, sedative and analgesic activity.
5. There is little evidence that any preparation can specifically facilitate expectoration.
6. Pulmonary surfactant increases surface tension in the alveoli.
7. Therapeutic surfactant is identical to natural human surfactant.
8. Doxapram should not be used in postoperative respiratory failure.
9. The mucolytic mecysteine acts by inhibiting the production of mucus.
10. Dornase alfa breaks down extracellular DNA in sputum.

True/false answers

1. **True.** Treatment of postviral cough should include increased humidity of inspired air and cough suppressants; other drugs are of little value.
2. **False.** Angiotensin II receptor antagonists do not cause cough. However, inhibitors of angiotensin-converting enzyme (ACE), which reduce the formation of angiotensin II, also prevent the breakdown of bradykinin and this causes cough in 15% of people.
3. **True.** Diphenhydramine and chlorpheniramine are common constituents of over-the-counter cough mixtures.
4. **False.** Dextromethorphan has the same cough suppressant potency as codeine but does not share its sedative or analgesic effects; dextromethorphan may act by blocking *N*-methyl-D-aspartate (NMDA) receptors.
5. **True.** Expectorants may nevertheless serve a useful placebo function.
6. **False.** Surfactant has a detergent-like action to lower surface tension, enabling the alveoli to expand and retain an expanded shape.
7. **False.** Therapeutic surfactants such as beractant and poractant alfa are animal products lacking the two hydrophilic surfactant proteins SP-A and SP-D.
8. **False.** Doxapram is sometimes used in hospitals for postoperative respiratory failure. It stimulates the respiratory centre and the carotid chemoreceptors, but its precise mode of action is unknown.
9. **False.** Mecysteine breaks the disulphide cross-bridges that maintain the polymeric gel-like structure of mucus.
10. **True.** Dornase alpha is a recombinant deoxribonuclease that digests DNA released by dying neutrophils in sputum; it is given by nebuliser to reduce viscosity of lung secretions in cystic fibrosis.

FURTHER READING

Cough

Bolser DC (2006) Current and future centrally acting antitussives. *Resp Physiol Neurobiol* 152, 349–355

Chang AB (2006) The physiology of cough. *Paediatr Resp Rev* 7, 2–8

Dicpinigaitis PV (2006) Current and future peripherally-acting antitussives. *Respir Physiol Neurobiol* 152, 356–362

Dicpinigaitis PV (2011) Cough: an unmet clinical need. *Br J Pharmacol* 163, 116–124

Irwin RS, Madison JM (2000) Primary care: the diagnosis and treatment of cough. *N Engl J Med* 343, 1715–1721

Cystic fibrosis

Boyle MP (2007) Adult cystic fibrosis. *JAMA* 298, 1787–1793

Cuthbert AW (2011) New horizons in the treatment of cystic fibrosis. *Br J Pharmacol* 163, 141–172

Davies JC, Alton EWFW, Bush A (2007) Cystic fibrosis. *BMJ* 335, 1255–1259

Elborn JS (2006) Practical management of cystic fibrosis. *Chron Resp Dis* 3, 161–165

Neonatal respiratory distress syndrome

Curstedt T, Johansson J (2005) New synthetic surfactants – basic science. *Biol Neonate* 87, 332–337

Pfister RH, Soll RF (2005) New synthetic surfactants: the next generation? *Biol Neonate* 87, 338–344

Whitsett JA, Weaver TE (2002) Mechanisms of disease: hydrophobic surfactant proteins in lung function and disease. *N Engl J Med* 347, 2142–2148

Compendium: drugs used to treat respiratory disorders

Drug	Kinetics (half-life)	Comment
Cough suppressants		
All cough suppressants given below are opioid derivatives (see Ch. 19 and its Compendium for details); usually given orally as a linctus. Sedating antihistamines (Ch. 39) are also sometimes given for their cough suppressant actions.		
Codeine	Metabolism (3–4 h)	Use is associated with constipation
Dextromethorphan	Extensive first-pass metabolism to dextrorphan, a non-opioid cough suppressant, and by glucuronidation (3 h)	Fewer unwanted effects than codeine; not used as an analgesic
Methadone	Metabolism and renal excretion (6–8 h)	Used mainly in palliative care for the distressing cough of terminal lung cancer (but less than other opioids)
Morphine	Metabolism and renal excretion (1–5 h)	Used in palliative care for the distressing cough of terminal lung cancer
Pholcodine	Slowly eliminated (32–43 h) due to high apparent volume of distribution (50 L·kg^{-1}); clearance by hepatic metabolism	Fewer unwanted effects than codeine
Mucolytics		
Given orally.		
Carbocisteine	Good oral absorption; eliminated unchanged and as metabolites in urine	Used in COPD and bronchiectasis
Dornase alfa	Few data available; not detectable in blood after inhalation administration; activity in sputum is measurable for at least 6 h	Recombinant human deoxyribonuclease preparation used for cystic fibrosis; given by nebuliser
Erdosteine	Undergoes first-pass metabolism to an active metabolite(s) containing a thiol group	Used in COPD and bronchiectasis
Mecysteine	Few kinetic data available	Used in COPD and bronchiectasis
Pulmonary surfactants		
Used for respiratory distress in preterm infants.		
Beractant	No human kinetic data available; the apparent half-life of the natural surfactant (phosphatidylglycerol) is about 30 h	Given by endotracheal tube; activity occurs at the alveolar surface without systemic absorption; respiratory distress syndrome may enhance permeability and uptake
Poractant alfa	See beractant	See beractant
Respiratory stimulants		
Given only under expert supervision.		
Doxapram	Hepatic metabolism (2–4 h)	Given by intravenous injection (over 30 s) or by continuous intravenous infusion

COPD, chronic obstructive pulmonary disease.

4

The renal system

14 Diuretics

Almost all diuretics act on the kidney to increase the tubular concentration and elimination of Na^+ ions (natriuresis), with a concurrent excretion of water. Loss of water with the Na^+ ions depletes intravascular volume. Diuretics are used in the management of a wide range of conditions that produce oedema (e.g. heart failure, cirrhosis of the liver and nephrotic syndrome) and for the treatment of hypertension.

FUNCTIONS OF THE KIDNEY

The kidney has several important functions:

- regulation of plasma electrolyte concentrations and fluid balance,
- regulation of acid–base balance,
- elimination of waste products,
- conservation of essential nutrients.

Of these, a basic knowledge of the mechanisms of electrolyte and fluid handling by the kidney is essential for understanding the uses and unwanted effects of diuretics.

THE KIDNEY AND MAINTENANCE OF SALT AND WATER BALANCE

Each day the renal glomeruli of a healthy adult filter about 180 L of fluid (about 20% of the plasma that enters the glomerular capillaries), together with its content of ions such as Na^+, K^+ and Cl^-. Since the urine output is only 1–2 L per day, it is clear that most of the filtered fluid is absorbed back from the tubule into the blood. Different regions of the tubule and collecting duct vary in their capacity to reabsorb water and solutes (Figs 14.1 and 14.2).

The proximal convoluted tubule

In the proximal convoluted tubule, about 65–70% of the filtered Na^+ is reabsorbed together with an equivalent (isosmotic) amount of water. Therefore, on leaving the proximal tubule, the tubular fluid still has the same osmolarity as plasma. Reabsorption of ions from the proximal tubule into the renal tubular cells is passive (Fig. 14.1, site 1). The activity of the Na^+/K^+-ATPase pump on the basolateral surface of the tubular cell (transporting three Na^+ out of the tubular cell in exchange for two K^+) helps to establish the electrochemical gradient for passive Na^+ reabsorption from the tubular lumen into the tubule cell. Water reabsorption by the proximal renal tubule is driven by the osmotic gradient across the tubular cells, which is created by the active transport of Na^+ out of the cell across the basolateral membrane. Water reabsorption occurs via transmembrane aquaporin (AQP) channels. The extent of the proximal tubular reabsorption of Na^+ and water is determined by two regulatory mechanisms: glomerulotubular feedback (enhanced tubular Na^+ reabsorption when the glomerular filtration rate rises), and various neural and hormonal influences such as the sympathetic nervous system, angiotensin II, endothelin, dopamine and parathyroid hormone.

The proximal tubule has transporters for the secretion of organic anions into the tubular lumen (Fig. 14.1, site 1; see also Ch. 2), and the reabsorption of water-soluble essential nutrients, such as glucose and amino acids, from the lumen. The organic anion transporters (OATs) are important for the transport of many drugs and their metabolites from the blood into the tubule (e.g. see acetazolamide and loop diuretics below). The inward Na^+ gradient provides the drive for several carriers, such as that for glucose. Bicarbonate is also reabsorbed from the proximal tubule by a mechanism dependent on the enzymatic activity of carbonic anhydrase (Fig. 14.1, site 2).

The loop of Henle

The descending limb of the loop of Henle is permeable to water, due to the presence of aquaporin channels, but not to Na^+. Water passes from the tubule into the interstitium of the renal medulla, where the fluid is hypertonic as a result of ion transport in the thick ascending limb of the loop of Henle (see below). Therefore, tubular fluid reaching the ascending limb of the loop of Henle is hypertonic.

The thick ascending limb of the loop of Henle is impermeable to water but has an active $Na^+/K^+/2Cl^-$ co-transporter complex (NKCC2) in the luminal (apical) membrane (Fig. 14.1, site 3). Na^+ is actively transported from the tubular cells to the interstitium by the Na^+/K^+-ATPase pump in the basolateral membrane. This creates a low intracellular Na^+

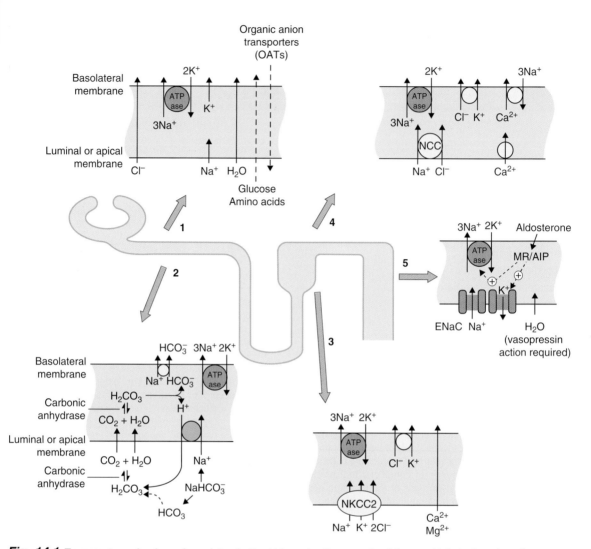

Fig. 14.1 Transport mechanisms for solutes in the kidney. In all segments of the renal tubule there is active transport of Na^+ out of and K^+ into the cell across the basolateral membrane using Na^+/K^+-ATPase proton pumps. This sets up electrochemical gradients for the transport of other ions. In the proximal tubule (sites 1 and 2), considerable amounts of Na^+, glucose and amino acids are taken up from the lumen, along with water which crosses via aquaporin channels. The principal function of the organic anion transporters (OATs) (site 1), including OAT1 and OAT3 (Ch. 2) is the elimination of metabolites of ingested xenobiotics. Transport by OATs also enables diuretic drugs such as furosemide and bendroflumethiazide to gain access to their sites of action on apical membranes in the tubule. Hydrogen ions are excreted in exchange for Na^+ uptake and this, in part, depends upon the activity of carbonic anhydrase (site 2). In the ascending limb of the loop of Henle (site 3), the luminal membrane has a $Na^+/K^+/2Cl^-$ co-transporter (NKCC2) but is impermeable to water. In the proximal part of the distal tubule (cortical diluting segment; site 4) Na^+ and Cl^- ions are reabsorbed by the Na^+/Cl^- co-transporter (NCC), but water is not reabsorbed. Ca^{2+} also exchanges with three Na^+ at the basolateral border at this site. In the distal part of the distal tubule and collecting duct (site 5) Na^+ is reabsorbed from the lumen via an epithelial Na^+ channel (ENaC), in exchange for loss of K^+ into the lumen. The expression and activity of ENaC and the basolateral Na^+/K^+-ATPase pump are regulated by aldosterone acting via mineralocorticoid receptors (MRs) and aldosterone-induced proteins (AIPs). Water is reabsorbed in the collecting duct under the influence of antidiuretic hormone (ADH, vasopressin) acting through vasopressin receptors in the basolateral membrane.

concentration in the tubular cells and generates the Na^+ ion gradient that drives the luminal NKCC2 co-transporter. The ascending limb of the loop of Henle can reabsorb up to 25% of the Na^+ filtered at the glomerulus. K^+ that is carried from the tubule into the cells of the loop by the NKCC2 co-transporter is recycled back into the tubular lumen, which ensures that there is always enough tubular K^+ to continue to favour Na^+ reabsorption. K^+ recycling creates a lumen-positive transepithelial voltage gradient, which drives a paracellular ionic current that is responsible for half the

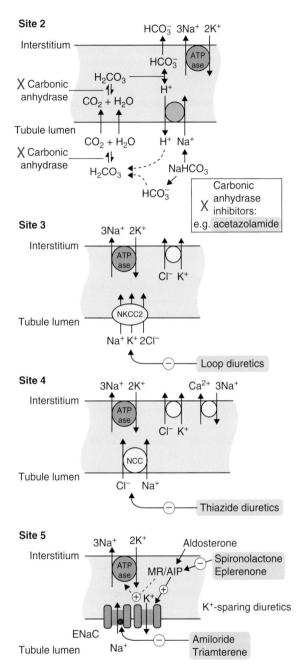

Site 2

Site 3

Site 4

Site 5

◄ ─────────────────────────

Fig. 14.2 **Sites of action of diuretics.** For location of these sites in the tubule, see Fig. 14.1. Osmotic diuretics increase osmotic pressure through the tubule, reducing electrolyte reabsorption across the luminal membrane. Other drugs gain access to their sites of action after secretion into the tubule by the organic anion transporters (OATs) in the proximal tubule. Acetazolamide inhibits carbonic anhydrase (site 2) and is a weak self-limiting diuretic, now largely used for other conditions such as glaucoma. Loop diuretics such as furosemide block the luminal $Na^+/K^+/2Cl^-$ co-transporter (NKCC2) and inhibit up to 25% of filtered Na^+ reabsorption (site 3). The thiazide diuretics inhibit the luminal Na^+/Cl^- co-transporter (NCC) (site 4) and can reduce reabsorption of 5–8% of filtered Na^+. The potassium-sparing diuretics spironolactone and eplerenone compete with aldosterone for the mineralocorticoid receptor (MR), blocking the induction by aldosterone of the expression and activity of the epithelial Na^+ channel (ENaC), the basolateral Na^+/K^+-ATPase pump and other aldosterone-induced proteins (AIP) (site 5). Amiloride and triamterene act directly on ENaC to block Na^+ reabsorption. Potassium-sparing diuretics inhibit the reuptake of less than 3% of filtered Na^+.

The proximal (cortical) diluting segment of the distal convoluted tubule

The filtrate leaving the loop of Henle is hypotonic and passes to the proximal part of the distal convoluted tubule (also known as the cortical diluting segment of the distal tubule). This part of the renal tubule is impermeable to water but has a luminal Na^+/Cl^- co-transporter (NCC) (Fig. 14.1, site 4). The driving force for this thiazide-sensitive co-transporter is again generated by the Na^+/K^+-ATPase pump in the basolateral membrane. About 5–8% of the filtered Na^+ load can be reabsorbed at this site. The rich blood supply to this region allows rapid diffusion of the reabsorbed ions into the plasma and prevents the interstitium from becoming hypertonic. Reabsorption of Ca^{2+} is also regulated at this site, under the influence of parathyroid hormone and calcitriol (Ch. 42). The rate of Ca^{2+} transport is inversely related to that of Na^+ transport; this is because Na^+ inside the tubular cell either inhibits luminal voltage-gated Ca^{2+} channels or reduces the activity of the basolateral Na^+/Ca^{2+} exchanger.

In the cortical diluting segment of the distal tubule the increased luminal concentration of Na^+ or Cl^- initiates two responses that limit Na^+ loss. The first is tubuloglomerular feedback, a mechanism (possibly mediated by adenosine) that constricts the afferent glomerular arteriole to that nephron. The second is secretion of renin, which, through activation of the renin–angiotensin system, eventually enhances the release of aldosterone from the adrenal cortex and increases Na^+ reabsorption at the distal part of the distal convoluted tubule (see Chs 6 and 44, and below).

total Na^+ reabsorbed by this region of the kidney, along with Ca^{2+} and Mg^{2+}.

The reabsorption of Na^+, but not water, by the thick ascending limb of the loop of Henle establishes the hypertonicity of the medullary interstitium (the corticomedullary concentration gradient). This interstitial hypertonicity is responsible for an osmotic gradient across the collecting ducts, which permits the formation of hypertonic urine (see below). There are various hormonal regulators of Na^+ reabsorption in the ascending limb of the loop of Henle, including calcitonin, parathyroid hormone and prostaglandin E_2.

The distal part of the distal convoluted tubule and the collecting duct

The tubular fluid that has become yet more hypotonic in the cortical diluting segment of the distal tubule is delivered to the distal part of the distal tubule and then to the collecting duct. There are two main cell types in this region, the principal cells and the intercalated cells.

In the principal cell, Na^+ is reabsorbed through a highly specific amiloride-sensitive epithelial Na^+ channel, known as ENaC, and this is accompanied by obligatory K^+ loss into the urine (Fig. 14.1, site 5). Aldosterone acts at this site at cytosolic mineralocorticoid receptors (MRs), inducing transcription of genes encoding components of ENaC and the basolateral Na^+/K^+-ATPase pump. Other aldosterone-induced proteins (AIPs) include serum- and glucocorticoid-regulated kinases (SGK) and channel-inducing factor, which further increase the activity of ENaC and the Na^+/K^+-ATPase. Together, these changes increase the reabsorption of Na^+ from the tubule and the concomitant loss of K^+ into the lumen.

Less important hormonal regulators of Na^+ reabsorption in the distal tubule and the collecting duct include calcitonin and bradykinin. The natriuretic peptides, atrial natriuretic peptide (ANP) and brain natriuretic peptide (BNP), also decreases Na^+ reabsorption by receptor-mediated phosphorylation of ENaC. Overall, only about 3–5% of filtered Na^+ is reabsorbed at the distal part of the distal tubule. However, the distal renal tubule is the primary site in the kidney responsible for maintenance of K^+ homeostasis. Relatively small changes in extracellular K^+ concentration can affect cardiac muscle, skeletal muscle and brain function, so the extracellular K^+ concentration is closely regulated.

The principal cell is also the site of action of antidiuretic hormone (ADH, vasopressin; Ch. 43). This hormone is secreted by the posterior pituitary gland and binds to receptors in the basolateral membrane, where it increases the permeability of the cell to water by upregulating aquaporin (AQP2) channels. In the presence of ADH, water reabsorption into the hypertonic medullary interstitium is increased, which concentrates the urine as it passes through the collecting duct.

Intercalated cells are the second important cell type in the distal part of the distal tubule and the collecting duct (not illustrated in Figs 14.1 and 14.2). Two subtypes of intercalated cells express H^+-ATPases that help to regulate acid–base balance by secreting or reabsorbing H^+ and HCO_3^-.

DIURETIC DRUGS

CARBONIC ANHYDRASE INHIBITORS

Example

acetazolamide

Mechanism of action

Acetazolamide interferes with the small proportion of Na^+ that is actively reabsorbed in the proximal tubule in exchange for H^+ (Fig. 14.2, site 2). This process is dependent on carbonic anhydrase, which is inhibited by acetazolamide. Acetazolamide increases HCO_3^-, Na^+ and K^+ secretion, causing alkaline urine. H^+ retention produces mild acidosis in the blood, but the fall in plasma HCO_3^- concentration stimulates carbonic anhydrase activity, which rapidly leads to tolerance to the diuretic action of acetazolamide. In consequence, acetazolamide does not have a clinically useful diuretic action. Its clinical use is restricted to treatment of altitude sickness (Ch. 13) and glaucoma (Ch. 50).

Pharmacokinetics

Acetazolamide is secreted into the proximal renal tubule by organic acid transporters (OATs) and works at the luminal surface of the proximal tubule. It is eliminated unchanged in the urine.

Unwanted effects

- Nausea, vomiting, anorexia, taste disturbance.
- Paraesthesia, dizziness, fatigue, irritability, ataxia, depression.
- Hypokalaemia (see loop diuretics).

OSMOTIC DIURETICS

Example

mannitol

Mechanism of action

Mannitol is filtered at the glomerulus but not reabsorbed from the renal tubule. It exerts osmotic activity within the proximal renal tubule and particularly in the descending limb of the loop of Henle, and limits passive tubular reabsorption of water. Water loss produced by mannitol is accompanied by a variable natriuresis (up to 25% of filtered Na^+). Unlike other diuretics, the osmotic action of mannitol produces an initial expansion of plasma and extracellular fluid volume, which limits its clinical uses.

Mannitol does not readily cross the blood–brain barrier. It is used to treat some forms of acute brain injury, when the main mechanism of action may be through haemodilution and reduced blood viscosity which may limit ischaemic damage, rather than a dehydrating action on cerebral tissues.

Pharmacokinetics

Mannitol is given by intravenous infusion and is excreted unchanged at the glomerulus. It has a half-life of 2 h, which is substantially increased in renal impairment.

Unwanted effects

- Expansion of plasma volume can precipitate heart failure.

- Urinary K^+ loss can lead to hypokalaemia (see loop diuretics).

LOOP DIURETICS

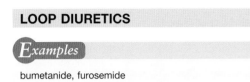

bumetanide, furosemide

Mechanism of action and effects

Loop diuretics, such as furosemide, must be secreted into the proximal kidney tubule by the tubular organic anion transporters to access their site of action. The extent of the natriuresis and diuresis is dependent on the rate of delivery of the drug to the renal tubule via this secretory mechanism. Once these transporters have been saturated, increasing the dose of the diuretic will not enhance its effect. Loop diuretics bind to the $Na^+/K^+/2Cl^-$ co-transporter complex (NKCC2) at the luminal border of the thick ascending limb of the loop of Henle, and inhibit Cl^- reabsorption. This diminishes the electrochemical gradient across the cell and reduces Na^+ reabsorption from the tubular fluid (Fig. 14.2, site 3). Loop diuretics therefore reduce the ability of the kidney to generate the medullary ionic concentration gradient and impairs generation of concentrated urine in the collecting duct. Loop diuretics also inhibit tubuloglomerular feedback and the afferent artery vasoconstriction in response to the increased tubular concentrations of Na^+ and Cl^-. They are powerful, 'high-ceiling' diuretics which can inhibit reabsorption of up to 25% of the Na^+ that appears in the glomerular filtrate.

The dose–response curves of loop diuretics are steep, but the doses required to achieve maximal inhibition of Na^+ reabsorption show wide inter-individual variation. Because they have a short duration of action, there is partial compensation for the natriuresis by subsequent rebound Na^+ uptake from the tubular fluid after their action has finished. Loop diuretics remain effective even in advanced renal failure, but larger doses are necessary to deliver an effective concentration of drug to the remaining renal tubules as the reduced tubular secretion results in greater metabolism of the drug in the liver.

When injected intravenously, furosemide releases vasodilator prostaglandins, such as prostacyclin, into the circulation and produces a short-lived venodilation. Pooling of blood in these capacitance vessels reduces central blood volume, which can be useful in the treatment of acute left ventricular failure (Ch. 7). Loop diuretics also produce arterial vasodilation (see thiazide diuretics), but because of their short duration of action they are not widely used to treat hypertension, except in renal failure when their diuretic action can be useful.

Pharmacokinetics

Furosemide is incompletely and erratically absorbed from the gut, with considerable inter-individual variation. Bumetanide is more completely and reliably absorbed. Furosemide and bumetanide can also be given intravenously.

Natriuresis and diuresis begin about 30 min after an oral dose and last up to 6 h; intravenous injection produces a more rapid effect, with an onset of diuresis within minutes. Loop diuretics are partially metabolised in the liver. They are highly protein bound in plasma and little drug is filtered at the glomerulus. Renal failure impairs the delivery of drug to the tubular fluid, since the ability of the kidney to secrete organic anions is reduced and other substrates compete with the diuretic for the organic anionic transporters.

Unwanted effects

- Excessive salt and water depletion can cause intravascular volume depletion, hypotension and renal impairment.
- Dilutional hyponatraemia can arise from excessive Na^+ loss that exceeds water loss. Hyponatraemia is far less common than with thiazide diuretics. Stimulation of ADH secretion in response to plasma volume contraction also contributes to hyponatraemia by promoting reabsorption of water from the collecting duct. Hyponatraemia can present with lethargy, impaired consciousness and eventually coma and seizures.
- Hypokalaemia is dose-related, but less severe than with diuretics such as thiazides which have a longer duration of action (see below). It arises from increased urinary K^+ loss from the distal part of the distal renal tubule. There are several contributory mechanisms:
  - loop diuretics increase the delivery of Na^+ to the distal convoluted tubule, so there is enhanced Na^+ reabsorption at this site. This creates a negative luminal gradient that promotes K^+ diffusion into the tubular lumen,
  - the dilute urine increases the K^+ gradient across the tubular membrane, which also favours K^+ diffusion into the tubular lumen,
  - diuretic-induced hypovolaemia stimulates release of renin and aldosterone. Aldosterone further enhances Na^+ reabsorption in the distal tubule at the expense of increased K^+ excretion.

    Obligatory urinary loss of Cl^- with the K^+ creates a mild metabolic alkalosis in the plasma. To counteract the alkalosis, H^+ is shifted out of cells in exchange for intracellular accumulation of K^+, which exacerbates the hypokalaemia.

The consequences and treatment of hypokalaemia are discussed below.

- Hypomagnesaemia can accompany hypokalaemia and makes the correction of hypokalaemia more difficult. About 70% of filtered Mg^{2+} is reabsorbed by paracellular diffusion in the loop of Henle, and this is impaired by loop diuretics, which inhibit the electrical gradient necessary for Mg^{2+} reabsorption. Hypomagnesaemia predisposes to cardiac arrhythmias.
- Increased urinary Ca^{2+} excretion from inhibition of paracellular reabsorption of Ca^{2+} at the loop of Henle. It does not produce hypocalcaemia, but this action can be helpful in the management of hypercalcaemia (Ch. 42).
- Hyperuricaemia arises from reduced glomerular filtration of uric acid following reduction of plasma volume. There may be an additional reduction of proximal tubular urate secretion as a result of competition between uric acid and the diuretic for organic anion transporters. Clinical

gout is unusual (Ch. 31) and less common with loop diuretics than with thiazide diuretics.

- Incontinence can result from the rapid increase in urine volume. In older males with prostatic hypertrophy retention of urine can occur.
- Ototoxicity with deafness can result from cochlear damage, especially when renal failure reduces the rate of drug excretion or when very large doses of a loop diuretic are used. Tinnitus and vertigo may result from vestibular damage; both are more common with furosemide and are usually reversible.

THIAZIDE AND RELATED DIURETICS

bendroflumethiazide, chlortalidone, hydrochlorothiazide, indapamide

Mechanisms of action and effects

The thiazides are structurally related to sulphonamides. They act at the luminal surface of the cortical (proximal) diluting segment of the distal convoluted tubule and inhibit the Na^+/Cl^- co-transporter (NCC) (Fig. 14.2, site 4). This prevents Na^+ and Cl^- from entering the tubular cell. Several structurally different 'thiazide-like' drugs, such as chlortalidone and indapamide, share this site of action. Thiazides and related diuretics have a lower efficacy than loop diuretics, achieving a maximum natriuresis of about 5–8% of the filtered Na^+ load, and have shallow dose–response curves. The onset of diuresis is slow, but they have a longer duration of action than loop diuretics, which varies among the drugs; for example, bendroflumethiazide produces a natriuresis for up to 6–12 h and chlortalidone for 48–72 h. Thiazide and related diuretics are less effective in renal failure (especially when the glomerular filtration rate is below 20 mL·min⁻¹). Thiazide and related diuretics, unlike the loop diuretics, reduce urinary Ca^{2+} loss by inhibiting Ca^{2+} transport in the proximal and distal tubules.

Thiazide and related diuretics produce arterial vasodilation during long-term use, which appears to be the basis of their hypotensive effect (Ch. 6), but the mechanism of vasodilation is incompletely understood. It may involve direct inhibition of agonist-induced contraction of vascular smooth muscle cells by Ca^{2+} desensitization linked to the Rho kinase pathway, a regulator of actin–myosin cross-bridging (Ch. 1). The vasodilator action of these drugs occurs at lower dosages than are required for significant diuresis.

Pharmacokinetics

The thiazide and related diuretics are fairly well absorbed from the gut and most are metabolised in the liver. They are highly protein-bound and therefore little is filtered at the glomerulus. Like the loop diuretics, thiazides act from within the renal tubular lumen after secretion by organic anion transporters in the proximal tubule. Thiazides generally have more prolonged durations of action than loop diuretics.

Unwanted effects

- Hypokalaemia. Clinically this is more important with thiazides than with loop diuretics. The greatest reduction in plasma K^+ usually occurs within 2 weeks of starting treatment.
- Hyponatraemia. Prolonged block by thiazides of Na^+/Cl^- co-transport in the distal convoluted tubule (where water cannot be reabsorbed) impairs free water clearance. The combination of a thiazide with amiloride (see below) is particularly associated with dilutional hyponatraemia (see loop diuretics).
- Hyperuricaemia (see loop diuretics). Gout occurs infrequently and is less common in women.
- Decreased urinary Ca^{2+} excretion. This is in contrast to loop diuretics and the mechanism is not well understood. This action of thiazides is useful for the treatment of renal stones due to hypercalciuria. Hypercalcaemia does not usually occur unless there is another underlying disturbance of Ca^{2+} metabolism, such as hyperparathyroidism.
- Glucose intolerance. This is dose-related, with a progressive increase in plasma glucose over many months. The major cause is prolonged hypokalaemia and the consequent reduced intracellular K^+ concentration. This inhibits insulin release and impairs tissue uptake of glucose in response to insulin. The glucose intolerance usually reverses over several months if the thiazide is stopped (see Ch. 40).
- Hyperlipidaemia. There is a dose-related increase in low-density lipoprotein cholesterol and triglycerides. The long-term effects (>1 year) are small, but there is a theoretical increased atherogenic risk if high doses of thiazides are used (Ch. 48).
- Impotence. This is reported by up to 10% of middle-aged hypertensive men treated with high doses of thiazides (Ch. 16).
- Nocturia and urinary frequency can result from prolonged diuresis.

POTASSIUM-SPARING DIURETICS

amiloride, eplerenone, spironolactone, triamterene

Mechanism of action and effects

Drugs in this class produce a diuresis while preventing urinary K^+ loss. All potassium-sparing diuretics act at the late distal convoluted tubule and cortical collecting duct. Spironolactone, its active metabolite canrenone, and eplerenone are the only diuretics that do not act at the luminal membrane of the tubular cells. They compete with aldosterone for the cytoplasmic MR in the distal convoluted tubular cells and block transcriptional upregulation of the ENaC, the basolateral Na^+/K^+-ATPase pump and AIPs. They therefore antagonise the effects of aldosterone on Na^+ reabsorption and K^+ excretion (Fig. 14.2, site 5). Spironolactone and eplerenone only work in the presence of aldosterone so their effect is enhanced in hyperaldosteronism.

Amiloride and triamterene have a different mechanism of action: they directly block the epithelial Na^+ channel (ENaC) at the luminal surface of the renal tubule (Fig. 14.2). Their action is independent of the presence of aldosterone.

The maximum natriuresis achieved by potassium-sparing diuretics is small (usually less than 2–3% of filtered Na^+) unless there is marked secondary hyperaldosteronism, when spironolactone and eplerenone are much more effective. With potassium-sparing diuretics the Na^+ and water loss is accompanied by preservation of plasma K^+, because the reduced Na^+ reabsorption limits ATP-dependent Na^+ exchange with K^+ at the basolateral membrane (Fig. 14.2, site 5). When used together with thiazide or loop diuretics, potassium-sparing diuretics reduce or eliminate the excess urinary K^+ loss.

Pharmacokinetics

All potassium-sparing diuretics are given orally. Spironolactone is metabolised in the wall of the gut and the liver to canrenone, which has a much longer half-life and is probably responsible for most of the diuretic effect. The onset of action of spironolactone or eplerenone is slow, starting after 1 day and becoming maximal by 3–4 days, largely a consequence of their transcriptional mechanism of action.

Triamterene is extensively metabolised in the liver, and tubular secretion of the sulphate ester metabolite is responsible for the diuretic action. Amiloride is secreted unchanged into the proximal renal tubule. The onset of action of both drugs is rapid.

Unwanted effects

- Hyperkalaemia. This is more common in the presence of pre-existing renal disease, in the elderly and during combination treatment with angiotensin-converting enzyme (ACE) inhibitors or angiotensin II receptor antagonists (Ch. 6). Retention of Mg^{2+} also occurs, in contrast to the loss of Mg^{2+} with the thiazides and loop diuretics.
- Hyponatraemia. This is more common with thiazide/amiloride combinations.
- Spironolactone has an anti-androgenic effect, a consequence of its ability to bind to androgen receptors and prevent their interaction with dihydrotestosterone. This causes gynaecomastia and impotence in males, and menstrual irregularities in women. The anti-androgenic effect is sometimes used in women to treat hirsutism (such as in polycystic ovary syndrome; Ch. 43), male-pattern hair loss and acne. Eplerenone has greater aldosterone receptor selectivity and does not have anti-androgenic actions.
- Gastrointestinal disturbances.

MANAGEMENT OF DIURETIC-INDUCED HYPOKALAEMIA

A modest reduction in plasma K^+ concentration is common during treatment with loop or thiazide diuretics. Marked hypokalaemia (below 3.0 $mmol \cdot L^{-1}$) predisposes to cardiac rhythm disturbances (including ventricular arrhythmias), particularly in the presence of acute myocardial ischaemia, during treatment with digitalis glycosides (Ch. 7), or with antiarrhythmic agents that prolong the Q–T interval on the electrocardiogram (Ch. 8). It may also precipitate encephalopathy in people with liver failure. The risk of hypokalaemia is greatest with:

- thiazide rather than loop diuretics, because of their longer duration of action,
- low oral intake of K^+,
- high doses of diuretic,
- hyperaldosteronism, for example in hepatic cirrhosis or nephrotic syndrome.

Both treatment and prevention of diuretic-induced hypokalaemia can be achieved with the addition of a potassium-sparing diuretic. It is unnecessary to routinely prescribe a potassium-sparing diuretic with a thiazide or loop diuretic. A pragmatic approach would be to reserve the use of combination treatment for those at high risk from hypokalaemia, or those who develop significant hypokalaemia during regular diuretic treatment.

Alternatively, oral K^+ supplements can be given to correct hypokalaemia, but these are less effective unless used in large quantities (greater than 30 mmol daily), which often cause gastric irritation. Modified-release tablets and effervescent formulations of K^+ are available to improve tolerability. Oral K^+ supplements should not be used together with potassium-sparing diuretics.

Intravenous K^+ treatment is rarely needed unless there is severe K^+ depletion. Rapid intravenous injection of K^+ can produce potentially lethal hyperkalaemia (provoking asystole), and a maximum infusion rate of 10 $mmol \cdot h^{-1}$ is recommended, with hourly monitoring of the plasma K^+ concentration if such a high infusion rate is necessary.

MAJOR USES OF DIURETICS

Diuretics can be used to treat a number of conditions.

Oedema in heart failure, nephrotic syndrome and hepatic cirrhosis

Mild oedema can sometimes be controlled by a thiazide diuretic, but more marked oedema usually requires the use of a loop diuretic (see Ch. 7 for oedema in heart failure). Modest doses of a loop diuretic provide a near-maximal response if renal function is normal, but large doses are sometimes necessary if there is renal failure (see above). Long-term use of a loop diuretic can occasionally produce tolerance, due to hypertrophy of epithelial cells of the cortical diluting segment of the distal convoluted tubule, which results in increased Na^+ reabsorption at this site. There are various strategies that can be tried if fluid retention is resistant to oral furosemide, as follows.

- Salt restriction and avoidance of salt-retaining drugs, such as non-steroidal anti-inflammatory drugs (Ch. 29). Water restriction may be necessary if there is dilutional hyponatraemia, since raising the serum Na^+ concentration improves diuretic responsiveness.

- Divided oral doses of a loop diuretic can be used to give more prolonged drug delivery to the kidney. This also reduces post-diuretic rebound Na$^+$ retention.
- Oral bumetanide can be used rather than furosemide, because of its more consistent oral absorption.
- A loop diuretic can be given by intravenous infusion (often over 24 h) to prolong the duration of action and give a more sustained natriuresis and diuresis. Slow intravenous infusion of higher drug doses will also help to avoid ototoxicity.
- The addition of a thiazide or related diuretic to a loop diuretic. Sequential inhibition of tubular Na$^+$ reabsorption can produce a dramatic diuresis and natriuresis. However, hyponatraemia, hypokalaemia, hypovolaemia and renal impairment are all more frequent with such combinations.
- If there is marked secondary hyperaldosteronism, for example in ascites associated with cirrhosis of the liver or caused by treatment with high doses of a loop diuretic, spironolactone or eplerenone can be particularly useful.

Hypertension

Low doses of a thiazide or related diuretic are usually used for hypertension. A loop diuretic or spironolactone can be useful for resistant hypertension or when there is renal impairment. See also Chapter 6.

Hypercalciuria with renal stone formation

Thiazides can be used to reduce urinary Ca^{2+} excretion.

Glaucoma

Acetazolamide can be used to reduce intraocular pressure (Ch. 50). Tolerance does not occur to this effect, unlike the diuretic action.

Altitude sickness

An unlicensed use for acetazolamide is the prevention and treatment of altitude sickness (Ch. 13). It should be taken for several days before ascending to altitude, and continued until descent. The mechanism is unclear but the drug may combat respiratory alkalosis produced by hyperventilation at high altitudes.

Hypoventilation in chronic obstructive pulmonary disease

Acetazolamide creates a mild metabolic acidosis. This can stimulate respiration in the short term, and reduce carbon dioxide retention (Ch. 12).

Acute brain injury

Mannitol is occasionally used to reduce ischaemic cerebral damage, for example after neurosurgery or in acute traumatic brain injury. Fluid loss via the kidney should be replaced with intravenous crystalloid to avoid dehydration.

SELF-ASSESSMENT

True/false questions

1. A fall in plasma K$^+$ concentration can affect cardiac muscle function.
2. The main renal site of K$^+$ loss in the urine is from the proximal convoluted tubule.
3. The Na$^+$/K$^+$-ATPase pump is only found on the basolateral membrane of the loop of Henle.
4. The thick ascending limb of the loop of Henle is impermeable to water.
5. Osmotic diuretics are poorly reabsorbed from the renal tubule.
6. Osmotic diuretics should not be given in heart failure.
7. The carbonic anhydrase inhibitor acetazolamide is used in the treatment of glaucoma.
8. All thiazide diuretics are shorter-acting than loop diuretics.
9. Thiazide diuretics act by inhibiting Na$^+$/Cl$^-$ co-transport in the basolateral membrane.
10. Thiazide diuretics increase urinary Ca^{2+} excretion.
11. Thiazide diuretics may exacerbate diabetes mellitus.
12. Spironolactone and amiloride act by the same mechanism to reduce K$^+$ loss.
13. Potassium-sparing diuretics and angiotensin-converting enzyme (ACE) inhibitors can cause a harmful interaction.
14. Thiazide or loop diuretics should not be given together with potassium-sparing diuretics.
15. Non-steroidal anti-inflammatory drugs (NSAIDs) reduce the response to diuretics.

One-best-answer (OBA) questions

1. Which of the following *best* describes the mechanism of action of triamterene?
   A. Antagonism of a cytosolic receptor
   B. Blockade of a Na$^+$/K$^+$/2Cl$^-$ co-transporter
   C. Blockade of a selective Na$^+$ channel
   D. Blockade of a Na$^+$/Cl$^-$ symporter
   E. Reduction in HCO$_3^-$ reabsorption
2. Which of the following is the *most accurate* statement about loop diuretics?

   A. Loop diuretics are useful in the treatment of acute pulmonary oedema.
   B. Loop diuretics and thiazide diuretics should not be taken together.
   C. Loop diuretics do not produce hypokalaemia.
   D. Loop diuretics increase the hypertonicity of the interstitium in the medullary region.
   E. Loop diuretics reduce the risk of ototoxicity with aminoglycoside antibacterial drugs.

Extended-matching-item question

Choose the *most likely* option (A–F) related to the case scenarios 1 to 3 below.

A. Raised serum K^+ concentration
B. Lowered serum K^+ concentration
C. Increased natriuresis
D. Reduced natriuresis
E. Raised plasma glucose
F. Lowered plasma glucose

Case 1. A 58-year-old woman was taken to the accident and emergency department with dyspnoea and bradycardia (40 beats·min^{-1}). She had previously had a myocardial infarction and coronary angioplasty. She was taking the diuretics bendroflumethiazide and amiloride, and had recently had her dose of the ACE inhibitor lisinopril increased.

Case 2. A 40-year-old man with type 1 diabetes mellitus and hypertension was being treated with insulin. He had started on the thiazide-related diuretic chlortalidone 2 months previously for his hypertension and was seeking medical advice about his increased tiredness and lethargy.

Case 3. A 55-year-old man with congestive heart failure was treated with digoxin and lisinopril. Furosemide was added because of oedema and he subsequently complained of palpitations. He was admitted to hospital and the electrocardiogram showed atrial tachycardia.

True/false answers

1. **True.** Hypokalaemia can also affect brain and skeletal muscle function.
2. **False.** Much of the filtered K^+ is reabsorbed in the proximal tubule and loop of Henle, and its loss into the urine occurs mainly in the collecting ducts.
3. **False.** The basolateral Na^+/K^+-ATPase pump is present throughout the renal tubule.
4. **True.** Impermeability to water and the NKCC2 transporter that co-transports Na^+, K^+ and Cl^- ions from the lumen into the tubular cell in the thick ascending limb together generate the hyperosmotic interstitium important in concentrating urine in the collecting duct.
5. **True.** Osmotic diuretics are retained within the tubule where their osmotic activity reduces passive reabsorption of water in the proximal tubule and descending limb of the loop of Henle.
6. **True.** By extracting water from intracellular compartments and expanding extracellular and intravascular fluid volumes, osmotic diuretics can precipitate pulmonary oedema.
7. **True.** Acetazolamide reduces the formation of aqueous humour.
8. **False.** Some thiazide diuretics such as chlortalidone can produce a diuresis for 48–72 h, while most loop diuretics are relatively short-lived.
9. **False.** Thiazide diuretics act from within the renal tubular lumen on the thiazide-sensitive Na^+/Cl^- co-transporter (NCC) on the luminal (apical) membrane.
10. **False.** The thiazide diuretics do not increase urinary Ca^{2+} excretion, unlike the loop diuretics.

11. **True.** Thiazide diuretics may exacerbate diabetes mellitus, probably through hypokalaemia reducing insulin release from pancreatic β-cells.
12. **False.** Amiloride blocks the epithelial Na^+ channel (ENaC) directly, whereas spironolactone competes with aldosterone at mineralocorticoid receptors, thus reducing the transcriptional expression of ENaC. The reduced Na^+ reabsorption produced by both drugs in the collecting duct reduces the loss of K^+ into the urine.
13. **True.** ACE inhibitors, by reducing angiotensin-induced aldosterone secretion, will reduce K^+ excretion and hence increase plasma K^+ concentration, particularly when combined with potassium-sparing diuretics.
14. **False.** Thiazides and loop diuretics increase Na^+ concentrations in the tubular fluid reaching the collecting duct; the excessive loss of K^+ that results can be reduced by combining the thiazide or loop diuretic with a potassium-sparing diuretic.
15. **True.** NSAIDs inhibit prostaglandin synthesis in the kidney and this reduces renal blood flow, leading to reduced natriuretic responses to thiazide and loop diuretics.

OBA answers

1. **Answer C** is correct. Triamterene is a potassium-sparing diuretic that directly blocks a selective Na^+ channel (ENaC) on the luminal membrane of tubule cells in the collecting duct. Answer A is the mechanism of action of aldosterone (mineralocorticoid) receptor antagonists such as spironolactone. Answers B, D and E are the mechanisms of action of loop diuretics, thiazides and carbonic anhydrase inhibitors respectively.
2. **Answer A** is correct.
   A. **Correct.** Loop diuretics are widely used in the control of oedema in heart failure for the elimination of excessive salt and water load. The direct venodilator activity of furosemide reduces central blood volume.
   B. Incorrect. A thiazide diuretic can be added to a loop diuretic to act sequentially at different sites in the nephron, thus producing a marked diuresis and natriuresis.
   C. Incorrect. Delivery of greater concentrations of Na^+ to the collecting ducts increases the exchange for K^+ at that site, thus increasing K^+ loss.
   D. Incorrect. By inhibiting the $Na^+/K^+/2Cl^-$ co-transporter (NKCC2), the medullary interstitial hypertonicity falls and this reduces the reabsorption of water in the collecting ducts (in the presence of antidiuretic hormone).
   E. Incorrect. Loop diuretics alone can cause ototoxicity (especially at high doses or in renal impairment) and also when taken with other ototoxic drugs such as aminoglycosides.

Extended-matching-item answers

Case 1. **Answer A**. The combination of a potassium-sparing diuretic (amiloride) and an ACE inhibitor (lisinopril) may have raised the plasma K^+ concentration and this may have been the cause of the profound bradycardia.

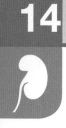

Case 2. **Answer E**. Thiazide-like diuretics can worsen insulin resistance, resulting in an increased plasma glucose concentration.

Case 3. **Answer B**. The loop diuretic may cause hypokalaemia. This enhances the toxicity of digoxin, resulting in arrhythmias.

FURTHER READING

Brater DC (2000) Pharmacology of diuretics. *Am J Med Sci* 319, 38–50

De Bruyne LKM (2003) Mechanisms and management of diuretic resistance in congestive heart failure. *Postgrad Med J* 79, 268–271

Duarte JD, Cooper-DeHoff RM (2010) Mechanisms for blood pressure lowering and metabolic effects of thiazide and thiazide-like diuretics. *Exp Rev Cardiovasc Ther* 8, 793–802

Greenberg A (2000) Diuretic complications. *Am J Med Sci* 319, 10–24

Krämer BK, Schweda F, Riegger GAJ (1999) Diuretic treatment and diuretic resistance in heart failure. *Am J Med* 106, 90–96

Shankar SS, Brater DC (2003) Loop diuretics: from the Na-K-2Cl transporter to clinical use. *Am J Physiol Renal Physiol* 284, F11–F21

Wright SH, Dantzler WH (2004) Molecular and cellular physiology of renal organic cation and anion transport. *Physiol Rev* 84, 987–1049

Compendium: diuretic drugs

All given orally unless otherwise stated

Drug	Kinetics (half-life)	Comment
Carbonic anhydrase inhibitors		
Acetazolamide	Eliminated unchanged in urine (6–9 h)	Little clinical value as a diuretic due to rapid tolerance; used in glaucoma (Ch. 50)
Osmotic diuretics		
Mannitol	Urinary excretion (2 h) very prolonged (36 h) in cardiac or renal failure	Given by rapid intravenous infusion in cerebral oedema; not used in heart failure
Loop diuretics		
Used for heart failure and oedema, and oliguria due to renal failure.		
Bumetanide	Well absorbed from the gut; 50% conjugated with glucuronic acid and excreted in urine and bile (1–2 h)	Given orally or by intravenous or intramuscular injection
Furosemide	Incomplete and erratic absorption from gut; limited metabolism (15%) by glucuronidation (1 h)	Given orally or by intravenous or intramuscular injection
Torasemide	Good oral absorption; about 25% cleared by kidney and remainder by metabolism; half-life unchanged in renal failure (2–4 h)	Known as torsemide in USA; little used in UK; given orally
Thiazide and related diuretics		
Given orally; used for heart failure, oedema and, in lower doses, for hypertension.		
Bendroflumethiazide	Complete absorption from gut; 30% excreted in urine unchanged (3–9 h)	
Chlortalidone	Incomplete oral absorption; long half-life (50–90 h) due to high volume of distribution and plasma protein binding	Thiazide-related diuretic
Cyclopenthiazide	Renal excretion	Offers no advantages over other thiazides and is now little used in UK
Hydrochlorothiazide	Renal excretion (8–12 h)	Offers no advantages over other thiazides and is now used in UK only in antihypertensive combined formulations; available as a single formulation in continental Europe
Indapamide	Rapidly absorbed from the gut; extensive hepatic metabolism; only 5% excreted unchanged (10–22 h)	Thiazide-related diuretic
Metolazone	Good oral absorption; 80% eliminated unchanged in urine (4–5 h)	Thiazide-related diuretic; effective even in advanced renal failure
Xipamide	Rapidly absorbed from the gut; renal excretion of parent drug and glucuronide conjugate (5 h)	Thiazide-related diuretic
Potassium-sparing diuretics		
Prevention of diuretic-induced hypokalaemia, hyperaldosteronism and ascites associated with liver cirrhosis.		
Amiloride	Excreted unchanged in urine (6–9 h)	Used in combination with thiazides and loop diuretics to conserve K^+
Eplerenone	Metabolised to inactive products (4–6 h)	Greater selectivity than spironolactone for mineralocorticoid receptor; reduced anti-androgenic effects; used in heart failure
Spironolactone	Variable absorption from gut; hepatic metabolism to active metabolite (canrenone), which is eliminated in urine (17–22 h)	Used in primary hyperaldosteronism (Conn's syndrome), liver cirrhosis (ascites), acne, female hirsutism
Triamterene	Variable absorption owing to first-pass metabolism; hepatic metabolism (2 h)	Used in combination with thiazides and loop diuretics to conserve K^+

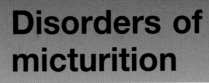

15 Disorders of micturition

PATHOPHYSIOLOGY OF MICTURITION

The urinary bladder is a smooth muscle organ, most of which is the detrusor muscle, that relaxes to allow bladder filling up to 500–600 mL. A smaller muscle, the trigone, is found between the ureteric orifices and bladder neck. Internal and external distal sphincter mechanisms are normally constricted to prevent bladder emptying and maintain continence (Fig. 15.1). Coordination of bladder filling, continence and bladder emptying are brought about by the frontal lobe of the cortex and the pontine micturition centre. Conscious sensations of bladder fullness are processed by the cerebral cortex, which then sends signals to the micturition centre.

During *bladder filling*, sympathetic nervous system stimulation via the hypogastric nerve relaxes the bladder smooth muscle (via β_2- and β_3-adrenoceptors in the detrusor which generate intracellular cAMP). At the same time sympathetic stimulation of α_1-adrenoceptors (α_{1A}- and to a lesser extent α_{1B}-adrenoceptor subtypes), via the vesical nerve, contracts the smooth muscle of the internal urethral sphincter. Stimulation of the striated muscle of the external urethral sphincter, which is under voluntary control via the pudendal nerve, and aided by pelvic muscle control in women, contributes to maintenance of internal urethral sphincter tone and continence. The sensation of urge to micturate occurs in adults at a bladder volume of 200–300 mL.

Bladder emptying is initiated by myogenic stretch receptor activity produced by distention of the trigone, and by sensory signals from the urothelium (the epithelial cell lining of the bladder). Release of ATP from the urothelium stimulates P2X purinoceptors which along with other local receptor modulators initiate sensory impulses in the afferent nerves (see Ch. 1). The afferent sensory nerves project to the pontine micturition centre, which then initiates activity in efferent motor pathways. Stimulation of the pelvic nerve, acting through parasympathetic muscarinic M_3 receptors in the detrusor muscle, leads to bladder contraction and voiding. Acetylcholine, acting through these receptors, leads to generation of intracellular inositol 1,4,5-triphosphate (IP_3) and diacylglycerol (DAG). At the same time, stimulation of muscarinic M_2 receptors on presynaptic nerve terminals inhibits intracellular cAMP production, and therefore opposes the effects of sympathetic activity. Non-cholinergic-mediated efferent impulses (ATP neurotransmission acting via P2X purinoceptors) also contribute to bladder contraction, and this component becomes more prominent in unstable bladders. Contraction of the detrusor is coordinated with inhibition of the tonic control of distal sphincter mechanisms and the bladder neck, thus relaxing the bladder outflow tract. Bladder emptying may be augmented by contraction of the diaphragm and abdominal muscles. M_3 and M_2 receptors are present in detrusor muscle but the M_3 subtype appears to be more important for detrusor contraction.

DISORDERS OF MICTURITION

Disorders of micturition can arise from a disturbance of bladder function or from abnormalities affecting bladder outflow. Although there are distinct clinical syndromes, many people with incontinence have mixed incontinence; for example, both stress and urge incontinence (see below). Management of disorders of micturition should also consider possible contributory factors, such as diuretics, α_1-adrenoceptor antagonists used for treatment of hypertension, and stool impaction, which inhibits sacral parasympathetic neurotransmission.

OVERACTIVE BLADDER SYNDROME

Detrusor instability produces uncontrolled bladder contractions during normal filling. Symptoms from this include urinary urgency, nocturia and frequency (overactive bladder syndrome), often accompanied by urge incontinence (a sudden compelling desire to urinate). Most cases in women are idiopathic but probably have a neurogenic component, while in men bladder outflow obstruction is the commonest cause. Upper motor neuron lesions, such as those produced by stroke, spinal cord injuries or multiple sclerosis, can also produce an overactive bladder. First-line approaches to management include reduction in excessive fluid intake, weight loss, smoking cessation and behavioural training that includes pelvic floor muscle rehabilitation and suppression of urge.

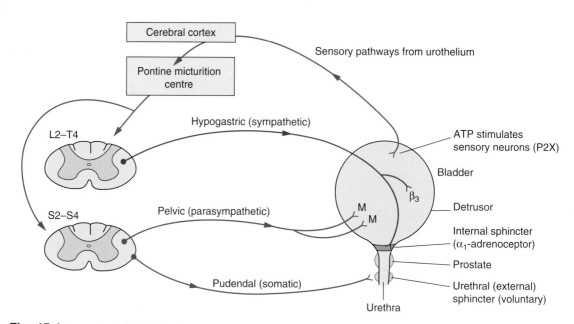

Fig. 15.1 **Aspects of the bladder/prostate structures and the innervation involved in the micturition reflex.**
Bladder filling provides neuronal signals to the micturition centre via sensory input from purinoceptors on neurons in the urothelium. To accommodate filling and continence, sympathetic stimulation both relaxes the smooth muscle of the bladder via β_2- and β_3-adrenoceptors and stimulates sphincter mechanisms through α_1-adrenoceptor subtypes. Somatic control of the external sphincter also aids continence. Voluntary urination involves parasympathetic stimulation of bladder smooth muscle through M_3 and M_2 muscarinic receptor subtypes (M) and inhibition of the sympathetic and somatic outflow. Aspects of bladder control may involve other less understood transmitter substances. For example, γ-aminobutyric acid (GABA) interneurons inhibit bladder contraction. P2X, purinergic receptors.

DRUGS FOR TREATMENT OF OVERACTIVE BLADDER SYNDROME

Increased understanding of the neural pathways involved in initiating micturition is opening up new avenues for drug therapy to augment the relatively ineffective treatments currently available. Those used at present to treat overactive bladder act at peripheral muscarinic receptors to decrease bladder activity.

Muscarinic receptor antagonists

Examples

darifenacin, fesoterodine, oxybutynin, solifenacin, tolterodine, trospium

These drugs act with various degrees of selectivity at muscarinic receptor subtypes. Antimuscarinic unwanted effects (Ch. 4) are most troublesome with oxybutynin, particularly central nervous system (CNS) effects such as sedation, insomnia, confusion and cognitive problems (from M_1 receptor blockade) and dry mouth (from M_3 receptor blockade in salivary glands). The need for continued use of these drugs should be reviewed after 6 months.

- Oxybutynin is a selective antagonist of M_1 and M_3 receptors and has additional weak muscle relaxant properties

through calcium channel blocking actions and local anaesthetic activity. Oxybutynin is rapidly absorbed from the gut and metabolised in the liver to an active metabolite. Modified-release and transdermal formulations are available because oxybutynin has a short half-life (1–3 h) and use of standard formulations can result in large fluctuations in plasma drug concentrations and increase the severity of unwanted effects.
- Tolterodine, fesoterodine and trospium are non-selective muscarinic receptor antagonists with no additional properties and less lipophilicity than oxybutynin. They cross the blood–brain barrier less readily and have fewer cognitive unwanted effects. Both tolterodine and trospium have short half-lives. Tolterodine is better tolerated in a modified-release formulation.
- Darifenacin and solifenacin are more selective antagonists of M_3 receptors and may have fewer CNS actions.

Beta3-adrenoceptor agonist

Example: mirabegron

Stimulation of β_3-adrenoceptors in the bladder trigone flattens and lengthens the bladder base, which facilitates urine storage. Mirabegron reduces symptoms of urinary frequency and urgency with similar efficacy when compared to the muscarinic receptor antagonists. The main adverse effects are an increase in blood pressure and heart rate. It may be an option for those who fail to respond to muscarinic receptor antagonists, or who cannot tolerate them.

Other drugs

- Topical vaginal oestrogen-replacement therapy (Ch. 45) reverses atrophic changes in the lower genital tract in postmenopausal women and may be helpful for overactive bladder syndrome.
- Desmopressin, a synthetic antidiuretic hormone (ADH) analogue (Ch. 43), is sometimes helpful to reduce nocturia in unstable bladder syndrome. It is taken orally; the nasal spray is no longer licensed for this indication because of the risk of water intoxication in children.

HYPOTONIC BLADDER

Hypotonic bladder is often a result of lower motor neuron lesions, or can arise from bladder distension following chronic urinary retention. Drugs with antimuscarinic properties (such as tricyclic antidepressants; Ch.22) and the specific antimuscarinic drugs above can make the symptoms worse. Hypotonic bladder leads to incomplete bladder emptying, with urinary retention and overflow incontinence. Treatment depends on the cause.

- Chronic urinary retention is often caused by bladder outlet obstruction. If renal function is impaired, it should be managed by bladder catheterisation and correction of the underlying cause.
- Neurogenic problems are sometimes treated with anticholinesterases (such as distigmine) which may increase the force of detrusor contraction (Ch. 4), although they are probably ineffective. Cholinergic drugs should not be used in the presence of urinary outflow obstruction.

URETHRAL SPHINCTER INCOMPETENCE

Urethral sphincter incompetence produces stress incontinence in women (urine leakage with effort, exertion, sneezing or coughing) or sphincter weakness incontinence in men. The most common cause in women is loss of collagenous support in the pelvic floor or perineum; it also arises from trauma to the membranous urethra (sphincter mechanism), such as may occur from pelvic trauma or following prostatectomy in males. Drugs such as α_1-adrenoceptor antagonists (see below) can make the symptoms worse. Pelvic floor muscle training may be helpful, while minimal access surgical sling procedures or colposuspension to provide urethral support are among the surgical options. Drug therapy is limited, and only recommended if surgical treatment is not suitable.

Duloxetine is a serotonin and noradrenaline reuptake inhibitor (SNRI; see Ch. 22). It is believed to augment sympathetic activity, which relaxes the detrusor, and to enhance external urethral sphincter activity by increasing efferent impulses in the motor neurons of the pudendal nerve when the bladder is placed under stress. It reduces the frequency of incontinence episodes significantly in about half of those treated.

Box 15.1 Symptoms of benign prostatic hypertrophy

Obstructive	Irritative
Hesitancy	Urgency
Poor stream	Frequency
Straining to pass urine	Nocturia
Prolonged micturition	Urge incontinence
Feeling of incomplete bladder emptying	
Urinary retention	

BENIGN PROSTATIC HYPERTROPHY

Benign prostatic hypertrophy (BPH) produces symptoms in more than 25% of men above the age of 60 years, and up to 70% of men over the age of 70 years. The spectrum of symptoms is often called prostatism (Box 15.1). Left untreated, spontaneous improvement occurs or symptoms remain stable in up to half of all those with prostatism. Acute urinary retention occurs at a rate of 1–2% per year. Scoring systems can reliably quantify the extent to which symptoms affect the quality of life and therefore as a guide to treatment.

DRUGS FOR PROSTATISM

Alpha₁-adrenoceptor antagonists

 Examples

doxazosin, tamsulosin

Selective α_1-adrenoceptor antagonists inhibit contraction in prostatic and bladder neck smooth muscle, without affecting the detrusor. Relaxation of these muscles improves urine flow rate and symptoms of BPH. Tamsulosin is claimed to be a more selective antagonist in the smooth muscle of the urinary tract and may produce fewer peripheral vasodilatory unwanted effects compared with many other α_1-adrenoceptor antagonists. This was assumed to be due to a selective action at the α_{1A}-adrenoceptor subtype found in the prostate, but is more likely to be due to selective access to the target tissue. More information about α_1-adrenoceptor antagonists is found in Chapter 6.

5α-Reductase inhibitors

 Examples

dutasteride, finasteride

Inhibition of 5α-reductase reduces the enzymatic conversion of testosterone to dihydrotestosterone (DHT) in prostatic cells, but does not affect circulating testosterone levels. DHT is involved in prostate growth, and inhibition of

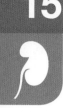

its production can reduce prostate volume by up to 30%. There are two isoenzymes of 5α-reductase, both found in the prostate. Finasteride only inhibits the type 2 isoenzyme, while dutasteride inhibits both the type 1 and 2 isoenzymes, but it is not yet known whether this confers any clinical advantage.

Pharmacokinetics

Both finasteride and dutasteride are well absorbed after oral administration and eliminated by hepatic metabolism. Finasteride has a half-life of about 6 h, whereas the half-life of dutasteride is extremely long at about 4 weeks.

Unwanted effects

These occur in up to 10% of people taking 5α-reductase inhibitors, and include:

- reduced libido,
- erectile impotence or decreased ejaculation,
- breast tenderness or enlargement,
- reduction of the plasma concentration of prostate-specific antigen by an average of 50%, which should be considered when screening for prostate cancer.

Plant extracts

saw palmetto plant extracts, β-sitosterol plant extract

These products are available direct to consumers, but their composition varies among suppliers. Very limited trial evidence suggests that they produce modest short-term improvements in symptoms of prostatism, but a more rigorous study found no benefit for a preparation of saw palmetto extract compared to placebo. It is uncertain how they might work, but these extracts may reduce the synthesis of DHT or inhibit expression of prostatic growth factors. Plant extracts are well tolerated, with unwanted effects mainly confined to gastrointestinal upset.

TREATMENT OF PROSTATISM

Many symptomatic individuals do not require or want treatment, and a policy of 'watchful waiting' will be appropriate. The aim of drug treatment is either to reduce prostatic size or to relax the smooth muscle that restricts urine outflow. There is no evidence that medical treatment avoids the need for surgery in the long term.

Selective α₁-adrenoceptor antagonists are the first-choice drugs for improving symptoms and urinary flow rates. Symptomatic improvement usually occurs within 1 month, and is seen in about two-thirds of those treated. 5α-Reductase inhibitors usually take 3–6 months to improve symptoms of prostatism, but the improvements are maintained. These drugs may be more effective with larger-volume prostates. Additional symptomatic benefit can be obtained from combining finasteride or dutasteride with an α₁-adrenoceptor antagonist.

Surgical treatment is usually required for severe symptoms or complications of BPH (Box 15.2). Transurethral

Box 15.2	Indications for surgery in patients with benign prostatic hypertrophy

Acute retention of urine
Chronic retention of urine
Recurrent urinary tract infection
Bladder stones
Renal insufficiency owing to benign prostatic hypertrophy
Large bladder diverticula
Severe symptoms

resection of the prostate improves symptoms in 70–90% of those with prostatism. Long-term sequelae include impotence (5–10%), retrograde ejaculation (80–90%) and incontinence (<5%). Several less invasive procedures are now available, but they may be less successful for relieving symptoms and do not reduce the risk of long-term consequences, although they produce fewer immediate postoperative complications.

SELF-ASSESSMENT

True/false questions

1. Urinary bladder function is controlled by both voluntary and involuntary nervous pathways.
2. The antimuscarinic drug darifenacin causes urinary frequency and urge incontinence.
3. The antidepressant drug duloxetine can be used to treat stress incontinence.
4. The anticholinesterase distigmine can be given safely if there is urinary outflow obstruction.
5. Blockade of α₁-adrenoceptors in the bladder neck smooth muscle improves urine flow rates.
6. Finasteride reduces prostate volume by blocking testosterone receptors.

Extended-matching-item questions

Choose the *most appropriate* pharmacological option A–F for each case scenarios 1–3 below.

A. Tamsulosin
B. Finasteride
C. Duloxetine
D. Amitriptyline
E. Bethanecol
F. Oxybutynin

1. A 50-year-old man with a 2-year history of difficulty in urinating and hesitancy was diagnosed with benign prostatic hypertrophy (BPH) and an enlarged prostate. He was given a 1-month trial of an α₁-adrenoceptor antagonist, which did not improve his symptoms. He did not at this stage want to undergo surgery. What pharmacological treatment might be of benefit?
2. A 30-year-old woman with normal bladder function complained of difficulty in urination after being prescribed new medication for her depression. She was

found to have urinary retention. What class of anti-depressant could cause this effect?

3. A 60-year-old woman had severe urge incontinence. She urinated 16–20 times a day and had leakage two to three times a day and at night. What treatment could she be given?

Case-based question

A 65-year-old man developed progressive urinary problems over a 5-year period. He had difficulty passing urine and was getting up three times in the night to pass urine. A rectal examination by his GP showed an enlarged prostate. Ultrasound, flow tests and prostate-specific antigen measurements suggested BPH.

A. What pharmacological approaches to the treatment of BPH could be considered?
B. What are the unwanted effects of these treatments?
C. What are the possible outcomes of not giving treatment?

True/false answers

1. **True.** Bladder function is controlled by involuntary parasympathetic and sympathetic innervation of the detrusor and sphincter muscles and by voluntary control via the somatic nervous system.
2. **False.** Darifenacin blocks muscarinic receptors with some selectivity for the M_3 subtype, inhibiting the parasympathetic effects on the detrusor muscle. It is used for treatment of overactive bladder.
3. **True.** Duloxetine inhibits the reuptake of serotonin and noradrenaline and increases the contractility of the urethral sphincters.
4. **False.** The anticholinesterase distigmine increases detrusor muscle contractility, which is undesirable in the presence of urinary outflow obstruction.
5. **True.** Selective antagonism of the α_{1A}-adrenoceptor subtype in bladder smooth muscle may reduce unwanted vasodilator effects.

6. **False.** Finasteride and dutasteride block the conversion of testosterone to dihydrotestosterone by inhibiting 5α-reductase in the prostate.

Extended-matching-item answers

1. Answer **B**. Finasteride inhibits the conversion of testosterone to dihydrotestosterone, which is a promoter of prostatic cell growth. A reduction of up to 30% in prostate size can be obtained. Symptomatic benefit may be increased if finasteride and an α_1-adrenoceptor antagonist are given together
2. Answer **D**. The tricyclic antidepressant amitriptyline is also an antagonist at muscarinic receptors and may inhibit the micturition reflex.
3. Answer **C**. Duloxetine could be tried if the condition were caused by sphincter incompetence. Duloxetine increases the levels of noradrenaline and serotonin in the synapse and the activity of the motor neurons in the pudendal nerve. Pelvic floor exercises should also be suggested as drug therapy is of limited benefit.

Case-based answers

A. Drugs may be used in mild disease and while awaiting a transurethral resection of the prostate. Selective α_1-adrenoceptor antagonists increase urine flow to a limited extent but also decrease urgency, frequency and hesitancy. The 5α-reductase inhibitor finasteride slowly reduces prostate size.
B. Alpha$_1$-adrenoceptor antagonists can cause postural hypotension, especially with the first dose. They cause dizziness and can interact with other drugs to lower blood pressure. Finasteride can reduce libido and cause impotence.
C. The outcome is variable; symptoms may not worsen appreciably for many years, but moderate symptoms can lead to a poor quality of life. Complications include urinary retention, incontinence and renal insufficiency owing to hydronephrosis.

FURTHER READING

Barendrecht MM, Oelke M, Laguna MP et al. (2007) Is the use of parasympathetics for treating an underactive urinary bladder evidence-based? *BJU Int* 99, 749–752

Connolly SS, Fitzpatrick JM (2007) Medical treatment of benign prostatic hyperplasia. *Postgrad Med J* 83, 73–78

Foley CL, Kirby RS (2003) 5-Alpha-reductase inhibitors: what's new? *Curr Opin Urol* 13, 31–37

Gerber GS (2002) Phytotherapy for benign prostatic hyperplasia. *Curr Urol Rep* 3, 285–291

Hashim H, Abrams P (2006) Pharmacological management of women with mixed incontinence. *Drugs* 66, 591–606

Marinkovic SP, Rovner ES, Moldwin RM et al. (2012) The management of overactive bladder syndrome. *BMJ* 344, e2365

Norton P, Brubaker L (2006) Urinary incontinence in women. *Lancet* 367, 57–67

Nygaard I (2010) Idiopathic urgency urinary incontinence. *N Engl J Med* 363, 1156–1162

Robinson D, Cardozo L (2012) Antimuscarinic drugs to treat overactive bladder. *BMJ* 344, e2130

Rogers RG (2008) Urinary stress incontinence in women. *N Engl J Med* 358, 1029–1036

Shamliyan TA, Kane RL, Wyman J et al. (2008) Randomised, controlled trials of non-surgical treatments for urinary incontinence in women. *Ann Intern Med* 148, 459–473

Thorpe A, Neal D (2003) Benign prostatic hyperplasia. *Lancet* 361, 1359–1367

Wilt TJ, Dow JN (2008) Benign prostatic hyperplasia. Part 2 – Management. *BMJ* 336, 206–210

Compendium: drugs used to treat disorders of micturition

Drug	Kinetics (half-life)	Comment
Drugs for urinary retention		
All drugs taken orally.		
α_1-Adrenoceptor antagonists		
Alfuzosin	Oral bioavailability about 50% with food; mainly hepatic metabolism (4–10 h)	Relative selectivity for α_{1A}-adrenoceptors in the genitourinary tract may reduce vasodilator effects at α_{1B}- and α_{1D}-adrenoceptors
Doxazosin	Oral bioavailability 65%; eliminated largely hepatic metabolism (10–20 h)	Relaxes bladder smooth muscle in BPH; also reduces blood pressure, including postural hypotension, especially with first dose
Indoramin	Oral bioavailability 10–20% due to extensive hepatic first-pass metabolism (2–10 h); longer half-life and fivefold higher blood levels in the elderly	As for doxazosin
Prazosin	Oral bioavailability about 60%; hepatic metabolism (2–4h)	As for doxasosin
Tamsulosin	Food reduces bioavailability to about 60%; eliminated by hepatic metabolism and renal excretion (15 h)	Relative selectivity for α_{1A}-adrenoceptors in the genitourinary tract; normally taken with food to reduce unwanted effects
Terazosin	High oral bioavailability (90%); hepatic metabolism; eliminated in faeces and urine as parent drug and metabolites (10–12 h)	As for doxazosin
Parasympathomimetics		
Bethanechol	Few kinetic data available; poorly absorbed	Muscarinic agonist; increases bladder detrusor activity; rarely used
Distigmine	Very poor oral bioavailability (5%), especially if taken with food; hydrolysed by plasma esterases with renal excretion (70 h)	Acetylcholinesterase inhibitor; increases detrusor contractility in hypotonic bladder of neurogenic origin
β_3-adrenoceptor agonist		
Mirabegron	Oral bioavailability 30%; eliminated by hepatic metabolism (50 h)	
5α-Reductase inhibitors		
Dutasteride	Oral bioavailability about 60%; hepatic metabolism; very long half-life (4–5 weeks); requires about 6 months to reach steady state	Similar profile to finasteride, but blocks 5α-reductase types 1 and 2
Finasteride	Oral bioavailability 60–80%; hepatic metabolism (3–16 h)	Reduces prostate growth by blocking synthesis of dihydrotestosterone by 5α-reductase type 2
Drugs for urinary frequency and incontinence		
All drugs taken orally.		
Muscarinic receptor antagonists		
Darifenacin	Low oral bioavailability; hepatic metabolism (13–19 h)	Selective M_3 receptor antagonist (about ninefold difference compared with M_1)
Flavoxate	Few kinetic data available; metabolised by carboxylation and also eliminated unchanged in urine	Fewer unwanted effects but also weaker clinical action
Fesoterodine	Prodrug converted by esterases to an active metabolite of tolterodine (4–20 h)	Non-selective muscarinic antagonist
Oxybutynin	Very low oral bioavailability (6%) owing to extensive first-pass metabolism (1–3 h), which generates an active metabolite	Antimuscarinic side-effects at M_1 receptors in CNS and M_3 receptors in salivary glands limit use of higher doses; delayed-release and transdermal preparations are better tolerated
Propantheline	Variable oral bioavailability (10–25%); undergoes first-pass metabolism to inactive products (1–2 h)	Quaternary amino compound; rarely used

Compendium: drugs used to treat disorders of micturition—cont'd

Drug	Kinetics (half-life)	Comment
Propiverine	Oral bioavailability about 50%; hepatic metabolism (4 h)	Non-selective muscarinic antagonist. modified-release preparation better tolerated
Solifenacin	High oral bioavailability; hepatic metabolism with <15% excreted in urine unchanged (55 h)	Selective M_3 receptor antagonist
Tolterodine	High oral bioavailability (about 75%); highly variable metabolism to an active product responsible for part of the therapeutic effect (2–10 h)	Non-selective muscarinic antagonist; modified release formulation available
Trospium	Very low oral bioavailability (<10%); partly eliminated by hepatic metabolism and partly by excretion (1–2 h)	Non-selective muscarinic antagonist; quaternary amino compound
Serotonin and noradrenaline reuptake inhibitor		
Duloxetine	Good oral absorption; hepatic metabolism (9–19 h)	Used for moderate to severe stress incontinence in women

Erectile dysfunction

PHYSIOLOGY OF ERECTION

Achieving and maintaining an erection is a spinal reflex that involves a complex series of interactions between the central nervous system, the autonomic nervous system and local mediators. Psychological, visual, olfactory and tactile stimuli are all important. The primary erectile innervation is the parasympathetic nervous system. There are four phases in achieving full penile erection.

Phase 1. Parasympathetic stimulation relaxes both arterial smooth muscle and the smooth muscle that forms bands (trabeculae) with connective tissue in the highly vascular erectile tissues of the penis (corpus cavernosa and corpus spongiosum). These actions increase the influx of blood into the sinusoidal spaces of the corpus cavernosa, which become engorged (Fig. 16.1). Conversely, sympathetic stimulation inhibits erection by increasing vascular smooth muscle tone.

Phase 2. Pressure rises within the corpus cavernosum and the sinusoids expand. The penis elongates and widens.

Phase 3. The rise in pressure in the sinusoids compresses the venous plexus and reduces venous outflow, thus maintaining the erection (the corporeal veno-occlusive mechanism).

Phase 4. The pudendal nerve (part of the parasympathetic innervation) stimulates the ischiocavernous muscle. This squeezes the crura at the base of the penis and stops both arterial inflow and venous outflow, maintaining full erection. Muscle fatigue eventually allows return of perfusion.

There are also many locally produced mediators that appear to be involved in achieving and maintaining an erection. Nitric oxide (NO) synthesised by blood vessel endothelial cells and released from non-adrenergic non-cholinergic (NANC) nerves in the corpora appears to be crucial for cavernosal smooth muscle relaxation. Nitric oxide generates intracellular cGMP, which activates protein kinase G. cGMP is degraded to GMP by phosphodiesterase type 5 (PDE5) (see Table 1.1), terminating its effects. Inhibition of PDE5 is a primary target for the pharmacological treatment of erectile dysfunction (see below). Other vasodilators that are involved in modulating penile vascular smooth muscle relaxation and blood flow include vasoactive intestinal peptide (VIP), calcitonin gene-related peptide (CGRP) and prostaglandin E_1, but their precise roles are less well understood. Numerous central facilitatory mediators have been identified, including dopamine, acetylcholine and a variety of peptides. These are involved in the psychological preparedness that is essential for an erection to occur.

ERECTILE DYSFUNCTION

Erectile dysfunction is defined as the consistent inability to achieve or sustain an erection of sufficient rigidity for sexual intercourse. It is a common problem, affecting up to 20% of adult men, with up to 10% over the age of 40 years having complete erectile dysfunction. Any disease process that affects penile neural supply, arterial inflow or venous outflow can produce erectile dysfunction. There is a physical cause in about 80% of cases (Box 16.1) but a psychological component often coexists. Psychogenic erectile dysfunction is more common in younger men. Drugs are an important cause of erectile dysfunction, particularly antihypertensive, psychotropic and 'recreational' drugs, and account for up to 25% of cases. Drugs can also affect libido and therefore arousal, or inhibit ejaculation in those who achieve an erection (Table 16.1).

MANAGEMENT OF ERECTILE DYSFUNCTION

A number of strategies can be used in the management of erectile dysfunction. Initially there should be an assessment and treatment of any underlying psychological cause or physical disease or if possible withdrawal of a causative drug. Treatment options for persistent dysfunction include:

- pharmacological, using the drugs described below,
- mechanical aids, such as the vacuum constriction device: these are usually advised for older people who do not respond to pharmacological treatment and do not wish to have surgery,
- penile implants using a malleable or inflatable prosthesis,
- testosterone-replacement therapy for hypogonadism (Ch. 46), an uncommon cause of impotence.

Hyperprolactinaemia impairs erection; it is most commonly caused by drug therapy (e.g. with phenothiazines) and can be improved by oral dopamine agonists (Ch. 43) if the cause cannot be treated.

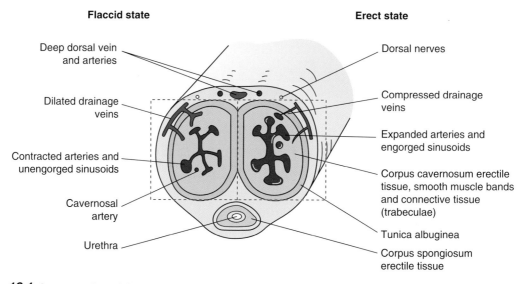

Fig. 16.1 Cross-section of the penis, showing structures involved in erection. This diagram shows only part of the rich nervous and vascular filling and drainage system in the penis. The left-hand area shows the situation in the flaccid penis and the right-hand area the erect penis. The rising pressure during erection limits the venous outflow, thus maintaining the erection. The penis contains three cylinders of erectile tissue: two corpora cavernosa and the corpus spongiosum. The corpus spongiosum contains the urethra. The cylinders of erectile tissue are divided into spaces known as sinusoids or lacunae, which are lined by vascular epithelium. The walls of these spaces are made up of thick bundles of smooth muscle cells within a framework of fibroblasts, collagen and elastin (trabeculae). The erectile tissues are supplied with blood from the cavernosal and helicine arteries, which drain into the sinusoidal spaces. Blood is drained from the sinusoidal spaces through emissary veins. The venules join together to form larger veins that drain into the deep dorsal vein or other veins at different parts of the penis. Arterial and sinusoid dilation is important for erection, while swelling is limited by the inelastic tunica albuginea.

| Box 16.1 | Common causes of erectile dysfunction |

Diabetes
Vascular disease
Prostate surgery
Drugs (see Table 16.1)
Substance abuse, e.g. nicotine, alcohol, recreational drugs
Testosterone deficiency, e.g. hyper- or hypothyroidism
Neurological disease, e.g. multiple sclerosis, Alzheimer's
   disease, epilepsy
Spinal cord injury
Psychological factors (20% as a primary cause, more
   commonly secondary to physical problems)

ORAL PHOSPHODIESTERASE INHIBITORS

 xamples

sildenafil, tadalafil, vardenafil

Endothelial-derived nitric oxide increases the synthesis of cGMP that acts via protein kinases to cause blood vessel dilation (see Ch. 5, Fig. 5.3). cGMP is broken down in penile tissue by PDE5. Sildenafil, tadalafil and vardenafil are orally active analogues of cGMP that selectively inhibit the enzyme. PDE5 is also found in lower concentrations in other vascular and visceral smooth muscles, and in skeletal muscle and platelets. Sexual stimulation resulting in the release of nitric oxide is a prerequisite for these drugs to produce an erection, and the drug will then prolong the vasodilator effect of nitric oxide on penile vascular smooth muscle. If an appropriate dose of the drug is used, about 60% of men with erectile dysfunction will achieve erections sufficient to permit intercourse. The response is often better if precipitating factors are also treated, such as depression or excess alcohol consumption.

Sildenafil and tadalafil are also used to treat pulmonary hypertension (Ch. 6).

Pharmacokinetics

Sildenafil is relatively well absorbed orally, but vardenafil and tadalafil are less well absorbed. The median time to onset of action for all is about 30 min. The absorption of sildenafil and vardenafil is delayed by a fatty meal, whereas the absorption of tadalafil is rapid and unaffected by food. All are eliminated by hepatic metabolism mediated primarily by CYP3A4. Sildenafil and vardenafil have half-lives of less than 6 h, and should be taken 30–60 min before sexual activity for maximum benefit. The half-life of tadalafil is longer (17 h), and its duration of action is up to about 24–36 h; therefore, planning of sexual activity (and its timing in relation to drug dosage) is less relevant with this drug.

Table 16.1 Drugs that commonly cause male sexual dysfunction

	Ejaculatory dysfunction	Erectile dysfunction	Loss of libido
Antihypertensives			
Beta-adrenoceptor antagonists		+	
Alpha-adrenoceptor antagonists	+		
Methyldopa	+	+	+
Thiazide diuretics		+	
Psychotropic drugs			
Phenothiazines	+	+	+
Benzodiazepines	+	+	+
Tricyclic antidepressants		+	+
Selective serotonin reuptake inhibitors (SSRIs)		+	+
Other prescription drugs			
Spironolactone			+
Digoxin		+	
Cimetidine/ranitidine		+	+
Metoclopramide		+	+
Carbamazepine		+	+
Recreational drugs			
Alcohol	+	+	
Marijuana		+	
Cocaine		+	+
Amfetamines	+	+	+
Anabolic steroids		+	+

Sildenafil and vardenafil both have active metabolites, but tadalafil does not.

Unwanted effects

- Dyspepsia, nausea, vomiting.
- Hypotension, dizziness, flushing, headache and nasal congestion from systemic vasodilation.
- Myalgia, back pain.
- PDE6 (involved in phototransduction in the eye) is inhibited by high doses of sildenafil, but less so by tadalafil or vardenafil. This can cause visual disturbance (enhanced perception of bright lights, or a 'blue halo' effect) and raised intraocular pressure. Ischaemic optic neuropathy can cause sudden visual impairment.
- Priapism, a painful and sustained erection, can occur rarely.
- Drug interactions: oral PDE5 inhibitors should not be used together with nitrates or nicorandil (see Ch. 5), because of a synergistic effect on vascular nitric oxide with exaggerated vasodilator effects. Several antiviral drugs, such as saquinavir (Table 2.7 and Ch. 51), inhibit the CYP3A4 isoenzyme that metabolises oral PDE5 inhibitors, and can potentiate their effects.

ALPROSTADIL

Intracavernosal injection of alprostadil is effective if arterial flow is normal, such as with neurogenic and psychogenic impotence. It should not be used if the person has bleeding tendencies, and may be problematic if there is poor manual dexterity or morbid obesity. The injection is made into the side of the penis, directly into the corpus cavernosum.

Alprostadil is a synthetic prostaglandin E_1 analogue. It vasodilates by acting on smooth muscle cell surface receptors to increase intracellular cAMP, which in turn reduces the intracellular Ca^{2+} concentration. Local pain after injection is a common unwanted effect, reported by one-third of users, and can be reduced by the addition of a local anaesthetic such as procaine (Ch. 18). Rapid local metabolism of alprostadil minimises unwanted systemic effects. Priapism (prolonged painful erection) is the most worrying complication, and may require aspiration and lavage of the corpora.

High doses of intra-urethral alprostadil can be given as a pellet using a plastic applicator, but are less effective than the injection. In responders, an erection develops within 15 min and lasts for 30–60 min. Because of the uterine-stimulant activity of alprostadil, a condom is recommended if the partner is pregnant.

SELF-ASSESSMENT

True/false questions

1. Sildenafil should not be taken by men already taking nitrates.
2. Sexual stimulation is a prerequisite for sildenafil to cause an erection.
3. Phosphodiesterase (PDE) type 5 is only found in the vasculature in the penis.
4. Increased parasympathetic outflow to the penis causes a failure of erection.
5. Erections caused by injected drugs such as alprostadil are not easy to control.
6. Impotence caused by hypogonadism can be treated with oestrogen.
7. Diabetes can cause impotence.
8. The duration of the biological actions of sildenafil and tadalafil is similar.
9. Sildenafil inhibits the breakdown of cAMP.
10. Alprostadil reduces prostaglandin synthesis by inhibiting cyclo-oxygenase-1.

One-best-answer (OBA) question

Which statement concerning drug action and erectile dysfunction is the *least accurate*?

A. Alcohol can cause erectile difficulties.
B. Cimetidine can exacerbate the potential for sildenafil to cause headache.
C. Nicorandil is safe when taken together with tadalafil.
D. Amitriptyline can cause impotence.
E. Sildenafil prevents the breakdown of cGMP.

Case-based questions

Mr JA, aged 56 years, presented with erectile dysfunction of gradual onset over the last 2–3 years. He was hypertensive, with a blood pressure of 160/96 mmHg, and was being treated with atenolol and bendroflumethiazide. There was a family history of coronary artery disease. He smokes 30 cigarettes a day and drinks four pints of beer a night. Investigation revealed that he was hypercholesterolaemic and there were signs of coronary artery disease. Tests for liver function and testosterone were normal and no organic reason for the dysfunction was found. Mr JA also has recurrent heartburn, for which he is taking cimetidine on most days.

It was decided not to prescribe a pharmacological agent for his erectile dysfunction at this stage, but a number of suggestions and recommendations were made.

After 3 months, during which time Mr JA followed the advice he was given, his blood pressure was within normal limits and his cholesterol was lower. He was regularly taking cimetidine. However, his erectile dysfunction persisted.

Following discussions, it was decided that Mr JA should try sildenafil.

A. Which of the above factors could contribute to his erectile dysfunction and what recommendations would you suggest?

B. From his history, what precautions should be taken in prescribing sildenafil and what advice should Mr JA be given?

True/false answers

1. **True.** Nitrates result in increased nitric oxide production and this elevates cGMP. Sildenafil elevates cGMP by blocking its breakdown, and the combination with nitrates can lead to additive unwanted effects, particularly hypotension.
2. **True.** Sildenafil and other PDE type 5 inhibitors prolong the vasodilator action of NO produced as a result of sexual stimulation..
3. **False.** PDE type 5 is found in some other blood vessels and tissues, which can result in unwanted effects when sildenafil is given.
4. **False.** Parasympathetic stimulation enhances erection, and drugs known to inhibit the parasympathetic outflow (e.g. tricyclic antidepressants) can cause erectile failure.
5. **True.** Painful priapism with erections lasting many hours can occur with intracavernosal drugs.
6. **False.** Testosterone can be useful if the impotence is due to hypogonadism.
7. **True.** Diabetes mellitus probably causes erectile problems through vascular dysfunction.
8. **False.** Tadalafil has a much longer biological half-life than sildenafil, allowing it to be taken up to 12 hours before sexual activity.
9. **False.** Sildenafil inhibits the breakdown of cGMP, not cAMP.
10. **False.** Alprostadil is a synthetic prostaglandin E_1 analogue, which vasodilates by increasing cAMP.

OBA answer

Answer C is the least accurate.

A. True. Alcohol use is a recognised cause of erectile dysfunction.
B. True. Cimetidine inhibits the isoenzyme CYP3A4 that metabolises sildenafil, enhancing its vasodilator effects, including headache.
C. **False.** Nicorandil is a K^+ channel opener (Ch. 5) that also has a nitrate structure; this increases cGMP formation and would add to the effects of tadalafil, with the potential for increased unwanted effects.
D. True. Amitriptyline has antimuscarinic actions that could decrease blood vessel dilation in the penis, thereby inhibiting erection.
E. True. Blocking the breakdown of cGMP is the main mechanism of action of sildenafil, leading to vasodilation.

Case-based answers

A. The contribution of psychological factors in Mr JA's erectile dysfunction needs to be assessed and dealt with if they are present. Vascular disease, smoking and alcohol consumption may also contribute and Mr JA should be helped to manage these. Because of the evidence of coronary artery disease, which is known to be associated with erectile dysfunction, it would be advisable to be more intensive in treating his high blood pressure and reducing his cholesterol levels. Although this is unlikely to restore erectile function, it may improve the patient's well-being and have a psychological benefit. Beta-adrenoceptor antagonists (atenolol) and thiazide diuretics (bendroflumethiazide) can contribute to erectile problems; Mr JA could be treated with an ACE inhibitor, such as enalapril, which has not been shown to contribute to impotence.

B. Cimetidine is an inhibitor of hepatic CYP3A4 (Table 2.7) that metabolises sildenafil, so the initial dose of sildenafil should be reduced. Alternatively, Mr JA could use ranitidine, which does not inhibit CYP3A4. Studies of sildenafil in patients with a history of cardiovascular disease have shown that the simultaneous use of nitrates is an absolute contraindication. Mr JA should be told about the dangers of drug interactions and possible unwanted effects.

FURTHER READING

Andersson K-E (2001) Pharmacology of penile erection. *Pharmacol Rev* 53, 417–450

Corbin JD, Francis SH (2002) Pharmacology of phosphodiesterase-5 inhibitors. *Int J Clin Pract* 56, 453–459

McVary KT (2007) Erectile dysfunction. *N Engl J Med* 357, 2472–2481

Morgentaler A (1999) Male impotence. *Lancet* 354, 1713–1718

Sivalingam S, Hashim H, Schwaibold H (2006) An overview of the diagnosis and treatment of erectile dysfunction. *Drugs* 66, 2339–2355

Compendium: drugs used to treat erectile dysfunction[a]

Drug	Kinetics (half-life)	Comments
Phosphodiesterase type 5 inhibitors		
All PDE5 inhibitors given orally.		
Sildenafil	Oral bioavailability about 40% due to first-pass metabolism; absorption delayed by fatty food; hepatic metabolism (2h)	Taken between 30 min and 4 h before sexual activity; also used for pulmonary hypertension
Tadalafil	Bioavailability not defined, but rapid absorption not affected by food; hepatic metabolism (17 h)	Long half-life and duration of action mean tadalafil can taken up to 12 h before sexual activity
Vardenafil	Low oral bioavailability (about 15%); absorption delayed by fatty food; hepatic metabolism (4–5 h)	Usually taken about 1 h before sexual activity
Other drugs used for erectile dysfunction		
Alprostadil	Metabolic pathways undefined; very short half-life (30 s)	Prostaglandin E_1 analogue; given by intracavernosal injection or urethral application; care needed if partner is pregnant; can cause priapism; can be given with papaverine (see below)
Apomorphine	Sublingual bioavailability is 10–20%; hepatic metabolism (0.5 h)	Increases erections via agonist activity on dopamine receptors in the hypothalamus and limbic system; stimulation of the chemoreceptor trigger zone (CTZ) produces potent emetic actions; taken sublingually 20 min before sexual activity; not licensed for this indication in UK
Papaverine	Hepatic metabolism (2 h); the 4-hydroxy metabolite is a phosphodiesterase inhibitor	Smooth muscle relaxant; given by intracavernosal injection; not licensed for this indication in the UK
Phentolamine	Partially hepatic metabolism, partially eliminated unchanged in urine (1.5 h)	An α_1-adrenoceptor antagonist; given by intracavernosal injection (unlicensed indication)

[a]All drugs in this table should be used with caution in people with cardiovascular disease.

5

The nervous system

17

General anaesthetics

● ●

General anaesthetics work in the brain to induce reversible unconsciousness with amnesia, akinesia and varying degrees of analgesia. This allows surgical or other painful procedures to be undertaken without the person being aware. General anaesthesia was introduced into clinical practice in the 19th century, with the inhalation of vapours such as diethyl ether and chloroform. Major drawbacks with such compounds included the time taken to cause loss of consciousness, slow recovery, unpleasant taste, irritant properties and their potential to explode. Cardiac and hepatic toxicity also limited the usefulness of chloroform. The perfect general anaesthetic would possess the properties shown in Box 17.1, but no single anaesthetic agent has all of these. Therefore, to produce general anaesthesia it is usual to use a combination of several drugs that have different desirable and unwanted effects. Each contributes in different degrees to sedation, analgesia and muscle relaxation, an approach known as 'balanced anaesthesia' (Table 17.1). Full general anaesthesia produces not only loss of consciousness, but also depresses brainstem reflexes with loss of spontaneous respiration and depression of heart rate and blood pressure, a state that is comparable to coma.

General anaesthesia for surgical procedures involves several steps, although not all are essential for successful anaesthesia:

- premedication,
- induction,
- muscle relaxation and intubation,
- maintenance of anaesthesia,
- analgesia,
- reversal.

Premedication is given to adults to reduce anxiety and produce amnesia, usually with a benzodiazepine such as diazepam (Ch. 20). In addition, an antiemetic such as metoclopramide (Ch. 32) may be used.

Anaesthesia was originally induced and maintained solely by inhalation of a volatile agent, when several stages of general anaesthesia are observed during induction in adults (Table 17.2). The stage of excitation with struggling can be overcome by using a bolus of intravenous anaesthetic for rapid induction, followed by an inhalational anaesthetic for maintenance. For short surgical procedures in adults, both induction and maintenance can be achieved with an intravenous anaesthetic alone (total intravenous anaesthesia). In children, excitation is less of a problem, and anaesthesia is often both induced and maintained with an inhalational anaesthetic agent. Full general anaesthesia produces depression of spontaneous respiration and blood pressure, requiring artificial ventilation and perhaps circulatory support. Some short procedures do not need full general anaesthesia, and can be carried out under sedation by an anaesthetic with preserved respiratory and cardiovascular function. The adequacy of general anaesthesia is assessed by monitoring the heart rate, blood pressure and other physiological functions. For example, it can be inferred that the level of anaesthesia is inadequate and that pain is being experienced if the heart rate rises, or the person develops perspiration, tears, return of muscle tone, movement or change in pupil size.

For abdominal and thoracic surgery, and for long operations, full skeletal muscle paralysis is produced by giving neuromuscular blocking drugs (Ch. 27), in which case endotracheal intubation and mechanical ventilation are essential. Analgesia can be provided by an intravenous opioid for systemic analgesia, or by a local anaesthetic (Ch. 18) to provide regional analgesia, such as into the epidural space (epidural analgesia) or around peripheral nerves.

At the end of an operation, resumption of consciousness (reversal of anaesthesia) occurs when intravenous anaesthetics are redistributed or metabolised, or when inhalational anaesthetics are redistributed or exhaled. Residual neuromuscular blockade by competitive blocking agents may need reversal with an anticholinesterase such as neostigmine (Ch. 27). Attentiveness, and therefore the ability to drive safely, may be impaired for up to 24 h after general anaesthesia.

MECHANISMS OF ACTION OF GENERAL ANAESTHETICS

General anaesthesia can be produced by compounds of widely differing chemical structure: simple gases such as nitrous oxide, volatile liquids such as isoflurane and non-volatile solids such as propofol (Fig. 17.1). They act at several sites in the brain, but particularly the brainstem arousal centres, frontal cortex and thalamus to produce unconsciousness, and the spinal cord, pons and medulla to produce muscle relaxation.

General anaesthetics act at cell membranes, and the relationship between lipid solubility and potency led to the Meyer–Overton hypothesis that their incorporation into lipids altered the properties and function of neuronal cell membranes. However, this does not account for many of the properties of general anaesthetics, including the differing anaesthetic potencies of the stereoisomers of some anaesthetic agents which suggests stereospecific interaction with target receptors. The general relationship between lipid solubility and anaesthetic potency is probably more important for determining the pharmacokinetic properties of the drug than for explaining its mode of action.

Although it is not known precisely how general anaesthetics work, there is increasing evidence that implicates actions at ligand-gated ion channels (Table 17.3). Individual intravenous or inhalational anaesthetic agents have diverse abilities to inhibit or enhance the functions of a number of ion channels, thus explaining the differences in their capacities to produce unconsciousness, amnesia, analgesia and muscle relaxation. This may be achieved by direct interaction with the ion channel or by modulation of the receptors that control these channels. In particular, their actions are to *inhibit* the functions of excitatory receptors (such as those for acetylcholine [nicotinic] and for glutamate (*N*-methyl-D-aspartate [NMDA] receptors) and to *enhance* the functions of inhibitory receptors (such as those for γ-aminobutyric acid [GABA$_A$] and possibly glycine), or to

(A) Nitrous oxide (gas)

$$N_2O$$

(B) Isoflurane (organic liquid)

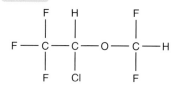

(C) Propofol (oil in water emulsion)

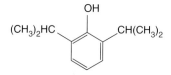

Fig. 17.1 Examples of general anaesthetics of different chemical natures.

Box 17.1 Properties of an ideal inhalational anaesthetic

Inherent stability
Non-flammable and non-explosive when mixed with air, oxygen or nitrous oxide
Potent, allowing the use of a high inspired oxygen concentration
Low blood solubility, allowing rapid induction (with minimal excitation stage); rapid emergence from anaesthesia, with no hangover; and rapid adjustment of the depth of anaesthesia
Non-irritant to the airways
Non-toxic
Lack of sensitisation of the heart to catecholamines
Analgesic
Easily reversible
Minimal interactions with other drugs
Inexpensive

Table 17.1 The concept of 'balanced anaesthesia'

	Sedation	Analgesia	Muscle relaxation
Drugs exerting a major effect	Intravenous anaesthetics Inhalational anaesthetics Premedicant benzodiazepines	Opioids Local anaesthetics	Neuromuscular blocking drugs (Ch. 27)
Drugs exerting a minor effect	Opioids Nitrous oxide	Nitrous oxide	Inhalational anaesthetics

Drugs are used in combination to produce the appropriate balance of sedation, analgesia and muscle relaxation while minimising unwanted effects; at particular doses and concentrations, each contributes minor or major effects to achieve this balance. Excessive or inadequate doses of any one agent could disturb the balance.

Table 17.2 The stages of anaesthesia

Stage	Description	Effects produced
I	Analgesia	Analgesia without amnesia or loss of touch sensation; consciousness retained
II	Excitation	Excitation and delirium with struggling; respiration rapid and irregular; frequent eye movements with increased pupil diameter; amnesia
III	Surgical anaesthesia	Loss of consciousness; subdivided into four levels or planes of increasing depth Plane I: decrease in eye movements and some pupillary constriction Plane II: loss of corneal reflex Planes III and IV: increasing loss of pharyngeal reflex, and progressive decrease in thoracic breathing and general muscle tone
IV	Medullary depression	Loss of spontaneous respiration and progressive depression of cardiovascular reflexes, no eye movements; requires respiratory and circulatory support

activate K$^+$ channels that are widely expressed in inhibitory GABA interneurons.

Receptor binding sites for general anaesthetics have not been fully characterised, but are probably on proteins associated with the receptors and ion channels. General anaesthetics may compete with endogenous ligands or modulate the effect of these ligands at the receptor. As a result, they inhibit both local and long-range (such as thalamocortical) neural circuits.

Table 17.3 Possible sites of action of inhalation and intravenous general anaesthetics[a]

Drug group	Properties of group	Receptor and channel targets
Etodimate, propofol, thiopental	Potent amnesics Potent sedatives Weak muscle relaxants	Enhance activity at GABA$_A$ receptors
Nitrous oxide, ketamine	Potent analgesics Weak sedatives Weak muscle relaxants	Inhibit glutamate NMDA receptors Inhibit ACh nicotinic receptors Open two-pore K$^+$ channels
Sevoflurane, isoflurane, desflurane	Potent amnesics Potent sedatives Potent muscle relaxants	Enhance activity at GABA$_A$ receptors Enhance activity at glycine receptors Inhibit glutamate NMDA receptors Inhibit ACh nicotinic receptors Open two-pore K$^+$ channels

ACh, acetylcholine; GABA, γ-aminobutyric acid; NMDA, N-methyl-D-aspartate.
[a]Information for this table is derived mainly from Solt and Forman (2007) and is based on data from *in vitro* studies and *in vivo* studies in transgenic animals.

The various stages of anaesthesia (Table 17.2) probably arise as a result of the different sizes of neurons affected by anaesthetics and their accessibility to the anaesthetic agent. A rapid action on small neurons in the dorsal horn of the spinal cord (nociceptive impulses; Ch. 19) and inhibitory cells in the brain (see effects of alcohol; Ch. 54) explain the early analgesic and excitation phases. By contrast, neurons of the medullary centres are less sensitive.

DRUGS USED IN ANAESTHESIA

General anaesthetics can be grouped according to their route of administration, which is either intravenous or inhalational.

INTRAVENOUS ANAESTHETICS

Examples

etomidate, ketamine, propofol, thiopental

Intravenous anaesthetics can be given by slow intravenous injection for rapid induction of anaesthesia and then replaced by inhalational anaesthetics for longer-term maintenance of anaesthesia. Both propofol and ketamine (but not etomidate or thiopental) can also be given by continuous infusion without inhalational anaesthesia for short operations (total intravenous anaesthesia) or for prolonged sedation. Ketamine is analgesic, unlike all other available intravenous anaesthetics, but it does not reliably suppress laryngeal reflexes, which can make endotracheal intubation more difficult. It is now rarely used, except for paediatric anaesthesia. Some properties of commonly used intravenous anaesthetics are shown in Table 17.4.

Table 17.4 Some properties of common intravenous anaesthetics

Drug	Type	Speed of induction	Recovery	Hangover effect	Analgesic	Comment
Thiopental	Barbiturate	Rapid	Slow, owing to redistribution; slow liver metabolism	Yes	No	Highly alkaline and causes tissue necrosis if extravasation occurs from the blood vessel at the site of injection; cannot be given by continuous infusion due to accumulation
Propofol	Phenol	Rapid	Rapid; liver metabolism	Low	No	Does not accumulate; continuous infusion can be used for total intravenous anaesthesia or for sedation of adults in intensive care
Etomidate	Imidazole	Rapid	Fairly rapid; liver metabolism	Low	No	Not infused continuously because repeated doses suppress adrenocortical function
Ketamine	Cyclohexanone	Slower	Slower	No	Yes	Can be given by continuous infusion; produces analgesia that outlasts anaesthesia; usually used for children

Pharmacokinetics

Thiopental is a thiobarbiturate that has a very rapid onset of action (within 30 s) owing to its high lipid solubility and ease of passage across the blood–brain barrier. The duration of action after a bolus dose is very short (about 2–5 min). Blood concentrations fall rapidly, initially because of distribution into tissues with greatest blood flow; distribution then occurs more slowly into the major muscle groups and into adipose tissue, which is lipid-rich but has poor blood flow (Fig. 17.2). With thiopental, total intravenous anaesthesia is not practicable, as during a lengthy procedure the brain and blood and slowly equilibrating tissues would reach equilibrium. Recovery from anaesthesia on cessation of anaesthetic administration would then depend on the elimination half-life (3–8 h for thiopental, related to hepatic metabolism) not the distribution half-life (about 3 min). Therefore, following induction of anaesthesia with thiopental, an inhalational agent is used for maintenance of anaesthesia.

Propofol has a slightly slower onset of action (about 30 s) compared with thiopental, but its duration of action is also limited by redistribution after a bolus dose. It can be given as an infusion for total intravenous anaesthesia (and for sedation in intensive care), but under these circumstances its duration of action is determined by a slower tissue distribution phase (half-life 0.5–1 h), whereas after prolonged use its duration of action is determined by

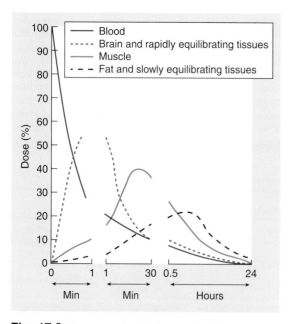

Fig. 17.2 The amounts of thiopental in blood, brain (and other rapidly equilibrating tissues), muscle, adipose tissue and other slowly equilibrating tissues after an intravenous infusion over 10 s. Note: the time axis is not linear: the continued uptake into muscle between 1 and 30 min lowers the concentration in the blood and in all rapidly equilibrating tissues (including the brain); the terminal elimination slopes are parallel for all tissues; metabolism removes about 15% of the body load per hour.

hepatic clearance (half-life about 6 h). Propofol is particularly useful for day surgery, because of its rapid distribution and absence of hangover effects. It can also be used by intravenous infusion for up to 3 days for sedation in conscious adults requiring controlled ventilation in an intensive care unit.

Ketamine can be given by intramuscular injection or intravenously by bolus injection or infusion. When used for induction or for total intravenous anaesthesia the anaesthetic action is terminated largely by distribution (half-life about 15 min). With prolonged infusion it becomes dependent on hepatic metabolism (half-life 2–4 h).

Etomidate has a rapid onset of action after intravenous injection, and its action is terminated by rapid metabolism in plasma and the liver, so that the duration of action is about 6–10 min with minimal hangover. It is not used to maintain anaesthesia because prolonged infusion can suppress adrenocortical function.

Unwanted effects

- On the central nervous system (CNS): general depression of the CNS can produce respiratory and cardiovascular depression. Slow release of thiopental distributed into tissues may result in some sedation for up to 24 h after use. Hallucinations and vivid dreams are common during recovery from ketamine (emergence reactions), but are less frequent in children. They can be reduced by giving a benzodiazepine (Ch. 20).
- On muscles: extraneous muscle movement is common with etomidate, and to a lesser degree with propofol. They can be reduced by a benzodiazepine or opioid analgesic given before induction. Ketamine increases muscle tone and can cause laryngospasm.
- On the heart: thiopental, propofol and to a lesser extent etomidate depress the heart, producing bradycardia and reducing blood pressure. By contrast, ketamine more often produces tachycardia and an increase in blood pressure.
- Nausea and vomiting during recovery are experienced by up to 40% of people but rarely persist for more than 24 h. Propofol has an anti-emetic action.
- Convulsions have been reported after propofol. These can be delayed, indicating the need for special caution after day surgery.
- Pain on injection with etomidate and propofol: this can be reduced by injecting into a large vein or by giving an opioid analgesic just before induction with etomidate, or giving intravenous lignocaine with propofol. Thiopental is an alkaline solution that is irritant if it extravasates outside the vein, causing tissue necrosis.
- Propofol is not used for continuous sedation in children because of the risk of propofol infusion syndrome, which includes metabolic acidosis, heart failure and rhabdomyolysis.

INTRAVENOUS OPIOIDS

Examples

fentanyl, remifentanil

Intravenous opioids are usually given at induction for intra-operative analgesia, therefore reducing the dose requirement of anaesthetic agents. They can also be used for sedation and respiratory depression during assisted ventilation in intensive care. In high doses, opioids stimulate the vagus and produce bradycardia; this can be helpful to reduce the tachycardia and hypertension produced by sympathetic nervous system activation during surgery. Details of the mechanism of action of opioids can be found in Chapter 19.

Pharmacokinetics

After intravenous injection, fentanyl has a rapid onset of action within 1–2 min. After a single dose the drug is distributed rapidly into skeletal muscle and fat (half-life about 15 min) and its duration of action is about 30–60 min. The effect is maintained by repeated injections or infusion, but with prolonged use tissue stores are saturated and fentanyl then has a long duration of action determined by its hepatic metabolism (half-life about 4 h). After repeated injections respiratory depression may become apparent during recovery from the anaesthetic.

Remifentanil is an opioid ester that has a similar rapid onset to fentanyl but a very short half-life of about 5 min, due to metabolism by tissue and plasma esterases. After an initial bolus dose of remifentanil continuous intravenous infusion is used to maintain its effects.

Unwanted effects

- Muscle rigidity: this particularly affects the chest wall and jaw and can be prevented during surgery with neuromuscular junction blocking drugs (Ch. 27). Myoclonus and rigidity can persist after recovery, and require reversal with the opioid antagonist naloxone (Ch. 19)
- Respiratory depression: this may be profound and means that assisted ventilation is usually necessary during surgery when large doses have been used.
- Nausea and vomiting.

INHALATIONAL ANAESTHETICS

Examples

desflurane, halothane, isoflurane, nitrous oxide, sevoflurane

Inhalational anaesthetics are either volatile liquids, which must be vaporised before administration, or gases. All inhalational anaesthetics must be given with adequate oxygen (usually a minimum 25% of the inspired gas mixture) to avoid hypoxia during anaesthesia.

Volatile liquid anaesthetics such as sevoflurane can be used for both induction and maintenance of anaesthesia, or for maintenance following induction with an intravenous anaesthetic. Sevoflurane is widely used for induction as well as maintenance in children as it has a pleasant odour. With some volatile liquid anaesthetics, such as desflurane and isoflurane, irritation of the mucous membranes makes them less suitable for induction. Recovery is rapid after sevoflurane, since it is eliminated more quickly than isoflurane, and therefore early postoperative analgesia may be necessary.

Nitrous oxide is a gaseous anaesthetic that is not sufficiently potent to be used alone (Table 17.5), but it has the advantage of producing analgesia (unlike the other inhalational anaesthetics). It is often used in combination with other anaesthetics, and reduces the required dose of the other agent. Nitrous oxide can only be used as the sole inhalational agent when combined with an intravenous opioid and a neuromuscular blocking drug (Ch. 27), but there is a risk of awareness during surgery. Nitrous oxide is also used in sub-anaesthetic doses for analgesia alone.

Pharmacokinetics

The concentration and duration of administration of inhaled anaesthetic required to give a sufficient concentration of the drug in the CNS for general anaesthesia will depend on the relationships shown in Figure 17.3 and Table 17.5. There are four factors to consider.

Table 17.5 Inhalational anaesthetics

Compound	Blood:gas partition coefficient	Induction time	Oil:gas partition coefficient	MAC (%)	Metabolism (%)
Nitrous oxide	0.5	Fast	1.4	>100	0
Isoflurane	1.4	Medium	91	1.12	0.2
Enflurane	1.9	Medium	96	1.7	2.10
Halothane	2.3	Medium	224	0.8	15
Sevoflurane	0.6	Fast	53	2.1	≈5
Diethyl ether	12.1	Slow	65	2	5–10

The blood:gas partition coefficient correlates closely with the time to induction when the drug is used as the sole anaesthetic. The oil:gas partition correlates with the potency of the anaesthetic, which correlates inversely with the minimum alveolar concentration (MAC) necessary for surgical anaesthesia. Nitrous oxide cannot produce anaesthesia alone so has a theoretical MAC of >100%. Metabolism is the percentage of drug eliminated as urinary metabolites, with the remainder eliminated mainly in the expired air. Halothane is no longer available in the UK, and diethyl ether is no longer used clinically but is included in the table for comparative purposes.

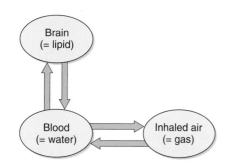

Fig. 17.3 Equilibration of inhalational general anaesthetics between air, blood and brain. The concentration ratio between blood and air at equilibrium is estimated from *in vivo* studies of the blood:gas partition coefficient and correlates with the induction time of the drug (Table 17.5). The concentrations in brain and blood at equilibrium reflect the different affinities of the two body compartments for general anaesthetics. The brain:blood ratio is 1–3:1 for all commonly used anaesthetics. The concentration in the inspired air required to give the necessary concentration in brain membranes (minimum alveolar concentration; MAC) correlates inversely with the blood:gas partition coefficient which is an indication of the potency of the compound.

1. The rate of absorption across the alveolar membranes. This depends on both the concentration of drug in the inspired air and the rate of drug delivery; that is, the rate and depth of inspiration. These factors are most important if an inhaled agent is used for induction, but less significant once equilibrium has been established between the inhaled concentration and that in the brain. Lung conditions such as emphysema, which result in poor alveolar ventilation, will slow the induction of anaesthesia.
2. The rate at which the anaesthetic concentration in the blood reaches equilibrium with that in the inspired air, which is affected by the solubility of the anaesthetic in blood and in rapidly equilibrating tissues. A high solubility in blood compared with the brain will slow the attainment of equilibrium.
3. The cardiac output, which will determine circulation time and drug delivery to the brain. This is not usually a limiting factor.
4. The relative concentrations of the drug in the brain and blood at equilibrium. The rate of entry of drug into the brain is not limiting for lipid-soluble drugs such as anaesthetics. The rate-limiting step is the rate of delivery via the inhaled gas compared with the total amount in the body at equilibrium.

Anaesthetic potency of the volatile anaesthetics is measured as the minimum alveolar concentration (MAC) of an agent necessary to immobilise 50% of subjects exposed to a noxious stimulus (which in humans is a surgical skin incision). Therefore, MAC is the equivalent of the ED_{50} (the 50% effective dose) for other drugs (Ch. 1). The MAC for inhaled anaesthetics correlates *inversely* with the oil:gas partition coefficient, which reflects the ratio between the concentration in the lipid membranes of brain cells (oil) and the

inhaled concentration (gas). A potent inhalational anaesthetic agent such as halothane has a high oil:gas ratio and this high lipid solubility means it has a low MAC (Table 17.5).

Another physicochemical property that affects the action of an inhaled anaesthetic agent is the blood:gas partition coefficient (or blood:gas ratio), which indicates the relative solubilities of the drug in blood and air. A high solubility in blood, and therefore in all rapidly equilibrating body tissues, means that a greater amount of the agent will need to be administered before its partial pressure in the blood equilibrates with that in the inspired air. The blood:gas ratio therefore correlates with the time to induction of anaesthesia. This conforms to the basic pharmacokinetic principle that compounds with a large apparent volume of distribution take longer to reach steady state during a constant rate of drug administration (Ch. 2). Table 17.5 shows that sevoflurane has a low blood:gas ratio and consequently a fast induction time, while induction with diethyl ether (which is no longer used clinically) is prolonged because of its high blood:gas ratio,

The major route of elimination of inhalational anaesthetics is via the airways in expired air. Factors that influence the duration of the induction phase, such as ventilation rate and the blood:gas partition coefficient, will also affect the time taken to eliminate the anaesthetic. Diethyl ether has a very long recovery time due its high blood:gas ratio (Table 17.5). The recovery time may also depend on the duration of inhalation, which can affect the extent to which the drug has entered slowly equilibrating tissues. Elimination from these tissues is also slow, which can maintain the plasma concentration of the drug and delay recovery. During recovery, the depth of anaesthesia reverses through the stages discussed above (Table 17.2) to consciousness; a rapid recovery which minimises stage II of anaesthesia (see Table 17.2) is beneficial.

General anaesthetics are also partly eliminated by metabolism, the extent of which depends on the time that the agent is retained in the body and is available to the metabolising enzymes. Thus, exhalation and metabolism can be regarded as alternative pathways of elimination, the proportions of which are determined largely by the volatility of the agent and its blood:gas partition coefficient (Table 17.5).

Unwanted effects

A number of unwanted effects are common to most clinically useful inhalational anaesthetics; however, each agent also has a unique profile of additional unwanted effects.

■ **Cardiovascular system.** The volatile liquid anaesthetics depress myocardial contractility and predispose to bradycardia by interfering with transmembrane Ca^{2+} flux, with a resultant decrease in cardiac output and blood pressure. Isoflurane is less cardiodepressant, but may reduce blood pressure by arterial vasodilation. Nitrous oxide also has less depressant effect on the heart and circulation and its use in combination with other agents that depress the heart may permit reduction in their dosage. Inhalational anaesthetics often increase cerebral blood flow, which can exacerbate an elevated intracranial pressure. Arrhythmias occasionally occur with volatile liquid anaesthetics.

- **Respiratory system.** All anaesthetic agents depress the response of the respiratory centre in the medulla to carbon dioxide and hypoxia. They also decrease tidal volume and increase respiratory rate. Desflurane and isoflurane are irritant to mucous membranes and can cause coughing, apnoea and laryngospasm if used for induction.
- **Liver.** Most agents decrease liver blood flow. Mild hepatic dysfunction, because of specific hepatic toxicity, is common after treatment with halothane. However, about 1 in 30 000 people will develop severe hepatic necrosis following the use of halothane, especially after repeat exposure within a short time interval. For this reason, halothane is only used after a careful anaesthetic history (especially in the preceding 3 months) and is avoided in those with a history of unexplained jaundice or pyrexia following exposure to halothane. Halothane is only available in the UK on special order. Hepatotoxicity is rare with other halogenated anaesthetics.
- **Uterus.** Relaxation of the uterus may increase the risk of haemorrhage when anaesthesia is used in labour. Nitrous oxide has less effect on uterine muscle than the volatile liquid anaesthetics.
- **Skeletal muscle.** Most agents produce some muscle relaxation, which enhances the activity of neuromuscular blocking drugs (Ch. 27). With sevoflurane this may be sufficient to enable tracheal intubation without the use of a neuromuscular blocker.
- **Chemoreceptor trigger zone.** Inhalational anaesthetics trigger postoperative nausea and vomiting. This may be most pronounced with nitrous oxide.
- **Postoperative shivering.** This occurs in up to 65% of those recovering from general anaesthesia. The aetiology is unclear.
- **Malignant hyperthermia.** This is a rare but potentially fatal complication of volatile liquid anaesthetics. It is genetically determined, and results from a defect in the ryanodine receptor (RyR1) that regulates release of Ca^{2+} from the sarcoplasmic reticulum in muscle cells (Ch. 5, Fig. 5.4). A sudden increase in intracellular Ca^{2+} produces tachycardia, unstable blood pressure, hypercapnoea, fever and hyperventilation, followed by hyperkalaemia and metabolic acidosis. Muscle rigidity may occur. Treatment is with dantrolene, which is an RyR1 receptor antagonist (Ch. 24).

SELF-ASSESSMENT

True/false questions

1. Inhalational anaesthetics may have their effect by interacting with specific receptors.
2. Inhalational anaesthetics are all gases.
3. Most inhalational anaesthetics are sulphur-containing compounds.
4. Halothane closely approaches the properties of an ideal inhalational anaesthetic.
5. The risk of hangover effects with inhalational anaesthetics increases if the operation is long.

6. The minimum alveolar concentration (MAC) of an inhalational anaesthetic required to produce surgical anaesthesia correlates inversely with the oil : gas partition coefficient of drug.
7. Nitrous oxide administered alone at a concentration of 50% in inspired air reaches the MAC necessary for surgical anaesthesia.
8. Nitrous oxide is frequently given with oxygen and a halogenated anaesthetic agent to produce effective surgical anaesthesia.
9. Isoflurane is metabolised as extensively as halothane.
10. The short duration of action of thiopental is due to its distribution into richly perfused tissues such as muscles.
11. The elimination half-life of thiopental is similar to the distribution half-life.
12. Propofol can be given alone by continuous intravenous infusion to maintain anaesthesia.
13. Accidental injection of thiopental into an artery can have serious consequences.
14. Ketamine is a sedative but is without analgesic action.
15. Fentanyl should not be administered concurrently with inhalational anaesthetics.
16. With modern anaesthetics the classical stages of anaesthesia induction are rarely seen.
17. When administering an inhalational anaesthetic, the excitement stage of anaesthesia may be prolonged if an intravenous anaesthetic is not given beforehand.
18. Most inhalational anaesthetics have a depressant effect on the cardiovascular system.
19. Inhalational anaesthetics increase the sensitivity of the respiratory centre to carbon dioxide and hypoxia.
20. Sevoflurane has the advantage of a fast onset of action and rapid elimination.

One-best-answer (OBA) question

1. Which the following is the *most accurate* statement concerning the pharmacology of agents used in anaesthesia?
   A. The respiratory medulla is particularly sensitive to the depressant action of general anaesthetics.
   B. The major route of elimination of most inhalational anaesthetics is via the liver.
   C. Metoclopramide is often given as a premedication before general anaesthesia.
   D. The intravenous opioid fentanyl should not be administered together with sevoflurane.
   E. Atropine is a commonly administered pre-operative agent.
2. Which of the following is *not* an ideal property of an inhalational anaesthetic?
   A. Stability
   B. Non-flammability
   C. Potency
   D. Analgesic action
   E. High blood : gas partition coefficient.

Case-based question

A 40-year-old woman is scheduled for a laparotomy because of an abdominal swelling. She has not had a previous operation and is otherwise healthy, with normal cardiovascular and respiratory function. She was premedicated with pethidine (meperidine) and atropine. The operation lasted 40 min. Refer to Ch.27 for information on neuromuscular junction blockers.

A. Why is atropine little used nowadays as pre-anaesthetic medication in adults?

B. Do the muscarinic receptor antagonists atropine and hyoscine have the same properties?

   The woman was intubated after the administration of thiopental, fentanyl and suxamethonium (succinylcholine).

C. Why has the routine use of suxamethonium to facilitate endotracheal intubation been reduced?

   Following intubation, pancuronium and fentanyl were given and she was ventilated with nitrous oxide, enflurane and oxygen. An ovarian cyst was removed and the operation took 40 min.

D. Is pancuronium the most suitable choice of muscle relaxant? What alternatives are available?

   After the operation, she did not breathe spontaneously, despite the administration of neostigmine and glycopyrronium.

E. What are the possible reasons for the apnoea and how could they be treated?

F. Would mivacurium (a short-duration muscle relaxant) have been a preferable muscle relaxant to use in this patient?

G. What is the reason for administering glycopyrronium with neostigmine at the end of the operation?

True/false answers

1. **True.** It is increasingly thought that general anaesthetics act at a number of excitatory and inhibitory receptors (Table 17.3).

2. **False.** Many inhalational anaesthetics are volatile liquids.

3. **False.** The main inhalational anaesthetics are halogenated compounds.

4. **False.** Halothane is potent but can cause cardiac arrhythmias, hepatotoxicity, hypotension and sensitisation of the heart to catecholamines.

5. **True.** In prolonged anaesthesia, lipid-soluble agents may accumulate in body fat stores and be slowly released after the operation.

6. **True.** The higher the oil : gas ratio, the lower the inhaled concentration of anaesthetic required to produce anaesthesia.

7. **False.** Even at concentrations higher than 50%, nitrous oxide is not potent enough to produce effective surgical anaesthesia on its own.

8. **True.** Nitrous oxide provides additional analgesic activity in combination with a fluorinated anaesthetic and oxygen.

9. **False.** Halothane undergoes substantial metabolism, but the other halogenated anaesthetics do not.

10. **True.** Rapid redistribution of thiopental from the CNS terminates its anaesthetic action.

11. **False.** The half-life of the thiopental redistribution is about 3 min, but its elimination from the body is much

slower (half-life 3–8 h), partially accounting for the hangover effect seen with this drug.

12. **True.** Propofol is useful for short operations, but its rapid elimination and little hangover effect mean that it can also be given by continuous infusion for maintenance anaesthesia, such as in intensive care units.

13. **True.** Extravascular or intra-arterial injection of thiopental can be damaging due its high pH (approximately 9–10).

14. **False.** Ketamine does have analgesic action, unlike other available intravenous anaesthetics.

15. **False.** Fentanyl is short-acting with a rapid recovery and is increasingly used for intraoperative analgesia with inhalation anaesthetics.

16. **True.** The classical stages of anaesthetic induction were originally described following the use of slower-acting anaesthetics than those used today.

17. **True.** The intravenous agent is used to provide rapid induction of anaesthesia.

18. **True.** Most are negatively inotropic and they depress myocardial function by interfering with Ca^{2+} fluxes. Halothane also sensitises the heart to catecholamines and can lead to arrhythmias.

19. **False.** Inhalational anaesthetics *reduce* the ventilatory response to carbon dioxide and hypoxia and increase the arterial partial pressure of carbon dioxide.

20. **True.** Sevoflurane is rapid in onset and more rapidly eliminated than halothane or isoflurane.

OBA answers

1. **Answer C** is correct as an anti-emetic such as metoclopramide is often used to reduce the risk of vomiting caused by general anaesthetics and opioid analgesics. Medullary centres are relatively *in*sensitive to anaesthetics (answer A). Inhalation anaesthetics are eliminated mainly by exhalation, not hepatic metabolism (answer B). Fentanyl is often used as an analgesic together with inhalational anaesthetics (answer D). With modern anaesthetic practice atropine is seldom needed to reduce bronchial and salivary secretions (answer E).

2. **Answer E** is correct as a high blood : gas ratio is associated with a long induction time, so it is *not* an ideal property of an inhalational anaesthetic. The other answers (A–D) are desirable properties of an ideal anaesthetic.

Case-based answers

A. Atropine (and hyoscine) block muscarinic receptors, reducing bronchial and salivary secretions, but modern anaesthetics have less irritant effect, thus reducing this problem. Muscarinic antagonists can reduce the bradycardia caused by some inhalation anaesthetics and by suxamethonium.

B. No. Atropine can cause CNS excitation, whereas hyoscine causes sedation and has anti-emetic properties.

C. Relatively minor but frequent complications occur with suxamethonium, including bradycardia, postoperative myalgia, transient hyperkalaemia and raised intraocular, intracranial and intragastric pressures. A rare, but potentially fatal, complication is malignant hyperthermia. The competitive blocking drug rocuronium has a short duration of action and does not cause these problems.

D. Pancuronium is probably not the ideal muscle relaxant to use as it can cause tachycardia and hypertension and is long-acting (Ch. 27). An alternative would be vecuronium, which has an intermediate duration of action and lacks cardiovascular effects. Rocuronium is more expensive but has a rapid onset and short duration of action and a low risk of cardiovascular effects.

E. There are at least three possible reasons for the postoperative apnoea. (1) Opioid-induced apnoea caused by the use of pethidine followed by fentanyl, resulting in respiratory depression. The effect could be reversed by the opioid antagonist naloxone. (2) The dose of neostigmine given may have been insufficient to reverse the competitive blockade induced by long-acting pancuronium. (3) The woman could have a genetically determined deficiency of pseudocholinesterase (plasma cholinesterase, butyrylcholinesterase), found in about 1 in 2000 individuals, which would normally metabolise suxamethonium. Administration of neostigmine would exacerbate the respiratory suppression. Fresh frozen plasma (containing pseudocholinesterase) could be given.

F. Although mivacurium is a short-acting muscle relaxant, it is metabolised by pseudocholinesterase and its effect would be greatly prolonged if the person has the genetic deficiency in this enzyme.

G. Neostigmine inhibits acetylcholinesterase, increasing acetylcholine concentrations at cholinergic synapses. It partially or fully reverses the actions of competitive blockers of N_2 receptors at the neuromuscular junction, but also enhances the activity of acetylcholine at muscarinic receptors, causing bradycardia and bronchoconstriction. Glycopyrronium is a selective muscarinic receptor antagonist used to prevent these muscarinic effects.

FURTHER READING

Brown EN, Lydic R, Schiff, ND (2010) General anesthesia, sleep, and coma. N Engl J Med 363, 2638–2650

Campagna JA, Miller KW, Forman SA (2003) Mechanisms of actions of inhaled anesthetics. N Engl J Med 348, 2110–2124

Chau P-L (2010) New insights into the molecular mechanisms of action of general anaesthetics. Br J Pharmacol 161, 288–307

Dodds C (1999) General anaesthesia: practical recommendations and recent advances. Drugs 58, 453–467

Fox AJ, Rowbottam DJ (1999) Anaesthesia. BMJ 319, 557–560

Litman RS, Rosenberg H (2005) Malignant hyperthermia. Update on susceptibility testing. JAMA 293, 2918–2924

Nathan N, Odin I (2007) Induction of anaesthesia. A guide to drug choice. Drugs 67, 701–723

Solt K, Forman SA (2007) Correlating the clinical actions and molecular mechanisms of general anesthetics. Curr Opin Anaesthesiol 20, 300–306

Compendium: general anaesthetics

Drug	Kinetics (half-life)	Comments
Intravenous anaesthetics		
Following a bolus dose, the duration of action depends on the rate of distribution and not the elimination half-life given below.		
Etomidate	Action of single dose terminated by rapid distribution; metabolism faster than thiopental (1–2 h)	Used for rapid induction (<30 s) without hangover; suppresses adrenocortical function on continuous dosage and should not be used for maintenance anaesthesia; may cause involuntary movements
Ketamine	Action of single dose terminated by rapid distribution; hepatic metabolism (2–4 h)	Analgesic activity at sub-anaesthetic doses; used for paediatric anesthesia; slower onset than other induction agents (2–5 min); transient psychotic effects (hallucinations, nightmares) may occur
Propofol	Hepatic metabolism; duration of action partly determined by distribution and partly by rapid glucuronidation in liver and other tissues; in prolonged use, drug has long half-life (3–12 h)	Most widely used intravenous anaesthetic; can be used for rapid induction (<30 s) or for maintenance; rapid recovery with little hangover
Thiopental	Action of single dose terminated by rapid distribution; on repeated dosing its slow hepatic metabolism (3–8 h) can cause accumulation in poorly perfused tissues	Reconstituted solution is highly alkaline; rapid induction (<30s) and recovery but may cause sedation up to 24 h due to slow metabolism
Intravenous opioids		
Provide analgesia and enhance anaesthesia.		
Alfentanil	Hepatic metabolism (0.7–2h)	Used especially during short procedures and for outpatient surgery; respiratory depression may persist after the end of the procedure if repeated doses are given
Fentanyl	Hepatic metabolism (1–6h)	Respiratory depression may persist after the end of the procedure if repeated doses are given
Remifentanil	Very rapid clearance by blood and tissue esterases (0.1h)	Given intra-operatively as an intravenous infusion; very rapid clearance minimises postoperative respiratory depression
Inhalational anaesthetics		
Desflurane	Eliminated by exhalation	Not recommended for induction in children; irritant, causing cough, laryngospasm and increased secretions; very rapid recovery (minutes)
Enflurane	Eliminated mainly by exhalation	Powerful cardiorespiratory depressant; largely superseded by isoflurane
Halothane	Eliminated by exhalation and significant hepatic metabolism (15%)	Potent and non-irritant but largely superseded due to risk of severe hepatotoxicity on repeated exposure; now available in the UK on special order only
Isoflurane	Eliminated mainly by exhalation	An isomer of enflurane; may decrease peripheral vascular resistance; potentiates effects of muscle relaxant drugs
Nitrous oxide	Eliminated rapidly by exhalation due to low blood:gas partition coefficient	Low potency compared with other inhaled agents precludes use as sole anaesthetic; rapid recovery owing to low potency and low tissue affinity; has analgesic activity
Sevoflurane	Eliminated rapidly by exhalation and some metabolism (≈5%)	Potent maintenance anaesthetic with rapid recovery; non-irritant so can also be used for inhalational induction

Various other drugs, such as analgesics (Chs 19 and 29) and anxiolytics (Ch. 20), are used in the perioperative period.

18

Local anaesthetics

• •

Local anaesthetics are drugs that reversibly block the transmission of pain stimuli locally at their site of administration.

Examples

bupivacaine, cocaine, lidocaine, ropivacaine

PHARMACOLOGY

MECHANISM OF ACTION

Local anaesthetics produce reversible blockade of nerve conduction and prevent impulse transmission in nerve fibres by inhibiting depolarisation of the cell. At rest, the neuronal cell membrane has only limited permeability to Na^+ but about 50–70 times greater permeability to K^+ because of the greater number of channels open for passive transport of K^+ out of the cell. The maintenance of a negative resting membrane electrical potential is largely determined by the K^+ gradient across the cell membrane, with a smaller contribution from the active Na^+/K^+-ATPase pump, which pumps out three Na^+ ions for every two K^+ ions it transports in. Conduction of a nerve action potential results from opening of voltage-dependent Na^+ channels, and rapid influx of Na^+ to depolarise the cell (see Fig. 18.2, below). Na^+ channels cycle between three states:

- **resting**, when the channel is closed but able to open in response to a change in transmembrane potential,
- **open**, when the channel opens in response to an action potential and allows the rapid influx of Na^+ ions through to the cytoplasm,

- **inactivated** due to a very rapid change in conformation at the cytoplasmic end of the channel that occurs very soon after the action potential has passed. During this stage the channel is resistant to depolarising influences, but sensitivity returns when the membrane potential is restored to the resting level.

There is considerable redundancy in the membrane Na^+ channels; as a consequence, nerve conduction can continue even when 90% of the channels are blocked.

Local anaesthetics block the voltage-dependent Na^+ channels that depolarise the cell. They bind to the Na^+ channel at a site on the inner surface of the membrane and hold them in an inactivated state. Local anaesthetics progressively interrupt Na^+ channel-mediated depolarisation until conduction fails. The probability that propagation of a nerve impulse will fail at a particular segment of the nerve is related to:

- the local concentration of the anaesthetic drug,
- the size of the nerve fibre,
- whether the nerve is myelinated,
- the length of the nerve exposed to the drug.

In general, nerve transmission is blocked in smaller-diameter fibres before that in larger fibres (Table 18.1). The myelinated Aδ and small non-myelinated C fibres that transmit pain (nociceptive fibres) are blocked before larger sensory and motor fibres. Therefore, pain pathways are most rapidly and intensely blocked by local anaesthetics (Table 18.1), and also show the longest duration of local anaesthetic effect. In myelinated nerves the drug penetrates at the nodes of Ranvier and must block at least three consecutive nodes to produce conduction block. Unmyelinated nerves must be blocked over a sufficient length and around the full circumference of the nerve.

Structural requirements of local anaesthetics

The action of local anaesthetics results mainly from binding of the ionised form of the anaesthetic to a site on the inside (cytoplasmic opening) of the Na^+ channel. Membrane penetration, however, is better in the non-ionised (lipid-soluble) form. The structural requirements for local anaesthetic activity appear to involve a minimum of a lipid-soluble hydrophobic aromatic ring structure connected to a hydrophilic amine group by a short ester or amide intermediate linkage (Fig. 18.1). Clinically used potent local anaesthetics are all secondary or tertiary amines with an intermediate amide or ester bond. The length of the intermediate bonding chain is critical to local anaesthetic activity and is optimal between three and seven carbon atoms or equivalent atoms. The lipophilic aromatic group enables

Table 18.1 Nerve fibres and their responsiveness to local anaesthetics

Fibre type	Site or function	Myelination	Diameter (μm)	Sensitivity to anaesthesia[a]
A				
Alpha	Motor Muscle sense	Yes	12–20	+
Beta	Motor (muscle spindle) Touch, proprioception	Yes	5–12	+
Gamma	Motor (muscle spindle)	Yes	3–6	++
Delta	Pain, temperature, crude touch, pressure	Yes	2–5	+++
B				
	Preganglionic autonomic	Yes	1–3	++++
C				
	Pain, temperature, touch, pressure, itch	No	0.4–1.2	+++
	Postganglionic autonomic	No	0.3–1.3	+++

[a]Increasing number of + indicates increasing sensitivity to local anaesthesia.

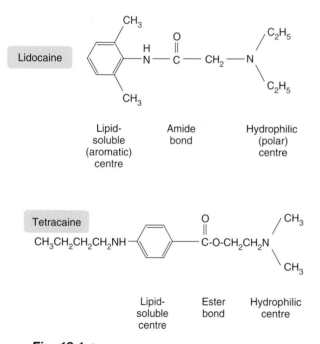

Lidocaine

Lipid-soluble (aromatic) centre | Amide bond | Hydrophilic (polar) centre

Tetracaine

Lipid-soluble centre | Ester bond | Hydrophilic centre

Fig. 18.1 General structure of local anaesthetics. All local anaesthetic structures contain a lipophilic centre and a hydrophilic centre linked by an amide or ester bond.

for longer and have a long duration of action. Thus, procaine, which has a low binding affinity (6% protein bound), has a very short duration of action, whereas bupivacaine has a high binding affinity (95% protein bound) and a long duration of action.

The pK_a of the drug determines the extent of ionisation at physiological pH and the speed of onset of the conduction block. All local anaesthetics are weak bases and will be relatively more ionised at a pH below the pK_a (which for most local anaesthetics is between 7.7 and 9.1). Because the water solubility of a local anaesthetic is greatest in the ionised form, injectable preparations are formulated as the hydrochloride salts with a pH of 5.0–6.0. However, the base (non-ionised) form is more lipid-soluble and more readily penetrates lipid membranes; therefore, after injection, the drug solution (pH 5.0–6.0) must be buffered in the tissues to physiological pH (7.4) before a significant amount of non-ionised local anaesthetic is available to penetrate the nerve and reach its site of action. A drug with a high pK_a will be more ionised at physiological pH, and the speed of onset of anaesthesia will be slower. Alkalinisation of the injected solution by adding bicarbonate will increase the proportion of the drug in its non-ionised lipid-soluble form and therefore increase the rate of absorption of the anaesthetic into the nerve which will accelerate the onset of action.

In contrast, it is the ionised form of the drug that binds to the receptor within the cytoplasmic opening of the Na^+ channel. Drugs with a higher pK_a will re-ionise to a greater extent within the cell (pH 7.4) and produce more effective blockade. The majority of the local anaesthetic molecules therefore pass across the cell membrane in their non-ionised form and enter the cytosol where they become ionised and available to bind to the protein receptor via the cytoplasm. The binding site is most accessible when the channel is in its open (activated) state (Fig. 18.2). For this reason the effectiveness of most local anaesthetics is dependent on the frequency of firing of the neuron (use-dependency), and a faster onset of local anaesthesia occurs in rapidly firing neurons. Once the local anaesthetic has

the molecule to cross the nerve membrane, and the potency of the drug is directly related to its lipid solubility.

Specific intraneuronal binding

Local anaesthetics bind to a receptor protein within the cytoplasmic opening of the Na^+ channel, and compounds with high protein-binding affinity stay at the site of action

INTRACELLULAR   EXTRACELLULAR

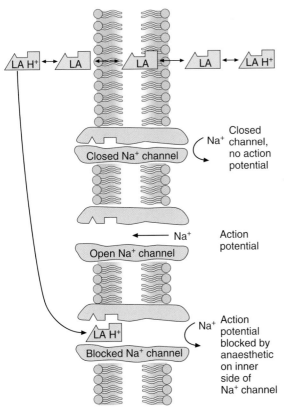

Fig. 18.2 Site and mechanism of action of local anaesthetics. Local anaesthetics are weak bases and exist in an equilibrium between ionised (LA + H⁺) and non-ionised (LA) forms. The non-ionised form is lipid-soluble and crosses the axonal membrane, allowing the ionised form to bind to the intracellular end of the receptor. Some non-ionised anaesthetic may reach the ion channel by diffusion within the cell membrane, become ionised within the Na⁺ channel and then bind to the receptor site.

bound to the channel, the influx of Na⁺ is blocked and the channel remains in the *inactivated* state and resistant to further depolarisation. The local anaesthetic does not dissociate from the channel when it is inactivated as it has a high affinity for the channel in this state. The local anaesthetic leaves the binding site when the membrane potential returns to its resting level, and the channel is in the *resting* state. This is further facilitated when the cytoplasmic concentration of the drug decreases as it diffuses away from the site of administration.

Local anaesthetics bind to K⁺ channels, but very weakly compared to Na⁺ channels. This binding may contribute to toxic effects of local anaesthetics in other organs such as the heart.

Local anaesthetics also bind to other ion channels and cell receptors, including presynaptic Ca^{2+} channels, tachykinin type 1 receptors, glutamate, bradykinin B_2 and acetylcholine receptors. These actions may be involved in

reducing nociceptive neurotransmission and in the production of spinal anaesthesia.

PHARMACOKINETICS

As seen above, the speed of onset of local anaesthetic action is largely determined by the physicochemical properties of the drug molecule. The duration of action of local anaesthetics is dependent on the degree of receptor binding (see above) and on their rate of removal from the site of administration, rather than their systemic elimination by metabolism. Most local anaesthetics cause vasodilation at the site of injection, which will enhance their removal. In contrast, cocaine, which blocks noradrenaline reuptake by noradrenergic neurons (Ch. 4), produces intense vasoconstriction. Because of the risk to local tissue integrity associated with the vasoconstriction, cocaine is never given by injection and its medical use is restricted to topical anaesthesia in otolaryngology. The duration of action of any local anaesthetic can be extended considerably by co-administration with a vasoconstrictor such as an α₁-adrenoceptor agonist, for example adrenaline (epinephrine). However, the pH of the solution must be 2.0–3.0 to prevent decomposition of the adrenaline (epinephrine). Local anaesthetic preparations with other vasoconstrictors such as phenylephrine or felypressin are also available.

Once the local anaesthetic has diffused away from the site of administration it enters the general circulation and undergoes elimination from the body. Most local anaesthetics have an intermediate amide bond, and are eliminated at least in part by hepatic hydrolysis of the amide bond. The half-life of amide local anaesthetics within the circulation is generally between 1 and 3 h. In contrast, the plasma half-lives of the ester drugs procaine and tetracaine are 3 min or less, since ester bonds are very rapidly hydrolysed by plasma esterases.

UNWANTED EFFECTS

Local effects

These occur at the site of administration and include irritation and inflammation. Local ischaemia can occur if local anaesthetics are co-administered with a vasoconstrictor; therefore this should be avoided in the extremities such as the digits. Tissue damage with necrosis can follow inappropriate administration (e.g. accidental intra-arterial administration or spinal administration of an epidural dose).

Systemic effects

These are related to the anaesthetic action, and usually result from excessive plasma concentrations that affect other excitable membranes such as the heart (see antiarrhythmic action of lidocaine; Ch. 8). After regional anaesthesia, the maximum plasma drug concentration occurs within 30 min, requiring close observation for toxic effects during this period. Toxic plasma concentrations of drug are more likely after accidental intravenous injection, or rapid absorption from highly vascular sites or from inflamed tissues. Intravenous lipid emulsions are a recommended adjunct to resuscitation when treating severe toxicity with circulatory arrest. Lipid emulsion probably works by partitioning the drug away from receptors within tissues.

- **Central nervous system (CNS) effects:** high concentrations of local anaesthetics can produce light-headedness, paraesthesia, dizziness, nausea and vomiting progressing to sedation and loss of consciousness. Severe reactions can be accompanied by convulsions and respiratory arrest. CNS toxicity tends to occur before cardiovascular toxicity, but this is not invariable.
- **Cardiovascular effects:** high plasma concentrations can cause tachycardia and arrhythmias. Serious arrhythmia is a particular problem with bupivacaine and is caused by its avid tissue binding in the heart. As a result of its high lipid solubility and high protein binding, it has a fast-in, slow-out kinetic pattern at the Na$^+$ channel. Bupivacaine (particularly the R(+)-isomer) blocks the normal cardiac conducting system and predisposes to ventricular re-entrant pathways and intractable ventricular arrhythmias, possibly a consequence of binding to ATP-sensitive K$^+$ channels (see Ch. 8). More profound toxicity can lead to cardiovascular collapse from systemic vasodilation and a negative inotropic effect. Levobupivacaine and ropivacaine have about the same local anaesthetic potency but less potential to produce cardiac effects, having less effect on cardiac Na$^+$ channels.
- **Allergy:** true allergy is rare, but can occur with ester agents due to their metabolism to p-aminobenzoic acid (PABA). For this reason, amide bond local anaesthetics are more commonly used.

TECHNIQUES OF ADMINISTRATION

The extent of local anaesthesia depends largely on the technique of administration.

SURFACE ADMINISTRATION

High concentrations (up to 10%) of drug in an oily vehicle can slowly penetrate the skin or mucous membranes to give a small localised area of anaesthesia. Lidocaine can be applied as a cream to an area before a minor skin procedure or venepuncture. Benzocaine is a relatively weak local anaesthetic that is included in some throat pastilles to produce anaesthesia of mucous membranes. Cocaine is restricted to topical use in otolaryngeal procedures, to produce vasoconstriction and reduce mucosal bleeding.

INFILTRATION ANAESTHESIA

A localised injection of an aqueous solution of local anaesthetic, sometimes with a vasoconstrictor, produces a local field of anaesthesia. The anaesthetic effect produced is more efficient than surface anaesthesia, but requires a relatively large amount of drug. Smaller volumes can be used for field-block anaesthesia, involving subcutaneous injection close to nerves around the area to be anaesthetised. This technique is used extensively in dentistry.

PERIPHERAL NERVE BLOCK ANAESTHESIA

Injection of an aqueous solution around a nerve trunk produces a field of anaesthesia distal to the site of injection. This can also be used for temporary sympathetic nerve block, such as the stellate ganglion, or for lumbar sympathectomy.

EPIDURAL ANAESTHESIA

Injection or slow infusion via a cannula of an aqueous solution adjacent to the spinal column, but outside the dura mater, produces anaesthesia both above and below the site of injection after 15–30 min. The extent of anaesthesia depends on the volume of drug administered and the rate of delivery. It is unaffected by the position of the person receiving the injection. Epidural anaesthesia is used extensively in childbirth for pain relief (using a local anaesthetic with an opioid) and for surgical anaesthesia, either alone or in combination with a general anaesthetic. The concentration of drug used is the same as that for spinal anaesthesia, but the volume (10–20 mL), and therefore the dose, is greater. For this reason, systemic unwanted effects are more frequent than with spinal anaesthesia. Sympathetic fibres are particularly sensitive to local anaesthetics (Table 18.1); this can result in hypotension that can be particularly exaggerated during pregnancy (probably related to the concurrent effects of high progesterone concentrations). Backache is a frequent postoperative complication with both epidural and spinal anaesthesia.

SPINAL ANAESTHESIA

This involves injection of an aqueous solution (1.5–2.5 mL) of local anaesthetic alone (often bupivacaine) or with an opioid into the lumbar subarachnoid space, usually between the third and fourth lumbar vertebrae. The spread of anaesthetic within the subarachnoid space depends on the density of the solution (a solution in 10% glucose is more dense than cerebrospinal fluid) and the posture of the person during the first 10–15 min while the solution flows up or down the subarachnoid space. Anaesthesia is produced after about 5 min and can be used for surgical procedures below the umbilicus lasting for up to 2 h. Spinal and epidural anaesthesia can be used together.

INTRAVENOUS REGIONAL ANAESTHESIA

This involves injection of a dilute solution of local anaesthetic into a limb after application of a tourniquet (Bier's block). It is used for manipulation of fractures and minor surgical procedures. Arterial blood flow must not be occluded for more than 20 min.

SELF-ASSESSMENT

True/false questions

1. The block produced by local anaesthetics is more rapid and complete when the nerve is actively firing.
2. Local anaesthetics have no systemic unwanted effects.
3. Local anaesthetics block smaller myelinated axons more effectively than larger myelinated axons.
4. The α_1-adrenoceptor antagonist prazosin is added to local anaesthetics to extend their duration of activity.
5. Local anaesthetics in their non-ionised form penetrate the axon more readily than in their ionised form.
6. Ropivacaine is a long-acting local anaesthetic.

One-best-answer (OBA) question

Which of the following is the *most accurate* statement about local anaesthetics?

A. Raising the pH of a local anaesthetic solution will increase its speed of onset.
B. Liver metabolism is the primary mechanism in terminating local anaesthetic action.
C. The effectiveness of a local anaesthetic is not altered by local tissue pH.
D. Direct effects on blood vessel diameter of most commonly used local anaesthetics prolong their duration of action.
E. Adrenaline (epinephrine) is given with a local anaesthetic injection in digits and appendages to increase the duration of anaesthesia.

Extended-matching-item question

Choose the *most appropriate* drug A–F for each situation 1–4 below.

A. Cocaine
B. Adrenaline (epinephrine)
C. Salbutamol
D. Tetracaine
E. Lidocaine
F. Benzocaine

1. A child needed a minor surgical procedure on her nasopharynx and you chose to use a single agent that could be administered topically to reduce mucous membrane bleeding.
2. An agent that would extend the duration and potency of a local anaesthetic.
3. An agent that could be applied topically to produce anaesthesia of the conjunctiva which would not cause vasoconstriction.
4. An agent that could be administered intravenously in the treatment of ventricular arrhythmias.

True/false answers

1. **True.** This is because most local anaesthetics gain better access to binding sites in Na^+ channels that are in the open state.
2. **False.** If absorbed, systemic high doses of local anaesthetics can produce cardiovascular collapse and CNS depression.
3. **True.** For example $A\delta$ axons (2–5 μm diameter) are blocked more readily than motor fibres (12–20 μm diameter).
4. **False.** Prazosin is a vasodilator and would increase removal of the local anaesthetic from its injection site; a vasoconstrictor like adrenaline (epinephrine) is necessary.
5. **True.** The non-ionised form is lipophilic and better able to cross the axon membrane.
6. **True.** Ropivacaine is a long-acting local anaesthetic (2–4 h) similar to bupivacaine but is less arrhythmogenic.

OBA answer

Answer A is correct.

A. Most local anaesthetics are weak bases (pK_a 7–9). Raising the pH will increase the amount of the non-ionised form and therefore enhance lipid solubility and membrane penetration.
B. Local anaesthetic action is terminated mainly by uptake from tissues into the systemic circulation, not by hepatic metabolism.
C. Altered local pH could change the ratio of the ionised and non-ionised forms of the local anaesthetic, affecting its potential to penetrate membranes (when non-ionised) and block Na^+ channels (as the ionised form).
D. With the exception of cocaine, local anaesthetics dilate blood vessels, hastening their removal from the site of injection and shortening their duration of action.
E. Adrenaline (epinephrine) should not be given with a local anaesthetic for injection in digits and appendages because of the risk of ischaemic necrosis.

Extended-matching answers

1. Answer **A**. Cocaine can be administered topically and, unlike other local anaesthetics, inhibits the neuronal uptake of released noradrenaline, resulting in vasoconstriction.
2. Answer **B**. Adrenaline (epinephrine) causes vasoconstriction and the administered local anaesthetic resides at its site of injection for a longer period.
3. Answer **D**. Tetracaine is poorly absorbed and is used topically for conjunctival anaesthesia.
4. Answer **E**. Lidocaine can be given intravenously for the treatment of ventricular arrhythmias (Ch. 8).

FURTHER READING

Heavner SE (2007) Local anaesthetics. *Curr Opin Anaesthesiol* 20, 336–342

Scholz A (2002) Mechanisms of (local) anaesthetics on voltage-gated sodium and other ion channels. *Br J Anaesth* 89, 52–61

Tetzlaff JE (2000) The pharmacology of local anesthetics. *Anesth Clin North Am* 18, 217–233

Veering BT (2003) Complications and local anaesthetic toxicity in regional anaesthesia. *Curr Opin Anaesthesiol* 16, 455–459

Wiklund RA, Rosenbaum SH (1997) Anesthesiology. Part II. *N Engl J Med* 337, 1215–1219

Yanagidate F, Strichartz GR (2007) Local anesthetics. *Handb Exp Pharmacol* 177, 95–127

Compendium: local anaesthetics

Drug	Kinetics (half-life)	Comments
Articaine	Half-life 1 h when used to produce regional anaesthesia; hydrolysed by plasma esterases	Used in dentistry; concentrations in tooth alveolus are 100 times those in circulation
Benzocaine	Minimal oral absorption; hepatic metabolism (<1 min)	Used in throat lozenges
Bupivacaine	Hepatic metabolism (2–4 h)	Used for local infiltration anaesthesia, peripheral nerve block, epidural block and sympathetic block; slow onset (1–10 min) and long duration of action (3–9 h); more cardiotoxic than lidocaine
Cocaine	Hepatic metabolism (1–2 h)	Very rapid onset of action; used topically on mucosal surfaces (the only legal route!); profound CNS effects limit clinical usefulness
Levobupivacaine	Hepatic metabolism (1–3 h)	The *S*(–)-isomer of bupivacaine; similar to bupivacaine but less cardiotoxic
Lidocaine	Hepatic metabolism (1–2 h)	Used for local infiltration anaesthesia, intravenous regional anaesthesia, nerve blocks and dental anaesthesia; also used topically; for use in ventricular dysrhythmia, see Chapter 8
Mepivacaine	Hepatic metabolism (2–3 h)	Used in dentistry
Prilocaine	Hepatic metabolism (1–2 h)	Used for local infiltration anaesthesia, intravenous anaesthesia, nerve blocks and dental anaesthesia; may cause methaemoglobinaemia (especially in infants)
Procaine	Very rapid ester hydrolysis at site of injection and in plasma (minutes)	Seldom used now; local infiltration anaesthesia
Ropivacaine	Hepatic metabolism (2–4 h)	Similar to bupivacaine but less cardiotoxic; used for epidural, major nerve block and field block
Tetracaine	Poorly absorbed; rapidly hydrolysed by pseudocholinesterase (3 min)	Mostly used topically

19 Opioid analgesics and the management of pain

PAIN AND PAIN PERCEPTION

Pain is a complex phenomenon that involves the person's awareness of, and response to, a noxious stimulus. Pain is highly subjective to the individual, and psychological factors will determine to what extent the individual experiences suffering or distress (Fig. 19.1). Pain can be *acute*, lasting only until the initiating trauma resolves, which is sometimes described as *nociceptive pain*. Pain can also become protracted and *chronic*, outlasting the original trauma, and can in some cases become intractable as a result of persistent pathological change in the way that the nociceptive (pain-carrying) neuronal pathways function (*neuropathic pain*).

Nociceptive pain is a defensive response to a variety of stimuli (e.g. mechanical, thermal or chemical) that activate nociceptor sensory units on nerve endings. It is defensive as it induces behaviour that avoids exacerbation of the pain, and allows us to protect a damaged part of the body while it heals. Painful stimuli are transmitted to the central nervous system (CNS) by two types of fibre. Fast fibres in the neospinothalamic pathways (mechanical and thermal stimuli) carry pain that is appreciated as sharp and localised, while slow fibres in the paleospinothalamic pathways (chemical stimuli) produce poorly localised aching, throbbing or burning pain (Fig. 19.2).

Neuropathic pain may result from abnormal neuronal activity that persists beyond the time expected for healing of the injury. Examples include phantom limb pain following amputation and shingles causing pain well beyond the healing of the injury. There are multiple pathophysiological mechanisms underlying neuropathic pain. Neuropathic pain can be spontaneous (stimulus-independent), when it is usually described by the sufferer as shooting or lancinating sensations, electric shock-like pain or an abnormal unpleasant sensation (dysaesthesia). Alternatively, it can be an exaggerated response to a painful stimulus (hyperalgesia) or a painful response to a trivial stimulus (allodynia).

Some pain states have mixed nociceptive and neuropathic elements, for example mechanical spinal pain with local nerve damage such as radiculopathy or myelopathy.

The pathophysiological and molecular explanations for nociceptive and neuropathic pain and the endogenous responses that modulate pain are complex and incompletely understood. In brief, the genesis of nociceptive pain results from initial stimulation of afferent sensory neurons (nociceptors) by thermal, mechanical or chemical stimuli sufficient to stimulate the nociceptors (free nerve endings responsive to high-threshold noxious stimuli) on Aδ and C axons (Fig. 19.3). Nociceptors carry many surface receptors that modulate their sensitivity to stimulation, such as those for γ-aminobutyric acid (GABA), opioids, bradykinin, histamine, serotonin (5-hydroxytryptamine, 5-HT) and capsaicin, and mechanosensitive ion channels (responsive to touch, pressure, etc.). The particular type of painful stimulus may determine which receptors or ion channels are activated. Activation of the ion channels or receptors results in an influx of Na^+/Ca^{2+} sufficient to generate action potentials in the nerve (Fig. 19.3). Most nociceptors are dormant (silent), but when tissue damage occurs nociceptors that were not normally active can be recruited and sensitise the area to painful stimuli. The afferent fibres from these nociceptors enter both the dorsal and ventral horns of the spinal cord, and link to ascending pathways. Chemical transmission of the afferent impulse travels across synapses in the spinal cord and in the projections of the ascending pathways to the thalamus, and from there to the reticular formation and the cortex. Transmitters in these central pathways include excitatory substances such as glutamate, tachykinins (neurokinins and substance P) and calcitonin gene-related peptide (CGRP). Synaptic transmission responsible for nociceptive pain can be reduced by local inhibitory neurons, mediated by GABA. There are also important descending modulatory pathways arising from the locus coeruleus that inhibit ascending pain pathways, with a further host of neurotransmitters including endogenous opioids, noradrenaline (acting on α_2-adrenoceptors) and serotonin. Activation of these systems produces hyperpolarisation of neurons in the pain pathways (by inhibiting Na^+/Ca^{2+} influx and enhancing K^+ efflux) and prevents generation of nociceptive action potentials (Figs 19.4 and 19.5). The endogenous cannabinoids (anandamide and 2-arachidonyl glycerol) may also have modulatory functions in the descending pathways.

Activation of pain pathways generates intracellular protein synthesis through stimulation of the proto-oncogene c-Fos and various inducible transcription factors in CNS neurons. These mediate the many changes in neuronal structure and the neuronal proliferation that occur with chronic pain.

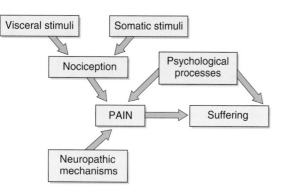

Fig. 19.1 The origin of pain and suffering.

Neuropathic pain may result from chronic hypersensitisation and phenotypic change in neurons. These changes can occur both peripherally and centrally, probably as a result of repetitive stimulation of synaptic transmission. In neuropathic and other chronic pain states, the following mechanisms may be important.

- **Sensitisation of afferent inputs**: this may include recruitment of silent nociceptors and a lower threshold for generation of action potentials in the spinal cord (through the action of cytokines released from glial cells), leading to enhanced action potential generation (Figs 19.3 and 19.5). Central sensitisation is also important with excessive neurotransmitter release. Abnormal voltage-gated Na^+ channel expression may also be important in both peripheral and central sensitisation.
- **Dysfunctional descending pain-modulatory and -facilitatory pathways**: the functioning of the descending modulatory pathway (Fig. 19.4) may become inadequate as a result of persistent nociceptive pain. Persistent painful stimuli may be related to the overactivity of endogenous pain facilitatory pathways that run in tracts from the medulla to the spinal dorsal horn. The imbalance in the pain pathways then maintains neuropathic pain states.
- **Loss of inhibitory neurons and generation of new synapses that act as nociceptive neurons (neuronal plasticity)**: in neuropathic pain, Aβ nerve fibres that normally transmit tactile stimuli can sometimes undergo phenotypic change and take on the properties of a nociceptive neuron.

ANALGESIC DRUGS

Non-steroidal anti-inflammatory drugs (NSAIDs; Ch. 29) and opioids are the major classes of pain-relieving (analgesic) drugs. They act at different levels in the pain-transmitting pathways to influence the production and recognition of pain as indicated in Figures 19.3 and 19.4.

Non-steroidal anti-inflammatory drugs

These act mainly by blocking the peripheral generation of the nociceptive impulses. Prostaglandins enhance

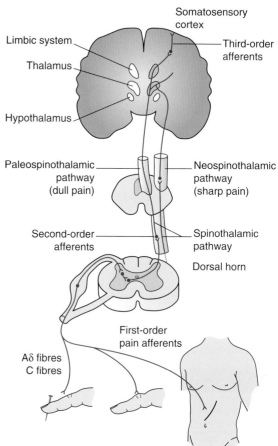

Fig. 19.2 Ascending pathways of pain perception. Ascending pathways are activated following stimulation of afferent sensory nociceptive nerve terminals. Many mediators and neurotransmitters are involved during afferent stimulation of the nociceptive pathway. Mediator release (bradykinin, serotonin, prostaglandins) and thermal and mechanical influences can stimulate and sensitise the sensory nerve terminals of pain fibres, resulting in increased cation influx, depolarisation and generation of action potentials (see Fig. 19.3). Onward afferent transmission of ascending nerve impulses at the synapses in the dorsal horn involves transmitters such as substance P, glutamate and calcitonin gene-related peptide (CGRP) (Fig. 19.5). Hyperexcitability of pain fibres can also be promoted by other mediators. Prolonged activation of the nociceptive pathways can produce pathophysiological and phenotypic changes resulting in neuropathic pain that persists when the original pathological cause of the pain has resolved, and generation of nociceptive signals can occur at low levels of axonal stimulation.

nociceptive impulses in peripheral afferent neurons by enhancing the ability of thermal, mechanical or chemical stimuli to increase Na^+/Ca^{2+} influx and thereby to generate action potentials in nociceptive afferent neurons. NSAIDs inhibit the production of prostaglandins by the cyclo-oxygenase type 1 and type 2 (COX-1, COX-2) isoenzymes and thereby reduce the sensitivity of sensory nociceptive

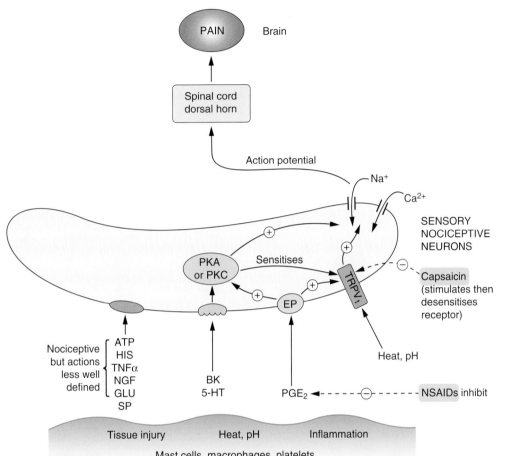

Fig. 19.3 **Mediators involved in the genesis and modulation of pain.** Numerous mediators are able to stimulate or sensitise primary sensory neurons (nociceptors), leading to activation of nociceptive fibres. Tissue injury and other noxious stimuli such as heat or extremes of pH can stimulate the release of substances that act to promote pain, such as bradykinin (BK) and serotonin (5-hydroxytryptamine, 5-HT). Prostaglandin E_2 (PGE$_2$) acting at prostaglandin E receptors (EP) sensitises the nerve endings to the actions of nociceptive mediators including BK and 5-HT. ATP and histamine (HIS) also have nociceptive actions, acting in poorly defined ways. Heat and H^+ stimulate the transient receptor potential vanilloid 1 (TRPV$_1$) receptor, producing pain. The TRPV$_1$ receptor is also sensitised by many other mediators. Capsaicin and other TRPV$_1$ receptor stimulants desensitise the receptor on persistent stimulation, resulting in an analgesic effect. Non-steroidal anti-inflammatory drugs (NSAIDs) inhibit the production of PGE$_2$. Overall the effect of nociceptive stimuli is to depolarise the neuron, setting up action potentials in the fibres to the dorsal horn and pain-perceiving areas of the brain. Substance P (SP) and calcitonin gene-related peptide (CGRP) may also be involved in nociception. GLU, glutamate; NGF, nerve growth factor; PKA, protein kinase A; PKC, protein kinase C; TNFα, tumour necrosis factor α.

nerve endings to agents released by injured tissue that initiate pain, such as bradykinin and substance P. NSAIDs may also act on pain pathways in the CNS. Paracetamol, although not usually considered to be an NSAID, may also work in part through the same pathways. These drugs are considered fully in Chapter 29.

Opioids

These act on the spinal cord and limbic system, and stimulate the long descending inhibitory pathways from the midbrain to the dorsal horn. They produce their effects via specific receptors that are closely associated with the neuronal pathways which transmit pain from the periphery to the CNS.

Non-opioid, non-NSAID analgesics

A variety of drugs that were developed for other purposes are being used increasingly for their analgesic actions when NSAIDs and opioids are less effective, for example in neuropathic pain (see Table 19.2, below).

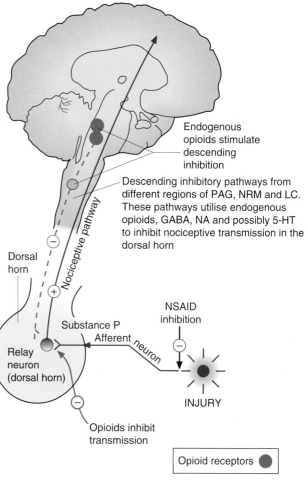

Fig. 19.4 Transmitters and receptors for pain perception and control. The afferent nociceptive pathways are subject to inhibitory control. Opioids act at opioid receptor-rich sites in the periaqueductal grey matter (PAG), the nucleus raphe magnus (NRM) and other midbrain sites to stimulate descending inhibitory fibres that inhibit nociceptive transmission in the dorsal horn. Descending pathways from the locus coeruleus (LC) that are noradrenergic are also involved. Opioids also act at a local level in the dorsal horn (Fig. 19.5). Inhibitory modulation of nociceptive transmission via local nerve networks also results from actions of other agents (Fig. 19.5). 5-HT, 5-hydroxytryptamine (serotonin); GABA, γ-aminobutyric acid; NA, noradrenaline; NSAID, non-steroidal anti-inflammatory drug.

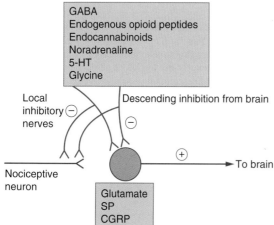

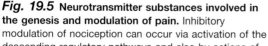

Fig. 19.5 Neurotransmitter substances involved in the genesis and modulation of pain. Inhibitory modulation of nociception can occur via activation of the descending regulatory pathways and also by actions of local interneurons. 5-HT, 5-hydroxytryptamine (serotonin); CGRP, calcitonin gene-related peptide; GABA, γ-aminobutyric acid; SP, substance P.

OPIOID ANALGESICS

Examples

buprenorphine, codeine, diamorphine (heroin), dihydrocodeine, fentanyl, methadone, morphine, oxycodone, tramadol

Opioid is a term used for both naturally occurring and synthetic molecules that produce their effects by an agonist action at opioid receptors. The terms opiate analgesic (specifically, a drug derived from the juice of the opium poppy, *Papaver somniferum*) and narcotic analgesic (which literally means a 'stupor-inducing pain killer') are no longer used.

Mechanism of action

The brain produces several endogenous opioid peptides, which are neurotransmitters that act via specific opioid receptors. Among these are the two pentapeptide enkephalins. These each contain the amino acid sequence Tyr-Gly-Gly-Phe as the message domain, linked to either leucine or methionine, and are called leu-enkephalin and

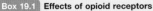

Box 19.1   **Effects of opioid receptors**

Mu (μ) or MOP
    Analgesia (supraspinal μ_1, spinal μ_2)
    Respiratory (μ_2)
    Euphoria
    Miosis
    Physical dependence
    Sedation
    Inhibition of gastrointestinal motility
Kappa (κ) or KOP
    Analgesia (spinal, peripheral)
    Sedation
    Miosis
    Dysphoria
Delta (δ) or DOP
    Analgesia (spinal)
    Respiratory depression
    Inhibition of gastrointestinal motility

met-enkephalin. Other agonists incorporating the same amino acid sequence are dynorphins A and B and the most potent agonist β-endorphin, a 31-amino acid peptide with met-enkephalin at its carboxyl end. Two further peptides, endomorphins 1 and 2, have been identified that have Tyr-Pro-Phe and Tyr-Pro-Trp message domain sequences. All opioid peptides are derived by selective cleavage of larger precursor molecules.

Opioid receptors are found on the presynaptic and postsynaptic membranes of neurons in CNS pain pathways, and also in the peripheral nervous system. Three major classes of opioid receptor have been identified, which mediate distinct effects: the μ (mu), κ (kappa) and δ (delta) receptors, also termed MOP, KOP and DOP, respectively (Box 19.1). There is a distinctive regional distribution of opioid peptides and their receptors in the CNS, with high concentrations in the limbic system and spinal cord. These regions also contain high concentrations of a neutral endopeptidase (enkephalinase), which rapidly hydrolyses the pentapeptides into fragments. The various endogenous opioid peptides show preferential receptor-binding affinities: β-endorphin binds equally to μ- and δ-receptors, endomorphins bind mainly to μ-receptors, dynorphins bind preferentially to κ-receptors and the enkephalins bind preferentially to δ-receptors. The different physiological effects produced by these receptors are due to their specific neuronal distributions. An 'orphan' opioid receptor has been identified that does not bind the major opioid peptides, which has been named the nociceptin receptor after its specific endogenous agonist. It is widely distributed in the brain and facilitates descending enkephalinergic pathways in the spinal cord.

Opioid receptors are found on both presynaptic and postsynaptic neurons. The postsynaptic actions inhibit neuronal depolarisation, and the presynaptic effect inhibits neurotransmitter release. All opioid receptors are coupled to inhibitory G-proteins (G_i/G_0), and receptor activation has many intracellular consequences:

■ inhibition of adenylyl cyclase with reduced intracellular generation of cAMP, which reduces neurotransmitter release,

■ phosphorylation of extracellular signal-regulated kinase (ERK) may be important in suppression of the immune system,

■ activation of voltage-gated inwardly rectifying K⁺ channels, which hyperpolarises the target cells, making them less responsive to depolarising impulses,

■ inhibition of voltage-gated N-type Ca^{2+} channels in target neurons, which reduces neurotransmitter release.

Morphine and synthetic opioid analgesics produce their effects largely by acting as agonists at specific opioid receptors in the CNS. Opioid drugs show receptor selectivity and can have agonist, partial agonist or antagonist properties at various opioid receptor types (Table 19.1). The analgesic action of opioids is the result of a complex series of neuronal interactions. In the nucleus raphe magnus of the brain, μ-receptor stimulation decreases activity in inhibitory GABA neurons that project to descending inhibitory serotonergic neurons in the brainstem. These neurons in turn connect presynaptically with afferent nociceptive fibres in the dorsal horn of the spinal cord. Inhibition of the GABA neurons permits increased firing of the descending inhibitory serotonergic neurons. Analgesia is produced by inhibition of the release of the pain pathway mediators, substance P, glutamate and nitric oxide from the afferent nociceptive neurons (Fig. 19.5). Activation of κ-receptors antagonises the analgesia produced by μ-receptor stimulation, by inhibiting the descending (pain-modulating) serotonergic neurons in the pain pathway. However, there is a paradoxical spinal analgesic effect from unopposed κ-receptor activation.

Opioid receptors are also present on peripheral nerves in the pain pathways, and a μ-receptor agonist reduces the sensitivity of peripheral nociceptive neurons to pain stimuli, particularly in inflamed tissues. Non-neuronal κ-receptors are involved in the inflammatory response, and are found on endothelial cells, T-lymphocytes and macrophages; κ-receptor agonists are being developed to modulate the inflammatory response orchestrated by these cells.

■ **Full agonists**: these act principally at μ-receptors and include morphine, diamorphine, fentanyl, pethidine, codeine and dihydrocodeine. They also have weak agonist activity at δ- and κ-receptors.

■ **Mixed agonist–antagonist**: pentazocine has agonist effects at the κ-receptor (and, to a lesser extent, the δ-receptor) and is a weak μ-receptor antagonist.

■ **Mixed partial agonist–antagonist**: buprenorphine is a potent partial agonist at the μ-receptor and has antagonist activity at κ-receptors. The latter action will enhance the analgesic action produced via the μ-receptors.

Some opioids have additional properties: meptazinol is a μ-receptor agonist with muscarinic receptor agonist activity; tramadol and methadone are μ-receptor agonists that also inhibit neuronal noradrenaline and serotonin uptake. These supplementary actions of tramadol and methadone contribute to their analgesic actions, since amine-mediated neurotransmission potentiates descending inhibitory pain pathways (Fig. 19.4). Methadone is also an antagonist at glutamate N-methyl-D-aspartate (NMDA) receptors, an action which can also inhibit pain transmission (Fig. 19.5).

Opioid receptor antagonists such as naloxone have no analgesic actions and are used in the treatment of opioid overdose (Ch. 53).

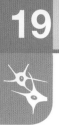

Table 19.1 Opioid analgesics

Compound	Analgesic potency	Tolerance and dependence	Actions and comments
Alfentanil	+++	–	Selective μ-receptor agonist; not used for management of *chronic* pain and therefore tolerance and dependence not relevant
Buprenorphine	++++	++	Partial μ-receptor agonist and κ-receptor antagonist; can precipitate withdrawal in individuals dependent on other opioids; action only partly reversed by naloxone (opioid antagonist)
Codeine	+	+	Selective μ-receptor agonist; antitussive and antidiarrhoeal actions; produces little respiratory depression
Dextropropoxyphene	(+)	+	Selective μ-receptor agonist; withdrawn in the UK in 2005; reports of fatalities with overdose, especially when taken with alcohol
Diamorphine (heroin)	++++	++++	Potent μ-receptor agonist; acetylated prodrug is more lipid-soluble than morphine
Dihydrocodeine	+	+	Similar profile to codeine
Dipipanone	++	++	Less sedating than morphine
Fentanyl	+++	+	Selective μ-receptor agonist; more potent than morphine
Hydromorphone	+++	+++	Selective μ-receptor agonist; similar to morphine in most properties
Meptazinol	+	–	Behaves as a mixed agonist/antagonist and lacks withdrawal and dependence symptoms
Methadone	+++	++	Potent and selective μ-receptor agonist; also a monoamine reuptake inhibitor; slow onset and long duration of action support major use for withdrawal from morphine/heroin dependence
Morphine	+++	+++	Strong μ-receptor agonist with weak agonism at κ-and δ-receptors; standard opioid against which other opioids are compared; potent analgesic; commonly causes euphoria, respiratory depression, nausea and vomiting
Nalbuphine	+++	+	Mixed action; μ-receptor antagonist, partial κ-receptor agonist and δ-receptor agonist; similar potency and efficacy to morphine but with fewer unwanted effects and a lower abuse potential; more effective in women than in men
Oxycodone	+++	++	Agonist of μ- and κ-receptors; similar pharmacological profile to morphine
Pentazocine	+++	++	κ-Receptor agonist, but weak antagonist at μ-receptors; will provoke a withdrawal syndrome in a morphine-dependent person; may cause hallucinations
Pethidine (meperidine)	++	+	Selective μ-receptor agonist; not useful for antitussive or antidiarrhoeal effects; less respiratory depression and less suppression of uterine contractility than other opioids; antimuscarinic activity may cause tachycardia
Remifentanil	+++	–	Selective μ-receptor agonist; used by injection for intraoperative analgesia; not used for management of *chronic* pain and therefore tolerance and dependence not relevant
Tramadol	+	+	Dual mechanism of action as μ-receptor agonist and as weak inhibitor of monoamine reuptake; opioid analgesia is enhanced by increased serotonergic and noradrenergic pathway activity; less potential for respiratory depression

Effects and clinical uses

Effects on the central nervous system

Analgesia

The analgesia produced by morphine is most effective for chronic visceral pain, but can still be helpful for some types of neuropathic pain. In addition to its antinociceptive effect, morphine alters the perception of pain, making it less unpleasant. This supraspinal effect, possibly at the limbic system, is less marked with some opioids such as pentazocine. Opioid analgesics have no anti-inflammatory effect. In fact, morphine can release the inflammatory mediator histamine locally at the site of an injection. Full μ-receptor agonists are the most powerful opioid analgesics (see Table 19.1 for list of full and partial agonists). However, some full μ-receptor agonists, for example codeine, have a low affinity for the receptors and have a limited analgesic effect. There is growing evidence that the antagonist action of methadone at NMDA receptors can produce effective analgesia in people who have become tolerant to high doses of morphine (see below). Short-acting opioids such as fentanyl and remifentanil are used for analgesia during general anaesthesia (Ch. 17).

The ceiling analgesic effect of a μ-receptor partial agonist is lower than that of a full agonist. If a person receiving high doses of a potent full μ-receptor agonist is given a μ-receptor partial agonist (e.g. buprenorphine) or a μ-receptor antagonist (e.g. pentazocine), then some of the full agonist molecules will be displaced from receptor sites by the less effective partial agonist molecules or antagonist molecules. The degree of analgesia may then be reduced, and in dependent individuals withdrawal symptoms can be produced (see below and Table 19.1).

Euphoria

The use of morphine is often associated with an elevated sense of well-being (euphoria, mediated by μ-receptors), an action that contributes considerably to its analgesic efficacy. The opposite effect (dysphoria, mediated by agonist activity at κ-receptors) counteracts the euphoric action, and the degree of euphoria produced will depend on the receptor-binding characteristics of the drug.

Respiratory depression

The sensitivity of the respiratory centre to stimulation by carbon dioxide is reduced by morphine at doses that produce analgesia. Respiratory depression is a common cause of death in opioid overdose. Occasionally, the effect on respiratory rate can be of clinical benefit; for example, intravenous morphine relieves the dyspnoea associated with acute pulmonary oedema, and morphine is used orally or by subcutaneous infusion for the treatment of breathlessness in palliative care. Meptazinol and tramadol are claimed to cause less respiratory depression than other opioids.

Suppression of the cough centre

Opioids possess an antitussive action. Compounds such as codeine and dextromethorphan are effective for cough suppression (Ch. 13), despite having relatively weak analgesic effects.

Vomiting

Opioids stimulate the chemoreceptor trigger zone and cause vomiting in up to 30% of people. Tolerance to the nausea and vomiting can occur with repeated doses. Powerful opioids such as morphine are usually given with an anti-emetic (Ch. 32), particularly when used for acute pain.

Miosis

Stimulation of the third-nerve nucleus results in pupillary constriction. Pinpoint pupils, together with coma and slow respiration, are signs of opioid overdose (Ch. 53).

Endocrine effects

Opioids inhibit the hypothalamic–pituitary–adrenal axis, leading to a progressive decline in plasma cortisol levels (Ch. 44). They also increase prolactin and decrease luteinizing hormone release, which leads to testosterone deficiency in men and a reduction in oestrogen synthesis in women (Chs 45 and 46). Men usually benefit from testosterone replacement during long-term opioid use (Ch. 46).

Peripheral effects

Gastrointestinal tract

There is a general increase in resting tone of the gut wall and sphincters. These effects arise from stimulation of μ- and κ-receptors on neuronal plexuses in the gut wall. An increase in biliary pressure caused by opioid-induced spasm at the sphincter of Oddi can exacerbate biliary colic. In the stomach, a decrease in motility and pyloric tone can produce anorexia, nausea and vomiting. In the small and large intestines there is increased segmenting activity and decreased propulsive activity. Thus, opioid administration is associated with constipation, and up to 80% of people who take opioids in the long term will need a laxative. Methylnaltrexone, a specific antagonist of peripheral opioid receptors, is used to treat opioid-induced constipation during palliative care when laxatives are inadequate. The effects of opioids on gastrointestinal motility make them useful in the treatment of diarrhoea (Ch. 35). Pethidine and tramadol have less effect on the gastrointestinal tract than do equi-analgesic doses of morphine.

Cardiovascular system

Opioids have little effect on the heart or circulation except at high doses that can depress the medullary vasomotor centre. Hypotension can occur with parenteral use of morphine, possibly because of histamine release.

Other systems

Opioids have minor effects on other systems. For example, there is an increase in tone of the bladder wall and sphincter, which can lead to urinary retention. There is increasing evidence that long-term use of opioids suppresses immune function by inhibiting the development and differentiation of many types of immune cells. The clinical relevance of this is not known.

Tolerance and dependence

Tolerance and dependence result from changes in the functioning of opioid receptors during continuous opioid administration. As a consequence of adaptive changes, more of the drug is necessary to produce the same effect (tolerance) and withdrawal of the drug produces adverse physiological effects until the compensatory changes are reset (dependence).

Tolerance to opioids occurs in two ways. Associative (learned) tolerance has a major psychological component. Non-associative (adaptive) tolerance involves downregulation or desensitisation of opioid receptors. This arises in response to increased firing of neurons in the noradrenergic pathways of the locus coeruleus (an area of the brain involved in the physiological response to stress, which is rich in inhibitory opioid receptors), and activation of the reward pathway in the brain (see Ch. 54). It may also involve increased activity at NMDA receptors for excitatory glutamate-mediated neurotransmission in spinal and supraspinal circuits. Tolerance to the analgesia, euphoria, respiratory depression and emesis develops rapidly during regular opioid administration, but much less to the constipation or miosis. A high degree of cross-tolerance is shown by many opioids; consequently, individuals who develop tolerance to one opioid are often (but not invariably) tolerant to another. Opioid-induced NMDA receptor activation can also produce abnormal pain sensitivity at spinal cord dorsal horn cells. This sensitisation process can be confused with tolerance and lead to opioid dose escalation. Methadone may be useful in this situation (see above).

Dependence manifests itself as a withdrawal syndrome, which can be precipitated when individuals who have taken the drug for a long period of time have their intake stopped or are given an opioid antagonist or partial agonist (Ch. 54). This is most often a problem for people who abuse the drug, but can occur from long-term intake of a prescribed opioid.

During the first 12 h after opioid withdrawal, effects such as nervousness, sweating and craving are largely psychological, because they can be alleviated by the administration of a placebo. Following this period the effects of physiological dependence manifest themselves; for example, dilated pupils, anorexia, weakness, depression, insomnia, gastrointestinal and skeletal muscle cramps, increased respiratory rate, pyrexia, piloerection with goose-pimples, and diarrhoea. The time course for the development and resolution of these symptoms varies among the opioids. In the case of morphine, the maximum intensity of withdrawal effects occurs quickly (after about 1–2 days) and subside rapidly (about 5–10 days), and often the intensity of the symptoms is intolerable.

In contrast to morphine, withdrawal from methadone is a slow process because of its very long half-life, but the effects are far less intense (peak effect at almost 1 week and symptoms persist for about 3 weeks). Therefore, morphine- or heroin-dependent individuals who have been abusing the drug are often transferred from their drug of abuse to methadone prior to withdrawal (opioid-substitution therapy). Methadone also produces less euphoria than morphine or heroin. After a period of treatment with methadone, the methadone dosage is gradually reduced and the person undergoes a more tolerable withdrawal. Buprenorphine is used as an alternative to methadone, and produces less sedation and a low intensity of withdrawal symptoms. It can be given for 6 days in a rapid detoxification programme, or for long-term maintenance for reducing relapse in people who are addicted to opioids, since its partial agonist activity blocks the 'high' from illicit opioid use.

Rapid in-hospital tapering of opioids over 2 weeks has an early 80% success rate. On an outpatient basis, slow tapering over 6 months is more successful than rapid withdrawal, but still leads to only a 40% success rate. Long-term buprenorphine therapy, combined with high-intensity psychosocial group therapy, has achieved up to 75% withdrawal rates after 1 year. Detoxification from opioids can be helped by the presynaptic α_2-adrenoceptor agonists clonidine or lofexidine (a clonidine analogue with fewer unwanted effects). These inhibit the excessive sympathetic nervous system activity associated with opioid withdrawal, such as lacrimation, rhinorrhoea, muscle pain, joint pain and gastrointestinal symptoms. However, the lethargy, insomnia and restlessness persist.

Naltrexone is a μ- and κ-receptor antagonist and a weak agonist at the δ-receptor. It blocks the effects of opioid agonists, and is used for prevention of relapse in people who were dependent on opioids, and who have withdrawn for at least 7–10 days.

Pharmacokinetics

The pharmacokinetic properties of individual opioid analgesics are summarised in the Compendium at the end of this chapter. Most opioids are available for oral use. However, buprenorphine is formulated for sublingual absorption, and fentanyl as a sublingual or buccal tablet or a nasal spray for rapid pain relief. Some opioids, such as morphine, buprenorphine, meptazinol, methadone, oxycodone and tramadol can be given by intravenous or intramuscular injection. Morphine and oxycodone can also be given by subcutaneous infusion in palliative care. Diamorphine is more potent than morphine and can be given by subcutaneous infusion in smaller volumes, which can be useful for emaciated people. Morphine and pentazocine are available as suppositories. Fentanyl and buprenorphine can be delivered transdermally via self-adhesive patches for prolonged analgesia.

Some opioids, such as morphine, have a low and variable absorption across the gut wall, and the dose should be reduced when given parenterally to achieve equivalent analgesia and avoid unwanted effects. Others, such as dihydrocodeine, have a low oral bioavailability due to extensive first-pass metabolism. Opioids are eliminated by hepatic metabolism. A metabolite of morphine, morphine 6-glucuronide, has more analgesic activity than the parent compound and is excreted by the kidney. The dose of morphine must therefore be reduced in renal failure. Diamorphine is an acetylated morphine derivative that is converted to morphine by hydrolysis in plasma and in most tissues, including the brain. Codeine is a prodrug that is metabolised by CYP2D6, which shows genetic polymorphism, to several active metabolites. Codeine 6-glucuronide is responsible for most of the analgesic activity, while about 5% is converted to morphine. About 10% of people have low CYP2D6 activity, and have a reduced analgesic response to codeine.

Most opioid analgesics have half-lives in the range of 1–6 h. For long-term pain control, morphine, and some other powerful opioids, is often given as a modified-release formulation to prolong the duration of action. Fentanyl has a short half-life (1–6 h) but can be given as a transdermal delivery patch, when pain relief lasts 12–24 h due to slow drug delivery (Ch. 2). In addition, the effect persists for several hours after removing the patch owing to build-up of a subcutaneous drug reservoir at the site of application. Care is necessary both to maintain analgesia and to avoid unwanted opioid effects if the dose of fentanyl is increased or fentanyl patches are changed for another opioid.

Unwanted effects

The unwanted effects of opioids are caused by their actions on those opioid receptors that are not the primary site for

Table 19.2 The mechanisms of action of some non-opioid, non-NSAID analgesics[a]

Drug	Mechanism[b]
Gabapentin, pregabalin	GABA concentrations increased
Carbamazepine, lamotrigine	Membrane stabilisation; Na^+ channel blockade; attenuation of glutamate-related synaptic transmission
Baclofen	$GABA_B$ receptor agonist; attenuation of glutamate-related synaptic transmission
Clonidine	α_2-Adrenoceptor agonist
Tricyclic antidepressants (imipramine, amitriptyline)	Increase noradrenaline availability
Ketamine, dextromethorphan	Glutamate NMDA receptor antagonists
Local anaesthetics	Neuronal transmission (Na^+ channel block)
Capsaicin	Substance P depletion, stimulation of vanilloid ($TRPV_1$) receptor followed by desensitisation
Cannabinoids	Stimulation of cannabinoid (CB) receptors

GABA, γ-aminobutyric acid; NMDA, *N*-methyl-D-aspartate; $TRPV_1$, transient receptor potential vanilloid 1.
[a]The mechanisms of pain control by these classes of drugs are imperfectly understood. Some are selective in their actions. For example, pain related to diabetic neuropathy and post-herpetic neuralgia (shingles), but not lower back pain, responds to tricyclic antidepressants.
[b]See also Fig. 19.3 for details about mechanism.

therapeutic benefit. For example, respiratory depression and constipation are unwanted effects when an opioid is used as an analgesic, but the same effects are therapeutically beneficial in the treatment of breathlessness or diarrhoea. Tolerance and dependence can also be regarded as unwanted problems associated with long-term use.

NON-OPIOID, NON-NSAID AGENTS USED FOR ANALGESIA

A diverse group of drugs are now being used for pain control in circumstances where opioids and NSAIDs are inadequate (Table 19.2). These are dealt with individually in the next section and the detailed pharmacology of the drugs is given in the chapters describing their main clinical uses.

PAIN MANAGEMENT

THE ANALGESIC LADDER

Appropriate management of pain depends on its origin and severity. The analgesic ladder developed by the World

Box 19.2   The analgesic ladder

Step 1   Non-opioid analgesics, e.g. paracetamol, NSAIDs
Step 2   Opioid suitable for moderate pain ± simple analgesics
Step 3   Opioid suitable for severe pain ± simple analgesics

Adjuvant analgesics (non-opioid, non-NSAID) may be required at any step (see text).

Health Organization (WHO) is useful for choosing drug therapy appropriate to the level of pain (Box 19.2).

Step 1 drugs

Paracetamol (Ch. 29) is suitable for mild pain. However, an NSAID (Ch. 29) may be more appropriate if there is local inflammation. The choice will be determined by the balance of benefits and risks of NSAIDs. Examples of pain that respond better to an NSAID are soft-tissue injury, tissue compression, visceral pain caused by pleural or peritoneal irritation and bone pain caused by metastatic deposits. Bone metastases cause local secretion of prostaglandins, and NSAIDs can be particularly effective. Individual responses to an NSAID vary; about 60% of people will respond to an alternative drug even if the first was ineffective.

Step 2 drugs

A weak opioid should be added to a step 1 drug for moderate pain, or when the response to a step 1 drug is inadequate. Opioids suitable for moderate pain include codeine and dihydrocodeine. These are often used in combination with paracetamol, such as the compound formulation co-codamol (codeine and paracetamol), although the dose of opioid in some combinations is too low to produce useful additional analgesia. Tramadol has been advocated at this stage, but it is no more effective than co-codamol, and claims that it has less effect on respiration and gastrointestinal motility are of uncertain clinical importance.

Step 3 drugs

The drug of choice for moderate to severe pain is morphine. It is usually effective orally, using a rapid-onset formulation for initial pain control. Doctors are often unwilling to give adequate doses of strong opioid because of concern about addiction. In severe chronic pain this is not an issue, and it should not be used as a reason for avoiding the use of morphine in non-cancer pain. Opioid addiction is not a problem when opioids are given appropriately for relief of pain.

ACUTE PAIN

Acute pain usually has an obvious cause and is often accompanied by anxiety. For rapid pain relief in a self-limiting condition, for example migraine, a readily absorbed, short-acting drug will be appropriate. For more protracted conditions, for example sprains, a long-acting drug may be helpful to improve adherence by reducing the frequency of administration.

The principles of the WHO analgesic ladder should be followed. Very severe acute pain, for example with myocardial infarction, will require a powerful opioid such as morphine given intravenously for rapid effect. Intramuscular injection should be avoided if possible, since severe pain is often accompanied by sympathetic nervous system stimulation which produces peripheral vasoconstriction and thereby delays drug absorption. Some acute severe pain, such as that arising postoperatively or from trauma, renal colic, cholecystitis, pancreatitis or sickle cell crisis, should be treated initially with a powerful analgesic, then less powerful analgesics as the condition resolves. This involves applying the principles of the WHO analgesic ladder in reverse.

Postoperative pain has many components, including hyperalgesia in the area of the incision, local ischaemia in the wound and central neuronal sensitisation in addition to the inflammatory response to surgery. Many studies have shown that the treatment of postoperative pain is often inadequate. There is some evidence that intraoperative and postoperative opioid use can increase the risk of hyperalgesia (acute opioid-induced hyperalgesia), an effect that can be modulated by the use of α_2-adrenoceptor agonists (such as clonidine), cyclo-oxygenase (COX)-2 inhibitors (Ch. 29) or glutamate NMDA receptor antagonists (such as ketamine or methadone).

Persistent postsurgical pain is common, and is usually considered to be present if symptoms continue for more than 2 months after the procedure. There are many surgical, psychosocial, genetic and environmental factors that predict the development of this condition. Postoperative regional anaesthesia and combination analgesic regimens can reduce the risk of developing the syndrome. Although the principles of the WHO pain ladder are still important for management of postoperative pain, it is clear that combinations of regional anaesthetic techniques (Ch. 18) and analgesics (including those more commonly used for neuropathic pain) after surgery may be important to ensure optimal outcomes.

CHRONIC PAIN

Chronic pain is usually defined as pain lasting for at least 3 months, or at least until acute tissue pathology that initiated the pain would have been expected to heal. It can be a result of persistent nociceptive stimulation or can have a neuropathic origin. There are numerous psychosocial contributors to the development of chronic pain as well as physical pathology, and therefore management of much chronic pain is more effective if facilitated by multidisciplinary pain teams. Drug therapy is not the only solution for chronic pain, and, depending on the cause, non-pharmacological or local treatments are often appropriate. Examples include:

- surgery for neoplastic, structural or ischaemic disorders,
- physical methods such as acupuncture, transcutaneous electrical nerve stimulation (TENS; which activates spinal inhibitory neurons by acting as a counter-irritant) and local anaesthetic nerve block (Ch. 18),

- behavioural modification, for example biofeedback, relaxation techniques, hypnosis,
- a corticosteroid (Ch. 44) for raised intracranial pressure or spinal cord compression, or to reduce inflammation which can be associated with a cancer.

As for neuropathic pain, many forms of chronic non-cancer pain, such as fibromyalgia, osteoarthritis or low-back pain respond better to adjuvant analgesics such as tricyclic antidepressants or anticonvulsant drugs (see below) than to conventional analgesics. Combinations of both adjuvant and conventional analgesics are often used. If conventional analgesia is needed (especially for nociceptive pain and several types of cancer-related pain) then the principles of escalation of analgesia described by the WHO analgesic ladder should be followed.

For most severe chronic nociceptive pain morphine is the treatment of choice. If pain remains severe with a low initial dosage of morphine, the dosage should be increased by 50–100% every 24 h. Once the pain is moderate in intensity, increments of 25–50% daily are usually sufficient to achieve control without excessive unwanted effects. A modified-release formulation of morphine can be substituted once a stable dosage has been determined, although a rapid-acting formulation may still be required to treat breakthrough pain. Oral administration may not be possible if there is vomiting, dysphagia or intestinal obstruction. In these circumstances, rectal administration of morphine or subcutaneous infusion of morphine using a syringe driver can be used. Diamorphine can also be given by epidural or intrathecal injection for intractable pain. Transdermal delivery of an opioid such as fentanyl from an adhesive patch is an alternative to modified-release oral morphine. There is substantial evidence that if a person is unable to tolerate a particular opioid then an alternative opioid may be better tolerated. The factors that predict intolerance to a particular agent are poorly understood, although it is now recognised that intolerance to morphine may be associated with a mutation in the multidrug resistance 1 transporter protein (Chs 2 and 52). Oxycodone is increasingly used as an alternative to morphine, and there is evidence that the response to methadone can persist when other μ-receptor agonists are ineffective.

NEUROPATHIC PAIN

Neuropathic pain, such as trigeminal neuralgia, post-herpetic neuralgia and phantom limb pain after an amputation, often responds less well than nociceptive pain to conventional analgesia. Although the mechanisms of neuropathic pain are now better understood there is still little agreement on how to use this knowledge to direct treatment. As with all forms of chronic pain a multidisciplinary approach that considers the psychosocial contributors to the pain and promotes appropriate physical activity is often necessary.

First-line treatment is usually with an anticonvulsant that binds to voltage-gated Ca^{2+} channels (such as gabapentin or pregabalin) (Ch. 23). Tricyclic antidepressants (Ch. 22) that increase synaptic noradrenaline and serotonin concentrations in the descending spinal inhibitory pathways are an alternative first-line approach (Figs 19.4 and 19.5). The importance of noradrenaline in modulating pain is shown by the lack of efficacy of selective serotonin reuptake inhibitor (SSRI) antidepressants for neuropathic pain. However, selective serotonin and noradrenaline reuptake inhibitors (SNRI) such as duloxetine (Ch. 22), which have fewer unwanted effects than tricyclic antidepressants, can be effective.

Opioids are useful in some cases of stimulus-independent pain when central mechanisms may be important. Other pharmacological treatments that are sometimes considered include baclofen (Ch. 24) and the NMDA receptor antagonist ketamine (Ch. 17), which modulate spinal transmission of the pain signal. The use of cannabinoids (the active components of cannabis; Ch. 54) for relief of hyperalgesia in conditions such as multiple sclerosis is receiving considerable attention. Stimulation of cannabinoid receptors produces an antinociceptive action and inhibits pain transmission in the spinal cord.

Stimulus-evoked pain may respond to topical treatment if it is localised and arises from peripheral mechanisms. Lidocaine cream or topical patches can be effective through its local anaesthetic actions (Ch. 18) for conditions such as mechanical allodynia in post-herpetic neuralgia. Alternatively, capsaicin, a derivative of red chilli peppers that stimulates C fibres in the afferent nociceptive pathway, can be applied topically as a counter-irritant. This releases substance P and stimulates the transient receptor potential vanilloid 1 (TRPV$_1$) receptor and initially provokes hyperalgesia by promoting depolarisation and action potential generation. Subsequent depletion of substance P and even nerve terminal degeneration then blocks nerve function (Fig. 19.3).

Trigeminal neuralgia is distinct from other forms of neuropathic pain. It can be treated surgically, but also responds well to carbamazepine (Ch. 23), which can reduce the frequency and intensity of attacks. Alternative treatments include phenytoin and lacosamide (Ch. 23).

SELF-ASSESSMENT

True/false questions

1. Opioids inhibit pain transmission in the dorsal horn of the spinal cord.
2. Opioids can cause euphoria or dysphoria.
3. Tolerance develops uniformly to all of the biological effects of the opioids
4. Morphine can cause itching and vasodilation at injection sites.
5. Methadone has a rapid onset of action and a short half-life.
6. Meptazinol is a pure μ-receptor agonist.
7. Naloxone is a short-acting opioid agonist.
8. Drugs that inhibit the reuptake of noradrenaline can be effective analgesics in neuropathic pain.
9. Anticonvulsants should not be used in the treatment of neuropathic pain.
10. Buprenorphine is a partial agonist at μ-opioid receptors.
11. Pentazocine can precipitate withdrawal symptoms in morphine addicts.
12. Pethidine (meperidine) is used in childbirth because of its short half-life.

One-best-answer (OBA) questions

1. Which of the following is the *most appropriate* statement about opioid analgesics?
   A. In the elderly, tolerance rapidly develops to the constipating effects of morphine.
   B. An opioid analgesic is the drug of choice for phantom limb pain following a below-knee amputation after a road traffic accident.
   C. The analgesic potency of codeine and dihydrocodeine are similar to that of morphine.
   D. Tolerance does not develop to the miotic effect of opioids.
   E. Fentanyl can be used for opioid withdrawal and maintenance of the chronically relapsing heroin addict.
2. Choose the *most accurate* statement about opioid drugs.
   A. Heroin (diamorphine) is too toxic for clinical use.
   B. Morphine suppresses pain by reducing histamine release in inflamed tissues.
   C. Fentanyl can be administered transdermally.
   D. Naloxone is used to treat opioid addiction.
   E. Morphine is acid-labile and must be given parenterally.

Case-based questions

Pain control in terminal cancer: a 60-year-old man was admitted to a hospice. He had previously had a left nephrectomy for renal cell carcinoma and now had intense metastatic bone pain in his ankles, right iliac crest and left upper arm. He was also having periods of dyspnoea. Prior to admission, his medication was co-codamol three times daily and diclofenac (150 mg) at night. He was also taking cimetidine (400 mg) twice daily. His pain was not well controlled on admission. After a week of assessment and optimisation of drug therapy, his treatment comprised the following drugs.

Morphine, modified release	260 mg	once or twice daily
Morphine, oral solution	50 mg	when required
Diclofenac, slow release	150 mg	at night
Dexamethasone	2 mg	three times daily
Metoclopramide	10 mg	three times daily
Lansoprazole	30 mg	once daily
Docusate sodium	100 mg	three times daily
Temazepam	20 mg	at night

1. Was this man taking an opioid analgesic before admission to the hospice?
2. How does morphine exert its pharmacological action as an analgesic?
3. Why was oral morphine solution (an immediate-release form) made available in addition to the slow-release formulation?
4. Was the dependence potential of morphine likely to present a problem in this man?
5. What alternative opioids might you consider as an immediate replacement for morphine?
6. How does diclofenac control inflammation and why was it useful in this man?
7. What was the rationale for the use of dexamethasone?

8. Metoclopramide is an anti-emetic. Why do you think that this man was likely to suffer from nausea and possibly vomiting?
9. How does metoclopramide act to alleviate nausea and what other anti-emetic drugs could be used?
10. Why might gastric or duodenal ulceration be a problem in this man?
11. Why was cimetidine given before admission and why was it replaced with lansoprazole?
12. Why was constipation likely to be a problem in this man?
13. What is the mechanism of action of docusate sodium and what alternative laxative agents could have been used?
14. Why was temazepam given?

True/false answers

1. **True.** Opioids act at opioid receptors to block transmitter release and postsynaptic trasmission in the dorsal horn.
2. **True.** In people who have pain, analgesia is often associated with well-being (μ-receptors), whereas in pain-free people dysphoria can occur (κ-receptors).
3. **False.** Much less tolerance to miosis and constipation develops than to the other biological effects of opioids, including analgesia and respiratory depression.
4. **True.** Morphine is an alkaloid which in parenteral doses may release histamine from mast cells, leading to itch, vasodilation and hypotension.
5. **False.** Methadone has good oral absorption and less potential to cause euphoria, so it is used in controlled withdrawal in people with opioid dependence. Its slow onset of action and long half-life mean that withdrawal symptoms are more gradual and less intense than with morphine or heroin.
6. **True.** Because the μ-opioid receptors produce analgesia and the κ-receptors are involved in respiratory depression, it is claimed that meptazinol has less respiratory depressant action.
7. **False.** Naloxone is a short-acting opioid *antagonist*, blocking μ-, κ- and δ-receptors. It is used in opioid overdose, although severe withdrawal symptoms can occur in people addicted to opioids following naloxone administration.
8. **True.** Tricyclic antidepressants can be effective for the treatment of some cases of neuropathic pain. They may act by enhancing amine levels in the descending inhibitory pathways that control the pain gate mechanism (see Table 19.2).
9. **False.** Anticonvulsants such as carbamazepine and lamotrigine can be of use in the treatment of neuropathic pain, probably by stabilising neuronal membranes and inhibiting release of excitatory neurotransmitters, while gabapentin and pregabalin increase levels of the inhibitory transmitter γ-aminobutyric acid (GABA).
10. **True.** The partial agonism of buprenorphine at μ-opioid receptors is associated with lower abuse potential than morphine.
11. **True.** A partial agonist (such as pentazocine) can reduce the effects of a full agonist (such as morphine) at the same receptor.

12. **True.** The short half-life of pethidine reduces respiratory depression in the neonate and allows rapid adjustment of dosage. Pethidine also has less suppressive effect on the uterine muscles than morphine.

OBA answers

1. **Answer D** is correct.
   A. Constipation continues to be a problem with long-term morphine treatment, and laxatives are often required.
   B. Chronic pain is usually less responsive to opioids, and non-opioid treatments (e.g. anticonvulsants) may be required.
   C. Codeine and dihydrocodeine are *less* potent analgesics than morphine.
   D. This is correct. Miosis is one of the signs of opioid abuse.
   E. Fentanyl is not suitable. Methadone can be used as a substitute in the detoxification process.
2. **Answer C** is correct
   A. Unlike the street drug, heroin for medical use is not contaminated and can be effective for severe pain in terminal cancer and acute myocardial infarction.
   B. Opioid analgesia occurs by central action and not by effects on histamine release in inflamed tissues.
   C. Fentanyl can be administered by transdermal patch due to its high potency and lipid solubility.
   D. The opioid antagonist naloxone can be used in opioid overdose but triggers severe withdrawal effects in opioid-addicted individuals.
   E. Although its oral bioavailability is relatively low, morphine can be administered by oral, rectal or parenteral routes.

Case-based answers

1. The simple analgesic paracetamol can be given in compound formulations with the opioid analgesic codeine (co-codamol) or with dihydrocodeine (co-dydramol). A non-steroidal anti-inflammatory drugs (NSAID) analgesic (diclofenac) was also given to this man. Although this regimen conforms to the WHO analgesic ladder principle of combining opioid, NSAID and simple analgesics, codeine lacks the efficacy of morphine and failed to provide adequate pain control before admission.
2. Morphine acts at specific opioid receptors at spinal and supraspinal sites to produce analgesia. Morphine is a strong agonist at μ-opioid receptors that produce analgesia, euphoria, sedation, respiratory depression, dependence and inhibition of gastrointestinal motility.
3. Oral morphine solution is used to control breakthrough exacerbations of pain on a patient-initiated basis. Repeated use of oral morphine solution should signal a reassessment of the dose of the long-acting morphine. When the person is unable to take oral medication because of weakness or vomiting, rectal or continuous subcutaneous infusion may be required. Normally, 80% of people require less than 200 mg morphine per day

to control severe pain. With terminally ill people having persistent severe pain, the dose is gradually increased over a period of 1–2 weeks until appropriate control is achieved. The maximum dose may be as high as 2–3 g per day. Unwanted effects can occur so close monitoring is needed when an opioid is initiated or its dosage altered.

4. For reasons that are not easily explained, dependence seldom occurs in people with a high degree of pain. Possible reasons include high levels of endogenous opioids or catecholamines.

5. Diamorphine can be used instead of morphine. It is more potent but no more efficacious. Its major advantage is its high solubility, which reduces the volume of intramuscular injections or continuous subcutaneous infusion if these are required. Infrequently, an unusual response to morphine may require its replacement by other opioids. Fentanyl delivered via a transdermal patch has fewer unwanted effects.

6. Diclofenac is an aspirin-like NSAID often used in the treatment of arthritic conditions (Ch. 29). Unlike opioids, it has both analgesic and anti-inflammatory actions, due to its inhibition of the synthesis of prostaglandins by cyclo-oxygenase. The pain from bone metastases is compounded by local inflammation. Prostaglandins sensitise nociceptors to pain stimuli, and inflammatory swelling triggers pain due to increased pressure. Inflammation is reduced by diclofenac, thereby reducing the requirement for morphine.

7. Dexamethasone is a potent glucocorticoid (Ch. 44), reducing inflammation and swelling at metastatic sites.

8. Nausea is an unwanted effect of morphine, occurring particularly during the first week of use, but it may also be a consequence of the cancer itself or related complications such as hypercalcaemia. Tolerance to the nausea induced by morphine occurs.

9. Metoclopramide is a dopamine antagonist that acts in the chemoreceptor trigger zone (CTZ) to reduce nausea caused by opioid analgesics, chemotherapy and radiotherapy. It also has prokinetic activity on the gut that reduces the risk of nausea and vomiting. Other dopamine antagonists such as prochlorperazine can also be used (Ch 32).

10. Gastric and/or duodenal inflammation (which may cause considerable discomfort) or even ulceration may occur with prolonged use of diclofenac and a corticosteroid, due to inhibition of the synthesis of protective prostaglandins in the gut wall.

11. Cimetidine is a histamine H_2 receptor antagonist that reduces histamine-mediated gastric acid secretion by the parietal cells (Ch. 33), and was used twice-daily to reduce the risk of NSAID-induced gastric or duodenal ulceration. Cimetidine inhibits the enzymes that convert codeine into morphine and may reduce its analgesic effect. After admission, cimetidine was replaced with the proton pump inhibitor lansoprazole, which is more effective in blocking acid secretion and can be given once daily (Ch. 33).

12. Constipation is a feature of morphine therapy. Tolerance does not develop to opioid-induced constipation. Peristalsis is reduced, while the tone of the intestinal muscle is increased.

13. Docusate sodium has some faecal-softening properties and is a stimulant of intestinal smooth muscle, which restores peristalsis. In practice, terminally ill people are often given danthron, in combination with either docusate sodium (co-danthrusate) or poloxamer (co-danthramer). Danthron is a stimulant drug and stool softener and is particularly useful when 'bowel movements must be by strain'. The irritant properties of danthron and its carcinogenic potential restrict its general use. The alternatives in use include senna preparations (stimulants) and magnesium sulphate (a bulk purgative).

14. Temazepam is a short-acting benzodiazepine anxiolytic sedative used to aid sleeping (Ch. 20).

Note. Pain control must also take note of the psychological, social and spiritual condition of the person. At all times, if pain control is inadequate, adjuvant treatments such as radiotherapy or transcutaneous electrical nerve stimulation (TENS) should be considered. Where neuropathic pain is evident, tricyclic antidepressants or anticonvulsants should also be considered.

FURTHER READING

Ballantyne JC, Mao J (2003) Opioid therapy for chronic pain. *N Engl J Med* 349, 1943–1953

Bennetto L, Patel NK, Fuller G (2007) Trigeminal neuralgia and its management. *BMJ* 334, 201–205

Berde CB, Sethna NF (2002) Analgesics for the treatment of pain in children. *N Engl J Med* 347, 1094–1103

Eisenberg E, McNicol ED, Carr DB (2005) Efficacy and safety of opioid agonists in the treatment of neuropathic pain of nonmalignant origin. *JAMA* 293, 3043–3052

Freynhagen R, Bennett MI (2009) Diagnosis and management of neuropathic pain. *BMJ* 339, 391–395

Gonzalez G, Oliveto A, Kosten TR (2002) Treatment of heroin (diamorphine) addiction. *Drugs* 62, 1331–1343

Holdcroft A, Power I (2003) Management of pain. *BMJ* 326, 635–639

Jensen TS (2002) Anticonvulsants in neuropathic pain: rationale and clinical evidence. *Eur J Pain* 6 (Suppl A), 61–68

Johnson RW, Dworkin RH (2003) Treatment of herpes zoster and postherpetic neuralgia. *BMJ* 326, 748–750

Lobmaier P, Gossop M, Waal H, Bramness J (2010) The pharmacological treatment of opioid addiction: a clinical perspective. *Eur J Clin Pharmacol* 66, 537–545

Mendell JR, Sahenk Z (2003) Painful sensory neuropathy. *N Engl J Med* 348, 1243–1255

O'Connor AB, Dworkin RH (2009) Treatment of neuropathic pain: an overview of recent guidelines. *Am J Med* 122 (Suppl 1), S22–S32

Portenoy RK (2011) Treatment of cancer pain. *Lancet* 377, 2236–2247

Somogyi AA, Barratt DT, Coller JK (2007) Pharmacogenetics of opioids. *Clin Pharm Ther* 81, 429–444

Turk DC, Wilson HD, Cahana A (2011) Treatment of chronic non-cancer pain. *Lancet* 377, 2226–2235

Vadalouca A, Siafaka I, Argyra E et al. (2007) Therapeutic management of chronic neuropathic pain: an examination of pharmacologic treatment. *Ann NY Acad Sci* 1088, 164–186

Vanderah TW (2007) Pathophysiology of pain. *Med Clin North Am* 91, 1–12

Wu CL, Raja SN (2011) Treatment of acute postoperative pain. *Lancet* 377, 2215–2225

Compendium: opioids and related drugs

Drug	Kinetics (half-life)	Comments
Opioids used primarily for analgesia		
Alfentanil	Hepatic metabolism (1–2 h)	Used by injection for intraoperative analgesia (Ch. 17); respiratory depression may persist after the end of the procedure if repeated doses are given
Buprenorphine	Sublingual bioavailability better than oral; hepatic metabolism (1–7 h)	Mixed agonist/antagonist properties; long duration of action; used as an alternative to morphine for analgesia, but nausea may limit its tolerability; given sublingually, by slow intravenous or intramuscular injection, or as transdermal patches
Codeine	Codeine is partially (5–15%) converted to morphine by CYP2D6; polymorphism in this enzyme linked to variability in response to drug; mostly eliminated by hepatic metabolism, with 10% excreted unchanged	Given orally for mild to moderate pain or by intramuscular injection; also used when antitussive and antidiarrhoeal actions required
Diamorphine	Readily crosses the blood–brain barrier; metabolised to morphine by hydrolysis (2–5 min)	Clinical uses restricted because of high abuse potential; given orally or by infusion for the pain of terminal cancer; given for acute severe pain, e.g. myocardial infarction; given by intramuscular or subcutaneous injection
Dihydrocodeine	Extensive first-pass metabolism; hepatic metabolism (3–5 h)	Similar potency to codeine; given orally or by intramuscular or subcutaneous injection for moderate pain
Dipipanone	Hepatic metabolism (3–4 h)	The only available formulation in the UK contains cyclizine (an anti-emetic), which makes it unsuitable for long-term use
Fentanyl	Rapid initial uptake from the blood into lungs, followed by tissue distribution and then hepatic metabolism (1–6 h); not metabolised in skin (transdermal)	Increasingly used by transdermal patch or buccal route for intractable pain; intravenous adjunct in anaesthesia (Ch. 17); respiratory depression may persist after the end of the procedure if repeated doses are given
Hydromorphone	Good oral bioavailability (60%); hepatic metabolism (2–3h)	Given orally; shorter duration of action (about 3–4 h); may limit usefulness in chronic pain compared with morphine
Meptazinol	Rapid absorption but low oral bioavailability (5–20%); hepatic metabolism (1–3 h)	Less potent than morphine with short duration of action and possibly a reduced risk of respiratory depression; given orally or by intramuscular or slow intravenous injection
Methadone	Good oral bioavailability (40–100%); hepatic metabolism (via CYP isoenzymes that may undergo autoinduction on repeated dosage) and renal excretion (6–8 h)	Potent μ-receptor agonist but less sedating than morphine; longer action with reduced excitation leads to its use in managing opioid withdrawal; given orally or by subcutaneous or intramuscular injection
Morphine	Low oral bioavailability (10–50%); hepatic metabolism (1–5 h) by conjugation to morphine 3-glucuronide (inactive major metabolite) and morphine 6-glucuronide (active minor metabolite)	Can be given orally, rectally as suppositories, or by subcutaneous, intramuscular or slow intravenous injection
Oxycodone	Bioavailability 50–90%; mainly hepatic metabolism (3–5 h)	Similar efficacy and adverse effect profile to morphine; used largely in palliative care as an alternative in people who cannot tolerate morphine; given orally (normal or modified-release tablets) or by subcutaneous or slow intravenous injection
Papaveretum	Preparation of morphine, papaverine and codeine	Rarely used combined formulation; not to be confused with papaverine alone
Pentazocine	Oral bioavailability 11–32%; hepatic metabolism (2–3 h)	Its weak antagonism or partial agonism at μ-receptor can precipitate withdrawal in people dependent on other opioids; given orally, rectally, or by slow intravenous injection; may cause irritation given subcutaneously

Compendium: opioids and related drugs—cont'd

Drug	Kinetics (half-life)	Comments
Pethidine (meperidine)	Oral bioavailability about 50%; metabolised (3–8 h) to active metabolite (norpethidine), which has long half-life (15–30 h) and may accumulate on repeated dosage	Produces rapid but short-lasting analgesia; frequently used in labour; given orally or by subcutaneous or slow intravenous injection
Remifentanil	Very rapid metabolism by blood and tissue esterases (0.1 h)	Used for intraoperative analgesia (Ch. 17); given as an infusion
Tramadol	Oral bioavailability 60–70%; converted in liver (5–6 h) to metabolite which is a more potent μ-receptor agonist, responsible for most of the activity of the drug	Obstetric use; WHO-classified step 2 agent; given orally or by intramuscular or intravenous injection
Opioid antagonists		
Methylnaltrexone	Quaternary ammonium compound; oral absorption is 40–50% and it does not cross the blood–brain barrier; renal excretion and some hepatic metabolism (2–3 h)	Peripheral μ-receptor antagonist; reduces opioid-induced constipation without affecting central actions including analgesia or inducing withdrawal symptoms; used in combination with laxatives in palliative care when laxatives alone have failed and also used to reduce postoperative paralytic ileus; unwanted effects include abdominal pain, flatulence, nausea, dizziness; given by subcutaneous injection
Naloxone	Hepatic metabolism (1–1.5 h)	Opioid antagonist used to treat opioid overdose (Chs 53 and 54); administered by injection, giving a rapid onset of action (1–2 min); short duration of action
Naltrexone	Oral bioavailability 100%. Slow absorption from intramuscular sites results in very long half-life if given by this route (5–10 days) metabolised in liver and elsewhere (4 h); an active metabolite has longer half-life (14 h)	Oral opioid receptor antagonist; longer duration of action than naloxone; oral, subcutaneous or intravenous administration. Also used for treatment of alcohol dependence (Ch. 54)
Opioids used primarily for non-analgesic effects		
Dextromethorphan	Rapidly absorbed orally; hepatic metabolism (11 h)	The antitussive action is the only opioid activity shown; antagonist to NMDA receptors; given orally
Diphenoxylate	Oral bioavailability may be limited due to incomplete dissolution in gut; hepatic metabolism (2–3 h); an active metabolite has long half-life (3–14 h)	Opioid agonist; used in acute diarrhoea (Ch. 35); may exert its effects locally on smooth muscle rather than via opioid receptors; given orally
Loperamide	Oral bioavailability 40%; hepatic metabolism (11 h)	Only opioid characteristic is an anti-diarrhoeal action (Ch. 35); tolerance does not develop; given orally
Related drugs or actions		
Lofexidine	Mainly hepatic metabolism	α_2-Adrenoceptor antagonist; useful in opioid withdrawal; given orally

There is considerable overlap in the pharmacology of drugs that have anxiolytic (anxiety-relieving) and hypnotic (sleep-inducing) properties. Compounds with sedative properties (moderating excitement and calming) at low doses often have hypnotic effects at higher doses. In addition, sedative drugs may have anxiolytic properties when used at doses that are too low to produce sedation. Compounds such as buspirone have been developed that have anxiolytic properties but do not sedate.

ANXIETY DISORDERS

BIOLOGICAL BASIS OF ANXIETY DISORDERS

Anxiety disorders are among the most common psychiatric syndromes and affect 15% of the general population at some time during their life. The clinical manifestations of anxiety are both psychological and physical. Anxiety is only pathological when it is inappropriate to the degree of stress to which the individual is exposed. A variety of anxiety disorders is recognised, of which the most common are generalised anxiety disorder, panic disorder, phobic disorder and obsessive compulsive disorder. Mixed anxiety and depressive disorder is the most common clinical presentation. Many anxiety syndromes present early in life, and tend to become chronic if untreated. They are often associated with substance abuse.

The symptoms vary among the anxiety disorders, but usually include apprehension, worry, fear and nervousness. Increased sympathetic nervous system activity frequently accompanies these feelings, causing sweating, tachycardia and epigastric discomfort. Sleep is often disturbed, with difficulty getting to sleep being a common feature. Physical symptoms can be prominent (somatisation) and disabling,

and are sometimes difficult to interpret because anxiety can coexist with an underlying chronic physical condition.

Dysfunction of neurotransmission in the limbic region of the brain underlies the genesis of anxiety. The amygdala is a central part of the system that processes a fear stimulus and selects a response based on previous experience. Implementation of the response is through the locus coeruleus (autonomic and neuroendocrine responses) and nucleus paragigantocellularis (autonomic responses) in the brainstem, and through the hypothalamus. There are many neurobiological theories that attempt to explain the origin of anxiety disorders. These try to integrate our understanding of the neurochemical disturbances with genetic predisposition and environmental triggers. It is now thought that generalised anxiety disorder and major depression may share a genetic basis, and that expression of the clinical syndrome is determined by environmental factors. Structural changes in the neural pathways from the amygdala to the cortex have been identified in anxiety disorders, which may underlie hyperactive sensory processing of threat stimuli. In addition, the cognitive control mechanisms that terminate the emotional response to the sensory cues is deficient.

Decreased serotonergic (5-hydroxytryptamine, 5-HT) neurotransmission in the limbic system has been implicated in many anxiety syndromes. Overactivity of noradrenergic systems may also be important. Deficient inhibition of limbic neurotransmission by γ-aminobutyric acid (GABA) interneurons is found in many anxiety disorders, with reduced sensitivity of postsynaptic $GABA_A$ receptors. Excessive activity in excitatory glutamatergic neurons at N-methyl-D-aspartate (NMDA) receptors in the amygdala has also been implicated, and may be responsible for fear conditioning. Supersensitivity of receptors for peptide neurotransmitters such as cholecystokinin and neuropeptide Y may also occur. There is increasing evidence for the central role of brain-derived neurotrophic factor (BDNF) in modulating neural plasticity in anxiety states (see Fig. 22.2). BDNF is regulated by most of the neurotransmitters implicated in the genesis of anxiety states, and a decrease in BDNF correlates with anxiety and memory deficits.

In some anxiety syndromes there is excess secretion of corticotropin-releasing hormone (CRH), but a low plasma cortisol concentration and upregulation of glucocorticoid receptors. CRH is a neurotransmitter in the limbic system, and upregulation may occur from early adverse experiences, leading to conditioning of those with a genetic predisposition to anxiety disorder in later life.

DRUG THERAPY FOR ANXIETY

Drugs used to treat anxiety are called anxiolytics.

Benzodiazepines

Examples

chlordiazepoxide, diazepam, lorazepam, midazolam, temazepam

In addition to their anxiolytic effect, benzodiazepines have several other properties that are clinically useful. This section also considers drugs that are not used primarily for treatment of anxiety.

Mechanism of action and effects

Benzodiazepines act by potentiating the actions of GABA, the primary inhibitory neurotransmitter in the central nervous system (CNS). They act at a regulatory site closely linked to the GABA$_A$ receptor which mediates fast inhibitory synaptic neurotransmission (Fig. 20.1). GABA increases the influx of Cl$^-$ into the neuron, hyperpolarises the cell membrane and decreases cell excitability. Binding of a benzodiazepine to subunits of the receptor induces a conformational change in the GABA receptor that enhances its affinity for the neurotransmitter (Fig. 20.1). Benzodiazepines act only in the presence of GABA to enhance GABA-mediated opening of the ion channel; they have no direct action on the channel (Fig. 20.1).

The GABA$_A$ receptor has α, β and γ subunits, arranged in a group of five (usually two α, two β and one γ, although only α and β are essential) around a central pore (see Fig. 20.1 and legend). There are many subtypes of each subunit, and therefore many receptor configurations that show differences in their regional distributions in the brain. Benzodiazepines bind between an α and γ subunit. The presence of an α$_1$- or α$_5$-subunit confers the sedative and amnesic properties of benzodiazepines, while both α$_2$ and α$_3$ appear to be involved in the anxiolytic and muscle relaxant effects. Anticonvulsant activity is conferred by several α subunits. The minority of GABA receptors with only α$_4$ or α$_6$ subunits do not bind benzodiazepines.

The increase in inhibitory neurotransmission produced by benzodiazepines has the following potentially useful effects:

- sedation from reduced sensory input to the reticular activating system,
- sleep induction at high drug concentrations,
- anterograde amnesia,
- anxiolysis from actions on the limbic system and hypothalamus,
- anticonvulsant activity (Ch. 23),
- reduction of muscle tone (Ch. 24).

Pharmacokinetics

Benzodiazepines are well absorbed from the gut and their lipid solubility ensures ready penetration into the brain. The pharmacokinetics of individual benzodiazepines determines their major clinical uses. Benzodiazepines that are useful for inducing sleep (e.g. temazepam) are rapidly absorbed from the gut. This produces a fast onset of sedation, then sleep. Metabolism of short-acting benzodiazepines produces inactive derivatives. A brief duration of action is desirable for hypnotics, to avoid hangover sedation in the morning

Long-acting benzodiazepines, such as diazepam, are metabolised in the liver to active compounds (see Fig. 2.12) that contribute to their duration of action through relatively slow elimination from the body. Repeated dosing with long-acting compounds, such as diazepam, increases the risk of accumulation and a prolonged sedative effect. The anxiolytic properties of benzodiazepines are best exploited by using a compound with a long duration of action. Smaller doses can then be used to minimise sedation, and the rebound in anxiety symptoms that can occur between doses of a short-acting drug is avoided.

Diazepam, lorazepam and midazolam can also be given by intravenous injection to provide rapid sedation pre-operatively or before procedures such as endoscopy. Intravenous lorazepam and diazepam are also given for emergency treatment of generalised seizures and status epilepticus (Ch. 23). Long-acting benzodiazepines, such as clobazam, clonazepam, diazepam and lorazepam, are used in the prophylaxis of epilepsy (see Ch. 23).

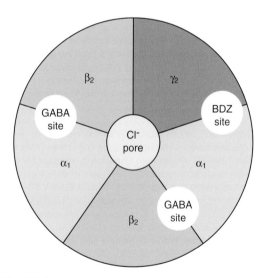

Fig. 20.1 The GABA$_A$ receptor. The GABA$_A$ receptor consists of five transmembrane subunits configured from the 19 possible subunits that have been identified; thus many configurations of the GABA receptor exist, which vary in their sensitivity to benzodiazepines. A common configuration comprises two α$_1$, two β$_2$ and one γ$_2$ subunit. Binding of GABA to the receptor at the interfaces of the α$_1$ and β$_2$ subunits mediates opening of the Cl$^-$ channel and an influx of Cl$^-$ ions, resulting in hyperpolarisation of the cell. This action is enhanced by drugs stimulating allosteric regulatory sites on the GABA receptor, distinct from the GABA-binding site. Diazepam, lorazepam and other 'classic' benzodiazepines (BDZs) bind at the interface of the α$_1$ and γ$_2$ subunits. Compounds such as zolpidem bind with high affinity for the α$_1$-subunits and also enhance Cl$^-$ ion influx. The intravenous anaesthetics propofol and etomidate bind to β$_2$- and β$_3$-subunits (Ch. 17).

Unwanted effects

- Drowsiness, which may cause problems with driving or operating machinery.
- Lightheadedness.
- Confusion, especially in the elderly.
- Paradoxical increase in aggression.
- Amnesia.
- Ataxia.
- Muscle weakness.
- Potentiation of the sedative effects of other CNS-depressant drugs, such as alcohol. In overdose, such combinations can lead to severe respiratory depression. Flumazenil is a competitive antagonist of benzodiazepines and can be used in acute overdose to reverse respiratory depression (Ch. 53)
- **Tolerance** to the therapeutic effects of benzodiazepines is common. There is widespread concern that their hypnotic effects are lost quite early, although there is little evidence to support this. However, rebound insomnia on withdrawal can perpetuate benzodiazepine use.
- **Dependence** with physical and psychological withdrawal symptoms occurs during long-term treatment. The risk is highest in people with personality disorders, or a previous history of dependence on alcohol or drugs, and is more likely to occur if high doses of benzodiazepines are used. Restricting use to a maximum of 4 weeks will minimise the risk of dependence. With long-acting drugs, withdrawal symptoms may be delayed by up to 3 weeks after stopping. Anxiety is the most frequent symptom, while insomnia, depression and abnormalities of perception, such as altered sensitivity to noise, light or touch, also occur. More severe reactions such as psychosis or convulsions arise occasionally. Some withdrawal symptoms may resemble those for which the drug was originally prescribed, encouraging continued use. Gradual withdrawal of a benzodiazepine over 4–8 weeks is desirable after long-term use, although complete withdrawal may take up to a year. Lorazepam is a potent benzodiazepine with a relatively short duration of action that proves particularly difficult to stop because of the intensity of withdrawal symptoms that begin a few hours after cessation of treatment. Substitution with the longer-acting drug diazepam may be helpful before withdrawal is attempted. There are no proven treatments for reducing symptoms associated with withdrawal. Beta-adrenoceptor antagonists (Ch. 5) are sometimes helpful, or an antidepressant (Ch. 22) if there are depressive symptoms or panic attacks.

Azapirones

buspirone

Mechanism of action and effects

Buspirone is a partial agonist at presynaptic 5-HT$_{1A}$ receptors, producing negative feedback to inhibit serotonin release. It has no effect on GABA receptors. Initial exacerbation of anxiety may occur, possibly caused by postsynaptic 5-HT$_{1A}$ receptor stimulation. The onset of the anxiolytic action of buspirone is slow, beginning after 2 weeks and reaching a maximum effect at approximately 4 weeks. The mechanism of action may involve gradual changes in neural plasticity (enhancement of neural performance or changes in neural connections; Ch. 22). Buspirone has no sedative action, and is ineffective for panic attacks.

Pharmacokinetics

Buspirone is well absorbed from the gut and undergoes extensive first-pass metabolism in the liver. The half-life is short (2–4 h).

Unwanted effects

- Nausea.
- Dizziness, lightheadedness and headache.
- Nervousness.

Neither tolerance nor dependence has been reported.

MANAGEMENT OF ANXIETY

If substance misuse is identified it should be treated first and may improve symptoms, while comorbid depression may require an antidepressant. Symptoms of anxiety, if mild, often respond to counselling or psychotherapy, using relaxation training or cognitive behavioural therapy without drug therapy.

Generalised anxiety disorder often requires long-term treatment, and there is now considerable evidence that antidepressants (Ch. 22) are useful in this situation. Selective serotonin reuptake inhibitors (SSRIs) such as sertraline are the treatment of choice, or a serotonin and noradrenaline reuptake inhibitor (SNRI) such as venlafaxine if an SSRI is ineffective. Antidepressants can initially exacerbate anxiety, and a benzodiazepine may be necessary for the first 2–3 weeks of treatment to prevent this. The optimal duration of antidepressant treatment in generalised anxiety disorder is uncertain, but similar treatment periods as for depression (Ch. 22) are usually recommended. Pregabalin, which increases inhibitory neurotransmission, is an effective alternative to antidepressants (Ch. 23).

Benzodiazepines can be considered as a short-term measure for anxiety to treat crises, since they have a rapid onset of action over 15–60 min. However, the potential for dependence should limit their use to a maximum of 4 weeks, and the dose should be gradually reduced after the first 2 weeks. Buspirone has similar efficacy to benzodiazepines, but the slow onset of action (3 days) makes it less versatile for managing short-term anxiety. In addition, anxiety that responds well to benzodiazepines often responds less well to buspirone, possibly due to a relative lack of effect of buspirone on somatic symptoms. Somatic symptoms of anxiety (e.g. tremor, palpitations) that are produced by overactivity in the sympathetic nervous system are often helped by a non-selective β-adrenoceptor antagonist such as propranolol (Ch. 5).

Social anxiety disorder responds to monoamine oxidase inhibitors (MAOIs; Ch. 22) better than to most other agents. Moclobemide is the treatment of choice, but phenelzine is also used. Phobic disorders usually need a different approach, and cognitive behavioural therapy is often most effective. Panic disorder is usually treated with tricyclic antidepressants or SSRIs, with MAOIs reserved for people who do not respond.

INSOMNIA

Defining insomnia is complicated by the considerable variability in the normal pattern of sleep. Most healthy adults sleep between 7 and 9 h per night, but much shorter or even longer periods can be normal. Insomnia is considered to be present if there is repeated inability to initiate or maintain sleep, despite adequate opportunity and time for sleep. There are three major categories of insomnia, defined by duration of symptoms (Table 20.1). Symptoms include sleep-onset insomnia (difficulty falling asleep, more common in younger people), frequent nocturnal awakening (difficulty maintaining sleep, more common in older people), early morning awakening (with difficulty getting back to sleep) and difficulty functioning in the daytime due to perceived poor sleep. Obstructive sleep apnoea is a common cause of sleep disturbance, affecting up to 10% of people who report insomnia.

The reticular formation in the midbrain, medulla and pons is responsible for maintaining wakefulness. Activity in the reticular formation is dependent on sensory input via collateral connections from the main sensory pathways. Neurotransmitter systems involved in the regulation of sleep are complex. Cortical arousal is regulated by noradrenergic pathways from the locus coeruleus, cholinergic ascending tracts from brainstem nuclei, histaminergic neurons from the tuberomammillary nucleus and serotonergic neurons from the raphe nuclei. Hypocretins are important neuropeptide transmitters found in the lateral hypothalamus which, through connections with other hypothalamic and brainstem nuclei, promote wakefulness (see also narcolepsy, Ch. 22). Sleep is induced by neurotransmission by GABA, melatonin and galanin (a predominantly inhibitory neuropeptide) from the anterior hypothalamus, which inhibits the arousal neurons.

SLEEP PATTERNS

The two main types of sleep pattern are non-rapid-eye-movement (non-REM) sleep and rapid-eye-movement (REM) sleep. These sleep patterns occur in cycles (Fig. 20.2), with non-REM sleep varying between light sleep (stages 1 and 2) and slow-wave sleep (stages 3 and 4). Two-thirds of sleep is usually spent in stages 2–4, characterised by continuous or intermittent delta waves (slow waves) on the electroencephalogram. These deeper stages of sleep are the recuperative phase, while most dreaming occurs during the REM sleep periods. Increasing age is associated with more nocturnal awakening and longer periods of REM sleep.

DRUGS FOR TREATING INSOMNIA (HYPNOTICS)

Benzodiazepines

Benzodiazepines have dose-related hypnotic effects. See above for details.

Non-benzodiazepine hypnotics that modulate the GABA$_A$/chloride channel

zaleplon, zolpidem, zopiclone

Mechanism of action and effects

Zaleplon, zolpidem and zopiclone (the so-called Z drugs) belong to different chemical classes but interact in a similar manner with the postsynaptic GABA$_A$ receptor on neuronal membranes. They bind to regulatory binding sites on the receptor that are close to, but distinct from, the benzodiazepine-binding site (Fig. 20.1). Like the benzodiazepines, they increase GABA-mediated Cl$^-$ influx into the cell, which inhibits neurotransmission. Zolpidem and zaleplon are selective for the α_1-subunit in the GABA receptor. Zopiclone also acts on the α_2-subunit of the GABA receptor. Although zopiclone also possesses anxiolytic and anticonvulsant activity, its short duration of action makes it unsuitable for these indications.

Table 20.1 Types of insomnia

Type of insomnia	Duration	Likely causes
Transient	2–3 days	Acute situational or environmental stress (e.g. jet lag, shift work)
Short-term	<3 weeks	Ongoing personal stress
Long-term	>3 weeks	Psychiatric illness, behavioural reasons, medical reasons

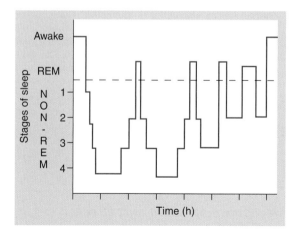

Fig. 20.2 Typical sleep pattern in a young adult. REM, rapid eye movement.

Pharmacokinetics

The Z drugs are rapidly absorbed from the gut, and are metabolised in the liver. They have short half-lives (1–6 h), which makes them well suited to their use as hypnotics.

Unwanted effects

- Bitter metallic taste (zopiclone).
- Gastrointestinal disturbances, including nausea and vomiting.
- Incoordination.
- Drowsiness, dizziness, headache and fatigue.
- Depression, confusion, amnesia.
- There is only anecdotal evidence for tolerance.
- Dependence with withdrawal symptoms has been reported.

MANAGEMENT OF INSOMNIA

Drugs play only a small part in the treatment of insomnia. Explanation of the normal variations in sleep patterns and avoidance of diuretics, drinks containing caffeine, cigarettes or alcohol in the hours before retiring can help. Eliminating excessive noise or heat in the bedroom, encouraging regular exercise in the day and minimising daytime napping may also be useful.

Hypnotic drugs are reserved for times when abnormal sleep markedly affects quality of life. The ideal hypnotic would induce good-quality prolonged sleep without disturbance of the normal sleep pattern. It should have a rapid onset of action, with no 'hangover' sedation in the morning, and should not produce tolerance or dependence. Few drugs come close to this ideal profile. Benzodiazepines reduce sleep latency (the time between settling down and falling asleep) and prolong sleep duration. However, they reduce the time spent in REM sleep, with more time spent in stage 2 sleep. Short-acting drugs (such as zolpidem) are preferred if there is delayed onset of sleep, and medium-acting drugs (such as temazepam or zopiclone) for those who wake in the middle of the night. Long-acting drugs are used to suppress daytime anxiety, but carry the risk of hangover sedation the following day. The Z drugs produce less disturbance of sleep 'architecture' than other drugs, having less effect on the amount of REM sleep while increasing the duration of deeper (slow-wave) sleep.

Hypnotic drugs should be used only for short periods and intermittently if possible, since tolerance to hypnotics frequently occurs after 2 weeks. If a benzodiazepine is used continuously for 4–6 weeks then rebound insomnia, caused by mild dependence, is common when the drug is stopped. Nevertheless, benzodiazepines are still widely used. The Z drugs carry a similar risk of dependence.

Of the other hypnotics, chloral derivatives and clomethiazole (see compendium) should usually be avoided. Compounds with sedative actions as a part of their therapeutic profile are sometimes used as hypnotics. For example, a sedative anti-histamine such as promazine (Ch. 39) can be helpful for children with somnambulism (sleep walking) or night terrors, but daytime sedation and weight gain can be a problem. Sedative tricyclic antidepressants (Ch. 22), such as amitriptyline, should be considered if there is an underlying depressive illness. If less-sedating antidepressants are used then short-term concurrent use of a benzodiazepine may be necessary while awaiting the onset of the antidepressant effect.

Melatonin is effective for insomnia caused by jet lag or shift work, but is ineffective for primary insomnia.

SELF-ASSESSMENT

True/false questions

1. Benzodiazepines with a medium to long duration of action are useful for treating anxiety states.
2. Long-term use of benzodiazepines is recommended in anxiety states.
3. Potentiation of the CNS effects of benzodiazepines occurs with concurrent use of alcohol.
4. The CNS-depressant effects of benzodiazepines can be reversed with flumazenil.
5. Lower doses of benzodiazepines should be used in the elderly.
6. Buspirone is more sedative than temazepam.
7. Benzodiazepines used to treat anxiety should be administered for as short a time as possible.
8. Benzodiazepines have no effect on sleep patterns as measured by the duration of REM sleep.

One-best-answer (OBA) question

Choose the *most correct* statement from the following.

A. Benzodiazepines act to potentiate the inhibitory actions of γ-aminobutyric acid (GABA) at its receptor.
B. Withdrawal symptoms abate within 3 weeks of abruptly stopping diazepam.
C. Barbiturates are the drugs of choice in patients with insomnia and anxiety.
D. Buspirone decreases anxiety by acting at the GABA receptor site.
E. If there is no response to one hypnotic, it is advisable to switch to another.

Case-based questions

Mrs FL is a 46-year-old mother of three who is finding it very hard to cope following the sudden death of her husband 3 months ago. She has returned to work but does not sleep properly, experiences occasional periods of anxiety during the day and feels that she is at risk of losing her job because tiredness and anxiety about her financial difficulties prevent her concentrating on her work.

A. What drug might you prescribe to help Mrs FL's insomnia, and what factors determine your choice of this drug?
B. How does your chosen drug work to reduce insomnia and anxiety?
C. What potential unwanted effects and drug interactions should you warn Mrs FL about?
D. Mrs FL returns 2 weeks later, saying that she regularly wakes at 4 a.m. and cannot get back to sleep; consider

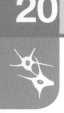

the advantages and disadvantages of changing her to a longer-acting drug or to another, 'newer' hypnotic.
E. What are the problems associated with long-term use of benzodiazepines?
F. What other options should be considered to help to manage Mrs FL's problems in the long term?

Extended-matching-item questions

Keeping in mind the equally important roles of psychological and psychiatric help, choose the *most appropriate* statement A–E for the next pharmacological course of action in the case scenarios 1 and 2 described below.

A. Gradual tapering of the medication over many months.
B. Gradual tapering of the medication over several days.
C. Prescribing another course of the same benzodiazepine.
D. Considering giving paroxetine.
E. Immediate withdrawal of all medications.

Scenario 1. A 54-year-old woman has a history of anxiety. Seven years earlier she had taken regular lorazepam and for the last 3 years her doctor had been refilling prescription requests without reassessing the clinical need. There is no indication of depressive illness. The woman now wishes to stop her medication.

Scenario 2. You have been treating a woman aged 25 for a year. She has been having up to 10 intense panic attacks a month. At any time of day, she suddenly develops a peculiar and very strong feeling of being lightheaded, jumpy and being smothered. Her heart rate increases dramatically and the episodes come on so quickly and severely that she feels she might be dying. She then feels shaky, sweaty and unsteady. Each attack quickly reaches such intensity that she is often unable to continue work and needs to go home. She has been treated with intermittent courses of diazepam for a year without improvement.

True/false answers

1. **True.** Benzodiazepines used in anxiety, such as diazepam, have long-lived metabolites that contribute to the duration of action.
2. **False.** Dependence, tolerance and withdrawal symptoms occur with long-term continuous use of benzodiazepines.
3. **True.** Alcohol, older anti-histamines and barbiturates can potentiate CNS depression by benzodiazepines.
4. **True.** Flumazenil is a competitive benzodiazepine antagonist used in acute overdose.
5. **True.** Hepatic metabolism of benzodiazepines is reduced in the elderly, who are also more sensitive to their effects.
6. **False.** Buspirone has less sedative action than benzodiazepines such as temazepam.
7. **True.** Using the lowest possible dose of benzodiazepine for the shortest duration reduces the risk of tolerance and withdrawal effects.
8. **False.** Benzodiazepines affect sleep structure, with loss of REM sleep. Zolpidem has less effect than benzodiazepines.

OBA answer

Answer A is correct.

A. **Correct.** Benzodiazepines potentiate the entry of Cl^- through the receptor-operated channel which is part of the $GABA_A$ receptor.
B. Incorrect. With long-acting benzodiazepines withdrawal symptoms may take more than 3 weeks to appear.
C. Incorrect. Barbiturates have been superseded as hypnotics because of unwanted effects, tolerance and dependence liability.
D. Incorrect. Buspirone acts at presynaptic $5\text{-}HT_{1A}$ receptors to reduce serotonin (5-HT) release.
E. Incorrect. An alternative hypnotic is unlikely to work and switching between hypnotics is not good practice.

Case-based answers

A. Mrs FL's insomnia and anxiety are a response to bereavement and might present fewer long-term problems than chronic 'endogenous' anxiety. Benzodiazepines and the newer hypnotics are safer than barbiturates. Nevertheless, the central concept in benzodiazepine therapy is to use the minimal effective dose for the shortest possible period. A short-acting benzodiazepine (e.g. temazepam) taken at night should help restore her sleep pattern and may improve her daytime tiredness. The relatively short half-life of temazepam (5–12 h) should minimise risk of sedation during the working day. However, if the daytime anxiety also warrants treatment, a long-acting benzodiazepine (e.g. diazepam) given at night may be the drug to choose. Only short or intermittent courses of treatment should be given. The anxiolytic buspirone is not sedative, but it is ineffective against panic attacks.
B. Benzodiazepines are $GABA_A$ agonists that enhance $GABA_A$-mediated inhibition of neuronal activity in the brain and spinal cord. Benzodiazepines bind to $GABA_A$ receptors at a site separate from GABA itself and increase the frequency of GABA-induced channel opening, enhancing Cl^- entry into the cell and neuronal hyperpolarisation.
C. Benzodiazepines are relatively free of serious unwanted effects if used correctly and are safe in overdose, but Mrs FL should be advised that they cause sedation and may interfere markedly with driving and operating machinery (worsened by interaction with alcohol, barbiturates and sedative anti-histamines). Other unwanted effects include headache, dry mouth, hypotension, anterograde amnesia, skin rashes and blood dyscrasias.
D. Rebound wakefulness may indicate a need for a longer-acting benzodiazepine such as nitrazepam or diazepam, which may also help to reduce Mrs FL's daytime anxiety and panic attacks. Conversely, daytime sedation may interfere with driving and work, exacerbated by long-acting metabolites of these drugs. An alternative may be to prescribe buspirone; however, this requires 1–2 weeks for a response. Switching to a newer hypnotic such as zolpidem is unlikely to make a difference.
E. Long-term use of a benzodiazepine is associated with dependence, manifested mainly as a withdrawal

reaction, which may include rebound anxiety, tremor, nausea, irritability, anorexia and dysphoria. Together with rapid development of tolerance (especially to hypnotic action), these contraindicate benzodiazepine treatment for more than 3 weeks.

F. In the longer term a course of antidepressants may be indicated. Mrs FL's recovery from bereavement may be aided by psychological counselling and support from family and employer.

Extended-matching-item answers

Scenario 1: Answer **A**. Withdrawal from long courses of benzodiazepines is difficult. She is liable to show withdrawal symptoms or return of the original complaints that determined the original prescription. Psychological and other forms of counselling may be advisable. Withdrawal should include gradual dosage reduction and anxiety management. Long-term psychological support is equally important for successful outcome, particularly for reducing the incidence and severity of post-withdrawal syndromes.

Scenario 2: Answer **D**. Continuing with a benzodiazepine is unlikely to improve matters after a year of treatment. The use of anxiolytics may be masking depression. An option might be to assess for depression and use a selective serotonin reuptake inhibitor (SSRI), such as paroxetine, licensed for the treatment of anxiety and panic disorders. General assessment is also recommended to rule out other disorders and non-pharmacological treatments should be considered.

FURTHER READING

Abramowitz JS, Taylor S, McKay D (2009) Obsessive compulsive disorder. *Lancet* 374, 491–499

Baldwin D, Woods R, Lawson R et al. (2011) Efficacy of drug treatment for generalized anxiety disorder: systematic review and meta-analysis. *BMJ* 342, d1199.

Ebert B, Wafford KA, Deacon S (2006) Treating insomnia: current and investigational pharmacological approaches. *Pharmacol Ther* 112, 612–629

Falloon K, Arroll B, Elley CR et al. (2011) The assessment and management of insomnia in primary care. *BMJ* 342, d2899

Fricehione G (2004) Generalized anxiety disorder. *N Engl J Med* 351, 675–682

Gale C, Davidson O (2007) Generalized anxiety disorder. *BMJ* 334, 579–581

Gottesmann C (2002) GABA mechanisms and sleep. *Neuroscience* 111, 231–239

Lader MH (1999) Limitations on the use of benzodiazepines in anxiety and insomnia: are they justified? *Eur Neuropsychopharmacol* 9 (Suppl 6), S399–S405

Lerch C, Park GR (1999) Sedation and analgesia. *Br Med Bull* 55, 76–95

Michels G, Moss SJ (2007) GABA_A receptors: properties and trafficking. *Crit Rev Biochem Mol Biol* 42, 3–14

Morin CM, Benca R (2012) Chronic insomnia. *Lancet* 379, 1129–1141

Roy-Byrne PP, Craske MG, Stein MB (2006) Panic disorder. *Lancet* 368, 1023–1032

Schenk CH, Mahowald MW, Sack RL (2003) Assessment and management of insomnia. *JAMA* 289, 2475–2479

Schneier FR (2006) Social anxiety disorder. *N Engl J Med* 355, 1029–1036

Szabadi E (2006) Drugs for sleep disorders: mechanisms and therapeutic prospects. *Br J Clin Pharmacol* 61, 761–766

Tyrer P, Baldwin D (2006) Generalised anxiety disorder. *Lancet* 368, 2156–2166

Wilson SJ, Nutt DJ, Alford C et al. (2010) British Association for Psychopharmacology consensus statement on evidence-based treatment of insomnia, parasomnias and circadian rhythm disorders. *J Psychopharmacol* 11, 1577–1601

Young C, Knudsen N, Hilton A, Reyes JG (2000) Sedation in the intensive care unit. *Crit Care Med* 28, 853–866

Compendium: anxiolytics, sedatives and hypnotics

Drug	Kinetics (half-life)	Comments
Anxiolytics		
Short-term use; given orally unless other otherwise indicated.		
Alprazolam	Almost complete oral bioavailability; hepatic metabolism (6–16 h)	Like all benzodiazepines, an allosteric GABA_A receptor agonist
Buspirone	Rapid absorption, but extensive first-pass metabolism reduces bioavailability to about 4%, improved if taken with food; hepatic metabolism (2–4 h)	Partial agonism at presynaptic 5-HT_{1A} receptors reduces 5-HT release; no effect on GABA_A receptors and no sedative action; anxiolytic onset after 2 weeks
Chlordiazepoxide	Complete oral bioavailability; slow hepatic metabolism to active metabolites with long half-lives (15–100 h)	Long-acting anxiolytic; also used as an adjunct in alcohol withdrawal

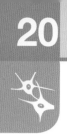

Compendium: anxiolytics, sedatives and hypnotics—cont'd

Drug	Kinetics (half-life)	Comments
Diazepam	Complete oral bioavailability; partially active N-desmethyl metabolite (nordiazepam) has longer half-life (30–200 h) than parent compound (20–100 h); other metabolites include temazepam and oxazepam	Long-acting benzodiazepine; may be given orally, rectally or by intramuscular or slow intravenous injection; also used for insomnia, status epilepticus and muscle spasm and in surgical premedication
Lorazepam	High bioavailability; hepatic conjugation (4–25 h)	Benzodiazepine anxiolytic; shorter-acting than diazepam; also anticonvulsant and for surgical premedication
Meprobamate	Good oral absorption; hepatic metabolism and some renal excretion of the parent drug (8–11 h)	Carbamate derivative with $GABA_A$ agonist and other CNS actions; not recommended because of potential toxicity and dependence
Oxazepam	High bioavailability; hepatic conjugation (4–25 h)	Benzodiazepine anxiolytic; shorter-acting than diazepam

Sedatives and hypnotics

All given orally and recommended for short-term use only (unless otherwise indicated).

Drug	Kinetics (half-life)	Comments
Chloral hydrate	Extensive first-pass metabolism; rapidly reduced to its active metabolite trichloroethanol (half-life 8–12 h)	Chlorinated derivative of ethanol; acts at $GABA_A$ receptor; formerly used as a hypnotic in children and the elderly; now rarely used
Clomethiazole	Rapid absorption but extensive (40–95%) first-pass metabolism; hepatic metabolism (4–6 h)	Derivative of chloral hydrate; acts at barbiturate site on $GABA_A$ receptor; used only for severe insomnia in the elderly (with little hangover) and for acute alcohol withdrawal (not preferred, as addictive)
Flurazepam	Good oral absorption; hepatic metabolism (2–3 h) to active metabolites with half-lives of 30–100 h and 2–4 h	Benzodiazepine hypnotic
Loprazolam	Good oral absorption; hepatic metabolism (7 h)	Benzodiazepine hypnotic
Lormetazepam	Eliminated as a glucuronic acid conjugate (8–10 h); about 10% metabolised in liver to lorazepam	Benzodiazepine hypnotic
Midazolam	Eliminated by hydroxylation in the liver (1–5 h)	Benzodiazepine used primarily in surgical premedication; given by slow intravenous or intramuscular injection
Nitrazepam	Rapid absorption but variable bioavailability (50–90%); hepatic metabolism (20–48 h) to inactive compounds	Benzodiazepine hypnotic
Promethazine	Oral bioavailability about 20%; hepatic metabolism (7–14 h)	H_1 anti-histamine that has prolonged sedative and hypnotic effects
Temazepam	High oral bioavailability; hepatic oxidation and glucuronidation (5–12 h) to inactive products	Benzodiazepine hypnotic; also used in surgical premedication
Zaleplon	Rapid absorption with bioavailability of 30%; oxidised to inactive products (1 h)	Z-drug hypnotic; binds to α_1-subunit of the $GABA_A$ receptor; used for up to 2 weeks
Zolpidem	Good oral bioavailability (about 70%); hepatic metabolism to inactive products (2–3 h)	Z-drug hypnotic; binds to α_1-subunit of the $GABA_A$ receptor; used for up to 4 weeks
Zopiclone	Rapid absorption and high bioavailability (about 80%); hepatic metabolism (4–6 h)	Z-drug hypnotic; binds to α_1- and α_2-subunits of the $GABA_A$ receptor; used for up to 4 weeks

Drugs that reverse sedative effects of benzodiazepines

Drug	Kinetics (half-life)	Comments
Flumazenil	Eliminated by hepatic metabolism (1 h); longer half-life (2–3 h) in severe hepatic dysfunction	Competitive antagonist of benzodiazepine binding site; given by intravenous injection or infusion in acute benzodiazepine overdose

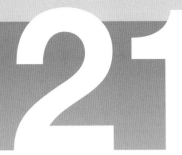

The major psychotic disorders: schizophrenia and mania

PSYCHOTIC DISORDERS

The term psychosis indicates a mental state in which the person affected has lost contact with reality. This is usually experienced as hallucination, delusion or disruption in thought processes often with lack of insight. The most profound 'functional' or primary psychotic condition is schizophrenia, but there is a continuum that embraces the so-called schizoaffective disorders. Mania and bipolar disorder can also have psychotic features. Organic disease caused by metabolic disturbance, toxic substances or psychoactive drugs can cause psychosis (Box 21.1).

SCHIZOPHRENIA

Clinical features of schizophrenia are categorised as positive or negative (Table 21.1), although none are pathognomonic of the disorder. The positive features are disordered versions of thinking, perception, formation of ideas or sense of self. They include hallucinations (false sensory perceptions) and delusions (false beliefs held with absolute certainty and unexplained by the person's socioeconomic background). The negative features, deficits in normal behaviour, are often the most debilitating in the long term. Schizophrenia is more common in males and usually presents relatively early in life. The onset is usually gradual but can be abrupt. Once established, it can have a relapsing or persistent course.

Biological basis of schizophrenia

There is a strong genetic component to schizophrenia with several risk genes that affect early brain development and predispose an individual to developing the condition. Triggers which impact further on neurodevelopment, such as prenatal exposure to viral infections or obstetric complications, probably only lead to the disease in those with a genetic predisposition. Many neurobiological abnormalities have been described in schizophrenia, including disturbances in neuronal numbers and synaptic connections in the cortical, thalamic and hippocampal areas. These disturbances become more marked as the illness progresses, but the heterogenous nature of the disease makes it difficult to determine the precise underlying neuropathology.

Dopamine–glutamate interactions and their possible involvement in schizophrenia

The limbic region and prefrontal cortex are involved in cognition, emotional memory and the initiation of behaviour. They are regulated by a complex interplay among their neuronal connections, with dopamine and glutamate as important neurotransmitters. Most dopaminergic pathways in the central nervous system (CNS) arise from the substantia nigra (among the basal ganglia) and the ventral tegmental area in the midbrain (Fig. 21.1). One major dopaminergic pathway has its origin in the substantia nigra and projects to γ-aminobutyric acid (GABA)-ergic inhibitory interneurons in the corpus striatum through the nigrostriatal pathway (Ch. 24). This pathway modulates motor and behavioural function through ongoing projections to the thalamus and cortex. The corpus striatum in turn receives glutamatergic inputs from the cortex. Other major pathways connect the ventral tegmental area via the mesolimbic projections to the limbic region (especially the hippocampus) and via the mesocortical projections to the prefrontal cortex (the reward pathway; see Ch. 54). The limbic region also receives cortical afferents.

Several receptors for the neurotransmitter dopamine are found in the brain (see table of receptor families at end of Ch. 1). CNS dopamine receptors belong to two families: D_1-like (which includes subtypes D_1 and D_5 that are coupled to a stimulatory G protein) and D_2-like (which includes subtypes D_2, D_3 and D_4 that are coupled to an inhibitory G protein). Postsynaptic D_1 and D_2 receptor subtypes are found in the dopaminergic pathways in the corpus striatum, limbic system, thalamus and hypothalamus. Postsynaptic D_2 receptors are also present in the pituitary. Presynaptic D_3 receptors are found on the dopaminergic neuronal terminals in the corpus striatum and limbic system, and their stimulation inhibits dopamine release in these areas.

Schizophrenia
Schizophreniform disorder
Schizoaffective disorders
Delusional disorders (includes persecutory, grandiose and other subtypes)
Brief psychotic disorder
Psychosis caused by organic disease
Manic episode
Bipolar affective disorder

Table 21.1 Clinical features of schizophrenia

Features	Characteristics
Positive features	
Hallucinations	Third-person auditory hallucinations (voices talking about the person as 'he' or 'she') Second-person commands Olfactory, tactile or visual hallucinations
Delusions	Thought withdrawal (thoughts being taken from the person's mind) Thought insertion (alien thoughts inserted in the person's mind) Thought broadcast (thoughts are known to others) Actions are caused or controlled from outside Bodily sensations are imposed from outside Delusional perception (a sudden, fully formed delusion, in the wake of a normal perception)
Negative features	
Loss of interest in others, initiative or sense of enjoyment Blunted emotions Limited speech	

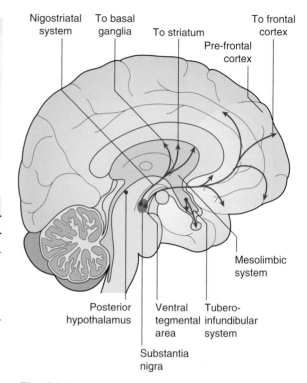

Fig. 21.1 **Dopamine pathways.** Major dopaminergic pathways in the central nervous system.

Postsynaptic D_4 receptors are found in the limbic system and prefrontal cortex.

Schizophrenia is believed to involve interconnected abnormalities of glutamatergic and dopaminergic neurotransmission. However, it is uncertain whether reduced glutamatergic activity at N-methyl-D-aspartate (NMDA) receptors or increased dopaminergic neurotransmission at D_2 receptors in the mesolimbic pathway is the primary abnormality. There are several pieces of evidence that support the involvement of defective glutamatergic and overactive dopaminergic neurotransmission in the genesis of schizophrenia:

- amfetamine-induced dopamine release is greater in people with schizophrenia,
- the dopamine concentration in the corpus striatum is higher in people with schizophrenia,
- blockade of the D_2 family of receptors produces antipsychotic effects,
- increased stimulation of D_2-like receptors worsens positive symptoms,

- glutamate NMDA receptor antagonists (ketamine, phencyclidine) produce positive and negative symptoms, similar to those of schizophrenia,
- NMDA receptor agonists such as glycine improve symptoms.

In schizophrenia there is downregulation of D_3 and D_4 receptors in the prefrontal cortex, which may be responsible for the negative symptoms, and downregulation of D_4 receptors in the limbic system. Dysfunction of other neurotransmitter systems utilising serotonin, GABA and neuropeptide Y may also be important in schizophrenia, but their precise roles are as yet unresolved.

MANIA AND BIPOLAR DISORDER

Mania is a disorder of elevated mood that can occur alone (unipolar mania) or is more usually interspersed with episodes of depression (bipolar affective disorder or manic-depressive illness). Mild mania is termed hypomania. Sometimes, the fluctuations of mood are less marked, and the disorder is termed cyclothymia.

The onset of mania can be gradual or sudden, most often between the ages of 15 and 25 years, and varies in severity from mild elation, increased drive and sociability, to grandiose ideas, marked overactivity, overspending and socially embarrassing behaviour. Onset is usually early in adult life. Mania and bipolar disorder have (and share) a stronger genetic component than any other grouping of major psychiatric disorders.

Biological basis of bipolar disorder

The biological basis of bipolar disorder is less well understood than that for unipolar depression. Susceptibility genes have been identified that are shared with those for schizophrenia, but the environmental stressors that result in expression of the disorder are poorly understood. The dysregulation of neuronal function is probably triggered by altered expression of critical neuronal proteins, determined by the genetic predisposition. In bipolar disorder there is increased CNS monoamine neurotransmitter activity (particularly serotonin and dopamine) and reduced acetylcholine and GABA neurotransmission. These may all be important in orchestrating changes in neuronal function within the prefrontal cortex, visual association cortex and limbic circuitry.

The changes in neurotransmitter regulation produce functional disruption in the target neurons. Reduced neuronal levels of brain-derived neurotrophic factor (BDNF) may be important in the genesis of bipolar disorder (see also depression, Ch. 22). BDNF regulates several intracellular signal transduction pathways, and dysregulation of these pathways may produce the neuroplastic changes (especially synaptic plasticity) and neuronal cell loss that are features of bipolar disorder.

ANTIPSYCHOTIC DRUGS

CLASSIFICATION

Antipsychotic drugs (also known as neuroleptics or major tranquillizers) have a common mechanism for their beneficial clinical effects, but belong to various chemical classes that differ in their propensity to cause sedation, and antimuscarinic or extrapyramidal effects (Table 21.2). They are commonly considered in two groups that differ in their unwanted effects: the conventional and atypical antipsychotics.

CONVENTIONAL ANTIPSYCHOTIC DRUGS

Examples

chlorpromazine, flupentixol, haloperidol, sulpiride

Table 21.2 Some unwanted effects of selected antipsychotic drugs

Drug type	Example	Sedative	Antimuscarinic	Extrapyramidal	Hypotension
Conventional antipsychotics					
Phenothiazines					
Group 1 (aliphatics)					
	Chlorpromazine	+++	++	++	+++
Group 2 (piperidines)					
	Pipotiazine	+	++	++	++
Group 3 (piperazines)					
	Fluphenazine	++	+	+++	+
Thioxanthenes					
	Flupentixol	+	+	+++	+
Butyrophenones					
	Haloperidol	+	+	+++	++
Diphenylbutylpiperidines					
	Pimozide	0	+	+++	+
Substituted benzamides					
	Sulpiride	+	+	+	0
Atypical antipsychotics					
	Clozapine	++	+	0	+
	Olanzapine	++	+	0	+
	Quetiapine	++	0	0	+
	Risperidone	+	0	+	+

+++, High; ++, moderate; +, low; 0, minimal.

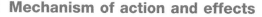

Mechanism of action and effects

The antipsychotic action of all conventional (or classical) antipsychotic drugs arises primarily from their antagonism of CNS dopamine D_2 receptors in the mesolimbic pathway. High affinity for the family of D_2 receptors is a common feature of all conventional antipsychotics, and the affinity of the drug for these receptors correlates well with its effective dose. Conventional antipsychotics have a higher affinity than dopamine for D_2 receptors, and dissociate slowly from the receptor. At least 65% D_2 receptor occupancy in the mesolimbic system is required for clinical benefit during long-term treatment of psychotic disorders. However, conventional antipsychotics also have D_2 receptor antagonist activity in other CNS pathways, and 80% or more D_2 receptor occupancy in the striatum will produce extrapyramidal unwanted effects (see below).

Many conventional antipsychotics also block serotonin 5-HT_{2A} and 5-HT_{2C} receptors, actions that may contribute to their clinical effects in suppressing negative symptoms. Antagonist activity at other receptors, including α_1-adrenoceptors and histamine H_1 receptors, does not influence their efficacy in psychotic illness but can produce unwanted effects (in which respect they resemble tricyclic antidepressants; Ch. 22). The severity of these unwanted effects varies considerably among the different drugs.

Clinical improvement with antipsychotic drugs develops slowly, despite an immediate antagonist action at dopamine receptors. There is increasing evidence that these drugs modulate complex intracellular pathways that affect neuroplasticity. This leads to changes in synaptic connections in areas of the brain known to be involved in psychotic illness which may be important for their long-term benefit. Clinically useful effects produced by antipsychotic drugs include the following.

■ A depressant action on conditioned responses and emotional responsiveness: in psychoses this is particularly helpful for the management of thought disorders, abnormalities of perception and delusional beliefs.
■ A sedative action, which is useful for the treatment of restlessness and confusion: sensory input into the reticular activating system is reduced by inhibition of collateral fibres from the lemniscal pathways. Spontaneous activity is preserved but arousal stimuli produce less response.
■ An anti-emetic effect through dopamine receptor antagonist activity at the chemoreceptor trigger zone (CTZ), which is useful to treat vomiting, such as that associated with drugs (e.g. cytotoxics, opioid analgesics) and uraemia: some antipsychotic drugs are also effective in motion sickness, through muscarinic receptor blockade (Ch. 32).
■ Antihistamine activity produced by histamine H_1-receptor antagonism can be used for treatment of allergic reactions (Ch. 39).

Pharmacokinetics

Conventional antipsychotics are rapidly absorbed from the gut but most undergo extensive first-pass metabolism. For some drugs, the plasma concentrations of active drug (including metabolites) can vary up to 10-fold among individuals, but there is not a close relationship between plasma drug concentration and clinical response. Elimination is by metabolism in the liver. Several antipsychotic drugs, such as chlorpromazine, haloperidol, perphenazine and zuclopenthixol, are metabolised predominantly by the polymorphic enzyme CYP2D6. There is a relationship between the steady-state plasma concentrations of these drugs (and therefore propensity to unwanted effects) and the CYP2D6 genotype (Ch. 2). Sulpiride does not undergo first-pass metabolism and is largely eliminated unchanged by the kidney. The half-lives of the antipsychotics vary widely; for example, that of sulpiride is 6–8 h, while the half-life of pimozide is very long, at 2 days. Some antipsychotics, such as chlorpromazine and haloperidol, can be given by intramuscular injection for more rapid onset of action.

Since adherence to treatment is often poor in psychotic disorders, depot formulations of many antipsychotics have been developed. They are given by intramuscular injection as a prodrug – which is the active compound esterified to a long-chain fatty acid and dissolved in a vegetable oil – that slowly releases the drug for between 1 and 12 weeks (depending on the formulation). When given as a depot preparation, or by deep intramuscular injection, the doses used are smaller than those for oral treatment, due to the absence of first-pass metabolism. The half-lives given in the Compendium at the end of this chapter do not reflect the slow absorption rate-limited half-life of the depot form (see Ch. 2). Examples of depot preparations are flupentixol decanoate and zuclopenthixol decanoate.

Unwanted effects

The antipsychotic drugs differ mainly in the degree of associated or unwanted effects (Table 21.2).

■ Extrapyramidal effects arise from D_2 receptor blockade in the nigrostriatal pathways, and take various forms: acute dystonias (tongue protrusion, torticollis, oculogyric crisis) are most common after the first dose or first few doses in children and young adults. Akathisia (restlessness) usually follows large initial doses, while parkinsonism has a gradual onset over several weeks usually in adults or the elderly. Extrapyramidal effects (Ch. 24) occur in more than half of those being treated with conventional antipsychotics, but are usually reversible if the drug is stopped. With prolonged use (several months to years) and especially in the elderly, tardive dyskinesias or tardive dystonias can develop. These consist of choreoathetoid and repetitive orofacial movements which often persist when the drug is withdrawn. Their aetiology is uncertain: upregulation of D_2 receptors may contribute, but damage to inhibitory GABAergic neurons and/or dysfunction in other neurotransmitter pathways is probably involved. Extrapyramidal effects are most common with piperazine phenothiazines (such as prochlorperazine), the butyrophenones (such as haloperidol) and depot preparations (Table 21.2).
■ Drowsiness and cognitive impairment can occur as a result of histamine and dopamine receptor antagonism.
■ Galactorrhoea, with gynaecomastia, amenorrhoea in women, impotence in men and reduced bone mineral density. These can arise when more than 70% D_2

receptor occupancy in hypothalamic pathways produces hyperprolactinaemia and reduced gonadotrophin secretion. Antimuscarinic activity and α_1-adrenoceptor antagonism also contribute.

- Antimuscarinic effects: peripheral antimuscarinic actions include dry mouth, constipation, micturition difficulties, blurred vision and reduced sexual arousal (Ch. 4). CNS muscarinic receptor blockade predisposes to acute confusional states.
- Postural hypotension, nasal stuffiness and impaired erection and ejaculation in men due to α_1-adrenoceptor antagonism.
- Hypothermia as a consequence of depressed hypothalamic function. Altered serotonergic neuronal activity may be responsible.
- Reduced seizure threshold.
- Hypersensitivity reactions include cholestatic jaundice, skin reactions and bone marrow depression.
- Weight gain, with an increased risk of insulin resistance and glucose intolerance.
- Gastrointestinal disturbances.
- Prolongation of the Q–T interval on the electrocardiogram, a particular problem with pimozide, predisposes to ventricular arrhythmias (Ch. 8).
- Neuroleptic malignant syndrome is a rare genetically determined disorder caused by a polymorphism in the D_2 receptor and consequent abnormal dopamine receptor antagonist activity in the corpus striatum and hypothalamus. In the presence of this polymorphism, antipsychotic drugs produce high fever, muscle rigidity, autonomic instability with hypertension, urinary incontinence and sweating, and altered consciousness. Immediate withdrawal of the antipsychotic and treatment with dantrolene or a dopamine receptor agonist (Ch. 24) may be life-saving. Symptoms can take up to 1 week to subside, or longer after a depot preparation. Cautious reintroduction of an antipsychotic may be possible without recurrence, but at least 2 weeks should be allowed after symptoms of the syndrome have resolved.
- Sudden withdrawal after long-term use can produce nausea, vomiting, anorexia, diarrhoea, sweating, myalgia, paraesthesia, insomnia and agitation. These symptoms usually subside within 2 weeks.

ATYPICAL ANTIPSYCHOTIC DRUGS

Examples

aripiprazole, clozapine, olanzapine, risperidone

Mechanism of action and effects

The antipsychotic action of atypical antipsychotic drugs, like that of conventional antipsychotics, arises primarily from blockade of CNS dopamine D_2 receptors in mesolimbic pathways. However, the atypical antipsychotic drugs have a lower affinity for D_2 receptors than dopamine and transient receptor occupancy. Since the receptor occupancy is much less than that of conventional antipsychotics, they are less likely to produce extrapyramidal

movement disorders at usual doses (Ch. 24). Antagonist activity at serotonin 5-HT_2 receptors may contribute to their antipsychotic action, particularly in improving the negative features such as apathy and blunted emotions.

- Aripiprazole has partial agonist activity at the D_2 and D_3 receptors, which limits the degree of receptor antagonism. It is also a partial agonist at 5-HT_{1A} and 5-HT_{2C} receptors, but an antagonist at 5-HT_{2A} receptors, and has moderate antagonist activity at histamine H_1 receptors and α-adrenoceptors.
- Clozapine is a relatively weak D_2 receptor antagonist with selective cortical receptor occupancy, and shows greater antagonist activity at D_1 and D_4 receptors. It has a much higher affinity for and antagonist activity at serotonin 5-HT_{2A} and 5-HT_{2C} receptors, α_1-adrenoceptors, H_1 histamine receptors and muscarinic receptors.
- Olanzapine has a similar profile to clozapine, with additional antagonist activity at serotonin 5-HT_3 receptors.
- Quetiapine has moderate affinity for D_2 receptors, and is an antagonist at 5-HT_{1A}, 5-HT_{2A} and 5-HT_{2C} receptors. It also has antagonist activity at α_1- and α_2-adrenoceptors and histamine H_1 receptors.
- Risperidone has higher-affinity for D_2 and D_4 receptors, with dose-dependent limbic selectivity. It also has antagonist activity at several 5-HT_1 and 5-HT_2 receptor subtypes, α_1- and α_2-adrenoceptors and histamine H_1 receptors. It does not bind to muscarinic receptors.

Adherence to treatment with atypical antipsychotics is greater than for conventional antipsychotics, probably as a result of less marked unwanted effects, which may explain their apparently greater efficacy. Clozapine, however, is uniquely superior to all other drugs for treatment of refractory schizophrenia.

Pharmacokinetics

Atypical antipsychotics are rapidly absorbed from the gut and most undergo extensive first-pass metabolism to inactive metabolites. The half-lives of the atypical antipsychotics vary widely. Some atypical antipsychotics, such as olanzapine and risperidone, can be given in a depot formulation.

Unwanted effects

The atypical antipsychotic drugs show some differences from conventional antipsychotics in their unwanted effects (Table 21.2).

- Extrapyramidal effects are less likely to be caused by atypical antipsychotics, except at high dosages, when the risk is similar to conventional antipsychotics.
- Drowsiness and cognitive impairment are less marked than with conventional antipsychotics. Risperidone can cause insomnia and agitation.
- Galactorrhoea and sexual dysfunction are less common with most atypical antipsychotics, except risperidone.
- Antimuscarinic effects are uncommon with atypical antipsychotics.
- Postural hypotension, especially during initial dose titration with clozapine and quetiapine.
- Reduced seizure threshold with clozapine.

- Agranulocytosis is a particular problem with clozapine (1–2% risk); regular blood tests are mandatory during treatment with this drug.
- Weight gain with clozapine and olanzapine.
- Hyperglycaemia is more common than with conventional antipsychotics.
- Neuroleptic malignant syndrome is rare.
- Sudden withdrawal syndrome.

MOOD-STABILISING DRUGS FOR BIPOLAR DISORDER

LITHIUM

Mechanism of action

The mechanism of action of lithium is not well understood, but it has multiple effects in the CNS.

- Lithium has complex effects on the generation of intracellular second messengers in cortical neuronal pathways. It attenuates the function of G_s proteins coupled to adenylyl cyclase but increases basal adenylyl cyclase activity, effects that alter cAMP synthesis. Lithium also inhibits intracellular inositol monophosphatase, and therefore interferes with substrate generation for second messengers involved in phosphoinositide pathway signalling. These actions affect several monoaminergic and cholinergic systems in the CNS. The overall action of lithium may be to stabilise intracellular signalling by enhancing basal activity but decreasing maximum activity.
- It suppresses pro-apoptotic genes and increases expression of anti-apoptotic genes, with consequent neuroprotection. Lithium inhibits the multifunctional enzyme glucose synthase kinase-3 (GSK-3), a regulator of many signal transduction pathways that are involved in neuronal apoptosis. Inhibition of the activity of the pro-apoptotic enzyme caspase-3 by lithium also confers neuroprotection.
- Increased neurogenesis has been found in the hippocampus after lithium treatment, which may be one consequence of the complex changes in intracellular signalling.

Pharmacokinetics

Lithium is given as a salt (e.g. carbonate, citrate), which is rapidly absorbed from the gut. To avoid high peak plasma concentrations (which are associated with unwanted effects), modified-release formulations are normally used. Lithium is widely distributed in the body but enters the brain slowly. It is selectively concentrated in bone and the thyroid gland. Excretion is by glomerular filtration, with 80% reabsorbed in the proximal tubule by the same mechanism as Na^+ although, unlike Na^+, lithium is not reabsorbed from more distal parts of the kidney. When the body is depleted of salt and water, for example by vomiting or diarrhoea, then enhanced reabsorption of Na^+ in the proximal tubule is accompanied by enhanced lithium reabsorption, which can produce acute toxicity. Lithium has a long half-life of about 1 day. Lithium has a narrow therapeutic index, and regular monitoring of serum concentrations is mandatory at least every 3 months during long-term treatment. The serum concentration should be measured 12 h after dosing, so that the absorption and distribution phases are completed, with the aim of maintaining a therapeutic plasma lithium concentration between 0.4 and 1.0 $mmol \cdot L^{-1}$.

Unwanted effects

- Nausea and diarrhoea can occur even at low plasma concentrations.
- CNS effects, including tremor, giddiness, ataxia, dysarthria and mild cognitive and memory impairment.
- Hypothyroidism can be caused by interference with thyroxine synthesis during long-term treatment. Thyroid function should be monitored every 6 months
- Reduced responsiveness of the distal renal tubule to antidiuretic hormone (ADH), which can produce a reversible nephrogenic diabetes insipidus with polyuria and consequent polydipsia.
- Overdosage usually produces symptoms with serum lithium concentrations above 1.5 $mmol \cdot L^{-1}$. Severe toxicity (serum lithium concentration above 2.0 $mmol \cdot L^{-1}$) can lead to coma, convulsions and profound hypotension with oliguria.

Drug interactions

Diuretics can reduce lithium excretion by producing dehydration (see pharmacokinetics above). This is most marked with thiazides (Ch. 14) because of their prolonged action. Angiotensin-converting enzyme inhibitors, angiotensin II receptor antagonists (Ch. 6) and some non-steroidal anti-inflammatory drugs (Ch. 29) also reduce the excretion of lithium. The risk of extrapyramidal effects may be increased when lithium is prescribed concurrently with antipsychotic drugs.

ANTICONVULSANTS

carbamazepine, lamotrigine, sodium valproate

Mechanism of action in bipolar disorder

The mode of action of the anticonvulsants carbamazepine, lamotrigine and sodium valproate in mania may be related to facilitation of GABAergic inhibitory neurotransmission and consequent modulation of excitatory glutamatergic neurons. Like lithium, anticonvulsants affect cAMP-mediated intracellular events, inhibit the phosphoinositide signalling pathway and activate neuroprotective anti-apoptotic genes. They also stimulate hippocampal neurogenesis. Anticonvulsant (antiepileptic) drugs are discussed in Chapter 23.

MANAGEMENT OF PSYCHOTIC DISORDERS

MANAGEMENT OF SCHIZOPHRENIA

Acute psychotic symptoms such as hallucinations and delusions can be controlled relatively rapidly with an antipsychotic drug such as haloperidol or chlorpromazine. The initial sedative actions of these drugs can be particularly helpful. However, reductions in thought disturbance, withdrawal and apathy are delayed and the clinical improvement is gradual over several weeks of treatment. Atypical antipsychotics should be considered in preference to conventional antipsychotics:

■ when choosing first-line treatment for newly diagnosed schizophrenia,
■ if there are unacceptable unwanted effects with a conventional drug,
■ during an acute schizophrenic episode when discussion with the person is not possible.

Treatment for schizophrenia is not curative and long-term maintenance therapy is usually required to prevent relapse. The optimal duration of this treatment is determined by the number of acute episodes, and is usually at least 2–5 years. Intermittent treatment that is only given for relapses is associated with a higher overall relapse rate of 50–80%, compared with 25–40% in those taking prophylactic therapy. The relapse rate is lower with atypical antipsychotics compared to conventional antipsychotics. Adherence to maintenance treatment is often poor in schizophrenia, and can be improved by depot injections given every 1–4 weeks. Continuous antipsychotic treatment provides relief of symptoms for more than 70% of people with schizophrenia but resistance to conventional antipsychotics is particularly common if negative symptoms predominate.

Atypical antipsychotic drugs produce greater relief of negative symptoms than the conventional antipsychotic drugs, although this may be due to better adherence to treatment. There is limited evidence to support the concurrent use of a selective serotonin reuptake inhibitor (SSRI; Ch. 22) with an atypical antipsychotic drug for those whose negative symptoms do not respond to the antipsychotic drug alone. Clozapine is the only antipsychotic drug that is effective in treatment resistance (incomplete recovery), but close monitoring is required because of the 1–2% risk of agranulocytosis. Clozapine should always be tried if symptoms have failed to respond to two antipsychotic drugs, at least one of which should be an atypical drug, each given for 6–8 weeks. Between 30 and 50% of those who are resistant to other treatments will respond to clozapine.

Various psychological treatments to improve social skills are important as an adjunct to drug treatment and should be provided along with social support.

MANAGEMENT OF MANIA AND BIPOLAR DISORDER

When symptoms of acute mania are mild or moderate, they can usually be controlled by lithium, although the therapeutic effect may be delayed for at least a week. For this reason, a benzodiazepine (Ch. 20) is usually given as well for the first 7 days. The anticonvulsant sodium valproate is an effective alternative to lithium for the acute phase, and its sedative action produces a response in 1–4 days when used alone. Carbamazepine can be used, but has a delayed onset of action and is given initially with a benzodiazepine.

If manic symptoms are more severe it is usually necessary to give an antipsychotic drug in combination with lithium, carbamazepine or sodium valproate and perhaps initially a benzodiazepine. Conventional antipsychotic drugs are only recommended for short-term use, because of their extrapyramidal unwanted effects, and an atypical drug such as olanzapine, quetiapine or risperidone is usually preferred.

Depression in bipolar disorder is often treated with a combination of lithium and an antidepressant. However, the response to antidepressant therapy is less satisfactory than with unipolar depression, and there is a risk of provoking a switch to mania. There is limited evidence that mania is less likely to be provoked by an SSRI than by a tricyclic antidepressant (Ch. 22). Alternative treatments include the atypical antipsychotic quetiapine, a combination of olanzapine with the SSRI fluoxetine, or the mood-stabilising anticonvulsant lamotrigine, which have all been reported to be effective for bipolar depression.

Treatment should be continued for at least two years from the last episode of mania. If a person with bipolar disorder has had at least two episodes of either mania or depression in five years then prophylactic therapy is recommended for at least five years. The optimal duration of prophylactic therapy is unknown. If a decision is made to discontinue treatment then gradual withdrawal is recommended to reduce the risk of relapse, especially of mania. Lithium is the conventional treatment of choice for prophylaxis (although the full prophylactic effect may not be apparent for 6–12 months), but carbamazepine or lamotrigine are equally effective. There is less evidence to support the use of sodium valproate, which is usually reserved for those who do not tolerate first-line treatments, or for when these are ineffective.

Electroconvulsive therapy is used for refractory episodes of both mania and depression, and has a much more rapid action than drug therapy. As for schizophrenia, psychological treatments are an important adjunct to drug therapy in bipolar disorder.

SELF-ASSESSMENT

True/false questions

1. It may take several weeks for the full beneficial effects of antipsychotics to be seen.
2. The positive symptoms of schizophrenia (e.g. delusions) are more readily controlled than negative symptoms (e.g. withdrawal).
3. There is a close correlation between plasma levels of chlorpromazine and its antipsychotic effect.
4. Antipsychotics are effective in treating about 70% of people with schizophrenia.
5. Some antipsychotic drugs can be given in a depot preparation injected at 6-monthly intervals.

6. The atypical antipsychotic drugs have relatively low affinity for dopamine D_2 receptors.
7. The atypical antipsychotic clozapine has greater antimuscarinic activity than chlorpromazine.
8. Clozapine causes agranulocytosis.
9. The atypical antipsychotic drugs have relatively few effects on the extrapyramidal system.
10. Group 2 phenothiazines cause fewer extrapyramidal symptoms than other conventional antipsychotics.
11. Lithium interferes with thyroxine synthesis.
12. Lithium is reabsorbed through the distal convoluted tubule in the kidney.

One-best-answer (OBA) question

Choose the *most accurate* statement about antipsychotic drugs.

A. Adherence to atypical antipsychotic drugs is generally worse than with conventional antipsychotics.
B. Depot antipsychotic injections reduce the risk of extrapyramidal effects.
C. Dopamine receptor agonists may be life-saving in neuroleptic malignant syndrome.
D. Haloperidol causes nausea.
E. Clozapine causes little sedation.

Extended-matching-item questions

Choose one mechanism from A to E below most likely to underlie each of the drug effects 1–5:

A. Blockade of dopamine receptors in the substantia nigra.
B. Blockade of muscarinic receptors.
C. Blockade of α_1-adrenoceptors.
D. Blockade of serotonin 5-HT$_2$ receptors.
E. Blockade of histamine receptors.

  1. Antipsychotic activity
  2. Postural hypotension
  3. Sedation
  4. Constipation
  5. Extrapyramidal movement disorders

Case-based questions

A 25-year-old man (Mr PS) with schizophrenia has been treated with high-dose oral chlorpromazine for 2 years. His main symptoms of auditory hallucinations and delusional thoughts ('The people in the flat above are broadcasting my thoughts on their radio') had improved, but he remained socially withdrawn and apathetic and described a number of problems, including feeling very tired, faintness on standing up, dry mouth, sexual problems, blurred vision, occasional difficulty with fine control of movement and weight gain. Mr PS has had two severe relapses requiring hospitalisation within the last 18 months and is vague on whether he always takes his medication as directed.

A. How might you improve adherence to treatment?
B. Consider alternative antipsychotic drugs that might help Mr PS.

True/false answers

1. **True.** Acute psychotic symptoms may respond relatively rapidly but further gradual improvement is seen over several weeks.
2. **True.** Negative symptoms are more difficult to treat, but may respond better to atypical antipsychotics.
3. **False.** The plasma levels of chlorpromazine are highly variable and do not correlate with clinical effect.
4. **True.** Schizophrenia is well controlled in about 70% of people taking continuous antipsychotic drug therapy.
5. **False.** Depot injections are usually given at 1- to 4-week intervals, depending on the drug dose and formulation.
6. **True.** The atypical antipsychotics have fewer extrapyramidal (movement) than the conventional drugs.
7. **True.** The atypical antipsychotics have lower affinity for D_2 receptors, and more transient D_2 receptor occupancy, than conventional antipsychotics.
8. **False.** The atypical antipsychotics such as clozapine have less antimuscarinic activity than most phenothiazines.
9. **True.** The 1–2% risk of agranulocytosis with clozapine necessitates regular blood monitoring.
10. **True.** Compared to other classical antipsychotic drugs, Group 2 phenothiazines have relatively high antimuscarinic activity, which may reduce unwanted extrapyramidal effects (see use of antimuscarinic drugs in parkinsonism, Ch. 24).
11. **True.** Hypothyroidism can occur with use of lithium and thyroid function should be monitored.
12. **False.** Lithium is reabsorbed through the proximal convoluted tubule in the kidney, at the same site that Na^+ is absorbed.

OBA answer

Answer C is correct.

A. Incorrect. Adherence is higher with atypical drugs, probably as a result of fewer unwanted effects.
B. Incorrect. The risk of extrapyramidal effects is increased with depot injections.
C. **Correct.** Dopamine receptor agonists reverse D_2 receptor blockade in neuroleptic malignant syndrome.
D. Incorrect. Antipsychotics do not cause nausea and some are used in the treatment of nausea and vomiting.
E. Incorrect. Clozapine has a sedative action.

Extended-matching-item answers

1. Answer **D** is correct. Serotonin (5-HT) receptor antagonism is most likely to contribute to antipsychotic activity.
2. Answer **C** is correct. Blockade of α_1-adrenoceptors on blood vessels produces hypotension.
3. Answer **E** is correct. Blockade of histamine H_1 receptors in the CNS causes sedation.
4. Answer **B** is correct. Antimuscarinic effects include constipation, dry mouth, blurred vision and problems with micturition.

5. Answer **A** is correct. Antagonism of nigrostriatal pathway dopamine D_2 receptors produces extrapyramidal disorders of movement.

Case-based answers

A. Approaches include the possible use of a depot preparation and stressing the importance of support from the patient's GP and family in maintaining adherence. A principal cause of poor adherence is the unwanted effects of antipsychotic therapy. Since unwanted effects vary widely from drug to drug, the choice of drug may have a major impact on adherence.

B. Mr PS may benefit from a different conventional antipsychotic drug, such as another phenothiazine that causes less sedation and fewer antimuscarinic effects than chlorpromazine, but extrapyramidal effects may be worse. An atypical drug may be more appropriate and Mr PS's adherence may increase as a result of fewer unwanted effects. Atypical antipsychotics may also be more effective on Mr PS's negative symptoms of apathy and withdrawal. Both positive and negative features may be particularly resistant in a proportion of people with schizophrenia; clozapine may be effective in unresponsive patients after failure of two or more antipsychotic drugs, one of which is an atypical drug, but the risk of blood disorders with clozapine makes blood monitoring mandatory.

FURTHER READING

Altamura AC, Sassella F, Santini A et al. (2003) Intramuscular preparations of antipsychotics. *Drugs* 63, 493–512

Belmaker RH (2004) Bipolar disorder. *N Engl J Med* 351, 476–486

Cipriani A, Barbui C, Salanti G et al. (2011) Comparative efficacy and acceptability of antimanic drugs in acute mania: a multiple-treatments meta–analysis. *Lancet* 378, 1306–1315

Frye MA (2011) Bipolar disorder – a focus on depression. *N Engl J Med* 364, 51–59

Geddes J, Freemantle N, Harrison P, Bebbington P (2000) Atypical antipsychotics in the treatment of schizophrenia: systematic overview and meta-regression analysis. *BMJ* 321, 1371–1376

Hartling L, Abou-Setta AM, Dursun S (2012) Antipsychotics in adults with schizophrenia: comparative effectiveness of first-generation versus second-generation medications: a systematic review and meta-analysis. *JAMA* 157, 498–511

Harwood AJ, Agam G (2003) Search for a common mechanism of action of mood stabilizers. *Biochem Pharmacol* 66, 179–189

Horacek J, Bubenikov-Valesova V, Kopecek M et al. (2006) Mechanism of action of atypical antipsychotic drugs and the neurobiology of schizophrenia. *CNS Drugs* 20, 389–409

Kane JM, Correll CU (2010) Past and present progress in the pharmacologic treatment of schizophrenia. *J Clin Psychiatry* 71, 1115–1124

Laruelle M, Kegele S, Abi-Darham A (2003) Glutamate dopamine and schizophrenia. From pathology to treatment *Ann NY Acad Sci* 1003, 138–158

Laruelle M, Frankle WG, Narenran R et al. (2007) Mechanism of action of antipsychotic drugs: from dopamine D_2 receptor antagonism to glutamate NMDA facilitation. *Clin Ther* 27 (Suppl A), S16–S24

Li X, Ketter TA, Frye MA (2002) Synaptic, intracellular, and neuroprotective mechanisms of anticonvulsants: are they relevant for the treatment and course of bipolar disorders? *J Affect Disord* 69, 1–14

Miyamoto S, Duncan GE, Marx CE et al. (2005) Treatments for schizophrenia: a critical review of pharmacology and mechanisms of action of antipsychotic drugs. *Mol Psychiatry* 10, 79–104

Möller H-J (2003) Management of the negative symptoms of schizophrenia. *CNS Drugs* 17, 793–823

Mueser KT, McGurk SR (2004) Schizophrenia. *Lancet* 363, 2063–2072

Müller-Oerlinghausen B, Berghöfer A, Bauer M (2002) Bipolar disorder. *Lancet* 359, 241–247

Picchioni MM, Murray RM (2007) Schizophrenia. *BMJ* 335, 91–95

Rochon PA, Stukel TA, Sykora A et al. (2005) Atypical antipsychotics and parkinsonism. *Arch Intern Med* 165, 1882–1888

Van Os J, Kapur S (2009) Schizophrenia. *Lancet* 374, 635–645

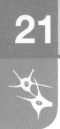

Compendium: antipsychotic drugs

Drug	Kinetics (half-life)	Comments
Conventional antipsychotics		
Benperidol	Oral bioavailability 40–50%; hepatic metabolism (5–7 h)	Butyrophenone antipsychotic; given orally; main indication is control of deviant antisocial sexual behaviour (but efficacy uncertain)
Chlorpromazine	Low oral bioavailability (10–33%); numerous pathways of metabolism, with some very long-acting metabolites (8–35 h)	Group 1 phenothiazine; oral, suppository and injection formulations available; marked sedative effect; also used as anti-emetic in palliative care
Flupentixol	Oral bioavailability 55%; half-life for release from depot injection is about 17 days; hepatic metabolism and mainly biliary excretion (35 h)	Thioxanthene; given orally, or by depot injection (as the decanoate ester)
Fluphenazine	Oral bioavailability about 50%; half-life for release from depot injection is about 26 days; hepatic metabolites responsible for about 50% of drug activity (16 h)	Group 3 phenothiazine; given orally, or by depot injection (as the decanoate ester)
Haloperidol	Oral bioavailability about 60%; half-life for release from depot injection is about 21 days; metabolism to an active metabolite in liver and extrahepatic tissues; undergoes enterohepatic circulation (9–67 h)	Butyrophenone; given orally and by injection, or by depot injection (as the decanoate ester)
Levomepromazine	Oral bioavailability about 50%; hepatic metabolism to numerous products and highly variable kinetics (15–70 h)	Group 1 phenothiazine; given orally or by injection (intramuscularly or intravenously); also used for pain relief and as anti-emetic in palliative care
Pericyazine	No kinetic data available	An early Group 2 phenothiazine; given orally
Perphenazine	Variable oral bioavailability due to first-pass metabolism by multiple pathways; hepatic metabolism (9 h)	Group 3 phenothiazine; given orally; also used as anti-emetic
Pimozide	Oral bioavailability 60–80%; hepatic metabolism to inactive products (55 h)	Diphenylbutylpiperadine; given orally; ECG monitoring mandatory before first use
Pipotiazine palmitate	Long half-life (15–16 days) results from slow release from depot injection; parent drug (pipotiazide) has an elimination half-life of a few hours	Group 2 phenothiazine; given only as a depot injection
Prochlorperazine	Variable absorption of oral doses; hepatic metabolism (6–7 h)	Phenothiazine antipsychotic; given orally, rectally or by deep intramuscular injection; also used as an anti-emetic
Promazine	Hepatic metabolism (>24 h?)	Group 1 phenothiazine; a low-potency metabolite of chlorpromazine with little antipsychotic activity; given orally, used as a sedative
Sulpiride	Low oral bioavailability (30–40%) owing to poor absorption; water-soluble compound eliminated largely unchanged in urine and faeces (6–8 h)	A substituted benzamide; given orally
Trifluoperazine	Low oral bioavailability due to first-pass metabolism in gut and liver; numerous hepatic metabolites (7–18 h)	Group 3 phenothiazine; given orally; also used as an anti-emetic
Zuclopenthixol	Oral bioavailability about 60%; hepatic metabolism (13–23 h); half-lives of the depot forms are about 19 days	Thioxanthene; given orally, or as deep intramuscular depot injection (as the decanoate or acetate)
Atypical antipsychotics		
Amisulpride	Oral bioavailability about 50%; largely renal elimination (12 h)	D_2 and D_3 antagonist with presynaptic and limbic system selectivity; given orally
Aripiprazole	High oral bioavailability; hepatic metabolism; one active metabolite produced by CYP2D6 (60 h)	Partial agonist at D_2 and 5-HT$_{1A}$ receptors and antagonist at 5-HT$_{2A}$ receptors; given orally

Compendium: antipsychotic drugs—cont'd

Drug	Kinetics (half-life)	Comments
Clozapine	Oral bioavailability 30–50%; hepatic metabolism (6–33 h)	High-affinity antagonist of D_1, D_4 and 5-HT$_2$ receptors; given orally
Olanzapine	Oral bioavailability 60%; hepatic metabolism (21–54 h)	Antagonist at D_1, D_2, D_4 and 5-HT$_2$ receptors; given orally
Paliperidone	Oral bioavailability 28%; renal elimination (80%), mainly of unchanged drug (23 h)	Hydroxylated metabolite of risperidone; antagonist at D_2 and 5-HT$_2$ receptors; given orally (as extended release formulation), or by depot injection (as palmitate ester)
Quetiapine	Good oral absorption; hepatic metabolism (6 h)	Antagonist at D_2 and 5-HT$_2$ receptors; given orally
Risperidone	Oral bioavailability about 70%; extensive hepatic metabolisers eliminate the drug 5–10 times more rapidly (2–4 h) than poor metabolisers (17–22 h)	Antagonist at D_2 and 5-HT$_2$ receptors; given orally or by deep intramuscular depot injection
Zotepine	Low oral bioavailability (7–13%); hepatic metabolism (12–24 h)	Antagonist at D_2 and 5-HT$_2$ receptors; given orally

Mood-stabilising drugs

Drug	Kinetics (half-life)	Comments
Lithium	Complete oral absorption; filtered at the glomerulus and about 80% reabsorbed in the proximal, but not distal, renal tubule	Given orally

DEPRESSION

Clinical depression is characterised by diverse psychological and physical symptoms. Major depressive disorder is considered to be present if there are at least five of the following symptoms present for at least two months, or producing marked functional impairment for at least two weeks: depressed mood, loss of interest and enjoyment of activities, loss of energy, loss of appetite or weight disturbance (significant weight loss or gain), sleep disturbance, psychomotor change, a sense of guilt and worthlessness, concentration difficulties or indecisiveness or thoughts of death or suicide. Depressed mood or loss of interest must be present, but otherwise depression can present with mainly physical rather than psychological symptoms. The existence of mixed anxiety–depression disorder is now also well accepted.

Major depressive disorder is an episodic illness that has a lifetime prevalence of about 15% of the population, and recurs in almost three-quarters of people who experience an episode. In about 25% of people with depression the condition may become chronic, with duration of symptoms of more than two years, while up to 40% of people report reduced psychosocial functioning even after recovery from a depressive episode. As the number of depressive episodes increases the threshold for precipitation of a further episode by life stresses appears to decrease, a process referred to as 'kindling'. Both a genetic predisposition and the effects of adverse events in early life may determine whether a person is susceptible to depressive illness in later life.

BIOLOGICAL BASIS OF DEPRESSION

The cause of depression is unknown and there may not be a single mechanism. The neurotrophic hypothesis postulates that there are changes in the connectivity between key structures in the brain that are involved in regulation of mood and the stress response, including limbic structures (amygdala, hippocampus and nucleus accumbens) and the prefrontal cortex. It has been suggested that disruption to limbic connections with the prefrontal cortex impairs the normal feedback from the cortex that regulates limbic activity. Depression involves a negative emotional bias that may lead the person to preferentially recall negative events. This negative information is processed in the amygdala, which is hyperactive in people with depression.

In people who are genetically predisposed to depression, stress can initiate remodelling and elimination of hippocampal circuits involved in regulation of mood, cognition and behaviour. High plasma concentrations of the stress peptide corticotropin-releasing hormone (CRH; also known as corticotropin-releasing factor) and the stress hormone cortisol lead to impaired neuroplasticity. Atrophy of the hippocampus blunts the negative feedback from this structure on neuroendocrine function and leads to a perpetuation of the stress response.

The monoamine theory, which has underpinned treatment of depression for many years, is complementary to the neurotrophic hypothesis. Depression is associated with reduced central nervous system (CNS) monoaminergic neurotransmission, possibly as a result of high monoamine oxidase A activity. This affects both serotonergic and noradrenergic pathways, which are closely involved in regulation of mood.

Corticotropin-releasing hormone in depression

In depression, there is hypersecretion of the 'stressor' peptide CRH (Ch. 43), which has detrimental effects on neural synaptic plasticity and neurogenesis, and promotes neuronal excitotoxicity. CRH depresses serotonergic neurotransmission and is also a neurotransmitter that orchestrates the CNS control of many behavioural, endocrine, autonomic and immunological responses. Many of these circuits involve glutamatergic neurotransmission via the excitatory N-methyl-D-aspartate (NMDA) receptor. Depressed neurotransmission in these pathways provides a potential target for the treatment of depression. CRH also increases cortisol secretion, which contributes to the loss of neuroplasticity.

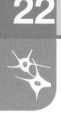

Serotonergic and noradrenergic pathways in the brain

Most serotonergic neurons are found in the raphe area of the midbrain, from where they project to the hippocampus in the limbic system and to the cerebral cortex. Presynaptic α_2-adrenoceptors and 5-hydroxytryptamine 1 (5-HT$_1$) autoreceptors (not shown in Fig. 22.1) inhibit serotonin release. Somatodendritic 5-HT$_1$, α_1- and β-adrenoceptor autoreceptors on the neuronal cell bodies of the raphe nuclei also regulate firing in serotonergic neurons. Postsynaptic 5-HT$_2$ receptors mediate the effects of serotonin and are widely distributed in the cerebral cortex, but especially the prefrontal cortex. A schematic of these mechanisms is shown in Figure 22.1.

In contrast, most noradrenergic neurons arise in the locus coeruleus and the lateral tegmental areas of the brainstem. The locus coeruleus and the raphe region have many reciprocal neural projections, and therefore the pathways are interdependent. For example, noradrenergic neurotransmission stimulates serotonergic neurons by activating somatodendritic α_1-adrenoceptors, but also inhibits serotonin synthesis and release through presynaptic α_2-adrenoceptors.

Pathways mediated by glutamate, γ-aminobutyric acid (GABA) and substance P also modulate monoaminergic neurotransmission.

Monoamine neurotransmitters and depression

Serotonergic pathways in the CNS are believed to be mainly involved in mood, while noradrenergic pathways are involved in stress systems, drive and energy state. These monoaminergic circuits in the brain are closely integrated. Simplistically, it has been hypothesised that the following biological changes in the monoamine system are important in depression:

- low levels of monoamine neurotransmitters,
- upregulation of postsynaptic monoamine receptors,
- upregulation of the inhibitory presynaptic and somatodendritic autoreceptors that control monoamine release.

There are increased 5-HT$_2$ receptor numbers in the frontal cortex of depressed suicide victims, whereas other studies have indicated that serotonin and noradrenaline concentrations in the brain are reduced in depression. Overall, evidence for the 'monoamine' theory as a molecular basis for depression is limited, but the response to drugs that increase monoamine neurotransmission supports the concept.

Regulation of brain-derived neurotrophic factor in depression

Most antidepressant drugs increase the CNS monoamine concentrations rapidly, but the clinical benefit of antidepressant therapy is delayed. This suggests that more gradual adaptive changes occur as a result of increased monoaminergic neurotransmission. These pharmacologically induced changes are incompletely understood, but

they may help to normalise the fundamental dysfunction in intracellular signalling pathways and transduction mechanisms that have been described in depression.

There is evidence for the central role of brain-derived neurotrophic factor (BDNF) in depression. Regulation of BDNF by monoamines is shown in Figure 22.2. BDNF expression is reduced when monoamine neurotransmission is impaired, but also in conditions of stress with elevated serum cortisol. Decreased expression of BDNF has adverse effects on neuronal plasticity can reduce neuronal networks, and may be a major factor in loss of neuronal circuitry and hippocampal atrophy. There is some evidence that successful antidepressant treatment is associated with increased BDNF expression and a restoration of hippocampal function and neuroendocrine regulation.

ANTIDEPRESSANT DRUG ACTION

Most of the antidepressant drugs currently used clinically target the mechanisms involved in the control of monoamine neurotransmitter turnover or monoamine receptor function. There seems to be little difference in efficacy between drugs that act predominantly on serotonergic or on noradrenergic pathways, although they differ in their side-effect profiles. The ways that major antidepressants work to modify monoamine turnover and function are shown in Figure 22.1.

Long-term treatment with antidepressants promotes both the structural and functional integrity of the neural circuits that regulate mood. The mechanisms by which they achieve this are complex.

- Enhanced CNS monoamine levels. The initial action of most drugs used in the treatment of depression is to enhance neurotransmission by CNS monoamines, particularly serotonin but also noradrenaline and dopamine. Increased noradrenergic activity further enhances serotonergic neurotransmission by stimulating somatodendritic α_1-adrenoceptors on serotonergic neurons. However, although antidepressants rapidly increase synaptic monoamine levels, clinical improvement is delayed. In part, this may be due to slow reduction in the number of upregulated somatodendritic and presynaptic 5-HT$_1$ inhibitory autoreceptors (see above), which is necessary before activity increases in serotonergic pathways.
- Effects on postsynaptic monoamine receptor expression and intracellular signal transduction. During treatment with antidepressants there is a gradual increase in responsiveness to serotonin in the prefrontal cortex. There is considerable evidence that antidepressants reverse the changes in intracellular signalling that are found in depression (Fig. 22.2). They enhance the response to monoamine receptor stimulation, which increases expression of BDNF and its receptor. As a result there is enhanced differentiation of progenitor cells into neurons and increased neuronal survival. Of note, electroconvulsive therapy can also increase the expression and activity of BDNF.
- Regulation of CRH production. During long-term treatment with antidepressants there is normalisation of overexpressed CRH secretion. This may be related to

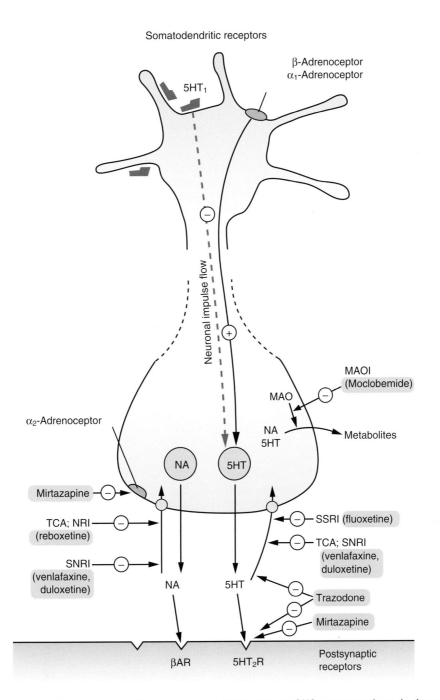

Fig. 22.1 **The actions of drugs used in the treatment of depression on CNS serotonergic and adrenergic functioning.** The primary action of many drugs in current clinical use is to enhance serotonin (5-HT, 5-hydroxytryptamine) and noradrenaline (NA) availability. The majority of released serotonin and noradrenaline is rapidly removed from the synapse by reuptake into the neuron (yellow circles). Antidepressants vary in their abilities to inhibit the reuptake of serotonin or noradrenaline, thus enhancing the synaptic concentrations of these transmitters. Stimulation of presynaptic α_2-adrenoceptors reduces monoamine release; mirtazapine, by blocking these presynaptic autoreceptors, increases noradrenaline and serotonin release and transmission. Other drugs act by significantly blocking postsynaptic receptors which are upregulated in depression. βAR, β-adrenoceptor; MAO, monoamine oxidase; MAOI, monoamine oxidase inhibitor; NA, noradrenaline; NRI, (selective) noradrenaline reuptake inhibitor; SNRI, serotonin and noradrenaline reuptake inhibitor; SSRI, selective serotonin reuptake inhibitor; TCA, tricyclic antidepressant.

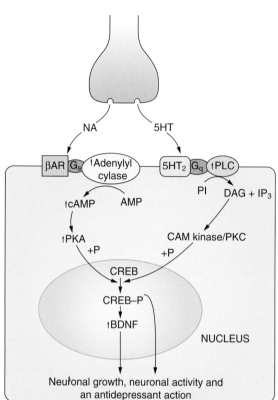

Fig 22.2 The regulation of neuronal growth and plasticity by monoamines and brain-derived neurotrophic factor (BDNF). Adequate levels of monoamines, cAMP response element-binding protein (CREB-P) and BDNF are considered necessary for neuronal growth and plasticity. An increase in cAMP can result from noradrenaline (NA) acting on β-adrenoceptor (βAR) subtypes, and an increase in diacylglycerol (DAG) signalling can result from serotonin (5-HT) acting on 5-HT$_2$ type receptors. There is also evidence that cAMP can be increased by serotonin acting on 5-HT$_4$ and 5-HT$_7$ receptors, and DAG by noradrenaline acting on α_1-adrenoceptors (not shown). Critical points in this cascade may be dysfunctional in depressed individuals, including reduced synthesis of the monamine transmitters, genetic polymorphism affecting the function or expression of monoamine receptors, anomalies in coupling of G$_s$ to adenylyl cyclase, reduced protein kinase A (PKA) activity and reduced phosphorylation of CREB. These may result in reduced BDNF activity, leading to neuronal atrophy and cell death in the hippocampus and cortex. CAM kinase, calmodulin-dependent protein kinase; IP$_3$, inositol triphosphate; PI, phosphatidylinositol; PKC, protein kinase C; PLC, phospholipase C.

upregulation of CNS glucocorticoid receptors, with feedback inhibition of CRH.
■ Antagonism of NMDA receptor action. Antidepressant drugs bind to a site in NMDA receptor-associated ion channels in the hippocampus and cerebral cortex, and may protect cells against stress-induced 'glutamate excitotoxicity'.

ANTIDEPRESSANT DRUGS

Tricyclic antidepressant drugs

Examples

amitriptyline, imipramine, lofepramine

Mechanism of action

Tricyclic antidepressants (TCAs) inhibit the reuptake of monoamine neurotransmitters into the presynaptic neuron by competitive inhibition of monoamine transporter (MAT) proteins, particularly the noradrenaline transporter NET and the serotonin transporter SERT (Fig. 22.1). Some drugs show little monoamine selectivity, while other compounds are more selective for one monoamine (Table 22.1). However, the degree of monoamine selectivity has not been shown to influence efficacy. The subsequent effects on the CNS are described above.

Many of the unwanted effects of these drugs are a consequence of blockade of other postsynaptic receptors (e.g. muscarinic and histamine H$_1$ receptors and α_1-adrenoceptors) (Table 22.1), which do not influence their antidepressant action.

Pharmacokinetics

All TCAs are well absorbed from the gut and highly protein bound in plasma. They undergo extensive first-pass metabolism in the liver, and active metabolites are formed which are partially responsible for the variable effective half-lives of these drugs (8–90 h; see Compendium at the end of this chapter). The combination of high first-pass metabolism and high clearance but a long elimination half-life is explained by high apparent volumes of distribution (10–50 L·kg^{-1} body weight). There is considerable inter-individual variability in the first-pass metabolism of most TCAs, leading to up to 40-fold differences in the plasma concentrations of the parent drug. There is no clear dose relationship for the therapeutic effects, although unwanted effects are dose-related. Dose titration is usually necessary to optimise the therapeutic response; this should be gradual over 1–2 weeks to minimise unwanted effects.

Unwanted effects

■ Sedation as a result of histamine H$_1$ receptor and α_1-adrenoceptor blockade (Ch. 39). Some compounds are highly sedative, for example amitriptyline, and others less so. Sedation can be useful to help restore sleep patterns in depression (using a larger dose of a sedative drug at night) but can be troublesome or even dangerous during the day.
■ Antimuscarinic effects (see Ch. 4): dry mouth is a frequent occurrence, and less commonly constipation, urinary retention, impotence and visual disturbance. Tolerance to these effects can occur and gradual increases in dose may reduce their incidence.
■ Excessive sweating and tremor.
■ Postural hypotension produced by peripheral α_1-adrenoceptor blockade (Ch. 4) can be particularly troublesome in the elderly, although tolerance can occur.

Table 22.1 Comparative properties of some commonly used antidepressant drugs

	Uptake inhibition	Muscarinic receptor blockade	Alpha₁-adrenoceptor blockade	Histamine H₁ receptor blockade	P450-related metabolism	Sedation
TCAs						
Amitriptyline	Serotonin = NA	+++	+++	++++	Inhibition	+++
Imipramine	Serotonin = NA	++	++	+++	Inhibition	++
Lofepramine	NA ≫ serotonin	+	+	+	?	+/–
SSRIs						
Citalopram	Serotonin ≫ NA	0	+	+	Weak inhibition	0
Fluoxetine	Serotonin ≫ NA	0	0	0	Inhibition	0
Paroxetine	Serotonin > NA	++	+	+	Inhibition	0
Sertraline	Serotonin ≫ NA	0	++	0	Weak inhibition	0
SNRIs						
Duloxetine	Serotonin ≥ NA	Low	Low	Low	Low	Low
Venlafaxine	Weak NA = serotonin	0	0	0	Weak inhibition	0
NRI						
Reboxetine	NA ≫ serotonin	Low	Low	Low	Weak inhibition	0
α₂-Adrenoceptor blocker						
Mirtazapine		+	+	+++++	Weak inhibition	+
5-HT₂ receptor blocker						
Trazodone	Weak serotonin	Low	+	+	Weak inhibition	+

The table is constructed from data in Richelson E (2002) The clinical relevance of antidepressant interaction with neurotransmitter transporters and receptors. *Psychopharmacol Bull* 36(4), 133–150 and other sources for approximate comparison only.
Drugs are listed under their conventional groupings but many have mixed or uncertain mechanisms of action. Differential blockade of muscarinic receptors, α₁-adrenoceptors and histamine H₁ receptors contributes to the side-effect profiles of antidepressant drugs. Other antidepressant drugs, including monoamine oxidase inhibitors (MAOIs), are listed in the Compendium at the end of the chapter. NA, noradrenaline; SSRI, selective serotonin reuptake inhibitor; SNRI, serotonin and noradrenaline reuptake inhibitor; NRI, noradrenaline reuptake inhibitor; TCA, tricyclic antidepressant.

■ Epileptogenic effects: TCAs lower the convulsive threshold, and seizures can be provoked, even when there is no previous clinical history.

■ Cardiotoxicity in overdose: most tricyclic drugs depress myocardial contractility. They can produce tachycardia and severe arrhythmias when taken in overdose, due to both antimuscarinic effects and excessive noradrenergic stimulation. Lofepramine is less cardiotoxic than other drugs in this class.

■ Weight gain: appetite stimulation is common, probably due to histamine H₁ receptor blockade.

■ Hyponatraemia from inappropriate antidiuretic hormone (ADH; vasopressin) secretion, leading to drowsiness, confusion and convulsions.

■ Sexual dysfunction with reduced interest in sex, erectile dysfunction in men and diminished arousal in women, and difficulty attaining orgasm.

■ Sudden withdrawal syndrome: during long-term treatment doses should be gradually reduced over four weeks to avoid agitation, headache, malaise, sweating and gastrointestinal upset, which can accompany sudden withdrawal. These may result from excessive cholinergic activity following prolonged muscarinic receptor blockade.

Drug interactions

Several important drug interactions are recognised. TCAs potentiate the central depressant activity of many drugs, including alcohol. A dangerous interaction can result from giving a monoamine oxidase (MAO) inhibitor (MAOI) (see below) and a TCA together due to prolonged action of the increased serotonin released from the neuron. The interaction can lead to hyperpyrexia, convulsions and coma, and can occur up to two weeks after stopping an MAOI due to the long duration of MAO inhibition.

The risk of serious arrhythmias is increased when TCAs are taken with drugs that prolong the Q–T interval on the electrocardiogram (Ch. 8). Such drugs include the class III antiarrhythmic sotalol, and all class I antiarrhythmics.

Selective serotonin reuptake inhibitors and related antidepressants

Examples

citalopram, fluoxetine, paroxetine, sertraline

Mechanism of action

Unlike the TCAs, the selective serotonin reuptake inhibitors (SSRIs) reduce the neuronal reuptake of serotonin by its presynaptic transporter protein (SERT), but have little or no effect on noradrenaline reuptake (Table 22.1). They have a more favourable profile of unwanted effects than TCAs because of their low affinity for muscarinic and histamine receptors and α_1-adrenoceptors. Paroxetine is unusual among SSRIs in having affinity for muscarinic M_3 receptors, found in the brain, salivary glands and smooth muscle.

The proposed mechanism of action of SSRIs is as follows.

- The increase in synaptic serotonin concentration as a result of reduced neuronal uptake leads to downregulation of the 5-HT_1 somatodendritic and axon terminal presynaptic inhibitory autoreceptors on serotonergic neurons.
- Reduced inhibitory autoreceptor activity increases serotonin release at the axon terminal. The prolonged increase in synaptic serotonin concentration (as a result of both increased release and reduced neuronal uptake) downregulates postsynaptic 5-HT_2 receptors.

Subsequent changes in intracellular function are described above.

Pharmacokinetics

SSRIs are well absorbed from the gut and metabolised in the liver. Paroxetine has a long half-life (10–20 h), which is greatest in poor metabolisers of CYP2D6 substrates (30–50 h). Citalopram, fluoxetine and sertraline have very long half-lives (23–75 h). The active metabolite of fluoxetine has a half-life of 6 days, and the resulting very long duration of action can be a disadvantage if an MAOI is used subsequently (see below).

Unwanted effects

In contrast to the TCAs, SSRIs have few antimuscarinic effects (apart from paroxetine), cause little sedation or weight gain and are not cardiotoxic in overdose. However, they may cause:

- nausea (frequent), dyspepsia, abdominal pain or diarrhoea (less frequent),
- insomnia, anxiety and agitation,
- anorexia with weight loss,
- rashes,
- hyponatraemia, due to inappropriate secretion of ADH and leading to drowsiness, confusion and convulsions, is more frequent than with TCAs,
- dry mouth and constipation with paroxetine,
- sexual dysfunction with reduced interest in sex, erectile dysfunction in men and diminished arousal in women, and difficulty attaining orgasm. This affects up to three-quarters of people taking SSRIs,
- increased risk of bleeding due to platelet dysfunction,
- SSRIs lower the convulsive threshold, and seizures can be provoked, even when there is no previous clinical history,
- sudden withdrawal syndrome after long-term use, which may be most troublesome with paroxetine; it presents with gastrointestinal symptoms, headache, anxiety, dizziness, paraesthesia, electric shock sensations in the head, neck and spine, sleep disturbance and sweating and usually begins 24–72 h after stopping treatment. The dose should be gradually reduced over at least 4 weeks,
- increase in suicidal thoughts and self harm in people aged under 25 years.

Drug interactions

The most serious interaction is with MAOIs (see TCAs above). An interval of five weeks is recommended after stopping fluoxetine, or two weeks after paroxetine or sertraline, before an MAOI (including selegiline, Ch. 24) is taken. Fluoxetine and other SSRIs inhibit hepatic CYP2D6 (Table 2.7), and this can increase the plasma concentration of drugs metabolised by this enzyme.

Serotonin and noradrenaline reuptake inhibitors

duloxetine, venlafaxine

Mechanism of action and uses

Venlafaxine and duloxetine are classified as serotonin and noradrenaline reuptake inhibitors (SNRIs) although at lower doses they have a greater effect on serotonin reuptake (Table 22.1). Like the TCAs, they inhibit neuronal reuptake of both serotonin and noradrenaline, but share with SSRIs a low affinity for muscarinic and histamine receptors and α_1-adrenoceptors. Their unwanted effect profiles are therefore closer to those of the SSRIs than those of the TCAs. There is some evidence that clinical improvement with venlafaxine may begin earlier than with other antidepressant drugs.

Duloxetine is also used as an adjunctive treatment for smoking cessation (Ch. 54), and in urinary stress incontinence (Ch. 15).

Pharmacokinetics

Venlafaxine and duloxetine are well absorbed from the gut and undergo extensive first-pass metabolism in the liver. The main active metabolite of venlaxafine has a long half-life (11 h) and the half-life of duloxetine is 9–19 h.

Unwanted effects

- Nausea, vomiting, anorexia, dyspepsia, constipation.
- Hypertension, palpitation.
- Dry mouth.
- Drowsiness, insomnia, dizziness, confusion, headache, tremor.
- Sexual dysfunction.
- QT segment prolongation on the ECG with venlafaxine, which predisposes to ventricular arrhythmias (see Ch. 8); it should be avoided in people at high risk of arrhythmias.
- Sudden withdrawal symptoms are more frequent than with other antidepressants, with gastrointestinal symptoms, headache, anxiety, dizziness, paraesthesia, tremor, sleep disturbance and sweating.

Selective noradrenaline reuptake inhibitors

reboxetine

Mechanism of action

Reboxetine is related to fluoxetine but is a selective noradrenaline reuptake inhibitor (NRI). Increased noradrenergic activity at somatodendritic α_1-adrenoceptors enhances serotonergic neurotransmission. Reboxetine, in common with the SSRIs, has little activity at muscarinic and histamine receptors and α_1-adrenoceptors. It therefore has fewer unwanted effects than do TCAs.

Pharmacokinetics

Reboxetine is rapidly absorbed orally. It is eliminated by hepatic metabolism and has a long half-life (15 h).

Unwanted effects

- Nausea, anorexia, constipation.
- Palpitation, postural hypotension.
- Dry mouth, urinary retention, blurred vision.
- Sweating.
- Headache, insomnia, dizziness, paraesthesia.

Presynaptic α_2-adrenoceptor blockers

mirtazapine

Mechanism of action

Mirtazapine is a tetracyclic drug unrelated structurally to the TCAs. In addition to potent postsynaptic 5-HT$_{2C}$ receptor-blocking activity in the cortex (see serotonin receptor blockers below), mirtazapine blocks presynaptic α_2-adrenoceptors (Fig. 22.1). This reduces negative feedback inhibition of serotonin release from raphe nucleus neurons in their terminal projections to regions such as the cortex and hippocampus. Mirtazapine blocks histamine H$_1$ receptors but has a low affinity for muscarinic receptors and postsynaptic α_1-adrenoceptors. It has minimal effects on monoamine reuptake.

Pharmacokinetics

Mirtazapine is well absorbed from the gut. It is metabolised in the liver and has a very long half-life (20–40 h).

Unwanted effects

- Drowsiness, especially at lower doses, due to histamine H$_1$ receptor blockade. At higher doses, increased noradrenergic neurotransmission offsets some of the sedative effects.

- Increased appetite and weight gain.
- Fatigue, tremor dizziness.
- Oedema.

Serotonin receptor blockers

trazodone

Mechanism of action

Trazodone is a tetracyclic compound. Its most significant antidepressant action is blockade of postsynaptic 5-HT$_{2C}$ receptors, which increases activity of dopamine and noradrenaline in the frontal cortex. It also produces weak inhibition of presynaptic serotonin reuptake, but does not inhibit noradrenaline reuptake. Trazodone blocks α_1-adrenoceptors and weakly blocks muscarinic and histamine H$_1$ receptors.

Pharmacokinetics

Trazodone is well absorbed orally and metabolised in the liver. The half-life is 7–13 h.

Unwanted effects

- These are similar to those of TCAs, but with fewer antimuscarinic and cardiovascular effects.
- Priapism.

Classic (non-selective) monoamine oxidase inhibitors

Examples

phenelzine, tranylcypromine

Mechanism of action

The mechanism of action of classic (non-selective) monoamine oxidase inhibitors (MAOIs) is complex, but their primary action is irreversible inhibition of intracellular MAO, which is the enzyme responsible for degrading free monoamines in the presynaptic nerve terminal. This leads to accumulation of monoamine neurotransmitters in the presynaptic neuron and increased release when the nerve is stimulated (Fig. 22.1). There are two MAO isoenzymes (Fig. 22.3). MAO-B is the predominant enzyme in many parts of the brain, but MAO-A is present in noradrenergic and serotonergic neurons, especially in the locus coeruleus and other cells of the brainstem, as well as being the main enzyme in peripheral tissues. Inhibition of MAO-A in the brain produces the therapeutic effects of these drugs, but classic inhibitors (MAOIs) are not selective for this isoenzyme. Inhibition of both MAO-A and MAO-B in the gut wall and liver has important consequences (see below). MAOIs also inhibit various drug-metabolising enzymes in the liver, which predisposes to drug interactions but does not contribute to clinical efficacy.

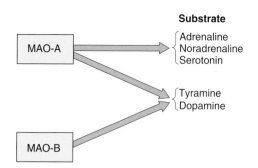

Fig. 22.3 **Actions of monoamine oxidase (MAO) and MAO inhibitors.** The relative selectivity of the substrates for MAO is shown. MAO-A is the target for drugs useful in treating depression. Non-selective inhibition of both MAO-A and MAO-B blocks the metabolism of tyramine, which is responsible for the adverse food reaction that occurs with these drugs. Reversible inhibitors of MAO-A (RIMAs) block only subtype A. Therefore, tyramine is still metabolised by subtype B and the food reaction is reduced. Selective inhibitors of MAO-B enhance CNS dopamine levels and are used in Parkinson's disease (Ch. 24).

Pharmacokinetics

All drugs in this class are well absorbed from the gut. They are irreversible enzyme inhibitors and therefore their prolonged duration of action is unrelated to the half-life of the drug. Drug withdrawal is followed by gradual restoration of normal MAO activity over about 2 weeks as new enzyme is synthesised.

Unwanted effects

- Compared with the TCAs, antimuscarinic effects are unusual and there is no predisposition to seizures (except in overdose; see below).
- Dose-related postural hypotension can occur. Unlike with the TCAs, tolerance does not develop. The mechanism may involve conversion of tyramine (normally degraded by MAO) to octopamine, a false neurotransmitter which competes with noradrenaline at sympathetic nerve terminals.
- Due to its structural similarity to amfetamine (Ch. 54), tranylcypromine causes CNS stimulation, leading to irritability and insomnia. Doses should be given early in the day to avoid disturbing sleep.
- Hepatitis is a rare idiosyncratic reaction to the hydrazine derivative phenelzine.
- Acute overdose produces delayed toxic effects after some 12 h. Excessive adrenergic stimulation leads to chest pain, headache and hyperactivity, progressing to confusion and severe hypertension, with eventually profound hypotension and seizures.
- Food interactions can occur because MAO in the gut wall and liver usually prevents the absorption of natural amines, particularly tyramine, which is an indirect-acting sympathomimetic (Ch. 4). If food containing tyramine, for example cheese, yeast extracts (such as Bovril, Oxo or Marmite), pickled herrings, chianti and caviar, or broad bean pods (which contain L-dopa) is eaten, the

increased absorption of tyramine and consequently greater release of noradrenaline result in vasoconstriction and severe hypertension. The first indication of this is a throbbing headache. A warning card should be supplied to people who take MAOIs.

Drug interactions

A number of drug interactions can occur. Indirect-acting sympathomimetics (Ch. 4) in cold remedies (e.g. ephedrine, phenylpropanolamine), and levodopa (treatment of Parkinson's disease, Ch. 24) will be more active, with a risk of hypertensive crisis. The toxicity of the triptans (5-HT$_1$ receptor agonists used for treatment of migraine, Ch. 26) will be potentiated. All these drugs should be avoided for two weeks after stopping an MAOI. The combination of MAOIs with TCAs or SSRIs (see above) can be dangerous. Other important interactions occur because MAOIs can impair the hepatic metabolism of certain drugs, especially opioid analgesics.

Reversible inhibitors of monoamine oxidase A (RIMAs)

moclobemide

Mechanism of action and effects

Moclobemide is a reversible inhibitor of MAO-A, the same isoenzyme target for the antidepressant action of classic MAOIs. However, moclobemide does not inhibit MAO-B, so tyramine absorbed from the gut can still be degraded and the food reaction described above for classic MAOIs is very unlikely to occur. Also, since the action of moclobemide on MAO-A is reversible, high concentrations of tyramine will displace the drug from the enzyme, further facilitating degradation of tyramine. If moclobemide is taken after meals, then inhibition of MAO-A in the gut during absorption of tyramine will be minimised, providing further protection. MAO-A inhibition by moclobemide lasts less than 24 h after a single dose.

Pharmacokinetics

Oral absorption of moclobemide is good but there is substantial first-pass metabolism, partially to an active metabolite. Moclobemide undergoes hepatic metabolism and has a short half-life (1–2 h).

Unwanted effects

- Sleep disturbance, agitation, confusion.
- Gastrointestinal upset.
- Dizziness, headache, paraesthesia.
- Dry mouth, visual disturbances.
- Oedema.

Drug interactions

Inhibition of cytochrome P450 activity in the liver by cimetidine (Ch. 33) substantially reduces the metabolism of moclobemide, and smaller starting doses are recommended in this situation. Moclobemide should not be given with other antidepressants, and the recommendations for stopping these drugs before prescribing moclobemide are the same as for classic MAOIs.

Melatonin receptor agonist and serotonin receptor antagonist

 Example

agomelatine

Mechanism of action and effects

Agomelatine is a synthetic agonist of the naturally occurring substance melatonin, which is secreted by the pineal gland and is involved in regulation of circadian rhythms and therefore sleep pattern. Agomelatine is an agonist at both melatonin MT_1 receptors (attenuating alerting signals to the cortex) and MT_2 receptors (producing a phase-shifting action on the circadian rhythm of sleep). Agomelatine significantly improves sleep quality when taken at night to mimic the natural rhythm of melatonin release. It is a weak antagonist at $5\text{-}HT_{2C}$ receptors (see serotonin receptor blockers above), and increases noradrenaline and dopamine release in the frontal cortex. The antidepressant efficacy of agomelatine is similar to that of SSRIs.

Pharmacokinetics

Agomelatine is almost completely absorbed from the gut. It is metabolised in the liver and has a short half-life of 1–2 h.

Unwanted effects

- Nausea, diarrhoea, constipation, abdominal pain.
- Headache, dizziness, drowsiness, insomnia, fatigue, anxiety.
- Back pain.
- Sweating.

MANAGEMENT OF DEPRESSION

Drugs form only part of the management of depression but are usually necessary for moderate, severe or protracted symptoms. However, in mild to moderate depression, cognitive therapy is as effective as drug treatment and should be tried first. The herbal remedy *Hypericum perforatum* (St John's wort) is comparable to antidepressant drugs for treatment of mild depression, but neither St John's wort nor antidepressant drugs show convincing efficacy compared to placebo in mild disease. St John's wort does not often cause unwanted effects, but concentrations of the active constituents vary among different preparations. St John's wort can induce cytochrome P450, and should not be taken with a prescribed antidepressant. All antidepressant drugs have a delayed onset of action, and people who are severely ill should be considered for electroconvulsive therapy (ECT), which gives a more rapid response.

The TCAs are now less frequently prescribed for depression. They have serious cardiotoxic effects when taken in overdose and should usually be avoided when treating people who are at high risk of attempting suicide. Encouraging adherence to treatment with TCAs may initially be difficult, since antimuscarinic unwanted effects can be troublesome before any benefit is perceived. Starting with a small dose of TCA followed by gradual dose titration can minimise unwanted effects. There is now evidence that large doses of a TCA do not necessarily enhance the treatment response but do increase unwanted effects, so the use of low dosages may therefore be preferred.

The newer drugs, for example SSRIs and SNRIs, are no more effective than TCAs and do not work any faster, but they are better tolerated. They are certainly safer than TCAs when there is a high risk of suicide. The use of SSRIs or SNRIs as the first-line treatment for depression is now well established.

Up to 70% of depressed people will respond to drug therapy if the dosage is adequate, compared with about 30% taking placebo. However, only 50% will respond to an individual drug, and up to a further 20% of people with depression will respond if the drug is changed after failure of the initial treatment. Responders show an initial improvement in sleep pattern within a few days. Psychomotor retardation responds more gradually over several days, leading to greater involvement with everyday activities and enjoyment of life. Improvement in the depressed mood is delayed, beginning up to two or more weeks after commencing treatment with an adequate drug dosage. The response of most symptoms tends to be erratic, with good and bad days.

Initial treatment with an antidepressant should be for 4–6 weeks. If there is no response after this time, and if it is believed that adherence to treatment is not a problem, then either the dose should be increased, if unwanted effects permit, or an alternative drug can be substituted. If there is a good response then the dosage can usually be reduced, but maintenance treatment should be continued for at least 4–6 months after the first episode of depression to minimise the risk of relapse. A longer period of maintenance treatment to prevent recurrence (at least one year and often longer) is often recommended for the elderly, for others who are at high risk of recurrence, and for people who have experienced two or more depressive episodes. About half of all people who experience depression only have a single episode. In individuals with recurrent illness, relapse occurs within a year in up to 65% of those who stop treatment, but only in 15% of people who continue treatment. Risk factors for relapse in major depression include:

- presence of residual symptoms,
- number of previous episodes,
- severity of most recent episode,
- duration of most recent episode,
- degree of treatment resistance in previous episode.

Classic MAOIs are usually reserved for atypical depression with hypochondriacal and phobic symptoms, or when SSRIs have failed. The therapeutic place of the newer antidepressants such as SNRIs and RIMAs in those who fail to respond to an SSRI has yet to be established. Small doses of the phenothiazine antipsychotic drug flupentixol (Ch. 21) are sometimes used for treatment of depressed elderly people. The evidence for a true antidepressant effect of flupentixol is slight, but some symptoms undoubtedly do improve.

Treatment is most difficult in severe depression, especially if there are psychotic features, or where depression forms part of a bipolar affective disorder (Ch. 21). ECT is used for treatment-resistant depression and in the elderly, who are particularly likely to show a response. Overall, ECT is probably more effective than drug therapy but does produce some lasting cognitive impairment, especially if given bilaterally rather than unilaterally, or given frequently or with high currents. ECT should be combined with prolonged antidepressant drug treatment. Lithium (Ch. 21) is used for people with severe recurrent depressive episodes and for prophylaxis of bipolar affective disorder. The effect of lithium can take several months to become fully established. The treatment of depression in bipolar disorder is discussed further in Chapter 21.

ATTENTION DEFICIT HYPERACTIVITY DISORDER AND NARCOLEPSY

Several drugs with similar mechanisms of action to antidepressants, as well as central stimulant drugs, have limited uses in the management of attention deficit hyperactivity disorder (ADHD) and narcolepsy.

ATTENTION DEFICIT HYPERACTIVITY DISORDER

ADHD is the most common behavioural and cognitive disorder in children of school age, but often remains a problem in adult life. The mechanism is poorly understood, but may involve dopamine deficiency in the prefrontal cortex. There are three subtypes:

- predominantly inattentive subtype: failing to pay attention to details, difficulty with sustained attention, disorganisation and forgetfulness,
- predominantly hyperactive-impulsive subtype: excessive fidgeting and squirming, restlessness, frequently interrupting and intruding on others,
- predominantly inattentive/hyperactive-impulsive subtype: features of both subtypes in two areas of life and causing dysfunction in at least one area.

Adults with ADHD often present with poor occupational performance, marital instability, poor self-discipline or self-organisation, and restlessness. Sleep disturbances may also be prominent.

NARCOLEPSY

Narcolepsy usually begins in adolescence and is characterised by overwhelming daytime sleepiness, even if nighttime sleep has been adequate. Sudden daytime naps are frequent and there may be prolonged periods of drowsiness. Hallucinations may be troublesome on falling asleep or awakening. The condition may coexist with cataplexy,

characterised by sudden loss of muscle function ranging from weakness to collapse that is often precipitated by laughter. People with narcolepsy have an abnormal sleep pattern, with rapid-eye-movement (REM) sleep at the onset of sleep rather than after a period of non-REM sleep (Ch. 20). Narcolepsy has a genetic predisposition and there may be an autoimmune component. There is loss of hypocretin-secreting neurons in the hypothalamus, possibly as a result of autoimmune-mediated cell destruction. Hypocretins are neurotransmitters that regulate wakefulness by releasing dopamine and noradrenaline in the hypothalamus, which excite histaminergic tuberomammillary neurons. The tuberomammillary nucleus is involved in control of arousal, sleep and circadian rhythms.

DRUGS FOR ATTENTION DEFICIT HYPERACTIVITY DISORDER AND NARCOLEPSY

Atomoxetine

Mechanism of action

Atomoxetine is a selective inhibitor of presynaptic neuronal uptake of noradrenaline. There is a secondary increase in dopaminergic activity in the prefrontal cortex. It has antidepressant activity, but the mechanism of action in ADHD is not known.

Pharmacokinetics

Atomoxetine is well absorbed from the gut. It is metabolised in the liver and has a half-life of 6 h in most individuals (extensive metabolisers), but 19 h in poor metabolisers of CYP2D6 substrates.

Unwanted effects

- Anorexia, dry mouth, nausea, vomiting, abdominal pain, constipation.
- Palpitation, hypertension, postural hypotension.
- Sleep disturbance, dizziness, headache, fatigue, irritability, depression, tremor.
- Urinary retention, sexual dysfunction.

Methylphenidate

Mechanism of action

Methylphenidate is an amfetamine derivative that activates the brainstem arousal system. Its mechanism is not established, but there is evidence that the drug blocks the presynaptic reuptake of noradrenaline and dopamine, and increases dopaminergic neurotransmission in the prefrontal cortex.

Pharmacokinetics

Methylphenidate is well absorbed from the gut. It is metabolised in the liver and has a short half-life of 3 h.

Unwanted effects

- Dry mouth, nausea, vomiting, abdominal pain.
- Palpitation, hypertension, postural hypotension.

- Sleep disturbance, dizziness, headache, fatigue, irritability, depression.
- Fever, arthralgia, rash.

Dexamfetamine

Dexamfetamine selectively releases monoamines such as noradrenaline, serotonin and dopamine from CNS neurons in the mesolimbic pathway and also the reticular formation that regulates alertness and sleep (see Ch.54).

Unwanted effects

- Sleep disturbance, dizziness, headache, fatigue, irritability, depression, tremor, seizures, psychosis.
- Anorexia, dry mouth, gastrointestinal upset.
- Palpitation, hypertension.
- Tolerance and dependence.

Modafinil

Mechanism of action

Modafinil blocks the presynaptic reuptake of noradrenaline and dopamine, increasing dopaminergic neurotransmission in the prefrontal cortex. It may also reduce inhibitory GABA-mediated neurotransmission. There is also evidence that modafinil activates hypocretin-releasing neurons in the hypothalamus.

Pharmacokinetics

Modafinil is well absorbed from the gut. It is metabolised in the liver and has a long half-life of 15 h.

Unwanted effects

- Anorexia, dry mouth, nausea, dyspepsia, abdominal pain, diarrhoea.
- Palpitation, chest pain.
- Sleep disturbance, dizziness, confusion, agitation, depression.

MANAGEMENT OF ATTENTION DEFICIT HYPERACTIVITY DISORDER

Behaviour management and psychotherapy have a role, but are more effective when combined with drug treatment. However, there is some concern that the benefits of the currently available compounds may be short-lived, with loss of efficacy after about three years. Methylphenidate is usually the first choice, while dexamfetamine can be tried if there is no improvement with methylphenidate. Atomoxetine is used when stimulant drugs are ineffective.

MANAGEMENT OF NARCOLEPSY

Planned short naps may avoid the need for drug treatment, but drowsiness may require use of a CNS stimulant. Dexamfetamine or modafinil are usually chosen, but methylphenidate may be helpful. Cataplexy can respond to a TCA or a SSRI.

SELF-ASSESSMENT

True/false questions

1. The processes underlying depression are all explained by the monoamine hypothesis.
2. Downregulation of serotonin (5-HT$_2$) receptors occurs during antidepressant treatment.
3. Most tricyclic antidepressants (TCAs) inhibit the reuptake of noradrenaline and serotonin equally.
4. TCAs have a less satisfactory therapeutic ratio than do selective serotonin reuptake inhibitors (SSRIs).
5. Selective inhibitors of noradrenaline or serotonin reuptake are equally effective as antidepressants.
6. TCAs potentiate the central depressant effects of alcohol.
7. Lofepramine is more cardiotoxic than amitriptyline.
8. Co-administration of an SSRI and a monoamine oxidase inhibitor (MAOI) can cause cardiovascular collapse.
9. The antidepressant activity of mirtazepine is related to blockade of serotonin receptors.
10. Trazodone is a potent inhibitor of monoamine reuptake.
11. Venlafaxine has marked sedative and antimuscarinic actions.
12. Venlafaxine has a low incidence of cardiovascular toxicity.
13. Only 30–40% of people with depression improve as a direct result of antidepressant drug treatment.
14. Lithium is only used for treatment of bipolar affective disorder.
15. Methylphenidate is an amfetamine derivative used in the management of ADHD.
16. Narcolepsy is associated with loss of neurons that secrete hypocretins.

One-best-answer (OBA) question

Which statement concerning antidepressant drugs is the *most accurate*?

A. A TCA would be more suitable than an SSRI for a patient with urinary outflow problems due to benign prostate hypertrophy.
B. The antidepressant action of trazodone is due mainly to muscarinic receptor blockade.
C. People taking moclobemide are likely to get an adverse reaction if they eat cheese.
D. An SSRI would be more suitable than a TCA to treat a person with serious depression and suicidal tendencies.
E. Increases in levels of brain monoamine levels occur only after 2–3 weeks of treatment with a TCA.

Case-based questions

JA, a 34-year-old female financier, is a former international athlete now working in the City of London. In 2006 she was appointed manager of the emerging countries fund of a large unit trust company. In early 2009 the company was taken over and JA had a new boss and was demoted to assistant manager of the fund. From 2009 to 2010 she had

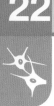

put on 10 kg in weight, and started a strict diet and worked out at a gym four times a week. She visited her GP with a 6-month history of increasing insomnia, lack of concentration, irritability and anxiety. She had begun to withdraw from a busy social calendar and was becoming indecisive. This was now affecting her work. For the previous four weeks she had had recurrent thoughts of suicide. She had also lost 4 kg in weight during that period. The GP diagnosed that she was depressed, arranged a psychiatric consultation for her and started her on a TCA.

A. What are the risk factors for depression? Was JA at risk prior to the diagnosis?
B. What neurochemical and receptor changes are associated with depressive illness?
C. How successful is treatment with TCAs and what are their unwanted effects?
D. Are TCAs an appropriate first choice for JA?

True/false answers

1. **False.** The monoamine hypothesis cannot alone explain all features of depression, including the slow onset of antidepressant action of drugs that can rapidly increase CNS levels of monamines.
2. **True.** Downregulation of 5-HT$_2$ receptors parallels the time course of improvement of clinical condition, whereas the time course of the increase in amine transmitters does not.
3. **False.** TCAs vary in their ability to affect noradrenaline and serotonin reuptake.
4. **True.** TCAs have a greater potential to produce serious unwanted effects, e.g. causing cardiac arrhythmias in acute overdose.
5. **True.** Antidepressant drugs differ more in their profiles of unwanted effects profile than in their clinical efficacy.
6. **True.** Alcohol should not be consumed by people taking TCAs.
7. **False.** Lofepramine is among the least cardiotoxic of the tricyclic and related antidepressants; it also causes little sedation.
8. **True.** An MAOI and an SSRI should not be combined. The combination can cause CNS excitation, tremor and hyperthermia. An MAOI should not be started until 2–3 weeks after stopping the SSRI, depending upon which SSRI has been taken. Conversely, other antidepressants should not be started until 2–3 weeks after stopping an MAOI.
9. **True.** The main action of mirtazepine is blockade of postsynaptic 5-HT$_2$ receptors and central presynaptic α_2-adrenoceptors.
10. **False.** Trazodone is only a weak inhibitor of serotonin reuptake, and does not block noradrenaline reuptake; its main action is blockade of postsynaptic 5-HT$_2$ receptors.
11. **False.** Like the TCAs, the SNRI drug venlafaxine inhibits both noradrenaline and serotonin reuptake, but it lacks the sedative and antimuscarinic effects of TCAs.
12. **False.** Venlafaxine causes QT segment prolongation and predisposes to ventricular arrhythmia in high-risk depressed people, such as those with uncontrolled blood pressure.

13. **True.** Depression improves in up to 70% of people taking antidepressants, compared with 30% on placebo.
14. **False.** Although most commonly used in bipolar affective disorder, lithium is also used in those with severe recurrent depressive episodes who do not respond to other treatment.
15. **True.** The amfetamine derivative methylphenidate is a first-line drug treatment in ADHD; dexamfetamine may be required in refractory ADHD.
16. **True.** Hypocretins promote wakefulness by releasing noradrenaline and dopamine.

OBA answer

Answer D is correct.

A. Incorrect. Many TCAs have antimuscarinic activity, which could exacerbate urinary retention.
B. Incorrect. Trazodone acts mainly by blockade of post-synaptic 5-HT$_{2C}$ receptors.
C. Incorrect. Moclobemide is a reversible inhibitor of MAO-A and has relatively little effect on MAO-B, which remains available to metabolise dietary tyramine. The 'cheese reaction' is therefore less likely than with classic (non-selective) MAO inhibitors.
D. **Correct**. An SSRI would be more suitable than most TCAs in severe depression with suicidal ideation because of their generally lower toxicity in overdose. The effectiveness of SSRIs and TCAs is similar.
E. Incorrect. The increase in brain monoamine levels following treatment with a TCA occurs within hours to days. However, the antidepressant effects on behaviour and mood may take 4–6 weeks or longer to become apparent.

Case-based answers

A. Risk factors include sex (more frequent in women), age (peak age 20–40 years), family history of depression, marital status (higher rates in separated and divorced people) and stress. It is possible, but we cannot be certain, that any of the circumstances in the clinical history were contributory to her depression.
B. There is a biological association of depression with reduced CNS monoaminergic neurotransmission, notably noradrenaline and serotonin, but it is still unclear whether this is cause or effect. Drugs that deplete monoamines can induce depression, and when monoamines are repleted, symptoms decrease. Probably because of the depletion of monoamines, there is an upregulation of postsynaptic monoamine receptors, including 5-HT$_2$ and β_1-adrenoceptors. There are also dysfunctions in other CNS signalling systems (see text). Drugs used to treat depression increase CNS serotonin and/or noradrenaline in the synaptic cleft, which eventually results in postsynaptic receptor downregulation.
C. The onset of antidepressant activity is delayed for at least 2–4 weeks. Two-thirds of depressed people improve, one-third do not. One-third of people with depression would improve spontaneously without drug therapy. Whether TCAs prevent recurrence is unknown.

Unwanted effects of TCAs include muscarinic receptor blockade (dry mouth, blurred vision, constipation), cardiotoxicity, sedation (variable) and postural hypotension.

D. TCAs may not be the most appropriate choice as JA was showing suicidal tendencies; the safety of TCAs in overdose is low. Another antidepressant drug such as an SSRI may have been a better choice as they are safer in overdose and have a generally better profile of unwanted effects, although nausea and sexual dysfunction are relatively common.

FURTHER READING

Depression

Alexopoulos GS (2005) Depression in the elderly. *Lancet* 365, 1961–1970

Belmaker RH, Agam G (2008) Major depressive disorder. *N Engl J Med* 358, 55–68

Donati RJ, Rasenick MM (2003) G-protein signaling and the molecular basis of antidepressant action. *Life Sci* 73, 1–17

Ebmeier, KB, Donaghey C, Steele JD (2006) Recent developments and current controversies in depression. *Lancet* 367, 153–167

Furukawa TA, McGuire H, Barbui C (2002) Meta-analysis of effects and side effects of low dosage tricyclic antidepressants in depression: systematic review. *BMJ* 325, 991–995

Geddes JR, Carney SM, Davies C et al. (2003) Relapse prevention with antidepressant drug treatment in depressive disorders: a systematic review. *Lancet* 361, 653–661

Hatcher S, Arroll B (2012) Newer antidepressants for the treatment of depression in adults. *BMJ* 344, d8300

Krishnan V, Nestler EJ (2010) Linking molecules to mood: new insights into the biology of depression. *Am J Psychiatry* 167, 1305–1320

Mann JJ (2005) The medical management of depression. *N Engl J Med* 353, 1819–1834

Millan MJ (2006) Multi-target strategies for the improved treatment of depressive states: conceptual foundations and neuronal substrates, drug discovery and therapeutic application. *Pharmacol Ther* 110, 135–370

Nair A, Vaidya VA (2006) Cyclic AMP response element binding protein and brain derived neurotrophic factor: molecules that modulate our mood. *J Biosci* 31, 423–443

Reid S, Barbui C (2010) Long term treatment of depression with selective serotonin reuptake inhibitors and newer antidepressants. *BMJ* 340, 752–756

Tanti A, Belzung C (2010) Open questions in current models of antidepressant action. *Br J Pharmacol* 159, 1187–1200

Timonen M, LiuKonen T (2008) Management of depression in adults. *BMJ* 336, 435–439

Narcolepsy and ADHD

Cao M (2011) Advances in narcolepsy. *Med Clin N Am* 94, 541–555

Jamdar S, Sathyamoorthy BT (2007) Management of attention deficit/hyperactivity disorder. *Br J Hosp Med* 68, 360–366

Kaplan G, Newcorn JH (2011) Pharmacotherapy for child and adolescent attention–deficit hyperactivity disorder. *Paed Clin N Am* 58, 99–120

Keam S, Walker MC (2007) Therapies for narcolepsy with or without cataplexy: evidence-based review. *Curr Opin Neurol* 20, 699–703

Pliszka SR (2007) Pharmacologic treatment of attention-deficit/hyperactivity disorder: efficacy, safety and mechanisms of action. *Neuropsychol Rev* 17, 61–72

Young TJ, Silber MH (2006) Hypersomnias of central origin. *Chest* 130, 913–920

Compendium: drugs used to treat depression

Drug	Kinetics (half-life)	Comments
Depression		
Tricyclic antidepressants (TCAs) and related compounds		
Given orally.		
Amitriptyline	Bioavailability 30–60%; hepatic metabolism to nortriptyline (see below) (10–28 h)	Particularly useful when sedation is required; hazardous in overdose; also used for nocturnal enuresis in children, for neuropathic pain and for prophylaxis of migraine
Clomipramine	Oral bioavailability about 50%; hepatic metabolism (12–36 h)	Relatively selective inhibitor of serotonin uptake; sedative effect; also used for phobic and obsessive states
Dosulepin	Bioavailability about 30%; hepatic metabolism (11–40 h)	Useful when sedation is required; hazardous in overdose; specialist use only
Doxepin	Bioavailability 25–32%; variable hepatic metabolism (8–25 h) to an active, long-lived desmethyl metabolite (30–50 h)	Useful when sedation is required
Imipramine	Bioavailability about 50%; hepatic metabolism to an active product (desipramine) (8–20 h)	Little sedative effect; also used for nocturnal enuresis in children
Lofepramine	Rapid oral absorption; prodrug converted rapidly in the liver (4–5 h) to active metabolite (desipramine) (21–23 h)	Relatively selective inhibitor of noradrenaline uptake; good side-effect profile, little sedation; risk of hepatotoxicity
Mianserin	Oral bioavailability 20–30%; hepatic metabolism; desmethyl metabolite is a weak α_2-adrenoceptor agonist (10–20 h)	Tetracyclic compound; noradrenaline reuptake inhibitor and also blocks postsynaptic 5-HT$_2$ receptors; particularly useful when sedation is required; risk of neutropenia and aplastic anaemia in elderly
Nortriptyline	Bioavailability 50–60%; variable hepatic metabolism (18–90 h)	Little sedative effect; also used for nocturnal enuresis in children and for neuropathic pain
Trazodone	Complete oral bioavailability (100%); hepatic metabolism; active metabolite (7–13 h)	Tetracyclic compound. Weak inhibitor of serotonin reuptake; main action is blockade of postsynaptic 5-HT$_{2C}$ receptors
Trimipramine	Bioavailability 40%; hepatic metabolism (20–26 h)	Useful when sedation is required
Selective serotonin reuptake inhibitors (SSRIs)		
Given orally.		
Citalopram	Oral bioavailability 80%; hepatic metabolism (80%) and renal clearance (20%) (23–75 h); weakly inhibits CYP2D6	Also used for panic disorder
Escitalopram	Oral bioavailability 80%; mainly hepatic metabolism (27–32 h)	Active isomer of citalopram; also used for panic disorder
Fluoxetine	Essentially complete bioavailability; variable hepatic metabolism (48–72 h) to active, long-lived metabolite (norfluoxetine) (6 days); parent drug and norfluoxetine inhibit CYP2D6	Long duration of action; also used for bulimia nervosa and obsessive compulsive disorder
Fluvoxamine	High oral bioavailability; hepatic metabolism (7–70 h)	Also used for obsessive compulsive disorder
Paroxetine	Good but variable absorption; variable hepatic metabolism (10–50 h)	Also used for obsessive compulsive disorder, panic disorder, social phobia, post-traumatic stress, and generalised anxiety disorder; some antimuscarinic effects; risk of sudden withdrawal syndrome
Sertraline	Low oral bioavailability increased if given with food; hepatic metabolism (26 h)	Also used for obsessive compulsive disorder and post-traumatic stress disorder

Compendium: drugs used to treat depression—cont'd

Drug	Kinetics (half-life)	Comments
Serotonin and noradrenaline reuptake inhibitors (SNRIs)		
Given orally.		
Duloxetine	Oral bioavailability about 50%; hepatic metabolism (9–19 h)	Also used in generalised anxiety disorder; diabetic neuropathy and stress urinary incontinence (Ch. 15)
Venlafaxine	Low oral bioavailability (10–45%) due to first-pass metabolism; hepatic metabolism (5 h) to long-lived active metabolite (10–11 h)	Risk of ventricular arrhythmia; risk of withdrawal effects; also used for generalised anxiety disorder
Classic (non-selective) monoamine oxidase inhibitors (MAOIs)		
Given orally.		
Isocarboxazid	Essentially complete bioavailability; hydrolysed by esterases (2–3 h); prolonged inhibition of MAO (days)	Used in refractory depression; slow onset of clinical action (weeks); risk of tyramine reaction
Phenelzine	Extensively absorbed; rapid hepatic metabolism (1 h); prolonged inhibition of MAO (weeks)	Used in refractory depression; slow onset of clinical action (weeks); risk of tyramine reaction; risk of hepatitis
Tranylcypromine	Extensively absorbed; hepatic metabolism (2–3 h); prolonged inhibition of MAO	Faster onset of clinical action than other classic MAOIs, but more hazardous due to stimulant action; risk of tyramine reaction
Reversible inhibitors of monoamine oxidase A (RIMAs)		
Given orally.		
Moclobemide	Bioavailability about 50%; numerous metabolic routes (1–4 h); short duration of action (<24 h)	Lower risk of tyramine reaction than with classic MAOI; used for refractory depression; also used for social phobia
Other antidepressant drugs		
Given orally.		
Agomelatine	Low bioavailability (<10%); hepatic metabolism (1–2 h)	Agonist at melatonin receptors and a weak antagonist at 5-HT$_{2C}$ receptors; also anxiolytic properties
Flupentixol	Bioavailability about 40%; hepatic metabolism; enterohepatic circulation of glucuronide conjugate (35 h)	Phenothiazone antipsychotic (Ch. 21); useful for depression with associated psychoses
Lithium	Complete oral absorption; filtered at glomerulus and 80% reabsorbed inproximal renal tubule (8–45 h)	Mechanism unknown; used for severe recurrent depressive episodes and for prophylaxis of bipolar affective disorder
Mirtazapine	Bioavailability about 50%; hepatic metabolism (20–40 h)	Principal action is blockade of central presynaptic α_2-adrenoceptors and postsynaptic 5-HT$_2$ receptors; tolerance develops to initial sedative effects
Reboxetine	Complete oral bioavailability; hepatic metabolism and some renal clearance (10%) (15 h)	Selective noradrenaline uptake inhibitor (NRI)
Tryptophan	Amino acid; active gut absorption and transport across blood–brain barrier; undergoes decarboxylation and deamination (2 h)	Very restricted hospital use as an adjunct to conventional treatments
Drugs used to treat attention deficit hyperactivity disorder (ADHD) and narcolepsy		
Given orally.		
Atomoxetine	Rapidly absorbed; hepatic metabolism (6–19 h)	Noradrenaline reuptake blocker; used for ADHD
Dexamfetamine	Rapidly and completely absorbed; eliminated unchanged in urine plus hepatic metabolism (6–12 h)	Blocks monoamine reuptake; used for narcolepsy and refractory ADHD

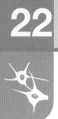
Compendium: drugs used to treat depression—cont'd

Drug	Kinetics (half-life)	Comments
Methylphenidate	Good oral absorption; de-esterified in liver (3 h)	Amfetamine derivative; blocks presynaptic reuptake of noradrenaline and dopamine; used for ADHD and narcolepsy
Modafinil	Oral bioavailability >80%; hepatic metabolism (10–15 h)	Blocks presynaptic reuptake of noradrenaline and dopamine; used for daytime sleepiness associated with narcolepsy or sleep apnoea
Sodium oxybate	Rapid but incomplete (25%) absorption, probably due to saturable first-pass metabolism; hepatic metabolism	Central stimulant; the sodium salt of γ-hydroxybutyric acid (GHB); used for narcolepsy with cataplexy

23 Epilepsy

PATHOLOGICAL BASIS OF EPILEPSY

Epilepsy affects up to 0.6% of the population and is characterised by recurrent epileptic seizures without any immediate provoking cause. Epileptic seizures are sudden, transient and usually unpredictable episodes of motor, sensory, autonomic or psychic disturbance triggered by abnormal neuronal discharges in the brain. The clinical manifestations depend on the site of the discharge.

■ In *partial or focal seizures* the discharge starts in a localised area of the brain and may remain localised or may secondarily spread to affect the whole brain.
■ In *generalised seizures* the abnormal discharge affects the whole of the brain (Table 23.1).

Identification of the type of seizure is important in the selection of the most appropriate therapy.

The origin of epilepsy is complex. For most people with epilepsy the initial focus of abnormal neuronal activity is structural damage in the brain such as that resulting from trauma, tumours, cerebrovascular disease or haemorrhage. Seizures can also be caused by metabolic disturbance, such as hypoglycaemia or alcohol abuse. In about 30% of cases of epilepsy where there is no identifiable structural or metabolic disorder (idiopathic epilepsy) there is an important genetic component.

NEUROTRANSMITTERS AND EPILEPSY

Coordinated activity among neurons depends on a controlled balance between excitatory and inhibitory influences on the electrical activity across neuronal cell membranes. Neuronal networks cooperate by oscillatory electrical activity between different parts of the brain. Generalised epilepsy involves a change from these oscillations to abnormally synchronised activity across large-scale neuronal networks, in particular involving both the cortex and subcortical structures such as the thalamus. Structural changes in neuronal networks in the brain are often found in people with epilepsy and this may provide the basis for generation of the abnormal discharges. These arise from focal lesions in the neocortex and limbic structures (especially hippocampus and amygdala) that promote formation of abnormal regional hyperexcitable circuits.

In healthy neuronal circuits, depolarising inward Na^+ and Ca^{2+} ionic currents are mainly activated by excitatory glutamate N-methyl-D-aspartate (NMDA) receptors. Depolarisation is followed by repolarising outward K^+ currents activated by $GABA_B$ receptors which act as a feedback inhibitory circuit in response to excitation. Influx of Cl^- ions into the neuron produced by $GABA_A$ receptor activation hyperpolarises the cell and inhibits impulse generation. Neuropeptide Y is co-released with γ-aminobutyric acid (GABA) and potentiates the inhibition. Membrane-bound ATPase pumps contribute to maintenance of the correct resting membrane potential by active transport of ions across the cell membrane in the resting phase (Ch. 8).

An epileptic seizure probably arises from a localised imbalance between excitatory neurotransmission, principally mediated by glutamate, and inhibitory neurotransmission, mediated by GABA, which leads to a focus of neuronal instability. In some forms of epilepsy there may be a defect in the neuronal currents that results in incomplete repolarisation of the cell. This will leave the neuron closer to its threshold potential for firing and create a hyperexcitable state. Such instability could initiate the burst of firing that produces epileptiform activity. Once an electrical discharge is triggered, spontaneous repetitive firing of the focus is maintained by a feedback mechanism known as post-tetanic potentiation. The synchronisation of the electrical charge that is necessary to generate a seizure may also be enhanced by neural plasticity. Remodelling of the neural connections of an individual GABA neuron can lead to simultaneous hyperpolarisation of a large group of glutamatergic neurons. Neurogenesis can be triggered by seizures and potentiate the development of this type of circuitry,

Table 23.1 Simplified classification of epileptic seizures

Seizure type	Characteristics
Partial (focal) seizures	
Simple partial seizures	Motor, somatosensory or psychic symptoms; consciousness is not impaired
Complex partial seizures	Temporal lobe, psychomotor; consciousness is impaired
Secondary generalised seizures	These begin as partial seizures
Generalised seizures	Affect whole brain with loss of consciousness
Clonic, tonic or tonic–clonic	Initial rigid extensor spasm, respiration stops, defaecation, micturition and salivation occur (tonic phase, ≈1 min); violent synchronous jerks (clonic phase, 2–4 min)
Myoclonic	Seizures of a muscle or group of muscles
Absence	Abrupt loss of awareness of surroundings, little motor disturbance (occur in children)
Atonic	Loss of muscle tone/strength
Unclassified seizures	

creating a group of hyperpolarised cells. Repolarisation activates currents that generate rebound excitation, producing a synchronised discharge. Generalisation of this discharge probably relies on increased synaptic connections from the excitatory cells.

Several inherited epilepsy syndromes have now been characterised at a cellular level, and arise from mutations of proteins involved in ion channel function. Reduction in the activity of membrane-bound ATPases linked to neuronal transmembrane ion pumps has also been found in the brains of people with primary generalised epilepsy. Ion channel dysfunction may therefore provide the basis for the genesis of many types of generalised seizures, but defective GABA-mediated inhibitory neurotransmission also appears to be a key factor. The genesis of partial seizures is less well understood. These circuits may be generated by disruption of glial cell function and changes in the neuronal microenvironment.

ANTIEPILEPTIC DRUGS

Most antiepileptic drugs produce their main antiepileptic effects either by blockade of depolarising ion channels, or by enhancing the inhibitory actions of GABA. Many drugs have multiple sites of action, so the drugs below are grouped by their principal mode of action.

SODIUM CHANNEL BLOCKERS

Carbamazepine, oxcarbazepine, eslicarbazepine

Mechanism of action and uses

Carbamazepine and oxcarbazepine are effective in most types of epilepsy, *except for myoclonic epilepsy and absences, which they can exacerbate*. Eslicarbazepine is the major active metabolite of oxcarbazepine, given as an acetate prodrug. Their mechanisms of action are incompletely understood but include:

- use-dependent blockade of Na^+ channels by stabilising them in the inactive state, which inhibits repetitive neuronal firing. This is the main mechanism of action,
- attenuation of the action of glutamate at NMDA receptors, and reduced glutamate release.

Carbamazepine and oxcarbazepine are also used in the management of trigeminal neuralgia (Ch. 19), and carbamazepine in the management of diabetic neuropathy (Ch. 19) and bipolar disorder (Ch. 21).

Pharmacokinetics

Carbamazepine is metabolised in the liver to an active epoxide metabolite. The half-life of carbamazepine is initially very long, at about 1.5 days, but decreases by about a half over the first 2–3 weeks of treatment because of 'autoinduction' of its own metabolism in the liver. Seizure control may then require an increase in dose. Transient unwanted neurological effects, which may occur in association with the peak plasma drug concentration when using the conventional formulation of carbamazepine, can be minimised by the use of a modified-release formulation.

Oxcarbazepine is well absorbed orally and is rapidly and extensively converted in the liver to active metabolites, including *S*-licarbazepine. Eslicarbazepine acetate is a prodrug converted rapidly to *S*-licarbazepine after oral administration, and is metabolised by glucuronidation and renal excretion.

Unwanted effects

The unwanted effects of oxcarbazepine and eslicarbazepine are less severe than those of carbamazepine.

- Nausea and vomiting (dose-related, and especially early in treatment), constipation, diarrhoea, anorexia.
- Rashes, especially transient generalised erythema but more severe reactions also occur. If a rash is produced by carbamazepine, oxcarbazepine can often be given without recurrence. Stevens–Johnson syndrome occasionally occurs with carbamazepine, and is more frequent in people with HLA-B*1502, who are most often of Han Chinese or Thai origin. Testing for this allele is recommended in such people before using carbamazepine.
- Central nervous system toxicity leads to headache, double vision, dizziness, drowsiness, confusion or ataxia. These are most common early in treatment and are dose-related.
- Transient leucopenia is common, especially early in treatment, but severe bone marrow depression is rare.

- Hyponatraemia, caused by potentiation of the action of antidiuretic hormone on the kidney, can lead to confusion and decreased control of seizures. This may be more pronounced with oxcarbazepine.
- Teratogenicity in the form of neural tube defects is common (see below).
- Induction of hepatic CYP3A4 (Table 2.7) by carbamazepine can lead to drug interactions. The most common interaction is with the oral combined contraceptive pill (Ch. 45) and the dose of oestrogen should be increased to avoid failure of contraception. The metabolism of warfarin (Ch. 11) and ciclosporin (Ch. 38) are also accelerated. Inhibition of CYP3A4 by erythromycin, clarithromycin or diltiazem can increase the plasma concentration of carbamazepine. Interactions of carbamazepine with other antiepileptic drugs are discussed below. Oxcarbazepine and eslicarbazepine have little effect on cytochrome P450 and therefore have few drug interactions.

Phenytoin and fosphenytoin

Mechanism of action and uses

Phenytoin and its prodrug fosphenytoin have a broad spectrum of activity and are effective against all forms of epilepsy, *except absences.* They have several actions that may contribute to the antiepileptic activity:

- use-dependent blockade of Na^+ channels, which reduces cell excitability, is the main mechanism of action,
- blockade of voltage-gated L-type Ca^{2+} channels,
- potentiation of the action of GABA at $GABA_A$ receptors.

Phenytoin is sometimes used in the management of trigeminal neuralgia (Ch. 19).

Pharmacokinetics

Phenytoin is well absorbed from the gut, but this is a slow process. Slow intravenous injection can be used if a rapid onset of action is needed. Intramuscular injection of phenytoin should be avoided since absorption by this route is erratic and muscle damage can occur. Phenytoin is eliminated by hepatic metabolism, but metabolism is readily saturated so its elimination changes from first-order (linear) kinetics to zero-order (non-linear) kinetics (Ch. 2; Fig. 23.1). This occurs in some individuals at plasma drug concentrations below or near the lower end of the therapeutic range. A small change in dose then produces a large change in the plasma concentration (Ch. 2) and the elimination half-life is increased from about 12 h to almost 2 days. Plasma phenytoin concentrations are closely correlated to the clinical effect, and their measurement is useful as a guide to dosing. When the plasma concentration is close to or within the therapeutic range then any increase in dose should be small. Phenytoin is highly protein-bound (about 90%) and can be displaced from its binding sites by sodium valproate and salicylates, which briefly enhance the clinical effect of phenytoin to an unpredictable extent. The concentration of phenytoin in saliva reflects the free drug concentration in plasma, and measurement of the salivary concentration can be useful to guide dose adjustment in pregnancy or renal failure, or to avoid blood sampling in children.

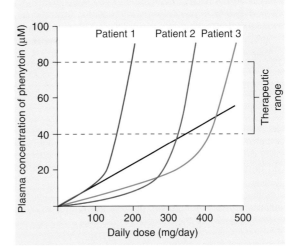

Fig. 23.1 **Inter-individual variation in the plasma concentration of phenytoin at steady state in relation to the daily dose.** The figure illustrates the relationship between daily dose and plasma concentrations in three different individuals. The straight line illustrates the increase in plasma concentrations of phenytoin in Patient 1 that would occur if the metabolism were not saturated (i.e. first-order kinetics). Non-linearity within the desired therapeutic range due to saturation of metabolism can lead to difficulties in dosage adjustment.

Fosphenytoin is a prodrug of phenytoin that is only available for parenteral use. It can be given by intramuscular injection (absorption from this route is good, unlike that of phenytoin) or by intravenous infusion, and is completely metabolised to phenytoin.

Unwanted effects

Most unwanted effects of phenytoin and fosphenytoin are dose-related.

- Nausea, vomiting, constipation, anorexia.
- CNS effects: impaired brainstem and cerebellar function, producing confusion, dizziness, tremor, nervousness or insomnia. Nystagmus, blurred vision, ataxia and dysarthria are signs of overdosage.
- Chronic connective tissue effects: gum hypertrophy, coarsening of facial features, hirsutism and acne. It is therefore usual to avoid phenytoin in young women or adolescents.
- Rashes. Stevens–Johnson syndrome occasionally occurs with phenytoin, and is more frequent in people with HLA-B*1502, who are most often of Han Chinese or Thai origin. Testing for this allele is recommended in such people before using phenytoin.
- Folic acid metabolism is increased by phenytoin, producing megaloblastic haemopoiesis, although anaemia with a macrocytic blood picture is rare.
- Increased vitamin D metabolism can produce vitamin D deficiency; in rare cases this results in osteomalacia.
- Teratogenicity with carbamazepine, including facial and digital malformations, occurs in up to 10% of pregnancies.

- Induction of hepatic cytochrome P450 enzymes (Ch. 2) predisposes to several drug interactions. In particular, the metabolism of warfarin and ciclosporin are increased; interactions with other antiepileptic drugs are discussed below.

Lacosamide

Mechanism of action and uses

Lacosamide is used for adjunctive treatment of refractory partial seizures with or without secondary generalisation. Its major mechanism of action is enhancing the slow inactivation of neuronal Na^+ channels, which stabilises cell membranes. It also binds to collapsing response mediator protein-2 (CRMP-2), which is involved in neuronal differentiation and axonal outgrowth, but it is not known whether this is important for the antiepileptic action.

Pharmacokinetics

Lacosamide is well absorbed from the gut and is eliminated by metabolism and also by the kidneys. It has a half-life of about 13 h.

Unwanted effects

- CNS effects: drowsiness, lethargy, dizziness, headache, confusion, ataxia, tremor, depression, impaired concentration.
- Nausea, vomiting, constipation.

Lamotrigine

Mechanism of action and uses

Lamotrigine has a wide spectrum of efficacy for partial and generalised seizures. It produces use-dependent inhibition of neuronal voltage-gated Na^+ channels. Unlike carbamazepine and phenytoin, it selectively targets dendrites of pyramidal neurons that synthesise glutamate and aspartate and lamotrigine reduces glutamate release.

Lamotrigine is also used for prophylaxis of depression in bipolar disorder (Ch. 21).

Pharmacokinetics

Lamotrigine is well absorbed orally and is metabolised in the liver. The half-life is long (15–60 h).

Unwanted effects

- Nausea, vomiting, diarrhoea, dry mouth.
- CNS effects: drowsiness, headache, fatigue, dizziness, double vision and ataxia; tremor can be troublesome at high dosages.
- Arthralgia, back pain.
- Hypersensitivity syndrome with fever, rash, lymphadenopathy and hepatic dysfunction. This is more common if lamotrigine is used together with sodium valproate.
- Rashes: some disappear despite continued treatment, but severe skin reactions, including Stevens–Johnson syndrome and toxic epidermal necrolysis, occasionally occur, particularly in children, following rapid dose escalation or with concurrent use of sodium valproate.
- Bone marrow suppression.

Zonisamide

Mechanism of action and uses

Zonisamide is used for adjunctive treatment of refractory partial seizures with or without secondary generalisation. Its mechanisms of action include:

- use-dependent blockade of neuronal Na^+ channels, which stabilises cell membranes. This is the most important effect,
- blockade of voltage-dependent T-type Ca^{2+} channels, which also stabilises cell membranes.

Pharmacokinetics

Zonisamide is well absorbed from the gut and is eliminated by metabolism. It has a very long half-life in plasma (about 60 h) and binds selectively to red blood cells.

Unwanted effects

- CNS effects: drowsiness, lethargy, dizziness, confusion, ataxia, emotional lability, psychosis, impaired concentration.
- Anorexia, weight loss, nausea, abdominal pain, diarrhoea.
- Rash.

GABA RECEPTOR AGONISTS

Benzodiazepines

Examples

clobazam, clonazepam, diazepam, lorazepam

Mechanism of action and uses

These drugs enhance the action of the inhibitory neurotransmitter GABA (Ch. 20). Clonazepam and clobazam are used orally for prophylaxis, usually as an adjunct to other drugs. Lorazepam, diazepam or clonazepam can be used intravenously to treat individual seizures, or if intravenous access is not available then rectal diazepam or buccal or intranasal midazolam can be used. Intravenous diazepam is formulated as an emulsion to reduce the incidence of thrombophlebitis.

Pharmacokinetics

These are long-acting benzodiazepines, discussed in detail in Chapter 20.

Unwanted effects

These are discussed in Chapter 20. Partial or complete tolerance to the antiepileptic action of benzodiazepines often occurs after about 4–6 months of continuous treatment.

Phenobarbital and primidone

Mechanism of action and effects

These drugs have a wide spectrum of activity and are effective in most forms of epilepsy, but unwanted effects limit their use. Phenobarbital is a barbiturate, and its major mechanism of action is activation of postsynaptic neuronal GABA$_A$ receptors (see also Ch. 20). This increases the duration of opening of the transmembrane Cl$^-$ channel associated with the receptor, and the neuronal membrane is therefore hyperpolarised and less likely to fire. In contrast to benzodiazepines, the GABA receptors are activated by phenobarbital independently of the presence of the inhibitory amino acid neurotransmitter, but phenobarbital will also potentiate the effect of GABA (Ch. 20). The action of primidone is due in part to its conversion to phenobarbital. Primidone has no advantage over phenobarbital and is generally less well tolerated. People with epilepsy who do not respond to phenobarbital or who tolerate it poorly are unlikely to benefit from primidone.

Pharmacokinetics

Oral absorption of phenobarbital is almost complete. Elimination is by hepatic metabolism and renal excretion. The half-life is very long, at about 4 days, but with considerable inter-individual variation. Primidone is well absorbed orally and is converted in the liver to two active metabolites, one of which is phenobarbital.

The plasma concentrations of phenobarbital and primidone relate poorly to the control of seizures; they are only useful as a guide to adherence to treatment. Control of seizures or unwanted effects should be used to determine dosages.

Unwanted effects

- CNS effects: sedation, fatigue and memory impairment are common in adults; paradoxical excitement, confusion and restlessness can occur in the elderly, and hyperactivity can occur in children.
- Folic acid metabolism is increased by phenobarbital, producing megaloblastic haemopoiesis, although anaemia with a macrocytic blood picture is rare.
- Increased vitamin D metabolism can produce vitamin D deficiency; in rare cases this results in osteomalacia.
- Tolerance to both unwanted and therapeutic effects occurs during long-term treatment.
- Dependence with a physical withdrawal reaction is seen after long-term treatment.
- Teratogenicity (see below).
- Induction of hepatic cytochrome P450 enzymes (Ch. 2) leads to increased metabolism of phenobarbital itself and warfarin, ciclosporin and oestrogen (reducing the effectiveness of oral contraception). Interactions with other antiepileptic drugs are considered below.

GABA REUPTAKE INHIBITOR

Tiagabine

Mechanism of action and uses

Tiagabine is used as an adjunctive therapy for partial seizures with or without secondary generalisation. It is a potent inhibitor of GABA transporter 1 (GAT-1) and decreases glial and presynaptic neuronal uptake of the inhibitory amino acid GABA. Uptake by GAT-1 is the mechanism that normally limits the duration of action of GABA at its receptor. The action of tiagabine is relatively selective for the hippocampus and thalamus.

Pharmacokinetics

Tiagabine is well absorbed from the gut. It is metabolised in the liver and has a half-life of 5–8 h.

Unwanted effects

- CNS effects: dizziness, lethargy, nervousness, impaired concentration, emotional lability, tremor.
- Nausea, diarrhoea.

GABA TRANSAMINASE INHIBITOR

Vigabatrin

Mechanism of action and uses

Vigabatrin is only used in combination with other drugs to treat epilepsy that is resistant to other drug combinations, or when they are poorly tolerated. It is effective in partial epilepsy with or without secondary generalisation, but its use is now restricted because of the unacceptably high risk of visual field defects (see below). It is, however, still useful for infantile spasms. Vigabatrin is a structural analogue of GABA and produces irreversible inhibition of GABA transaminase (GABA-T), the enzyme that inactivates GABA. The generalised increase in CNS concentrations of GABA inhibits the spread of epileptic discharges.

Pharmacokinetics

Vigabatrin is rapidly absorbed from the gut and is excreted unchanged by the kidney. Irreversible drug binding to its target enzyme GABA-T means that its duration of action is determined by the time required for GABA-T synthesis, rather than the half-life of elimination of the drug. GABA-T activity recovers to about 60% of baseline after 5 days. The efficacy of vigabatrin, therefore, is unrelated to the plasma drug concentration, and blood concentration monitoring is of no value.

Unwanted effects

- CNS effects: sedation and fatigue, dizziness, nervousness, irritability, depression, impaired concentration, headache, blurred vision, diplopia, nystagmus and tremor.
- Nausea, abdominal pain.
- Psychotic reactions, especially if there is a history of psychiatric disorder.
- Severe peripheral visual field defects during prolonged use; they can arise from 1 month to several years after starting treatment, and are usually irreversible; regular monitoring of visual fields at 6-month intervals is recommended.
- Alopecia, rash.
- Weight gain, oedema.

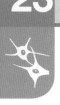

DRUGS WITH A POTENTIAL GABA-RELATED MECHANISM OF ACTION

Sodium valproate

Mechanism of action and uses

Sodium valproate has a wide spectrum of antiepileptic activity, and suppresses the initial seizure discharge as well as the spread of seizure activity. It is effective for all forms of epilepsy. The mechanisms of action of sodium valproate are uncertain, but include:

- potentiation of the effect of the inhibitory amino acid GABA, by enhancing the activity of glutamic acid decarboxylase (GAD), which converts glutamate to GABA.
- use-dependent blockade of transmembrane Na^+ channels, thus stabilising neuronal membranes.

The immediate antiepileptic effects may be due to extracellular actions on neuronal ion channels, but slow diffusion into neurons produces delayed intracellular effects. Inhibition of histone deacetylase (HDAC) by valproate modulates the transcription of multiple genes encoding signalling proteins and ion channels. The full benefit of treatment may not be apparent for several weeks. Valproate is also used for the management of neuropathic pain (Ch. 19) and bipolar disorder (Ch. 21) and the prophylaxis of migraine (Ch. 26).

Pharmacokinetics

Sodium valproate is well absorbed from the gut. Conventional-formulation tablets should be taken with food to reduce gastric upset. Valproate is highly protein-bound in plasma (90–95%) at low to moderate drug concentrations, but the proportion of free drug rises with increasing drug concentration. Valproate is highly ionised at physiological pH but is rapidly transported across the blood–brain barrier via an anion exchange transporter. Subsequent diffusion into and out of neurons is slow, partly explaining why the drug concentration in plasma does not correlate well with its therapeutic effect. The monitoring of blood concentrations is only useful to assess compliance.

Unwanted effects

- Gastrointestinal upset: nausea, vomiting, anorexia, abdominal pain and bowel disturbance. These can be minimised by gradual dosage titration. Valproate may rarely cause pancreatitis, and serum amylase should be measured if symptoms such as abdominal pain or nausea and vomiting arise.
- Weight gain caused by appetite stimulation.
- Transient hair loss, with hair regrowth being curly.
- Ataxia, tremor, confusion and, rarely, encephalopathy and coma. These can be minimised by slow dosage titration.
- Thrombocytopenia or impaired platelet activity.
- Severe hepatotoxicity can develop but is rare, and usually occurs in the first six months of therapy. This is most frequent in children under three years of age or in people with organic brain disorders who are receiving multiple drug therapy for seizures. Transiently raised liver enzymes are common but usually do not progress to more serious liver dysfunction.

- Teratogenicity in the form of neural tube defects (see below).
- Inhibition of hepatic cytochrome P450 enzymes, leading to interactions with other antiepileptic drugs (see below).

Gabapentin and pregabalin

Mechanism of action and uses

The major use of gabapentin and pregabalin is in partial seizures with or without secondary generalisation. Although designed as a structural analogue of GABA, gabapentin does not mimic GABA in the brain. The mechanisms of action of gabapentin and pregabalin are unclear, but probably include:

- potentiation of the inhibitory effect of GABA by enhancing activity of GAD, which converts glutamate to GABA,
- reduced synthesis of the excitatory neurotransmitter glutamate,
- inhibition of P/Q-type voltage-gated Ca^{2+} channels in the neocortex and hippocampus. The drugs reduce Ca^{2+} entry into neurons, which may inhibit release of excitatory neurotransmitters such as glutamate.

Gabapentin and pregabalin are also used in the management of neuropathic pain (Ch. 19), and pregabalin for generalised anxiety disorder (Ch. 20).

Pharmacokinetics

Gabapentin is incompletely absorbed from the gut via a saturable transport mechanism, while pregabalin is better absorbed. Both drugs are excreted largely unchanged by the kidney with half-lives of about 6 h.

Unwanted effects

- Nausea, vomiting, dry mouth, dyspepsia, diarrhoea, constipation, abdominal pain.
- CNS effects, including drowsiness, dizziness, ataxia, fatigue, headache, tremor, diplopia, dysarthria, confusion and emotional lability.
- Weight gain from stimulation of appetite.
- Rhinitis, cough, dyspnoea.
- Myalgia, arthralgia.
- Rashes.

GLUTAMATE RECEPTOR ANTAGONIST

Topiramate

Mechanism of action and uses

Topiramate is used alone or as an add-on treatment for drug-resistant partial or generalised seizures. Various mechanisms of action have been proposed:

- antagonist activity at the α-amino-3-hydroxy-5-methyl-4-isoxazole propionic acid (AMPA)/kainite subtype of receptor for the excitatory amino acid glutamate,
- use-dependent blockade of neuronal Na^+ channels,
- enhancement of the action of GABA at $GABA_A$ receptors, although the mechanism of this interaction is unknown,

- inhibition of carbonic anhydrase isoenzymes, producing multiple effects on transmembrane ionic fluxes.

Topiramate is also used for prophylaxis of migraine (Ch. 26).

Pharmacokinetics

Topiramate is rapidly absorbed orally and up to 70% is eliminated unchanged by the kidney, while the rest is metabolised in the liver. It has a long half-life (20–30 h).

Unwanted effects

- CNS effects, including impaired concentration, cognitive impairment, confusion, dizziness, ataxia, headache agitation, emotional lability or depression.
- Gastrointestinal upset, with nausea, dyspepsia, taste disturbance, abdominal pain, anorexia, dry mouth and weight loss.
- Nephrolithiasis.
- Myalgia, muscle weakness.
- Rash, alopecia.
- Teratogenicity with increased risk of cleft palate.

NEURONAL CALCIUM CHANNEL BLOCKER

Ethosuximide

Mechanism of action and uses

Ethosuximide is a drug of choice in absence seizures, and may be effective for myoclonic seizures, and tonic or atonic seizures. It is ineffective in other types of epilepsy. In absence seizures, T-type Ca^{2+} channels are believed to be responsible for generating excessive activity in thalamocortical relay neurons. Ethosuximide blocks these channels and prevents synchronised neuronal firing.

Pharmacokinetics

Absorption of ethosuximide from the gut is almost complete. Metabolism in the liver is extensive and the half-life is very long, at 2–3 days, although it is shorter in children. Plasma and salivary drug concentrations correlate well with control of seizures and can be used to monitor treatment.

Unwanted effects

- Nausea, vomiting, anorexia (less frequent if the drug is taken with food and if the dose is gradually increased).
- Drowsiness, dizziness, ataxia, dyskinesias, photophobia, headache and depression.

NEURONAL POTASSIUM CHANNEL OPENER

Retigabine

Mechanism of action and uses

Retigabine is used as an adjunctive (add-on) therapy for partial seizures with or without secondary generalisation. It is an activator of neuronal voltage-receptor K^+ channels, which hyperpolarises neurons. It may also enhance GABA-mediated neurotransmission, and reduce the release of the excitatory neurotransmitter glutamate.

Pharmacokinetics

Absorption of retigabine from the gut is almost complete. It is metabolised in the liver and the half-life is 8–11 h.

Unwanted effects

- Increased appetite with weight gain, nausea, constipation, dyspepsia, dry mouth.
- Drowsiness, dizziness, vertigo, amnesia, paraesthesia, tremor, impaired concentration, confusion, diplopia, myoclonus.
- Haematuria.

DRUGS WITH OTHER MECHANISMS OF ACTION

Levetiracetam

Mechanism of action and uses

Levetiracetam is used for adjunctive treatment of partial seizures with or without secondary generalisation. Its mechanisms of action remain uncertain, although levetiracetam binds to a protein (synaptic vesicle protein 2A) on the presynaptic neuronal plasma membrane and modulates release of excitatory neurotransmitters, such as glutamate. It produces selective inhibition of synchronised epileptiform burst firing and propagation of seizure activity in the hippocampus, without affecting neuronal excitability.

Pharmacokinetics

Levetiracetam is rapidly absorbed after oral administration. It is largely eliminated unchanged by the kidney; the half-life is 7 h.

Unwanted effects

- CNS effects: drowsiness, lethargy, dizziness, ataxia, headache, tremor, insomnia, emotional lability, impaired concentration.
- Anorexia, nausea, vomiting, dyspepsia, diarrhoea, weight changes.
- Cough.
- Myalgia.
- Rash.

INTERACTIONS AMONG ANTIEPILEPTIC DRUGS

Many antiepileptics affect hepatic drug-metabolising enzymes, especially cytochrome P450 isoenzymes (see Ch. 2, Table 2.7); therefore, drug interactions are frequent. Interactions when two or more antiepileptics are used together can have major clinical implications for seizure control and/or toxicity. However, the extent of the interaction is variable and unpredictable. Common interactions are listed below.

Carbamazepine is an enzyme inducer that often lowers the plasma concentrations of clobazam, clonazepam, lamotrigine, tiagabine, topiramate, sodium valproate, zonisamide and an active metabolite of oxcarbazepine.

Phenobarbital and *primidone* are enzyme inducers that often lower the plasma concentrations of clonazepam, lamotrigine, phenytoin, sodium valproate, tiagabine, zonisamide and an active metabolite of oxcarbazepine.

Phenytoin is an enzyme inducer and it often lowers the plasma concentrations of carbamazepine, clonazepam, lamotrigine, tiagabine, topiramate, sodium valproate, zonisamide and an active metabolite of oxcarbazepine.

Valproate inhibits hepatic drug metabolism which often increases the plasma concentrations of phenobarbital and lamotrigine, as well as those of an active metabolite of carbamazepine. Sodium valproate can displace phenytoin from plasma protein binding sites but also inhibits the metabolism of phenytoin, and the net result is an increase in the active free component.

Vigabatrin often reduces plasma phenytoin concentration by an unknown mechanism.

MANAGEMENT OF EPILEPSY

TREATMENT OF INDIVIDUAL SEIZURES

The initial management of a seizure involves positioning the person to avoid injury. Particular attention must also be given to maintaining the airways and ensuring adequate oxygenation. A correctable cause such as hypoglycaemia should be sought and treated, and intravenous thiamine given if alcohol abuse is suspected.

Prolonged or repetitive seizures (status epilepticus) usually require urgent parenteral drug treatment. Intravenous lorazepam is the drug of choice, with clonazepam as an alternative. Diazepam can be used, but it can cause thrombophlebitis and has a shorter duration of action owing to more rapid tissue distribution. A second dose of benzodiazepine can be given if necessary after 10 min. If intravenous access is not available, then midazolam can be given by the buccal or intranasal routes. Diazepam is available as a rectal solution, which may be particularly useful for children or for initial treatment out of hospital. Close observation for signs of drug-induced respiratory depression should be maintained after giving a benzodiazepine.

If there is no response after 25 min, or seizures recur, then a slow intravenous injection of phenytoin, or a more rapid injection of fosphenytoin or phenobarbital, should be given. If seizures are still not controlled with these measures, then full anaesthesia using thiopental or propofol (Ch. 17) with assisted respiration in an intensive care unit will be necessary.

PROPHYLAXIS FOR SEIZURES

A diagnosis of epilepsy requires two or more spontaneous seizures. After a single event, up to 80% of people will have a second fit within three years. If a predisposing cause cannot be identified and avoided (e.g. alcohol withdrawal, photosensitive epilepsy precipitated by viewing a television from too close a distance), drug treatment will usually be recommended after a second seizure, unless the seizures were separated by very long intervals or were mild.

Table 23.2 Drug choice in the treatment of epilepsy

Type of seizure	First-line drugs	Second-line drugs
Partial seizures	Carbamazepine Lamotrigine Oxcarbazepine Sodium valproate	Clobazam Gabapentin Levetiracetam Pregabalin Tiagabine Topiramate Zonisamide
Generalised seizures		
Tonic–clonic (grand mal)	Carbamazepine Lamotrigine Sodium valproate	Clobazam Levetiracetam Oxcarbazepine Topiramate
Myoclonic	Sodium valproate	Clonazepam Levetiracetam Lamotrigine Topiramate
Absence	Ethosuximide Sodium valproate	Clonazepam Lamotrigine
Atonic	Sodium valproate Lamotrigine Clonazepam	Clobazam Ethosuximide Levetiracetam Topiramate

Occasionally, treatment will be recommended after a first fit, such as when there is structural brain damage.

Treatment should begin with a single drug, the choice depending on the type of epilepsy and relative toxicity of the drugs (Table 23.2). For generalised seizures or unclassifiable seizures, in the absence of factors that would lead to an alternative choice, sodium valproate is often recommended since it has the broadest spectrum of activity. Lamotrigine is usually considered the drug of first choice for partial seizures. The initial drug dose should be low, with gradual titration to minimise unwanted effects. If seizures continue, then the maximum tolerated dose should be taken. If seizures are not controlled with the first-choice drug it becomes more important to accurately identify the type of seizure. A second single drug should then be introduced and titrated to an adequate dose before the first drug is gradually withdrawn (Table 23.2). A single drug will usually control seizures in up to 90% of people with epilepsy, although this may not be achieved with the first drug chosen. However, if the first drug does not control the seizures, then the chance of a second single drug being successful is 13%, and with a third only 4%.

Refractory epilepsy can indicate poor adherence to treatment, inappropriate drug choice or dosage, or that the seizures are 'pseudoseizures' (non-epileptic attack disorder) rather than true epilepsy. Multiple drug treatment (initially with two first-line drugs, or a first- and a second-line drug) should be reserved for seizures that have not been controlled by treatment with two or three first- or second-line drugs given alone. Drugs like tiagabine, vigabatrin and zonisamide are usually used in combination with other agents.

Combination therapy at maximally tolerated doses does not control the seizures in some people with epilepsy, even when there is good adherence to treatment recommendations. Lack of seizure control is more frequent if the onset was at an early age, if there are generalised, atonic or absence seizures, or if there is underlying structural brain damage. Some data suggest that resistance can arise from overexpression of proteins that transport drugs out of the CNS, such as P-glycoprotein, but the evidence for this is conflicting. Alternatively, resistance may arise from genetic variation affecting targets for drug action. For temporal lobe epilepsy there is now good evidence that surgical treatment should be considered if more than two consecutive antiepileptic drugs fail to control the seizures. Surgery for other forms of epilepsy may provide some amelioration of seizure frequency.

It is not usually necessary to monitor plasma drug concentrations unless seizure control is poor, or if poor adherence or drug toxicity is suspected. Good seizure control will often be achieved at plasma drug concentrations that are below the accepted therapeutic range, and under such circumstances an increase in dosage would not be necessary. Conversely, people who continue to have seizures may need plasma drug concentrations above the standard therapeutic range to achieve seizure control, provided the drug is well tolerated. The only drug for which monitoring is of proven benefit for dosage adjustment is phenytoin, primarily because metabolism may be saturated at therapeutic doses and the kinetics become non-linear (Fig. 23.1). Adjustment of the dosages of carbamazepine or ethosuximide may be easier if the plasma concentration is known; however, for other drugs monitoring is only of value to confirm that the drug is being taken.

In the UK, a driving licence is revoked until the individual has been seizure-free for one year, or has suffered only nocturnal seizures for three years. Driving is not advisable during withdrawal of antiepileptic drugs, or for six months afterwards.

Once started, treatment should usually be continued for at least 2–3 years after the last seizure. Treatment should probably be lifelong if there is a continuing predisposing condition or the person wishes to continue to drive. If a decision is made to withdraw treatment then it should be gradual over at least 2–3 months to minimise the risk of rebound seizures. When several drugs are used, one should be withdrawn at a time.

Prophylaxis for seizures is often given for up to three months following neurosurgical procedures or head injury, particularly if there was a depressed skull fracture or an associated intracranial haematoma. Evidence that such routine use is beneficial is not secure.

Febrile convulsions occur commonly in infancy and usually do not lead to epilepsy or produce CNS damage. About 4% of children have them and they recur in about one-third. It is important to reduce pyrexia during subsequent febrile episodes, such as by removal of clothes and use of paracetamol (Ch. 29). Routine prophylaxis with antiepileptic drugs is not recommended, but rectal diazepam is sometimes given when a child who has previously had a febrile convulsion becomes pyrexial.

ANTIEPILEPTIC DRUGS IN PREGNANCY

No antiepileptic drug has a proven safety record in pregnancy and their use may carry a high risk of teratogenesis if the fetus is exposed in the first trimester (see Table 56.1). Fetal abnormalities are most frequent if more than one drug is used. Neural tube defects and other problems are particularly common with sodium valproate (malformations in about 10% of pregnancies), and to a lesser extent with carbamazepine and oxcarbazepine (2–4%). Developmental abnormalities also occur with phenobarbital, phenytoin, lamotrigine and topiramate, but there is too little information about many of the other drugs. There is also increasing evidence of language and neurocognitive defects in children born to mothers who are taking antiepileptic drugs.

Women of child-bearing age who are taking antiepileptic drugs should be given contraceptive advice. If they wish to become pregnant they should be counselled about the risk and offered antenatal screening during pregnancy, with α-fetoprotein measurement (to detect neural tube defects) and second-trimester ultrasound scanning. Folic acid supplements may reduce the risk of neural tube defects and should be recommended before and during pregnancy. It is important to advise a potential mother with epilepsy that the risks of uncontrolled seizures during pregnancy, to both her and the fetus, may be greater than the risk associated with drug therapy.

When the mother is taking carbamazepine, phenobarbital or phenytoin there is an increased risk of neonatal bleeding. Prophylactic vitamin K_1 should be given to the mother from 36 weeks of pregnancy, and to the newborn immediately after birth.

SELF-ASSESSMENT

True/false questions

1. Generalised seizures include tonic–clonic and absence seizures.
2. Absence seizures occur mainly in adults.
3. Partial seizures cause motor, sensory or psychic symptoms without loss of consciousness.
4. Generalised muscle contractions do not occur in partial seizures.
5. The excitatory amino acid glutamate is increased in some seizures.
6. There are currently no antiepileptic drugs that act by reducing excessive glutamatergic activity.
7. Antiepileptic drugs that stimulate γ-aminobutyric acid (GABA) receptors or enhance GABA stability act by inhibiting Na^+ influx in neurons.
8. A major mechanism of antiepileptic drug action is the inhibition of Na^+ channels.
9. The metabolism of carbamazepine diminishes with regular use.
10. Activation of K^+ channels by retigabine hyperpolarises neurons.
11. Ethosuximide blocks neuronal Ca^{2+} channels.
12. The plasma concentrations of phenytoin increase in a linear manner with increasing dosage of the drug.
13. Vigabatrin is a first-line drug for the treatment of all types of epilepsy.
14. Tiagabine enhances GABA levels in synapses by reducing its reuptake.

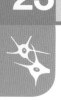

15. The abrupt withdrawal of antiepileptics should be avoided.
16. The antiepileptic drug gabapentin is also used for neuropathic pain.

One-best-answer (OBA) question

Which of the following is the *most accurate* statement about antiepileptic drugs?

A. Phenytoin causes hair loss.
B. The use of diazepam in epilepsy is confined to long-term prophylaxis in tonic–clonic seizures.
C. Valproate induces drug-metabolising enzymes in the liver.
D. The effectiveness of phenobarbital diminishes with time.
E. The risk of teratogenicity can be reduced in pregnancy by combining antiepileptic drugs.

Case-based questions

Case 1: a 7-year-old boy was described as 'dreamy' by his mother. He was making slow progress at school and his mother and teachers commented that he could not concentrate and had frequent episodes of staring vacantly for a few seconds, then carrying on as normal. Following an electroencephalogram (EEG) a synchronised electrical discharge characteristic of an absence form of epilepsy was demonstrated.

A. Which of the following would be suitable as a drug of first choice: phenytoin, phenobarbital, sodium valproate, ethosuximide?
B. What are the major unwanted effects of the drug(s) you have chosen?
C. If control of absence seizures is inadequate with your chosen antiepileptic, can combination therapy be given?

Case 2: a 19-year-old woman had a long-term history of epilepsy of the complex partial seizure type, which often gravitated to generalised seizures. For several years her epilepsy had been well controlled with a stable drug regimen. She now sought advice on contraception.

A. What antiepileptic drugs might be effective in the type of epilepsy this woman has?
B. What suitable options are available for contraception?
C. What potential problems can arise if the woman takes the combined oral hormonal contraceptive?
D. Would an injected progestogen contraceptive be worth considering?
E. If the combined oral hormonal contraceptive were the chosen method, what strategies should be adopted to ensure its efficacy?
F. Would the oral progestogen-only contraceptive be a suitable method of contraception?

True/false answers

1. **True.** Tonic–clonic seizures (formerly termed grand mal) and absence seizures (formerly petit mal) are two types of generalised seizure affecting the whole brain.

2. **False.** Absences, manifested by transient unawareness of surroundings and generally without motor disturbance, occur in children.
3. **False.** Simple partial (or focal) seizures do not cause loss of conciousness, but consciousness can be impaired in complex partial seizures and in secondary generalised seizures that arise from partial seizures.
4. **False.** In 'Jacksonian epilepsy' an epileptic focus in the primary motor cortex causes jerking localised to a specific group of muscles, which gradually spreads to involve many other muscle groups.
5. **True.** Glutamatergic over-activity is implicated in some types of epilepsy and may cause neuronal excitotoxicity.
6. **False.** Reducing glutamatergic activity may account in part for the action of antiepileptic drugs such as topiramate, which can block glutamate AMPA receptors, and others such as lamotrigine, levetiracetam and retigabine, which decrease glutamate release.
7. **False.** GABA hyperpolarises neurons by increasing the influx of Cl^- ions.
8. **True.** Blockade of Na^+ channels reduces repetitive neuronal firing and is a major mechanism of action of many antiepileptic drugs.
9. **False.** The sodium channel blocker carbamazepine induces its own metabolism (autoinduction), so its elimination accelerates with regular use.
10. **True.** The K^+ channel activator retigabine hyperolarises neurons and modulates GABA and glutamate release.
11. **True.** The action of ethosuximide in absence seizures rests on its blockade of T-type Ca^{2+} channels in thalamocortical relay neurons.
12. **False.** Phenytoin exhibits first-order kinetics at low doses, but at higher doses it has zero-order kinetics because the liver drug-metabolising enzymes become saturated.
13. **False.** Vigabatrin is effective in all types of epilepsy, inhibiting the breakdown of GABA by GABA transaminase, but due to the risk of irreversible narrowing of the visual field it is reserved for people who are resistant to other drugs.
14. **True.** Tiagabine reduces GABA reuptake by glial cells and presynaptic neurons by inhibiting the GABA transporter GAT-1.
15. **True.** Withdrawal of an antiepileptic drug should be gradual over 2–3 months to prevent rebound seizures.
16. **True.** Gabapentin and pregabalin are inhibitors of glutamic acid decarboxylase used for epilepsy and neuropathic pain.

OBA answer

Answer D is correct.

A. Incorrect. Phenytoin causes hair growth (hirsutism); other unwanted effects include gingival hyperplasia, acne and facial coarsening.
B. Incorrect. Diazepam is used as an adjunct to other treatments for prophylaxis but also alone in status epilepticus.
C. Incorrect. Valproate *inhibits* drug-metabolising enzymes in the liver, increasing plasma concentrations of many other drugs.

D. **Correct**. Tolerance to the therapeutic effects and unwanted effects of phenobarbital develops with time.

E. Incorrect. The risk of teratogenesis is increased if more than one drug is given.

Case-based answers

Case 1

A. The absence seizures experienced by this boy should respond well to sodium valproate or ethosuximide; phenytoin and phenobarbital are ineffective in absence seizures.

B. Sodium valproate causes nausea, reversible hair loss and weight gain. Uncommonly, liver damage can occur. Ethosuximide causes nausea, anorexia and headache.

C. Monotherapy with ethosuximide or sodium valproate should be tried, and adherence with monotherapy checked, before combining drugs. Sodium valproate reduces the clearance of ethosuximide and may cause toxicity.

Case 2

A. A variety of antiepileptic drugs could be used by this woman with complex partial seizures. First-line drugs usually include carbamazepine, oxcarbazepine, lamotrigine or sodium valproate.

B. Non-hormonal contraceptives such as barrier methods or intra-uterine devices, are effective and do not carry the risk of drug interactions. However, many women will want to use a hormonal method.

C. Carbamazepine, phenytoin, phenobarbital and topiramate all induce liver enzymes that increase the metabolism of sex steroids and reduce the efficacy of oral contraceptives.

D. The metabolism of injected medroxyprogesterone acetate (MPA) is affected less than that of sex steroids taken orally. The interval between MPA injections should nevertheless be reduced to 10 weeks. MPA may also reduce the incidence of seizures.

E. Because oestrogen metabolism is enhanced by several antiepileptic drugs, it is recommended that, if one of these drugs needs to be prescribed, formulations containing a high concentration of oestrogen (at least 50 µg) should be used. Sometimes more than 100 µg oestrogen daily in split doses may be required to prevent breakthrough bleeding. The pill-free period can also be reduced. If any change in medication for her epilepsy is made, additional barrier methods of contraception should be used until medication is stabilised.

F. The progestogen-only oral contraceptive would be unsafe, as its metabolism is increased.

FURTHER READING

Duncan JS, Sander JW, Sisodiya SM et al. (2006) Adult epilepsy. *Lancet* 367, 1087–1100

French JA, Pedley TA (2008) Initial management of epilepsy. *N Engl J Med* 359, 166–176

Guerrini R (2006) Epilepsy in children. *Lancet* 367, 499–524

Kalviainen R, Tomson T (2006) Optimising treatment of epilepsy during pregnancy. *Neurology* 67, S59–S63

Lason W, Dudra-Jastzebska M, Rejdak K et al. (2011) Basic mechanisms of antiepileptic drugs and their pharmacokinetic/pharmacodynamic interactions: an update. *Pharmacol Rep* 63, 271–292

Marson AG, Al-Kharusi AM, Alwaidh M et al. (2007) The SANAD study of effectiveness of carbamazepine, gabapentin, lamotrigine, oxcarbazepine, or topiramate for treatment of partial epilepsy: an unblinded randomised controlled trial. *Lancet* 369, 1000–1015

Marson AG, Al-Kharusi AM, Alwaidh M et al. (2007) The SANAD study of effectiveness of valproate, lamotrigine, or topiramate for generalised and unclassified epilepsy: an unblinded randomised controlled trial. *Lancet* 369, 1016–1026

Perruca E (2005) Birth defects after prenatal exposure to antiepileptic drugs. *Lancet Neurol* 4, 781–786

Perruca E, Tomson T (2011) The pharmacological treatment of epilepsy in adults. *Lancet Neurol* 10, 446–456

Pohlmann-Eden B, Beghi E, Camfield C et al. (2006) The first seizure and its management in adults and children. *BMJ* 332, 339–342

Rugg-Gunn FJ, Sander JW (2012) Management of chronic epilepsy. *BMJ* 345, e4576

Shorvon S (2011) The treatment of status epilepticus. *Curr Opin Neurol* 4, 165–170

Tatum WO IV, Liporace J, Benbadia SR et al. (2004) Updates on the treatment of epilepsy in women. *Arch Intern Med* 164, 137–146

Torbjorn T, Hiilesmaa V (2007) Epilepsy in pregnancy. *BMJ* 335, 769–773

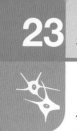

Compendium: drugs used to treat epilepsy and status epilepticus

Drug	Kinetics (half-life)	Comments
Drugs used for epilepsy		
Drugs given orally, usually once or twice daily, to encourage better compliance.		
Acetazolamide	Negligible metabolism; renal excretion (6–15 h)	Carbonic anhydrase inhibitor; low efficacy, but specific role in epilepsy associated with menstruation; also used as adjunctive drug for partial and tonic–clonic seizures
Carbamazepine	Good oral bioavailability; hepatic metabolism; epoxide metabolite has antiepileptic activity; wide inter-individual variation in cytochrome P450 induction and drug interactions; autoinduction of its metabolism reduces initial half-life (15–65 h) after repeated dosage (12–17 h)	Sodium channel blocker; used for partial and secondary generalised tonic–clonic seizures, some primary generalised seizures; also used for neuropathic pain control (Ch.19) and for bipolar disorder unresponsive to lithium (Ch. 21); given orally or rectally
Clobazam	High oral bioavailability; hepatic metabolism (10–50 h); high plasma levels of active N-desmethyl metabolite	Benzodiazepine GABA$_A$ receptor agonist; used as adjunctive therapy in epilepsy; also used short term for anxiety
Clonazepam	High oral bioavailability (80%); hepatic metabolism (18–45 h)	Benzodiazepine GABA$_A$ receptor agonist; used in all forms of epilepsy; also used in myoclonus
Eslicarbazepine acetate	High oral bioavailability; prodrug rapidly deacetylated to eslicarbazepine, an active metabolite of oxcarbazepine; does not cause autoinduction of metabolism; eliminated by hepatic glucuronidation and renal excretion (20–24 h)	Sodium channel blocker; related to carbamazepine and oxcarbazepine; used for adjunctive treatment of partial seizures in adults with or without secondary generalisation
Ethosuximide	Hepatic metabolism (50–60 h); half-life shorter in children (30 h)	Blocks neuronal T-type Ca^{2+} channels; used for absence seizures, myoclonic seizures and some atypical seizures
Gabapentin	Rapid oral bioavailability (60%) decreases at high doses due to saturable gut absorption; renal excretion (5–7 h)	Increases GABA by activating glutamic acid decarboxylase; used as adjunctive treatment in partial epilepsy with or without secondary generalised tonic–clonic seizures; also used for neuropathic pain and migraine
Lacosamide	Rapid and complete absorption; renal excretion of parent drug and hepatic metabolism (13 h)	Slow inactivator of neuronal sodium channels; used as adjunctive treatment of refractory partial seizures with or without secondary generalisation; given orally or intravenously
Lamotrigine	Rapid absorption; high bioavailability (85%); hepatic metabolism (15–60 h)	Sodium channel blocker; used for partial and primary and secondary generalised tonic–clonic seizures; long-acting, can be given once daily
Levetiracetam	Rapid absorption and 100% bioavailability; eliminated largely by glomerular filtration and some hepatic metabolism (6–8h)	Uncertain action, but may reduce glutamate release; used for partial seizures and generalised myoclonic or atonic seizures
Oxcarbazepine	Oxcarbazepine is the keto analogue of carbamazepine; rapid and complete oral absorption; reduced in the liver (2 h) to the active metabolite (S-licarbazepine), which has a longer half-life (9 h) and is responsible for most of the anti-seizure activity	Sodium channel blocker; used for partial seizures with or without secondary generalised tonic–clonic seizures
Phenobarbital	Oral bioavailability >90%; eliminated by hepatic oxidation and renal excretion (50–150 h); potent inducer of cytochrome P450 isoenzymes, leading to numerous drug interactions	Barbiturate GABA$_A$ receptor agonist; can be used for all forms of epilepsy except absence seizures, but no longer front-line drug due to sedation and drug interactions
Phenytoin	Complete oral bioavailability; dose-dependent elimination because of saturation of hepatic metabolism, with wide inter-subject variation (7–60 h); potent inducer of cytochrome P450 isoenzymes, leading to numerous drug interactions	Sodium channel blockade and other antiepileptic actions; can be used for all forms of epilepsy except absence seizures but now little used
Pregabalin	High oral bioavailability (90%); mainly renal elimination of parent drug (6 h)	Structural analogue of gabapentin; used as an adjuvant for partial seizures; also used for neuropathic pain and generalised anxiety disorder

Compendium: drugs used to treat epilepsy and status epilepticus—cont'd

Drug	Kinetics (half-life)	Comments
Primidone	Hepatic metabolism (4–22 h); active metabolites (including phenobarbital) have longer half-lives and account for most activity; potent inducer of cytochrome P450 isoenzymes, leading to numerous drug interactions	Prodrug of phenobarbital; used for all forms of epilepsy except absence seizures; also used for essential tremor
Retigabine	Oral bioavailability 50–60%; hepatic metabolism not dependent on cytochrome P450 (8–11 h)	Neuronal potassium channel activator; used as adjunctive therapy for partial seizures with or without secondary generalisation
Rufinamide	Good oral bioavailability (85%); hepatic metabolism (6–10 h); clearance increased by cytochrome P450 inducers	Sodium channel blocker; used as adjunctive drug in Lennox–Gastaut epilepsy syndrome in children and adults
Tiagabine	Rapidly and completely absorbed; hepatic metabolism (5–8 h) enhanced by cytochrome P450 inducers	Blocks GABA reuptake transporter GAT-1; used as adjunctive treatment in partial epilepsy with or without secondary generalised tonic–clonic seizures
Topiramate	Rapid absorption with high bioavailability; 70% eliminated unchanged (20–30 h) but also hepatic metabolism which is enhanced by cytochrome P450 inducers	Glutamate AMPA receptor antagonist; used as monotherapy or adjunctive treatment in generalised tonic–clonic seizures and in partial epilepsy with or without secondary generalisation; also used in migraine
Valproate sodium	High oral bioavailability (>95%); highly protein bound (81–90%); heaptic metabolism (9–21 h)	Sodium channel blocker and activator of glutamic acid decarboxylase; used in all forms of epilepsy; available in modified-release and intravenous formulations
Vigabatrin	Oral bioavailability 80–90%; excreted unchanged; duration of action exceeds the drug half-life (7–8 h) due to irreversible binding to enzyme target (GABA transaminase)	Increases GABA by irreversibly inhibiting GABA transaminase; used under specialist supervision as adjunctive treatment in refractory partial epilepsy with or without secondary generalised tonic–clonic seizures
Zonisamide	Good oral absorption; hepatic metabolism (60 h)	Sodium channel blocker; used as an adjunct for refractory partial seizures

Drugs used primarily for status epilepticus

These drugs may also be used for other forms of epilepsy.

Drug	Kinetics (half-life)	Comments
Clonazepam	See above	Benzodiazepine GABA$_A$ receptor agonist; given by intravenous injection or infusion; see above for other information
Diazepam	See Ch. 20 for details	Benzodiazepine GABA$_A$ receptor agonist; given rectally or by intravenous injection; see Ch. 20 for other details
Fosphenytoin sodium	Rapidly metabolised by hydrolysis to phenytoin (0.15–0.25 h)	Ester prodrug of phenytoin; given by intravenous injection or infusion
Lorazepam	See Ch. 20 for details	Benzodiazepine GABA$_A$ receptor agonist; given by intravenous injection; see Ch. 20
Midazolam	See Ch. 20 for details	Benzodiazepine GABA$_A$ receptor agonist; given orally; see Ch. 20
Paraldehyde	Mainly hepatic metabolism, with up to 30% excreted in exhaled breath	Trimer of acetaldehyde; sedation, but little respiratory depression; given rectally using a glass syringe (it reacts with plastic and rubber); oxidises in air
Phenobarbital sodium	See above	Barbiturate; given by intravenous injection
Phenytoin sodium	See above	Sodium channel blocker; given by intravenous injection or infusion; solution for injection is alkaline and venous irritation is reduced by injecting saline before and after drug administration

Extrapyramidal movement disorders and spasticity

The group of nuclei in the area of the brain known as the basal ganglia (Fig. 24.1) are part of an integrative loop motor circuit (the cortico-basal ganglia-thalamo-cortical loop). This loop is intimately involved in the coordination of motor function. Nuclei in the basal ganglia feed neuronal output to the cortex and receive input from the cortex. Degeneration of vital neurons in the basal ganglia produces disordered regulation of neuronal activity and dysfunctional motor activity. Treatment for these disorders is directed at restoring the balance among the neurotransmitters in the basal ganglia.

PARKINSON'S DISEASE AND PARKINSONISM

Parkinson's disease and parkinsonism arise from dysfunction in the part of the brain called the basal ganglia, which is involved in the control of movement. The basal ganglia system includes several nuclei such as the substantia nigra, the striatum, the globus pallidus and the subthalamic nucleus (Fig. 24.1). Between these nuclei there are many complex *internal neuronal loop circuits* that use glutamate, dopamine, acetylcholine or γ-aminobutyric acid (GABA) as neurotransmitters. In addition there are *external neuronal loop circuits* that integrate neurons outside of the basal ganglia with the internal circuits of the basal ganglia. For example, basal ganglia nuclei feed into and receive information from the cortex (via the cortico-basal ganglia-thalamo-cortical loop). The precise details of the complex interplay

between the neuronal circuits are beyond the scope of this book and only general principles are given.

Parkinson's disease is a disorder characterised by a triad of:

- resting tremor,
- skeletal muscle rigidity,
- bradykinesia (poverty of movement).

There are two clinical subtypes of Parkinson's disease: the akinetic-rigid form and the tremor-dominant type. The trigger for the condition is unknown, but environmental toxins have been implicated in a small and specific gene mutations may be responsible in a small proportion of cases.

The underlying pathology involves loss of neurons in the substantia nigra pars compacta and deposition of intracytoplasmic Lewy bodies. Lewy bodies are complex structures that produce functional changes in dopaminergic neurons of the nigrostriatal pathway, possibly involving impaired handling of free radicals generated during dopamine metabolism. This ultimately leads to progressive neuronal death and degeneration of the nigrostriatal pathway (Fig. 24.1). More than 50% of substantia nigra pars compacta neurons must undergo degeneration before symptoms are apparent.

In Parkinson's disease, as a result of degeneration of the nigrostriatal dopaminergic pathways, there is destabilisation of the motor control networks. The basal ganglia normally provide a persistent inhibitory influence on the initiation of movement through GABAergic inhibition of the thalamus. When movement is required, the nigrostriatal dopaminergic pathways act to release the relevant thalamic and cortical motor systems from this inhibition. Denervation of the substantia nigra results in reduced stimulation of D_1 and D_2 receptors in the striatum. The consequence of this is excessive GABAergic inhibition of the thalamus and reduced glutamatergic activation of cortical systems (Fig. 24.1B shows changes in Parkinson's disease relative to normal function in Fig. 24.1A). At the same time, hyperactivity in the glutamatergic pathways that connect the cortex to the basal ganglia exacerbates the predominant inhibitory influence of the basal ganglia on movement. Cholinergic transmission in the basal ganglia is also enhanced in Parkinson's disease, contributing particularly to tremor.

In some conditions that have clinical similarities to Parkinson's disease, for example the Steele–Richardson–Olszewski (progressive supranuclear palsy) and Shy–Drager syndromes, the GABA neurons also degenerate, which explains the poor response of these conditions to treatment with dopamine-replacement therapy. Drugs that block striatal dopamine receptors, such as antipsychotic drugs (Ch. 21), can produce a parkinsonian syndrome which also responds poorly to dopamine-replacement therapy.

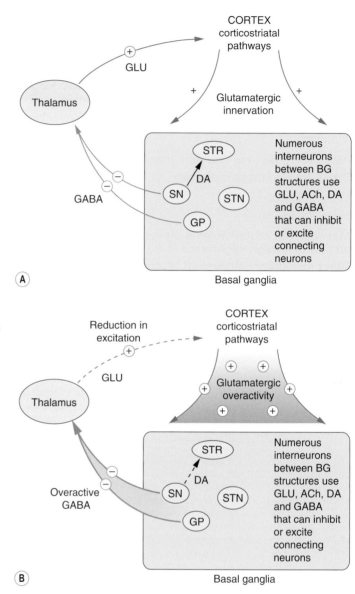

Fig. 24.1 The cortico-basal ganglia-thalamo-cortical loop. (A) Main pathways connecting the basal ganglia, the thalamus and the cortex involved in movement; (B) indicates how they are disordered in Parkinson's disease relative to (A). In Parkinson's disease the pathological changes in the basal ganglia, principally the loss of dopaminergic activity required to initiate movement, result in increased inhibitory γ-aminobutyric acid (GABA) transmission in pathways from the substantia nigra and the globus pallidus to the thalamus; consequently there is excessive inhibition of thalamic-cortical brainstem motor networks. Hyperactivity in the glutamatergic cortico-basal ganglia pathways and also in cholinergic pathways within the basal ganglia exacerbates the predominant inhibitory influence of the basal ganglia on movement. BG, basal ganglia; DA, dopamine; GLU, glutamate; GP, globus pallidus; SN, substantia nigra; STN, subthalamic nucleus; STR, striatum; −, inhibition; +, stimulation; dashed line, reduced activity compared to normal function in control (A).

DRUGS FOR PARKINSON'S DISEASE

Targets for drug therapy in Parkinson's disease are:

- enhancement of dopaminergic activity,
- inhibition of cholinergic activity.

Glutamatergic dysregulation has not yet provided suitable targets for drug therapy.

DOPAMINERGIC DRUGS

Levodopa

Mechanism of action

Dopamine cannot be given to replace the underlying deficiency in the basal ganglia because it does not cross the blood–brain barrier. However, levodopa (L-DOPA) is the immediate precursor of dopamine that is carried by the large neutral amino acid transporter into the brain. It is taken up into dopaminergic neurons and converted to dopamine by L-aromatic amino acid decarboxylase, also known as DOPA decarboxylase (Ch. 2).

Pharmacokinetics

Levodopa is absorbed from the small intestine by an active transport mechanism for large neutral amino acids. A similar transport system transfers levodopa across the blood–brain barrier. When it is given alone, levodopa is extensively decarboxylated to dopamine in peripheral tissues such as the gut wall, liver and kidney. This reduces the amount of levodopa that reaches the brain to about 1% of an oral dose, while the peripheral dopamine that is generated produces unwanted effects. Therefore, levodopa is given in combination with a peripheral dopa decarboxylase inhibitor (with carbidopa as co-careldopa or with benserazide as co-beneldopa). Inhibition of the peripheral metabolism of levodopa increases the amount that crosses the blood–brain barrier to 5–10% of the oral dose. The dopa decarboxylase inhibitor *does not* cross the blood–brain barrier and therefore does not inhibit the required conversion of levodopa to dopamine by DOPA decarboxylase within the central nervous system (CNS).

The half-life of levodopa is short (about 1 h). In the early stages of Parkinson's disease synthesis and storage of dopamine in striatal neurons is sufficient to ensure a stable response despite infrequent doses of levodopa. This becomes less reliable as the disease progresses and more neurons are lost. Modified-release formulations of levodopa provide a more continuous supply of drug to the neurons and can be useful to treat 'end-of-dose' deterioration in symptoms. Transition from conventional levodopa to a modified-release formulation requires care, because the latter has a lower bioavailability which makes it difficult to estimate the equivalent dose.

Unwanted effects

- Peripheral formation of dopamine produces nausea and vomiting due to stimulation of the chemoreceptor trigger zone (CTZ) of the medullary vomiting centre which lies outside the blood–brain barrier. Nausea and vomiting are rarely dose-limiting but can be reduced by domperidone, a peripheral dopamine antagonist (Ch. 32). Peripheral dopamine may also cause arrhythmias, and vasodilation may cause postural hypotension and flushing.
- Excessive dopamine generation within the CNS can produce dyskinetic involuntary movements, especially of the face and neck, or akathisia (restlessness). Psychological disturbance can also occur, including hallucinations, anxiety, confusion, pathological gambling, increased libido and psychosis.
- Sedation, sudden onset of sleep.

Dopamine receptor agonists

Examples

apomorphine, pramipexole, ropinirole, rotigotine

Mechanism of action

In contrast to levodopa, these drugs are direct agonists at central dopaminergic receptors (Ch. 4). They have a longer duration of action than levodopa. The orally active drugs act with varying patterns of selectivity on dopamine receptors of the D_1-like family (D_1, D_5) and the D_2-like family (D_2, D_3, D_4); activity at receptors of the D_2-like family is thought to underlie their therapeutic effect in Parkinson's disease (Fig. 24.2). Dopamine agonists that are structurally related to ergot alkaloids (Ch. 26), such as bromocriptine and pergolide, have been associated with fibrotic reactions (see below) and these drugs are now rarely used. The non-ergot drugs ropinirole, pramipexole and rotigotine are also used to treat restless legs syndrome.

Pharmacokinetics

Pramipexole is well absorbed from the gut and is eliminated by hepatic metabolism. It has a half-life of 8–12 h. Ropinirole has a lower bioavailability and is eliminated by the kidneys, with a half-life of 6 h. Rotigotine is only formulated for delivery via a transdermal delivery patch to provide a more continuous supply of the drug.

Apomorphine is given parenterally by subcutaneous injection or continuous infusion, giving a very rapid onset of action. It has a short duration of action because of rapid hepatic metabolism.

Unwanted effects

Gradual dosage titration over several months may limit unwanted effects, which may include:

- nausea, vomiting, dyspepsia, abdominal pain,
- dyskinesias,
- dizziness, nervousness, fatigue,
- neuropsychiatric effects with hallucinations and confusion which are more frequent than with levodopa,
- sedation, sudden onset of sleep,
- skin reactions (with transdermal patches),
- postural hypotension, peripheral oedema,
- ergot-derived drugs such as bromocriptine and pergolide (now rarely used) may cause peripheral vasospasm, especially in people with Raynaud's phenomenon,
- ergot-derived drugs may also cause pulmonary, pericardial and retroperitoneal fibrosis, and cardiac valve lesions,
- respiratory depression with high dosages of apomorphine (an opioid derivative), which is antagonised by naloxone (Ch. 19).

Amantadine

Mechanism of action and uses

Amantadine is believed to act in Parkinson's disease by stimulating release of dopamine stored in nerve terminals and by reducing reuptake of released dopamine by the presynaptic neuron (Fig. 24.2). It is also a weak glutamate *N*-methyl-D-aspartate (NMDA) receptor antagonist. Its effectiveness tends to be short-lived because of the development of tolerance, but it can be beneficial for treatment of levodopa-induced dyskinesias. Amantidine is also used as an antiviral drug (Ch. 51).

Pharmacokinetics

Amantadine is well absorbed from the gut and is excreted unchanged by the kidneys. It has a long half-life (10–15 h).

Unwanted effects

Most are mild and dose-related. They include:

- anorexia, nausea,
- peripheral oedema,
- nervousness, insomnia, hallucinations, seizures with high doses,
- livedo reticularis (skin vasoconstriction caused by local catecholamine release).

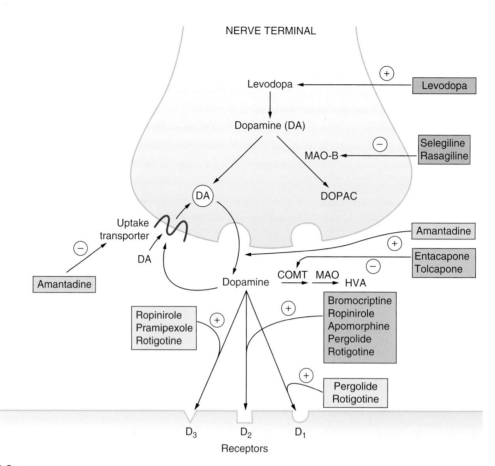

Fig. 24.2 **The major effects of drugs on the dopaminergic nerve terminal in the CNS.** Drugs act at a number of different sites to amplify dopaminergic signalling. COMT, catechol-O-methyltransferase; DA, dopamine; DOPAC, 3,4-dihydroxyphenylacetic acid; HVA, homovanillic acid; MAO-B, monoamine oxidase B; +, stimulation; −, inhibition.

Selective monoamine oxidase type B inhibitors

rasagiline, selegiline

Mechanism of action and effects

These drugs are irreversible inhibitors of the enzyme monoamine oxidase (MAO), which is responsible for the intraneuronal degradation of monoamine neurotransmitters (Ch. 4 and Fig. 22.3). They are relatively selective at low doses for the isoenzyme (MAO-B) found in the striatum. This isoenzyme is distinct from MAO-A, which is also present in the gut wall and other peripheral tissues. Interactions with drugs and foods containing tyramine, which is a problem with conventional non-selective MAO inhibitor (MAOI) antidepressants (Ch. 22), do not occur with these MAO-B-selective drugs. Selective MAO-B inhibitors prolong the duration of action of dopamine and reduce the levodopa dosage requirement by about one-third, but only produce modest clinical benefit when used alone.

Pharmacokinetics

Selegiline and rasagiline have relatively low oral bioavailability (20–40%) and both drugs have short half-lives (1–3 h) due to rapid hepatic metabolism, but their duration of action is longer due to irreversible inhibition of their enzyme target. Selegiline undergoes metabolism in part to the L-isomers of amfetamine and metamfetamine, which have long half-lives and may contribute to unwanted neuropsychiatric effects.

Unwanted effects

- Nausea, dry mouth, dyspepsia, constipation, diarrhoea.
- Transient dizziness or lightheadedness is common; vertigo.
- Insomnia, agitation, confusion, hallucinations.
- Arthralgia, myalgia.

Catechol-O-methyltransferase inhibitors

Examples

Entacapone, tolcapone

Mechanism of action and effects

Catechol-O-methyltransferase (COMT) is responsible for breakdown of between 10 and 30% of levodopa, both peripherally and in the CNS (Ch. 4), but, in the presence of a peripheral dopa decarboxylase inhibitor, COMT is responsible for most of the peripheral metabolism of levodopa. Inhibition of COMT doubles the half-life of levodopa (when it is used with a dopa decarboxylase inhibitor) and produces a 50% increase in the motor response to any given dose, and reduces end-of-dose deterioration. The dose of levodopa may therefore need to be reduced when a COMT inhibitor is started.

Pharmacokinetics

Entacapone and tolcapone are rapidly but variably absorbed from the gut. They are metabolised in the liver and have short half-lives of 2–3 h. Entacapone does not cross the blood–brain barrier, and therefore only inhibits peripheral COMT. Tolcapone crosses the blood–brain barrier and has greater efficacy but causes more unwanted effects.

Unwanted effects

- Dry mouth, nausea, vomiting, anorexia, abdominal pain, diarrhoea, constipation.
- Dyskinesias, hallucinations, confusion, insomnia.
- Reddish discoloration of urine.
- Risk of hepatotoxicity limits tolcapone to specialist use.

ANTIMUSCARINIC DRUGS

Examples

orphenadrine, procyclidine, trihexyphenidyl hydrochloride

Mechanism of action and effects

Drugs that block central muscarinic receptors (Ch. 4) help to restore the balance between CNS cholinergic and dopaminergic activity. They have little effect on bradykinesia, and are less effective than levodopa for treating tremor and rigidity.

Pharmacokinetics

Antimuscarinic drugs used for parkinsonian symptoms are well absorbed from the gut and undergo hepatic metabolism. They have half-lives in the range of 3–16 h.

Unwanted effects

These result from blockade of peripheral muscarinic receptors (Ch. 4) causing constipation, dry mouth, urinary retention and blurred vision. Reduced saliva production can be helpful in some people with Parkinson's disease, in whom sialorrhoea is a problem. Blockade of CNS muscarinic receptors can produce confusion, memory impairment and restlesness in the elderly. Tolerability of the antimuscarinic drugs varies, and changing to an alternative may be helpful if there are unwanted effects.

MANAGEMENT OF PARKINSON'S DISEASE AND PARKINSONIAN SYNDROMES

Treatment is usually delayed in Parkinson's disease until symptoms affect quality of life. Levodopa (with a peripheral decarboxylase inhibitor) is still widely used for the initial treatment of Parkinson's disease, and a useful clinical response is achieved in about 70% of those treated. Levodopa is particularly useful for reducing bradykinesia. Poor responses to individual doses of levodopa may be due to interference with its absorption by a high-protein meal or by delayed gastric emptying, and the response may be improved by taking the drug before meals. There is increasing reluctance to use levodopa in the early stages of Parkinson's disease, since it is possible that pulsatile dopaminergic stimulation produced by oral doses of levodopa, with its short half-life, may increase the risk of dyskinesias and response fluctuations developing later in treatment. Various strategies to reduce this problem are under investigation.

If a dopamine receptor agonist, such as pramipexole, is used as initial treatment of Parkinson's disease there is significantly less risk of response fluctuation or dyskinesias with levodopa in advanced disease. Therefore a dopamine receptor agonist is often preferred for treatment of younger people. Levodopa is still preferred to a dopamine receptor agonist for older people (over 65 years) or those with cognitive impairment, because of its lower propensity to cause confusion.

Levodopa can produce disabling motor complications immediately on starting treatment, but they become progressively more likely with prolonged use. These complications are due to a change from a long-duration response to levodopa to a short-duration response as the population of dopaminergic neurons reduces and their dopamine storage capacity is limited. The duration of symptomatic benefit after each dose may be reduced ('wearing off'), the dose may take longer to work ('delayed on') or it may sometimes fail to produce any improvement ('no on'). The 'on–off' phenomenon with rapid swings between severe bradykinesia and toxic dyskinesias should be treated by a reduction in total levodopa dosage and by adding another drug with the aim of maintaining more stable delivery of levodopa to the neurons. Successful combinations include levodopa and a peripheral decarboxylase inhibitor with either an MAO-B inhibitor such as selegiline or a COMT inhibitor such as entacapone. Alternatively, a dopaminergic receptor agonist could be added. The rapid action of subcutaneous apomorphine can be invaluable to abort the 'off' state. Apomorphine is highly emetogenic and may need to be given with domperidone, an anti-emetic dopamine receptor blocker that does not cross the blood–brain barrier (Ch. 32). Domperidone should be taken 30 min before apomorphine, but it is often necessary to 'load' with domperidone for 24 h before starting apomorphine. Infusion of levodopa gel into the jejunum via a gastrostomy tube can improve motor function in late-stage disease. The addition of amantadine may reduce levodopa-associated dyskinesias.

High-frequency bilateral electrical stimulation of the subthalamic nuclei via implanted electrodes is used to switch off their activity. This strategy is effective for people who respond to levodopa but continue to have marked motor complications despite optimising therapy. It is used as an alternative to surgical ablation of the nuclei since it allows the clinician to vary the site and area of the stimulation with time. Depression may be a problem with this treatment. Surgical treatment is sometimes advocated in advanced Parkinson's disease. Severe tremor may respond to stereotactic thalamotomy or pallidotomy. Pallidotomy can also be helpful for severe dyskinesias.

Antimuscarinic agents are rarely used for idiopathic Parkinson's disease, but may be given for tremor that responds inadequately to levodopa. They can also be helpful in reducing excessive salivation.

Symptomatic treatment for a variety of associated symptoms may be necessary in Parkinson's disease. These include treatment of autonomic symptoms such as postural hypotension, vomiting, constipation, urinary frequency and impotence. Parkinsonian psychosis should be treated with an atypical antipsychotic drug, such as clozapine or quetiapine (Ch. 21).

Drugs improve symptoms and quality of life in idiopathic Parkinson's disease, but there is little evidence that they alter the underlying rate of neuronal degeneration. Levodopa therapy increases life expectancy, probably by reducing complications such as aspiration pneumonia. Several studies are underway to look at a potential neuroprotective effect of dopamine receptor agonists. However, neuroprotective strategies have so far proved disappointing.

Drug-induced parkinsonism (e.g. with antipsychotics; Ch. 21) responds poorly to levodopa because the causative drug occupies the D_2 receptors. Parkinsonism resulting from antipsychotic drug therapy responds best to withdrawal of the drug. If this is not possible, then an atypical antipsychotic drug should be used and an antimuscarinic drug used to treat residual symptoms.

OTHER INVOLUNTARY MOVEMENT DISORDERS (DYSKINESIAS)

Dyskinesias are abnormal involuntary movement disorders that can present in several ways.

- **Tremor** is a rhythmic sinusoidal movement caused by repetitive muscle contractions. It may be an exaggeration of the normal physiological tremor, or an abnormal movement such as is seen in Parkinson's disease.
- **Akathisia** is a compulsive need to move, often in stereotyped patterns.
- **Chorea** is irregular, unpredictable, jerky and non-stereotyped movement that involves several different parts of the body.
- **Myoclonus** is rapid shock-like movements that are often repetitive.
- **Tics** are rapid repetitive movements that can sometimes be controlled voluntarily, but with difficulty, for short periods.
- **Dystonias** are sustained spasms of muscle contraction that distort a part of the body into a dystonic posture. The dystonia is often exaggerated by voluntary movement. Examples include spasmodic torticollis (twisted neck) and oculogyric crisis.

Movement disorders have numerous causes, and can be precipitated by drug therapy. For example, a tremor can be caused by lithium, sodium valproate, tricyclic antidepressants and sympathomimetics. Antipsychotic drugs (Ch. 21) are associated with a wide variety of movement disorders, ranging from acute dystonia to akathisia, and tardive dyskinesias (involving choreodystonic movements often of the face and mouth). The dopamine receptor antagonist metoclopramide (Ch. 32) can produce acute dystonias, especially in children and young adults, and occasionally tardive dyskinesias.

Some movement disorders have a genetic origin. An example is Huntington's disease, an autosomal dominant hereditary condition, which presents in adult life with progressive impairment of motor coordination, bizarre limb movements and dementia. The pathology is a loss of GABA inhibitory neurons within the neostriatum, which connect with the substantia nigra. There is a consequent reduction of inhibitory activity on dopaminergic cells in the substantia nigra and cells in the globus pallidus. Therefore, these cells generate uncoordinated discharges that produce bursts of excess motor activity.

DRUG TREATMENT

Tetrabenazine

Mechanism of action

Tetrabenazine inhibits the vesicular monamine transporter 2 protein (VMAT2) in CNS neurons that transports newly synthesised monoamines from the cytosol into synaptic vesicles for storage and later release. The monamines, including dopamine, are instead degraded prematurely by MAO. Tetrabenazine is mainly used for Huntington's disease and related disorders.

Pharmacokinetics

Tetrabenazine has a low oral bioavailability. It is extensively metabolised by first-pass metabolism in the liver to an active derivative. The half-lives of parent drug and metabolite are 7 and 12 h, respectively.

Unwanted effects

- Gastrointestinal disturbances.
- Drowsiness.
- Postural hypotension.
- Depression.
- Dysphagia, which may be caused by extrapyramidal dysfunction.

MANAGEMENT OF DYSKINESIAS AND DYSTONIAS

Treatment options depend on the cause. Some common strategies are listed below.

- Withdrawal of a provoking drug. Symptoms may initially be exacerbated but then usually settle. Withdrawal dyskinesias usually respond to gradual drug discontinuation. Tardive dyskinesias associated with antipsychotic treatment may become worse on drug withdrawal, but then slowly improve over many months.

- Exaggerated physiological tremor (e.g. anxiety tremor or tremor of thyrotoxicosis) may respond to a non-selective β-adrenoceptor antagonist such as propranolol (Ch. 5). Benign essential tremor is an action tremor that may be suppressed by a β-adrenoceptor antagonist or by primidone (Ch. 23). Gabapentin is an alternative second-line treatment (Ch. 23).
- Tetrabenazine is sometimes effective for treatment of choreiform movements.
- Many acute dystonias will respond to an antimuscarinic drug such as trihexyphenidyl given orally, or procyclidine given by intramuscular or intravenous injection for more severe symptoms.
- Enhancing inhibitory GABA neurotransmitter activity with baclofen (see below), sodium valproate or clonazepam (Ch. 23) may help some dystonias.
- Botulinum toxin (Ch. 27), which impairs acetylcholine release from cholinergic nerve endings, can be injected into dystonic muscles to provide temporary relief by blocking transmission at the neuromuscular junction. Spread of the paralytic effect to adjacent muscles can cause problems; for example, dysphagia after injection of neck muscles for torticollis. There are two serologically distinct types of botulinum toxin used therapeutically; some people who are refractory to botulinum toxin A may respond to botulinum toxin B.

SPASTICITY

Spasticity is a state of sustained muscle tone or tension which is often associated with an increase in stretch reflexes. The increase in muscle tone can arise from continued spinal reflex activity in the absence of inhibitory input from the motor cortex, such as can result from a stroke or spinal cord injury or in multiple sclerosis. Spasticity in skeletal muscles is often associated with partial or complete loss of voluntary movement and can produce painful and deforming shortening of the muscle (contractures).

DRUGS FOR SPASTICITY

Diazepam

Diazepam (and other benzodiazepines) enhances spinal inhibitory pathways by facilitating GABA-mediated opening of Cl^- channels (Ch. 20). The main disadvantage is sedation, a result of inhibitory activity in higher centres at the doses necessary for a spasmolytic action.

Baclofen

Mechanism of action

Baclofen is an analogue of GABA that inhibits excitatory activity at mono- and polysynaptic reflexes at the spinal level. Its precise mechanism of action is uncertain. However, it binds stereoselectively to $GABA_B$ receptors, and has an agonist action which hyperpolarises neurons by increasing K^+ conductance. This inhibits reflex pathways by blocking presynaptic Ca^{2+} influx and thus reducing excitatory neurotransmitter release. Baclofen also has an analgesic effect, probably by inhibition of the release of substance P in pain pathways (Ch. 19).

Pharmacokinetics

Baclofen is absorbed rapidly from the gastrointestinal tract. It has a short half-life (3–4 h) and is eliminated largely unchanged in the urine. It can be given by intrathecal infusion using an implantable pump if severe spasticity is resistant to oral therapy.

Unwanted effects

- Sedation and drowsiness are common. Other CNS effects include lightheadedness, confusion, dizziness, ataxia, seizure, headache.
- Nausea, gastrointestinal disturbances.
- Urinary disturbances.
- Sudden withdrawal can precipitate hyperactivity, autonomic dysfunction and seizures.

Tizanidine

Mechanisms of action

Tizanidine is an α_2-adrenoceptor agonist that increases presynaptic inhibition of motor neurons in the spinal cord via descending noradrenergic pathways. Inhibition is greatest in polysynaptic rather than monosynaptic pathways. Tizanidine has only 10% of the antihypertensive activity of the α_2-adrenoceptor agonist clonidine.

Pharmacokinetics

Tizanidine is well absorbed from the gut but undergoes extensive first-pass metabolism in the liver. Its elimination half-life is 2–4 h.

Unwanted effects

These are mainly dose-related, and can be minimised by slow dose titration. They include:

- drowsiness, fatigue, dizziness,
- dry mouth, gastrointestinal disturbances,
- hypotension.

Dantrolene

Mechanism of action and uses

Dantrolene is an antagonist at the ryanodine receptor (RyR1) that inhibits the release of Ca^{2+} from the sarcoplasmic reticulum of skeletal muscles (Ch. 5) and uncouples muscle excitation from activation of the contractile apparatus.

Dantrolene is also used for the treatment of malignant hyperthermia (Ch. 17) and as an adjunctive treatment in neuroleptic malignant syndrome (Ch. 21).

Pharmacokinetics

Dantrolene is absorbed slowly from the gut and metabolised in the liver. It has a variable and unpredictable half-life (2–24 h).

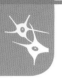

Unwanted effects

- Drowsiness, dizziness, weakness and malaise (usually transient).
- Anorexia, nausea, diarrhoea, abdominal pain.
- Headache, drowsiness, dizziness, seizures.
- Pericarditis, pleural effusion.
- Rash.
- Dose-related risk of hepatitis.

MANAGEMENT OF SPASTICITY

Mild spasticity can be useful, since the increased tone may provide support for a weak limb and should not be treated with drugs. Excessive spasticity following a stroke or in multiple sclerosis is most effectively prevented by adequate physiotherapy, and can be helped with orthoses that support the limb and correct deformities.

Drugs are most useful for deforming or painful spasticity, particularly if the person is not ambulant, since muscle hypotonia is a common problem in the drug therapy of spasticity. The primary sites of action of these agents are the spinal reflexes or the release of Ca^{2+} in the muscle fibre, rather than the neuromuscular junction. Drugs that block the neuromuscular junction (Ch. 27) are not used to treat spasticity, because their main effect would be a further loss of voluntary movement. Baclofen is usually the drug of first choice, and is most often required for spasticity associated with multiple sclerosis or spinal cord injury. Cannabis extract (Ch. 54) is used for spasticity in multiple sclerosis that does not respond to standard treatments. Intramuscular injection of botulinum toxin (see above, and Ch. 27) produces 'chemodenervation' and is used for severe focal spasticity. It produces an effect after 24–72 h, which is maximal after 2 weeks and lasts for 2–3 months. In severe spasticity that fails to respond to standard treatments, intrathecal baclofen infusion can provide relief.

SELF-ASSESSMENT

True/false questions

1. In Parkinson's disease, there is abnormally low dopaminergic activity and increased GABAergic and cholinergic activity.
2. Symptoms of Parkinson's disease become apparent when approximately 25% of dopaminergic neurons have been lost.
3. Glutamate receptor antagonists are being investigated for use in Parkinson's disease.
4. Levodopa has a half-life of 24 h.
5. Treatment with levodopa may lead to dyskinesias and on–off fluctuations.
6. In early Parkinson's disease the dopamine receptor agonist ropinirole is as effective as levodopa.
7. Antimuscarinic drugs such as trihexyphenidyl have a low incidence of unwanted effects.
8. Pramipexole is a potent agonist at dopamine D_3 receptors.

9. Some of the movement disorder in Parkinson's disease arises from abnormalities in non-dopaminergic innervated areas of the brain.
10. The chemoreceptor trigger zone (CTZ) is stimulated by peripheral dopamine generated from levodopa.
11. The monoamine oxidase inhibitor (MAOI) selegiline causes the 'cheese' reaction with ingestion of tyramine-containing foods.
12. Entacapone is a direct dopamine receptor agonist.
13. Tetrabenazine may cause depression.
14. Dantrolene is useful in spasticity as it reduces the Ca^{2+} release that contributes to contraction of skeletal muscle.
15. Baclofen enhances muscle tone.
16. Botulinum toxin has a duration of action of up to three months.

One-best-answer (OBA) questions

1. Which is the *most accurate* statement about drugs used for Parkinson's disease?
   A. Levodopa does not slow the progress of Parkinson's disease.
   B. Selegiline is a selective MAO-A inhibitor used for Parkinson's disease.
   C. More than 50% of oral levodopa enters the brain unaltered.
   D. Currently used drugs for Parkinson's disease selectively stimulate D_1-type dopamine receptors.
   E. Carbidopa is a CNS dopamine decarboxylase inhibitor.
2. Which one of the following adjunctive therapies *will not* increase dopamine levels in the brain when given together with levodopa?
   A. Entacapone
   B. Benserazide
   C. Carbidopa
   D. Procyclidine
   E. Rasagiline
3. Which one of the following unwanted effects is *least likely* to occur following levodopa administration?
   A. Nausea and vomiting
   B. Arrhythmias
   C. Orthostatic hypotension in the elderly
   D. Slowing of heart rate
   E. Dyskinesia

Case-based questions

Case 1: a 75-year-old woman had been suffering from progressive symptoms of Parkinson's disease for 5 years. From the outset she had been treated continuously with levodopa, but problems had developed in controlling the symptoms with this drug.

A. What is the cause of Parkinson's disease?
B. What symptoms is this woman likely to have?
C. Levodopa was given as co-beneldopa; what are the benefits of this formulation compared with levodopa alone?
D. What difficulties can arise in controlling symptoms with co-beneldopa in the later stages of treatment?
E. What changes in therapy could then be considered?

Case 2: a married man aged 40 years was newly diagnosed as suffering from Parkinson's disease. His symptoms were tremor, bradykinesia, hypokinesia and rigidity, which were sufficiently mild that he was still able to carry out his work and pursue his hobbies. He was a security guard and had previously fought as a relatively unsuccessful professional boxer for 10 years, before retiring from the ring at the age of 35.

A. What are the optimal treatment regimens for this man?

True/false answers

1. **True**. Loss of dopaminergic neurons creates abnormal activity within GABAergic and cholinergic pathways.
2. **False**. Symptoms usually develop when more than 50% of neurons have been lost.
3. **True**. There is over-activity of some glutamatergic neurons in parkinsonism.
4. **False**. The short half-life of levodopa (1–2 h) may contribute to end-of-dose deterioration; modified-release formulations provide a more continuous supply of the drug.
5. **True**. About 50% of people will experience these complications after 5 years treatment with levodopa.
6. **True**. In very early Parkinson's disease clinical trials up to six months' duration indicate ropinirole is as effective as levodopa.
7. **False**. Trihexyphenidyl (benzhexol) can cause minor unwanted effects but also severe confusion, particularly in the elderly.
8. **True**. Pramipexole is a potent D_3 agonist, but also a full agonist at D_2 receptors.
9. **True**. Tremor and rigidity in particular may occur because of transmitters other than dopamine.
10. **True**. The CTZ in the area postrema of the medulla is outside the blood–brain barrier and can be activated by peripheral dopamine.
11. **False**. Selegiline only inhibits MAO-B, leaving MAO-A intact to metabolise tyramine in cheese and other foods (see Ch. 22).
12. **False**. Entacapone is a peripheral inhibitor of catechol-O-methyltransferase (COMT), so it preserves levodopa for access to the brain and subsequent conversion to dopamine.
13. **True**. The risk of depression with tetrabenazene is consistent with its depletion of CNS monamines (see Ch. 22).
14. **True**. Dantrolene blocks Ca^{2+} release from sarcoplasmic reticulum so it reduces excitation/contraction coupling in skeletal muscle.
15. **False**. Baclofen improves spasticity by inhibiting excitatory synapses, probably acting at $GABA_B$ receptors.
16. **True**. Botulinum toxin is used in spasticity by intramuscular injection and inhibits local acetylcholine release for up to three months.

OBA answers

1. **Answer A** is correct.
   A. **Correct.**
   B. Incorrect. Selegiline and rasagiline are selective inhibitors for MAO-B, not MAO-A.
   C. Incorrect. Only 1–2% of an oral dose of levodopa enters the brain in the absence of a peripheral decarboxylase inhibitor.
   D. Incorrect. Drugs for Parkinson's disease are thought to act mainly by agonism of the D_2-like receptor family (D_2, D_3, D_4).
   E. Incorrect. Carbidopa is a peripheral dopa decarboxylase inhibitor; it does not cross the blood–brain barrier.
2. **Answer D** is correct.
   A. Entacapone inhibits peripheral catechol-O-methyltransferase (COMT), increasing the amount of levodopa crossing into the brain and its subsequent conversion to dopamine.
   B. Benserazide is a peripheral decarboxylase inhibitor that increases the amount of levodopa crossing into the brain and its subsequent conversion to dopamine.
   C. Carbidopa is a peripheral decarboxylase inhibitor that increases the amount of levodopa crossing into the brain and its subsequent conversion to dopamine.
   D. Procyclidine is a muscarinic receptor antagonist and will not affect dopamine levels.
   E. Rasagiline is an irreversible selective MAO-B inhibitor that will reduce the breakdown of dopamine within the brain.
3. **Answer D** is correct.
   A. Dopamine is a neurotransmitter in the chemoreceptor trigger zone and stimulates nausea and vomiting.
   B. Dopamine can stimulate β-adrenoceptors in the heart, increasing the likelihood of arrhythmias.
   C. Orthostatic hypotension is common, particularly in the elderly.
   D. Dopamine may increase myocardial contractility, but without affecting the heart rate.
   E. Excessive CNS dopamine concentrations are associated with involuntary movements.

Case-based answers

Case 1

A. Parkinson's disease results from degeneration of more than 50% of dopaminergic neurons in the substantia nigra. The cause of this degeneration is unknown but hypotheses include the actions of reactive oxygen species, neurotoxins, immune disturbances and specific gene mutations. The consequent neurochemical disturbances include over-activity of cholinergic, GABAergic and glutamatergic pathways. Current therapies aim to supplement dopaminergic activity or decrease cholinergic activity.

B. People with Parkinson's disease have akinesia, rigidity and tremor, possibly from inhibition of the motor cortical system, whereas the descending inhibition of the brainstem locomotor areas may contribute to abnormalities of gait and posture.

C. Levodopa is the immediate precursor of dopamine and is transported into the CNS by the large neutral amino acid transporter and converted into dopamine, while dopamine itself cannot cross the blood–brain barrier.

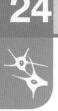

Levodopa causes nausea and vomiting because it is also metabolised to dopamine in the periphery, which activates the chemoreceptor trigger zone (CTZ). Co-beneldopa is a combination of levodopa with benserazide, a peripheral decarboxylase inhibitor, which prevents the breakdown of levodopa to dopamine in the periphery. The peripheral dopamine receptor antagonist domperidone can also be used to protect against nausea and vomiting.

D. Levodopa remains the most effective treatment for Parkinson's disease but there considerable debate about when to start levodopa therapy. There is no convincing evidence that levodopa accelerates neurodegeneration, and survival is reduced if treatment is delayed until greater disability is present. In time, and despite long-term treatment with levodopa, there is an increasing incidence of dyskinesias and on–off fluctuations of effect, although most people continue to derive benefit throughout the duration of their illness. At the end of five years of treatment approximately 50% of those treated will be experiencing reduced effectiveness with levodopa. These motor fluctuations can be a result of unpredictable pharmacokinetic changes, such as unpredictable absorption across the blood–brain barrier or delayed gastric emptying, or because further loss of dopaminergic neurons during disease progression further reduces neuronal storage capacity for dopamine.

E. Resolving these problems is highly individual, but dyskinesia and on–off effects may be helped by dosage adjustment (up or down), by shortening the dose interval or by using modified-release formulations. An antimuscarinic drug can be given with levodopa and may be useful in the treatment of tremor, but could cause confusion and hallucinations, particularly in this elderly person. Other drugs which inhibit dopamine metabolism can also be introduced. The selective MAO-B inhibitors selegiline or rasagiline are far more effective as adjuncts to levodopa than as monotherapy. The COMT inhibitor entacapone reduces the peripheral breakdown of levodopa and dopamine and prolongs the benefits of levodopa therapy. A direct dopamine receptor agonist could also be added to levodopa treatment for this woman; non-ergot derivatives including ropinirole, rotigotine (as a transdermal patch) or pramipexole are preferred. Apomorphine, a D_2 receptor agonist, given subcutaneously can also be used to counteract the off periods in advanced disease, with domperidone given to reduce its emetic effects.

Case 2

A. There is considerable debate about when to commence levodopa therapy in early-onset Parkinson's disease. The goal should be to improve quality of life and limit long-term unwanted effects. If the degree of disability is not severe there may be no immediate need for therapy, but this is controversial as survival is reduced if treatment with levodopa is delayed until disability develops. If treatment is required in this man, dopamine receptor agonists could be started. These are less likely to produce dyskinesias and could delay the need for levodopa until progressive disabilities start to occur. The possibility of brain damage caused by boxing injury should also be considered; this responds poorly to standard treatments for Parkinson's disease.

FURTHER READING

Parkinson's disease

Bhidayasiri R, Truong DD (2008) Motor complications in Parkinson's disease: clinical manifestations and management. *J Neurol Sci* 266, 204–215

Biglan KM, Ravina B (2007) Neuroprotection in Parkinson's disease: an elusive goal. *Semin Neurol* 27, 106–112

Blanchet PJ (2003) Antipsychotic drug-induced movement disorders. *Can J Neurol Sci* 30 (suppl 1), S101–S107

Clarke CE (2007) Parkinson's disease. *BMJ* 335, 441–445

Gerfen CR (2000) Molecular effects of dopamine on striatal-projection pathways. *Trends Neurosci* 23 (suppl), S64–S70

Hauser RA, Zesiewicz TA (2007) Advances in the pharmacological management of early Parkinson disease. *Neurologist* 13, 126–132

Hermanowicz N (2007) Drug therapy for Parkinson's disease. *Semin Neurol* 27, 97–105

Hirose G (2006) Drug induced parkinsonism: a review. *J Neurol* 253 (suppl 3), iii22–iii24

Lewitt PA (2008) Levodopa for the treatment of Parkinson's disease. *N Engl J Med* 359, 2468–2476

Obeso JA, Rodriguez-Oroz MC, Rodriguez M et al. (2002) The basal ganglia and disorders of movement: pathophysiological mechanisms. *News Physiol Sci* 17, 51–55

Schapira AH (2007) Treatment options in the modern management of Parkinson's disease. *Arch Neurol* 64, 1083–1088

Dyskinesias, dystonias and spasticity

Jancovic J (2006) Treatment of dystonia. *Lancet Neurol* 5, 864–872

Louis ED (2001) Essential tremor. *N Engl J Med* 345, 887–891

Meleger AL (2006) Muscle relaxants and antispasticity agents. *Phys Med Rehab Clin North Am* 17, 401–413

Papapetropoulos S, Singer C (2007) Botulinum toxin in movement disorders. *Semin Neurol* 27, 183–194

Rekand T (2010) Clinical assessment and management of spasticity: a review. *Acta Neurol Scand Suppl* 190, 62–66

Tarsey D, Simon DK (2006) Dystonia. *N Engl J Med* 355, 818–829

Compendium: drugs used to treat extrapyramidal movement disorders

Drug	Kinetics (half-life)	Comments
Drugs used for Parkinson's disease		
Given orally unless otherwise stated.		
Dopamine receptor agonists		
Apomorphine	Hepatic metabolism (0.5–1 h)	D_2 receptor agonist; opioid derivative given by subcutaneous injection; not effective orally, probably as a result of first-pass metabolism
Bromocriptine	Low oral bioavailability (about 10%) due to poor absorption and first-pass metabolism; hepatic metabolism (3 h)	D_2 receptor agonist; ergot derivative, risk of fibrotic reactions
Cabergoline	Hepatic metabolism (60–90 h)	D_2 receptor agonist; used as an adjunct to levodopa; ergot derivative, risk of fibrotic reactions
Levodopa (L-DOPA)	Complete absorption; metabolised by DOPA decarboxylase to dopamine and by methylation (1.3 h)	Precursor of dopamine; normally given with carbidopa or benserazide (see peripheral decarboxylase inhibitors below) to reduce first-pass metabolism and increase duration of action
Pergolide	Rapid absorption but high first-pass metabolism; hepatic metabolism (27 h)	Agonist at D_2 and D_1 receptors; ergot derivative, risk of fibrotic reactions
Pramipexole	High oral bioavailability; eliminated by renal tubular secretion and filtration (8–12 h)	Selective agonist at D_3 receptors, some activity at D_2 receptors
Ropinirole	Bioavailability about 50%; hepatic metabolism (6 h)	Agonist at D_3 and D_2 receptors
Rotigotine	Steady-state plasma levels achieved after 2–3 days; hepatic metabolism (5–7 h)	Agonist at D_3, D_2 and D_1 receptors; administered via a transdermal patch
Peripheral decarboxylase inhibitors used in combination with oral levodopa therapy		
Benserazide	Incomplete absorption; metabolised by hydrolysis	Combination of benserazide with levodopa (in ratio 1:4) is co-beneldopa
Carbidopa	Variable bioavailability (40–90%); limited metabolism (1–3 h)	Combination of carbidopa with levodopa (in ratio of 1:4 or 1:10) is co-careldopa
Monoamine oxidase (MAO) type B inhibitors		
Rasagiline	Bioavailability about 40%; hepatic metabolism; no correlation between half-life (3 h) and duration of action	Irreversible inhibitor; used alone or in combination with levodopa
Selegiline	Bioavailability variable ($\approx$20%), improved with food; hepatic metabolism to active metabolite and amfetamine analogues; no correlation between half-life (1–2 h) and duration of action	Irreversible inhibitor; used alone or in combination with levodopa; amfetamine metabolites may contribute to unwanted neuropsychiatric effects; oral and buccal formulations
Catechol-O-methyltransferase (COMT) inhibitors		
Entacapone	Oral bioavailability 30–50%; does not cross blood–brain barrier; hepatic conjugation (2–3 h)	Used as adjunct to levodopa for end-of-dose deterioration
Tolcapone	Rapidly absorbed with bioavailability 65%; crosses blood–brain barrier; hepatic metabolism (2–3 h)	Specialist use as adjunct to levodopa for end-of-dose deterioration; risk of hepatotoxicity
Other dopaminergic drugs		
Amantadine	Complete oral bioavailability; renal elimination; half-life (10–15 h) increases in elderly, related to renal function	Enhances dopamine release and blocks dopamine reuptake; also used as antiviral agent
Antimuscarinic drugs		
Orphenadrine	Bioavailability about 70%; hepatic metabolism (14–16 h)	Efficacy of the antimuscarinic drugs used in Parkinson's disease is similar
Procyclidine	Bioavailability about 75%; hepatic metabolism (13 h)	Given orally or by intramuscular or intravenous injection

Compendium: drugs used to treat extrapyramidal movement disorders—cont'd

Drug	Kinetics (half-life)	Comments
Trihexyphenidyl hydrochloride	High bioavailability; hepatic metabolism and renal excretion (3–7 h)	Also known as benzhexol

Drugs used for essential tremor, chorea, tics and related disorders

Given orally.

Drug	Kinetics (half-life)	Comments
Chlorpromazine	—	Antipsychotic; see Ch. 21
Clonidine	—	α_2-Adrenoceptor agonist; see Ch. 6
Haloperidol	—	Antipsychotic; see Ch. 21
Pimozide	—	Antipsychotic; see Ch. 21
Piracetam	Mostly eliminated by glomerular filtration (4 h)	Mechanism uncertain; used as adjunctive treatment for cortical myoclonus
Primidone	—	Barbiturate; see Ch. 23
Propranolol	—	β-Adrenoceptor antagonist; see Ch. 8
Sulpiride	—	Antipsychotic; see Ch. 21
Tetrabenazine	Oral bioavailability 5%; hepatic metabolism; active dihydro metabolite has longer half-life (12 h) than parent drug (7 h)	Vesicular monamine transporter (VMAT2) inhibitor; depletes monoamines from CNS neurons
Trihexyphenidyl	—	Antimuscarinic; see above

Drugs used to treat spasticity

Given orally.

Drug	Kinetics (half-life)	Comments
Baclofen	Good oral bioavailability (95%); mainly renal excretion (3–4 h)	GABA$_B$ receptor agonist, suppresses spinal reflexes; given orally or by intrathecal injection
Dantrolene	Oral bioavailability 40–80%; hepatic metabolism (4–24 h)	Ryanodine receptor antagonist, blocks excitation/contraction coupling in skeletal muscle; also used for malignant hyperthermia and neuroleptic malignant syndrome
Diazepam	—	Benzodiazepine; see Ch. 20
Tizanidine	Oral bioavailability about 20–40% because of first-pass metabolism; hepatic metabolism (2–4 h)	α_2-Adrenoceptor agonist; inhibits polysynaptic motor neuron transmission

Other drugs affecting movement

Drug	Kinetics (half-life)	Comments
Botulinum toxins A and B	Probably proteolysed locally	Block acetylcholine release; used for torsional dystonias and other involuntary movements; specialist use; given by local intramuscular injection; onset and duration of action depend on the clinical use of the drug
Methocarbamol	Complete absorption; hepatic metabolism (1 h)	Carbamate; centrally acting muscle relaxant; used for short-term symptomatic relief of muscle spasm; given orally; efficacy uncertain
Quinine	Almost complete absorption; hepatic metabolism (8–21 h)	Used for nocturnal leg cramps; given orally

Other neurological disorders: multiple sclerosis, motor neuron disease and Guillain–Barré syndrome

MULTIPLE SCLEROSIS

Multiple sclerosis is characterised by an immunologically mediated inflammatory demyelination of the central nervous system (CNS). The cause is unknown, but it may be initiated by exposure of genetically susceptible individuals to an infective agent with an antigenic structure similar to myelin basic protein (molecular mimicry). This trigger initiates a peripheral immune response and the blood–brain barrier is then breached by primed T- and B-lymphocytes and macrophages. The initiating agent may also upregulate adhesion molecules (integrins) on T-lymphocytes, promoting their adhesion to cerebrovascular endothelium and transport across the blood–brain barrier. The inflammation in the brain has the characteristics of a Th1-lymphocyte autoimmune response (Ch. 38), with the T-cells secreting inflammatory cytokines such as interferon-γ, interleukin (IL)-17 and lymphotoxin (or tumour necrosis factor β, TNFβ). The destruction of myelin is probably initiated by B-cell-derived autoantibodies. Deficient numbers of regulatory T-cells may also contribute to the lack of tolerance to self-antigens.

The T-cell cytokines activate macrophages that phagocytose myelin coated with antimyelin antibody, and destroy the myelin sheath around nerves, particularly in white matter. The immunological damage also affects oligodendrocytes, the cells that produce the myelin. The result of these processes is the generation of demyelinated plaques that disturb normal conduction of electrical impulses in the CNS. However, the long-term disability in multiple sclerosis is mainly due to axonal damage, which occurs most extensively in the acute stages of the disease. Demyelination may predispose axons to damage from upregulation of Na^+ channels, with subsequent reversal of the Na^+–Ca^{2+} exchanger and Ca^{2+}-induced cytotoxicity. Axon degeneration may also be enhanced by oligodendrocyte dysfunction and failure to remyelinate the nerves.

Multiple sclerosis usually begins in the second or third decades of life and in 85% of cases presents with relapsing and remitting symptoms and signs of multifocal CNS dysfunction. The usual clinical course is initially one of stepwise deterioration, but eventually there is progressive deterioration (secondary progressive multiple sclerosis). In the other 15%, the course is slowly progressive from the outset (primary progressive multiple sclerosis). To secure the diagnosis, episodes of neurological dysfunction must be separated in both time and place (more than one episode in more than one area of the brain). A single clinical episode of demyelination with several areas of demyelination on magnetic resonance scanning of the brain that have not caused symptoms is known as clinically isolated syndrome. The areas of the CNS most often involved in multiple sclerosis are the optic nerves, spinal cord, brainstem and cerebellum. Common clinical presentations are optic neuritis, weakness with spasticity, ataxia, and bladder and bowel dysfunction.

DRUG TREATMENT

There is no cure for multiple sclerosis, but drugs can be used to reduce the symptoms. In relapsing–remitting disease there is increasing evidence that modulating the immune response as early as possible in the disease process may reduce disability. By contrast, most treatments are ineffective in primary or secondary progressive multiple sclerosis.

- **Corticosteroids** (Ch. 44) are often used to treat an acute relapse (e.g. intravenous methylprednisolone for 3 days or oral prednisolone for 3 weeks). They probably shorten the duration of an attack but have no effect on long-term outcome.
- **Interferon beta-1a or -1b** reduces the inflammatory response in an acute attack and can reduce the frequency of relapses. Interferons are translocated to cell nuclei and act as transcription factors by binding to enhancer elements, where they stimulate gene expression. Proposed mechanisms for the clinical effect include decreased expression of major histocompatibility complex molecules on antigen-presenting cells (Ch. 38), inhibition of T-cell activation, decreased release of inflammatory cytokines and enhanced activity of suppressor T-cells. After a single episode of demyelination about 50% of people will subsequently develop the clinical syndrome of multiple sclerosis. The use of interferon beta at the time of this clinically isolated syndrome significantly reduces the risk of developing multiple sclerosis two years after treatment. Otherwise, the use of interferon beta is reserved for ambulant individuals who have had at least two attacks of relapsing and remitting disease over the previous 2 or 3 years. However, although the drug may reduce relapses by about one-third, it does not prevent ultimate disability.

Interferon beta is given by intramuscular or subcutaneous injection. The most frequent unwanted effects are influenza-like symptoms, which occur commonly and may persist for several months, and pain or ulceration at the injection site. Neutralising antibodies are produced during repeated administration in 5% of people, which leads to treatment failure within two years of starting treatment.

- **Glatiramer acetate** is a synthetic tetrapeptide immunomodulator that has some structural similarities to myelin basic protein. It may produce immunological tolerance by increasing the number of regulatory T-cells. Its use may reduce the frequency of relapses but, like interferon beta, it does not influence long-term disability. Glatiramer acetate is mainly used when antibodies reduce the effectiveness of interferon beta. It is given by subcutaneous injection. Unwanted effects include flushing, chest pain, palpitation and dyspnoea immediately after injection, and reactions at the injection site.
- **Mitoxantrone**, a cytotoxic antibiotic (Ch. 52), has shown encouraging results in reducing disability when given at 1–3-monthly intervals. It is not licensed for this use in the UK, but is an option when people do not respond to interferon beta or glatiramer acetate.
- **Natalizumab** is a monoclonal antibody that selectively inhibits the α_4-integrin adhesion molecule on the surface of T-lymphocytes. This prevents T-cells from interacting with receptors on the vascular endothelium and crossing the blood–brain barrier. Natalizumab reduces relapse rate in relapsing–remitting multiple sclerosis. It increases the risk of infection, and there is a small risk of developing the brain disease *progressive multifocal leucoencephalopathy* when it is used in combination with interferon beta. Natalizumab is currently used when interferon beta or glatiramer acetate have failed.
- **Fingolimod** is an oral prodrug that undergoes reversible phosphorylation to an agonist of sphingosine 1-phosphate receptors on lymphocytes, causing their internalisation. This inhibits lymphocyte egress from lymph nodes and therefore reduces their migration into demyelinating lesions in the CNS. It is used for relapsing–remitting disease that remains active despite use of interferon beta.
- Other agents that modify the behaviour of lymphocytes have shown promising results in the treatment of relapsing–remitting disease. These include the cancer chemotherapeutic drugs cladribine and alemtuzumab (Ch.52), as well as several newer drugs currently under investigation.
- A new voltage-gated potassium channel blocker, fampridine, blocks exposed K^+ channels in demyelinated axons and inhibits repolarisation. This prolongs the nerve action potential and improves walking time. However, fewer than 50% of people with multiple sclerosis will respond. The main unwanted effects are gastrointestinal disturbances, urinary tract infection, insomnia, ataxia, dizziness, paraesthesia, tremor, headache and seizures. Symptomatic treatment of spasticity may be necessary, for example with baclofen (Ch. 24). A multidisciplinary team approach is essential for the management of the numerous disabling symptoms that may occur in multiple sclerosis.

MOTOR NEURON DISEASE

Motor neuron disease is an uncommon, rapidly progressive disorder of motor neurons that occurs most often in middle-aged males. The most common form, amyotrophic lateral sclerosis, leads to both upper motor neuron signs and symptoms (hypertonia, impaired fine movement and hyperreflexia) and lower motor neuron signs and symptoms (fasciculations, muscle cramps, weakness and muscle atrophy). Other forms affect either upper or lower motor neurons. Up to half of affected people develop cognitive impairment. Death from respiratory failure usually occurs 2–5 years from the onset of symptoms. The pathophysiology involves neuronal loss among the anterior horn cells of the spinal cord, motor cortex and hypoglossal nucleus in the lower medulla. The cause is unknown, but recent evidence suggests that there is dysfunction in a nuclear RNA splicing factor known as TDP-43, leading to aberrant mRNA splicing. There is evidence of excessive activation of excitatory glutamate receptors in the CNS which may lead to prolonged depolarisation of motor neurons, intracellular Ca^{2+} overload, mitochondrial damage and cell death (excitotoxicity). Oxidative stress from excessive free radical generation may be important, and familial forms of the disease are associated with mutations of genes coding for the free radical-scavenging enzyme, superoxide dismutase.

DRUG TREATMENT

Riluzole is the only available agent that alters the course of motor neuron disease. It crosses the blood–brain barrier and inhibits the release of glutamate, as well as acting as an indirect antagonist at glutamate *N*-methyl-D-aspartate (NMDA) receptors on damaged neurons. These actions may inhibit glutamate-induced excitotoxicity. Treatment with riluzole does not arrest the disease but may slow its progression to a modest extent, improving survival by an average of three months after 18 months of treatment. Unwanted effects of riluzole include nausea, vomiting, diarrhoea, lethargy and dizziness.

Physiotherapists can help with advice on posture and exercise early in the disease, and later with passive movement to reduce musculoskeletal pain. Symptomatic treatment is often necessary for complications such as pain, breathlessness or dysphagia.

GUILLAIN–BARRÉ SYNDROME

Guillain–Barré syndrome is an autoimmune acute inflammatory demyelinating polyradiculopathy, triggered in about three-quarters of cases by infection, of which *Campylobacter jejuni* infection is the most frequent. It only affects the peripheral nervous system and it produces rapid onset of limb weakness with loss of tendon reflexes and autonomic dysfunction, with variable sensory signs. In about 5% of cases the problem arises from acute axonal neuropathy. About 10% of affected people die in the acute illness phase and a further 10% have incomplete recovery and are left with severe long-term disability.

The immunological response is probably due to shared antigens on the infecting organism and the peripheral nerve tissue. In many cases, antiganglioside antibodies are present. The autoantibodies fix complement, and attract lymphocytes and then macrophages, which invade the myelin sheaths. Axonal degeneration may result from matrix metalloproteinases and toxic nitric oxide radicals released from the macrophages, and frequently results in long-term disability.

MANAGEMENT

There are several aspects to the management of Guillain–Barré syndrome.

- Supportive treatment may be life-saving and is the cornerstone of management. For example, ventilatory support is necessary for respiratory muscle weakness or paralysis. Haemodynamic disturbance, including significant bradycardia and asystole, can result from autonomic involvement and may require cardiovascular support. Prophylaxis for deep venous thrombosis with subcutaneous heparin (Ch. 11) should be given. Pain may require analgesia, or the use of gabapentin or carbamazepine (Ch.23), and can be reduced by passive limb movement.
- High-dose intravenous immunoglobulin (IgG) given within the first 2 weeks is equally effective as plasma exchange, and is now the preferred treatment. It may work by blocking macrophage receptors, inhibiting antibody production and complement binding and neutralising the pathological antibodies. Unwanted effects include malaise, chills and fever. IgG reduces the need for supported ventilation, and the time taken to recover walking.
- Plasma exchange, when used within 4 weeks of the onset of symptoms, improves the long-term outcome. The benefit is probably due to removal of autoantibodies.
- Corticosteroids are of no benefit, either alone or in combination with immunoglobulin.

SELF-ASSESSMENT

True/false questions

1. Treatment with interferon beta is of benefit in reducing relapses in multiple sclerosis.
2. Multiple sclerosis is characterised in the early years by a steady progressive worsening of symptoms in the majority of people.
3. Glutamate can cause neuronal damage.
4. Riluzole is of benefit in motor neuron disease by blocking the release of γ-aminobutyric acid (GABA).
5. Natalizumab is used in multiple sclerosis as it enhances the action of adhesion molecules, increasing the passage of lymphocytes into the CNS.
6. Fingolimod is a produg activated by phosphorylation.

One-best-answer (OBA) question

Which of the following is the *most accurate* statement about the treatment of multiple sclerosis?

A. Interferon beta causes influenza-like symptoms in 1% of those who receive it.
B. Expert opinion does not recommend glatiramer acetate as a first-line drug for use in multiple sclerosis.
C. Glatiramer acetate causes few unwanted effects following injection.
D. Corticosteroid treatment is of benefit in reducing the progression of multiple sclerosis.
E. Neuronal conduction is unimpaired in multiple sclerosis.

True/false answers

1. **False.** Interferon beta is used in multiple sclerosis and may diminish the production of inflammatory interferon-γ.
2. **False.** Multiple sclerosis is usually characterised by relapses and remissions over a number of years, although after about 10 years a steady decline sets in.
3. **True.** Glutamate is an excitatory amino acid neurotransmitter but can cause cell damage and death (excitotoxicity) by a number of mechanisms, including an uncontrolled increase in intracellular Ca^{2+}.
4. **False.** Riluzole is the only drug that will alter the course of motor neuron disease; it inhibits glutamate release and action, thereby reducing its toxicity.
5. **False.** Natalizumab is an inhibitor of the α_4-integrin adhesion molecule and reduces the migration of lymphocytes into the CNS.
6. **True.** Fingolimod is rapidly phosphorylated by sphingosine kinases.

OBA answer

Answer B is correct.

A. Incorrect. Influenza-like symptoms can occur in about 50% of people.
B. **Correct**. The use of glatiramer acetate is usually restricted to people who cannot tolerate interferon beta, or who have developed antibodies to interferon beta.
C. Incorrect. Glatiramer acetate can cause flushing, chest tightness, palpitations, anxiety and breathlessness.
D. Incorrect. Corticosteroids may shorten the duration of acute attacks but have no effect on progression of multiple sclerosis.
E. Incorrect. Long-term disability is due to demyelination of nerves and consequent further axonal damage. Demyelination of nerves results in disordered neuronal conduction.

FURTHER READING

Compston A, Coles A (2008) Multiple sclerosis. *Lancet* 372, 1502–1517

Howard RS, Orrell RW (2002) Management of motor neurone disease. *Postgrad Med J* 78, 736–741

Javed A, Reder AT (2006) Therapeutic role of beta-interferons in multiple sclerosis. *Pharmacol Ther* 110, 35–56

Kiernan MC, Vucic S, Cheah B et al. (2011) Amyotrophic lateral sclerosis. *Lancet* 377, 942–955

Kieseier BC, Wiendl H, Hemmer B, Hartung H-P (2007) Treatment and treatment trials in multiple sclerosis. *Curr Opin Neurol* 20, 286–293

Killestein J, Rudick RA, Polman CH (2011) Oral treatment for multiple sclerosis. *Lancet Neurol* 10, 1026–1034

Murray TJ (2006) Diagnosis and treatment of multiple sclerosis. *BMJ* 332, 525–527

Ransohoff RM (2007) Natalizumab for multiple sclerosis. *N Engl J Med* 356, 2622–2629

Winer JB (2008) Guillain-Barré syndrome. *BMJ* 337, 227–231

Compendium: drugs used to treat multiple sclerosis, motor neuron disease and Guillain–Barré syndrome

Drug	Kinetics (half-life)	Comments
Corticosteroids	See Ch. 44	Corticosteroids such as methylprednisolone or prednisolone may be of benefit for acute relapse in people with multiple sclerosis (see Ch. 44)
Glatiramer acetate	Hydrolysed locally at the site of injection; absorbed parent compound and fragments enter the blood and lymphatic system; metabolised by proteolysis	A tetrapeptide that may act as an immunological decoy for myelin basic protein; given by subcutaneous injection to treat multiple sclerosis
Fingolimod	Prodrug with high oral bioavailability; rapidly phosphorylated to active metabolite; highly sequestered in tissues; hepatic metabolism (4–9 days)	Sphingosine analogue; phosphorylated form prevents lymphocyte egress from lymph nodes; given orally
Interferon beta	Rapid elimination due to tissue uptake and catabolism (especially in the liver); metabolised by proteolysis (2–4 h)	Anti-inflammatory cytokine given by subcutaneous or intramuscular injection for relapsing–remitting multiple sclerosis
Mitoxantrone	Metabolism and renal excretion; long terminal half-life (5–18 days)	A cytotoxic antibiotic given by intravenous infusion for the treatment of cancer (Ch. 52); not currently licensed for multiple sclerosis
Natalizumab	Protein clearance (11 days); clearance increased in the presence of natalizumab antibodies	A monoclonal antibody that blocks lymphocyte adhesion; given as an intravenous infusion for relapsing–remitting multiple sclerosis
Riluzole	High oral bioavailability (90%); hepatic metabolism (12 h)	A glutamate receptor antagonist used for motor neuron disease; given orally

26

Migraine and other headaches

Headache has many causes and most headaches are not produced by any structural abnormality or metabolic disturbance (primary headache; see Box 26.1). Tension is by far the most common primary cause, accounting for about two-thirds of cases, while migraine is the second most frequent cause. When headache is present for a prolonged time, or is recurrent, secondary causes may need to be excluded by a full history and examination for associated neurological symptoms and signs.

Migraine is an episodic headache, typically lasting 4–72 h. The diagnostic features of migraine are listed in Box 26.2. These are the only symptoms in the majority of migraineurs. However, in up to one-third the headache is preceded or accompanied by focal neurological symptoms (migraine with aura), usually visual disturbances but occasionally more severe focal neurological episodes such as hemiparesis.

PATHOGENESIS OF MIGRAINE

The pathogenesis of migraine is imperfectly understood but involves both neuronal and vascular dysfunction (Fig. 26.1). Headache in people with migraine is associated with sensitisation of the pain pathways in both the meninges (peripheral sensitisation) and the central processing of sensory stimuli in the brainstem (central sensitisation). Genetic predisposition is a factor in migraine, and abnormal function of voltage-dependent ion channels in cortical and brainstem structures may provide the basis for increased excitability in the neuronal circuits that are responsible for the headache.

An aura precedes a migraine attack in 15% of cases with transient visual symptoms (such as flashing or jagged lights) or sensory symptoms. Visual symptoms are probably caused by an initial intense but brief neuronal excitation producing cortical hyperaemia. This is followed by a slowly propagated wave of cortical depolarisation that transiently depresses spontaneous and evoked neuronal activity (cortical spreading depression). The depressant wave is associated with vasoconstriction, which may produce focal neurological symptoms and signs. The majority of migraineurs who do not experience an aura appear to have 'silent' cortical spreading depression and this suppression of electrical activity may therefore be the trigger for the migraine headache.

The hallmark of the migraine process is activation of the trigeminal nerve pathway (Fig. 26.1). Increased dopaminergic and glutamatergic neurotransmission, with reduced serotonergic neurotransmission, are all thought to contribute to this activation.

The migraine process involves vasodilation and inflammation of the dural blood vessels and dura mater (neurogenic inflammation). This results from activation of afferents in the trigeminal pathway from the trigeminocervical complex in the brainstem to the dural blood vessels. The triggers that activate the pathway are unknown, but are probably chemical. Activation of the pathway releases vasoactive peptides such as calcitonin gene-related peptide (CGRP) and substance P from the perivascular axons in the dura mater. As a result, the local concentrations of cytokines, serotonin, histamine and nitric oxide increase, producing vasodilation and activating endothelial cells, mast cells and platelets. Mediators released from these cells further contribute to neurogenic inflammation. Sensory nociceptors on the trigeminal nerves in the dura are stimulated, and the nociceptive impulses are relayed from the dura through the trigeminocervical complex in the brainstem, from where they are transmitted to the thalamus. Thalamic stimulation produces pain, nausea and vomiting. Monoaminergic pathways in the trigeminocervical complex modulate the nociceptive pain (Ch. 19) via afferent nerves to intra- and extracranial blood vessels. There are also reflex parasympathetic connections back to the dural vessels that potentiate vasodilation (Fig. 26.1). The trigeminocervical complex is rich in serotonin $5-HT_{1B/1D}$ receptors, and their stimulation (particularly $5-HT_{1B}$ receptors) inhibits neurotransmission to the thalamus.

DRUGS FOR MIGRAINE

SPECIFIC DRUGS FOR THE ACUTE MIGRAINE ATTACK

Triptans

Examples

frovatriptan, naratriptan, sumatriptan, zolmitriptan

Mechanisms of action and effects

The triptans are serotonin 5-HT$_{1B/1D}$ receptor agonists, which may alter the pathophysiology of migraine (Fig. 26.2) by:

- intracranial vasoconstriction (5-HT$_{1B}$),
- inhibition of neurotransmission in the trigeminocervical complex and inhibition of release of pro-inflammatory and vasoactive mediators from perivascular trigeminal neurons (5-HT$_{1B/1D}$).

Sumatriptan does not easily cross the blood–brain barrier since it is water-soluble, but this barrier may be impaired during a migraine attack. Naratriptan, zolmitriptan and other 'second-generation' triptans penetrate the blood–brain barrier more readily. These drugs directly inhibit excitability of the trigeminocervical complex in the brainstem and relieve both the pain and the nausea associated with migraine.

Pharmacokinetics

Absorption of sumatriptan from the gut is rapid but erratic, whereas second-generation triptans such as naratriptan and zolmitriptan have better absorption. Effective plasma concentrations of these drugs are usually reached within 30 min of oral administration. Sumatriptan and zolmitriptan undergo first-pass metabolism by monoamine oxidase A (MAO-A) and have a low oral bioavailability. Subcutaneous injection or administration by nasal spray avoid first-pass metabolism with these drugs and relieves symptoms within 15 min. These routes can be more effective if the headache is accompanied by nausea, because gastric stasis often delays oral drug absorption during a migraine attack. Naratriptan is not a substrate for MAO-A, which gives it high oral bioavailability. Elimination of most triptans is partially by

hepatic metabolism and partially by renal excretion. Most triptans have short half-lives of between 2 and 6 h, but the half-life of frovatriptan is longer, at 26 h.

Unwanted effects

The frequency and intensity of unwanted effects is highest after subcutaneous use of sumatriptan:

- tingling, pressure, tightness, heaviness or sensation of warmth in the head, neck, chest and limbs,
- flushing,
- dizziness or vertigo,
- drowsiness,
- nausea or vomiting,
- angina caused by coronary artery vasoconstriction (via 5-HT$_{1B}$ receptor stimulation),
- pain or irritation at the injection site, or in the nose after local use.

Ergotamine

Mechanism of action

Ergotamine probably has an antimigraine action similar to the triptans by stimulating 5-HT$_1$ receptors. Unwanted effects arise from agonist activity at several other receptors, including α_1-adrenoceptors and dopamine D$_2$ receptors.

Pharmacokinetics

Oral administration is often accompanied by nausea, and absorption is poor, erratic and delayed. Ergotamine undergoes extensive metabolism in the liver and has a short half-life (2 h). However, tight receptor binding produces a longer duration of action.

Unwanted effects

- Nausea and vomiting are caused by dopamine receptor stimulation at the chemoreceptor trigger zone (Ch. 32).
- Abdominal cramps.
- Dizziness.
- Severe vasoconstriction as a result of α_1-adrenoceptor stimulation can lead to peripheral gangrene (acute ergotism). Ergotamine should be avoided in people with known atheromatous vascular disease (including ischaemic heart disease).
- Chronic intoxication with dependence can occur after prolonged use. Withdrawal then produces nausea and headache similar to an acute migraine attack. For this reason, ergotamine treatment should not be repeated at intervals of less than 4 days.

PROPHYLACTIC DRUGS

Beta-adrenoceptor antagonists

In migraine, β-adrenoceptor antagonists without intrinsic sympathomimetic activity, such as propranolol, timolol and metoprolol, have the greatest evidence for efficacy, while drugs with partial agonist activity that cause vasodilation (e.g. pindolol) are ineffective. The antagonist action at β_1-adrenoceptors is complemented by 5-HT receptor antagonist activity with some β-adrenoceptor antagonists. Effects

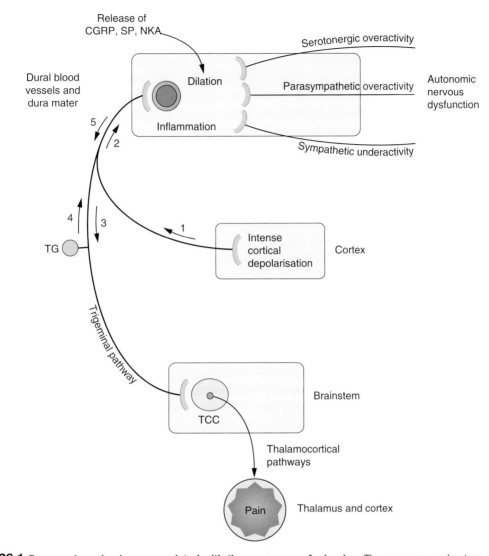

Fig. 26.1 **Proposed mechanisms associated with the processes of migraine.** The sequence and nature of neurogenic and vascular involvement in migraine are vigorously debated and may vary in different kinds of migraine-type headache. One scenario is that the trigger is a wave of cortical depression (1) which sensitizes and stimulates the trigeminal pathway in either direction (2, 3). This results in stimulation of the trigeminocervical complex (TCC) (3) in the brainstem, and onward stimulation of the thalamus and other areas can cause pain and nausea. Other reflex pathways from the brainstem via the superior salivatory nucleus to the dural blood vessels, which result in vasodilation, can also be activated at this stage. The stimulation of trigeminal nerves innervating the dural blood vessels (2, 4) results in the release of mediators such as calcitonin gene-related peptide (CGRP), substance P (SP) and neurokinin A (NKA), which cause vasodilation and participate in inflammation. CGRP and possibly other mediators are able to stimulate nociceptors in the trigeminal nerve endings, resulting in further activation of the pathways to the TCC and thalamus (5) and consequently further pain. The control of vascular tone in the dural blood vessels is complex, with sympathetic, parasympathetic and serotonergic systems contributing to the migraine process. Vasoconstrictor innervation of these vessels is by sympathetic nerves and vasodilation occurs by parasympathetic innervation. Serotonergic pathways produce vasoconstriction by stimulation of 5-HT$_{1B}$ receptors and vasodilation via 5-HT$_2$ receptors. TG, trigeminal ganglion.

on central nervous system function include reduced neuronal firing in noradrenergic neurons in the locus coeruleus and inhibition of cortical potentials evoked by auditory and visual stimuli, suggesting a modulation of neuronal excitability. Full details of β-adrenoceptor antagonists can be found in Chapter 5.

Antiepileptic drugs

The mechanism of action of sodium valproate, gabapentin and topiramate in the prophylaxis of migraine is not well understood. They almost certainly work by multiple mechanisms, including γ-aminobutyric acid (GABA)-mediated

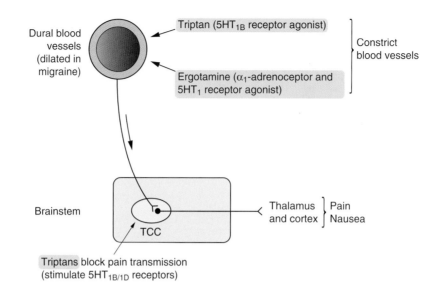

Fig. 26.2 **Possible mechanisms of action of 5-HT receptor agonists in migraine.** The trigeminocervical complex (TCC) is rich in 5-HT$_{1B/1D}$ receptors and stimulation of these receptors by so-called second-generation triptans inhibits neurotransmission to the thalamus and cortex. Triptans also cause vasoconstriction acting at 5-HT$_{1B}$ receptors on blood vessels.

suppression of neurotransmission through the trigeminocervical complex in the brainstem, and modulating neuronal excitability through effects on voltage-gated Na$^+$ channels. Blockade of P/Q-type Ca^{2+} channels may also contribute by reducing glutamate release. Antiepileptic drugs with a predominant single mechanism of action seem to be ineffective in treatment of migraine. Full details of these drugs can be found in Chapter 23.

Amitriptyline

The mechanism of action of amitryptiline in migraine is unknown, but probably relates to multiple neurotransmitter–receptor interactions that modulate the processing of nociceptive impulses. In addition to reducing neuronal reuptake of noradrenaline and serotonin, amitriptyline is also a 5-HT$_2$ receptor antagonist, and may enhance the pain threshold by α_2-adrenoceptor activation. Amitriptyline works in migraine at lower doses than those used to treat depression. Several other antidepressants have been studied but, with the possible exception of fluoxetine, they are ineffective. Full details of amitriptyline can be found in Chapter 22.

MANAGEMENT OF MIGRAINE AND OTHER HEADACHES

THE ACUTE MIGRAINE ATTACK

Withdrawal of possible triggers such as cheese, chocolate, citrus fruits or alcoholic drinks may reduce the frequency of attacks by up to 50%. The combined oral hormonal contraceptive is a potential exacerbating factor, although it can be helpful for prevention of menstrual-related migraine.

Simple analgesia with a non-steroidal anti-inflammatory drug (NSAID) such as aspirin or ibuprofen (Ch. 29) may be sufficient for the relief of a mild acute attack of migraine. Nausea frequently accompanies a migraine attack and delays gastric emptying. If this occurs, absorption of the analgesic will be more rapid if an anti-emetic such as metoclopramide or domperidone (Ch. 32) is given concurrently. If the person is vomiting, rectal or intramuscular analgesia, for example with an NSAID such as diclofenac or naproxen, can be used combined with rectal domperidone. Analgesics are usually more effective when given early after the onset of pain. Opioid analgesics are not recommended as they are short-acting, produce dependence and frequent use can also promote medication-overuse headaches (see below).

If attacks are poorly controlled by simple analgesics or are moderate to severe in intensity, a triptan is usually highly effective. It can relieve pain even if taken more than 4 h after the onset of an attack, but is less effective in those migraineurs who have developed cutaneous allodynia (a form of neuropathic pain; Ch. 19) in the trigeminal nerve distribution in association with the headache. Subcutaneous sumatriptan or intranasal sumatriptan or naratriptan are useful if a rapid response is required or if nausea precludes oral therapy. The response of individuals varies to the different triptans and it is worth changing to an alternative after two unsuccessful attempts at treatment with one drug. Headache recurs in about 40% of those who initially gain relief from a triptan, although the risk of recurrence may be less with frovatriptan, which has a long half-life. A second dose of a triptan can be used for recurrent headache if there was a good response to the first dose. If migraine headaches are prolonged or recur frequently despite treatment with a triptan then the combination of a triptan with an NSAID can be tried.

Ergotamine can be used to treat acute attacks, but is not recommended concurrently with a triptan. The risk of vasospasm and habituation means that ergotamine should be avoided in older people (who may have cardiovascular disease) and in those with frequent attacks. For these reasons, and because of the frequency of other unwanted effects, ergotamine is now infrequently used.

PROPHYLAXIS OF MIGRAINE

Prophylaxis is usually recommended for people experiencing at least two attacks of migraine each month that significantly interfere with the person's daily routine. Beta-adrenoceptor antagonists are widely held to be the best choice, providing there are no contraindications. The antiepileptic drugs sodium valproate and topiramate are effective second-line alternatives. There is less consistent evidence for the use of gabapentin, which is used as a third-line option. The major disadvantage of these agents is the risk of teratogenicity in women of childbearing age. Amitriptyline may be particularly effective when tension headache coexists with migraine. Methysergide and pizotifen (see the Compendium at the end of this chapter) are less commonly used.

Botulinum toxin type A (Ch. 24), by injection into sites such as the forehead, temporalis, cervical and trapezius muscles may reduce symptoms for up to 3 months. The mechanism in unclear, but inhibition of peripheral sensory neurons may indirectly reduce central neuronal sensitisation. Some evidence suggests that people who describe their headache as 'being crushed from the outside' or have 'eye-popping' headache (imploding or ocular headaches) respond better than those who describe a build-up of pressure inside the head (exploding headache). This suggests that botulinum toxin works best if there is an extracranial trigger for the pain.

The efficacy of all current prophylactic treatments is limited. Although the response to an individual drug class is unpredictable, only about half of all migraineurs can expect to have a 50% reduction in the frequency of attacks.

MEDICATION-OVERUSE HEADACHE

Regular use of opioids or compound analgesic drugs, especially those containing caffeine, to treat any type of headache, or triptans for migraine, can lead to a chronic daily headache known as medication-overuse headache (also called analgesic or rebound headache). It is the third most common cause of headache. The mechanisms underlying this are not well understood, but probably involve downregulation of receptor or enzyme targets of the drugs with consequent sensitisation of the pain pathways. Medication-overuse headache is most common in women aged between 30 and 60 years, and is diagnosed when headache is present for at least 15 days each month for at least 3 months in someone who is taking regular medication to treat headache. The person experiencing the headache is often reluctant to consider that the drugs are the cause, but abrupt withdrawal of the causative treatment is advised to achieve resolution. NSAIDs can be used for withdrawal headaches, and prophylactic treatment for the underlying tension or migrainous headache given prior to withdrawal.

MANAGEMENT OF OTHER HEADACHES

Most other primary headaches are managed as for any other form of acute pain, usually using step 1 of the World Health Organization (WHO) analgesic ladder (Ch. 19). Care must be taken to avoid medication-overuse headache. Tension-type headache is usually bilateral and not disabling. Frequent tension headaches may respond to prophylactic treatment with amitriptyline at low dosage. Cluster headache is characterised by severe attacks of unilateral pain in the distribution of the trigeminal nerve that are associated with autonomic features on the side of the headache (such as ptosis, miosis, conjunctival injection, lacrimation and rhinorrhoea). Cluster headache usually responds to a triptan, but if prophylaxis is needed for recurrent episodes, then the calcium channel blocker verapamil (Ch. 5) is the drug of choice.

Suspected secondary headache requires treatment of the precipitating cause. Red flag features include thunderclap headache with peak severity achieved in seconds or minutes (usually primary headache but possible subarachnoid haemorrhage), focal neurological signs or new cognitive disturbance (possible intracranial pathology) and headache worse on standing (possible low-pressure headache due to cerebrospinal fluid leak). Other symptoms suggesting raised intracranial pressure are headache that wakes the person from sleep or worsening of headache with coughing, laughing or straining. Meningitis and temporal arteritis can also present with headache. Headache due to focal intracerebral pathology that is causing raised intracranial pressure is often alleviated by dexamethasone (Ch. 44), which reduces cerebral oedema.

SELF-ASSESSMENT

True/false questions

1. Diet plays little part in the precipitation of migraine attacks.
2. Serotonin is released in a migraine attack.
3. Agonists at $5\text{-}HT_{1B/1D}$ receptors are used for the treatment of migraine.
4. Ergotamine is used prophylactically for migraine.
5. Sumatriptan is not useful for acute attacks of migraine as it is slow-acting.
6. Sumatriptan causes chest discomfort in 40% of people as a result of coronary vasoconstriction.
7. Regular use of triptans can cause rebound headache.
8. Pizotifen is used prophylactically and blocks $5\text{-}HT_2$ receptors.
9. Ergotamine is safe to use in ischaemic heart disease.
10. Tricyclic antidepressants and β-adrenoceptor antagonists may be useful in prophylaxis of migraine.
11. Where migraine is associated with vomiting, metoclopramide and paracetamol given together is a useful combination.
12. Pindolol is effective in prophylaxis of migraine.
13. The combined oral contraceptive pill reduces the frequency of migraine attacks in women.
14. Prophylactic treatment for migraine is highly effective.
15. Injections of botulinum toxin may reduce migraine symptoms.

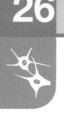

True/false answers

1. **False.** In some people, stress and dietary items like chocolate, cheese and alcohol may provoke migraine attacks.
2. **True.** Serotonin, histamine, nitric oxide and other vasoactive mediators contribute to neurogenic inflammation in migraine.
3. **True.** The triptans are 5-HT$_{1B/1D}$ agonists used in acute migraine.
4. **False.** Because of unwanted effects, ergotamine should not be used prophylactically, or more than twice a month for acute attacks.
5. **False.** Oral sumatriptan acts within 30 min, and more quickly when given by subcutaneous or nasal routes of administration.
6. **False.** Although sumatriptan causes chest discomfort and is contraindicated in people with ischaemic heart disease, chest discomfort in people without ischaemic heart disease is probably caused by oesophageal spasm, not myocardial ischaemia.
7. **True.** Medication-overuse headache may occur with triptans, opioids and compound analgesics when used regularly for headache.
8. **True.** Pizotifen is not commonly used but reduces perivascular inflammation, vasodilation and pain by blocking 5-HT$_2$ receptors.
9. **False.** Ergotamine causes vasoconstriction and should be avoided in people with vascular diseases.
10. **True.** Beta-adrenoceptor antagonists like propranolol are first-line drugs for migraine prophylaxis.
11. **True.** Metoclopramide is an anti-emetic and increases gastric emptying, so improving the rate of absorption of paracetamol.
12. **False.** Beta-adrenoceptor antagonists with partial agonist activity like pindolol are not effective as they may exacerbate vasodilation.
13. **False.** The combined oral hormonal contraceptive may exacerbate migraine, although it can be helpful in women with menstrual-related migraine.
14. **False.** The prophylaxis of migraine is effective in only about half of those who are treated.
15. **True.** Pericranial injections of botulinum toxin type A can reduce the frequency of migraine attacks.

FURTHER READING

Drug and Therapeutics Bulletin (2010) Management of medication overuse headache. *BMJ* 340, 968–972

Fenstermacher N, Levin M, Ward T (2011) Pharmacological prevention of migraine. *BMJ* 342, 540–543

Galletti F, Cupini LM, Corbelli P et al. (2009) Pathophysiological basis of migraine prophylaxis. *Prog Neurobiol* 89, 176–192

Goadsby PJ (2006) Recent advances in the diagnosis and management of migraine. *BMJ* 332, 25–29

Loder E (2010) Triptan therapy in migraine. *N Engl J Med* 363, 63–70

Nesbitt AD, Goadsby PJ (2012) Cluster headache. *BMJ* 344:e2407

Silberstein SD (2004) Migraine. *Lancet* 363, 381–391

Compendium: drugs used to treat migraine

Drug	Kinetics (half-life)	Comments
Analgesics		
Most migraine headaches respond to non-steroidal anti-inflammatory drugs, but reduced gastric emptying and peristalsis may slow the rate of oral absorption; tolfenamic acid is licensed specifically for oral treatment of acute attacks; see Ch. 29.		
Anti-emetics		
Anti-emetics (see Ch. 32) such as metoclopramide or domperidone are often given to relieve the nausea associated with migraine attacks.		
5-HT$_1$ receptor agonists (triptans)		
Act on 5-HT$_{1B}$ and 5-HT$_{1D}$ receptors; may be used during the acute headache phase; preferred treatment for those who fail to respond to analgesics		
Almotriptan	High oral bioavailability (70%); hepatic metabolism via monoamine oxidase and P450 and also by renal tubular secretion (3–4 h)	Given orally
Eletriptan	Good oral bioavailability (50%); hepatic metabolism (4–5 h)	Given orally
Frovatriptan	Oral bioavailability 20–30%; hepatic metabolism and renal excretion (26 h)	Given orally; long-acting
Naratriptan	High oral bioavailability (70%); hepatic metabolism; 50% excreted unchanged (6 h)	Given orally
Rizatriptan	More rapid absorption than sumatriptan; good oral bioavailability (45%); hepatic metabolism and renal excretion (2–3 h)	Given orally
Sumatriptan	Low oral bioavailability (15%) but complete availability after subcutaneous injection; hepatic metabolism and renal excretion of parent drug (2 h)	First-generation triptan; given orally, intranasally or by subcutaneous injection; also used for cluster headaches
Zolmitriptan	Oral bioavailability about 40%; the N-desmethyl metabolite is a 5-HT$_{1D}$ agonist and probably contributes to activity; also renal excretion of parent drug (3 h)	Given orally or intranasally; also used for cluster headaches (nasal route only)
Ergot alkaloids and related compounds		
Ergotamine	Very low oral bioavailability (2%); hepatic metabolism and biliary excretion (2 h)	5-HT$_1$ and α_1-adrenoceptor agonist; given orally or as suppositories
Methysergide	Rapid and complete absorption but bioavailability is about 15% due to first-pass metabolism; hepatic metabolism and renal excretion (10 h)	Synthetic ergot alkaloid; used orally for prophylaxis; risk of retroperitoneal fibrosis; should only be prescribed under hospital supervision
Other drugs for migraine		
Amitriptyline	See Ch. 22	Tricyclic antidepressant used for migraine prophylaxis; see Ch. 22
Antiepileptic drugs	See Ch. 23	Some antiepileptic drugs are used for migraine prophylaxis; see Ch. 23
Beta-adrenoceptor antagonists	See Ch. 8	Some β-adrenoceptor antagonists are used for migraine prophylaxis; see Ch. 8
Clonidine	See Ch. 6	Used orally for prophylaxis but is not recommended; see Ch. 6
Isometheptene	Metabolised in animals but kinetic data in humans not available	Indirectly acting sympathomimetic that constricts dilated cranial and cerebral arterioles; used orally for acute attacks in combination with paracetamol
Pizotifen	Good oral bioavailability (80%); metabolised to unusual polar quaternary N-glucuronide product (26 h)	5-HT$_2$ antagonist and antihistamine; given orally for prophylaxis, but rarely used

6

The musculoskeletal system

The neuromuscular junction and neuromuscular blockade

• •

NEUROMUSCULAR TRANSMISSION

The neuromuscular junction is a specialised synapse of a somatic neuron with the sarcolemma of skeletal muscle, termed the motor endplate (Fig. 27.1A). In mammals, depolarisation of the postsynaptic membrane at the motor endplate causes contraction of the muscle fibre in an all-or-nothing response. Greater contractility is achieved by the stimulation of more motor endplates.

The neurotransmitter at the neuromuscular junction is acetylcholine (ACh), acting at postsynaptic nicotinic N_2 receptors. The processes of synthesis and release of ACh are described in Chapter 4 in relation to the general properties of neurotransmitters in the nervous system. The presynaptic nerve terminal at the neuromuscular junction contains 300 000 or more vesicles, each of which may contain up to 5000 molecules of ACh (known as a quantum). In response to an action potential, up to 500 vesicles discharge their contents into the synapse over a very short period (0.5 ms). Each N_2 receptor has two binding sites for ACh, and the Na^+ channel in the centre of the receptor opens when both sites are occupied (Ch. 1). This allows an influx of Na^+ into the muscle cell and depolarisation of the motor endplate. If depolarisation is sufficient to reach the firing threshold potential for the cell then voltage-gated Na^+ channels open, full depolarisation of the muscle cell is triggered and an action potential is generated and propagated along the postsynaptic membrane. Initiation of an action potential requires the release of 50–200 quanta of ACh, which will activate 10–15% of motor endplate N_2 receptors (Fig. 27.1b).

The action potential generated in the skeletal muscle cell passes along the sarcolemma into the T tubules, where Ca^{2+} is released from the sarcoplasmic reticulum. The increased availability of intracellular Ca^{2+} brings about the processes that result in muscle contraction.

The action of ACh on N_2 receptors is very short-lived (about 0.5 ms) because the synaptic cleft contains large amounts of the extremely potent enzyme acetylcholinesterase (AChE), which rapidly degrades ACh (Ch. 4). An esterase called pseudocholinesterase (butyrylcholinesterase, plasma cholinesterase) in plasma hydrolyses any ACh that escapes from the synaptic cleft; it acts more slowly than AChE. Pseudocholinesterase is important pharmacologically because of its ability to metabolise several drugs with ester bonds. Tissue esterases that break down ACh are also present in many cells, notably in the liver.

Although ACh is the neurotransmitter responsible for contraction of both skeletal muscle and most smooth muscles, the basic organisation and functioning of these neuroeffector systems are very different, as shown in Table 27.1.

DRUGS ACTING AT THE NEUROMUSCULAR JUNCTION

Acetylcholinesterase inhibitors

AChE inhibitors block the breakdown of ACh following its release in neuronal synapses and at neuroeffector junctions. The mechanisms of action of different types of AChE inhibitor are described in Chapter 4; they are non-selective and prolong the availability and actions of ACh at all its receptors (nicotinic N_1 and N_2 and muscarinic). Full details of AChE inhibitors in the treatment of myasthenia gravis are given in Chapter 28.

Inhibitors of acetylcholine release

Botulinum toxin from the anaerobic bacillus *Clostridium botulinum* decreases the release of ACh from vesicles. It binds selectively to cholinergic nerve terminals and, after internalisation via a cell membrane vesicle, is released into the cell cytoplasm. The toxin cleaves cytoplasmic proteins (SNARE proteins) on the cell membrane that are essential for docking and fusion of vesicles with the neuronal membrane, and this inhibits neurotransmitter release. This chemical denervation stimulates collateral axon growth which eventually results in the formation of a new neuromuscular junction. Botulinum toxin is extremely dangerous, as evidenced by the consequences of botulinum poisoning, but it also has clinical roles when injected locally. Two toxin serotypes, A and B, are used in clinical practice as botulinum toxin–haemagglutinin complex. Injection into skeletal muscles produces local muscle paralysis for many weeks until new nerve terminals develop. Botulinum toxin is used to treat involuntary movements such as blepharospasm (spasm of the eyelids) or torticollis (wry-neck) and to

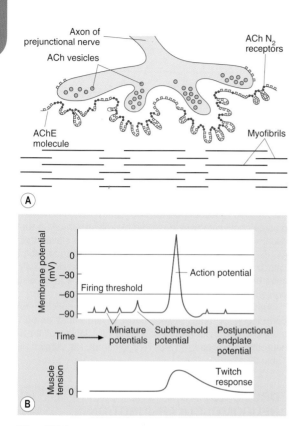

Fig. 27.1 Acetylcholine (ACh) at the neuromuscular junction. (A) The released ACh acts upon postsynaptic nicotinic N_2 receptors on the motor endplate, opening cation channels and an influx of Na^+ occurs, resulting in depolarisation. (B) At rest, insignificant amounts of ACh are released, and miniature endplate potentials generated are insufficient to reach the threshold potential to cause a propagated action potential. If sufficient ACh is released, an action potential is propagated, causing muscle contraction. Non-depolarising muscle relaxants prevent the generation of the action potential by blocking N_2 receptors. AChE, acetylcholinesterase.

relieve spasticity (Ch. 24). It is also used by local injection to reduce excessive sweating, because it inhibits ACh release at sweat glands, and is occasionally injected into facial muscles for the prophylaxis of migraine (Ch. 26). Botulinum toxin is increasingly being used for cosmetic reasons to temporarily remove frown lines and wrinkles.

Antagonists/blockers at the neuromuscular junction

Skeletal muscle relaxation is achieved by drugs that specifically and reversibly block the actions of ACh on nicotinic N_2 receptors at the neuromuscular junction; they do not affect autonomic nervous system function (i.e. the actions of ACh on nicotinic N_1 receptors in ganglia or on muscarinic receptors at postganglionic nerve endings). Drugs that block the neuromuscular junction almost all resemble ACh in that they have a quaternary ammonium (N^+) group that binds strongly to the anionic site of the nicotinic N_2 receptor (Fig. 27.2).

A neuromuscular blocker must occupy more than 75% of postsynaptic N_2 receptors before it can start to produce neuromuscular blockade. The potency of a neuromuscular blocker is measured by the ED_{95}, which is the dose required to produce 95% depression of muscular twitch (Table 27.2). About twice this dose is required for muscle relaxation adequate to permit tracheal intubation. The laryngeal muscles are more rapidly paralysed than other skeletal muscle groups, but the effect is often of shorter duration. This may reflect either the higher blood flow to this muscle, or the greater density of N_2 receptors.

Recovery of muscle action depends on the rate of clearance of the drug from the plasma. After a bolus injection of many neuromuscular blockers, this is largely a result of redistribution to tissues, rather than metabolism. Redistribution lowers the plasma concentration and consequently the concentration at the motor endplate. For those drugs which undergo rapid redistribution, the duration of neuromuscular blockade will be more prolonged after repeated boluses or infusions; this is because when equilibrium between plasma and tissue concentrations has been reached the duration of effect then becomes mainly dependent on metabolism.

Table 27.1 Comparison of skeletal and smooth muscle innervation

Property	Skeletal muscle fibre	Smooth muscle fibre
Nerves supplying fibre	Single	Multiple
Junction	Highly organised motor endplate	Simple
Neurotransmitter	Acetylcholine	Acetylcholine
Receptor subtype	Nicotinic N_2	Muscarinic (mainly M_3)
Receptor distribution	Only at motor endplate; only one motor endplate per muscle fibre	Widely on the muscle surface
Effects of stimulation	Single nerve contracts the whole muscle fibre (all-or-none response)	Each nerve contracts part of muscle fibre (graded response)
Effect of overdose with acetylcholinesterase inhibitor	Flaccid paralysis	Spasticity

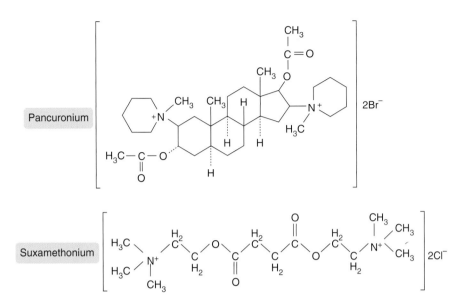

Fig. 27.2 Structures of pancuronium, a non-depolarising blocking drug, and suxamethonium (succinylcholine),
a depolarising blocker. Suxamethonium resembles two molecules of acetylcholine, each with a quaternary ammonium
(N^+) group, linked back-to-back. Pancuronium was designed to have a similar spatial arrangement of quaternary
nitrogens, but held rigidly in place by a steroid bridge that is resistant to pseudocholinesterase.

Competitive N_2 receptor antagonists (non-depolarising blockers)

atracurium, cisatracurium, mivacurium, pancuronium,
rocuronium, vecuronium

Mechanism of action and effects

Competitive N_2 receptor antagonists bind to the nicotinic
N_2 receptor at the neuromuscular junction without causing
depolarisation of the postsynaptic membrane. This blocks
the depolarising effect of ACh and leads to muscle relaxation. Whereas it takes two ACh molecules to activate the
N_2 receptor, only one molecule of a non-depolarising neuromuscular blocker at each receptor will prevent neurotransmission. Inhibition of ACh hydrolysis by an AChE
inhibitor (usually neostigmine, see Ch. 28) will prolong the
action of ACh and rapidly reverse competitive neuromuscular junction blockade. This principle is used at the end of
an operation to aid recovery of the paralysed person.

Pharmacokinetics

Because of their high polarity, conferred by the quaternary
ammonium (N^+) group (Fig. 27.2), non-depolarising neuromuscular blockers are not absorbed from the gastrointestinal tract and are given by intravenous injection. They have
a low apparent volume of distribution and do not cross the
blood–brain barrier. Vecuronium is partially metabolised in
the liver but largely excreted unchanged in the bile. Pancuronium and rocuronium are eliminated by a combination
of metabolism and renal excretion of unchanged drug. Atracurium (a mixture of 10 isomers) and cisatracurium (a single

isomer of atracurium) undergo non-enzymatic spontaneous
degradation as well as hydrolysis by non-specific esterases
in the plasma, which is an advantage in hepatic or renal
impairment. Mivacurium, like suxamethonium (see below),
is metabolised by pseudocholinesterase.

The speed of onset of action and duration of action of
competitive blockers differ (Table 27.2). Rocuronium has
the fastest onset of action, within 2 min, which can be
useful during endotracheal intubation. With the exception
of atracurium and cisatracurium, the duration of action of
competitive antagonists at the neuromuscular junction
(from about 30 min for vecuronium up to 75 min for pancuronium) is mainly determined by redistribution of the drug
into the body tissues. This leads to prolonged action with
repeated doses (see above). The duration of effect of atracurium and cisatracurium is about 40 min. This is slightly
longer than predicted from their plasma half-lives and may
be a consequence of high-affinity binding sites close to the
ACh receptor acting as a reservoir for the drug.

Unwanted effects

See Table 27.2.

Depolarising neuromuscular-blocking drugs

suxamethonium (succinylcholine)

Mechanism of action and effects

Suxamethonium is succinic acid with a choline molecule
attached at each carboxylic acid group; it therefore

Table 27.2 Properties of some neuromuscular junction-blocking drugs

Muscle relaxant	ED_{95} (mg·kg^{-1})[a]	Time to maximum block (min)[b]	Duration (min)[c]	Unwanted effects
Pancuronium	0.06	4–5	90	Tachycardia, hypertension due to sympathetic stimulation; increase in cardiac output
Vecuronium	0.05	3–4	45	Allergy
Atracurium	0.25	3–4	40	Histamine release; increase in heart rate and decrease in systemic vascular resistance, tachycardia, bronchospasm
Cisatracurium	0.05	4.5–5.5	30–40	Low incidence of unwanted effects
Rocuronium	0.4	2–3	30	Increase in heart rate; allergy
Mivacurium	0.08	2–3	15–20	Histamine release; increase in heart rate and decrease in systemic vascular resistance, tachycardia, bronchospasm; prolonged block in people lacking pseudocholinesterase (butyrylcholinesterase, plasma cholinesterase)
Suxamethonium (succinylcholine)		Fast	3–12	Muscle fasciculation; postoperative muscle pain; bradycardia, hyperkalaemia, malignant hyperthermia; after approximately 20 min, some elements of block are those of non-depolarising type; prolonged block in people lacking pseudocholinesterase

[a]ED_{95} is the effective dose required to suppress muscle twitch by 95%.
[b]Time to maximum block following administration of the dose used for intubation (double the ED_{95}).
[c]Time taken to recover to 25% of the original twitch height after an intubation dose (double the ED_{95}).

resembles two ACh molecules joined back to back (Fig. 27.2). When two molecules of suxamethonium bind to the nicotinic N_2 receptor it acts as an agonist and depolarises the motor endplate. However, suxamethonium is not hydrolysed by AChE and therefore produces more prolonged depolarisation than ACh. This probably leads to a conformational change in the receptor that allows the Na^+ channel to close despite the continued presence of an agonist, a process of desensitisation. As a result, the muscle repolarises and, although it can respond to direct electrical stimulation, it can no longer be stimulated via the neuronal release of ACh. Indeed, if the amount of available synaptic ACh is enhanced (such as occurs with the use of an AChE inhibitor), it will intensify a partial depolarising blockade rather than reverse it. After about 20 min of depolarising blockade, suxamethonium exhibits the properties of a 'dual block', with the onset of a non-depolarising competitive type of blockade. At this stage, a partial blockade can be partially reversed by an AChE inhibitor.

Pharmacokinetics

Suxamethonium is a highly polar molecule, is not absorbed orally and must be given intravenously. It has a low volume of distribution and does not cross the blood–brain barrier. Suxamethonium has an onset of action within 1 min, but is rapidly hydrolysed by pseudocholinesterase, which results in a very short duration of action (about 3–12 min). An infusion is therefore necessary to produce a prolonged effect. A very prolonged paralysis occurs in about 1 in 2000–3000 individuals, who have a genetically determined deficiency of pseudocholinesterase (see Ch. 2). In this population, the action of suxamethonium is terminated after some 2–3 h by renal excretion.

Unwanted effects

- There is an initial depolarisation of the motor endplates prior to blockade, which results in muscle fasciculation.
- Postoperative muscle pain is common, possibly due to muscle damage caused by fasciculation.
- Prolonged neuromuscular blockade and apnoea occur if there is a low circulating concentration of pseudocholinesterase, through either a genetic deficiency or a decreased synthesis of the enzyme in severe liver disease.
- The use of suxamethonium during anaesthesia has been linked with the development of a rare but potentially fatal disorder of muscles known as malignant hyperthermia, with a rapid rise in temperature, muscle rigidity, tachycardia and acidosis. Predisposition to this condition has an autosomal dominant inheritance and is associated with mutations in the ryanodine receptor RyR1. Treatment is with dantrolene (Ch. 24).
- Stimulation of nicotinic N_1 receptors at autonomic ganglia and muscarinic receptors produces bradycardia, especially with repeated doses.
- Hyperkalaemia, probably due to persistent activation of of N_2 receptors resulting in escape of intracellular K^+ ions from skeletal muscle fibres. This is especially marked in the presence of prolonged immobilisation, major tissue trauma and severe burns.

INDICATIONS FOR NEUROMUSCULAR-BLOCKING DRUGS

The neuromuscular-blocking drugs are used in both surgical procedures and intensive care. Their administration forms part of the achievement of balanced anaesthesia described in Chapter 17.

ENDOTRACHEAL INTUBATION

Relaxation of the vocal cords allows easy passage of an endotracheal tube. A rapid onset of action is essential to minimise the risk of aspiration of gastric contents. This is the only current major use for suxamethonium. Because of frequent unwanted effects, suxamethonium is largely superseded by rapidly acting non-depolarising blockers such as rocuronium.

DURING SURGICAL PROCEDURES

Neuromuscular blockade produces muscle relaxation for procedures such as abdominal incisions. Selective skeletal muscle relaxation reduces the concentrations of general anaesthetic needed for deep anaesthesia. It can be achieved by either a single injection of a drug or intravenous infusion for more prolonged surgery. At the end of the operation the effect of a non-depolarising blocker can be reversed within 1 min by intravenous injection of neostigmine. A muscarinic receptor blocker such as glycopyrrolate or atropine (Ch. 4) is given before neostigmine to prevent bradycardia or excessive salivation produced by stimulation of muscarinic receptors.

IN INTENSIVE CARE

Neuromuscular blockade is used in addition to analgesia and sedation during mechanical ventilation, particularly if respiratory drive is suppressed (e.g. in adult respiratory distress syndrome), in status asthmaticus, for status epilepticus or tetanus and for people with raised intracranial pressure.

SELF-ASSESSMENT

For a case-based question on the use of neuromuscular junction-blocking drugs in surgery, see the Self-assessment section of Ch. 17.

True/false questions

1. A skeletal muscle fibre is innervated by a single motor endplate.
2. The nicotinic receptors at skeletal muscle and autonomic ganglia are identical.
3. Suxamethonium is a competitive antagonist of nicotinic N_2 receptors.
4. Vecuronium has no haemodynamic effects.
5. Malignant hyperthermia is a rare, genetically determined reaction to suxamethonium.
6. The duration of action of all non-depolarising neuromuscular junction-blocking drugs is limited by redistribution.
7. Suxamethonium is the only muscle relaxant used for tracheal intubation.
8. Cisatracurium is well absorbed orally.
9. Botulinum toxin acts postsynaptically to block depolarisation induced by acetylcholine.
10. Botulinum toxin can be used to treat excessive sweating.

One-best-answer (OBA) question

Which statement about neuromuscular junction-blocking drugs is the *most accurate*?

A. Rocuronium crosses the blood–brain barrier and has direct effects on the central nervous system.
B. Pancuronium is the neuromuscular-blocking drug of choice for a surgical procedure that will take less than 30 min.
C. Suxamethonium is the only muscle relaxant that can be used for electroconvulsive therapy.
D. About 50% of nicotinic N_2 receptors must be occupied by a non-depolarising neuromuscular-blocking drug to produce complete block of an evoked twitch.
E. Atracurium causes the release of histamine.

True/false answers

1. **True.** Contraction of a skeletal muscle fibre is an all-or-none response to nerve stimulation at the motor endplate.
2. **False.** The nicotinic N_2 receptor at skeletal muscle is selectively blocked by non-depolarising and depolarising muscle relaxants, while the N_1 receptor at autonomic ganglia is selectively blocked by ganglion-blocking drugs (which now have little clinical application).
3. **False.** Suxamethonium is a nicotinic N_2 receptor *agonist* that causes persistent depolarisation then desensitisation of the receptor.
4. **True**. Unlike atracurium and mivacurium, vecuronium does not cause histamine release so it does not have significant haemodynamic effects.
5. **True.** Malignant hyperthermia in response to suxamethonium, halothane and some other drugs is associated with mutations in the ryanodine receptor RyR1, and is treated with dantrolene, a ryanodine receptor antagonist.
6. **False.** Atracurium and cisatracurium undergo spontaneous hydrolysis and mivacurium is hydrolysed by pseudocholinesterase.
7. **False.** Short-acting non-depolarising neuromuscular blockers such as rocuronium can also be used for intubation. The use of suxamethonium is declining because of the occurrence of malignant hyperthermia.
8. **False.** Because of the quaternary nature of their structures, neuromuscular junction-blocking drugs are not absorbed orally and do not cross the blood–brain barrier or placenta.

9. **False.** Botulinum toxin binds pre-synaptically to cause long-lasting block of ACh release.
10. **True.** Local injections of botulinum toxin can reduce activity of sweat glands, which are innervated by post-synaptic cholinergic fibres of the *sympathetic* nervous system.

OBA answer

Answer E is correct.

A. Incorrect. All non-depolarising neuromuscular-blocking drugs have a quaternary ammonium in their structure and will not cross the blood–brain barrier.

B. Incorrect. Pancuronium is a long-acting blocking drug and is used for procedures taking longer than 90 min.

C. Incorrect. Short-acting non-depolarising blocking drugs such as rocuronium or mivacurium are viable alternatives.

D. Incorrect. More than 90% of receptors need to be occupied to produce a complete block of skeletal muscle contractility.

E. **Correct**. Atracurium is one of the most potent neuromuscular-blocking drugs causing the release of histamine.

FURTHER READING

Bowman WC (2006) Neuromuscular block. *Br J Pharmacol* 147, S277–S286

Denborough M (1998) Malignant hyperthermia. *Lancet* 352, 1131–1136

Fagerlund MJ, Eriksson LI (2009) Current concepts in neuromuscular transmission *Br J Anaesth* 103, 108–114

Moore EW, Hunter JM (2001) The new neuromuscular blocking agents: do they offer any advantages? *Br J Anaesth* 87, 912–925

Münchau A, Bhatia KP (2000) Uses of botulinum toxin injection in medicine today. *BMJ* 320, 161–165

Compendium: drugs acting at the neuromuscular junction

Drug	Kinetics (half-life)	Comments
Acetylcholinesterase inhibitors		
Distigmine, edrophonium, pyridostigmine		See Ch. 28
Neostigmine	See Ch. 28	Given intravenously to reverse the effects of a non-depolarising blocker (with atropine to minimise effects of enhanced acetylcholine on the parasympathetic system); also used in myasthenia gravis (Ch. 28)
Non-depolarising blockers		
All are used for muscle relaxation for surgery; all have negligible oral absorption and are given by intravenous injection or infusion.		
Atracurium	Spontaneous hydrolysis; very rapidly breaks down within blood (0.3 h); unaffected by hepatic or renal failure	Also used for muscle relaxation during intensive care; a complex mixture of 10 isomers; cardiovascular effects due to histamine release
Cisatracurium	Spontaneous degradation (0.5 h); unaffected by hepatic or renal failure	Also used for muscle relaxation during intensive care; a single isomer of atracurium; does not cause histamine release
Mivacurium	Hydrolysed by pseudocholinesterase (2–60 min); prolonged effect in rare individuals with genetic deficiency of this enzyme	Consists of three isomers, two of which are responsible for the clinical response
Pancuronium	Hydrolysed to an active product (0.5 h); eliminated by renal and biliary routes	Often used for long-term muscle relaxation during mechanical ventilation in intensive care; sympathomimetic effects can cause tachycardia and hypertension
Rocuronium	Hepatic metabolism and renal elimination (1.2 h)	Also used for muscle relaxation during intensive care; most rapid onset of action of drugs in this class; minimal cardiovascular effects
Vecuronium	Hepatic metabolism; biliary excretion (1 h)	Lacks cardiovascular effects
Depolarising blocker		
Suxamethonium (succinylcholine)	Hydrolysed by pseudocholinesterase (2–5 min); prolonged effect in the rare individuals with genetic deficiency of this enzyme	Given intravenously for blockade of rapid onset and short duration of action (e.g. intubation); paralysis preceded by painful fasciculations.

28 Myasthenia gravis

Myasthenia gravis is a comparatively rare autoimmune disease in which there is an autoantibody to the acetylcholine nicotinic N_2 receptor system. The autoantibody can impair the responsiveness of the neuromuscular junction to acetylcholine (ACh; Ch. 27) by three distinct mechanisms:

- increased receptor destruction by complement binding,
- crosslinking of receptors, which causes increased receptor internalisation,
- receptor blockade by steric hindrance.

The result is that fewer functional receptors are available for ACh, which is therefore less likely to depolarise the muscle cell sufficiently to reach its threshold firing potential. Consequently, in myasthenia gravis there is skeletal muscle weakness. In healthy skeletal muscle, repetitive nerve stimulation leads to a reduction in the numbers of sensitive receptors, but this causes no physiological reduction in muscle activity due to the large number of spare receptors. However, in myasthenia gravis, with repetitive stimulation the smaller receptor pool reduces receptor availability to a level at which increasing numbers of muscle fibres fail to fire. This produces the characteristic rapid muscle fatigue on exertion. The earliest symptoms of myasthenia gravis are often diplopia, which arises from weakness of the extraocular muscles, or ptosis. In 85% of cases the symptoms progress to involve many other muscle groups, particularly producing bulbar, facial and proximal limb weakness.

The thymus gland plays a part in the genesis of the immune response in myasthenia gravis, although its precise role remains uncertain. About 80% of people with myasthenia gravis have an abnormality in the thymus, which is usually lymphoreticular hyperplasia if the onset of the condition is at an early age or a thymoma if the onset is over the age of 40 years.

Symptomatic treatment of the weakness in myasthenia gravis is achieved by prolongation of the action of ACh through inhibiting acetylcholinesterase, the enzyme responsible for its hydrolysis. However, immunosuppression is also important for disease control.

ACETYLCHOLINESTERASE INHIBITORS

Examples

edrophonium, neostigmine, pyridostigmine

MECHANISM OF ACTION AND EFFECTS

Acetylcholinesterase (AChE) inhibitors block the breakdown of ACh released from presynaptic neurons. Details of their mechanisms of action are found in Chapter 4. They enhance the effect of ACh at all synaptic connections at which it is the neurotransmitter, but their therapeutic actions in myasthenia gravis are by increasing the longevity of ACh at nicotinic N_2 receptors (Ch. 4). Unwanted effects arise from the excessive actions of ACh at nicotinic N_1 receptors in autonomic ganglia and at muscarinic receptors in postganglionic nerve endings in the parasympathetic nervous system and in sweat glands in the sympathetic nervous system.

PHARMACOKINETICS AND CLINICAL USES

Neostigmine and pyridostigmine are quaternary amines that are slowly and incompletely absorbed from the gut. As a result, oral doses need to be approximately 10 times greater than parenteral doses to be effective. They have short elimination half-lives (1–2 h) due to a combination of renal tubular secretion and some hepatic metabolism. They do not readily cross the blood–brain barrier (see Ch. 9 for AChE inhibitors that cross the blood–brain barrier and are used in Alzheimer's disease). Both neostigmine and pyridostigmine can be used to treat myasthenia gravis, but pyridostigmine is preferred because of its longer duration of action. Neostigmine has a faster onset of action, and is also used by intravenous injection to reverse the effect of competitive neuromuscular blockers (Ch. 27).

Edrophonium has a very short duration of action (2–5 min), owing largely to rapid tissue distribution. It is given as an intravenous bolus to test the therapeutic response to AChE inhibitors in myasthenia gravis (see below) but is of no value in treatment.

UNWANTED EFFECTS

Unwanted effects arise because the AChE inhibitors are effective at all sites where ACh is released. They are experienced by up to one-third of people treated and are more

troublesome with neostigmine than with pyridostigmine. Peripheral muscarinic receptor agonist effects, which can be blocked by co-administration of a muscarinic receptor antagonist such as propantheline, include:

- diarrhoea, abdominal cramps, excessive salivation,
- bradycardia, hypotension (uncommon),
- miosis and lacrimation,
- bronchoconstriction (see Ch. 12),
- nausea.

Excessive dosage of AChE inhibitors will lead to a depolarising neuromuscular blockade by ACh. Initially there may be muscle twitching and cramps, followed by weakness through the build-up of excess ACh (see below).

MANAGEMENT OF MYASTHENIA GRAVIS

DIAGNOSIS

When the diagnosis of myasthenia gravis is suspected, useful diagnostic information can be obtained rapidly by pharmacological testing. In untreated people with myasthenia an intravenous injection of the short-acting AChE inhibitor edrophonium will produce clinical improvement within 1 min that lasts for about 5 min. Detection of circulating N_2 receptor antibodies, and electromyographic tests that demonstrate abnormal fatigability in multiple muscle fibres, are used to confirm the diagnosis.

TREATMENT

Symptomatic treatment of myasthenia gravis is with an AChE inhibitor, which inhibits the normal rapid breakdown of ACh and thereby enhances the activity of ACh released by nerve stimulation. Pyridostigmine is commonly used since its action is more consistent than that of neostigmine, the dosing frequency is less, and there are fewer muscarinic unwanted effects. The onset of action of pyridostigmine is after about 30–45 min with a duration of action of 3–6 h. An antimuscarinic agent (such as propantheline) may be necessary to block any parasympathomimetic actions of pyridostigmine, especially if large doses are given. The type of interaction between the autoantibody and the receptor probably determines the effectiveness of treatment in an individual. Some individuals do not respond well to AChE inhibitors, while unwanted effects may preclude the use of adequate doses in others. In addition, muscle groups do not all respond equally well to AChE inhibitors; ptosis and diplopia are the most resistant to treatment.

Excessive dosage of an AChE inhibitor can lead to prolonged stimulation of the N_2 receptors by ACh, resulting in a depolarising blockade of the neuromuscular junction similar to that produced by suxamethonium (succinylcholine; Ch. 27). Therefore, muscle weakness in myasthenia gravis can be the result of either inadequate dosage ('myasthenic crisis') or excessive dosage ('cholinergic crisis') with an AChE inhibitor. The safest way to distinguish these problems is to use assisted ventilation and temporarily withdraw the AChE inhibitor.

Generalised myasthenia is usually treated by immunosuppression with a corticosteroid such as prednisolone (Ch. 44). Corticosteroids are also used for those who are severely ill. They probably act by suppressing T-cell proliferation and reducing antibody synthesis. Initial high-dose corticosteroid therapy can make the weakness worse, particularly in the first few hours, possibly due to a direct effect on neuromuscular transmission. A clinical response is usually apparent after one month, but maximum benefit is delayed for up to 9 months. Ciclosporin (alone or with a corticosteroid) or cyclophosphamide with a corticosteroid (Ch. 38) are used if there is a poor response to a corticosteroid alone, but the dosage of ciclosporin is usually limited by nephrotoxicity. Long-term immunosuppression is usually necessary, since relapse frequently occurs on withdrawal of therapy.

Plasma exchange to remove circulating ACh receptor antibodies can produce a short-term response in severe disease. With repeated plasma exchanges improvement is seen after one day, with a maximum response after 1–2 weeks that is sustained for 2–8 weeks. An alternative is the use of intravenous immunoglobulin, of which IgG is the active component. It produces improvement after about 4 days, and an optimal response after 1–2 weeks that is sustained for 6–15 weeks. Immunoglobulin treatment is usually better tolerated than plasma exchange.

Thymectomy can induce remission in myasthenia gravis, although this can be delayed for up to five years. It is most effective for early onset disease with lymphoreticular hyperplasia and positive receptor antibodies, when it produces complete remission within five years in about 40% and significant improvement in a further 35%. Thymectomy is also used to remove a thymoma, although the clinical benefit is often less clear-cut.

Some drugs can interfere with neuromuscular transmission and exacerbate the symptoms of myasthenia gravis. Those most often implicated include aminoglycoside antibiotics (Ch. 51), β-adrenoceptor antagonists (Ch. 5), phenytoin (Ch. 23), chloroquine and penicillamine (Ch. 30). There is also altered sensitivity to neuromuscular junction blockers, with increased response to competitive (nondepolarising) neuromuscular junction blockers but resistance to depolarising neuromuscular junction blockers (Ch. 27).

LAMBERT–EATON MYASTHENIC SYNDROME

Lambert–Eaton myasthenic syndrome (LEMS) is a clinical syndrome that resembles myasthenia gravis. It is often a paraneoplastic syndrome, with about 60% associated with malignancy (often small-cell lung cancer). LEMS is caused by antibodies to P/Q-type voltage-gated Ca^{2+} channels on the presynaptic membrane of motor nerves at the neuromuscular junction. These channels are responsible for Ca^{2+} influx into the neuron that initiates ACh release. LEMS presents with leg and arm weakness and autonomic disturbance such as postural hypotension. While it can involve bulbar muscles, eye muscles are less often affected.

When LEMS is related to cancer, treatment of the malignancy leads to resolution. The potassium channel blocker amifampridine is the first choice drug for symptom relief. It delays repolarisation of the nerve terminal after an action potential giving more time for Ca^{2+} to accumulate in the neuron, and the prolonged depolarisation allows greater ACh release. Pyridostigmine can help the symptoms by prolonging the action of released ACh at the motor end plate. Immunosuppression is relatively ineffective in the treatment of LEMS.

SELF-ASSESSMENT

True/false questions

1. In myasthenia gravis autoantibodies develop to nicotinic N_1 receptors.
2. Acetylcholinesterase inhibitors may cause bronchoconstriction.
3. Pyridostigmine produces fewer muscarinic effects than neostigmine.
4. In myasthenia gravis there is increased sensitivity to suxamethonium.
5. A cholinergic crisis should be confirmed by giving pyridostigmine.

One-best-answer (OBA) question

Which statement about myasthenia gravis is the *most accurate*?

A. People diagnosed with myasthenia gravis invariably have a thymoma.
B. Acetylcholinesterase (AChE) inhibitors must cross the blood–brain barrier to be effective in treating myasthenia gravis.
C. Glucocorticoids can be of benefit in myasthenia gravis because of their anti-inflammatory actions.
D. The unwanted effects of AChE inhibitors include diarrhoea, urination, miosis, bradycardia, nausea, lacrimation and salivation.
E. Plasmapheresis reduces plasma levels of pseudocholinesterase, thereby reducing breakdown of acetylcholine.

Case-based questions

A 35-year-old woman with no previous illness noticed that she had ptosis and occasional diplopia. Over a period of time she became aware that she suffered from leg weakness on exertion, although her coordination was normal. Following a sustained upward gaze for a minute, ptosis and diplopia could be elicited. Myasthenia gravis was suspected.

A. What tests should be performed to verify the diagnosis?
B. What is the pathogenesis of myasthenia gravis?
C. Why is edrophonium injection used as a test for myasthenia gravis?
D. If myasthenia gravis is confirmed, what principles should treatment follow?

True/false answers

1. **False.** Skeletal muscle weakness in myasthenia gravis is due to autoimmunity to nicotinic N_2 receptors in the neuromuscular junction.
2. **True.** Increased ACh at muscarinic receptors in the parasympathetic nervous system can cause bronchoconstriction; such effects can be blocked with antimuscarinic drugs such as propantheline.
3. **True.** Neostigmine has greater potency and a shorter duration of action than pyridostigmine so is more likely to cause muscarinic effects; pyridostigmine is therefore preferred in the treatment of myasthenia gravis.
4. **False.** Due to the loss of nicotinic N_2 receptor function people with myasthenia gravis are less sensitive to the depolarising neuromuscular junction blocker suxamethonium but more sensitive to competitive blockers such as vecuronium.
5. **False.** The cholinergic crisis results from the excessive effects of an AChE inhibitor and would be exacerbated by the long-acting pyridostigmine; assisted ventilation and withdrawal of the treatment should be performed.

OBA answer

Answer D is the most accurate.

A. Incorrect. About 15% have a thymoma and 60–80% have hyperplasia of the thymus.
B. Incorrect. The main anticholinesterases used in treating myasthenia gravis are quaternary amines and do not cross the blood–brain barrier; they act at the neuromuscular junction.
C. Incorrect. Glucocorticoids work by suppressing production of autoantibodies to nicotinic N_2 receptors.
D. **Correct.** These parasympathomimetic effects are caused by excess ACh activity at muscarinic receptors.
E. Incorrect. Plasmapheresis reduces the levels of circulating autoantibodies to nicotinic N_2 receptors.

Case-based answers

A. Tests include electromyography (Jolly test), single muscle fibre electromyography (SFEMG), anti-acetylcholine receptor (AChR) antibody titres and injection of a short-acting inhibitor of AChE (the Tensilon test, named after the proprietary name of edrophonium).
B. Autoantibody blocks nicotinic N_2 receptors; receptors are destroyed by complement activation and receptors are crosslinked, which causes them to be destroyed more rapidly. The decrease in functional receptors impairs motor endplate potentials and reduces the likelihood of the muscle contracting.
C. It is short-acting, giving an improvement in muscle strength within 30–60 s, subsiding in 4–5 min.
D. An AChE inhibitor, most commonly pyridostigmine, is used for symptomatic treatment; an antimuscarinic drug may be needed to reduce unwanted effects. Immunosuppression may be required with a corticosteroid, or with immunosuppressants such as ciclosporin or azathioprine. Plasmapheresis, intravenous immunoglobulins or thymectomy may also be considered.

FURTHER READING

Conti-Fine BM, Milani M, Kaminski HJ (2006) Myasthenia gravis: past, present, and future. *J Clin Invest* 116, 2843–2854

Hart IK, Sathasivam S, Sharshar T (2007) Immunosuppressive agents for myasthenia gravis. *Cochrane Database Syst Rev* 4, CD005224

Newsom-Davis J (2003) Therapy in myasthenia gravis and Lambert–Eaton myasthenic syndrome. *Semin Neurol* 23, 191–197

Schwendimann RN, Burton E, Minagar A (2005) Management of myasthenia gravis. *Am J Ther* 12, 262–268

Compendium: acetylcholinesterase inhibitors used in myasthenia gravis

Drug	Kinetics (half-life)	Comments
Distigmine	Very poor oral bioavailability (<5%), especially if taken with food; hydrolysed by plasma esterases with renal excretion (70 h)	Rarely used due to risk of accumulation causing cholinergic crisis; used for urinary retention (Ch. 15); given orally
Edrophonium	Kinetics poorly defined, but mainly renal elimination (1.8 h)	Very short duration of action (<5 min); mainly used for diagnosis; given intravenous over 30 s; not given orally
Neostigmine	Very low oral bioavailability (1–2%); absorption delayed by food; elimination after intravenous dosage (0.4–1.7 h) probably slower after oral dosage; metabolised by plasma and hepatic esterases	Given orally or by subcutaneous or intravenous injection
Pyridostigmine	Low oral bioavailability (10–20%); absorption delayed by food; elimination after intravenous dosage (0.4–1.9 h) probably slower after oral dosage; mainly excreted in the urine unchanged; longer-acting than neostigmine	Given orally

Drug used for Lambert–Easton myasthenic syndrome (LEMS)

Drug	Kinetics (half-life)	Comments
Amifampridine	Hepatic metabolism (6 h)	Acetylcholine release enhancer; specialist use for symptomatic LEMS; given orally

29

Non-steroidal anti-inflammatory drugs

● ●

THE ROLE OF COX ENZYMES IN THE ACTIONS OF NSAIDS

The major therapeutic and unwanted actions of non-steroidal anti-inflammatory drugs (NSAIDs) are achieved by inhibition of cyclo-oxygenase (COX) enzymes. COX enzymes are essential in the production of the prostanoids (prostaglandins, prostacyclins and thromboxanes), the most active of which are generated from the 20-carbon, polyunsaturated (ω-6) fatty acid arachidonic acid (Fig. 29.1). Arachidonic acid can also be converted via the 5-lipoxygenase pathway to leukotrienes, some of the actions of which are blocked by leukotriene receptor antagonists (Ch. 12). These classic eicosanoid families are local mediators that are generally synthesised and catabolised close to their site of action, and have numerous physiological actions. Arachidonic acid and other essential fatty acids are also the precursors of novel families of lipid mediators including lipoxins, resolvins, protectins, hepoxilins and endocannabinoids.

Arachidonic acid is mostly derived from dietary linoleic acid, which is found in vegetable oils such as sunflower oil. Linoleic acid is converted in the liver in several steps to arachidonic acid, which is then incorporated into glycerophospholipids in cell membranes. Arachidonic acid is released from membrane phospholipids by lipases such as phospholipase A_2. In the COX pathways, the initial products of arachidonic acid metabolism are unstable intermediates known as cyclic endoperoxides. These are converted by cell-specific synthases and isomerases to various receptor-active prostanoids (Fig. 29.1). The products of the COX pathway therefore differ among various tissues depending upon the synthases present, generating a diverse range of actions tailored to the individual requirements of each cell type. Most cell types can form different prostanoids simultaneously and in different quantities, with the pattern of production modulated by regulatory influences on the cell.

There are three COX isoenzymes: COX-1, COX-2 and COX-3. COX-1 is constitutively expressed in the endoplasmic reticulum of most cell types. Prostanoids generated via the COX-1 enzyme are produced in small amounts by many cells in the resting state and contribute to the regulation of several homeostatic processes such as renal and gastric blood flow, gastric cytoprotection and platelet aggregation (Table 29.1). COX-2 is present in greater concentrations in the nuclear envelope than in the endoplasmic reticulum. It is found in many cells such as endothelial cells, macrophages, synovial fibroblasts, mast cells, chondrocytes and osteoblasts. Its expression in these cells is induced by cytokines and other inflammatory stimuli, so that COX-2-derived prostanoids are formed in large amounts in response to inflammation, pain and fever. However, the concept that there is only a pathological role for inducible COX-2-derived prostanoids and a 'housekeeping' physiological role for the constitutive COX-1 enzyme is now recognised as too simplistic. In many organs, particularly the kidney, central nervous system (CNS), cardiovascular system and reproductive system, there is no clear separation between the functions of COX-1 and COX-2. Either isoform may be involved in the production of 'physiological' or 'pathological' prostanoids (Table 29.1).

COX-3 is a splice variant of COX-1 that retains the entire COX-1 transcript and has an additional conserved intronic sequence. It is mainly expressed in the brain and spinal cord and to a lesser extent in the heart, endothelial cells and monocytes. COX-3 may have a role in pain perception, but its precise functions are uncertain.

The actions of prostaglandins and thromboxanes depend upon the circumstances and site of their formation, and whether they are formed in excessive amounts. For example, prostaglandin E_2 (PGE_2) is generated in low physiological amounts by COX-1 in gastric mucosa where it is important for maintaining mucosal integrity by a variety of mechanisms, including bicarbonate and mucus production and maintaining mucosal blood flow. In contrast, damage to many tissues leads to increased PGE_2 synthesis via enhanced COX-2 expression. This contributes to inflammation and pain by vasodilation, increased vascular permeability and sensitisation of pain fibre nerve endings to the nociceptive action of bradykinin, serotonin and other mediators (Ch. 19). However, in the later stages of repair following tissue damage, COX-2-derived prostanoids may contribute to the processes of wound healing.

Prostanoids act via five main classes of G-protein-coupled receptors on cell surfaces (Fig. 29.1). Some of the actions of prostaglandins are shown in Table 29.2.

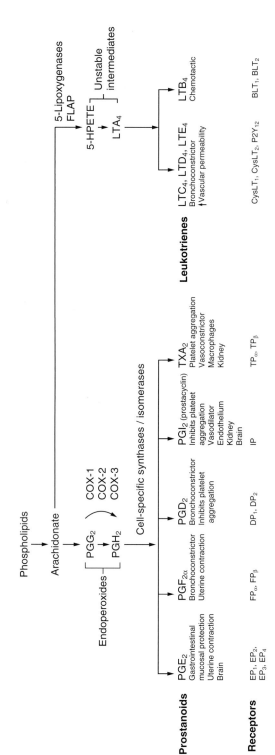

Fig. 29.1 The arachidonic acid cascade of eicosanoid synthesis. Arachidonic acid liberated from membrane phospholipids can be utilised by cyclo-oxygenases (COX-1, COX-2, COX-3) to form prostanoids (prostaglandins, prostacyclin and thromboxane) or by the 5-lipoxygenase pathway to form leukotrienes. The types and amounts of these eicosanoid products that are generated depend on the relative expression of the COX isozymes, 5-lipoxygenase and their respective downstream synthases in different cell types. After release from the cell, the eicosanoids have a multitude of actions via their selective G-protein-coupled receptors on the surface of target cells, such as bronchial, uterine and vascular smooth muscle cells, endothelial cells, platelets and leucocytes (Table 29.2). FLAP, five-lipoxygenase activating protein; 5-HPETE, 5-hydroperoxyeicosatetraenoic acid; LT, leukotriene; PG, prostaglandin; TX, thromboxane.

Table 29.1 Some biological roles of cyclo-oxygenase (COX) 1 and 2

COX-1 homeostatic roles	COX-2 homeostatic roles
Gastrointestinal protection	Renal function
Platelet aggregation	CNS function
Blood flow regulation	Tissue repair and healing (including gastrointestinal)
CNS function	Reproduction
	Uterine contraction
	Blood vessel dilation
	Pancreas
	Inhibition of platelet aggregation
	Airways
COX-1 pathological roles	**COX-2 pathological roles**
(Possible involvement in inflammation)	Inflammation
Chronic pain	Chronic pain
Raised blood pressure	Fever
	Blood vessel permeability
	Reproduction
	Alzheimer's disease
	Angiogenesis, inhibition of apoptosis
	Tumour cell growth

The second route for arachidonic acid metabolism is via the 5-lipoxygenase pathway to produce leukotrienes (Fig. 29.1). These are also involved in the inflammatory process by enhancing vascular permeability and smooth muscle contraction (particularly the cysteinyl-leukotrienes LTC_4, LTD_4 and LTE_4; see also Ch. 12) and through chemotactic attraction of leucocytes (particularly LTB_4) (Table 29.2).

NSAIDS

NSAIDs have three major therapeutic activities: anti-inflammatory, analgesic and antipyretic.

MECHANISMS OF ACTION

All NSAIDs share a common mode of action by inhibition of the COX isoenzymes (Table 29.3). Most NSAIDs bind reversibly to the site in the COX enzymes that accepts arachidonic acid, but the irreversible inactivation produced by aspirin (acetylsalicylic acid) involves acetylation of a serine residue in the enzyme. This mechanism of action is important in the use of aspirin as an antiplatelet drug (see below and Ch. 11).

Different NSAIDs inhibit the two main isoenzymes (COX-1 and COX-2) to varying extents. The degree of COX selectivity of each NSAID will also depend on the dosage used. The clinical responses and unwanted effect profiles of individual NSAIDs reflect the ability of the drug to inhibit the diverse biological actions of each isoenzyme (Tables 29.1 and 29.2). Highly selective inhibitors of COX-2 (coxibs) have been developed with the aim of reducing the unwanted effects associated with concomitant inhibition of COX-1 by the non-selective NSAIDs (see below). Neither the non-selective NSAIDs nor the selective COX-2 inhibitors directly affect the production of leukotrienes by 5-lipoxygenase. However, PGE_2 normally inhibits leukotriene synthesis and reduced PGE_2 generation as a consequence of NSAID use may increase leukotriene synthesis.

NSAIDs have additional anti-inflammatory effects that appear to be independent of COX inhibition. These effects may be mediated by actions on peroxisome proliferator-activated receptors (PPARs), particularly PPAR-γ. PPARs have key roles in modulating immune responses by suppressing transcription of pro-inflammatory genes, such as those encoding tumour necrosis factor α (TNFα), interleukin-1 (IL-1) and inducible nitric oxide synthase (iNOS) in macrophages. NSAIDs also have complex effects on lymphocytes, including inhibition of T-cell activation and increased T-cell apoptosis, which may reflect PPAR-mediated actions. NSAIDs may also modulate inflammatory gene transcription via actions on the nuclear transcription factor nuclear factor κB (NF-κB) and on other cell-signalling proteins including mitogen-activated protein (MAP) kinases. Some of these COX-independent actions only occur *in vitro* at NSAID concentrations higher than those required for anti-inflammatory activity or analgesia *in vivo*, and their clinical relevance remains to be determined.

CLASSIFICATION OF NSAIDS

Table 29.3 shows the principal chemical types of NSAIDs with an indication of their selectivity in inhibiting COX-1 or COX-2. Many classical NSAIDs produce greater inhibition of COX-1 than of COX-2, although at clinical doses this selectivity may not be apparent and both isoenzymes will be effectively inhibited. The coxibs are highly selective inhibitors of COX-2 at clinical doses.

ACTIONS AND EFFECTS OF NON-SELECTIVE NSAIDS

Some of the properties and actions of a selection of commonly used analgesic drugs are compared in Table 29.4.

Analgesic effect

The analgesic action of NSAIDs is in part a peripheral action at the site of pain and is most effective when the pain has an inflammatory origin (see Ch. 19). It is achieved predominantly through inhibition of COX-2-derived prostaglandins in inflamed or injured tissues. The main pain-inducing action of prostanoids is at sensory nerve endings on first-order

Table 29.2 Main biological actions of the eicosanoids

Tissue	Effect	Eicosanoid
Platelets	Increased aggregation	TXA_2
	Decreased aggregation	PGI_2, PGD_2
Vascular smooth muscle	Vasodilation	PGI_2, PGE_2, PGD_2
	Vasoconstriction	TXA_2, LTC_4, LTD_4
Other smooth muscle	Bronchodilation	PGE_2
	Bronchoconstriction	LTC_4, LTD_4, LTE_4, PGD_2, PGF_2, TXA_2
	Gastrointestinal tract (contraction/relaxation, depends on muscle type)	PGF_2, PGE_2, PGI_2, PGD_2
	Uterine contraction	PGE_2, $PGF_{2\alpha}$
Vascular endothelium	Increased permeability	LTC_4, LTD_4, LTB_4
	Potentiates histamine/bradykinin	PGE_2, PGI_2
Leucocytes	Chemotaxis of neutrophils, monocytes, lymphocytes	LTB_4
	Chemotaxis of eosinophils, basophils	LTE_4, PGD_2
Gastrointestinal mucosa	Reduced acid secretion	PGE_2, PGI_2
	Increased mucus secretion	PGE_2
	Increased blood flow	PGE_2, PGI_2
Nervous system	Inhibition of noradrenaline release	PGD_2, PGE_2, PGI_2
	Endogenous pyrogen in hypothalamus	PGE_2
	Sedation, sleep	PGD_2
Endocrine/metabolic	Secretion of ACTH, GH, prolactin, gonadotrophins	PGE_2
	Inhibition of lipolysis	PGE_2
Kidney	Increased renal blood flow	PGE_2, PGI_2
	Antagonism of ADH	PGE_2
	Renin release	PGI_2, PGE_2, PGD_2
Pain	Potentiates pain through bradykinin, serotonin	PGE_2, PGD_2

Only the main eicosanoids are shown. Inhibition of COX isoenzymes by NSAIDs reduces the synthesis only of prostanoids. Synthesis of leukotrienes is reduced by 5-lipoxygenase inhibitors (zileuton, not available in UK). Antagonists of the cysteinyl-leukotriene (LTC_4, LTD_4, LTE_4) receptor 1 are used in asthma prophylaxis (Ch. 12).
ACTH, adrenocorticotrophic hormone (corticotropin); ADH, antidiuretic hormone (vasopressin); GH, growth hormone; LT, leukotriene; PG, prostaglandin; TX, thromboxane.

neurons in peripheral tissues. PGE_2 enhances the ability of several mediators (serotonin, substance P, bradykinin) to stimulate $A\delta$ and C nociceptive fibres. There is also a CNS component to the analgesic action of NSAIDs which is due to inhibition of COX isoenzymes and reduction of prostaglandin production within the CNS pain pathways. COX inhibition decreases PGE_2 production in the dorsal horn of the spinal cord, which inhibits neurotransmitter release and reduces the excitability of second-order neurons in the pain relay pathway. The analgesic action of NSAIDs is apparent after the first dose, but does not reach its maximal effect until about 1 week with repeated dosing.

Anti-inflammatory effect

Inhibition of vasodilation and oedema is partly related to a reduction in peripheral COX-2-generated prostaglandin synthesis. However, NSAIDs also affect several other inflammatory processes unrelated to their effects on prostaglandins. For example, they probably reduce harmful superoxide free radical generation by neutrophils. They may also uncouple G-protein-regulated processes in the cell membrane of inflammatory cells, which reduces their responsiveness to a variety of agonists released by damaged tissues. The anti-inflammatory effects of NSAIDs develop gradually over about 3 weeks.

Antipyretic effect

Fever is reduced through inhibition of hypothalamic COX-2. Circulating pyrogens such as interleukin-1 enhance PGE_2 production in the hypothalamus, which depresses the response of temperature-sensitive neurons. NSAIDs do not affect normal body temperature.

Table 29.3 Selectivity of some NSAIDs for inhibition of COX-1 compared with COX-2

Drug	Class	
Flurbiprofen	Propionic acid	Increasing selectivity for inhibition of COX-1 compared with COX-2
Ketoprofen	Propionic acid	
Ketorolac	Heterocyclic acetic acid	
Aspirin	Salicylate	
Indometacin	Indole	
Ibuprofen	Propionic acid	
Naproxen	Propionic acid	
Fenoprofen	Propionic acid	Approximately equal inhibition of COX-1 and COX-2
Salicylate	Salicylate	
Meloxicam	Enolic acid	
Piroxicam	Enolic acid	
Sulindac	Indole	
Diclofenac	Phenyl acetic acid	
Celecoxib	Sulphonamide (coxib)	Increasing selectivity for inhibition of COX-2 compared with COX-1
Etoricoxib	Bipyridine (coxib)	

Table 29.4 Properties of some commonly used analgesic drugs

	Aspirin (moderate doses)	Paracetamol	Indometacin	Ibuprofen	Celecoxib
Analgesic	++	++	++	+	+
Anti-inflammatory	+	−	+++	+	+
Antipyretic	+	+	+	+	+
Gastrointestinal bleeding	+	−	+	Low	Low

Reduction of platelet aggregation

This action is mediated by inhibition of the synthesis of thromboxane A_2 (TXA_2), a potent platelet-aggregating agent, by platelet COX-1 (Ch. 11). This effect is most marked for aspirin, because it has an irreversible action on COX, and platelets are unable to synthesise more enzyme during their life span. The reversible action of most other NSAIDs produces weaker platelet inhibition (with the exception of naproxen), and selective COX-2 inhibitors do not inhibit platelet aggregation (Table 29.3).

PHARMACOKINETICS

Most NSAIDs are weak acids that undergo some absorption from the stomach due to pH partitioning (Ch. 2). This explains the relatively high drug concentration in cells of the gastric mucosa. However, the majority of the drug is absorbed via the larger surface area of the small bowel.

Absorption of NSAIDs from the gut is usually fairly rapid from conventional formulations. Some NSAIDs with short half-lives, such as diclofenac, are available as modified-release formulations to prolong their duration of action. Certain NSAIDs can be given by intramuscular or intravenous injection for rapid onset of postoperative analgesia (such as ketorolac), or rectally to achieve a prolonged action (such as diclofenac and ketoprofen). Transcutaneous delivery of several NSAIDs, usually as a gel formulation, was introduced with the intention of providing high local drug concentrations while attempting to minimise systemic unwanted effects. However, once the drug has penetrated the skin it is widely distributed, and this route has little advantage for reducing systemic toxicity.

Most NSAIDs undergo hepatic metabolism to inactive compounds and differ widely in their elimination half-lives.

Short-acting drugs require frequent dosing to maintain continuous therapeutic effect, although synovial fluid concentrations in joint disease fluctuate less than the plasma concentrations. Piroxicam undergoes enterohepatic cycling, which contributes to its long half-life.

Aspirin (acetylsalicylic acid) is initially converted to an active metabolite, salicylic acid, and finally inactivated by conjugation with glycine and, to some extent, glucuronic acid. Conjugation with glycine is saturable at higher doses and the metabolism of salicylate then changes from first-order to zero-order elimination kinetics (Ch. 2). This has important implications for aspirin overdose (Ch. 53).

UNWANTED EFFECTS

Most unwanted effects arise in part from the inhibition of prostaglandin synthesis throughout the body. They are usually dose-related.

Gastrointestinal effects

- Nausea, dyspepsia, gastric irritation and gastric ulceration are the most frequent unwanted effects. They occur principally as a result of inhibition of mucosal production of COX-1-generated PGE_2 and PGI_2, although inhibition of COX-2 may interfere with some aspects of tissue healing. PGE_2 has several actions that confer cytoprotection in the stomach (Ch. 33). There are many mechanisms by which NSAIDs cause gastric irritation, as follows.
  - Mucus secretion and bicarbonate secretion are reduced and acid secretion is increased as a result of inhibition of prostaglandin synthesis
  - Inhibition of prostaglandin synthesis also reduces mucosal blood flow, which probably enhances cytotoxicity by producing tissue hypoxia and enhanced local generation of free radicals.
  - The mucus gel layer is rendered less hydrophobic due to the acidic nature of NSAIDs and their local concentration in gastric mucosal cells; this reduces the barrier effect of the surface layer.
  - Uncoupling of cellular oxidative phosphorylation by NSAIDs increases mucosal cell permeability, with consequent back-diffusion of H^+ ions, which are trapped in the mucosal epithelium and lead to cytotoxicity.

  NSAIDs accumulate within gastric mucosal cells by direct absorption of the drug from the gastric lumen and also by systemic delivery of the drug to the mucosa. Consequently, rectal or transdermal administration or the use of a prodrug may reduce, but will not eliminate, the risk of gastric damage. Occult blood loss from the bowel is increased during regular treatment with NSAIDs and the risk of overt gastrointestinal bleeding is greater. The highest risk of gastrointestinal bleeding is with piroxicam and ketoprofen, while indometacin, diclofenac and naproxen carry an intermediate risk. Ibuprofen has the lowest risk. Management of NSAID-induced gastric damage is considered in Chapter 33.
- Exacerbation of inflammatory bowel disease (Ch. 34).
- Lower gastrointestinal bleeding or perforation.
- Local irritation and bleeding from rectal administration.

Renal effects

- NSAIDs can produce a reversible decline in renal function, with a rise in serum creatinine. Inhibition of prostaglandins (PGE_2, PGI_2) generated by both COX-1 and COX-2 reduces renal medullary blood flow (Ch. 14). An effect of NSAIDs on renal function is more likely if there is underlying chronic kidney disease (as is often the case in the elderly). There is also an increased risk in the presence of heart failure or cirrhosis, conditions that are associated with reduced effective circulating blood volume, when prostaglandins play a greater role in the maintenance of renal blood flow. NSAIDs are the second most common cause of drug-induced acute kidney injury after aminoglycoside antimicrobials, and this most often occurs during the first few weeks of treatment.
- NSAIDs can produce renal salt and water retention even when renal function is normal. Reduced prostaglandin synthesis in the ascending limb of the loop of Henle increases expression of the $Na^+/K^+/2Cl^-$ co-transporter complex, and prostaglandins antagonise the action of vasopressin (antidiuretic hormone, ADH; see Ch. 14). Water retention due to the unopposed action of ADH may exceed retention of Na^+, resulting in dilutional hyponatraemia. Salt and water retention produced by NSAIDs can exacerbate heart failure and raises blood pressure by an average of 3–5 mmHg. In addition, the efficacy of drug treatments for these conditions (e.g. diuretics, angiotensin-converting enzyme inhibitors, β-adrenoceptor antagonists) is blunted by NSAIDs.
- Suppression of prostaglandin-mediated renin secretion by NSAIDs can lead to hypoaldosteronism and hyperkalaemia.
- Acute interstitial nephritis is a less common cause of renal impairment and can occur with any NSAID. It often becomes apparent after many months of NSAID use.

Hypersensitivity

Hypersensitivity reactions occasionally produce asthma, urticaria, angioedema and rhinitis. People with nasal polyps and known allergic disorders appear to be most susceptible. NSAIDs can also precipitate 'pseudo-allergic' asthma in a subgroup of people with asthma, through inhibition of COX-1-generated PGE_2 production in the lung. PGE_2 has an inhibitory effect on leukotriene synthesis and mast cell degranulation. A reduction in PGE_2 leads to an increased synthesis of bronchoconstrictor cysteinyl-leukotrienes (LTC_4, LTD_4, LTE_4) (Ch. 12). It is suggested that as many as one in five people with asthma may be sensitive to NSAIDs.

Other unwanted effects

Other unwanted effects are unrelated to prostaglandin inhibition and are sometimes specific for individual compounds.

- CNS unwanted effects such as headache, dizziness, drowsiness, insomnia and confusion, particularly in the elderly.
- Rashes.
- Tinnitus in toxic doses; overdose of aspirin can be particularly hazardous (Ch. 53).

- Aspirin can cause Reye's syndrome in children, a rare condition producing acute encephalopathy and fatty degeneration of the liver. Aspirin should be avoided in children under the age of 12 years.
- The risk of myocardial infarction and stroke is increased by most NSAIDs, especially in people with known ischaemic heart disease or at high risk of a cardiovascular event. Naproxen may be associated with a lower risk than other NSAIDs.

COX-2-SELECTIVE INHIBITORS

 Examples

celecoxib, etoricoxib, parecoxib

Mechanism of action

Selective COX-2 inhibitors have less inhibitory action on COX-1, but the degree of selectivity for COX-2 varies among the drugs in this class. Selective COX-2 inhibitors have anti-inflammatory actions similar to conventional non-selective NSAIDs, but there is some evidence that they may be less effective analgesics. This may possibly be due to less inhibition of COX-3 in the brain and spinal cord. Selective COX-2 inhibitors have little direct effect on platelet TXA_2 production and do not impair platelet aggregation; however, they suppress the production of the anti-aggregatory and vasodilator PGI_2 by blood vessels, which may allow TXA_2 to exert unopposed aggregatory effects on platelets. Selective COX-2 inhibitors also interact with PPARs and impair macrophage activity and T-cell-mediated immune responses (see above).

Pharmacokinetics

Celecoxib and etoricoxib are well absorbed from the gut. They are eliminated by hepatic metabolism. The half-life of celecoxib is 11 h, while that of etoricoxib is longer (25 h). Parecoxib can be given by intramuscular or intravenous injection for control of postoperative pain and has a half-life of 5–9 h.

Unwanted effects

- COX-2-selective inhibitors produce fewer upper gastrointestinal unwanted effects, and celecoxib, but not etoricoxib, reduces the risk of ulcers and ulcer complications by up to 50% compared with conventional NSAIDs. However, if low-dose aspirin is taken concurrently for its antiplatelet benefit, this negates the gastrointestinal-sparing benefits of celecoxib.
- Exacerbation of inflammatory bowel disease (Ch. 34).
- Stomatitis or mouth ulcers.
- Fatigue, influenza-like symptoms.
- Palpitation.
- Selective COX-2 inhibitors rarely induce asthma attacks in NSAID-sensitive individuals.
- Selective COX-2 inhibitors increase the risk of myocardial infarction in people with known ischaemic heart disease or those who are at high risk of a cardiovascular event. The risk is similar to most non-selective NSAIDs.
- Renal effects, including salt and water retention and acute kidney injury, are similar for selective COX-2 inhibitors and non-selective NSAIDs.

PARACETAMOL

Mechanism of action

Paracetamol (acetaminophen in the USA) is an analgesic without anti-inflammatory activity and is not an NSAID. It has very little inhibitory effect on COX-1 or COX-2 in peripheral tissues. In the CNS, paracetamol inhibits COX-2 by reducing the availability of an essential co-substrate for the action of COX-2. In peripheral tissues, hydroperoxides generated during the metabolism of arachidonic acid by lipoxygenases may impair the action of paracetamol. There is weak inhibition of COX-3 in the CNS by paracetamol, but this may not be clinically important.

Other effects may contribute to the analgesic action of paracetamol, such as stimulation of spinal serotonergic neurotransmission via $5-HT_{1A}$ receptors and modulation of cannabinoid (CB_1) receptors (see also Ch. 19). Paracetamol is converted to a metabolite that inhibits neuronal reuptake of the endogenous cannabinoid anandamide. Anandamide acts at cannabinoid CB_1 receptors and transient receptor potential vanilloid 1 ($TRPV_1$) receptors, and high concentrations stimulate then desensitize the receptors in a similar manner to capsaicin (Ch.19). Lastly, a different metabolite of paracetamol (*N*-acetyl-*p*-benzoquinone imine, NAPQI) stimulates transient receptor potential ankyrin 1 ($TRPA_1$) receptors in the spinal cord, which inhibits voltage-gated Ca^{2+} and Na^+ channels in primary sensory neurons.

Pharmacokinetics

Paracetamol is rapidly absorbed from the gut. It is metabolised mainly by conjugation, but the minor metabolite NAPQI is produced by cytochrome P450 in the liver and kidneys. NAPQI is detoxified by a limited supply of glutathione in these organs. In paracetamol overdose, failure to conjugate this potentially toxic metabolite can lead to liver and renal damage (Ch. 53).

Unwanted effects

- Paracetamol is usually well tolerated, and because it does not inhibit peripheral prostaglandin synthesis it does not cause problems with homeostatic functions of prostanoids, for example gastrointestinal disturbances.
- Hepatic damage and renal failure in overdose (Ch. 53).

INDICATIONS FOR USING NSAIDS

NSAIDs are useful for pain relief, particularly for:

- inflammatory conditions affecting joints, soft tissues, etc.,
- postoperative pain,
- renal colic,

- headache,
- primary dysmenorrhoea; stimulation of the uterus by prostaglandins can be responsible for the pain in this condition.

About 60% of people will respond to any one NSAID, but those who fail to respond to one may derive benefit from another. Adequate time must be allowed for the full analgesic or anti-inflammatory effect to develop (see above). The initial choice of NSAID is mainly determined by unwanted effects, particularly on the stomach and the cardiovascular system. For these reasons, ibuprofen is often the NSAID of first choice.

NSAIDs are also used for other conditions not associated with pain:

- as an antipyretic in febrile conditions,
- to achieve closure of a patent ductus arteriosus in a neonate where patency may be inappropriately maintained by prostaglandin production; NSAIDs should not be given to a pregnant mother in the third trimester, to avoid premature closure of the ductus,
- for modest reduction of menstrual blood loss in menorrhagia (excessive blood loss at menstruation),
- for prevention of vascular occlusion by inhibition of platelet aggregation (low-dose aspirin; Ch. 11),
- aspirin and other NSAIDs reduce the risk of developing colorectal cancer, oesophageal and gastric cancer, breast cancer, bladder cancer and adenocarcinoma of the lung by about 30%. Aspirin also reduces the risk of metastasis from adenocarcinoma by 50%. The effect of NSAIDs may depend on inhibition of COX isoenzymes or actions on other nuclear transcription and cell signalling pathways that result in reduced cellular proliferation, migration and angiogenesis and enhanced apoptosis.

Selective COX-2 inhibitors should be used in preference to standard NSAIDs only in people who are at high risk of developing serious gastrointestinal adverse effects and when an NSAID is clearly indicated as part of the management.

SELF-ASSESSMENT

True/false questions

1. Three cyclo-oxygenase (COX) isoenzymes can synthesise prostanoids.
2. Gastrointestinal complications are the most common unwanted effects of NSAIDs.
3. COX-2 is not found constitutively in cells.
4. Prostaglandin E_2 (PGE_2) does not cause pain directly.
5. Non-steroidal anti-inflammatory drugs (NSAIDs) inhibit COX-1 and COX-2 isoenzymes with equal potency.
6. Paracetamol is a potent analgesic and anti-inflammatory drug.
7. Aspirin is a suitable analgesic for infants.
8. NSAIDs reduce gastric blood flow.
9. Celecoxib causes a greater incidence of gastrointestinal symptoms than naproxen.
10. Misoprostol reduces the gastric damage caused by diclofenac.

11. Antiplatelet doses of aspirin (75 mg per day) can compromise renal function.
12. The elderly have a greater risk of gastrointestinal adverse events when given NSAIDs.
13. Ibuprofen is an effective first-choice NSAID in severe rheumatoid arthritis.
14. Aspirin is a good choice of analgesic therapy for people with asthma.
15. Celecoxib is an antipyretic.
16. NSAIDs increase the risk of colorectal cancer.

Extended-matching-item questions

Choose the *most appropriate* NSAID from options A–E to be given initially in the case scenarios 1–3 below.

A. Aspirin
B. Celecoxib
C. Diclofenac plus misoprostol
D. Paracetamol
E. Indometacin

Case 1. An elderly man with a long history of hypertension, congestive heart failure with oedema, and chronic gastritis, has chronic mild knee pain, due to osteoarthritic changes. The pain is interrupting his sleep.

Case 2. A 38-year-old severely asthmatic woman with a history of nasal polyposis and recurrent dyspepsia, a diagnosis of rheumatoid arthritis and no history of heart disease.

Case 3. A 45-year-old man who recently had a myocardial infarction. He was prescribed an angiotensin-converting enzyme (ACE) inhibitor and simvastatin.

True/false answers

1. **True.** The isoenzymes are COX-1, COX-2 and COX-3 (a splice variant of COX-1).
2. **True.** Gastric irritation, ulceration and bleeding caused by inhibition of gastroprotective prostanoid synthesis are common unwanted effects of NSAID use.
3. **False.** COX-2 is present constitutively in some cells such as in blood vessels, but can be markedly induced in these cell types and others by cytokines and inflammatory stimuli.
4. **True.** PGE_2 generated by COX-2 does not directly stimulate sensory pain fibres but sensitises them to bradykinin and other mediators.
5. **False.** There is a wide range in the selectivity of NSAIDs for inhibition of COX-1 and COX-2. Their anti-inflammatory potency relates broadly to their potency in inhibiting COX-2, and their unwanted gastrointestinal effects to their potency in inhibiting COX-1.
6. **False.** Paracetamol is analgesic and antipyretic but has only a weak anti-inflammatory effect. The reasons for this are imperfectly understood but it may act by COX-independent mechanisms on pain pathways within the CNS.
7. **False.** Aspirin can precipitate Reye's syndrome and should not be used in children under 12 years old.
8. **True.** Reduced blood flow contributes to the gastric damage caused by NSAIDs; they also inhibit bicarbonate and mucus secretion.

9. **False.** The COX-2-selective inhibitor celecoxib is associated with fewer gastrointestinal unwanted effects than the non-selective NSAID naproxen, although this difference declines with continued use.

10. **True.** Misoprostol is a PGE_1 analogue, also available in combination formulations with diclofenac or naproxen; its use can limit the risk of gastric damage by restoring gastroprotective prostanoid activity.

11. **False.** Low doses of aspirin are safe, but long-term use of high doses can result in renal ischaemia, sodium and water retention, papillary necrosis and chronic renal failure.

12. **True.** Gastrointestinal unwanted effects are particularly common in those over 75 years of age and in those with a history of peptic ulcer.

13. **False.** Ibuprofen is effective in mild-to-moderate arthritis but other NSAIDs such as indometacin or diclofenac have greater anti-inflammatory potential, although a greater propensity to cause unwanted effects.

14. **False.** In a subgroup of people with asthma, aspirin and most other non-selective NSAIDs can induce an asthmatic episode through the formation of bronchoconstrictor cysteinyl-leukotrienes (LTC_4, LTD_4). Selective COX-2 inhibitors have less potential to cause asthma attacks in NSAID-intolerant asthmatics.

15. **True.** Pyrexia is caused by elevation of PGE_2 levels synthesised in the CNS by COX-2.

16. **False.** Increasing evidence suggests that NSAIDs reduce the risk of many cancers, most probably by inhibiting PGE_2 synthesis by COX-2, or by COX-independent pathways.

Extended-matching-item answers

Case 1: **Answer D** is correct. Paracetamol is a good choice for this man's mild osteoarthritic pain. His hypertension and heart failure mean that he should not be given an NSAID that may result in salt and water retention. Both the COX-2-selective and non-selective NSAIDs contribute to salt and water retention.

Case 2: **Answer B** is correct. The selective COX-2 inhibitor celecoxib could be prescribed as these are less likely than non-selective NSAIDs such as aspirin or diclofenac to precipitate a hypersensitive asthmatic attack. Paracetamol would not be useful as it has little anti-inflammatory action.

Case 3: **Answer A** is correct. This man should be given low-dose aspirin (75 mg daily) as it prevents platelet aggregation by inhibiting thromboxane A_2 (TXA_2) synthesis while having a minimal effect on the production of the vasodilator and anti-aggregatory PGI_2 (prostacyclin). This low dose has been shown to reduce the risk of another infarction.

FURTHER READING

Bleumink GS, Feenstra J, Sturkenboom CJM et al. (2003) Nonsteroidal anti-inflammatory drugs and heart failure. *Drugs* 63, 525–534

Burian M, Geisslinger G (2005) COX-dependent mechanisms involved in the antinociceptive action of NSAIDs at central and peripheral sites. *Pharmacol Ther* 107, 139–154

Epstein M (2002) Non-steroidal anti-inflammatory drugs and the continuum of renal dysfunction. *J Hypertens* 20 (suppl 6), S17–S23

Farooque SP, Lee TH (2009) Aspirin-sensitive respiratory disease. *Annu Rev Physiol* 71, 465–487

Högestätt ED, Jönsson BA, Ermund A et al. (2005) Conversion of acetaminophen to the bioactive N-acylphenolamine AM404 via fatty acid amide hydrolase-dependent arachidonic acid conjugation in the nervous system. *J Biol Chem* 280, 31405–31412

James MW, Hawkey CJ (2003) Assessment of non-steroidal anti-inflammatory drug (NSAID) damage in the human gastrointestinal tract. *Br J Clin Pharmacol* 56, 146–155

Micklewright R, Linley SLW, McQuade C et al. (2003) NSAIDs, gastroprotection and cyclo-oxygenase-II-selective inhibitors. *Aliment Pharmacol Ther* 17, 321–332

Paccani SR, Boncristiano M, Baldari CT (2003) Molecular mechanisms underlying suppression of lymphocyte responses by nonsteroidal antiinflammatory drugs. *Cell Mol Life Sci* 60, 1071–1083

Parente L, Perretti M (2003) Advances in the pathophysiology of constitutive and inducible cyclooxygenases: two enzymes in the spotlight. *Biochem Pharmacol* 65, 153–159

Peters-Golden M, Henderson WR (2007) Leukotrienes. *N Engl J Med* 357, 1841–1854

Serhan CN, Chiang N, Van Dyke TE (2008) Resolving inflammation: dual anti-inflammatory and pro-resolution lipid mediators. *Nat Rev Immunol* 8, 349–361

Stevenson DD (2009) Aspirin sensitivity and desensitization for asthma and sinusitis. *Curr Allergy Asthma Rep* 9, 155–163

Szallasi A, Cruz F, Geppetti P (2006) TRPV1: a therapeutic target for novel analgesic drugs? *Trends Mol Med* 12, 545–554

Trelle S, Reichenbach S, Wandel S et al. (2011) Cardiovascular safety of non-steroidal anti-inflammatory drugs: network meta-analysis. *BMJ* 342, c7086

Wang D, Dubois RN (2006) Prostaglandins and cancer. *Gut* 55, 115–122

Compendium: non-steroidal anti-inflammatory drugs (NSAIDs) and related drugs

Drug	Kinetics (half-life)	Comments
NSAIDs		
All drugs are given orally and have broad indications for pain relief unless stated otherwise below.		
Aceclofenac	Slow and incomplete absorption; bioactivated by hydrolysis to diclofenac; hepatic metabolism	Prodrug of diclofenac
Acemetacin	High oral bioavailability; converted to indometacin (1 h)	Prodrug of indometacin
Aspirin	Completely absorbed; hydrolysed rapidly (0.25 h) to salicylic acid, an active metabolite (3–20 h)	Not suitable for children under 12 years (risk of Reye's syndrome); for antiplatelet use, see Ch. 11
Celecoxib	Good oral absorption; hepatic metabolism (11 h)	Selective COX-2 inhibitor; used for pain and inflammation in osteoarthritis and rheumatoid arthritis
Dexibuprofen	Good oral bioavailability (80%); mainly hepatic metabolism (2–4 h)	The active enantiomer of ibuprofen
Dexketoprofen	High oral bioavailability (90%); hepatic glucuronidation (1–3 h)	Isomer of ketoprofen; used for short-term treatment of mild to moderate pain
Diclofenac	Oral bioavailability about 60%; hepatic metabolism (1–2 h)	Given orally, rectally, by deep intramuscular injection or intravenous infusion, transdermally, or topically to the eye; available orally in combined formulation with misoprostol for gastric protection (see Ch. 33)
Etodolac	Good oral bioavailability (80%); hepatic metabolism (6–7 h)	Used for pain and inflammation in osteoarthritis and rheumatoid arthritis
Etoricoxib	Good oral bioavailability (90%); hepatic metabolism (25 h)	Selective COX-2 inhibitor; used for pain and inflammation in osteoarthritis, rheumatoid arthritis and in acute gout; not approved for use in USA
Felbinac		Available for topical application
Fenoprofen	Rapidly and completely absorbed; hepatic metabolism (2–3 h)	Used for pain and inflammation in osteoarthritis and rheumatoid arthritis
Flurbiprofen	Rapidly and completely absorbed, hepatic metabolism and renal excretion (3–9 h)	Given orally, rectally, as lozenge for local treatment of sore throat, or topically to the eye
Ibuprofen	Good oral bioavailability (80%); mainly hepatic metabolism (2–4 h)	Modest anti-inflammatory action; given orally or transdermally for mild–moderate pain and inflammation
Indometacin	Rapidly and completely absorbed; hepatic metabolism and renal excretion (3–5 h)	Given orally or rectally
Ketoprofen	High oral bioavailability (90%); hepatic glucuronidation (1–3 h)	Given orally, rectally, by deep intramuscular injection or transdermally; also available in oral formulation with omeprazole
Ketorolac	Rapid and complete absorption; mainly renal excretion, also hepatic metabolism (3–9 h)	Used in short-term management of postoperative pain; given orally, by intramuscular or slow intravenous injection or topically to the eye
Mefenamic acid	Rapid and complete absorption, reduced if taken with food; hepatic metabolism (3–4 h)	Weak anti-inflammatory action
Meloxicam	Slow but complete absorption; hepatic metabolism (12–20 h)	Used for pain and inflammation in rheumatoid arthritis, osteoarthritis (short-term) and in ankylosing spondylitis; given orally or rectally
Nabumetone	Undergoes complete first-pass metabolism by hydrolysis to an active derivative that is eliminated by hepatic metabolism (24h)	Used for pain and inflammation in osteoarthritis and rheumatoid arthritis
Naproxen	Rapidly and completely absorbed; hepatic metabolism (12–15 h)	Given orally or rectally; also available in oral formulations with misoprostol or esomeprazole

Compendium: non-steroidal anti-inflammatory drugs (NSAIDs) and related drugs—cont'd

Drug	Kinetics (half-life)	Comments
Parecoxib	Hepatic metabolism, partially to active derivatives (5–9 h)	Selective COX-2 inhibitor; used in short-term management of postoperative pain; given by deep intramuscular or intravenous injection
Piroxicam	Rapid absorption; highly plasma protein bound; hepatic metabolism and undergoes enterohepatic circulation (30–60 h)	Given orally, rectally or by deep intramuscular injection; restricted use because of incidence of gastrointestinal unwanted effects and serious skin reactions; also unrestricted transdermal use
Sulindac	Good oral absorption; oxidised to an inactive sulphone then reduced in liver and gut to an active metabolite (7–8 h)	Prodrug for active thioether metabolite
Tenoxicam	Slow absorption after oral dosage; hepatic metabolism (44–100 h)	Similar profile to naproxen; given orally (once daily) or by intramuscular or intravenous injection
Tiaprofenic acid	Good oral bioavailability; hepatic oxidation and conjugation, renal excretion (2–4 h)	Not suitable for people with urinary tract disorders (risk of cystitis)
Tolfenamic acid	Complete oral bioavailability; biliary excretion (2 h)	Licensed for the treatment of migraine (see Ch. 26)

Related drugs

Given orally.

Drug	Kinetics (half-life)	Comments
Paracetamol (acetaminophen)	Rapidly and completely absorbed; hepatic conjugation (3–4 h); in overdose an oxidative metabolite (*N*-acetyl-*p*-benzoquinone imine, NAPQI) leads to hepatotoxicity (see Ch. 53)	The most widely used non-opioid analgesic

30 Rheumatoid arthritis, other inflammatory arthritides and osteoarthritis

RHEUMATOID ARTHRITIS

Rheumatoid arthritis is a chronic systemic inflammatory autoimmune condition to which some people are genetically predisposed. The symptoms of rheumatoid arthritis usually appear gradually and most often involve the proximal interphalangeal joints of the fingers, metacarpophalangeal joints and wrists. Inflammation of other joints such as the ankles and hips may be the presenting complaint, or they may become involved later. The affected joints are warm, swollen and painful. Stiffness is troublesome, particularly in the morning, as a result of an increase in extracellular fluid in and around the joint. Systemic disturbance is common, including general fatigue, malaise and weight loss, while extra-articular manifestations such as vasculitis and neuropathy can occur.

Autoimmune processes contribute to the maintenance of the rheumatoid arthritis, but it is uncertain whether it is initiated by an autoimmune reaction or by an exogenous antigen. Two autoantibodies, rheumatoid factor (IgM autoantibodies reactive with IgG) and anti-citrullinated protein antibodies, may be detected, but are absent in about one-third of cases. The initiating antigen is believed to bind to Toll-like receptors (TLRs) – pattern-recognition molecules that bind to both foreign and self structures – on dendritic cells and macrophages, which then initiate a response by the innate immune system (Ch. 38). The primary response is lymphoid cell infiltration of the synovium around the joint, formation of new blood vessels and a proliferation of the synovial membrane. The synovium becomes locally invasive (pannus) and osteoclasts destroy joint cartilage and bone. Apart from psoriatic arthritis, other forms of inflammatory arthritis do not produce erosive changes in periarticular bone or marked joint destruction to the same degree.

The chronic inflammatory process is initiated by T-helper 1 (Th1) lymphocytes that migrate into the joint. Failure of suppression of Th1 cells by regulatory T-cells may be important in the pathogenesis of the disease. Activated T-cells produce a gamut of pro-inflammatory cytokines, including tumour necrosis factor α (TNFα) and interleukin-1 (IL-1). These cytokines stimulate B-lymphocytes, macrophages, fibroblasts, chondrocytes and osteoclasts (Fig. 30.1). B-cells play an important role in the pathology of rheumatoid arthritis. They act as antigen-presenting cells that co-stimulate T-cells, generate inflammatory cytokines such as TNFα and produce rheumatoid factor antibody. Antigen-presenting cells express CD20, CD80 and CD86 surface markers and are involved in the activation of T-cells (Fig. 30.1). TNFα has a prominent role in orchestrating the production of other inflammatory mediators and the recruitment of further immune and inflammatory cells into the joint. This pattern of inflammation differs from most other immune-mediated diseases. The ubiquitous gene transcription factor nuclear factor κB (NF-κB) is also thought to be involved at many steps in cell activation and cytokine production in the destructive cycle of events.

TNFα and IL-1 aid the recruitment of inflammatory cells such as leucocytes by increasing the expression of adhesion molecules (integrins) on vascular endothelial cells. These cytokines also stimulate synovial fibroblasts, osteoclasts and chondrocytes to release tissue-destroying matrix metalloproteinases (MMPs) and to express chemokine receptors. Activated macrophages, lymphocytes and fibroblasts stimulate angiogenesis in the synovium.

Antibodies are produced to the collagen exposed in the damaged cartilage. Rheumatoid factor forms complexes with collagen in damaged cartilage, which then activate the complement pathway. The relevance of this to joint damage

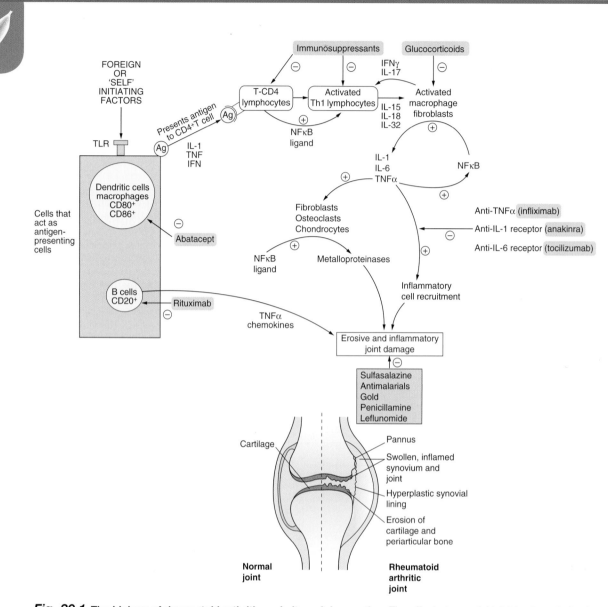

Fig. 30.1 **The biology of rheumatoid arthritis and sites of drug action.** The affected synovial joint is characterised by inflamed and swollen synovium with angiogenesis and increased presence of fibroblasts, osteoclasts, plasma cells, mast cells and B-lymphocytes. The synovial fluid contains increased numbers of neutrophil leucocytes and there is erosion of cartilage and adjacent bone. The cascade of self-perpetuating inflammatory events involves many factors, including upregulation of the ubiquitous nuclear transcription factor NF-κB and generation of cytokines including IL-1, IL-6 and TNFα. Some of the drugs shown act at multiple sites. APCs, antigen-presenting cells; IFN, interferon; IL, interleukin; NF-κB, nuclear factor κB; TLR, Toll-like receptor; TNFα, tumour necrosis factor α.

is not known. The activated osteoclasts increase bone resorption. The result of this complex inflammatory process is irreversible destruction of cartilage and erosion of periarticular bone.

The plethora of cells that enter the synovium, and the bewildering array of cytokines that are involved, provide a large number of potential targets for disease-modifying antirheumatic drugs affecting the immune system (Fig. 30.1).

OTHER TYPES OF INFLAMMATORY ARTHRITIS: THE SPONDYLOARTHRITIDES

There are many types of inflammatory arthritis that have a pattern of joint involvement different from that of rheumatoid arthritis. They involve the sacroiliac joints and can affect small or large joints peripherally. Collectively they are called the spondyloarthritides, and include ankylosing spondylitis, psoriatic arthritis, arthritis associated with inflammatory bowel disease and some juvenile idiopathic arthritis. There is a genetic predisposition to this type of arthritis, varying from a single genetic risk factor such as HLA-B27 in ankylosing spondylitis to polygenic influences in other disorders.

Spondyloarthritides are considered to be autoinflammatory syndromes and probably arise from activation of innate immune processes in response to bacterial or mechanical stress. This distinguishes them from autoimmune conditions that are triggered by activation of the adaptive immune system (Ch. 38). A variety of cytokines appear to be involved in the inflammatory response, including TNFα, and various interleukins such as IL-1, IL-6, IL-17 and IL-23. The inflammation is characteristically associated with enthesopathy (inflammation at the bone insertion of tendons and ligaments) and formation of new endochondral bone.

The presence of different pathophysiological mechanisms in rheumatoid arthritis and the spondyloarthritides explains the different responses to treatments designed to modify disease progression.

CONVENTIONAL DISEASE-MODIFYING ANTIRHEUMATIC DRUGS FOR RHEUMATOID ARTHRITIS

Non-steroidal anti-inflammatory drugs (NSAIDs; Ch. 29) provide symptomatic relief but do not alter the long-term progression of joint destruction in rheumatoid arthritis. A diverse group of compounds can reduce the rate of progression of joint erosion and destruction, leading to improvement both in symptoms and in the clinical and serological markers of rheumatoid arthritis activity. These drugs produce long-term depression of the inflammatory response even though they have little direct anti-inflammatory effect. They all have a slow onset of action, with many producing little improvement until about 3 months after starting treatment. Such drugs are grouped together and known as disease-modifying antirheumatic drugs (DMARDs).

SULFASALAZINE

The action of sulfasalazine in arthritis is poorly understood. It is cleaved in the colon by bacterial enzymes to 5-aminosalicylic acid (which is not believed to contribute to the antirheumatic action) and sulfapyridine. Sulfapyridine in the colon may reduce the absorption of antigens that promote joint inflammation. However, sulfasalazine and sulfapyridine are both absorbed and are found at similar concentrations in synovial fluid. Sulfasalazine can suppress several signal transduction pathways involved in the synthesis of pro-inflammatory cytokines, which may contribute to its efficacy.

High doses of sulfasalazine are required for the treatment of rheumatoid arthritis and these often produce gastrointestinal upset. This can be minimised by increasing the dose slowly and by using an enteric-coated formulation. Other problems include reversible oligospermia (therefore sulfasalazine should be avoided in males who wish to have a family) and blood dyscrasias. Sulfasalazine is discussed more fully in Chapter 34.

ANTIMALARIALS

hydroxychloroquine

Hydroxychloroquine is weakly basic, which permits its uptake and concentration in a non-ionised form within cells. Having entered the lysosomes inside the cell, the acidic environment traps and concentrates the drug in its ionised state. Macrophages depend on acid proteases in their lysosomes for digestion of phagocytosed protein. Hydroxychloroquine slightly increases the pH inside the macrophage lysosomes, which alters the processing of peptide antigens and reduces their subsequent presentation on the cell surface. Thus, the interaction between T-helper cells and antigen-presenting macrophages responsible for joint inflammation is reduced, with a reduction in the inflammatory response. Hydroxychloroquine also reduces the activation of plasmacytoid dendritic cells by blocking Toll-like receptors on their cell membrane.

Retinal toxicity is a potential problem due to selective binding to photoreceptor cells in the macula and subsequent disruption of lysosomal function. It is rare with recommended doses of hydroxychloroquine, but specialist assessment of the eyes is recommended before treatment and again during treatment if there is a change in visual acuity or blurring of vision or if treatment continues for more than five years. The pharmacokinetics and other unwanted effects of hydroxychloroquine can be found in Chapter 51.

LEFLUNOMIDE

Mechanism of action and uses

Leflunomide is an isoxazole derivative that inhibits dihydroorotate dehydrogenase, a key mitochondrial enzyme in the *de novo* synthesis of the pyrimidine ribonucleotide uridine monophosphate (UMP). Activated lymphocytes require an eightfold increase in their pyrimidine pool to proliferate. Inadequate provision of UMP increases the expression of the tumour-suppressor molecule p53 which translocates to the cell nucleus and arrests the cell cycle in the G_1 phase. This cytostatic action reduces the expansion of the activated autoimmune T- and B-lymphocyte pool, thereby suppressing immunoglobulin production and cellular immune processes. Other dividing cells can obtain adequate pyrimidines from a separate salvage pathway that reuses existing ribonucleotides and is not affected by leflunomide.

There are other potential mechanisms of immunomodulation by leflunomide, such as inhibition of tyrosine kinases and suppression of transcription factors that stimulate osteoclast formation, but they are probably of lesser importance.

Pharmacokinetics

Leflunomide is a prodrug. It is well absorbed from the gut and is converted non-enzymatically, mainly in the intestinal mucosa and plasma, to its active metabolite. The metabolite is excreted via the bile, and enterohepatic circulation contributes to its very long plasma half-life (15 days).

Unwanted effects

- Gastrointestinal upset, especially diarrhoea.
- Increase in blood pressure.
- Headache, dizziness, lethargy.
- Leucopenia, anaemia or thrombocytopenia.
- Rash, dry skin and pruritus.
- Alopecia.
- Hepatotoxicity, especially in the first 6 months.
- Teratogenicity: it is advised that conception should be avoided for two years after stopping treatment in women and for three months in men.

Prevention and management of unwanted effects

Monitoring of full blood count and liver function should be carried out regularly during treatment. If serious unwanted effects occur, elimination of the drug can be increased by the use of colestyramine (Ch. 48) or activated charcoal to bind the active metabolite present in the gut after biliary excretion, thereby interrupting its enterohepatic circulation (Ch. 2).

IMMUNOSUPPRESSANT DRUGS

Several drugs with immunosuppressant actions have been shown to be effective in rheumatoid arthritis. These include:

- antimetabolites: methotrexate, azathioprine (Ch. 38),
- calcineurin inhibitor: ciclosporin (Ch. 38).

Methotrexate is one of the most effective antirheumatic drugs. Although its primary mechanism of action is by folate antagonism, co-administration of folic acid supplements prevents much of the mucosal and gastrointestinal toxicity of the drug but does not reduce its immunomodulatory effect. A possible additional mechanism of action to explain the effect of methotrexate in arthritis is inhibition of the deamination of adenosine, causing its accumulation. Adenosine is an intermediate in purine biosynthesis and a potent anti-inflammatory mediator. It suppresses neutrophil adhesion and cytokine production, reduces macrophage function and impairs the expression of endothelial adhesion molecules. Methotrexate is usually given orally once a week for the treatment of inflammatory arthritis. It can be given intramuscularly if oral use produces intractable gastrointestinal symptoms or if absorption by the oral route is inadequate.

GOLD

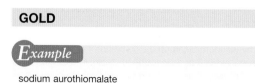

Example

sodium aurothiomalate

Mechanism of action

The precise mechanism by which gold compounds act is unknown. A popular concept is that the compound is taken up by mononuclear cells and inhibits their phagocytic function. This will reduce the release of inflammatory mediators and inhibit inflammatory cell proliferation. Production of inflammatory cytokines such as IL-1, IL-6 and TNFα is inhibited, and superoxide generation by neutrophils is reduced. There is also evidence for inhibition of other cell signalling pathways involved in inflammation, including NF-κB.

The advent of more effective and less toxic drugs has reduced the use of gold salts in current clinical practice.

Pharmacokinetics

Sodium aurothiomalate is given by deep intramuscular injection. An initial test dose is given to screen for acute toxicity (see below), followed by injections at weekly intervals to gradually achieve a therapeutic concentration in the tissues. Subsequently, a smaller dose is used to maintain remission. Gold binds readily to albumin and several tissue proteins and accumulates in many tissues such as the liver, kidney, bone marrow, lymph nodes and spleen. Accumulation also occurs in the synovium of inflamed joints. Elimination is largely renal. Gold has a half-life of several weeks, probably as a result of its extensive tissue binding.

Unwanted effects

The unwanted effects can be serious and all but the most minor effects should lead to immediate cessation of treatment:

- oral ulceration,
- proteinuria from membranous glomerulonephritis: this can develop after several weeks of treatment, sometimes progressing to nephrotic syndrome; recovery can take up to two years following drug withdrawal,
- blood disorders, especially thrombocytopenia but also agranulocytosis and aplastic anaemia,
- rashes,
- pulmonary fibrosis.

Prevention and management of unwanted effects

Urine should be checked for protein and a full blood count obtained before each injection of gold, and regularly during oral therapy. Major complications may require treatment with dimercaprol or penicillamine to chelate the gold (Ch. 53) and increase its elimination. Corticosteroids can be helpful to treat blood dyscrasias. Gold should not be used if there is a history of renal or hepatic disease, blood dyscrasias or severe rashes. Gold should be stopped if stomatitis, a pruritic rash, neutropenia, thrombocytopenia or significant proteinuria (>1 g in 24 h) develops.

PENICILLAMINE

Mechanism of action and uses

The mechanisms of action of penicillamine are uncertain. Modulation of the immune system is believed to be important, including a reduction in the number of activated lymphocytes, reduced synthesis of immunoglobulins and stabilisation of lysosomal membranes in inflammatory cells. Penicillamine has not been shown to slow the progression of joint erosions and is no longer widely used for rheumatoid arthritis.

Penicillamine is a thiol compound that can chelate many metals. This is probably of little relevance to its use in arthritis but has given the drug a role in the management of poisoning (Ch. 53) and in Wilson's disease, a genetically determined illness that is associated with copper overload.

Pharmacokinetics

Penicillamine is well absorbed from the gut, although oral iron supplements substantially reduce its absorption.

Unwanted effects

Unwanted effects occur frequently and are responsible for cessation of treatment in about 30% of people. They can be reduced by slow increases in dose. Many unwanted effects resemble those of gold:

- nausea, vomiting, abdominal discomfort and rashes (often with fever), especially early in treatment,
- loss of taste is common, but may resolve despite continued treatment,
- oral ulceration,
- proteinuria, which is caused by immune-complex glomerulonephritis and is dose-related; nephrotic syndrome can occur,
- blood disorders, especially thrombocytopenia, but also neutropenia and, rarely, aplastic anaemia.

Regular monitoring of urine, protein and blood counts should be carried out during treatment.

BIOLOGICAL DRUGS FOR RHEUMATOID ARTHRITIS

ANTIBODIES AGAINST TUMOUR NECROSIS FACTOR α

adalimumab, certolizumab, etanercept, golimumab, infliximab

Mechanism of action

TNFα stimulates several inflammatory processes (see above and Fig. 30.1). It acts by binding to one of two cell surface receptors, type 1 (p55) and type 2 (p75), which are found in several tissues. There are several antibody derivatives available that block the action of TNFα.

- Adalimumab and golimumab are fully humanised monoclonal antibodies specific for TNFα.
- Certolizumab pegol is a pegylated Fab fragment of a humanized monoclonal antibody for TNFα.
- Etanercept is a fusion protein consisting of two recombinant soluble extracellular portions of the human Type 2 (p75) TNF receptor, fused to the constant (Fc) domain of human immunoglobulin (IgG₁). It binds to TNFα and the cytokine lymphotoxin α (also known as TNFβ).
- Infliximab is a chimaeric monoclonal antibody comprising the variable region of a murine antibody, which neutralises TNFα, spliced to the constant region of a human antibody.

Pharmacokinetics

Adalimumab, certolizumab pegol, etanercept and golimumab are given by subcutaneous injection and infliximab by intravenous infusion. The mechanism of elimination of these recombinant compounds is poorly defined but likely to be by proteolysis. They have very long half-lives between 5 and 20 days, enabling dosing at frequencies ranging from twice weekly to monthly.

Unwanted effects

- All these biological drugs can produce gastrointestinal upset, decompensation of heart failure, hypersensitivity reactions, injection-site reactions, fever, headache and depression. Blood disorders, including anaemia, leucopenia and thrombocytopenia, also occur.
- Increased risk of pulmonary tuberculosis: screening for evidence of tuberculosis is recommended before initiation of therapy. Septicaemia and reactivation of hepatitis B virus occur more frequently.

INTERLEUKIN-1 RECEPTOR ANTAGONIST

anakinra

Mechanism of action

Anakinra is a recombinant human IL-1 receptor antagonist (Fig. 30.1). IL-1 is actually a family of three cytokines, comprising two IL-1 receptor antagonists (IL-1α and IL-1β) and an IL-1 receptor antagonist. The theoretical basis for the use of anakinra is that joint destruction arises from an imbalance between the agonists and the antagonist. IL-1 agonists are pro-inflammatory cytokines released by macrophages and fibroblasts in inflamed synovium, and by neutrophils in synovial fluid. The IL-1 peptides compete for occupancy of the IL-1 receptor on the membrane of synovial cells, and as little as 2–3% occupancy by the agonists produces

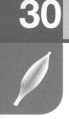

maximal pro-inflammatory cell activation. Anakinra blocks the receptors and suppresses the inflammatory response. In the UK anakinra is not currently recommended for routine use in rheumatoid arthritis.

Pharmacokinetics

Anakinra is given by daily subcutaneous injection. Elimination is via the kidneys and it has a short half-life (4–6 h).

Unwanted effects

- Injection-site reactions.
- Increased risk of serious infections, particularly in people with asthma.
- Neutropenia.

INTERLEUKIN-6 RECEPTOR ANTAGONIST

Example

tocilizumab

Mechanism of action

Tocilizumab is a recombinant humanized monoclonal antibody that acts as a competitive antagonist at the IL-6 receptor. IL-6 is a pro-inflammatory cytokine produced by a variety of cell types including T- and B-lymphocytes, monocytes and fibroblasts. IL-6 is involved in T-cell activation, immunoglobulin secretion and stimulation of hematopoietic precursor cell proliferation and differentiation. IL-6 is also produced by synovial and endothelial cells leading to local production of IL-6 in joints affected by inflammatory processes such as rheumatoid arthritis.

Pharmacokinetics

Tocilizumab is given by intravenous infusion every 4 weeks. It has a long half-life of 6 days, and is probably cleared by proteolysis.

Unwanted effects

- Abdominal pain, mouth ulceration, dyspepsia.
- Increased risk of infections, particularly upper respiratory tract infections.
- Oedema, hypertension.
- Dizziness, headache.

T-CELL CO-STIMULATION MODULATOR

Example

abatacept

Mechanism of action and uses

T-lymphocyte activation requires recognition of a specific antigen carried by an antigen-presenting cell, and a second co-stimulatory signal. A major co-stimulatory signal involves binding of CD80 and CD86 molecules on the surface of antigen-presenting cells to the CD28 receptor on T-cells. Abatacept is a monoclonal antibody that selectively binds to CD80 and CD86 and blocks the co-stimulatory signal. It therefore reduces the subsequent production of inflammatory mediators and pro-inflammatory cytokines. Abatacept is used for people who have failed to respond to, or are intolerant of, a TNFα inhibitor, but is not currently recommended in the UK. Another co-stimulation inhibitor, belatacept, is used as an immunosuppressant in renal transplantation (Ch. 38).

Pharmacokinetics

Abatacept is given by intravenous infusion. Its metabolism is unknown, and it has a very long half-life of about 14 days.

Unwanted effects

- Headache, dizziness, fatigue.
- Nausea, abdominal pain, diarrhoea.
- Rash.
- Upper respiratory tract infection and, less commonly, other infections.

ANTI-CD20 B-CELL DEPLETER

Example

rituximab

Mechanism of action and uses

Rituximab specifically depletes CD20+ B-lymphocytes by binding to the CD20 antigen expressed on the cell surface (Fig. 30.1). The depletion of mature and differentiating B-cells will reduce antigen presentation, stimulation of T-lymphocytes, cytokine production and production of autoantibodies. Responses usually last for up to six months, and relapse corresponds with B-cell repopulation.

Pharmacokinetics

Rituximab is given by intravenous infusion. Its metabolism is unknown, and it has a very long half-life of about 3–8 days.

Unwanted effects

- Cytokine release syndrome with fever, chills, nausea, vomiting and allergic reactions occurs in about one-third of people with the first infusion. Premedication with an anti-histamine and sometimes a corticosteroid will reduce these reactions.

- Exacerbation of angina, arrhythmia or heart failure can occur in people with cardiovascular disease.

MANAGEMENT OF RHEUMATOID ARTHRITIS

Progressive joint damage is common in rheumatoid arthritis. There is now a substantial body of evidence that early use of DMARDs (within three months of the onset of symptoms) leads to a better long-term outcome.

DMARDs do not have significant anti-inflammatory action and require 2–3 months before an effect is established. Therefore, they are almost always used initially in combination with a corticosteroid or an NSAID. Methotrexate, given with folic acid supplementation, is the first-choice DMARD. It is usually taken orally, but parenteral use can be considered if gastrointestinal tolerability is a problem. A combination of two DMARDs is now recommended as standard first-line therapy and is more effective than a single drug. Sulfasalazine, leflunomide or hydroxychloroquine are most frequently used in combination with methotrexate. Immunosuppressant drugs such as ciclosporin or azathioprine are generally reserved as third-line agents. Gold and penicillamine are less widely used due to toxicity and, in the case of penicillamine, limited efficacy. If disease activity cannot be suppressed by two DMARDs then a combination of three DMARDs (such as methotrexate, sulfasalazine and hydroxychloroquine) can be tried. Cyclophosphamide is useful for the management of extra-articular manifestations of rheumatoid disease, such as vasculitis, pericarditis or pleurisy.

Intra-articular injections of corticosteroid are used for individual inflamed joints (especially knee and shoulder). Pulsed intramuscular corticosteroid therapy can be given for disease flares, or to ameliorate symptoms in the first few weeks after initiating DMARD therapy (because of the slow response). In early rheumatoid disease a low dose of corticosteroid, given for six months in combination with DMARDs, retards bone destruction and slows disease progression. Intramuscular methylprednisone is often used and is preferred to oral prednisolone, which can be difficult to withdraw (Ch. 44).

Anti-TNFα drugs such as etanercept (the most frequently used biological agents for rheumatoid arthritis) are usually reserved for those who fail to respond to combination therapy with DMARDs, or who are intolerant of several DMARDs. They are typically used in combination with methotrexate, or leflunomide if methotrexate is not tolerated, which produces a better response than the biological agent given alone. The combination produces remission and halts disease progression in up to 60% of people who are treated. If one anti-TNFα drug is ineffective or poorly tolerated, then a different drug from the same class should be tried. Abatacept, tocilizumab and rituximab have been shown to be effective for people with rheumatoid arthritis who fail to respond to, or who cannot tolerate, TNFα blockers. Anakinra is less effective than anti-TNFα drugs and is currently not recommended in the UK.

NSAIDs (Ch. 29) are useful for symptomatic treatment of all types of inflammatory arthritis since they reduce both pain and stiffness. However, they do not affect the long-term course of the disease, and DMARDs have superseded them as the mainstay of treatment of rheumatoid arthritis. There is considerable variation in responses to different NSAIDs, and there is no way of predicting effectiveness in an individual. Propionic acid derivatives, such as ibuprofen, are often used first. They have a weaker anti-inflammatory activity than other classes of NSAID, but generally have fewer unwanted effects. More powerful drugs such as naproxen can be used when ibuprofen fails to control symptoms, although the increased risk of gastrointestinal irritation and cardiovascular events limit their use, especially in the elderly. Morning stiffness is often disabling in inflammatory arthritis. This is helped by giving a late-evening dose of an NSAID with a long half-life, a modified-release formulation of a compound with a short half-life or an NSAID suppository. Topical NSAIDs applied over the affected joint(s) are not usually recommended. Selective cyclo-oxygenase (COX)-2 inhibitors are usually reserved for people who are intolerant of NSAIDs, or who have a higher risk of serious gastrointestinal complications with an NSAID (Ch. 29).

Physical aids such as splinting and bed rest can help acute flares of joint inflammation. There is an increased risk of cardiovascular disease in people with rheumatoid arthritis, and attention to the conventional risk factors for prevention of atherosclerosis is important (Ch. 5).

MANAGEMENT OF SPONDYLOARTHRITIDES

NSAIDs remain the first-line treatment for this group of disorders, and will relieve pain and improve function. This should be combined with a tailored exercise regimen. Although most evidence for the use of DMARDs has been obtained in the treatment of rheumatoid arthritis, there is limited evidence for their efficacy in the seronegative spondyloarthritides. Sulfasalazine and methotrexate give some benefit for peripheral joint disease in these forms of inflammatory arthritis, but do not improve axial joint inflammation or enthesitis. Anti-TNFα agents can produce remission of disease in ankylosing spondylitis and psoriatic arthritis in about one-third of those treated, with considerable symptomatic benefit in others. Unlike DMARDs, these agents can help most aspects of the disease, with the exception of new bone formation. If treatment with an anti-TNFα agent is stopped after remission is achieved then relapse usually occurs within 6–12 months. The efficacy of biological agents that block other cytokines is unproven, and T- or B-lymphocyte targeted therapies are ineffective.

OSTEOARTHRITIS

Osteoarthritis is the clinical manifestation of joint degeneration that results from loss of articular cartilage and becomes more common with increasing age. Most osteoarthritis is idiopathic (when it can be localised or generalised) but a small proportion is secondary to other conditions such as joint injury or chondrocalcinosis. The cardinal symptom of osteoarthritis is pain in the affected joint during physical activity, which is relieved by rest. Pain also occurs at rest with advanced disease. Stiffness may be troublesome for a few minutes after rest. Various small joints can be involved, particularly the distal interphalangeal joints of the fingers and the carpometacarpal joint of the thumb. Large joints such as the knee, hip, elbow and shoulder are often asymmetrically affected.

The integrity of articular cartilage depends on the balance of synthetic and catabolic activity of the chondrocytes embedded in the cartilage matrix. Mechanical compression of cartilage produces many physical and biochemical stimuli that influence chondrocyte metabolism. Mechanical overload, the principal cause of secondary osteoarthritis, produces changes that promote matrix destruction and apoptotic chondrocyte death. Osteoarthritis is caused by an imbalance of cartilage degradation compared to synthesis of cartilage, with loss of the normal cartilage matrix. Synovial inflammation results from release of cartilage debris into the joint accompanied by catabolic mediators and results in joint swelling.

Synthesis of cartilage is promoted by the expression of growth factors by chondrocytes, particularly insulin-like growth factor 1 and transforming growth factor β (TGFβ). Degradation of cartilage proteins is carried out by matrix metalloproteinases (MMPs), particularly stromelysin 1 (MMP-3) in early osteoarthritis and gelatinase A (MMP-2) and MMP-13 in late disease. MMPs are synthesised by chondrocytes in response to stimulation by the pro-inflammatory cytokines IL-1β and TNFα released by inflammatory cells. Synovial inflammation often occurs adjacent to the damaged cartilage. Chondrocytes produce a chemokine, RANTES (regulated upon activation, normal T-cell expressed and secreted), and synovial fluid cells express chemokine receptors including CXC chemokine receptor type 4 (CXCR4), which may have a role in recruiting inflammatory cells to the joint.

Loss of matrix leads to disruption of the cartilage, with swelling and fissuring of the surface. Subchondral bone becomes increasingly vascular and new bone is laid down. It is uncertain whether the initiating factors for osteoarthritis originate in the articular cartilage or subchondral bone. However, recent evidence suggests that stiffening of subchondral bone, with less effective shock absorption, may be the trigger for cartilage loss.

MANAGEMENT OF OSTEOARTHRITIS

Treatment of osteoarthritis currently remains symptomatic. Non-pharmacological therapy such as weight loss, exercise, physical therapy and orthotics is often useful. Glucosamine sulphate or chondroitin sulphate supplements (over-the-counter preparations in the UK) are often used by people with osteoarthritis, but there is conflicting evidence of benefit. If pain is troublesome, simple analgesics such as paracetamol should usually be considered as first-line treatment. NSAIDs may be helpful for inflammatory episodes or if paracetamol is ineffective. *In vitro* studies suggest that some NSAIDs may accelerate the loss of articular cartilage in osteoarthritis. Clinical studies are inconclusive, but avoidance of powerful NSAIDs is probably desirable. The risks of gastrointestinal and cardiac toxicity may also limit the value of NSAIDs.

Intra-articular or periarticular injection of a corticosteroid (Ch. 44) can provide short-term symptomatic relief in osteoarthritis, even if there is little clinical evidence of joint inflammation. Corticosteroids inhibit pro-inflammatory mediators in synovial tissue, such as IL-1 and TNFα. Joint injection with hyaluronic acid remains a controversial treatment, with conflicting evidence of efficacy from clinical trials.

The recognition that osteoarthritis involves inflammatory flares and that cartilage repair can occur has opened up potential new approaches to management. However, there is no proven disease-modifying therapy currently available for the treatment of osteoarthritis. Long-term management of osteoarthritis may eventually require surgical joint replacement.

SELF-ASSESSMENT

True/false questions

1. The action of most disease-modifying antirheumatic drugs (DMARDs) is slow in onset.
2. Non-steroidal anti-inflammatory drugs (NSAIDs) reduce the symptoms of rheumatoid disease and retard its progress.
3. If penicillamine does not lead to clinical benefit within six months, it should be stopped.
4. Intramuscular gold can cause proteinuria.
5. Methotrexate has a rapid onset of action (4–6 weeks).
6. During methotrexate therapy, folic acid is contraindicated.
7. Methotrexate has relatively few unwanted effects compared with other DMARDs.
8. The active component of sulfasalazine in rheumatoid disease is 5-aminosalicylic acid.
9. Combination therapy with DMARDs should not be used in rheumatoid arthritis.
10. Leflunomide selectively inhibits pyrimidine synthesis in lymphocytes.
11. Intra-articular injections of corticosteroids slow the progression of erosions.
12. Prolonged treatment with high doses of corticosteroids can cause adrenal atrophy.
13. The antimalarial hydroxychloroquine is of little benefit in rheumatoid arthritis.
14. Rituximab depletes B-cells.
15. Adalimumab and golimumab are fully humanised anti-tumour necrosis factor α (TNFα) monoclonal antibodies.
16. Abatacept blocks antigen presentation to T-lymphocytes
17. Anakinra and tocilizumab activate cytokine receptors.
18. DMARDs are effective treatments for ankylosing spondylitis.

Case-based questions

A 30-year-old woman had developed painful wrists gradually over four weeks; she had not experienced similar episodes of pain before. On examination, both wrists and the metacarpophalangeal joints of both hands were tender but not deformed.

A. What course of treatment would you suggest?

There was some initial symptomatic improvement, but subsequently the pain, stiffness and swelling of the hands persisted and eight weeks later both knees became similarly affected. She saw a rheumatologist, who confirmed that she was suffering from rheumatoid arthritis and altered her treatment.

B. What treatment option would now be appropriate?

She was commenced on treatment that required folic acid supplements to counteract folate depletion.

C. What drug treatment had been started?

True/false answers

1. **True.** Most DMARDs take several weeks to show a clinical improvement.
2. **False.** NSAIDs do not slow disease progression; indeed, some evidence suggests they may hasten progress of the disease.
3. **True.** The second-line drugs take a long time to act (4–6 months) but they should be discontinued if there is no sign of improvement by that time.
4. **True.** Proteinuria occurs associated with immune-complex nephritis. Only 15% of people continue with gold treatment after 5–6 years because of unwanted effects.
5. **True.** Methotrexate is an immunosuppressant often chosen as initial disease-modifying therapy for rheumatoid arthritis because of its rapid onset of action.
6. **False.** Methotrexate inhibits reduction of folic acid to dihydrofolate and tetrahydrofolate, which are essential for nucleotide synthesis. Folic acid can be given daily to prevent gastrointestinal and haematological complications of methotrexate.
7. **True.** More than 50% of people who take methotrexate for rheumatoid arthritis continue taking the drug for five years or more, but a similar proportion have to cease treatment with most other DMARDs within two years.
8. **True.** Sulfasalazine is converted in the colon to 5-aminosalicylic acid, which is the active moiety in the treatment of inflammatory bowel disease, and to sulfapyridine, which is probably the main active moiety in rheumatoid arthritis.
9. **False.** The combination of methotrexate with ciclosporin, sulfasalazine or hydroxychloroquine has shown significant benefit in people with severe rheumatoid disease.
10. **True.** The active metabolite of leflunomide inhibits synthesis of uridine monophosphate and this slows the proliferation of T- and B-lymphocytes.
11. **False.** Corticosteroids can give dramatic relief of symptoms in rheumatoid arthritis, but there is no evidence they slow progression of the disease.
12. **True.** Adrenal atrophy caused by negative feedback on the hypothalamo–pituitary–adrenal axis can last for many months following prolonged treatment.
13. **False.** Hydroxychloroquine can cause remission of rheumatoid arthritis but does not slow the progression of joint damage.
14. **True.** Rituximab depletes B-lymphocytes by binding to their CD20 surface antigen.
15. **True.** Adalimumab, golimumab and other TNFα inhibitors are the most commonly used biological agents for moderate–severe rheumatoid arthritis, usually in combination with methotrexate or other DMARDs.
16. **True.** Abatacept blocks the CD80 and CD86 co-stimulatory molecules on antigen-presenting cells, preventing them interacting with CD28 on T-lymphocytes.
17. **False.** They are cytokine receptor antagonists; anakinra is an interleukin (IL)-1 receptor antagonist and tocilizumab blocks IL-6 receptors.
18. **False.** There is limited evidence for efficacy of DMARDs in the spondyloarthritides; TNFα inhibitors may be effective in inducing remission.

Case-based answers

A. The brief duration of the symptoms and their mild nature warrant the initial administration of an NSAID, such as ibuprofen, and follow-up.

B. The persistence of the symptoms and their spread to the knees suggest that a DMARD should be started. Guidelines now advise that DMARDs should be considered for persistent inflammatory joint disease of more than 8 weeks' duration.

C. Methotrexate is a DMARD that requires folate supplements (see answer to question 6, above). Methotrexate takes 4–6 weeks for its onset of action. Methotrexate and an NSAID (or a corticosteroid) should be given together to cover this interim period.

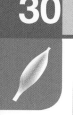

FURTHER READING

Rheumatoid arthritis and other inflammatory arthritides

Braun J, Sieper J (2007) Ankylosing spondylitis. *N Engl J Med* 369, 1379–1390

Brockbank J, Gladman D (2002) Diagnosis and management of psoriatic arthritis. *Drugs* 62, 2447–2457

Donahue KE, Gartlehner G, Jonas DE et al. (2008) Systematic review: comparative effectiveness and harms of disease-modifying medications for rheumatoid arthritis. *Ann Intern Med* 148, 162–163

Dougados M, Baeten D (2011) Spondyloarthritis. *Lancet* 377, 2127–2137

Emery P (2006) Treatment of rheumatoid arthritis. *BMJ* 332, 152–155

Goldblatt F, Isenberg DA (2008) Anti-CD20 monoclonal antibody in rheumatoid arthritis and systemic lupus erythematosus. *Handb Exp Pharmacol* 2008, 163–181

Katz WA (2002) Use of nonopioid analgesics and adjunctive agents in the management of pain in rheumatic diseases. *Curr Opin Rheumatol* 14, 63–71

Klarenbeek NB, Kerstens PJSM, Huizinga TWJ et al. (2010) Recent advances in the management of rheumatoid arthritis. *BMJ* 341, c6942

Klareskog L, Catrina AI, Paget S (2009) Rheumatoid arthritis. *Lancet* 373, 659–672

Olsen NJ, Stein CM (2004) New drugs for rheumatoid arthritis. *N Engl J Med* 350, 2167–2179

Scott DL, Kingsley GH (2006) Tumour necrosis factor inhibitors for rheumatoid arthritis. *N Engl J Med* 355, 704–712

Scott DL, Wolfe F, Huizinga TW (2010) Rheumatoid arthritis. *Lancet* 376, 1094–1108

Smolen JS, Aletaha D, Weisman MH et al. (2007) New therapies for the treatment of rheumatoid arthritis. *Lancet* 370, 1861–1874

Osteoarthritis

Bijlsma JW, Berenbaum F, Lafeber FP (2011) Osteoarthritis: an update with relevance for clinical practice. *Lancet* 377, 2115–2126

Dieppe P, Brandt KD (2003) What is important in treating osteoarthritis? Whom should we treat and how should we treat them? *Rheum Dis Clin North Am* 29, 687–716

Felson DT (2006) Osteoarthritis of the knee. *N Engl J Med* 354, 841–848

Hunter DJ, Felson DT (2006) Osteoarthritis. *BMJ* 332, 639–642

Sharma S (2002) Nonpharmacological management of osteoarthritis. *Curr Opin Rheumatol* 14, 603–607

Compendium: disease-modifying antirheumatic drugs (DMARDs)

Drug	Kinetics (half-life)	Comments
Aurothiomalate (sodium salt)	Data available for gold (not the drug form) suggest extensive tissue binding; probably metabolised and eliminated in urine and faeces (250 days)	Gold compound used for active progressive rheumatoid arthritis and juvenile arthritis; given by deep intramuscular injection
Chloroquine	See Ch. 51 for details	Used for moderate active rheumatoid arthritis and juvenile arthritis; given orally; also used for malaria (see Ch. 51)
Hydroxychloroquine	Extensive oral absorption; hepatic metabolism and renal excretion (18 days)	Used for moderate active rheumatoid arthritis and juvenile arthritis; given orally
Penicillamine	Incomplete oral absorption; hepatic metabolism, faecal and renal excretion (1–6 h)	Used for active progressive rheumatoid arthritis; given orally
Sulfasalazine	Sulfasalazine is reduced in the colon to 5-aminosalicylate (5-ASA) and sulfapyridine (see Ch. 34); sulfapyridine is the better-absorbed product and is metabolised by acetylation; renal elimination (5-ASA, 4–10 h; sulfapyridine, 6–17 h)	Used to suppress the inflammatory activity of rheumatoid arthritis; also used for ulcerative colitis; see Ch. 34 for details
Drugs suppressing the immune response		
Azathioprine	See Ch. 38 for details	Used for moderate to severe rheumatoid arthritis in people who have not responded to other DMARDs; more toxic than methotrexate and used for those who have not responded to methotrexate; given orally; see Ch. 38 for other details
Ciclosporin	See Ch. 38 for details	Used for severe active rheumatoid arthritis when conventional second-line therapy is inappropriate or ineffective; given orally or intravenously; see Ch. 38 for other details

Compendium: disease-modifying antirheumatic drugs (DMARDs)—cont'd

Drug	Kinetics (half-life)	Comments
Cyclophosphamide	See Ch. 52 for details	Used for rheumatoid arthritis with severe systemic manifestations when response to other DMARDs has been inadequate; given orally; see Ch. 52 for other details
Leflunomide	Prodrug converted to active metabolite with very long and variable half-life (2 weeks); hepatic metabolism and biliary excretion	Used for moderate to severe rheumatoid arthritis; more toxic than methotrexate and used for people who have not responded to methotrexate; given orally
Methotrexate	See Ch. 52 for details	Used for moderate to severe rheumatoid arthritis; given orally, subcutaneously or intramuscularly; see Ch. 52

Cytokine modulators and other immunobiological drugs

Recombinant human proteins; should be used under specialised supervision.

Drug	Kinetics (half-life)	Comments
Abatacept	Pathways of metabolism have not been defined; protein clearance (14 days)	Monoclonal antibody against CD80/CD86 co-stimulatory molecules; given by intravenous infusion; not currently recommended in UK
Adalimumab	Protein clearance (12 days)	Fully humanised monoclonal antibody against TNFα; used in combination with methotrexate for moderate to severe active rheumatoid arthritis when response to other DMARDs has been inadequate; given by subcutaneous injection
Anakinra	Renal elimination (4–6 h)	IL-1 receptor antagonist; given by daily subcutaneous injection; not recommended for routine use in UK
Certolizumab pegol	Protein clearance (14 days)	Pegylated Fab fragment of monoclonal antibody against TNFα; used in combination with methotrexate for moderate to severe active rheumatoid arthritis when response to other DMARDs has been inadequate; given by subcutaneous injection
Etanercept	Protein clearance (5 days)	Recombinant protein that inhibits TNFα; used for severe, active and progressive rheumatoid arthritis in people who have failed to respond to at least two standard DMARDs; given by weekly or twice weekly subcutaneous injection
Golimumab	Protein clearance (7–20 days)	Fully humanised monoclonal antibody against TNFα; used in combination with methotrexate for moderate to severe active rheumatoid arthritis when response to other DMARDs has been inadequate; given by monthly subcutaneous injection
Infliximab	Protein clearance (8–10 days)	Monoclonal antibody against TNFα; used for severe, active and progressive rheumatoid arthritis in people who have failed to respond to at least two standard DMARDs; given by intravenous infusion
Rituximab	Protein clearance (3–8 days)	Monoclonal antibody against CD20 that depletes B-lymphocyte precursors and mature B-cells; used in people with moderate–severe active rheumatoid arthritis who have an inadequate response to DMARDs and a TNFα inhibitor; given by intravenous infusion
Tocilizumab	Protein clearance (6 days)	Monoclonal antibody against IL-6 receptors; used in people with moderate–severe rheumatoid arthritis when response to at least one DMARD or TNFα inhibitor has been inadequate; given by monthly intravenous infusion

Unlike non-steroidal anti-inflammatory drugs, DMARDs may require 4–6 months for a full response.

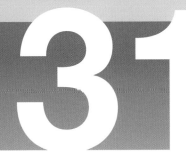

Hyperuricaemia and gout

THE PATHOPHYSIOLOGY OF GOUT

Gout is an inflammatory arthritis produced when monosodium urate crystals are deposited in synovial fluid. It is associated with a raised plasma uric acid (urate) concentration. Uric acid is a relatively insoluble product of catabolism of the nucleic acid purine bases guanine and adenine (Fig. 31.1). The immediate precursors of uric acid are xanthine and hypoxanthine, which are more water soluble. Uric acid is normally eliminated by the kidney. It is filtered at the glomerulus and then reabsorbed from the proximal tubule, and subsequently there is net secretion into the late proximal tubule.

Hyperuricaemia results from the following factors.

- Overproduction of uric acid, which this can arise from:
    - excessive cell destruction (e.g. lymphoproliferative or myeloproliferative disorders, especially during treatment for cancer, Ch. 52),
    - inherited defects that increase purine synthesis,
    - high purine intake (such as meat, fish and beer),
    - obesity.
- Reduced renal excretion of uric acid: more than 90% of filtered uric acid is reabsorbed in the early proximal tubule, but an amount equivalent to 6–10% of the filtered load is secreted by an active organic acid transporter in the second part of the proximal tubule (Ch. 14). Renal failure and certain drugs (e.g. loop and thiazide-type diuretics, low-dose aspirin, ciclosporin and lactate formed from excess alcohol) will reduce the tubular secretion of uric acid. Reduced uric acid excretion accounts for at least 80% of cases of gout.

A high plasma concentration of uric acid is often an incidental finding and does not lead to symptoms, but when the plasma concentration exceeds about 0.42 mmol·L^{-1} monosodium urate crystals can be deposited in tissues, forming a tophus. If these crystals are shed from a tophus in the synovial membrane or cartilage of a joint they produce an extremely painful acute arthritis that presents with the clinical syndrome of gout. In brief, the crystals are phagocytosed by macrophage cells within the synovium, which release mediators such as interleukin-1β. These mediators activate mast cells and endothelial cells with expression of adhesion molecules and chemokines. Uric acid crystals also provide a surface on which complement C5 is cleaved, with formation of complement membrane attack complex. The activated endothelial cells and complement membrane attack complex attract neutrophil leucocytes which release proteolytic and lysosomal enzymes that enhance tissue inflammation, destroy cartilage and damage the joint. Most attacks of gout are self-limiting, probably in part due to coating of the uric acid crystals with protein, which reduces their irritant properties. Acute gout usually presents with rapid onset of severe joint pain that reaches maximum intensity within 24 h. Pseudogout, due to deposition of calcium pyrophosphate crystals, has a similar clinical presentation.

Gout in younger people usually affects a single joint, with repeated acute attacks if the underlying cause is not treated. In the elderly, a chronic arthritis affecting multiple joints can occur. The diagnosis of gout is confirmed by the finding of monosodium urate crystals in the affected joint. With persistent hyperuricaemia, chronic urate deposits are sometimes found in tendon sheaths and soft tissues. Excess uric acid can also be deposited in the interstitium of the kidney or form stones in the renal calyces, both of which can produce progressive renal damage.

There are two components of drug treatment:

- treatment of an acute attack of gout,
- reduction of plasma uric acid concentration for prophylaxis against recurrent attacks of gout or to prevent kidney damage.

DRUGS FOR THE TREATMENT OF GOUT AND PREVENTION OF HYPERURICAEMIA

COLCHICINE

Mechanism of action

Colchicine interferes with several steps in the inflammatory cascade, particularly inhibiting recruitment and actions of neutrophil leucocytes in the gouty joint:

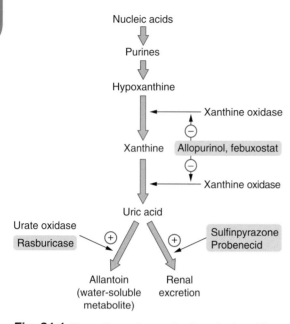

Fig. 31.1 The pathway for production of uric acid from purines and the sites of action of some of the drugs used in gout and hyperuricaemia.

- it reduces the production of inflammatory mediators by macrophages and downregulates their receptors on synovial and endothelial cells. Colchicine also inhibits the production of chemotaxins, which attract leucocytes into inflamed tissue,
- colchicine disrupts the assembly of microtubules in neutrophil leucocytes by forming a complex with tubulin in the cell. This impairs the adhesion of neutrophils to endothelial cells, which reduces their recruitment into the inflamed joint, and also impairs phagocytosis of crystals if the neutrophil does enter the joint. In addition, if crystals are phagocytosed into the neutrophil colchicine inhibits the subsequent release of enzymes and free radicals that damage the joint.

All of these actions give colchicine a specific anti-inflammatory effect in the gouty joint; it is ineffective in other forms of inflammatory arthritis. Other uses of colchicine include the management of recurrent pericarditis and familial Mediterranean fever.

Pharmacokinetics

Colchicine is well absorbed from the gut. It is usually given every 6–12 h until symptomatic relief is achieved or unwanted effects occur. Pain relief usually begins after about 18 h and is maximal by 48 h.

Unwanted effects

Colchicine has a low therapeutic index. Unwanted effects include:

- gut toxicity caused by inhibition of mucosal cell division, which produces abdominal pain, nausea, vomiting and diarrhoea; these effects are common and often dose-limiting,
- rash.

XANTHINE OXIDASE INHIBITORS

Examples

allopurinol, febuxostat

Mechanism of action

Allopurinol is an analogue of hypoxanthine, which is an intermediate in the pathway that generates uric acid. Both allopurinol and its major metabolite competitively inhibit the enzyme xanthine oxidase for which hypoxanthine is the natural substrate, thereby reducing uric acid formation (Fig. 31.1). Febuxostat is a non-purine selective xanthine oxidase inhibitor. Although plasma xanthine and hypoxanthine concentrations increase when these drugs are given, they do not crystallize. Because of their greater water solubility, their concentrations remain well below saturation levels even with maximal xanthine oxidase inhibition. Xanthine and hypoxanthine are reincorporated into the purine synthetic cycle, and this decreases the need for *de novo* purine formation.

Pharmacokinetics

Allopurinol is well absorbed from the gut and converted in the liver to an active metabolite with a long half-life, oxipurinol (alloxanthine). Febuxostat is well absorbed from the gut; it is eliminated by both metabolism and renal excretion and has a variable half-life (1–15 h).

Unwanted effects

- Gastrointestinal upset.
- An increased risk of acute gout during the first few weeks of treatment; this may be caused by fluctuations in plasma uric acid, possibly through uric acid release from tissue deposits.
- Hypersensitivity reactions with allopurinol, especially in people with renal impairment. These reactions include serious rashes such as Stevens–Johnson syndrome or toxic epidermal necrolysis.
- Drug interactions: allopurinol and febuxostat inhibit the metabolism of the cytotoxic drugs mercaptopurine and azathioprine (Ch. 52) because these are also metabolised by xanthine oxidase.

RASBURICASE

Mechanism of action

Rasburicase is a recombinant version of the enzyme urate oxidase which catalyses the oxidation of uric acid to a soluble metabolite, allantoin. This enzyme is present in mammals other than humans; the recombinant version is produced by a genetically modified strain of the fungus *Aspergillus flavus*. Rasburicase is used for prophylaxis of hyperuricaemia during treatment of malignancies with chemotherapy.

Pharmacokinetics

Rasburicase is given intravenously and is metabolised by peptide hydrolysis in plasma.

Unwanted effects

- Fever.
- Nausea, vomiting, diarrhoea.
- Hypersensitivity reactions: rasburicase induces antibody responses in about 10% of those treated, although allergic reactions such as rash, bronchospasm and anaphylaxis are rare.
- Haemolysis from the production of hydrogen peroxide as a by-product of the formation of allantoin.

URICOSURIC AGENTS

 Example

sulfinpyrazone

Mechanism of action

Sulfinpyrazone competitively inhibits transporters responsible for reabsorption of uric acid in the proximal tubule, therefore increasing urate concentrations in urine and reducing levels in plasma. There is a risk of precipitation of uric acid crystals in the kidney, particularly during the early stages of treatment, which can be prevented by maintaining a high fluid intake and alkaline urine (using potassium citrate or sodium bicarbonate) and by slowly titrating the dose. Aspirin and other salicylates should not be given with uricosuric drugs, because low doses of salicylates inhibit tubular uric acid secretion.

Probenecid used to be used as a uricosuric agent, but is now only available in the UK by special order for prevention of nephrotoxicity caused by the antiviral drug cidofovir.

Pharmacokinetics

Sulfinpyrazone is well absorbed from the gut. It is eliminated by hepatic metabolism and has a half-life of 4–5 h.

Unwanted effects

- Gastrointestinal upset.
- Renal uric acid deposition; deterioration of renal function can occur, especially if there is pre-existing impairment.
- Allergic rashes.

TREATMENT OF GOUT

ACUTE GOUT

Efforts should always be made to identify and remove precipitating causes of gout, particularly enquiring about alcohol intake and reviewing concurrent drug therapy. For acute attacks, non-steroidal anti-inflammatory drugs (NSAIDs; Ch. 29) are the treatment of choice. Aspirin should be avoided because at low doses it can inhibit renal excretion of uric acid and increase plasma urate concentration. Cyclo-oxygenase 2 (COX-2)-selective anti-inflammatory drugs are as effective as classic NSAIDs (Ch. 29). Colchicine is usually reserved for people who are intolerant of NSAIDs, or who have a contraindication to their use. Intra-articular injection of corticosteroid can be very effective if a single joint is involved, especially if other treatments are contraindicated. Oral corticosteroids, for example prednisolone (Ch. 44), are reserved for resistant episodes of gout. A 5-day high-dose regimen can be used, or two days of a high dose followed by a gradual reduction over 8–12 days to minimise the risk of a rebound flare of symptoms.

PREVENTION OF GOUT ATTACKS

Allopurinol is given for prophylaxis against recurrent attacks of acute gout, for chronic tophus formation in the tissues, or for the prevention of uric acid-induced renal damage. It is also given prophylactically before cytotoxic chemotherapy, when tissue breakdown releases purines, which generate large amounts of uric acid. To prevent gout, the serum uric acid concentration should be reduced to less than 0.36 mmol·L^{-1}, although it may be necessary to go below 0.3 mmol·L^{-1} to reabsorb gouty tophi.

Allopurinol should not be used during an acute attack of gout since it can prolong the attack, so waiting 1–2 weeks after symptoms have settled is advisable. There are two strategies to reduce the risk of provoking an attack when allopurinol is started in someone with hyperuricaemia. First, a low dosage of allopurinol can be given initially with slow dose titration until the target plasma uric acid concentration is achieved. Secondly, low dosage of an NSAID or colchicine can be given during the first 3 months of treatment. Febuxostat or sulfinpyrazone are reserved for people who do not tolerate allopurinol. Sulphinpyrazone is also used in combination with allopurinol for resistant hyperuricaemia. Low-dose NSAIDs or colchicine are sometimes used long term to prevent gout, although good data on their efficacy are lacking.

Prophylactic treatment should usually be life-long, since recurrence of gout or tophi frequently occurs if treatment is stopped. Short-term prophylaxis is possible when allopurinol is used during cytotoxic chemotherapy.

Rasburicase is used when intravenous prophylaxis against gout is required during cancer chemotherapy.

SELF-ASSESSMENT

One-best-answer (OBA) question

Choose the *most appropriate* statement below concerning drugs used in the treatment of gout.

A. Sodium urate is more water soluble than its precursor hypoxanthine.
B. Febuxostat is a purine analogue.
C. Allopurinol enhances the renal secretion of uric acid.
D. Colchicine inhibits the release of neutrophil proteases that cause joint damage.
E. Aspirin is safe to use in acute attacks of gout to reduce the pain and inflammation.

Case-based questions

A 56-year-old man awoke in the night with sudden severe pain in his first metatarsophalangeal joint, which lasted for a week. Over the next few months, he had similar acute episodes of pain in his ankles and knees, as well as his big toe. He had hypertension but no other vascular disease. The GP suspected gout and referred him to a specialist.

A. What treatment should the GP institute for the acute attacks, prior to the specialist diagnosis?
B. What test could the rheumatologist do to confirm the suspected diagnosis?
C. The diagnosis of gout was confirmed. What is the cause of gout?
D. What would you prescribe for prophylaxis to reduce recurrent attacks and how does this agent act?
E. The chosen treatment was only partially effective; what additional treatment could you prescribe?
F. What might be the consequences of inadequate treatment of this man?

OBA answers

Answer D is correct.

A. Incorrect. Hypoxanthine is more water soluble than urate; this is the rationale for the use of allopurinol, which inhibits conversion of hypoxanthine to urate by inhibiting xanthine oxidase.
B. Incorrect. Febuxostat is a non-purine inhibitor of xanthine oxidase.
C. Incorrect. Allopurinol prevents uric acid formation; the renal secretion of urate is enhanced by sulfinpyrazone and other uricosuric drugs.
D. **Correct.** Reducing neutrophil leucocyte activity is one of the anti-inflammatory mechanisms of colchicine in gout.
E. Incorrect. Unlike non-steroidal anti-inflammatory drugs (NSAIDs) used in acute gout, aspirin can inhibit the renal secretion of urate, exacerbating the gout.

Case-based answers

A. The treatment of choice for an acute attack is an NSAID to reduce pain and inflammation. Indometacin is often used and is effective within two days. Colchicine or glucocorticoids can be used in people intolerant to NSAIDs, but both have significant unwanted effects. Aspirin and other salicylates should be avoided as at low doses they reduce uric acid excretion, although at high doses they are uricosuric.
B. Plasma uric acid will be raised. An arthrocentesis sample will show sodium urate crystals. Infection should be excluded in an acutely inflamed joint.
C. Gout is caused by relatively insoluble sodium urate, a product of purine metabolism, crystallising in the joint space. People who develop gout have had hyperuricaemia for years. Overproduction of uric acid due to dietary purines (e.g. in meat and fish) or excessive alcohol consumption can contribute to gout, but in most people hyperuricaemia is caused by impaired renal clearance of uric acid.
D. Hyperuricaemia is treated after resolution of the acute attack. People who overproduce uric acid are best treated with allopurinol, which reduces plasma uric acid by inhibiting xanthine oxidase. This increases concentrations of hypoxanthine and xanthine, which are more water soluble than urate.
E. A low renal excretion of uric acid may be treated with a uricosuric drug (sulfinpyrazone); this inhibits the reabsorption of uric acid in the proximal convoluted tubule.
F. Untreated gout can lead to chronic joint damage and formation of kidney stones. A significant number of people with gout will have hypertension and increased risk of cardiovascular and renal disease.

FURTHER READING

Burns CM, Wortmann RL (2011) Gout therapeutics: new drugs for an old disease. *Lancet* 377, 165–177

Keith MP, Gilliland WR (2007) Update in the management of gout. *Am J Med* 120, 221–224

Neogi T (2011) Gout. *N Engl J Med* 364, 443–452

Underwood M (2006) Diagnosis and management of gout. *BMJ* 332, 1315–1319

Compendium: drugs used for gout and hyperuricaemia

Drug	Kinetics (half-life)	Comments
Allopurinol	High oral bioavailability; eliminated by metabolism to oxipurinol (0.5–2.0 h), which is less potent but has longer half-life (10–40 h) and may accumulate; both compounds are renally excreted	Xanthine oxidase inhibitor; used for prophylaxis of gout and of hyperuricaemia associated with cancer chemotherapy; given orally
Colchicine	Good oral absorption; rapidly eliminated from plasma (<1 h) but may be sequestered in leucocytes with a half-life of about 60 h	Anti-inflammatory drug used for acute gout and short-term prophylaxis during initial therapy with other drugs; given orally
Febuxostat	Eliminated by glucuronide conjugation and renal excretion (45–50%); highly variable half-life (1–15 h)	Non-purine xanthine oxidase inhibitor; used for prophylaxis in patients intolerant to allopurinol or when allupurinol is contraindicated; given orally
Probenecid	Complete oral bioavailability; hepatic metabolism and renal excretion (4–17 h); some active metabolites	Uricosuric drug; used to prevent nephrotoxicity associated with the use of the antiretroviral drug cidofovir; given orally; only available on special order in the UK
Rasburicase	Recombinant peptide eliminated by proteolysis (18–22 h)	Recombinant form of fungal urate oxidase which converts urate to soluble allantoin; used for hyperuricaemia during initial chemotherapy of haematological malignancy; given intravenously
Sulfinpyrazone	Good oral absorption; metabolised to an inactive sulphone and a sulphide analogue that inhibits platelet aggregation (4–5 h)	Uricosuric drug; used for gout prophylaxis and hyperuricaemia; given orally

For non-steroidal anti-inflammatory drugs (NSAIDs), see Ch 29.

7

The gastrointestinal system

32

Nausea and vomiting

NAUSEA AND VOMITING

Nausea, retching and vomiting (emesis) are part of the body's defence against ingested toxins. Vomiting is a reflex that is integrated by a loose neuronal network known as the 'vomiting centre' in the medulla oblongata of the brainstem. The exact location of the vomiting centre is unclear. It is composed of a series of nuclei in the nucleus tractus solitarius and the dorsal motor nucleus of the vagus. The afferent input to the vomiting centre comes from several sources (Fig. 32.1).

- Abdominal and cardiac vagal afferents are activated by mechano- or chemosensory receptors. Chemosensory receptors respond to several agonists such as acetylcholine, dopamine, serotonin, histamine and neurokinins. Some drugs induce vomiting by an effect on gastric chemosensory receptors.
- The area postrema in the floor of the fourth ventricle is the location of the chemoreceptor trigger zone (CTZ). This lies outside the blood–brain barrier and responds to stimuli from the cerebrospinal fluid and the systemic circulation. The CTZ has many receptors for neurotransmitters (such as dopamine, serotonin and substance P) and hormones and it has numerous afferent and efferent connections with the underlying nucleus tractus solitarius.

Other sources include:

- the vestibular nuclei, which are involved in the emetic response to motion,
- other brainstem structures, such as the amygdala,
- higher centres of the cortex and intracranial pressure receptors.

Several neurotransmitter receptors are involved in direct activation of the vomiting centre including those for dopamine (D_2), serotonin, acetylcholine (muscarinic), histamine (H_1) and substance P (neurokinin 1, NK_1) (Fig. 32.1).

The roles of these multiple receptors in the triggering of nausea and vomiting are complex. For example, $5-HT_3$ receptor antagonists will provide protection against nausea and vomiting induced by cytotoxic drugs and radiation but not by motion or by apomorphine. Vomiting can result from the summation of several sub-emetic stimuli, for example in the genesis of postoperative nausea and vomiting.

Efferent connections from the vomiting centre include the vagus and phrenic nerves. When stimulated these nerves relax the fundus and body of the stomach and the lower oesophageal sphincter, and retrograde giant contractions occur in the small intestine. Diaphragmatic and abdominal muscle contractions compress the stomach, and together these factors produce vomiting.

Many drugs produce vomiting by stimulating the CTZ and they do not have to cross the blood–brain barrier for this action (Box 32.1).

ANTI-EMETIC AGENTS

Antihistamines

Examples

cyclizine, promethazine

Mechanism of action and clinical use

Antihistamines prevent and treat vomiting by their antagonist action at histamine H_1 receptors (Ch. 39), and many also have antimuscarinic effects. Promethazine also blocks some 5-HT receptor subtypes. Antihistamines are effective against most causes of vomiting but, apart from the use of cyclizine for drug-induced vomiting, they are rarely treatments of choice. Promethazine is used to treat vomiting in pregnancy since it appears to be free from teratogenic effects.

Pharmacokinetics

These drugs are well absorbed orally; both promethazine and cyclizine can also be given by intramuscular or intravenous injection. After oral dosing, promethazine undergoes extensive first-pass metabolism.

Unwanted effects

- Sedation (particularly with promethazine) and headache.
- Antimuscarinic effects (Ch. 4), especially dry mouth, urinary retention and blurred vision.

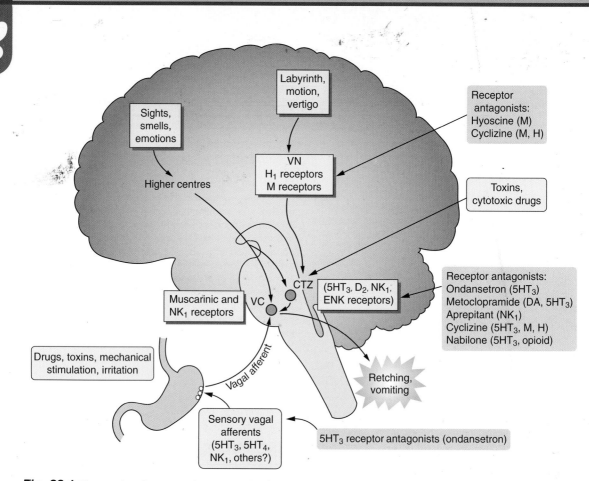

Fig. 32.1 **Neuronal pathways and receptors involved in the control of nausea and vomiting.** The pathways and neurotransmitter receptors involved in nausea and vomiting are complex and only those underpinning the mechanisms of action of the anti-emetic drugs are shown. The chemoreceptor trigger zone (CTZ) has neuronal connections to the vomiting centre (VC), which is a collection of nuclei including the dorsal motor nucleus of the vagus and the nucleus tractus solitarius. $5HT_3$, 5-Hydroxytryptamine type 3 receptor; DA, dopamine receptor; ENK receptor, enkephalin (opioid) receptor; H_1, histamine type 1 receptor; M, muscarinic receptor (possibly M_2); NK_1, neurokinin 1 receptor; VN, vestibular nuclei. Other mediators such as glutamate may also be involved.

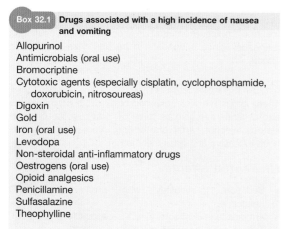

Box 32.1 **Drugs associated with a high incidence of nausea and vomiting**

Allopurinol
Antimicrobials (oral use)
Bromocriptine
Cytotoxic agents (especially cisplatin, cyclophosphamide, doxorubicin, nitrosoureas)
Digoxin
Gold
Iron (oral use)
Levodopa
Non-steroidal anti-inflammatory drugs
Oestrogens (oral use)
Opioid analgesics
Penicillamine
Sulfasalazine
Theophylline

Antimuscarinic agent

Example

hyoscine

Mechanism of action and clinical use

Muscarinic receptors are involved in the visceral afferent input from the gut to the vomiting centre and in the tract that the eighth cranial nerve takes from the labyrinth to the CTZ via the vestibular nucleus. Hyoscine (known as scopolamine in the USA) is used for the treatment of motion sickness and postoperative vomiting. Some antihistamines such as promethazine and cyclizine (see above), and dopamine receptor antagonists such as prochlorperazine (see below), also have antimuscarinic activity.

Pharmacokinetics

Hyoscine is available for oral, parenteral or transdermal use. Oral absorption is good. The adhesive patch for transdermal delivery can be placed behind the ear and delivers a therapeutic dose for 72 h.

Unwanted effects

- Typical antimuscarinic actions such as dry mouth, urinary retention and blurred vision (Ch. 4).
- Sedation.

Dopamine receptor antagonists

 Examples

domperidone, metoclopramide, prochlorperazine

Mechanism of action and clinical use

Domperidone, metoclopramide and the antipsychotic drugs are antagonists at dopamine D_2 receptors and inhibit dopaminergic stimulation of the CTZ (Fig. 32.1).

Anti-emetic doses of antipsychotic drugs are generally less than one-third of those used to treat psychoses. The pharmacology of the antipsychotic drugs is discussed in Chapter 21.

Domperidone acts solely by dopamine receptor blockade. Metoclopramide is a dopamine antagonist at usual oral doses, but it also acts as a 5-HT_3 receptor antagonist at higher doses. This enhanced efficacy is utilised by intravenous administration of high doses of metoclopramide to treat the vomiting induced by cytotoxic agents such as cisplatin.

Metoclopramide also has prokinetic actions on the gut including increased tone of the gastro-oesophageal sphincter and enhanced gastric emptying and small intestinal motility. These effects arise from agonist activity at the 5-HT_4 receptor subtype in the enteric nervous system, which leads indirectly to cholinergic stimulation.

Dopamine receptor antagonists are mainly used to reduce vomiting induced by drugs and surgery. Pure dopamine receptor antagonists are ineffective in motion sickness. Antipsychotic drugs such as prochlorperazine are effective for vestibular disorders and motion sickness as a result of their antimuscarinic activity.

Pharmacokinetics

Metoclopramide and domperidone are well absorbed orally, but have limited bioavailability due to extensive first-pass metabolism in the liver. Metoclopramide is also available for intravenous or intramuscular use, while domperidone can be given rectally by suppository. Metoclopramide has a shorter half-life (3–5 h) than domperidone (12–16 h).

Unwanted effects

Central nervous system (CNS) unwanted effects are produced by metoclopramide and the antipsychotics, but to a lesser extent by domperidone as a result of its lower CNS penetration.

- Acute and chronic extrapyramidal effects from dopamine receptor blockade in the basal ganglia can lead to acute dystonias (especially in children and young adults), akathisia and a parkinsonian-like syndrome. Tardive dyskinesias can develop with prolonged use (see also Ch. 24).
- Galactorrhoea and amenorrhoea caused by hyperprolactinaemia from pituitary dopamine receptor blockade.

5-HT_3 receptor antagonists

Examples

granisetron, ondansetron, palonosetron

Mechanism of action and clinical use

The 5-HT_3 receptor antagonists block the 5-HT_3 receptors in the CTZ and in the gut (Fig. 32.1). They are particularly effective against the acute vomiting induced by highly emetogenic chemotherapeutic agents used for treating cancer (e.g. cisplatin; Ch. 52) and for postoperative vomiting that is resistant to other agents. They are also used for prophylaxis when the consequences of retching and vomiting could be particularly deleterious, for example after eye surgery.

Pharmacokinetics

Oral absorption of ondansetron is rapid, and it can also be given by intravenous or intramuscular injection or by rectal suppository. Granisetron has a similar profile and is available for oral or intravenous use. Palonosetron has a long half-life and is given intravenously.

Unwanted effects

- Headache is common.
- Constipation, probably caused by 5-HT_3 receptor blockade in the gut.
- Flushing.
- Ondansetron prolongs the Q-T interval on the ECG at high doses, which predisposes to arrhythmias.

Neurokinin 1 receptor antagonists

Examples

aprepitant, fosaprepitant

Mechanism of action

Aprepitant and its prodrug fosaprepitant are antagonists at NK_1 receptors in the CNS, inhibiting the action of substance P. They augment the effects of 5-HT_3 receptor antagonists and corticosteroids in preventing the acute and delayed emetic response to the cancer chemotherapeutic agent cisplatin.

Pharmacokinetics

Aprepitant is well absorbed from the gut and has a long half-life. Fosaprepitant is given by intravenous infusion.

Unwanted effects

- Fatigue, dizziness, headache, hiccups.
- Anorexia, abdominal pain, diarrhoea.
- Drug interactions: aprepitant is an inhibitor of the liver enzyme CYP3A4 and an inducer of CYP2C9. It may decrease the clinical effect of warfarin.

Cannabinoids

 Example

nabilone

Mechanism of action and clinical use

Nabilone, a synthetic derivative of tetrahydrocannabinol (a psychoactive substance in cannabis; Ch. 54), is effective in combating vomiting induced by cytotoxic drugs, providing it is given before chemotherapy is started. The mechanism is uncertain, but it may involve inhibition of cortical activity and anxiolysis. Cannabinoid CB_1 receptors are found in several areas of the CNS and the action of nabilone at these receptors may inhibit neuronal serotonin release in the dorsal vagal nucleus.

Pharmacokinetics

Nabilone is well absorbed from the gut. It is metabolised extensively in the liver and has a short half-life, but some of its metabolites have long half-lives and may contribute to the activity.

Unwanted effects

- Sedation, vertigo, ataxia, sleep disturbance.
- Dry mouth.
- Dysphoric reactions with hallucinations and disorientation are most disturbing to older people. These may be reduced by concurrent use of prochlorperazine (see above).

Corticosteroids

Dexamethasone and methylprednisolone are weak anti-emetics. However, they produce additive effects when given with high-dose metoclopramide or with a 5-HT_3 receptor antagonist such as ondansetron. High doses of dexamethasone can be given intravenously before cancer chemotherapy, with subsequent oral doses to prevent delayed emesis. The mechanism of action is unknown but may involve reduction of prostaglandin synthesis or release of endorphins. The pharmacology of corticosteroids is discussed in Chapter 44.

Benzodiazepines

Benzodiazepines, such as lorazepam, have no intrinsic anti-emetic activity. They are given orally or intravenously before cancer chemotherapy to sedate and produce amnesia. They are especially useful if there has previously been vomiting with a cytotoxic treatment, since anticipatory nausea

Table 32.1 Common indications for various anti-emetic agents

Cause of vomiting	Treatment
Motion sickness	Hyoscine, cyclizine, promethazine
Postoperative vomiting	Hyoscine, metoclopramide, domperidone, prochlorperazine, ondansetron (reserved for resistant vomiting)
Drug-induced vomiting	Prochlorperazine, metoclopramide, cyclizine (particularly for opioid-induced vomiting)
Cytotoxic drug-induced vomiting	Prochlorperazine, metoclopramide, nabilone, ondansetron, aprepitant Adjunctive treatment, e.g. dexamethasone, benzodiazepines
Pregnancy-induced vomiting	Promethazine, metoclopramide, pyridoxine

and vomiting are then common with subsequent courses. Benzodiazepines are discussed in Chapter 20.

MANAGEMENT OF NAUSEA AND VOMITING

Anti-emetics are used in a number of situations where nausea and vomiting can be troublesome. Some specific clinical uses are considered in more detail (Table 32.1).

Drug-induced vomiting

It is sometimes necessary to use drugs that carry a high risk of inducing nausea and vomiting (Box 32.1). Cyclizine, prochlorperazine and metoclopramide are often effective for prevention of opioid-induced vomiting.

More problematic are the highly emetogenic agents used for cancer treatment. Cancer chemotherapy is accompanied by an increase in serotonin release in the gut and the brainstem. Serotonin in the gut probably stimulates vomiting via vagal afferent nerve fibres. For treatments that carry a low risk of vomiting, routine prophylaxis is not needed. For moderately emetogenic treatments, a 5-HT_3 receptor antagonist such as ondansetron, possibly combined with a corticosteroid (such as dexamethasone), is usually recommended. For highly emetogenic chemotherapy, a 5-HT_3 receptor antagonist combined with dexamethasone and aprepitant can achieve control in up to 80% of cases. Prochlorperazine, domperidone and nabilone can be used when there is intolerance of 5-HT_3 receptor antagonists or corticosteroids.

Delayed emesis, occurring at least 16 h after the chemotherapy, may be mediated by CNS 5-HT_3 and NK_1 receptors. Dexamethasone combined with aprepitant is recommended for control of delayed emesis, with a 5-HT_3 receptor antagonist being an alternative to aprepitant.

Anticipatory vomiting prior to cycles of chemotherapy usually occurs if previous cycles have been accompanied by nausea and vomiting. It is most effectively prevented by including a benzodiazepine such as lorazepam with the chemotherapy regimen from the start of treatment, to produce amnesia.

Postoperative vomiting

Postoperative nausea and vomiting frequently occur in the first 24 h after anaesthesia and surgery. They are more common in women, in non-smokers and after a previous episode of postoperative nausea and vomiting. They are provoked by inhalational rather than intravenous anaesthesia, more often by abdominal, ophthalmic or ear, nose and throat procedures, by the use of opioid analgesics, and by postoperative pain, hypotension and gastric stasis.

Dexamethasone, prochlorperazine, hyoscine (using a transdermal patch), promethazine and haloperidol are all effective for preventing postoperative vomiting. Antihistamines may be effective in emesis associated with surgery to the middle ear. If vomiting is severe, or if it carries high risk for the individual (e.g. after eye surgery), then a 5-HT$_3$ receptor antagonist such as ondansetron is particularly effective.

Motion sickness

Motion sickness arises from a mismatch between sensory inputs from the visual and vestibular systems. Behavioural treatments such as habituation or coping strategies involving distraction can be effective. If a drug is needed an antimuscarinic such as hyoscine or an antihistamine such as cyclizine are effective, with promethazine as an alternative. Antimuscarinic unwanted effects or drowsiness may be troublesome with each of these agents.

Vomiting in pregnancy

Nausea is common in pregnancy. High doses of pyridoxine (vitamin B$_6$) or of ground ginger may be effective, and counselling or hypnotism can also be tried.

Hyperemesis gravidarum, severe morning sickness which begins in the first trimester, can lead to marked maternal weight loss, dehydration, electrolyte disturbances and vitamin deficiencies. There is a natural desire to avoid drugs whenever possible if vomiting arises in pregnancy. However, for more severe vomiting, in addition to rehydration and nutritional supplementation, drugs will be necessary. Cyclizine and metoclopramide are the drugs of choice, with prochlorperazine, domperidone, ondansetron or a corticosteroid as second-line options. All these drugs appear to be safe in early pregnancy.

VERTIGO

Vertigo is an hallucination of motion, usually perceived as spinning, which is generated in the vestibular system of the inner ear. It is frequently accompanied by nausea and vomiting. There are several causes of vertigo (Box 32.2). The mechanisms of vertigo are poorly understood. Treatment is empirical and involves modulation of neurotransmitters and receptors involved in the vestibular sensory pathway to the

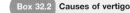

Box 32.2 **Causes of vertigo**

Ménière's disease
Benign positional vertigo
Migraine
Vestibular neuronitis
Multiple sclerosis
Brainstem ischaemia
Temporal lobe epilepsy
Cerebellopontine angle tumours

oculomotor nucleus. The neurochemistry of vertigo overlaps with that of vomiting, and involves:

- glutamate: excitatory, acting through N-methyl-D-aspartate (NMDA) receptors on both peripheral and central neurons,
- acetylcholine: excitatory, acting through muscarinic M$_2$ receptors on peripheral and central neurons,
- gamma-aminobutyric acid (GABA): inhibitory, acting through GABA$_A$ and GABA$_B$ receptors on central neurons,
- histamine: excitatory, acting through H$_1$ and H$_2$ receptors on central neurons,
- noradrenaline: involved in central modulation of vestibular sensory transmission,
- dopamine: excitatory at central neurons.

Ménière's disease is one of the causes of vertigo for which the pathogenesis is better understood. It usually presents with episodic vertigo and associated signs of vagal overactivity such as pallor, sweating, nausea and vomiting. Tinnitus and eventually sensorineural deafness are common. The basic defect is an excess of endolymph in the membranous labyrinth of the middle ear. There may be a genetic predisposition, while anatomical abnormalities in the middle ear and various immunological, vascular or viral precipitating insults may be involved.

DRUGS FOR TREATMENT OF VERTIGO

- **Antihistamines** (histamine H$_1$ receptor blockers), e.g. cyclizine, promethazine. These are the most widely used drugs for vertigo.
- **Antimuscarinic agents**. Vestibular suppression can be achieved with hyoscine, and the mechanism of action may be similar to that involved in the treatment of motion sickness.
- **Benzodiazepines**. The use of these agents for short periods may help in severe attacks of vertigo.
- **Cimetidine**. This drug probably produces symptom relief by blockade of histamine H$_2$ receptors in the CNS (Ch. 33).
- **Histamine receptor agonists**. The use of betahistine to treat Ménière's disease illustrates a paradox that both histaminergic and antihistaminic drugs have been advocated for treatment of this condition. Betahistine is an analogue of L-histidine, the metabolic precursor of histamine. It is a partial agonist at postsynaptic histamine H$_1$ receptors and an antagonist at presynaptic H$_3$ receptors, an action that facilitates central histaminergic neurotransmission. Betahistine also increases blood flow to

the inner ear. It is metabolised to an active derivative in the liver. The main unwanted effects are headache and nausea.

- **Dopamine receptor antagonists**. Several antipsychotic drugs such as prochlorperazine are used in vertigo, mainly to treat the associated nausea. Their use for treatment of dizziness in the elderly is not recommended because of the risk of extrapyramidal effects.

MANAGEMENT OF VERTIGO

Many forms of vertigo are brief and self-limiting. Acute vertigo, such as that caused by vestibular neuronitis, is often treated with anti-emetic agents until vestibular compensation occurs, which is usually encouraged by maintaining activity. The anti-emetic drug should usually be withdrawn as soon as the acute symptoms subside.

Benign paroxysmal positional vertigo responds poorly to drugs and is most effectively treated by vestibular exercises. Drug therapy should be avoided if possible, since it can blunt the effectiveness of the exercises by inhibiting vestibular compensation.

Ménière's disease is often treated initially with lifestyle changes, such as avoidance of excess caffeine, chocolate, alcohol and salt. Modification of the endolymph production in the inner ear with diuretics such as bendroflumethiazide (Ch. 14) is often attempted for persistent symptoms, although clear evidence of efficacy is lacking. Betahistine is often co-prescribed with a diuretic, again with little evidence of benefit. Oral or intratympanic injection of corticosteroid is an alternative to a diuretic. Sedative anti-emetic drugs such as promethazine, cinnarizine or prochlorperazine should only be used for very short periods since they impair vestibular rehabilitation. For refractory symptoms, the vestibular apparatus can be ablated, for example using local delivery of gentamicin (Ch. 51), which is toxic to the inner ear. Surgical treatment is also used for refractory disease.

Several drugs can cause dizziness or a sensation similar to vertigo and recent changes in drug therapy should be considered when a person presents with a new onset of dizziness. Examples of drugs that commonly cause dizziness are antihypertensive agents, vasodilators and antiparkinsonian agents. A more serious degree of vestibular toxicity can be produced by aminoglycosides such as gentamicin (Ch. 51) and high doses of loop diuretics such as furosemide (Ch. 14). This type of vestibular toxicity can be reversible, but is often permanent.

SELF-ASSESSMENT

True/false questions

1. Emetogenic toxins cross the blood–brain barrier to stimulate the chemoreceptor trigger zone (CTZ).
2. Some antihistamines are used for motion sickness.
3. Dopamine antagonists such as metoclopramide can cause movement abnormalities.
4. Metoclopramide decreases intestinal motility.
5. Aminoglycoside antibiotics may cause vertigo.

One-best-answer (OBA) question

Which statement concerning nausea and vomiting is the *most accurate*?

A. Afferents from the stomach to the vomiting centre inhibit vomiting when stimulated.
B. Selective 5-HT$_3$ receptor antagonists are effective against motion sickness.
C. Nabilone is derived from a psychoactive component of cannabis.
D. Stimulation of neurokinin 1 (NK$_1$) receptors in the CTZ inhibits nausea.
E. Digoxin inhibits nausea.

Case-based questions

A 35-year-old man was diagnosed with non-Hodgkin's lymphoma requiring many sessions of treatment with combined cytotoxic therapy, including cyclophosphamide and vincristine.

A. Why was this man likely to experience nausea and vomiting?

   Nausea and vomiting started several hours after each course of treatment and continued for 4–5 days.

B. What planned anti-emetic treatment prior to the first course of chemotherapy could be beneficial?
C. How do the treatments you have chosen work?

   This man became very distressed by the severity of the nausea and vomiting and developed intense nausea and vomiting prior to the administration of the chemotherapeutic agents.

D. What treatment could be given to reduce the anticipatory nausea and vomiting?

True/false answers

1. **False.** The CTZ (area postrema) is outside the blood–brain barrier. Some toxins can also cause vomiting by stimulating vagal afferents in the stomach.
2. **True.** Common antihistamines like promethazine have antimuscarinic activity and inhibit activity in the vomiting centre and in the vestibular nuclei. It is not certain whether the antihistamine component plays a role.
3. **True.** Dopamine antagonists used as anti-emetics are given at lower doses than in antipsychotic treatment, but they carry a risk of extrapyramidal movement disorders, particularly in the elderly.
4. **False.** Metoclopramide increases stomach and intestinal motility (prokinetic activity), which can add to its anti-emetic effects.
5. **True.** Aminoglycosides (such as gentamicin) and loop diuretics (furosemide) may cause vestibular damage, leading to vertigo.

OBA answer

Answer C is correct.

A. Incorrect. The vagal afferents from the stomach respond to toxins and are emetogenic.

B. Incorrect. Selective 5-HT$_3$ receptor antagonists are not effective against motion sickness, for which a drug with antimuscarinic actions, e.g. hyoscine or promethazine, should be used.

C. **Correct.** Nabilone is a derivative of tetrahydrocannabinol and an agonist at cannabinoid CB$_1$ receptors.

D. Incorrect. The effect of stimulating NK$_1$ receptors in the CTZ is to cause vomiting.

E. Incorrect. Digoxin causes nausea and vomiting.

Case-based answers

A. Cyclophosphamide induces nausea and vomiting in almost all people, but vincristine is much less emetogenic. The vomiting arises from stimulation of the CTZ.

B. A selective 5-HT$_3$ receptor antagonist such as ondansetron, alone or together with a corticosteroid, would be beneficial.

C. Ondansetron inhibits 5-HT$_3$ receptors in the CTZ and also in the stomach. In the stomach, some cancer chemotherapeutic agents can cause damage and release of serotonin, which stimulates vagal afferents to the vomiting centre. It is uncertain how corticosteroids work, but they have an anti-emetic effect which is additive with ondansetron.

D. Anticipatory nausea and vomiting is poorly treated with anti-emetic drugs. Treatment with benzodiazepine anxiolytic drugs prior to the course of chemotherapy can be helpful.

FURTHER READING

Baloh RW (2003) Vestibular neuritis. N Engl J Med 348, 1027–1032

Gan TJ, Meyer T, Apfel CC et al. (2003) Consensus guidelines for managing postoperative nausea and vomiting. Anesth Analg 97, 62–71

Hain TC, Uddin M (2003) Pharmacological treatment of vertigo. CNS Drugs 17, 85–100

Hesketh PJ (2008) Drug therapy-chemotherapy-induced nausea and vomiting. N Engl J Med 358, 2482–2494

Jarvis S, Nelson-Piercy C (2011) Management of nausea and vomiting in pregnancy. BMJ 342, d3606

Jordan K, Sippel C, Schmoll HJ (2007) Guidelines for antiemetic treatment of chemotherapy-induced nausea and vomiting: past, present, and future recommendations. Oncologist 12, 1143–1150

Nurdin L, Golding J, Bronstein A (2011) Managing motion sickness. BMJ 343, d7430

Niebyl JR (2011) Nausea and vomiting in pregnancy. N Engl J Med 363, 1544–1550

Sajjadi H, Paparella MM (2008) Ménière's disease. Lancet 372, 406–414

Wilhelm SM, Dehoorne-Smith ML, Kale-Pradhan PB (2007) Prevention of postoperative nausea and vomiting. Ann Pharmacother 41, 68–78

Compendium: anti-emetic agents

Drug	Kinetics (half-life)	Comments
Antihistamines		
These drugs have sedating properties.		
Cinnarizine	Very variable absorption; renal and faecal elimination (3 h)	Used for vestibular disorders and motion sickness; also used for peripheral vascular disease; given orally
Cyclizine	Few data available (20 h)	Used for a wide range of indications; given orally or by intramuscular or intravenous injection
Promethazine	Low bioavailability (25%); biliary elimination (7–14 h)	Given orally, by deep intramuscular injection or by slow intravenous injection for a wide range of indications
Dopamine receptor antagonists		
Phenothiazine and related drugs (see also Ch. 21)		
Chlorpromazine	Low oral bioavailability (10–33%); hepatic metabolism (8–35 h)	Used for nausea and vomiting associated with terminal illness; given orally, rectally or by deep intramuscular injection
Droperidol	Hepatic metabolism (2 h)	Used for postoperative nausea and vomiting; given by intavenous injection
Perphenazine	Low oral bioavailability (30–40%); hepatic metabolism (9 h)	Given orally for severe nausea and vomiting
Prochlorperazine	Variable oral absorption; hepatic metabolism (6–7 h)	Given orally or by deep intramuscular injection for severe nausea and vomiting
Trifluoperazine	Variable oral absorption; hepatic metabolism (7–18 h)	Given orally for severe nausea and vomiting

Compendium: anti-emetic agents—cont'd

Drug	Kinetics (half-life)	Comments
Domperidone and metoclopramide		
Domperidone	Low bioavailability (about 15%); hepatic metabolism, faecal and urinary excretion (12–16 h)	Used for a wide range of indications; given orally or rectally
Metoclopramide	Variable oral bioavailability (40–100%); hepatic metabolism and renal excretion (3–5 h)	Used for a wide range of indications; given orally or by intramuscular injection or intravenous injection over 1–2 min
5-HT_3 receptor antagonists		
Granisetron	Oral bioavailability 40–70%; hepatic metabolism and renal excretion (3–9 h)	Used to prevent nausea and vomiting induced by cytotoxic chemotherapy or radiotherapy; given orally or by intravenous injection or infusion
Ondansetron	Oral bioavailability 60%; hepatic metabolism (3 h)	Used to prevent nausea and vomiting induced by cytotoxic chemotherapy or radiotherapy; given orally, rectally, by intramuscular injection or by slow intravenous infusion
Palonosetron	Eliminated slowly by hepatic metabolism and renal excretion (40 h)	Given by intravenous injection for nausea and vomiting associated with severely emetogenic chemotherapy
Neurokinin 1 (NK_1) receptor antagonists		
Aprepitant	Good oral bioavailability (65%); hepatic metabolism (9–13 h)	Given orally as an adjunct for preventing nausea and vomiting associated with severely emetogenic chemotherapy
Fosaprepitant	Metabolised to aprepitant	Prodrug of aprepitant; given by intravenous infusion as an adjunct for preventing nausea and vomiting associated with severely emetogenic chemotherapy
Cannabinoids		
Nabilone	Completely absorbed; hepatic metabolism (2 h) to products that may contribute to the long duration of action	Given orally to prevent nausea and vomiting induced by cytotoxic chemotherapy which is unresponsive to conventional anti-emetics
Antimuscarinics		
Hyoscine (scopolamine)	Incomplete oral absorption; hepatic metabolism (8 h)	Given orally or as a transdermal patch for motion sickness and as premedication; also given by subcutaneous or intramuscular injection
Other drugs used for treatment and prevention of nausea and vomiting		
Benzodiazepines	–	See Ch. 20
Betahistine	Almost complete first-pass metabolism to active product which has a half-life of 5 h	Given orally for vertigo and tinnitus associated with Ménière's disease
Corticosteroids	–	See Ch. 44

33 Dyspepsia and peptic ulcer disease

THE SPECTRUM OF DISEASE

Dyspepsia is the term used for a group of symptoms that arise from the upper gastrointestinal tract. They include heartburn, abdominal pain or discomfort, fullness, bloating, early satiety, belching and nausea. Dyspepsia can occur alone (non-ulcer dyspepsia) or in association with various upper gastrointestinal disorders such as gastritis, peptic ulcer disease or gastro-oesophageal reflux disease.

NON-ULCER DYSPEPSIA

Several functional abnormalities in gastrointestinal motility, increased gastroduodenal sensitivity to mechanical distention and increased acid sensitivity in the duodenum have been described in people with non-ulcer dyspepsia.

PEPTIC ULCER DISEASE

Peptic ulceration is used to describe both gastric and duodenal ulcers. The characteristic symptom is epigastric pain, but other dyspeptic symptoms also occur. Symptoms are not a reliable guide to the location of an ulcer. However, the pain with duodenal ulceration is usually worse when fasting and at night and is relieved by antacids or by food. By contrast, with gastric ulcer the pain may be made worse by food and it is more likely than duodenal ulcer to be associated with weight loss, anorexia and nausea. Chronic ulcers at either site may be asymptomatic. Peptic ulcer disease is twice as frequent in males and more common in smokers, and there is often a family history of the disorder. There is also a higher incidence in people who use non-steroidal anti-inflammatory drugs (NSAIDs), including low-dose aspirin (Ch. 29), or who have a high alcohol intake. Women more often develop gastric rather than duodenal ulceration.

Complications of peptic ulcers include bleeding, perforation and – if close to the pylorus – scarring with gastric outlet obstruction.

Mechanisms of protection of gastric and duodenal mucosa

The healthy stomach mucosa is able to resist acid digestion. There is an adherent layer of viscoelastic mucus that acts as a physical barrier, and HCO_3^- is secreted into the mucus to neutralise acid locally. In addition, there is a high electrical resistance of, and tight junctions between, gastric mucosal cells, which make the mucosa relatively impermeable to luminal contents. Gastric mucosal blood flow provides an extra layer of defence, delivering HCO_3^- to buffer any H^+ ions that penetrate the mucosa, and also regulating acid secretion. Many of these protective functions are dependent on the synthesis by gastric mucosal cells of the prostaglandins PGE_2 and PGI_2 (Ch. 29) (Table 33.1).

The duodenal mucosa is protected by a layer of viscoelastic mucus, but the mucosal cells are highly permeable, permitting absorption of luminal nutrients. The mucosal cells secrete HCO_3^-, which accumulates in the mucus layer (the mucosal barrier) and buffers the pulses of gastric acid released from the stomach.

Aetiology of peptic ulceration

The precise aetiology of peptic ulceration is not known but there are many contributory factors. Gastric acid is essential for ulceration to arise, and there is often a failure of normal luminal acid concentration to inhibit further gastric acid secretion. Pepsin secretion is also enhanced in people with peptic ulceration. Accelerated gastric emptying is a factor in promoting duodenal ulceration, with entry of gastric contents at a lower pH into the duodenum. Prostaglandins increase mucosal protection against ulceration, and deficient production of prostaglandin E_1 is a factor in reducing

Table 33.1 Factors associated with protection and damage of the intestinal mucosa

Factors associated with peptic ulcer disease	Factors associated with peptic ulcer protection and healing
Thin or breached mucus layer	Intact mucus layer
Helicobacter pylori and host immune response	Adequate blood flow
Reduced bicarbonate secretion	Bicarbonate in mucus layer
Reduced mucosal blood flow	Prostaglandins (generated by cyclo-oxygenase COX-1 and COX-2 isoenzymes)
Stress	Hydrophobicity of phospholipid layer of epithelial cells
Smoking	Regrowth of epithelial cell layer following damage (restitution)
Alcohol	Growth factors
Acid	Nitric oxide
Pepsin	
Iatrogenic, e.g. NSAIDs.	

resistance to mucosal erosion in both the stomach and duodenum.

A major risk factor associated with peptic ulceration is gastric and duodenal infection with the Gram-negative bacterium *Helicobacter pylori*. The organism penetrates the mucus lining of the stomach and attaches to epithelial cells. The incidence of *H. pylori* in the gastric mucosa varies widely in the adult population in different countries, being highest in those who have poorer living conditions. About 10–15% of the UK population is infected. Infection is usually acquired in childhood and persists unless treated. Infection with *H. pylori* is an acknowledged risk factor for gastritis, peptic ulcer, gastric cancer and mucosa-associated lymphoid tissue (MALT) lymphoma. Only a small percentage of those who carry the bacteria develop *H. pylori*-associated disease, perhaps reflecting different host responses to the infection and whether the infecting strain carries particular factors for high virulence. Infection with *H. pylori* is found in about 80% of people with duodenal ulcer and somewhat fewer with gastric ulcer. *H. pylori* secretes the enzyme urease, which contributes to its survival during exposure to gastric acid by producing ammonia from urea. Ammonia is toxic to mucosal cells, and an immune response to the bacterial proteins also contributes to development of chronic gastritis.

H. pylori *and gastric ulceration*

If a gastric ulcer is present it is often associated with *H. pylori* infection of the corpus of the stomach or both the corpus and antrum (pangastritis). Moreover, unlike the situation in duodenal ulceration there is a decrease or at least no increase in acid secretion. The reason for this is that infection of the corpus is associated with atrophy of acid-secreting cells and metaplasia of the gastric mucosa, which lead to gastric ulceration and increase the risk of gastric cancer.

NSAIDs are the most frequent cause of gastric ulceration in the absence of *H. pylori*. The mechanisms are distinct, and relate to inhibition of prostaglandin formation and intracellular trapping of NSAID in the gastric mucosa (Ch. 29).

The prevalence of non-*H. pylori*, non-NSAID-associated gastric ulcers appears to be increasing in Western societies. The pathogenesis of these ulcers is poorly understood.

H. pylori *and duodenal ulceration*

In people who develop duodenal ulceration *H. pylori* infection is predominantly found in the stomach and confined to the antral mucosa. Antral mucosal cells secrete gastrin, which stimulates excess acid secretion from the body of the stomach. Exposure of duodenal cells to excess acid alters the structure of some of them, making them gastric-like (gastric metaplasia) and allowing them to be colonized by *H. pylori*.

As with gastric ulceration, NSAIDs are the most frequent cause of duodenal ulceration in the absence of *H. pylori* infection.

GASTRO-OESOPHAGEAL REFLUX DISEASE

Gastro-oesophageal reflux disease (GORD) can produce heartburn from regurgitation of gastric contents into the oesophagus (reflux), pain or difficulty in swallowing, and even the regurgitation of gastric contents into the mouth. If reflux is associated with inflammation of the oesophageal mucosa (oesophagitis), there may be more prolonged chest pain and even chronic bleeding. Gastro-oesophageal reflux is produced by the generation of transient lower oesophageal sphincter relaxations (TLOSRs) in the absence of swallowing. TLSORs arise from stimulation of gastric vagal mechanoreceptors and allow gastric acid, pepsin and bile to come into contact with the vulnerable epithelium of the oesophagus. Oesophageal hypomotility and abnormal patterns of oesophageal contractility often coexist with GORD, and reduce the clearance of refluxed material. The disturbance of normal motility may reflect a sensory abnormality in the oesophageal mucosa.

Oesophageal spasm is a distinct disorder, in which oesophageal pain is often not accompanied by any change in luminal pH. The pain frequently occurs in people who have no evidence of obvious dysmotility, and this syndrome is probably due to a combination of local mucosal sensory disturbances and psychological factors.

There is little correlation between the presence of oesophagitis at endoscopy and the severity of symptoms. Up to 50% of people with symptoms of GORD have no apparent oesophagitis, whereas severe oesophagitis may be asymptomatic unless complications such as stricture or anaemia arise. GORD has an association with asthma, through microaspiration of gastric contents into the lungs and triggering of vagal oesophago-bronchial reflexes. Microaspiration is also associated with chronic cough.

The relationship of *H. pylori* infection to GORD is not straightforward: antral infection appears to predispose to GORD by promoting greater amounts of gastric acid secretion, while corporal gastritis is protective partly because the acid content of the stomach may be reduced. Symptoms in GORD are usually chronic and relapsing, with at least two-thirds of those diagnosed still taking continuous or intermittent treatment after 10 years. It is now believed that there are three distinct clinical groups of GORD rather than a steady progression of severity. These are possibly determined by genetic factors and the immunological response to reflux. The groups are:

- non-erosive reflux disease,
- erosive oesophagitis, an acute inflammatory T-helper cell 1 (Th1) response (Ch. 38),
- Barrett's oesophagus (intestinal metaplasia of oesophageal mucosal cells) with increased risk of cancer; this is a Th2-type immunological response (Ch. 38).

CONTROL OF GASTRIC ACID SECRETION

Acid secretion into the canaliculi of gastric parietal cells is initiated by the activity of a membrane-bound proton pump which exchanges H^+ and K^+ across the cell membrane (H^+/K^+-ATPase). Hydrogen ions are obtained from carbonic acid (H_2CO_3) by carbonic anhydrase, and HCO_3^- enters the plasma in exchange for Cl^-. Chloride ions are then secreted into the stomach lumen with H^+ via a symport carrier. The activity of the proton pump is influenced by several mediators, including histamine, gastrin and acetylcholine (Fig. 33.1).

DRUGS FOR TREATING DYSPEPSIA, PEPTIC ULCER AND GASTRO-OESOPHAGEAL REFLUX DISEASE

ANTISECRETORY DRUGS

It is only necessary to raise intragastric pH above 3 for a few hours each day to promote healing of most peptic ulcers. However, rapid healing requires acid suppression for a minimum of 18–20 h per day. The duration of acid suppression determines the rate of healing but not the eventual proportion of ulcers healed. Several classes of drug have antisecretory actions on the gastric mucosa.

Proton pump inhibitors

Examples

esomeprazole, lansoprazole, omeprazole, pantoprazole

Mechanism of action

Since the proton pump (H^+/K^+-ATPase) is the final common pathway for acid secretion in gastric parietal cells, inhibition of the pump almost completely blocks acid secretion (Fig. 33.1). Proton pump inhibitors are irreversible inhibitors of H^+/K^+-ATPase and the return of acid secretion is dependent on the synthesis of new proton pumps. Proton pump inhibitors are weak bases that are selectively concentrated from the circulation into the acid environment of the secretory canaliculi of the gastric parietal cell. The drugs are then protonated and structurally transform into active derivatives that covalently bind to and irreversibly inhibit the proton pump. Because protonation to the active derivatives only takes place at acid pH, these drugs have a selective action on gastric cells, and proton pumps elsewhere in the body are not inhibited. Acid production is inhibited by about 90% for approximately 24 h following a single dose.

Pharmacokinetics

Proton pump inhibitors are prodrugs that are unstable in acid. They are given orally as enteric-coated formulations; esomeprazole, omeprazole and pantoprazole are also available as intravenous formulations. Elimination is by hepatic metabolism. They have short plasma half-lives (1–2 h) but, because of the irreversible mechanism of action, these bear no relationship to the long biological duration of action. Esomeprazole is the S-isomer of omeprazole that has lower clearance and therefore achieves slightly higher plasma concentrations.

Unwanted effects

- Gastrointestinal upset, such as nausea, vomiting, abdominal pain, diarrhoea, constipation.
- Headache.
- Omeprazole and esomeprazole are inhibitors of CYP2C9 and CYP2C19 in the liver. This can give rise to drug interactions with other substrates of these isoenzymes, for example decreasing the metabolism and increasing the clinical effects of warfarin, phenytoin and several antiviral drugs (see Table 2.7).

Concerns that substantial reductions of gastric acid, and the associated rise in gastrin secretion, might increase the risk of gastric cancer (comparable to the increased risk in pernicious anaemia) appear to be unfounded. These drugs do not completely abolish acid secretion and intragastric pH can still fall below 4 during part of the day, the critical pH below which bacterial populations that predispose to cancer are thought not to become established. However, symptomatic improvement following treatment with a proton pump inhibitor can mask the symptoms of gastric cancer.

Histamine H₂ receptor antagonists

Examples

cimetidine, ranitidine

Mechanism of action

Histamine H_2 receptor antagonists act competitively at receptors on gastric parietal cells. They reduce basal acid secretion and pepsin production, and prevent the increase in secretion that occurs in response to several secretory

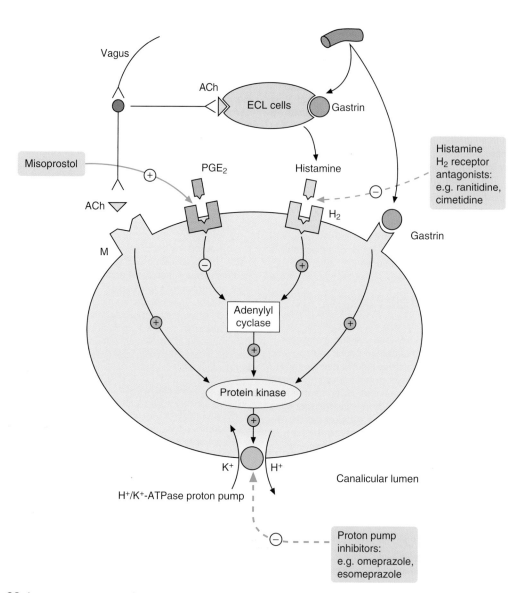

Fig. 33.1 Control of gastric acid secretion from the parietal cell. Acid secretion from the parietal cell is stimulated by acetylcholine (ACh), histamine and gastrin. Gastrin and ACh also reinforce acid secretion by causing the release of histamine from the enterochromaffin-like (ECL) cells which lie close to the parietal cells in the gastric pits. Prostaglandin E_2 (PGE_2) reduces acid secretion. The sites of action of the main drugs used to inhibit acid secretion from the parietal cell are shown. There are no useful inhibitors of gastrin action, and the gastric-selective muscarinic receptor (M) antagonist pirenzepine is no longer available in the UK. H_2, histamine type 2 receptor.

stimuli. Overall, acid secretion is reduced by about 60% (Fig. 33.1).

Pharmacokinetics

Absorption of cimetidine and ranitidine from the gut is almost complete but both undergo limited first-pass metabolism. The drugs are mainly eliminated unchanged by the kidney, in part through active tubular transport. Their half-lives are between 1 and 4 h.

Unwanted effects

- Diarrhoea and other gastrointestinal disturbances.
- Headache, dizziness, tiredness.
- Rash.
- Drug interactions: cimetidine is an inhibitor of hepatic P450 isoenzymes (see Table 2.7) and can increase the plasma concentrations and actions of drugs such as warfarin, phenytoin and theophylline.

ANTACIDS

xamples

aluminium hydroxide, magnesium trisilicate

Mechanism of action

Antacids neutralise gastric acid; magnesium salts do so much more rapidly than aluminium salts. They have a more prolonged effect if taken after food. If used without food, the effect lasts no more than an hour because of rapid gastric emptying. Antacids quickly produce symptom relief in peptic ulcer disease, but large doses are required to heal ulcers. Liquid preparations work more rapidly, but tablets are more convenient to use. Most antacids are relatively poorly absorbed from the gut. Simeticone is sometimes added to an antacid as an antifoaming agent. The combination may reduce flatulence, or relieve hiccups in palliative care.

Unwanted effects

- Constipation can occur with aluminium salts, and diarrhoea with magnesium salts; mixtures of aluminium and magnesium salts may have less effect on stool consistency.
- Systemic alkalosis can occur with very large doses.
- In advanced renal failure, retention of absorbed aluminium may contribute to metabolic bone disease and encephalopathy. Magnesium salts can also cause toxicity, and the dose should be reduced in renal failure.
- Drug interactions: aluminium salts can bind to NSAIDs and tetracyclines in the gut and reduce their absorption.

Antacids with alginic acid

Alginic acid is an inert substance. It is claimed that it forms a raft of high-pH foam which floats on the gastric contents and protects the oesophageal mucosa during reflux. All proprietary preparations combine alginic acid with an antacid, which is probably responsible for much of the clinical effect. Some formulations contain a high Na$^+$ concentration and these should be used with caution in people with fluid retention or hypertension.

CYTOPROTECTIVE DRUGS

Sucralfate
Mechanism of action

Sucralfate is a complex of aluminium hydroxide and sucrose octasulphate. It dissociates in the acid environment of the stomach to its anionic form, which binds to the ulcer base. This creates a protective barrier to pepsin and bile and inhibits the diffusion of gastric acid. Sucralfate also stimulates the gastric secretion of bicarbonate and prostaglandins.

Pharmacokinetics

Sucralfate is only slightly absorbed from the gut (<2%).

Unwanted effects

- Constipation.
- Bezoar formation (a mass trapped in the gut, usually the stomach), especially if gastric emptying is delayed.

Bismuth salts

xample

tripotassium dicitratobismuthate

Mechanism of action

Bismuth salts precipitate in the acid environment of the stomach and then bind to glycoprotein on the base of an ulcer. The resulting complex adheres to the ulcer and has similar local effects to sucralfate. Bismuth salts, in combination with antibiotics, were the first effective anti-*Helicobacter* agents and this effect may have accounted for their ulcer-healing properties. They have now largely been superseded by proton pump inhibitor combinations for this purpose; however, when triple therapy with two antibacterials and a proton pump inhibitor fails, bismuth is included as part of the treatment regimen (see below).

Pharmacokinetics

Bismuth compounds are poorly soluble and only slightly absorbed from the gut.

Unwanted effects

- Blackened stools and darkened tongue.

Prostaglandin analogues

xample

misoprostol

Mechanism of action

Misoprostol is an analogue of PGE$_1$ and has several actions that protect the gastric and duodenal mucosae (see Ch. 29). Misoprostol limits the damage to superficial mucosal cells caused by agents such as acid and alcohol. It is most widely used to prevent NSAID-associated ulcers, and is available in combination products with diclofenac or naproxen (Ch. 29).

Pharmacokinetics

Misoprostol is an ester that is well absorbed from the gut and undergoes essentially complete first-pass metabolism to an active acid metabolite. Elimination of the acid is mainly by hepatic metabolism and it has a very short half-life (<1 h).

Unwanted effects

- Diarrhoea and abdominal cramps are common.
- Uterine contractions: therefore, avoid in pregnancy. Misoprostol can be used to induce labour (Ch. 45).
- Menorrhagia and postmenopausal bleeding.

PROKINETIC DRUGS

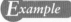 *Example*

metoclopramide

Mechanism of action

Metoclopramide is a dopamine receptor antagonist and is discussed in Chapter 32. It enhances gastric motility, increases the rate of gastric emptying and increases lower gastro-oesophageal sphincter tone.

MANAGEMENT OF DYSPEPSIA, PEPTIC ULCER AND GASTRO-OESOPHAGEAL REFLUX DISEASE

NON-ULCER DYSPEPSIA

Most people with dyspepsia do not have significant underlying disease (i.e. they have non-ulcer or functional dyspepsia). In all cases, efforts should be made to remove causative agents, for example smoking, excess alcohol or NSAIDs. For persistent symptoms, antacids provide symptomatic relief. Eradication of *H. pylori* does not usually reduce symptoms, although it can be effective for about 15% of people who probably have undiagnosed peptic ulceration.

Upper gastrointestinal endoscopy may be indicated to assess the cause of symptoms. However, younger people (especially those under 55 years of age) who do not have ALARM symptoms (**a**naemia, **l**oss of weight, **a**norexia, **r**ecent onset of progressive symptoms, **m**elaena, haematemesis or dysphagia) are often treated initially without investigation.

A proton pump inhibitor is more effective than a histamine H_2 receptor antagonist for symptom relief in non-ulcer dyspepsia. Treatment should be given for 4–6 weeks, followed by clinical review with the intention of reducing the dose of drug or moving to intermittent or on-demand therapy for symptom relief. Recurrent symptoms may prompt further investigation to exclude peptic ulceration or GORD.

CONFIRMED PEPTIC ULCERATION

Proton pump inhibitors produce the fastest rate of ulcer healing (over 90% of ulcers heal within four weeks). Histamine H_2 receptor antagonists usually give symptomatic relief for both gastric and duodenal ulcers within a week, but healing of the ulcer is much slower, requiring up to eight weeks for duodenal ulcer or 12 weeks for gastric ulcer. Other agents such as bismuth salts and sucralfate will heal ulcers in a similar proportion of people, but are used less often, since they do not improve symptoms as quickly.

Identification and eradication of *H. pylori* infection enhances ulcer healing and reduces relapse, so that maintenance therapy with acid-suppressing drugs is often unnecessary for uncomplicated ulcers. If *H. pylori* is not eradicated, 80% of ulcers will reoccur within a year, whereas following successful eradication the recurrence is less than 20%.

ERADICATION OF *H. PYLORI*

Several indications for *H. pylori* eradication have been proposed (Box 33.1). Many eradication regimens are available: the highest eradication rates are achieved by treatment with high dosage of a proton pump inhibitor combined with two antibacterials (to maximise efficacy and minimise resistance) given for one week. The first choice antibacterials are clarithromycin with either amoxicillin or metronidazole, but it important to avoid an antibacterial that has been used recently for treatment of other infections. Treatment for two weeks has a higher eradication rate, but unwanted effects often reduce adherence to the regimen, which limits the success rate. The incidence of *in vitro* resistance of *H. pylori* to metronidazole and to clarithromycin is increasing. If *in vitro* clarithromycin resistance is detected it is always reflected in a reduced ability to eliminate the bacterium clinically. By contrast, eradication may be successful even when laboratory resistance to metronidazole is demonstrated. Resistance to amoxicillin is less common, and resistance to tinidazole is currently lower than to metronidazole.

Eradication with a triple regimen is successful in about 85% of cases, and failure usually reflects antibacterial resistance or poor adherence to treatment. However, resistance to triple therapy is now widespread in some localities, with a failure to eradicate *H. pylori* in up to 20% of people treated. Quadruple therapy can be used for resistant bacteria. One recommended regimen is a proton pump inhibitor plus tripotassium dicitratobismuthate plus metronidazole plus tetracycline for 7 days (Fig. 33.2). Other regimens are used following the results of microbiological sensitivity tests on biopsy specimens. These quadruple-therapy regimens achieve an eradication rate of 93–98%.

Box 33.1 Indications for eradication of *H. pylori*

Eradication recommended
Proven peptic ulcer
Low-grade mucosa-associated lymphoid tissue (MALT) gastric lymphoma
Severe gastritis
After resection of early gastric cancer

Eradication suggested (less certain indications)
Functional dyspepsia
Family history of gastric cancer
Non-steroidal anti-inflammatory drug (NSAID) therapy
Intended long-term proton pump inhibitor therapy

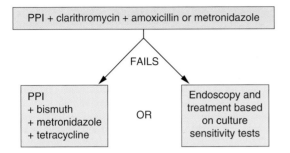

Fig. 33.2 Recommended regimens for the eradication of *H. pylori*. Many regimens exist, dictated by local patterns of sensitivity and resistance. Increasing resistance to metronidazole and clarithromycin is reducing the success rate of the triple regimen. If the proton pump inhibitor (PPI) is not tolerated, a histamine H$_2$ receptor antagonist can be substituted.

After *H. pylori* eradication, maintenance therapy with acid-suppressant treatment is only required if symptoms continue and after exclusion of more serious conditions.

BLEEDING FROM PEPTIC ULCERS

Active bleeding from a peptic ulcer is a medical emergency. Endoscopic treatment applied to a visible vessel in the ulcer base using diathermy, clipping, laser coagulation or injection with adrenaline may stop the bleeding. Even after achieving haemostasis, recurrent bleeding occurs in up to 20% of cases. Endoscopic treatment is followed by intravenous high-dose proton pump inhibitor for 72 h before changing to oral tharapy, which reduces the rebleeding rate and the need for surgery by 30–40%. The efficacy of proton pump inhibitors in this situation may be related to reversal of the deactivation of the coagulation system and platelet aggregation that occurs when the local pH falls below 4.

PEPTIC ULCERATION ASSOCIATED WITH NON-STEROIDAL ANTI-INFLAMMATORY DRUGS

If the NSAID cannot be withdrawn, then NSAID-associated ulcers will often heal if an ulcer-healing agent is co-prescribed. Continued use of NSAIDs can slow ulcer healing by histamine H$_2$ receptor antagonists, but probably not by proton pump inhibitors. Eradication of *H. pylori* infection is recommended if an NSAID must be continued in someone who has had previous peptic ulceration, although this may be more effective in preventing ulcers early in treatment with NSAIDs and less effective during long-term use.

When an NSAID is first used, careful assessment is recommended to decide whether prophylaxis against ulceration is given in the absence of upper gastrointestinal symptoms. Those at higher risk of NSAID-induced ulceration are the elderly (>65 years), smokers, heavy alcohol users and those taking concomitant treatment with medicines that cause gastrointestinal irritation, such as corticosteroids. People with a history of previous ulceration or those who have serious comorbidities, such as cardio-vascular disease, diabetes or renal or hepatic impairment, are also at higher risk.

Misoprostol provides effective prophylaxis against NSAID-induced gastric or duodenal ulceration. However, the high dosage necessary for prevention of ulcer recurrence and ulcer complications is often poorly tolerated due to colic or diarrhoea. Standard doses of a histamine H$_2$ receptor antagonist protect against NSAID-induced duodenal ulcers, but not against gastric ulceration. Double the usual doses of a histamine H$_2$ receptor antagonist or standard doses of a proton pump inhibitor protect against both gastric and duodenal ulceration, and are better tolerated than misoprostol. The use of a cyclo-oxygenase 2 (COX-2)-selective inhibitor has been advocated for people at higher risk of ulceration, but is no more effective than a conventional NSAID with a proton pump inhibitor. There is limited evidence to support the use of a COX-2-selective inhibitor with a proton pump inhibitor as a strategy to further reduce the risk of peptic ulceration in people at highest risk of ulceration. The combination of a COX-2 inhibitor with low-dose aspirin carries the same risk of ulceration as a conventional NSAID and should be avoided.

GASTRO-OESOPHAGEAL REFLUX DISEASE

Initial measures against GORD include avoidance of tight clothing around the waist, smoking, alcohol and caffeine, and encouraging weight loss. Raising the head of the bed on wooden blocks by 15 cm can promote symptom relief and mucosal healing. For mild persistent symptoms, reduction of gastric acid with antacids, with or without the addition of an alginate to provide a mechanical barrier, is often helpful. Alginates should be taken after meals to reduce their clearance by rapid gastric emptying. Proton pump inhibitors are the most effective treatment for severe resistant or relapsing GORD. They will rapidly ease symptoms and heal oesophagitis in up to 85% of those treated by eight weeks. Acid secretion may break through at night during treatment with a proton pump inhibitor. This may be important in severe erosive oesophagitis or Barrett's oesophagus, and in this situation esomeprazole may be more effective than other proton pump inhibitors. Failure to heal oesophagitis with a proton pump inhibitor often indicates bile rather than acid reflux. Histamine H$_2$ receptor antagonists often relieve troublesome symptoms, with relief of heartburn in up to 50% of cases after four weeks. However, mucosal repair is less likely, with healing of oesophagitis in about 20% of cases. Better response rates can often be achieved by using a histamine H$_2$ receptor antagonists at double the standard dosages, which will produce healing in 70–80% of cases by 8–12 weeks.

An alternative approach to the relief of symptoms is to enhance oesophageal motility with a prokinetic drug such as metoclopramide. Metoclopramide encourages normal peristalsis in the upper gastrointestinal tract and produces similar symptomatic relief to histamine H$_2$ receptor antagonists. However, it does not heal oesophagitis, and should only be used alone for non-erosive disease. Eradication of *H. pylori* in GORD does not improve symptoms.

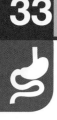

Intermittent therapy with healing agents, or use of an alginate after healing, often controls recurrent symptoms. For severe or resistant reflux disease, long-term use of a proton pump inhibitor is the only effective drug treatment, although about 60% of people will need only a low maintenance dose after healing has occurred. Laparoscopic anti-reflux surgery is increasingly used for resistant GORD, particularly if there is high-volume reflux.

Pain due to oesophageal spasm sometimes responds to smooth muscle relaxants such as calcium channel blockers (Ch. 5), nitrates (Ch. 5) or sildenafil (Ch. 16). Local injection of botulinum toxin (Ch. 24) has also been successful in limited studies.

SELF-ASSESSMENT

True/false questions

1. Histamine acts on H_1 receptors on the parietal cell to stimulate acid secretion.
2. Vagal stimulation of the parietal cell increases acid secretion.
3. An unwanted effect of antacids containing magnesium salts is diarrhoea.
4. Antacids are not effective in healing peptic ulcers.
5. Cimetidine can potentiate the effects of other drugs by inhibiting cytochrome P450 enzymes.
6. Ranitidine is associated with a lower incidence of gynaecomastia than cimetidine.
7. Cimetidine reduces acid secretion by more than 90%.
8. Omeprazole is a prodrug.
9. The active metabolite of lansoprazole is a reversible proton pump inhibitor.
10. Omeprazole inhibits the cytochrome P450 system in the liver.
11. Prostacyclin (prostaglandin I_2, PGI_2) reduces gastric mucosal blood flow.
12. Misoprostol causes constipation.
13. Histamine H_2 receptor antagonists and proton pump inhibitors are not useful for treatment of ulcers induced by non-steroidal anti-inflammatory drugs (NSAIDs).
14. Metoclopramide increases the rate of gastric emptying.
15. Sucralfate and bismuth bind to the ulcer base and promote ulcer healing.

One-best-answer (OBA) question

Which of the following statements about *Helicobacter pylori* is the *least accurate*?

A. *H. pylori* infection in the gastric antrum reduces acid secretion.
B. *H. pylori* infection can be found in the duodenum in people with duodenal ulcers.
C. If *H. pylori* is not eliminated, a duodenal ulcer is likely to recur.
D. *H. pylori* is a risk factor for the development of gastric cancer.
E. *H. pylori* frequently develops resistance to antibacterial treatment.

Case-based questions

A 47-year-old man, Mr TK, was newly appointed as headmaster of a large comprehensive school and was experiencing some difficulties with the increasing demands of the job. He increased his smoking from five to 20 cigarettes a day and he drank 10 units of alcohol a week. He had a good, varied diet. He had suffered intermittently from dyspepsia for some years, taking proprietary antacids when required. His symptoms then increased and the pain caused him to wake most nights. He bought a supply of ranitidine from the local chemist without consultation with the pharmacist. Following two weeks of treatment, his symptoms were successfully relieved and he was symptom-free for three months. His symptoms then returned and he took further treatment with ranitidine for two weeks. He was symptom-free for a further month, but when symptoms returned again he consulted his GP.

A. Why did his symptoms return?
B. Would his symptoms have been less likely to return following a short course of a proton pump inhibitor?
C. What should be the GP's course of action?

An endoscopic examination revealed a duodenal ulcer.

D. Why do some people infected with *H. pylori* develop gastric ulcer and some duodenal ulcer?
E. What eradication therapy for *H. pylori* should be given, and is a proton pump inhibitor beneficial when given with antibacterial therapy?

The eradication therapy given was 7 days with omeprazole, amoxicillin and clarithromycin. Mr TK was symptom-free for six weeks but then his symptoms returned.

F. What were the possible reasons for the return of the symptoms?
G. What treatment could be given?

True/false answers

1. **False.** The histamine receptors on parietal cells that stimulate acid secretion are H_2 receptors, which are selectively antagonised by ranitidine and cimetidine.
2. **True.** The vagal neurotransmitter acetylcholine stimulates muscarinic receptors, which increases acid secretion. Selective vagotomy has been used to treat ulcer disease.
3. **True.** Magnesium salts may cause diarrhoea, and antacids containing aluminium salts may cause constipation.
4. **False.** Antacids can heal peptic ulcers but their effects are slower than with proton pump inhibitors or histamine H_2 receptor antagonists.
5. **True.** Cimetidine, but not famotidine, nizatidine or ranitidine, inhibit cytochrome P450 isozymes and should be avoided in people taking warfarin, phenytoin or theophylline.
6. **True.** Cimetidine is more likely than other histamine H_2 receptor antagonists to cause galactorrhoea in women or gynaecomastia in men by inhibiting oestrogen metabolism.
7. **False.** Histamine H_2 antagonists reduce acid secretion by only about 60%, because these drugs do not block

other stimuli for acid secretion, such as gastrin and acetylcholine.

8. **True.** Omeprazole has to be converted to its active form by protonation in acid. It is therefore selectively active on the proton pump in the gastric parietal cell but not on proton pumps in other tissues that operate at higher pH.

9. **False.** The active metabolites of proton pump inhibitor prodrugs are irreversible inhibitors and fresh protein must be synthesised to replace the inhibited proton pump.

10. **True.** Omeprazole can inhibit the metabolism of drugs such as warfarin or phenytoin by both CYP2C9 and CYP2C19. Proton pump inhibitors differ in their inhibitory activity on cytochrome P450 isozymes, with pantoprazole and rabeprazole thought to have the least effect.

11. **False.** Part of the gastroprotective action of PGI_2 and PGE_2 is by increasing gastric mucosal blood flow, removing back-secreted H^+ and providing HCO_3^- to buffer the H^+ ions. They also increase mucus secretion and decrease acid secretion.

12. **False.** Prostaglandins (particularly PGI_2) in large doses can increase gastrointestinal motility and secretions and cause diarrhoea.

13. **False.** Both these classes of anti-ulcer drug can cause healing of NSAID-induced ulcers. Proton pump inhibitors may produce more rapid healing as this is probably related to the degree of acid suppression.

14. **True.** Metoclopramide increases lower oesophageal tone and rate of gastric emptying. This is the rationale for its use in treating oesophageal reflux disease, most effectively as an adjunct to proton pump inhibitors and H_2 receptor antagonists.

15. **True.** Sucralfate and bismuth salts have been largely superseded, although bismuth salts still have a place as quadruple therapy with PPIs and antibacterials' when triple therapy fails.

OBA answer

Answer A is the least accurate statement.

A. **Incorrect**. Acid secretion is enhanced by *H. pylori* infection in the antrum, while infection in the corpus is associated with reduced or unchanged acid secretion.

B. Correct. Although *H. pylori* lives mainly in the gastric mucosa, changes in the duodenal mucosa occur in response to low pH, enabling duodenal colonisation.

C. Correct. Following healing with a proton pump inhibitor, approximately 80% of duodenal ulcers will recur within a year if *H. pylori* is not eradicated.

D. Correct. *H. pylori* infection increases the risk of developing gastric adenocarcinoma by five- to sixfold.

E. Correct. In some countries *H. pylori* resistance to metronidazole is as high as 90%.

Case-based answers

A. This man could have non-ulcer dyspepsia or peptic ulceration. Ranitidine for only two weeks of treatment is available without prescription; if it had been continued, the symptoms would probably have been suppressed for longer. If he is *H. pylori*-positive and has non-ulcer dyspepsia, it is likely that he will develop peptic ulcer disease in the future. If he is *H. pylori*-positive and has peptic ulceration, failure to eradicate *H. pylori* is likely to result in a recurrence of peptic ulcer within a year.

B. If *H. pylori* is present, the symptoms will still recur in a high percentage of individuals.

C. It is recommended that any person over 45 years of age should be referred for endoscopic examination. *H. pylori* infection can be detected non-invasively using a blood test (antibody to urease), a stool antigen test or a radiolabelled (^{13}C) urea breath test. In a gastric antral biopsy, it can be detected using bacterial culture, histopathology or a rapid urease (CLO) test. Use of NSAIDs, tobacco and alcohol should be assessed, as these are strongly contributory to ulcer disease.

D. The reasons why some people develop gastric ulcer and others develop duodenal ulcer are imperfectly understood. If there is only antral inflammation and *H. pylori* is present, more gastrin and therefore excess acid is produced, resulting in duodenal ulcers. If a pangastritis exists it is associated with corporal atrophy, lower levels of acid secretion, and gastric ulcers.

E. Numerous treatment regimens have been evaluated. Seven days' therapy with a proton pump inhibitor (or ranitidine, if intolerant) plus two antimicrobials (clarithromycin and either metronidazole or amoxicillin, in a combination dictated by local sensitivities) results in a 70–90% eradication rate.

F. It is possible that the strain of *H. pylori* was resistant to the antibiotics used. In some places, clarithromycin resistance is 17%. Tests should be carried out to see whether *H. pylori* is still present after treatment. If necessary, quadruple therapy or longer treatment periods should be used.

G. Culture sensitivities of the *H. pylori* in a biopsy specimen could be sought. Quadruple therapy, which has 93–98% success, could be used; for example, a proton pump inhibitor (or ranitidine) plus bismuth salts plus metronidazole plus tetracycline (Fig. 33.2).

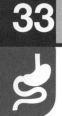

FURTHER READING

Coron E, Hatlebakk JG, Galmiche JP (2007) Medical therapy of gastroesophageal reflux disease. *Curr Opin Gastroenterol* 23, 434–439

Fass R (2007) Erosive and nonerosive reflux disease (NERD): comparison of epidemiologic, physiologic, and therapeutic characteristics. *J Clin Gastroenterol* 41, 131–137

Fuccio LL, Zagari RM, Cennamo V et al. (2008) Treatment of *Helicobacter pylori* infection. *BMJ* 337, 746–750

Gralnek IM, Barkun A, Bardou M (2008) Mangement of acute bleeding from a peptic ulcer. *N Engl J Med* 359, 928–937

Hawkey CJ, Langman MJS (2003) Non-steroidal anti-inflammatory drugs: overall risks and management. Complementary roles for COX-2 inhibitors and proton pump inhibitors. *Gut* 52, 600–608

Kahrilas PJ (2008) Gastroesophageal reflux disease. *N Engl J Med* 359, 1700–1707

Malfertheiner P, Chan FKL, McColl KEL (2009) Peptic ulcer disease. *Lancet* 374, 1449–1461

McColl KEL (2010) *Helicobacter pylori* infection. *N Engl J Med* 362, 1597–1604

Parfitt JR, Driman DK (2007) Pathological effects of drugs on the gastrointestinal tract: a review. *Hum Pathol* 38, 527–536

Seager JM, Hawkey CJ (2001) Indigestion and non-steroidal anti-inflammatory drugs. *BMJ* 323, 1236–1239

Stanghellini V, De Ponti F, De Giorgio R et al. (2003) New developments in the treatment of functional dyspepsia. *Drugs* 63, 869–892

Storr M, Allescher H-D, Classen M (2001) Current concepts on pathophysiology, diagnosis and treatment of diffuse oesophageal spasm. *Drugs* 61, 579–591

Compendium: drugs used for dyspepsia and peptic ulcer disease

Drug	Kinetics (half-life)	Comments
Antisecretory agents		
H₂ receptor antagonists		
Cimetidine	Oral bioavailability 60–70%; cleared by renal tubular secretion and hepatic metabolism (1–3 h); inhibits cytochrome P450 enzymes	Given orally; risk of drug interactions
Famotidine	Relatively low oral absorption (50%); mainly excreted in urine unchanged (3–4 h); does not affect cytochrome P450 enzymes	Given orally
Nizatidine	Oral bioavailability >70%; mostly eliminated by glomerular filtration and tubular secretion (1–2 h); does not affect cytochrome P450 enzymes	Given orally or by intravenous infusion
Ranitidine	Oral bioavailability 40–90%; elimination by renal tubular secretion and hepatic metabolism (2–3 h); no effect on cytochrome P450 enzymes	May be given orally, by intramuscular injection, or by slow intravenous injection or infusion
Proton pump inhibitors		
Due to the irreversible mechanism of action of the active metabolites the proton pump inhibitors have much longer durations of action than indicated by the half-life of the parent compound.		
Esomeprazole	Kinetics similar to omeprazole but higher plasma levels and slightly longer half-life (1–2 h); may cause drug interactions by inhibition of CYP2C19	The S-isomer of omeprazole (both isomers are active); given orally, or by intravenous injection or infusion
Lansoprazole	High oral bioavailability (80%); hepatic elimination (1–2 h); possibly fewer drug interactions than omeprazole	Given orally
Omeprazole	Oral bioavailability about 60%; metabolised by CYP2C19 (1 h); 3–4% of Caucasians are poor metabolisers; potent inhibitor of CYP2C19	Given orally or by slow intravenous injection (over 5 min) or infusion
Pantoprazole	Well absorbed with about 20% hepatic first-pass metabolism; half-life (1 h) is longer (4–10 h) in poor metabolisers; lower affinity for CYP2C19 and possibly fewer drug interactions than omeprazole	Given orally or by slow intravenous injection (over 2 min) or infusion
Rabeprazole	Bioavailability about 50%; hepatic metabolism to inactive products (1–2 h); fewer drug interactions than omeprazole	Given orally

Compendium: drugs used for dyspepsia and peptic ulcer disease—cont'd

Drug	Kinetics (half-life)	Comments
Cytoprotective agents		
Given orally.		
Misoprostol	Essentially complete first-pass metabolism to active misoprostol acid; renal elimination (0.3 h)	Prostaglandin E_1 analogue; prodrug of misoprostol acid
Sucralfate	Minimal absorption (2% or less)	Forms ulcer-adherent complex
Tripotassium dicitratobismuthate	Minimal absorption; absorbed bismuth is eliminated slowly in urine (5 days)	Used in quadruple therapy
Prokinetic drugs		
Metoclopramide	Oral bioavailability variable (40–100%); renal excretion (3–5 h)	Used for a wide range of indications; given orally or by intramuscular injection or slow intravenous injection
Other drugs		
Alginic acid	Not absorbed	Produces local effects within the stomach
Antacids	Absorption and systemic fates are not of therapeutic importance	Antacids include aluminium hydroxide, magnesium trisilicate, hydrocalcite and sodium carbonate; neutralise acid within the stomach
Antimicrobials	See Ch. 51	Used to eliminate *H. pylori*

34 Inflammatory bowel disease

· ·

Crohn's disease and *ulcerative colitis* are the two types of chronic inflammatory disorder of the gastrointestinal tract which together are termed 'inflammatory bowel disease' (IBD). This common terminology conceals many differences in predisposition and pathogenesis between the two conditions. It is also likely that within each category there are different individual disease phenotypes.

Ulcerative colitis is a disorder that is confined to the mucosa and submucosa, with inflammation usually confined to the large bowel, although when the whole of the colon is involved there can also be inflammation in the terminal ileum. The extent of colonic involvement varies, but the rectum is always involved and mucosal inflammation is continuous, not patchy. Symptoms include bloody diarrhoea, fever and weight loss. Ulcerative colitis can be associated with extracolonic manifestations such as uveitis, sacroiliitis and various skin disorders (Box 34.1).

Crohn's disease is a transmural granulomatous condition that can involve any part of the gut. The bowel involvement is discontinuous and segmental, most frequently found in the terminal ileum and colon but often sparing the rectum. Fistula formation, small-bowel strictures and perianal disease such as abscesses and fissures are common. Clinical features of colonic involvement include diarrhoea, abdominal pain and fatigue. Involvement of more proximal parts of the gut produces various symptoms depending on the site of the disease, and diarrhoea need not be present (Box 34.1).

The aetiologies of IBD are unclear, although several susceptibility genes have been identified (Fig. 34.1). The genetic predisposition is stronger in Crohn's disease, but both conditions can occur in the same families. Cigarette smoking increases the risk of Crohn's disease and the frequency of exacerbations, but slightly decreases the risk of ulcerative colitis. The trigger for disease in susceptible individuals is unknown but a failure of development of immune

tolerance in the gut may be important, and IBD may arise from impaired handling of microbial antigens by the intestinal immune system. Cells involved in innate immunity contribute to the inflammation, including natural killer T-cells, neutrophil leucocytes, macrophages and dendritic cells. These secrete tumour necrosis factor α (TNFα) and a variety of pro-inflammatory interleukins and chemokines. The abnormal immune response also involves an excess number of adaptive immune cells. In Crohn's disease these are T-helper type 1 (Th1) lymphocytes while in ulcerative colitis they are T-helper type 2 (Th2) lymphocytes, leading to different patterns of cytokine release (Ch. 38). T-helper type 17 (Th17) lymphocytes are also involved in the pathogenesis of both Crohn's disease and ulcerative colitis. Regulatory T-cells are probably deficient. There is a close interaction between the immune system and the enteric nervous system that contributes to initiation and maintenance of inflammation, motility disturbance in the bowel and pain. Inflammatory bowel disease can undergo periods of relapse and remission over many years.

Treatment of both types of IBD is intended to induce and maintain remission. The drugs used for these two conditions are broadly similar, but Crohn's disease is less responsive to some of the widely used drugs, especially when it involves the small intestine. Better understanding of the pathogenic mechanisms in IBD has resulted in advances in treatment, although much still needs to be learned.

DRUGS FOR INFLAMMATORY BOWEL DISEASE

AMINOSALICYLATES

Examples

balsalazide, mesalazine, olsalazine, sulfasalazine

Mechanism of action and effects

The active anti-inflammatory constituent of all the aminosalicylates is 5-aminosalicylic acid (5-ASA). The different aminosalicylate drugs are formulated in a variety of ways, but they are all designed to deliver 5-ASA to the lumen of the colon (see Pharmacokinetics). Sulfasalazine was the first aminosalicylate shown to be effective in treating IBD. Colonic bacteria cleave sulfasalazine into its constituent parts: 5-ASA and sulfapyridine. Sulfapyridine is responsible for many of the unwanted effects of this drug, but in contrast to its role in inflammatory arthritis (Ch. 30) it has no therapeutic value in IBD. The mechanisms of action of aminosalicylates are not clear, but they may involve inhibition of leucocyte chemotaxis by reducing cytokine formation, reduced free radical generation and inhibition of the production of lipid inflammatory mediators (such as prostanoids, leukotrienes and platelet-activating factor). Aminosalicylates are increasingly used as first-line prophylaxis of mild to moderate ulcerative colitis, and are highly effective for reducing relapse rates. Their efficacy in Crohn's disease is less well established, particularly for non-colonic disease. They are less effective in treatment of acute exacerbations of IBD.

Pharmacokinetics

Sulfasalazine is partially absorbed from the gut intact, but most reaches the colon, where it undergoes reduction by

gut bacteria to sulfapyridine and 5-ASA. Sulfapyridine and about 20% of the 5-ASA are absorbed from the colon, and then metabolised in the liver. Both have plasma half-lives of 5–20 h. There are several ways of delivering 5-ASA to the mucosa of the lower gut without also giving sulfapyridine. Mesalazine (the 5-ASA molecule itself) is given as an enteric-coated or modified-release formulation to limit absorption from the small bowel and deliver adequate drug to the colon. Olsalazine is a drug comprising two 5-ASA molecules joined by an azo bond. It is not absorbed from the upper gut and 5-ASA is released after reductive splitting of the azo bond by colonic flora. Balsalazide is a prodrug in which 5-ASA is linked to a carrier molecule (4-amino-benzoyl-β-alanine) by an azo bond, which is cleaved by bacterial reduction in the large bowel.

Mesalazine and sulfasalazine can be given rectally (by suppository or enema) to treat distal disease in the colon.

Box 34.1	Indicators of severity of ulcerative colitis and colonic Crohn's disease

More than 6–10 stools per day
Fever
Tachycardia
Anaemia
Nausea, vomiting
Abdominal tenderness
Abdominal distension with high-pitched bowel sounds
Rebound tenderness and reduction in bowel movements
   (toxic megacolon)

Unwanted effects

These occur in up to 45% of people treated with sulfasalazine, but only 15% of those who take mesalazine. They include:

- nausea, vomiting, diarrhoea, abdominal pain,
- headache,
- rashes,
- blood dyscrasias, especially agranulocytosis and thrombocytopenia,
- cough, insomnia, fever, oligospermia with sulfasalazine.

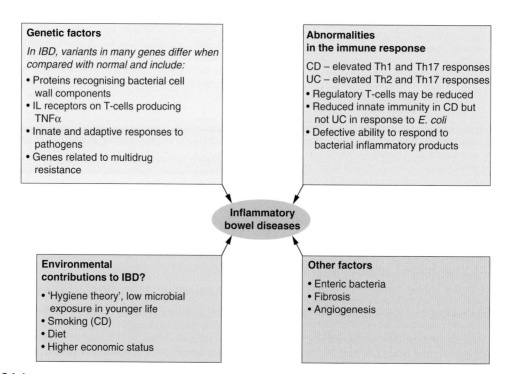

Genetic factors

In IBD, variants in many genes differ when compared with normal and include:

- Proteins recognising bacterial cell wall components
- IL receptors on T-cells producing TNFα
- Innate and adaptive responses to pathogens
- Genes related to multidrug resistance

Abnormalities in the immune response

CD – elevated Th1 and Th17 responses
UC – elevated Th2 and Th17 responses
- Regulatory T-cells may be reduced
- Reduced innate immunity in CD but not UC in response to *E. coli*
- Defective ability to respond to bacterial inflammatory products

Inflammatory bowel diseases

Environmental contributions to IBD?

- 'Hygiene theory', low microbial exposure in younger life
- Smoking (CD)
- Diet
- Higher economic status

Other factors

- Enteric bacteria
- Fibrosis
- Angiogenesis

Fig. 34.1 **Factors associated with inflammatory bowel disease.** Investigations into the aetiology of inflammatory bowel disease have confirmed the multiplicity of factors that might be involved. The association of some events is strong while others are weak. Some changes may occur as a consequence of the disease rather than being involved in the cause. CD, Crohn's disease; IBD, inflammatory bowel disease; IL, interleukin; TNFα, tumour necrosis factor α; UC, ulcerative colitis.

CORTICOSTEROIDS

Examples

budesonide, hydrocortisone, prednisolone

Corticosteroids (Ch. 44) are very effective for inducing remission in active IBD; however, there is little evidence that they prevent relapse when used at doses that do not produce significant unwanted effects. Newer corticosteroids formulated for topical use, such as budesonide (see also Ch. 44), have limited systemic unwanted effects and are useful alternatives to the older drugs. Topical treatment with liquid or foam enemas or suppositories is used for localised rectal disease, but oral or parenteral administration is needed for more severe or extensive disease.

CYTOKINE INHIBITORS (ANTI-TNFα ANTIBODIES)

Examples

adalimumab, infliximab

Mechanisms and uses

Infliximab was the first monoclonal antibody to be approved for the treatment of Crohn's disease. Adalimumab is effective when infliximab is poorly tolerated or for those who have become refractory to treatment. Inhibition of the binding of TNFα to its receptors reduces production of pro-inflammatory cytokines (e.g. IL-1 and IL-6), leucocyte migration and infiltration, and activation of neutrophils and eosinophils. Infliximab may also be useful for treatment of severe attacks of ulcerative colitis. Unwanted effects of TNFα antibodies are discussed in Chapter 30.

IMMUNOSUPPRESSANTS

Azathioprine and, less often, mercaptopurine are useful in some people with active IBD and may enable corticosteroid doses to be reduced. Mercaptopurine is more frequently used in North America; it may be a little less effective than azathioprine but perhaps with a lower rate of nausea. Maximal efficacy is not achieved with either drug for about 6–12 weeks. Nausea, vomiting, rashes and a hypersensitivity syndrome affect about 10% of people during the first 6 weeks of therapy. Pancreatitis and liver toxicity are rare but serious complications.

Methotrexate is useful in Crohn's disease. It is given subcutaneously or intramuscularly and is only used when azathioprine has failed. Ciclosporin can induce remission in corticosteroid-resistant ulcerative colitis but has no long-term efficacy. More details of these drugs are found in Chapter 38.

ANTIBACTERIALS

Metronidazole (Ch. 51) is moderately effective for treatment of some aspects of Crohn's disease, particularly perianal disease, although the mechanism of action is uncertain. Ciprofloxacin probably has similar efficacy.

MANAGEMENT OF INFLAMMATORY BOWEL DISEASE

ULCERATIVE COLITIS

Treatment is determined by the extent and severity of disease. Non-steroidal anti-inflammatory drugs (NSAIDs) and also selective cyclo-oxygenase 2 (COX-2) inhibitors (Ch. 29) can exacerbate symptoms in severe colitis and should not be used. Opioids (Ch. 35) should be avoided in the treatment of diarrhoea in extensive colitis since they can precipitate the life-threatening complication toxic megacolon.

Rectal drug delivery is often successful if the disease is limited to the rectum or left side of the colon (distal colitis). For mild symptoms, topical mesalazine is more effective than topical corticosteroid. Foam enemas or suppositories will treat inflammation up to 12–20 cm from the anus, while liquid enemas are effective up to 30–60 cm (i.e. to the splenic flexure). Oral aminosalicylate can be combined with rectal administration to improve efficacy. For more severe disease an oral corticosteroid may be necessary to induce remission, with gradual dosage reduction to minimise unwanted effects once control is achieved.

More extensive colitis will settle with an oral aminosalicylate if symptoms are mild to moderate, but the response can take 6–8 weeks. Oral corticosteroids such as prednisolone induce remission more quickly. Severe colitis requires intensive fluid and electrolyte replacement; anaemia should be corrected by transfusion, and large doses of parenteral corticosteroid should be given. Infliximab can be used for severe refractory disease. Surgery is required in about 20% of people with ulcerative colitis.

Once symptoms are quiescent, maintenance treatment with topical mesalazine or an oral aminosalicylate should be life-long and reduces the relapse rate by two-thirds. It also reduces the risk of developing colorectal cancer by up to 75%.

The indications for immunosuppressants in the treatment of ulcerative colitis are the same as for Crohn's disease (see below). Azathioprine is the only immunosuppressant agent with a good evidence base for long-term therapy of ulcerative colitis. Intravenous ciclosporin may induce remission in refractory cases.

CROHN'S DISEASE

Smoking cessation reduces the risk of relapse in Crohn's disease by 65%, an effect comparable in size to that achieved with an immunosuppressant. Corticosteroid therapy is the mainstay of medical treatment for active Crohn's disease, usually with oral prednisolone. Maintenance corticosteroid therapy does not reduce the risk of relapse, and every effort should be made to withdraw the drug once the disease activity has been controlled. Immunosuppressant drugs such as azathioprine may be useful to aid this process, especially in chronically active Crohn's disease, where corticosteroid dependence occurs in 40–50% of people who take the drug to induce remission. Azathioprine should be considered if control of Crohn's disease requires more than two 6-week courses of oral corticosteroid therapy per year, or if the disease relapses as the dose of corticosteroid is reduced. Azathioprine can also be used to induce remission. Methotrexate can induce and maintain remission in Crohn's disease, but is usually used when there is intolerance to azathioprine or mercaptopurine. Intramuscular or subcutaneous injections may be more effective than oral methotrexate due to greater bioavailability.

Disease confined to the distal colon can respond to topical therapy with a corticosteroid, and an oral aminosalicylate such as mesalazine can also have a modest benefit in colonic Crohn's disease (see management of ulcerative colitis, above). For Crohn's disease outside the colon, aminosalicylates are generally ineffective.

The antibacterial drugs ciprofloxacin and metronidazole are particularly useful for perianal disease. They probably have both an antibacterial and anti-inflammatory effect. Infliximab or adalimumab are used to induce and maintain remission in Crohn's disease that is resistant to conventional therapy. A single infusion can induce remission in Crohn's disease for up to 3 months, and subsequent intermittent 2-monthly maintenance infusions can reduce the severity of the disease. Antibody formation, which may cause allergic reactions and/or loss of efficacy, is less likely to occur with this regimen, and can be further reduced by corticosteroid pretreatment and maintenance immunosuppressant therapy.

Surgery may be necessary for disease that is refractory to medical therapy. Intestinal obstruction can require bowel resection, or abscesses may need drainage. A defunctioning ileostomy to 'rest' the bowel may allow active inflammation to settle with medical therapy in refractory disease, but colonic disease usually recurs after closure of the stoma. Surgery should be an integral part of the management plan, and is required in up to 80% of people with Crohn's disease.

SELF-ASSESSMENT

True/false questions

1. Crohn's disease lesions are transmural and confined to the small bowel.
2. Cigarette smoking increases the risk of Crohn's disease.
3. In inflammatory bowel disease (IBD) the main active constituent of sulfasalazine is sulfapyridine.
4. Mesalazine (5-aminosalicylic acid; 5-ASA) can be given rectally.
5. Mesalazine is equally useful in the treatment of Crohn's disease involving the colon or the small bowel.
6. Corticosteroids are effective for maintaining remission in ulcerative colitis.
7. Immunosuppressants such as azathioprine are ineffective for the treatment of Crohn's disease.
8. Infliximab can induce remission even in refractory IBD.

9. Non-steroidal anti-inflammatory drugs (NSAIDs) should be avoided in IBD.
10. Diarrhoea in IBD can be treated with the opioid loperamide.

One-best-answer (OBA) question

Choose the *most accurate* statement concerning IBD drugs from A–E below.

A. 5-Aminosalicylic acid given orally or rectally is well absorbed.
B. Balsalazide comprises two molecules of 5-ASA joined by an azo bond.
C. Azathioprine is the first-line drug of choice in treating mild Crohn's disease.
D. Adalimumab is an antibody directed against interleukin-6.
E. Metronidazole can be used in the treatment of inflammatory bowel disease.

Case-based questions

A 35-year-old man presented with a 3-week period of frequent diarrhoea with mucus but no blood in the stool. Stool analysis for infective agents was negative. Sigmoidoscopy indicated gross thickening of the mucosa, with inflammation and linear ulcers. Changes were present in restricted areas (skip lesions) with intervening normal mucosa. Histology was diagnostic of Crohn's disease and investigation suggested that the condition was confined to the sigmoid and part of the ascending colon.

A. What is the cause of Crohn's disease?
B. How should this man be treated initially?
C. How do corticosteroids act in Crohn's disease?
D. How should the corticosteroid be given, and why?
E. Why should the corticosteroid dosage be reduced slowly at the end of treatment?
F. How can remission be maintained in this man?
G. What alternative therapies can be given to try to reduce the risk of corticosteroid dependence?

True/false answers

1. **False.** Crohn's disease is transmural but can affect any part of the gastrointestinal tract.
2. **True.** There is increased risk of Crohn's disease in smokers but a slightly decreased risk of ulcerative colitis.
3. **False.** Sulfasalazine is broken down in the colon to 5-ASA, which is responsible for the beneficial effects in IBD, and sulfapyridine, which causes most of the unwanted effects.
4. **True.** Modified-release formulations of mesalazine are available for rectal administration to deliver the drug to the distal colonic mucosa.
5. **False.** Although mesalazine may be of some benefit in colonic Crohn's disease, it is not very effective for small-bowel Crohn's disease.
6. **False.** Although they are effective for inducing remission, there is little evidence that corticosteroids prevent relapse.

7. **False.** People with chronic Crohn's disease can become corticosteroid-dependent, and immunosuppressants such as azathioprine can be useful in reducing this dependence. Many months of treatment are required before they are fully effective.
8. **True.** A single infusion of infliximab can induce remission for up to 3 months; remission may be maintained by further infusions at 2-monthly intervals.
9. **True.** NSAIDs and selective cyclo-oxygenase 2 (COX-2) inhibitors (coxibs) can exacerbate symptoms in severe disease.
10. **False.** Opioids should be avoided as they can precipitate toxic megacolon.

OBA answer

Answer E is the most accurate.

A. Incorrect. 5-ASA is poorly absorbed by either route and acts locally within the gut.
B. Incorrect. The 5-ASA dimer is olsalazine, while balsalazide is a molecule of 5-ASA linked to an inert carrier molecule; in both cases the active 5-ASA is released by colonic bacterial reduction.
C. Incorrect. Azathioprine is usually given in corticosteroid-refractory disease or when people are having frequent courses of corticosteroids for treatment (more than two 6-week courses per year).
D. Incorrect. Adalimumab is a fully humanised monoclonal antibody against TNFα and is given subcutaneously for the treatment of refractory disease.
E. **Correct.** Antibacterials such as metronidazole can be useful in treating Crohn's disease, particularly if there is perianal disease.

Case-based answers

A. The cause of Crohn's disease is unknown. Several hypotheses have implicated a number of risk factors, including infection, altered immune response to infection and environmental factors (see Fig. 34.1).

B. Initial treatment is with corticosteroids. Because the Crohn's disease is confined to the distal colon, topical treatment with a corticosteroid such as budesonide could be used to limit systemic unwanted effects. If, however, there was involvement of the proximal large bowel or small bowel it would be necessary to give an oral corticosteroid, such as prednisolone.
C. Corticosteroids have a variety of actions. They can alter the release of inflammatory mediators such as arachidonic acid metabolites, kinins and cytokines. They can alter cell-mediated cytotoxicity, antibody production, adhesion molecule expression, phagocytic function, leucocyte chemotaxis and leucocyte adherence.
D. Corticosteroids should be given until remission occurs. If possible, the corticosteroid should be administered locally to keep the plasma concentration low, but for individuals who experience systemic symptoms of IBD (such as fatigue, anorexia or weight loss) oral therapy is indicated.
E. Systemic corticosteroids suppress the hypothalamo–pituitary–adrenal axis and can reduce the circulating levels of endogenous adrenal glucocorticoids (see Ch. 44). Gradual reduction of the dose of therapeutic corticosteroid allows recovery of the production of endogenous glucocorticoids.
F. If the colitis is restricted to the distal colon, topical administration of mesalazine or an oral formulation that delivers 5-ASA to the colon could be used. 5-ASA is, however, less effective in Crohn's disease, particularly if it involves the small bowel.
G. Continuous corticosteroid therapy for periods of 6 months or longer is eventually required in 40–50% of people with Crohn's disease. If more than two 6-week courses of corticosteroid per year are required to maintain control of symptoms, immunosuppressive therapy should be considered. Immunosuppressive therapy is usually with azathioprine or 6-mercaptopurine; prolonged treatment with these drugs is usually required (up to 6 months) before a clinical response occurs. TNFα antibody treatment is also of benefit in severe disease that is not responsive to other therapies.

FURTHER READING

Baumgart DC, Sandborn WJ (2007) Inflammatory bowel disease: clinical aspects and established and evolving therapies. *Lancet* 369, 1641–1657

Collins P, Rhodes J (2006) Ulcerative colitis: diagnosis and management. *BMJ* 333, 340–343

Cummings JFR, Keshav S, Travis SPL (2008) Medical management of Crohn's disease. *BMJ* 336, 1062–1066

Katz JA (2007) Management of inflammatory bowel disease in adults. *J Dig Dis* 8, 65–71

Mowat C, Cole A, Windsor A et al. (2011) Guidelines for the management of inflammatory bowel disease in adults. *Gut* 60, 571–607

Panés J, Gomollón F, Taxonera C et al. (2007) Crohn's disease: a review of current treatment with a focus on biologics. *Drugs* 67, 2511–2537

Peyrin-Biroulet L, Desreumaux P, Sandborn WJ et al. (2008) Crohn's disease: beyond antagonists of tumour necrosis factor. *Lancet* 372, 67–81

Scaldaferri F, Fiocchi C (2007) Inflammatory bowel disease: progress and current concepts of etiopathogenesis. *J Dig Dis* 8, 171–178

Compendium: drugs used in inflammatory bowel disease

Drug	Kinetics (half-life)	Comments
Aminosalicylates		
Balsalazide	Prodrug cleaved by bacterial azoreductases in the colon to release 5-ASA and an inactive metabolite; half-life not reported due to wide inter-individual variations	Used for mild to moderate ulcerative colitis and maintenance of remission
Mesalazine (5-ASA)	Uncoated tablets are absorbed in upper intestine; poor absorption after rectal administration; eliminated in faeces and urine (0.5–1 h)	Used for mild to moderate ulcerative colitis and maintenance of remission; given orally, or rectally as a foam enema or suppository; may be more effective than sulfasalazine in the presence of diarrhoea, because there is no requirement for reduction by the gut flora
Olsalazine	Only 3% absorbed in the upper intestine; colonic bacterial azoreduction generates 5-ASA (see mesalazine below); elimination in faeces and urine (1 h)	Used for mild ulcerative colitis and maintenance of remission
Sulfasalazine	About 20–30% absorbed in the small intestine and eliminated (3–11 h); remainder passes down to colonic bacteria which convert it to 5-ASA and sulfapyridine; 5-ASA is poorly absorbed and largely acetylated within colon and in liver (4–10 h); sulfapyridine is absorbed and undergoes hepatic metabolism (6–17 h)	Used for mild to moderate and severe ulcerative colitis and for Crohn's disease; given orally, or rectally as a retention enema or a suppository; active metabolite 5-ASA has local actions; sulfapyridine is probably the cause of many of the unwanted effects
Cytokine modulators		
Other than adalimumab and infliximab, TNFα inhibitors used for rheumatoid arthritis (see Ch. 30) are not currently approved for IBD.		
Adalimumab	Protein clearance (12 days)	Monoclonal antibody against TNFα; used in severe Crohn's disease unresponsive to other treatments; given by subcutaneous injection
Infliximab	Metabolised by cellular uptake and proteolysis (8–10 days);	Monoclonal antibody against TNFα; used in severe Crohn's disease and ulcerative colitis unresponsive to other treatments; given by intravenous infusion
Immunosuppressants		
Azathioprine	Bioactivated by metabolism to 6-mercaptopurine (3–5 h); see Ch. 38	Used in resistant and frequently relapsing cases of ulcerative colitis or Crohn's disease
Ciclosporin	See Ch. 38	Used for short-term treatment of ulcerative colitis (an unlicensed indication in the UK); given intravenously
Corticosteroids	See Ch. 44	Beclometasone dipropionate, budesonide, hydrocortisone and prednisolone; not suitable for maintenance treatment because of unwanted effects (see Ch. 44)
Mercaptopurine	See Ch. 52	Used in resistant and frequently relapsing cases of ulcerative colitis or Crohn's disease; main use is as an anti-cancer drug (see Ch. 52)
Methotrexate	See Ch. 52	May be given weekly in unresponsive or chronically active Crohn's disease; see Ch. 52 for other details
Antibiotics		
Metronidazole	Complete oral bioavailability; renal elimination (6–9 h)	May be beneficial for the treatment of active Crohn's disease; used in people who fail to respond to sulfasalazine; see Ch. 51

All given orally, unless otherwise indicated.

35 Constipation, diarrhoea and irritable bowel syndrome

CONSTIPATION

Humans normally defaecate with a frequency ranging from three times a day to once every 3 days (or sometimes less often). Maintenance of 'regular' bowel habits is a preoccupation of Western societies, and is best achieved by increasing dietary fibre. Nevertheless, laxative drugs are widely prescribed or taken without prescription and are frequently abused.

Frequent constipation affects 10% of the population, and is the passage of hard, small stools less frequently than the patient's own normal function and is often associated with straining. There are many causes (Box 35.1). Underlying organic disease should be excluded when there is persistent constipation or if there has been a recent change in bowel habit.

LAXATIVES

The mechanisms of action of common laxatives are shown in Figure 35.1. Some drugs have more than one mechanism, and they are classified by their principal action.

Bulk-forming laxatives

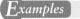

Examples

bran, ispaghula husk, methylcellulose, sterculia

Bulking agents include various natural polysaccharides, usually of plant origin, such as unprocessed wheat bran, ispaghula husk, sterculia and methylcellulose, all of which are poorly broken down by digestive processes. They have several mechanisms of action:

- a hydrophilic action causing retention of water in the gut lumen, which expands and softens the faeces,
- proliferation of colonic bacteria, which further increases faecal bulk,
- stimulation of colonic mucosal receptors by the increased bulk, promoting peristalsis,
- sterculia also contains polysaccharides which are degraded to substances that have an osmotic laxative effect.

Bulking agents take at least 24 h after ingestion to work. A liberal fluid intake is important to lubricate the colon and minimise the risk of obstruction. Bulking agents are useful for establishing a regular bowel habit in chronic constipation, diverticular disease and irritable bowel syndrome (IBS), but they should be avoided if the colon is atonic or there is faecal impaction.

Unwanted effects include a sensation of bloating, flatulence or griping abdominal pain.

Osmotic laxatives

Examples

lactulose, macrogols, magnesium salts, sodium acid phosphate

Magnesium compounds such as the sulphate (Epsom salts) and the hydroxide are poorly absorbed from the gut and act as osmotically active solutes that retain water in the colonic lumen. They may also stimulate cholecystokinin release from the small-intestinal mucosa, which increases intestinal secretions and enhances colonic motility (Fig. 35.1). These actions result in more rapid transit of gut contents into the large bowel, where distension promotes evacuation within 3 h. About 20% of ingested magnesium is absorbed and inhibits central nervous system, cardiovascular and neuromuscular activity if it is retained in the circulation in large enough amounts, as can occur in renal failure. Magnesium hydroxide is a mild laxative, while the action of magnesium sulphate can be quite fierce, associated with considerable abdominal discomfort.

Lactulose is a disaccharide of fructose and galactose. In the colon, bacterial action releases fructose and galactose, which are fermented to lactic and acetic acids with release of gas. The fermentation products are osmotically active. They also lower intestinal pH, which favours overgrowth of some selected colonic flora but inhibits the proliferation of ammonia-producing bacteria. This is useful in the treatment of hepatic encephalopathy (Ch. 36). Unwanted effects include flatulence and abdominal cramps. Lactulose can take more than 24 h to act.

Diet low in fibre or fluid
Drug-induced, e.g. colonic cancer, myxoedema,
    hypercalcaemia
Drug-induced – frequent causes include:

■ opioid analgesics (this chapter and Ch. 19)
■ antimuscarinic agents, e.g. oxybutynin (Ch. 15),
    orphenadrine (Ch. 24), cyclizine (Ch. 32)
■ antacids containing calcium or aluminium salts (Ch. 33)
■ calcium channel blockers (Ch. 5)
■ iron salts (Ch. 47)
■ tricyclic antidepressants (Ch. 22)
■ phenothiazines (Ch. 21)

Slow gut transit, especially in young women
Immobility
Hypotonic colon in the elderly

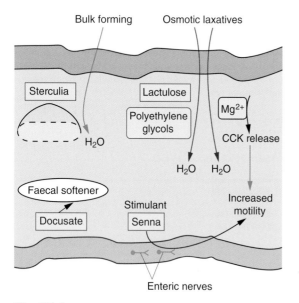

Fig. 35.1 Sites of action of the major classes of
laxative drug. Some laxative drugs have more than one
mechanism of action. CCK, cholecystokinin.

Macrogols (polyethylene glycols) are large, inert molecules that are not absorbed from the gut and exert an
osmotic effect in the colon. They are as effective as other
osmotic agents, but their Na^+ content may be hazardous
for people with impaired cardiac function.

Sodium acid phosphate and sodium citrate are osmotic
preparations that are given as an enema or suppository,
usually for bowel preparation before local procedures or
surgery.

Irritant and stimulant laxatives

Examples

bisacodyl, dantron, docusate sodium, senna, sodium
picosulfate

Irritant and stimulant laxatives include the anthraquinones
senna and dantron, and the polyphenolic compounds bisacodyl and sodium picosulfate. They act by a variety of
mechanisms, including stimulation of local reflexes through
myenteric nerve plexuses in the gut, which enhances gut
motility and increases water and electrolyte transfer into the
lower gut. Stimulant laxatives are useful for more severe
forms of constipation, but tolerance is common with regular
use and they can produce abdominal cramps. Given orally,
they stimulate defecation after about 6–12 h.

■ Senna has the most gentle purgative action of this
    group. Given orally, it is hydrolysed by colonic bacteria
    to release the irritant derivatives sennosides A and B.
■ Dantron is available as co-danthramer, a combination
    with the surface wetting agent poloxamer 188, and as
    co-danthrusate, a combination with the mildly stimulant
    and faecal-softening agent docusate (see below).
    Dantron is carcinogenic at high doses in animals, and it
    is recommended that its use in humans should be
    limited to the elderly or terminally ill.
■ Bisacodyl can be given orally or, for a more rapid
    action (15–30 min), rectally; it undergoes enterohepatic
    circulation.
■ Sodium picosulfate is a powerful irritant and is given
    orally to prepare the bowel for surgery or colonoscopy.
    It generally acts in less than 6 h.
■ Docusate sodium has some stimulant activity as well as
    detergent properties which may soften stools by increas-
    ing fluid and fat penetration into hard stool. It is a rela-
    tively ineffective laxative that is given rectally or orally.

The chronic use of stimulant laxatives has been suspected
to cause progressive deterioration of normal colonic function, with eventual atony ('cathartic colon'). It is now recognised that the condition probably arises from severe,
refractory constipation rather than from the treatment.

Faecal softeners

Example

arachis oil

Arachis oil can be given rectally to soften impacted faeces.
Other drugs with faecal-softening actions include bulk-
forming laxatives and docusate sodium. Liquid paraffin can
be given orally, but is not recommended since it impairs the
absorption of fat-soluble vitamins and can cause anal
seepage with anal pruritus, and lipoid pneumonia after accidental inhalation.

MANAGEMENT OF CONSTIPATION

For simple constipation adopting a high-fibre diet, supplemented by bulking agents when necessary, is recommended. Exercise and an adequate fluid intake are also
important. For short-term use, a stimulant laxative such as
senna or bisacodyl can be taken orally at night to give a
morning bowel action. Suppositories will give a more rapid
effect. For longer-term therapy, regular magnesium salts or
macrogols are usually well tolerated and effective.

Senna, magnesium salts and docusate appear to
be safe in pregnancy. Bisacodyl, co-danthramer and

co-danthrusate are suitable for the elderly or for the terminally ill with opioid-induced constipation. For opioid-induced constipation in terminal care, the peripheral opioid receptor antagonist methylnaltrexone can be added if laxatives are ineffective (Ch. 19). Lactulose is useful as a second-line agent and specifically to treat constipation associated with hepatic encephalopathy (Chs 36 and 56). For people in whom neurological disease affecting bowel motility is the cause of constipation, a faecal softener should be used, with regular enemas or rectal washouts.

Refractory idiopathic constipation is a condition almost exclusively found in women, starting at a young age. Long-term use of stimulant laxatives, often at high dosage, may be necessary. Bulk-forming laxatives are ineffective, and a high-fibre diet usually increases abdominal distension and discomfort. Prucalopride, a 5-HT4 receptor agonist (see compendium) is sometimes used for refractory chronic constipation. Biofeedback can help in up to 80% of people with the condition. For those who fail with these approaches, surgical intervention with colectomy may be the only option.

DIARRHOEA

Diarrhoea is frequent watery bowel movements, with or without gas and cramping. Severe acute diarrhoea is usually a result of gastrointestinal infection, and it can be the consequence of both reduced absorption of fluid and an increase in intestinal secretions. Viral gastroenteritis is much more common than bacterial causes of diarrhoea in children, but viral and bacterial causes are both important in adults. Traveller's diarrhoea is a particularly common problem because of exposure of the traveller to organisms which have not been encountered before. Common causes include enterotoxin-producing *Escherichia coli*, *Clostridium jejuni* and *Salmonella* and *Shigella* species. Parasites such as *Giardia lamblia*, *Cryptosporidium* species and *Cyclospora cayetanensis* are less commonly involved. Diarrhoea may result from local release of bacterial enterotoxins, which have a variety of actions on gut mucosal cells, including stimulation of intracellular cAMP synthesis, which causes excess Cl^- secretion into the bowel.

Drugs that can produce diarrhoea include magnesium salts (see above), cytotoxic agents (Ch. 52), α- and β-adrenoceptor antagonists (Chs 5 and 6) and broad-spectrum antibacterial drugs, which produce diarrhoea by altering colonic flora (Ch. 51). Antibacterial treatment can be associated with *Clostridium difficile* colitis.

Chronic diarrhoea requires full investigation for non-infectious causes such as carcinoma of the colon, inflammatory bowel disease and coeliac disease. Irritable bowel syndrome is often accompanied by increased frequency of defaecation, loose stool and a sensation of incomplete evacuation (see below).

DRUGS FOR TREATING DIARRHOEA

Opioids

codeine phosphate, diphenoxylate, loperamide

The anti-motility action of opioids is a result of binding to μ-receptors on neurons in the submucosal neural plexus of the intestinal wall (Ch. 19). This enhances segmental contractions in the colon, inhibits propulsive movements of the small intestine and colon and prolongs the transit time of intestinal contents. These actions provide the opportunity for prolonged contact of intestinal contents with the gut mucosa and enhanced absorption of fluids.

The opioids most often used to treat diarrhoea are codeine, loperamide and diphenoxylate (used in combination with atropine as co-phenotrope). Most have short half-lives (<5 h). Loperamide has a more rapid onset of action, and a longer half-life (11 h), giving it a longer duration of action. It is more selective for the gut because high first-pass metabolism limits systemic absorption and, in contrast to other opioids, dependence is not a problem. Loperamide has additional antimuscarinic activity that also inhibits peristalsis (also achieved by atropine in co-phenotrope) and it increases anal tone. Morphine is sometimes used to treat diarrhoea in combination with kaolin (see below), but is not generally recommended. Unwanted effects of opioid drugs are discussed in Chapter 19.

Adsorbent and bulk-forming agents

Kaolin is an adsorbent that is relatively ineffective, and is not recommended for the treatment of acute diarrhoea. Ispaghula, methylcellulose and sterculia are bulking agents that can help to control faecal consistency in diarrhoea-predominant irritable bowel syndrome, or for people with an ileostomy or colostomy. They are not recommended for treatment of acute diarrhoea.

MANAGEMENT OF DIARRHOEA

In developed countries, most people with acute infective diarrhoea who are otherwise fit generally require only high oral fluid and electrolyte intake. Fluid and electrolyte balance are particularly important in young children and the elderly, as they can dehydrate more quickly. Specially formulated powders containing electrolytes (particularly Na^+ and K^+) and glucose (to enhance electrolyte absorption) are available (oral rehydration therapy, ORT). When correctly reconstituted with clean water they provide a balanced rehydration solution that should be given rapidly over 3–4 h, and then continuing need reassessed. Intravenous fluids may be required in severe dehydration.

If drug treatment is required, an opioid is useful for mild to moderate diarrhoea. Opioids should be avoided in dysentery, when prolonging contact of the organism with the gut mucosa can be detrimental. In young children, ileus with severe abdominal distention can occur with opioids, and it is recommended that they are not used in this age group.

Antibacterial prophylaxis can be used to prevent traveller's diarrhoea in people visiting high-risk areas. Ciprofloxacin or azithromycin are most often recommended (Ch. 51), depending on the area to which the person is travelling. Alternatively, an antibacterial can be taken at the first sign of illness, and it will usually shorten the duration of the attack to less than 24 h. Ciprofloxacin is often recommended for empirical treatment if there is fever or bloody diarrhoea to suggest invasive disease (such as produced by *Campylobacter* or *Shigella* species). If these are not present then rifaximin, a non-absorbable antimicrobial, can be used.

Diarrhoea in inflammatory bowel disease should be treated by management of the underlying condition. Antidiarrhoeals should not be used in active inflammatory bowel disease because of the risk of precipitating toxic megacolon (see Ch. 34).

Clostridium difficile-associated diarrhoea

Antibacterial-induced diarrhoea usually resolves rapidly on stopping the provoking drug. *Clostridium difficile*-associated diarrhoea produces more prolonged and severe diarrhoea. Any broad-spectrum antibacterial can promote colonisation with *C. difficile* in the colon, but cephalosporins, penicillins and clindamycin are the most frequent causes. *C. difficile* colonisation does not necessarily produce symptoms, which arise from toxin production by the bacteria. The diagnosis is confirmed by detection of toxin in the stool. *C. difficile*-associated diarrhoea fails to settle with conservative treatment in 80% of cases, and can produce fatal colitis. Treatment with oral metronidazole or alternatively oral vancomycin should be given (Ch. 51).

IRRITABLE BOWEL SYNDROME

Irritable bowel syndrome (IBS) is said to occur in 15% of the population. It is characterised by abdominal distension, bloating and alteration in bowel habit. There are two overlapping clinical presentations: constipation-predominant and diarrhoea-predominant. Abdominal discomfort may be relieved by defecation, but there is a sensation of incomplete evacuation and mucus is often passed per rectum. The cause is unknown, but a generalised motor and/or sensory disorder of the gastrointestinal tract is likely. A strong psychological component is also evident and the brain–gut axis is thought to play an important role.

Confirming the diagnosis of IBS involves exclusion of more serious bowel pathology. Screening should include inflammatory markers, coeliac disease immunology and excluding anaemia, which may indicate alternative diagnoses. Faecal calprotectin (a marker of inflammatory bowel disease) may also be part of a screening workup.

DRUGS FOR TREATING IRRITABLE BOWEL SYNDROME

Antimuscarinic drugs

dicycloverine, propantheline

Mechanism of action

Antimuscarinic drugs reduce colonic motility by inhibiting parasympathetic stimulation of the myenteric and submucosal neural plexuses. They also inhibit gastric emptying.

Pharmacokinetics

Oral absorption of dicycloverine is good and it is metabolised in the liver. Propantheline is a poorly absorbed quaternary amine and most is hydrolysed in the bowel.

Unwanted effects

- Constipation.
- Transient bradycardia, followed by tachycardia.
- Urinary retention.
- Blurred vision.
- Dry mouth.

Other antispasmodic agents

Examples

alverine citrate, mebeverine, peppermint oil

Mechanism of action

These antispasmodic agents have direct smooth muscle-relaxant properties (possibly by phosphodiesterase inhibition). They can relieve gut spasm and the associated pain.

Pharmacokinetics

Oral absorption of mebeverine is rapid and it undergoes extensive first-pass metabolism. Little is known about the pharmacokinetics of alverine citrate and peppermint oil.

Unwanted effects

These are rare but include:

- nausea with alverine citrate, heartburn and perianal irritation with peppermint oil,
- headache,
- allergic reactions.

MANAGEMENT OF IRRITABLE BOWEL SYNDROME

Drug therapy should form only part of the treatment of IBS, supplemented by cognitive behavioural therapy, relaxation and hypnotherapy where appropriate. Hypnotherapy is effective in up to 60% of people, but should be given by a properly trained therapist. Reductions in tea and coffee consumption and smoking, and modification of diet, may be helpful.

Constipation can be treated with bulking agents such as ispaghula husk or, if colonic transit time is very prolonged, an osmotic laxative may be effective. Lactulose is not recommended. Linaclotide, is a guanylate cyclase 2C agonist (see compendium) that activates the enzyme on the luminal surface of intestinal epithelial cells and increases anion and fluid secretion. It is used to reduce abdominal pain in refractory constipation-predominant irritable bowel syndrome. Loperamide is the first-choice drug for diarrhoea because it has a rapid onset of action and enables people to control their bowels, particularly when out of their normal environment or in other circumstances where diarrhoea would be socially disruptive. Care has to be taken with other opioids because of the risks of dependency and opioid-induced abdominal pain. Regular use of small doses of a laxative or antidiarrhoeal drug may be preferable to intermittent use. The non-absorbable antibacterial rifaximin can reduce symptoms in diarrhoea-predominant IBS.

Treatments for diarrhoea in IBS do not usually reduce the abdominal pain. There may be benefit from antispasmodic agents or a low-dose of a tricyclic antidepressant for analgesic effect (Ch. 19). Selective serotonin reuptake inhibitors are only recommended if a tricyclic antidepressant is ineffective (Ch. 22). Proton pump inhibitors (Ch. 33) may relieve diarrhoea by reducing the gastro-colic reflex.

Overall, current treatment of IBS is unsatisfactory. Serotonin 5-HT$_3$ receptor antagonists (for diarrhoea-predominant IBS) and 5-HT$_4$ receptor agonists (for constipation-predominant IBS) are available in some countries, but currently not in the UK.

SELF-ASSESSMENT

True/false questions

1. Constipation is when defaecation is less frequent than once daily.
2. Most cases of simple constipation can be treated by lifestyle changes.
3. Chronic intake of senna causes progressive hyperactivity of colonic motility.
4. Antacids containing aluminium salts can cause constipation.
5. Laxatives invariably induce bowel movements within 6 h.
6. Diarrhoea can be largely of psychological origin in some people.
7. In infants (<2 years) diarrhoea is mainly caused by bacterial infection.
8. Broad-spectrum antibacterial drugs may cause pseudomembranous colitis.
9. The use of antibacterial drugs to treat acute episodes of diarrhoea is rarely necessary.
10. Oral rehydration powders are reconstituted to give a hypertonic solution.

One-best-answer (OBA) questions

1. Choose the *correct* statement below concerning laxatives.
   A. Bulk laxative use should be accompanied by drinking plenty of water.
   B. Magnesium sulphate inhibits cholecystokinin release.
   C. Lactulose acts by stimulating the enteric nerves.
   D. Aluminium hydroxide can cause diarrhoea.
   E. Sterculia acts as a laxative within 12 h.
2. Which of the following statements about diarrhoea is *incorrect*?

   A. Rotavirus is an uncommon cause of diarrhoea in adults.

B. Kaolin is not recommended for acute diarrhoea.
C. *Campylobacter jejuni* is a common cause of bacterial gastroenteritis in the UK.
D. Loperamide decreases the gut residence time of the infective organism.
E. Antibacterial drugs can be used prophylactically for traveller's diarrhoea.

True/false answers

1. **False.** Normal bowel habit varies widely, with defaecation between three times daily and once every 3 days (or longer) regarded as normal.
2. **True.** Increased fibre intake and exercise help most cases of 'simple' constipation.
3. **False.** Chronic use of senna has been associated with loss of colonic function and damage to the myenteric plexus (cathartic colon), but it is now thought to be due to the refractory constipation itself rather than to inappropriate use of stimulant laxatives.
4. **True.** Aluminium salts cause constipation, as do other drugs including opioid analgesics, calcium channel blockers and some antidepressants.
5. **False.** Some laxatives (such as magnesium salts) can act within 6 h, whereas others including lactulose and docusate take considerably longer to exert their activity.
6. **True.** There is a psychological component to diarrhoea and other symptoms in irritable bowel syndrome, which may respond to counselling or hypnotherapy.
7. **False.** Viral gastroenteritis, especially rotavirus, is the major cause of infant diarrhoea.
8. **True.** Broad-spectrum antibacterials may cause colitis due to overgrowth of the anaerobe *Clostridium difficile*; it is treated with metronidazole or vancomycin.
9. **True.** In developed countries antibacterial drugs are rarely necessary for acute diarrhoea in otherwise healthy individuals; fluid and electrolyte replacement are appropriate.
10. **False.** The osmotic action of a hypertonic solution would draw water into the bowel, exacerbating diarrhoea; oral rehydration solution should be isotonic or slightly hypotonic.

OBA answers

1. **Answer A** is correct.
   A. **Correct.** Adequate water intake is necessary to hydrate bulk-forming laxatives.
   B. Incorrect. Magnesium sulphate is an osmotic laxative that also induces cholecystokinin release, stimulating enteric nerves.
   C. Incorrect. Lactulose is an osmotic laxative.
   D. Incorrect. Aluminium salts can cause constipation.
   E. Incorrect. The bulk-forming laxative sterculia takes more than 24 h to act.
2. **Answer D** is the incorrect statement.
   A. Correct. Rotavirus causes diarrhoea in young children but very rarely in adults.

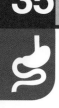

B. Correct. Kaolin is an adsorbent with limited effectiveness.
C. Correct. *C. jejuni* is one of the commonest causes of gastroenteritis in adults in developed countries.

D. **Incorrect.** Loperamide inhibits gut contractility by its opioid and antimuscarinic actions, and this may increase the residence of invasive organisms.
E. Correct. Ciprofloxacin or co-trimoxazole can be used prophylactically in travellers to high-risk areas.

FURTHER READING

DuPont HL (2009) Bacterial diarrhea. *N Engl J Med* 361, 1560–1569

Ford AC, Talley NJ (2012) Irritable bowel syndrome. *BMJ* 345, e5836

Kelly CP, LaMont JT (2008) *Clostridium difficile* – more difficult than ever. *N Engl J Med* 359 1932–1940

Lembo A, Camilleri M (2003) Chronic constipation. *N Engl J Med* 349, 1360–1368

Mayer EA (2008) Irritable bowel syndrome. *N Engl J Med* 358, 1692–1699

Spiller R (2007) Clinical update: irritable bowel syndrome. *Lancet* 369, 1586–1588

Spiller R, Aziz Q, Creed F et al. (2007) Guidelines on the irritable bowel syndrome: mechanisms and practical management. *Gut* 56, 1770–1798

Thielman NM (2004) Acute infectious diarrhea. *N Engl J Med* 350, 38–47

Thomas J, Karver S, Cooney GA (2008) Methylnaltrexone for opioid-induced constipation in advanced illness. *New Engl J Med* 358, 2332–2343

Wald A (2007) Appropriate use of laxatives in the management of constipation. *Curr Gastroenterol Rep* 9, 410–414

Compendium: drugs used in constipation, diarrhoea and irritable bowel syndrome

Drug	Kinetics (half-life)	Comments
Constipation		
Bulk-forming laxatives	Generally not absorbed	Bran, ispaghula husk, methylcellulose (also a faecal softener), sterculia; may affect the absorption of nutrients and minerals
Osmotic laxatives	Generally not absorbed	Lactulose, macrogols, magnesium salts; may affect the absorption of nutrients and minerals; phosphates (rectal), sodium citrate (rectal)
Irritant and stimulant laxatives	Some gut stimulants may undergo significant absorption and produce unwanted systemic effects; e.g. dantron produces liver damage	Bisacodyl (oral or rectal), dantron, docusate sodium (oral or rectal), glycerol (rectal), senna, sodium picosulfate
Faecal-softening agents	–	Glycerol (rectal), arachis oil (rectal); bulk-formating laxatives and docusate sodium (see above) also have faecal-softening properties; oral liquid paraffin is not recommended

Prucalopride

Rapidly absorbed; renal elimination by filtration and active secretion (24–30 h)

Serotonin 5-HT4 receptor agonist; used for chronic constipation to improve colonic motility

Diarrhoea

Anti-motility drugs such as opioids can be used for treatment of acute uncomplicated diarrhoea in adults but not in young children.

Drug	Kinetics (half-life)	Comments
Codeine phosphate	See Ch. 19	Opioid
Diphenoxylate	Oral bioavailability limited; hepatic metabolism (2–3 h), see Ch. 19	Opioid; given as co-phenotrope (co-formulation with atropine)
Kaolin	Not absorbed systemically	Adsorbs fluid within gut
Loperamide	Oral bioavailability 40%; hepatic metabolism (11 h); see Ch. 19	Opioid, with some antimuscarinic activity; action is due to parent drug before absorption
Morphine	Oral bioavailability 10–50%; hepatic metabolism (1–5 h); see Ch. 19	Opioid; available in combination with kaolin for short-term treatment of diarrhoea

Irritable bowel syndrome

Antispasmodic drugs and antimuscarinic drugs, some used for irritable bowel syndrome

Drug	Kinetics (half-life)	Comments
Alverine citrate	Few kinetic data available	Smooth muscle relaxant used for irritable bowel syndrome, as an adjunct in disorders characterised by spasm, and for dysmenorrhoea
Atropine	Rapidly absorbed; crosses the blood–brain barrier and the placenta; hepatic metabolism and renal excretion (12 h)	Antimuscarinic used for symptom relief in disorders characterised by gastrointestinal spasm; also used in the eye (Ch. 50), and as a surgical premedication (Ch. 17); unwanted effects limit use
Dicycloverine	Rapidly absorbed; oral bioavailability about 50%; eliminated in urine (9–10 h)	Antimuscarinic used for disorders characterised by gastrointestinal spasm, including irritable bowel syndrome; less severe antimuscarinic unwanted effects than atropine
Hyoscine	Incomplete oral absorption; hepatic metabolism (8 h)	Antimuscarinic used for disorders characterised by gastrointestinal spasm and for smooth muscle spasm in genitourinary disorders; also used as surgical premedication (Ch. 50) and for motion sickness (Ch. 32); unwanted effects limit use
Linaclotide	Minimal absorption; converted to active metabolite in the small intestine; subsequently degraded by proteolysis	peptide agonist of guanylate cyclase 2C which increases intracellular cGMP in intestinal epithelial cells and stimulates fluid secretion into the gut; relieves constipation and associated pain in irritable bowel syndrome

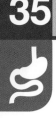

Compendium: drugs used in constipation, diarrhoea and irritable bowel syndrome—cont'd

Drug	Kinetics (half-life)	Comments
Mebeverine	Complete oral absorption; rapid first-pass metabolism	Smooth muscle relaxant used in disorders characterised by gastrointestinal spasm, including irritable bowel syndrome
Peppermint oil	Enteric-coated capsules delay release beyond stomach and upper small bowel	Used for gastrointestinal spasm in irritable bowel syndrome; local irritant if capsule not swallowed whole
Propantheline	Incomplete oral absorption (10–25%); hepatic glucuronide conjugation (1.5–2 h)	Antimuscarinic used for symptom relief in disorders characterised by gastrointestinal spasm, including irritable bowel syndrome; also used in urinary incontinence (Ch. 15)

All given orally unless otherwise indicated.

36 Liver disease

ACUTE AND SUBACUTE LIVER FAILURE

Liver failure arises from a number of insults to liver cells, principally viral infections or the toxic effects of drugs and chemicals. In the UK, paracetamol poisoning (Ch. 53) is the most common cause of acute liver failure.

Presenting symptoms of liver failure are often non-specific, with malaise, nausea and abdominal pain. As the syndrome progresses, signs of impairment of brain function occur (hepatic encephalopathy) with initial confusion followed by drowsiness and coma. These clinical features reflect alterations in neurotransmitter synthesis and increased central nervous system neuroinhibition with astrocyte swelling, caused by endogenous toxins that the liver fails to remove. Failure of coagulation and progressive multi-organ failure often follow.

The syndrome of liver failure can be categorised by the speed of onset of encephalopathy after the onset of jaundice:

- hyperacute: onset within 7 days, typically due to paracetamol or hepatitis A or E virus,
- acute: onset between 7 and 28 days, typically due to hepatitis B virus,
- subacute: onset between 29 days and 12 weeks; in this form, ascites and renal failure may also be prominent: typically due to non-paracetamol drug-induced injury.

MANAGEMENT

Acetylcysteine should be given if paracetamol was the precipitant (Ch. 53) and it may be useful in other forms of acute liver failure if treatment is started early when there is only low-grade encephalopathy. Other management is supportive and includes:

- prevention of bacterial and fungal infection with broad-spectrum antibacterial and antifungal agents,
- prevention of cerebral oedema by appropriate fluid management and particularly correction of hyponatraemia and the consequent hypo-osmolality. Cerebral oedema can be reduced by sedation and mechanical ventilation. Cerebral oedema is usually associated with encephalopathy, and is most marked in those who develop systemic infection, probably due to the interaction between pro-inflammatory mediators and circulating neurotoxins such as ammonia,
- prevention of hypoglycaemia with intravenous glucose,
- control of coagulopathy with intravenous vitamin K (Ch. 11), or fresh frozen plasma or cryoprecipitate if there is active bleeding,
- treatment of shock, often with a vasoconstrictors such as terlipressin (see below),
- artificial support for renal failure by maintaining circulating blood volume and, if necessary, with haemofiltration or haemodialysis,
- emergency liver transplantation is necessary for many people.

CHRONIC LIVER DISEASE

There are many causes of chronic liver disease, most of which ultimately lead to fibrotic changes in the liver that eventually alter the liver architecture and lead to distortion of the vasculature within the liver. This advanced change is called cirrhosis, and in the UK is most often caused by alcohol or hepatitis C virus. Hepatitis B virus is the most common cause in many developing countries. Other causes include autoimmune liver disease, haemochromatosis, Wilson's disease and α_1-antitrypsin deficiency. The diagnosis of liver cirrhosis is often made when complications arise (often referred to as decompensated cirrhosis), which include development of ascites, variceal haemorrhage, spontaneous bacterial peritonitis and hepatic encephalopathy (see below).

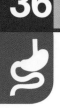

AUTOIMMUNE LIVER DISEASE

There are three principal forms of autoimmune liver disease: autoimmune hepatitis (AIH), primary biliary cirrhosis (PBC) and primary sclerosing cholangitis (PSC). The pathogenesis of these diseases is poorly understood, but the occurrence of circulating autoantibodies (antinuclear antibodies and smooth muscle antibodies, antibodies to liver/kidney microsome type 1 in AIH, antimitochondrial antibodies in PBC and low titres of several autoantibodies in PSC) and T-lymphocytes in the inflammatory infiltrate in the liver has encouraged the use of immunosuppressant treatments. Without treatment, AIH usually progresses to cirrhosis.

MANAGEMENT

Autoimmune hepatitis

- Corticosteroids, usually prednisolone (Ch. 44), induce remission in 85% of people with AIH, but, when used alone, up to 50% of those treated will still have developed cirrhosis after 10 years.
- Azathioprine (Ch. 38) has a corticosteroid-sparing action in AIH and is widely used in combination with corticosteroids, both to induce remission and for maintenance therapy. Treatment is usually required for up to 2 years.
- Mycophenolate mofetil or possibly ciclosporin (Ch. 38) are used for AIH that has not responded to corticosteroids. Evidence for their effectiveness is limited.
- Liver transplantation is necessary for end-stage disease.

Primary biliary cirrhosis

- Treatment of PBC is less satisfactory because immunosuppression is ineffective. Ursodeoxycholic acid is the only drug licensed for use with PBC in the UK. This is a bile acid that is produced by bacterial oxidation of chenodeoxycholic acid. It retards progression of the disease possibly by reducing apoptosis of hepatocytes and suppression of the cytotoxic effects of other bile acids. The main unwanted effect is diarrhoea. About one-third of people treated will have a response, with reduction in elevated liver enzymes, and a reduced risk of either death or the need for liver transplantation.
- Supportive therapy is necessary to reduce the complications that can arise from malabsorption of fat-soluble vitamins. Vitamin D (Ch. 42) and calcium supplements should be given to reduce the risk of osteomalacia and osteoporosis.
- Treatment of pruritis with colestyramine (Ch. 48), which binds bile acids in the gut.
- Liver transplantation is necessary for end-stage disease.

Primary sclerosing cholangitis

- There are no recognised medical treatments that alter the course of PSC. Ursodeoxycholic acid and immunosuppression are ineffective.
- Liver transplantation is necessary for end-stage disease.

CHRONIC VIRAL HEPATITIS

There are two important hepatic viral infections that can cause chronic hepatitis: hepatitis B virus (HBV; a DNA virus) and hepatitis C virus (HCV; an RNA virus). The result of the chronic inflammation produced by these viruses is cirrhosis.

DRUGS FOR TREATMENT OF VIRAL HEPATITIS

Interferon alfa

Mechanism of action and effects

Interferons are glycoprotein cytokines produced by virus-infected cells that protect uninfected cells of the same type. Interferon alfa binds to cell surface receptors and stimulates production of enzymes in the host cell that impair viral mRNA translation by host ribosomes. This inhibits viral replication and augments viral clearance from infected hepatocytes (Ch. 51). There are two forms of interferon alfa: interferon alfa-2a has lysine in position 23 and interferon alfa-2b has methionine in this position. Interferons are obtained either by recombinant DNA technology or from virus-stimulated leucocytes.

Pharmacokinetics

Interferon alfa is given by subcutaneous injection three times a week for 4–6 months. It is metabolised in the kidney and has a short half-life (3–4 h). Polyethylene glycol-conjugated (pegylated) derivatives of interferon alfa are available that increase the persistence of the interferon in the blood and these are given once weekly.

Unwanted effects

- Immediate effects are almost universal and include headache, myalgia, fever and rigors, usually occurring 4–6 h after injection. Tolerance to these effects occurs with repeated use.
- Delayed effects include fatigue, anorexia, nausea and diarrhoea.
- Depression.
- Bone marrow suppression, especially affecting granulocytes.

Nucleoside analogues

entecavir, lamivudine, ribavirin, tenofovir disoproxil

Mechanism of action and uses

Analogues of nucleosides and nucleotides (phosphorylated nucleosides) inhibit viral polymerase, reduce RNA and protein synthesis, and suppress viral replication (Ch. 51).

- Entecavir is a guanosine nucleoside analogue.
- Lamivudine is a cytosine nucleoside analogue.

- Ribavirin is a synthetic nucleoside analogue with activity against some RNA and DNA viruses. It inhibits viral RNA synthesis by blocking incorporation of uridine and cytidine. It also increases the production of antiviral cytokines. Ribavirin has little effect on viral replication when used alone, but it enhances the efficacy of interferon alfa against HCV. Ribavirin is also used by inhalation to treat respiratory syncytial virus infection.
- Tenofovir is a nucleotide analogue of adenosine 5′-monophosphate.

Pharmacokinetics

Nucleoside analogues are well absorbed from the gut. They are inactive prodrugs that are phosphorylated intracellularly to the active nucleotide derivatives, and then eliminated by the kidney. See Compendium at the end of the chapter for further details.

Unwanted effects

- Anorexia, abdominal pain, nausea, vomiting, diarrhoea.
- Cough, dyspnoea.
- Headache, dizziness, insomnia, fatigue.
- Rashes.
- Lactic acidosis with hepatic steatosis.
- Accumulation of ribavirin in red cells produces haemolysis.
- Interstitial pneumonitis, palpitation, chest pain, syncope with ribavirin.

Protease inhibitors

boceprevir, telaprevir

Mechanism of action

Boceprevir and telaprevir are specific inhibitors of the HCV serine protease. The protease is responsible for the cleavage of viral polyprotein that is an essential process in viral replication. The protease may also aid the virus in evading the normal inflammatory response of the host cell, so protease inhibitors may enhance the host response to infection.

Resistance

Viral resistance is due to emergence of mutations that interfere with the ligand-binding site on the protease.

Pharmacokinetics

Boceprevir and telaprevir are well absorbed from the gut and are metabolized in the liver with half-lives of about 3 and 10 h respectively.

Unwanted effects

- Nausea, vomiting, abdominal pain, diarrhoea, altered taste.
- Rash is common, including Stevens–Johnson syndrome with telaprevir.
- Anaemia, neutropenia.
- Syncope, oedema.

- Paraesthesia, dizziness, headache, anxiety, depression, insomnia with boceprevir.
- Drug interactions (Ch. 56): inhibition of the P450 enzyme CYP3A4 and P-glycoprotein by these drugs can lead to several potential drug interactions. Drugs that inhibit the activity of CYP3A4 can enhance the unwanted effects of protease inhibitors, whereas the concurrent use of inducers of CYP3A4 can lower plasma concentrations of the protease inhibitor and encourage viral resistance.

MANAGEMENT OF CHRONIC VIRAL HEPATITIS

Chronic hepatitis B

There is no role for drug treatment in acute hepatitis B, which usually resolves spontaneously. Chronic infection is characterised by persistence of hepatitis B surface antigen (HBsAg) and other immunological markers at least 6 months after the acute infection. Antiviral treatment should be used if there is evidence of active chronic infection with ongoing liver damage and high viral replication (high titre of HBV DNA). This is usually, but not always, associated with hepatitis Be antigen (HBeAg) in plasma as a marker of active viral replication. The criteria for successful treatment are a matter of debate. Seroconversion to HBe antibody only occurs in a minority of those who are treated, and even fewer seroconvert to HBs antibody, which is the ideal outcome. Measurement of HBV DNA is a sensitive way to monitor treatment and detect drug resistance.

The optimal choice of antiviral treatment is contentious. Lamivudine has been advocated, but complete eradication of the virus by lamivudine is unusual, and the relapse rate on withdrawal is high, with only about 10% of people showing long-term responses once treatment is discontinued. Emergence of viral strains with drug resistance to lamivudine is common and occurs progressively, with a 15–30% prevalence of resistant strains after 1 year of treatment. Increasingly, entecavir or tenofovir are becoming first-choice antiviral drugs, either alone or with tenofovir given in combination with lamivudine. Viral resistance to entecavir or tenofovir is unusual.

Interferon alfa is now less commonly used. It achieves seroconversion in about one-third of cases, with no difference between the pegylated and non-pegylated forms of the drug. About 40% of those treated will show a conversion to low viral replication, and about 10% will have complete eradication. Relapse is frequent when treatment is stopped.

Chronic hepatitis C

The aim of treatment is eradication of the virus. If left untreated about 85% of people who are infected develop chronic infection and of these up to 30% will develop cirrhosis. Treatment with pegylated interferon alfa alone can eradicate the virus, with a 15% sustained response rate. It can also prevent liver damage even if eradication is not successful. Treatment duration and success depend on the viral strain, or genotype, of which three are found in Europe. The addition of ribavirin to pegylated interferon alfa increases the overall response rate to 45% for genotype 1 and 80% for genotypes 2 or 3, and the combination is standard therapy for all people who can tolerate both drugs. For genotypes 2 or 3, treatment for 24 weeks is sufficient for a maximal response, while treatment for genotype 1 (the most common type in developed countries) should be continued for 48 weeks in those who have a response in the first 24 weeks. Pegylated interferons produce up to a 10% higher response rate than the conventional interferons.

The addition of viral protease inhibitors such as boceprevir or telaprevir to the combination of interferon alfa and ribavirin is more effective than dual therapy in genotype 1 infection, but with a higher incidence of anaemia and other unwanted effects.

CHRONIC HEPATIC ENCEPHALOPATHY

Many chronic liver diseases predispose to the neuropsychiatric disturbance known as chronic hepatic encephalopathy. The clinical features are similar to those occurring in acute liver failure. Spontaneous bacterial peritonitis is a common cause of deterioration in previously compensated liver failure. In people with chronic encephalopathy nutritional support may be necessary, and malabsorption of fat-soluble vitamins can be a particular problem if there is cholestasis. Osteoporosis can result, made worse by the use of corticosteroids.

MANAGEMENT

- Treatment of infections, constipation and electrolyte disturbances (particularly hypokalaemia), and avoidance of sedative drugs will help to prevent symptomatic encephalopathy.
- Lactulose (Ch. 35) can be given orally to reduce colonic production of neurotoxins (particularly ammonia) by decreasing intestinal transit time and increasing nitrogen fixation by colonic bacteria. It may also reduce bacterial translocation form the colon and prevent episodes of spontaneous bacterial peritonitis. Lactulose is effective for both treatment and prevention of encephalopathy.
- Low-absorption oral antibacterials such as neomycin, metronidazole or rifaximin (Ch. 51) reduce bacterial ammonia production in the colon. They are usually used only for short periods. Neomycin is less favoured because of its potential to cause nephrotoxicity and ototoxicity, even though little is absorbed from the gut.
- Careful attention to nutrition is required, especially a balanced carbohydrate and protein intake. Branched-chain amino acids should be consumed in preference to aromatic amino acids.
- Fat malabsorption can be treated with medium-chain triglyceride supplements, and sufficient calorie intake should be ensured. Supplements of fat-soluble vitamins (A, D, E, K) may be needed. Metabolic bone disease may require treatment with bisphosphonates (Ch. 42).
- Sepsis, including spontaneous bacterial peritonitis, is often due to bowel flora and should be treated with intravenous broad-spectrum antibacterial drugs, such as cefuroxime with metronidazole (Ch. 51).

VARICEAL HAEMORRHAGE

Varices are large collateral venous communications that develop in portal hypertension, most frequently at the gastro-oesophageal junction but also at other places such as the rectum. They arise from a combination of increased splanchnic blood flow and increased resistance to portal blood flow within the liver. Varices are found in 70% of people with cirrhosis and they carry a high risk of haemorrhage, from which mortality is 30–50%. Normal portal vein pressure is about 9 mmHg, while that in the inferior vena cava is 2–6 mmHg. The hepatic venous pressure gradient is therefore between 3 and 7 mmHg. Varices form when the venous pressure gradient rises above 10 mmHg. The probability of rupture is increased when the pressure gradient reaches 12 mmHg, and greatly increased when above 20 mmHg.

MANAGEMENT

Management of bleeding gastro-oesophageal varices

- Repletion of blood volume can be carried out with colloid solution, or preferably with whole blood. Impaired coagulation and thrombocytopenia are common findings in advanced liver disease, and transfusion of platelet concentrates and fresh frozen plasma may be necessary.
- The risk of bacterial infections is high in acute variceal bleeding, and short-term antibacterial prophylaxis with an agent such as ciprofloxacin or ceftriaxone (Ch. 51) should be given.
- Endoscopic variceal band ligation or injection with a sclerosant is successful in up to 95% of cases. The main complications are oesophageal ulceration, increased risk of infections and pleural effusions.
- Endoscopic variceal injection of a cyanoacrylate tissue adhesive is effective for bleeding gastric varices, and is successful in 80% of cases. It is also an option for oesophageal varices. These compounds are tissue glues that polymerise on contact with water or blood.
- Balloon tamponade to compress the bleeding point achieves control in 80–90% of bleeding varices. It can be used to treat re-bleeding after endoscopic sclerosant therapy or as a holding measure, but is rarely used as a first-line treatment.
- A transjugular intrahepatic portosystemic shunt (TIPS) is used as rescue therapy in the 10–20% of cases when sclerosant therapy has failed.
- Terlipressin (N-triglycyl-8-lysine-vasopressin) is a prodrug that is slowly converted to lysine-vasopressin, a synthetic vasopressin analogue (Ch. 43). Given intravenously by bolus injection, it produces splanchnic vasoconstriction, reduces portal pressure and limits bleeding from varices. Unwanted effects are uncommon. It is mainly used when endoscopic sclerosant therapy is not immediately available. Vasopressin has been used to treat bleeding varices, but has a shorter duration of action than terlipressin and must be given by

intravenous infusion. Systemic vasoconstriction causes ischaemic complications in up to 50% of those treated with vasopressin which is therefore little used.

- Octreotide (Ch. 43) and somatostatin (Ch. 43) are probably as effective as vasopressin for stopping haemorrhage, but there is less convincing evidence compared with terlipressin. They also work by reducing portal venous pressure.

Prevention of variceal re-bleeding

- Splanchnic vasoconstrictors that lower portal flow and reduce portal pressure by at least 20% will reduce the risk of re-bleeding to about 10% at 2 years. This is most often achieved by the use of a non-selective β-adrenoceptor antagonist such as propranolol (Ch. 5). Sometimes, isosorbide mononitrate (Ch. 5) is added to vasodilate the portal circulation and further reduce portal flow. However, this can produce systemic hypotension and promote renal salt and water retention.
- Local treatment of the varices, for example by endoscopic band ligation, will reduce the risk of re-bleeding, but does not reduce portal pressure. In about 50% of cases, the varices will recur within 2 years. Banding should therefore be followed by drug therapy to lower portal pressure.
- A TIPS is most commonly used when re-bleeding follows endoscopic variceal ligation and drug therapy to lower portal pressure. It can lead to chronic encephalopathy and other significant adverse effects. Surgical creation of a portosystemic shunt is an alternative to TIPS.

ASCITES

Ascites in chronic liver disease arises largely as a result of splanchnic vasodilation. Portal hypertension results in local production of vasodilators, which reduce effective circulating blood volume. This promotes salt and water retention in the kidney due to activation of the renin–angiotensin system. The increased portal pressure combined with vasodilation leads to transudation of fluid into the peritoneal cavity. Spontaneous bacterial peritonitis can complicate ascites associated with liver disease and make the ascites resistant to treatment.

MANAGEMENT

The presence of ascites in chronic liver disease is associated with a poor prognosis, with a 5-year survival of 30–40%, unless liver transplantation is carried out. Management of ascites includes:

- reduction of salt intake,
- diuretic therapy, starting with a potassium-sparing diuretic such as spironolactone (Ch. 14) together with a low dose of furosemide, with care taken to avoid hypovolaemia and consequent pre-renal failure,
- drainage by paracentesis is usually required in large-volume ascites in addition to diuretics as maintenance

therapy; paracentesis should be accompanied by plasma expansion with intravenous albumin to maintain circulating blood volume. Refractory ascites that fails to respond to high doses of diuretics or recurs rapidly after paracentesis may need repeated large-volume paracentesis with intravenous albumin replacement,
- a TIPS can be used to lower portal pressure for refractory ascites.

SELF-ASSESSMENT

One-best-answer (OBA) questions

1. Identify the *inaccurate* statement below concerning antiviral treatments.
   A. Interferon alfa protects against viral hepatitis.
   B. Pegylated and non-pegylated versions of interferon alfa are cleared from the plasma at the same rate.
   C. Boceprevir is an inhibitor of hepatitis C virus (HCV) serine protease.
   D. Lamivudine is a prodrug.
   E. Combination therapy with ribavirin and interferon alfa is recommended for the treatment of hepatitis C.

2. A 45-year-old woman was admitted to the accident and emergency department with acute liver failure. Identify the *inaccurate* statement below concerning her condition.
   A. Paracetamol overdose should be excluded.
   B. Paracetamol-induced hepatocellular liver damage is not reversible.
   C. Mannitol could be used to reduce the cerebral oedema associated with acute liver failure.
   D. Warfarin could be used to manage coagulopathy.
   E. Terlipressin could be given as a vasoconstrictor to treat shock.

Case-based questions

Mr SA was a 61-year-old publican who presented 'feeling as though I am 9 months pregnant'. His abdominal swelling was caused by ascites, which was drained. A liver biopsy was performed, which showed micro-nodular cirrhosis. He commenced treatment with oral spironolactone.

A. Was this a good choice of diuretic?

He remained well on this regimen for 5 years but continued to imbibe large quantities of alcohol. He re-presented as an emergency, having had a haematemesis and melaena. At the time he was slightly jaundiced and demonstrated signs of hepatic encephalopathy. In addition, there was gynaecomastia and testicular atrophy. The liver edge was palpable 8 cm below the right costal margin. Investigations showed a bilirubin level of 27 mmol·L^{-1} (normal <17 mmol·L^{-1}) and albumin of 30 g·L^{-1} (normal 32–50 g·L^{-1}). A gastroscopy was performed under sedation with intravenous diazepam and revealed oesophageal varices.

B. What evidence was there to indicate diminished hepatic reserve in this man?

C. Was diazepam a good choice during gastroscopy?

D. It has been shown that the incidence of re-bleeding from oesophageal varices can be reduced by oral propranolol (by reducing portal venous pressure). What effect is this man's liver disease likely to have on the pharmacodynamics and pharmacokinetics of propranolol?

E. People with hepatic cirrhosis are often treated with colestyramine and/or lactulose. How do these drugs work and what benefits are produced?

F. What would you use for pain relief in someone with established liver cirrhosis?

OBA answers

1. **Answer B** is the inaccurate statement.
   A. True. Interferon alfa prevents virus replication (Ch. 52) and can augment immune responses.
   B. **False**. Interferon alfa conjugated with polyethylene glycol (pegylated interferon alfa) has a longer plasma half-life (about 80 h) than the non-conjugated form (3–4 h).
   C. True. Boceprevir and telaprevir inhibit HCV serine protease and reduce viral replication.
   D. True. Lamivudine is converted to its active triphosphate form by phosphorylation by viral enzymes.
   E. True. Combined ribavirin and interferon alfa are recommended for the treatment of hepatitis C, giving better results than either treatment alone.

2. **Answer D** is the inaccurate statement.
   A. True. Paracetamol poisoning is the most common cause of acute liver failure in the UK.
   B. True. Liver damage induced by paracetamol is irreversible.
   C. True. Mannitol is an osmotic diuretic with relatively few uses (Ch. 14), but is effective for the reduction of cerebral oedema.
   D. **False**. The coagulopathy is due to a reduction in vitamin K-dependent clotting factors. Warfarin, a vitamin K antagonist, would make the problem worse, and vitamin K should be given.
   E. True. Terlipressin, an analogue of vasopressin that causes vasoconstriction, can be given to treat shock.

Case-based answers

A. Mr SA is at risk of encephalopathy/coma from electrolyte imbalances. Spironolactone, a potassium-sparing diuretic, would avoid changes in serum K^+ such as might be caused by loop diuretics or thiazides; these diuretics could be given cautiously after a few days. There is an increase in circulating aldosterone probably contributing to fluid retention, so spironolactone is usually chosen.

B. Diminished hepatic reserve is indicated by (i) increased plasma bilirubin, which will be a combination of unconjugated bilirubin, because of impaired glucuronidation, plus conjugated bilirubin, because of impaired biliary excretion; (ii) decreased plasma albumin, caused by decreased synthesis, which will lower the osmotic pressure of blood and lead to oedema/ascites; (iii) decreased clotting factors, caused by decreased synthesis, which may contribute to oesophageal bleeding; (iv) increased oestrogenic activity, as evidenced by gynaecomastia and testicular atrophy, possibly caused by decreased sex steroid inactivation in the liver.

C. Reduced hepatic cytochrome P450 metabolism might cause increased plasma levels of diazepam, a long-acting benzodiazepine. A shorter-acting benzodiazepine without active metabolites, such as midazolam, would be a better choice.

D. Reduced plasma protein concentration means that less propranolol is bound and free drug is increased. This will result in an increased response. Reduced hepatic P450 activity will decrease first-pass metabolism of propranolol and increase its bioavailability, while reduced clearance will increase its elimination half-life.

E. In liver cirrhosis, decreased bile outflow leads to accumulation of bile salts in the blood and their deposition in the skin, which causes itching. Colestyramine, an anion-exchange resin, adsorbs bile salts within the gut and reduces their enterohepatic circulation. Lactulose is a laxative (Ch. 35) and its fermentation products in the lower gastrointestinal tract reduce microbial formation of ammonia and tyramine, which may otherwise contribute to encephalopathy.

F. Analgesia in cirrhosis can be difficult. Opioids should usually be avoided because of the risk of encephalopathy, but low doses could be given. Non-steroidal anti-inflammatory drugs (NSAIDs) are best avoided to reduce the risk of haemorrhage from oesophageal varices. Paracetamol is potentially hepatotoxic, but it is well tolerated in cirrhosis, probably because decreased perfusion of hepatocytes and reduced activity of cytochrome P450 outweigh the impaired inactivation by conjugation.

FURTHER READING

Bernal W, Auzinger A, Dhawan A et al. (2010) Acute liver failure. *Lancet* 376, 190–201

Chapman R, Fevery J, Kalloo A et al. (2010) Diagnosis and management of primary sclerosing cholangitis. *Hepatology* 51, 660–678

Cooke GS, Main J, Thursz MR (2009) Treatment for hepatitis B. *BMJ* 339, b5429

Dienstag JL (2008) Drug therapy: hepatitis B virus infection. *N Engl J Med* 359, 1486–1500

Garcia-Tsao G, Bosch J (2010) Management of varices and variceal hemorrhage in cirrhosis. *N Engl J Med* 362, 823–832

Krawitt EL (2006) Autoimmune hepatitis. *N Engl J Med* 354, 54–66

Liaw Y-F, Chu GM (2009) Hepatitis B virus infection. *Lancet* 373, 582–592

Manns MP, Czaja AJ, Gorham JD et al. (2010) Diagnosis and management of autoimmune hepatitis. *Hepatology* 51, 1–31

Nash KL, Bentley I, Hirschfield GM (2009) Managing hepatitis C virus infection. *BMJ* 338, b2366

Rosen HR (2011) Chronic hepatitis C infection. *N Engl J Med* 364, 2429–2438

Rowe IA, Mutimer DJ (2011) Protease inhibitors for treatment of genotype 1 hepatitis C virus infection. *BMJ* 343, d6972

Runyon BA (2009) Management of adult patients with ascites due to cirrhosis: an update. *Hepatology* 49, 2087–2105

Schuppan D, Afdhal NH (2008) Liver cirrhosis. *Lancet* 371, 838–851

Selmi C, Bowlus CL, Gershwin ME et al. (2011) Primary biliary cirrhosis. *Lancet* 377, 1600–1609

Shah VH, Kamath P (2006) Management of portal hypertension. *Postgrad Med* 119, 14–18

Compendium: drugs used in liver disease

Drug	Kinetics (half-life)	Comments
Autoimmune liver disease		
Azathioprine	Converted to active 6-mercaptopurine (3–5 h) (see Ch. 38)	Has a corticosteroid-sparing action and is used in combination with corticosteroids; oral or intravenous dosage
Corticosteroids	See Ch. 44	Usually prednisolone is used
Ursodeoxycholic acid	Most absorbed in the small intestine; metabolised and eliminated in bile as glycine and taurine conjugates (like a bile acid); slow elimination due to enterohepatic circulation (days)	The only drug licensed for use in primary biliary cirrhosis; produced by bacterial oxidation of chenodeoxycholic acid; given orally
Other drugs	–	Ciclosporin, tacrolimus or mycophenolate (see Ch. 38) are used for autoimmune hepatitis that has not responded to corticosteroids
Viral hepatitis		
Interferons		
Interferon alfa	Catabolised in kidney (3–4 h)	Used in the treatment of chronic hepatitis B infection; given by subcutaneous, intramuscular or intravenous injection
Peginterferon alfa	Polyethylene glycol-conjugated form of interferon alfa; gives more prolonged blood levels (80 h)	Used in combination with ribavirin for chronic hepatitis C infection; given by subcutaneous injection
Nucleoside analogues		
Adefovir dipivoxil	Prodrug that undergoes hydrolysis to adefovir, then intracellular phosphorylation to the active diphosphate; eliminated by the kidneys (8 h)	Used in chronic hepatitis B infection with *either* compensated liver disease with evidence of viral replication and histologically documented active liver inflammation and fibrosis, *or* decompensated liver disease; given orally
Entecavir	Complete oral bioavailability; eliminated by glomerular filtration and tubular secretion (130 h)	Used in chronic hepatitis B infection with compensated liver disease, evidence of viral replication and histologically documented active liver inflammation or fibrosis
Lamivudine	Rapid absorption with about 70% bioavailability; undergoes intracellular phosphorylation to an active triphosphate; eliminated mainly by the kidneys and by sulphoxidation (5–7 h)	Antiviral reverse transcriptase inhibitor used in the initial treatment of hepatitis B infection, and for decompensated liver disease; given orally
Ribavirin	Oral bioavailability 50%; hepatic metabolism; cleared slowly from erythrocytes and tissues (7–21 days)	Used with pegylated interferon alfa for chronic hepatic C infection; given orally
Tenofovir disoproxil	Oral bioavailability about 25%; intracellular phosphorylation to diphosphate; eliminated by glomerular filtration and tubular secretion (17 h)	Used for people requiring treatment for both HIV and chronic hepatitis B; given orally
Protease inhibitors		
Boceprevir	Well absorbed; hepatic metabolism (3 h)	Specific hepatitis C virus serine protease inhibitor; used with ribavirin and pegylated interferon alfa for HCV genotype 1; given orally
Telaprevir	Well absorbed; hepatic metabolism (10 h)	Specific hepatitis C virus serine protease inhibitor; used with ribavirin and pegylated interferon alfa for HCV genotype 1; given orally
Drugs used for oesophageal varices		
Octreotide	Eliminated by renal excretion (about 40%) and probably by tissue uptake and metabolism (1.7 h)	Somatostatin analogue; given by subcutaneous injection, or by intravenous injection if a more rapid response is required
Terlipressin	Triglycyl prodrug hydrolysed to lysine-vasopressin (0.5 h)	Vasopressin prodrug; given by intravenous injection

37

Obesity

● ●

Obesity is defined as a body mass index (BMI) above 30 kg·m^{-2}, compared with the ideal range of 18.5–24.9 kg·m^{-2}. A BMI of 25–29.9 kg·m^{-2} is considered overweight. The prevalence of obesity is increasing in the Western world; it varies from less than 10% in the Netherlands to about 50% in some parts of Eastern Europe. In the UK it is currently about 15%, but over half the British population is now overweight.

The health consequences of obesity are considerable (Box 37.1). Obesity decreases life expectancy by 7 years at the age of 40 years. Recent data suggest that waist circumference above 102 cm in males or 88 cm in females is more closely correlated than BMI with the cluster of atherogenic risk factors known as the metabolic syndrome. Metabolic syndrome is the presence of at least two of the following characteristic features in association with large waist circumference:

■ abnormally raised triglyceride,
■ decreased high-density lipoprotein (HDL) cholesterol,
■ raised fasting blood glucose (as a result of insulin resistance),
■ hypertension.

Excess dietary calories are stored as fat in adipose tissue. Intra-abdominal (visceral) fat is most closely associated with the metabolic and atherogenic consequences of obesity. The association between central obesity and atherothrombosis is related to enlarged visceral adipocytes. These adipocytes secrete numerous inflammatory, pro-atherogenic and procoagulant cytokines such as interleukin-6, tumour necrosis factor α and plasminogen activator inhibitor-1, but secrete reduced amounts of the anti-inflammatory and anti-atherogenic hormone adiponectin. Cytokines produced by fat-laden omental adipocytes enter the portal circulation and influence many aspects of hepatic metabolism.

PATHOGENESIS OF OBESITY

Food intake is controlled by numerous hormonal, societal, genetic and psychological factors. Obesity usually develops gradually, and results when energy input exceeds output for a prolonged period. A small imbalance between energy intake and exercise or muscular work is all that is required for progressive weight gain. There are polygenic influences that determine who is more susceptible to weight gain. However, the recent epidemic of obesity in the Western world suggests that major environmental factors (reduced activity and dietary changes) are responsible, rather than biological causes.

For a few individuals, obesity arises from hormonal disturbances, or from neurological conditions that lead to behavioural change. Several drugs can produce weight gain, such as antipsychotics, tricyclic antidepressants, corticosteroids, antiepileptics, antihistamines and antidiabetic drugs.

There are two types of adipose tissue: brown adipose tissue is responsible for thermogenesis and white adipose tissue for energy storage. White adipose tissue is a target for insulin and in obese people there is resistance to the action of insulin, leading to accumulation of intracellular fat.

Energy balance is regulated in the hypothalamus, which integrates neural, hormonal and circulating nutrient stimuli, and sends signals to higher centres to trigger feelings of satiety or hunger. The hypothalamus also regulates sympathetic nervous system function (which controls lipolysis for release of fatty acids as an energy source, and also thermogenesis) and pituitary hormones that help to regulate energy expenditure.

The biochemical factors that underlie the regulation of weight are increasingly well characterised (Fig. 37.1). Signals to the hypothalamus that reduce food intake (satiety signals) are provided by a number of hormones produced by the endocrine cells of the gut, adipose tissue and the pancreas. Leptin, which is released from adipocytes, and insulin both signal via specific hypothalamic receptors to indicate the degree of filling of adipocytes and induce the sensation of satiety.

Several gut-derived peptides act as short-term appetite regulators. Ghrelin is released by the stomach preprandially, and *stimulates* orexigenic (appetite-stimulating) peptides. Oxyntomodulin, glucagon-like peptide-1 (GLP-1), cholecystokinin and peptide YY$_{3-36}$ (PYY) are released from the small intestine and colon in response to the presence of carbohydrates and lipids, and *inhibit* release of orexigenic peptides in the hypothalamus.

When energy levels are low, ghrelin release and reductions in leptin, insulin and other gut-derived peptides act on the hypothalamus to stimulate key hypothalamic neurotransmitters, including neuropeptide Y (NPY) and agouti-related protein (AgRP). This decreases activity in the melanocortin system which releases signalling by the orexigenic hormones melanin-concentrating hormone (MCH) and orexin (ORX) to stimulate appetite. Following a meal, high plasma concentrations of insulin, glucose, cholecystokinin and leptin stimulate the hypothalamic appetite-suppressing substances pro-opiomelanocortin (POMC) and cocaine- and amfetamine-regulated transcript (CART). These mediators increase α-melanocyte-stimulating hormone (α-MSH) release which inhibits MCH/ORX activity and signal satiety.

Unexpectedly, the circulating concentration of leptin is usually high in obesity. This may reflect the excess fat accumulation and hypothalamic resistance to satiety cues such as leptin.

Other neurotransmitters and hormones that influence appetite include the appetite inhibitors serotonin and dopamine, while cannabinoids, cortisol and growth hormone-releasing hormone stimulate appetite. The role of the endocannabinoid system in regulating appetite has received increased attention in recent years. Acting via CB$_1$ receptors, the natural agonists such as anandamide and 2-arachidonylglycerol have both CNS and peripheral

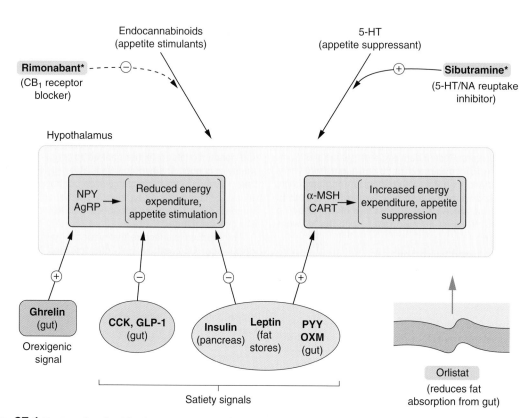

Fig. 37.1 **Factors involved in the regulation of food intake.** Feedback loops between the periphery and the brain control food intake. Peripheral signals stimulate or inhibit transmitters in the arcuate nucleus of the hypothalamus (shown in yellow) that control appetite and energy expenditure. The hypothalamus sends signals to higher centres, indicating satiety or hunger. The peripheral orexigenic (appetite-stimulating) signals include ghrelin, released preprandially from the gut, and satiety signals include insulin, leptin, peptide YY$_{3-36}$ (PYY) and oxyntomodulin (OXM). Other hypothalamic signalling mechanisms are described in the text. Endocannabinoid pathways are involved in stimulating appetite, and serotonin acts on the hypothalamus to suppress appetite. *Centrally acting appetite-suppressant drugs have been withdrawn due to unwanted effects, but rimonabant and sibutramine are shown to illustrate mechanisms. Orlistat reduces fat absorption from the gut by inhibiting pancreatic lipase. AgRP, agouti-related protein; CART, cocaine- and amfetamine-regulated transcript; CCK, cholecystokinin; GLP-1, glucagon-like peptide-1; α-MSH, α melanocyte-stimulating hormone; NA, noradrenaline; NPY, neuropeptide Y.

actions. Endocannabinoids in the CNS are released from postsynaptic neurons, and act on presynaptic receptors to inhibit neurotransmitter release. They stimulate appetite by actions at the hypothalamus and nucleus accumbens. Peripherally, endocannabinoids have effects on gastrointestinal motility that reduce satiety signals.

Improved understanding of the biochemical signals that regulate appetite has led to a search for more effective appetite-suppressant drugs. So far there has been little translation into clinical practice.

DRUGS FOR TREATMENT OF OBESITY

DRUGS ACTING ON THE GASTROINTESTINAL TRACT

Examples

methylcellulose, orlistat

Mechanisms of action

Orlistat acts by binding to pancreatic lipase in the gut and inhibiting its action. It reduces triglyceride digestion and, therefore, energy intake from dietary fat. An effect on energy intake is seen after 24–48 h, and orlistat achieves sustained weight loss when used as an adjunct to dietary restriction and exercise. However, only about 20% of people will lose more than 5% of body weight. Continuous use of orlistat for more than 2 years is not recommended.

Methylcellulose is taken before meals and swells when hydrated and produces a sense of satiety. There is little evidence to support its ability to reduce appetite, and it has little use in the treatment of obesity. It is also used in constipation as a bulk-forming laxative (Ch. 35).

Pharmacokinetics

Methylcellulose and orlistat undergo minimal absorption after oral administration, and are largely excreted unchanged in the faeces.

Unwanted effects

- Orlistat produces gastrointestinal upset, including flatulence, faecal urgency and faecal soiling. These are most common with poor adherence to a low-fat diet while taking the drug, and result in discontinuation of treatment by one-third of people. There is also impaired absorption of fat-soluble vitamins, especially vitamin D.
- Methylcellulose swells rapidly when hydrated and should be taken with water to avoid oesophageal obstruction. It may have a laxative effect.

CENTRALLY ACTING APPETITE SUPPRESSANTS

All centrally acting appetite suppressants, such as dexfenfluramine, fenfluramine, phentermine and sibutramine, have been withdrawn because of the increased risks of valvular heart disease and pulmonary hypertension. The selective CB_1 receptor antagonist rimonabant that suppresses appetite by an effect on the hypothalamus has been withdrawn due to psychological disturbances.

Centrally acting drugs that work by different mechanisms are under development, but none are available for clinical use.

MANAGEMENT OF OBESITY

Weight loss reduces the morbidity associated with obesity, but it is not known whether it prolongs life. Weight loss can be difficult to achieve and to maintain. Obesity is not usually caused by psychological disturbances, but these commonly arise in obese people. The social prejudice against obesity, concern about body image and the depression and irritability that arise from dieting are all contributory factors.

The cornerstone of management of obesity is to reduce energy intake by 500–600 kcal below daily requirements. Fat is 'energy dense' and should be particularly restricted. However, dietary restriction alone is usually inadequate to achieve weight loss, and increased exercise combined with diet is more effective than either alone. Exercise need not be vigorous, provided it is maintained long-term; walking or cycling is usually enough if performed daily. Behaviour modification is essential for long-term adherence to treatment.

Drug treatment should be restricted to individuals with a BMI of more than 30 $kg \cdot m^{-2}$, or a BMI of more than 28 $kg \cdot m^{-2}$ in the presence of diabetes, hypertension or hypercholesterolaemia. Currently orlistat is the only licensed available agent. A major disadvantage is that weight gain often follows cessation of drug therapy. The use of thyroxine to encourage weight loss by increasing metabolic rate is not recommended due to long-term risks such as osteoporosis. Bulking agents such as methylcellulose are usually ineffective for reducing food intake. Specialist clinics will consider the use of metformin (Ch. 40), selective serotonin reuptake inhibitors (Ch. 22), GLP-1 inhibitors such as liraglutide (Ch. 40) or topiramate (Ch. 23). Treatments under investigation that interfere with the many neurotransmitter systems that regulate weight promise to offer more effective pharmacotherapy than the current limited range of options.

Bariatric surgery to restrict the size of the stomach (gastroplasty: gastric banding or vertical sleeve gastrectomy) or gastric bypass (such as Roux-en-Y) are used in the morbidly obese (BMI >40 $kg \cdot m^{-2}$), or those with a BMI over 35 $kg \cdot m^{-2}$ and an obesity-related medical condition.

Current drug and lifestyle treatments for obesity can be expected to produce weight loss of about 10–15%, which is often enough to ameliorate obesity-related metabolic disorders and their accompanying clinical manifestations. Bariatric surgery produces an average weight loss of 25–30%. The management of obesity should be carried out by a multidisciplinary team who can advise on lifestyle and other treatment options.

SELF-ASSESSMENT

True/false questions

1. The posterior pituitary is the main central nervous system site of appetite control.
2. Ghrelin is an orexigenic hormone.
3. Satiety signals include insulin and leptin.
4. Orlistat acts centrally to inhibit release of orexigenic neurotransmitters.
5. Vitamin D deficiency can occur with orlistat treatment.
6. Methylcellulose should be taken with water.
7. Drug treatment for obesity should be restricted to individuals with a body mass index (BMI) of more than 30 kg·m⁻².
8. Weight loss is usually sustained after 12 months of orlistat treatment.

True/false answers

1. **False.** The hypothalamus and higher brain centres are most important in regulating food intake.
2. **True.** Ghrelin is produced by the gut pre-prandially and has an orexigenic (appetite-stimulating) action on the hypothalamus.
3. **True.** Satiety signals to the hypothalamus include insulin (from the pancreas), leptin (from fat stores) and gut peptides such as cholecystokinin, oxyntomodulin and peptide YY_{3-36}.
4. **False.** Orlistat reduces fat absorption in the gut by inhibiting pancreatic lipase.
5. **True.** People taking orlistat may unduly restrict their fat intake to avoid steatorrhoea, leading to reduced absorption of fat-soluble vitamin D.
6. **True.** Methylcellulose produces satiety by swelling rapidly when hydrated and should be taken with water.
7. **True.** Drug treatment should be restricted to obese people with BMI over 30 kg·m⁻² (or >28 kg·m⁻² in those with Type 2 diabetes, hypertension or hypercholesterolaemia).
8. **False.** Weight loss with orlistat often reverses gradually after stopping the drug; lifestyle measures including diet and exercise are important in long-term weight control.

FURTHER READING

Eckel RH (2008) Non-surgical management of obesity. *N Engl J Med* 358, 1941–1950

Haslam DW, James WPT (2005) Obesity. *Lancet* 366, 1197–1209

Mingfang L, Cheung BMY (2009) Pharmacotherapy for obesity. *Br J Clin Pharmacol* 68, 804–810

Padwal RS, Majumdar SR (2007) Drug treatments for obesity: orlistat, sibutramine, and rimonabant. *Lancet* 369, 71–77

Sargent BJ, Moore NA (2009) New central targets for the treatmengt of obesity. *Br J Clin Pharmacol* 68, 852–860

Compendium: drugs used in obesity

Drug	Kinetics (half-life)	Comments
Methylcellulose	Not absorbed	Bulk-forming agent taken before meals to produce satiety; taken with water to avoid oesophageal obstruction; little evidence of efficacy in obesity; also used as laxative (Ch. 35)
Orlistat	Negligible absorption (about 1%) and low systemic exposure in clinical use	Pancreatic lipase inhibitor; acts within intestine; taken orally before, during or immediately after a meal

8

The immune system

38 The immune response and immunosuppressant drugs

BIOLOGICAL BASIS OF THE IMMUNE RESPONSE

The immune system is composed of innate (natural) and adaptive components, which protect the host against a wide variety of pathogens and also tumour cells. The adaptive system is further divided into humoral and cell-mediated immunity. Overall the immune system has the ability to distinguish between self and non-self proteins and to protect the host (self) against non-self infectious and other pathogenic agents.

INNATE IMMUNITY

The term *innate immunity* (sometimes called *natural immunity*) was used because it is an inherited system and is part of our genetic make-up. It is made up of several generally *non-specific* protective mechanisms, some of which do not involve the immune system. All foreign pathogens are recognised approximately equally by pattern-recognition receptors on cells involved in the innate immune system. Pattern-recognition receptors identify pathogenic 'groups' such as bacterial lipopolysaccharides and bacterial DNA rather than responding to individual antigens. The innate immune system has an important role in processing foreign pathogens and triggering the highly selective adaptive system described below.

The innate immune system incorporates the following processes:

- physicochemical barriers, e.g. intact skin and mucous membrane, low stomach pH, antibacterial agents (lysozyme) in skin and tear secretions,
- macrophages and dendritic cells, particularly in lungs, liver, lymph nodes and spleen, phagocytose pathogenic material and produce antigen fragments (short peptides of approximately 8–25 amino acids) from the pathogenic material, which they then display on their surfaces. The cells are then described as antigen-presenting cells (APCs) and are necessary for the presentation of the antigen to T-lymphocytes and the triggering of the adaptive immune system (see below),
- attraction of immune cells to sites of inflammation by substances released from cells such as cytokines,
- phagocytosis of bacteria and parasites by granulocytes, including neutrophils, monocytes and macrophages,
- actions of natural killer cells (large granular lymphocytes),
- binding of antigens to IgE antibody on mast cells and basophils and the subsequent release of inflammatory mediators from the cell,
- fever,
- complement activation.

The innate immune system may be an adequate defence to deal with many pathogens but, unlike adaptive immunity, long-term specific immune protection following initial exposure to a pathogen does not occur.

ADAPTIVE IMMUNITY

Adaptive immunity is superimposed upon the innate mechanisms. It differs from innate immunity in that it is slower to respond, offers long-term specific protection and has exquisite specificity in recognising individual non-self molecules. Adaptive immunity has two basic complementary and interacting mechanisms: *cell-mediated immunity* and *humoral immunity* (Figs 38.1 and 38.2).

Essential components of the adaptive system are the two populations of lymphocytes:

- *T-lymphocytes* are produced in the bone marrow and migrate to the thymus, where they mature, express receptors for antigens and interact with immunogenic self peptides. T-cells are selected in the thymus for low or high avidity for self peptides, and those showing high avidity are destroyed. The surviving T-cells retain the potential to cross-react with multiple foreign non-self antigens but not self molecules.
- *B-lymphocytes* make up about 10% of the lymphocyte population and mature in the bone marrow.

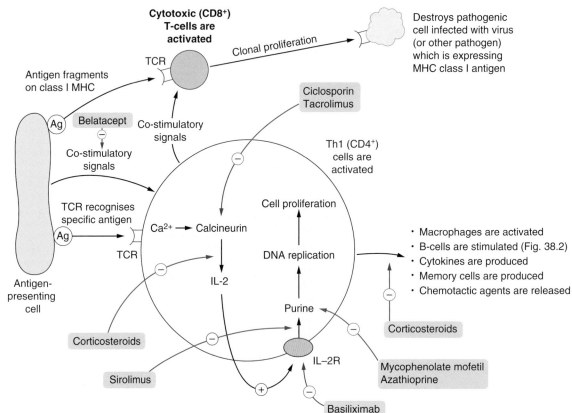

Fig. 38.1 **Aspects of cell-mediated immunity.** This shows in simplified form some steps in T-cell activation following antigen presentation to the T-cell receptor (TCR). Pathogenic antigens are presented by antigen-presenting cells to the uncommitted CD4$^+$ lymphocyte which carries the specific receptor to the antigen, in association with major histocompatibility complex (MHC) class I and co-stimulatory molecules. Under the influence of interleukin-2 (IL-2), Th1 cells undergo clonal proliferation and play a variety of roles in cell-mediated immunity, including activation of macrophages and other cells. Antigens can also be presented to CD8$^+$ lymphocytes, which mature into cytotoxic T-cells. Drugs used as immunosuppressants (red arrows) act at the sites shown. Corticosteroids act at many sites (see also Fig. 38.2 and Ch. 44). Ag, antigen; IL-2R, interleukin-2 receptor; Th, T-helper cell.

T-cells and B-cells are coated with vast numbers of proteins which act as receptors or as ligands for other receptors. These proteins can be defined by antibody typing (immunophenotyping) and are given cluster of differentiation (CD) numbers such as CD4, CD8, etc. When T-cells leave the thymus they are considered naïve or uncommitted since they have not yet been exposed to the non-self antigens. At this stage, naïve T-cells consist of two major populations, known as helper (Th; CD4$^+$) and cytotoxic or killer (Tc; CD8$^+$) T-cells (Fig. 38.1). Immunogenic peptides are presented to T-cells within the cleft of major histocompatibility complex (MHC) class II molecules on the surface of APCs from the innate immune system. The CD4$^+$ (Th) cells have surface receptors with a high affinity for class II MHC which binds antigenic peptides on APCs. The CD8$^+$ (Tc) cells have an affinity for class I MHC, which displays specific antigens on the surface of tumour cells or infected host cells.

The CD4$^+$ Th-cell is activated if its receptors recognise and bind avidly to an antigen, but only if the antigen is processed and presented on an APC. This triggers a series of complex activation pathways which prepare the Th-cell

for its immune role. Acivated Th-cells secrete the T-cell growth factor interleukin-2 (IL-2), which acts in an autocrine fashion on the Th-cells and causes them to proliferate. The Th-cells are then committed to become a type 1 Th-cell (Th1) or a type 2 Th-cell (Th2). The pattern of differentiation may be determined by the type of antigen or possibly the concentration of antigen presented to the Th-cell. Differentiated Th-cells orchestrate the immune response by secretion of specific cytokines (Figs 38.1 and 38.2). Th1-cells interact with macrophages to enhance their phagocytic activity and stimulate the proliferation of cytotoxic Tc-cells. Th2-cells stimulate B-cells to grow and divide, and activate humoral immune responses. The details of these responses are not well understood, and the existence of other Th-cell populations (such as Th3 and Th17) adds to the complexity of this cell family. The activities of Th-cells and APCs are modulated by regulatory T-cells (Treg).

Co-stimulatory signals involving cell surface CD proteins are important processes in immune cell function. For example, CD40 protein on APCs interacts with Th-cell proteins and has a co-stimulatory role in APC activation. The

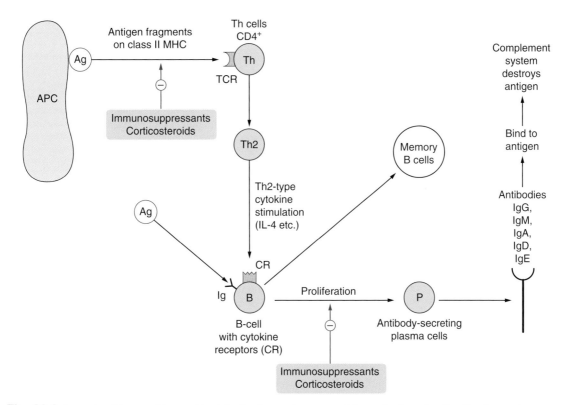

Fig. 38.2 Aspects of humoral immunity. Adaptive immunity can result in production of antibodies (humoral response) or a cell-mediated response (Fig. 38.1). Antigens on bacteria or bacterial toxins bind to immunoglobulins on B cells. Before proliferation and antibody production can occur, the B-cell also has to be stimulated by activated T-cell cytokine production, usually of the Th2 type. Antigen fragments can be presented with major histocompatibility complex (MHC) class II molecules to T-cells via a T-cell receptor (TCR) that recognises the antigen. T-cells undergo clonal proliferation and produce cytokines that stimulate B-cells to produce humoral antibodies (IgG, IgM, IgA, IgD and IgE). In atopic individuals, the T-cells are tipped towards the Th2 type and produce interleukins IL-4, IL-5, IL-10 and transforming growth factor β (TGFβ), which induce the B-cells to produce IgE. Ag, antigen; APC, antigen-presenting cell; CR, cytokine receptor; P, plasma cell; Th, T-helper cell.

CD80 and CD86 proteins on APCs interact with CD28 proteins on Th- and Tc-cells to co-activate them together with Th-cell cytokines. The expression of CD20 protein on B-cells enables an optimum immune response against T-cell-independent antigens (antigens that elicit a full humoral immune response without participation of T-cell cytokines).

Immature B-cells can bind antigen with the cooperation of T-cells, but on subsequent exposure antigen binds directly to immunoglobulins on the B-cell (Fig. 38.2)

Cell-mediated immunity

Cell-mediated immunity is largely T-cell-driven, utilising Th1 (CD4⁺) and cytotoxic T-cell (CD8⁺) subtypes, and is involved in responses to viral infection, graft rejection, chronic inflammation and tumour immunity. Figure 38.1 shows schematically the basic processes occurring in cell-mediated immunity. T-cells that possess the receptor to the antigen of the invasive pathogen that is presented on APCs are stimulated to express IL-2 and the IL-2 receptor. For clarity, the many co-stimulatory processes that are described in the text above are not shown in the figure.

Stimulation of the IL-2 receptor induces the Th-cell to:

- activate macrophages to phagocytose the pathogen,
- stimulate cytotoxic T-cells to proliferate,
- stimulate B-cells to proliferate,
- attract macrophages and neutrophils to the site,
- produce memory B-cells that respond rapidly to the pathogen on future exposure.

Cytotoxic T-cells that recognise the foreign antigen presented on MHC type I on APCs are activated to proliferate and attack pathogens expressing the antigen. When cytotoxic cells bind to an antigen on a pathogenic cell they release a variety of proteases or lysins to destroy the cell.

Humoral immunity

Figure 38.2 illustrates the basic processes in humoral immunity. The foreign antigen is recognised by immunoglobulin (Ig) molecules or specific receptors to that antigen on the surface of a specific clone of B-cells. The presence of nearby Th2-cells that have been activated to secrete IL-5 and IL-10 is required for initial antigen recognition by B-cells. The secreted interleukins cause B-cell clonal proliferation, and convert B-cells into active plasma cells that can secrete antibodies of the IgG, IgM, IgA, IgD and IgE classes which bind to and destroy pathogenic antigens.

On encountering an antigen, the primary immune response consists of IgM, replaced later by IgG. B-cells that are primed to produce specific antibodies survive as memory B-cells. On a further encounter with the antigen, the secondary immune response occurs more rapidly and consists of large amounts of IgG produced by plasma cells derived from reactivation of memory B-cells.

UNWANTED IMMUNE REACTIONS

The processes of inflammation and immunity described above are essential to protect the host against pathogens and other damage, but excessive, inappropriately prolonged or misdirected immune responses can cause disease, including hypersensitivity reactions, graft rejection and autoimmune diseases.

It is not always easy to decide whether predominantly Th1- or Th2-mediated immune responses are involved in a particular disease; in part this is due to the fact that Th2 cytokines can inhibit Th1-cell functions. Th1-mediated immune responses are significantly involved in rheumatoid arthritis (Ch. 30) and in the formation of atheroma (Ch. 48). Th2-mediated responses are important in mild to moderate asthma but with increasing participation of Th1-mediated responses in severe asthma (Ch. 12).

Hypersensitivity reactions

Hypersensitivity reactions were classified by Gell and Coombs in the late 1950s.

Type 1 (acute, immediate)

This category includes hay fever and acute asthma. IgE molecules on the surface of mast cells and basophils are crosslinked by harmless antigens (allergens such as pollens or house dust mites), leading to the synthesis and/or release of inflammatory mediators. These include cysteinyl-leukotrienes, prostaglandins, histamine, platelet-activating factor, proteases and cytokines.

Type 2 (cytotoxic)

Cell surface antigens, including microbial proteins and drug molecules haptenised onto cell surfaces, are recognised and bound by IgG and IgM antibodies (opsonisation), leading to activation of complement (classic pathway) and cytolysis of the target cell. Examples include destruction of red cells after incompatible blood transfusion, and haemolytic anaemia caused by binding of some drugs to host cells (see Ch. 53).

Type 3 (complex-mediated)

Soluble antigens react with excess circulating antibodies to form complexes that precipitate in small blood vessels, causing vasculitis and organ damage. The various forms of extrinsic allergic alveolitis, caused by exposure to animal or vegetable dusts, are systemic type 3 reactions, while the Arthus reaction is a local response to an injected antigen (e.g. non-human insulins).

Type 4 (cell-mediated, delayed-type hypersensitivity)

Inappropriate regulation of cell-mediated immunity may cause damaging chronic inflammation, leading to fibrosis and granuloma formation. Cell-mediated immunity misdirected against harmless foreign proteins (allergens) can lead to chronic allergic inflammation (such as occurs in eczema), or cause contact sensitivity in the skin to haptenising metals and chemicals. In allergy, Th2-cells secrete cytokines, including IL-4, IL-5 and IL-13, which promote eosinophilic inflammation and overproduction of IgE by B-cells.

Transplant rejection

In blood transfusion, rejection usually occurs because non-self antigens on the transfused red blood cells (ABO system) trigger a type 2 hypersensitivity reaction in the recipient. In immunodeficient people, transfused T-cells react against recipient antigens (graft-versus-host reactions).

For organ transplants, hyperacute rejection can occur if there is ABO incompatibility, or host-versus-graft reactions can arise later with foreign MHC molecules (human leucocyte antigens, HLA). The latter can be reduced by HLA tissue typing to increase the chance of selecting a graft that is compatible with the host tissues. This will reduce the rate of tissue destruction but not prevent chronic rejection. The immune response and its place in the rejection of a transplanted organ are complex. The antigens on the graft are recognised as foreign, and the cascaded responses outlined in Figures 38.1 and 38.2 occur, with increased production of B-cells, cytotoxic T-cells and monocyte/macrophages. Graft destruction occurs from antibody production against the graft, lysis of graft cells and delayed hypersensitivity responses. Rejection can be immediate (days), acute (weeks) or chronic (years).

Autoimmunity

Normally the immune system is tolerant of self antigens. T-cells in the thymus that express receptors with high avidity for self peptides are normally destroyed in a process known as negative selection (see above). If this self-tolerance breaks down, autoimmune disorders result. Numerous mechanisms can trigger autoimmune diseases, including viral infection of host cells, binding of drug molecules to host cells (e.g. penicillin), sharing of antigens between host cells and microbes and sequestration of antigens liberated by cell damage. Examples of autoimmune disease include haemolytic anaemia, type 1 diabetes mellitus, Addison's disease, rheumatoid arthritis, myasthenia gravis, systemic lupus erythematosus and Graves' disease.

IMMUNOSUPPRESSANT DRUGS

The immune system presents a large number of potential molecular targets for therapeutic intervention. Drugs currently used to suppress the immune response tend to be non-specific immunosuppressants with a range of unwanted effects. Immunosuppressant drugs are widely used in many diseases; examples include rheumatoid arthritis, psoriasis and inflammatory bowel disease. Their benefit is achieved both through modulation of the immune system and, in some cases, through their anti-inflammatory properties. Drug such as methotrexate and cyclophosphamide which are used for their cytotoxic actions in cancer chemotherapy (Ch. 52), are also used for their immunosuppressant properties in various disease states. Methotrexate and cyclophosphamide have immunosuppressant properties at doses much lower than those required to treat malignancy (Ch. 52). Corticosteroids (e.g. dexamethasone and prednisone; Ch. 44) are highly effective anti-inflammatory drugs that can be used systemically to suppress type 4 hypersensitivity reactions, autoimmune diseases and graft rejection. They are also used topically for inflammatory skin disease (Ch. 49), inflammatory bowel disease (Ch. 34) and allergic rhinitis (Ch. 39), and by inhalation for asthma (e.g. beclometasone, fluticasone; Ch. 12).

Co-stimulatory molecules on immune cells have recently been targeted in the development of drugs for the treatment of autoimmune disease: belatacept is an antibody that binds to CD80 and CD86 proteins on APCs and rituximab is an antibody that binds to CD20 on B-cells, thus modulating the destructive immune responsiveness against self molecules in disease (Ch. 30, Fig. 30.1).

As an alternative to immunosuppression, inflammatory mediators released during immune reactions can be blocked by antagonists at their receptors on target cells, or by inhibiting their synthesis. This is a useful strategy for management of allergic disorders and some inflammatory conditions. Anti-mediator drugs include histamine H_1 receptor antagonists (antihistamines), cysteinyl-leukotriene receptor antagonists (LTRAs) and cyclo-oxygenase inhibitors (non-steroidal anti-inflammatory drugs, NSAIDs). Antihistamines (e.g. loratadine and cetirizine) are used in the control of hay fever and other allergic disorders (Ch. 39), while oral LTRAs (e.g. montelukast and zafirlukast) are used in asthma (Ch. 12). Oral NSAIDs block the synthesis of prostaglandins and are used in inflammatory soft-tissue disorders and arthritis (Chs 29 and 30).

CALCINEURIN INHIBITORS

Examples

ciclosporin, tacrolimus

Ciclosporin

Mechanism of action

Ciclosporin is a fungal cyclic peptide which inhibits T-cell division. It binds in the cell cytoplasm to the protein cyclophilin to form a complex that inhibits calcineurin. Calcineurin is a calmodulin-/Ca^{2+}-dependent phosphatase which is a key component in T-cell activation (Fig. 38.1). Activated calcineurin is produced in response to an antigenic signal at T-cell receptors and dephosphorylates nuclear factor of activation in T-cells (NFAT). NFAT then enters the cell nucleus and binds to a promoter region of the IL-2 gene. IL-2 stimulates T-cell division. By inhibiting calcineurin, ciclosporin prevents dephosphorylation of NFAT, which remains in the cytoplasm. This inhibits IL-2 production, and the T-cell division cycle is arrested between G_0 and G_1.

Ciclosporin also inhibits various cellular mitogen-activated protein kinases (such as c-Jun N-terminal kinase and p38 kinases) which are triggered by inflammatory cytokines such as tumour necrosis factor α (TNFα) and IL-1. These protein kinases phosphorylate transcription factors involved in upregulation of *c-Fos*-mediated gene transcription, a process that is involved in activation of many cell types in response to inflammation.

Ciclosporin also stimulates the production of transforming growth factor β (TGFβ), possibly by releasing an inhibitory effect of calcineurin on TGFβ gene transcription. This may be responsible for some of the nephrotoxicity that occurs with the drug.

Pharmacokinetics

Oral absorption of ciclosporin is variable and incomplete, requiring initial dispersion by bile salts. To overcome this, a microemulsion formulation is used which disperses when it comes into contact with water in the gut so that absorption is independent of bile production. However, different formulations have varying absorption characteristics and switching between formulations should be avoided. Ciclosporin can also be given by intravenous infusion. Ciclosporin selectively concentrates in some tissues, including liver, kidney, several endocrine glands, lymph nodes, spleen and bone marrow. It is extensively metabolised in the liver by the CYP3A4 isoenzyme and has a long half-life (27 h). Monitoring of trough plasma drug concentration has traditionally been used to guide dosage for optimal effectiveness and to minimise toxicity. However, recent evidence suggests that a blood concentration 2 h post-dose may be a better guide to kidney graft survival and minimising toxicity.

Unwanted effects

- Nephrotoxicity almost always occurs, with a dose-dependent increase in serum creatinine in the first few weeks. The acute effect is due to intrarenal vasoconstriction that may persist and contribute to the less common long-term sequelae, which include interstitial fibrosis and tubular atrophy. Induction of TGFβ may be a contributory factor in the nephrotoxic effects. The decline in renal glomerular function is usually reversible, but permanent renal impairment can result.
- Hypertension, often associated with fluid retention, occurs in up to 50% of people, and especially after heart transplantation. It usually responds to standard antihypertensive drug treatment.
- Hepatic dysfunction.
- Tremor, headache, paraesthesia, fatigue, myalgia.
- Hypertrichosis (excessive hair growth) and gum hypertrophy are common.
- Gastrointestinal disturbances, including anorexia, nausea and vomiting, abdominal pain.
- Hyperlipidaemia, hyperuricaemia, hypomagnesaemia, hypokalaemia.

■ Drug interactions can be dangerous and caution should be taken when ciclosporin is used with other nephrotoxic drugs, such as aminoglycoside antimicrobials and amphotericin (Ch. 51) or NSAIDs (Ch. 29). Drugs that induce hepatic CYP3A4, such as phenytoin and carbamazepine, can reduce the plasma concentrations of ciclosporin to sub-therapeutic levels. Drugs that inhibit cytochrome P450, such as erythromycin and ketoconazole (Ch. 51), can increase ciclosporin plasma concentration and provoke toxicity.

Tacrolimus

Mechanism of action and effects

Tacrolimus inhibits calcineurin, and therefore T-cell proliferation, by arresting the cell cycle between G_0 and G_1 in a similar manner to ciclosporin. After binding to a receptor protein called FK-binding protein-12, the complex binds to calcineurin and inhibits Ca^{2+}-dependent calcineurin activation. Tacrolimus also inhibits c-Jun N-terminal kinase and p38 kinases. Unlike ciclosporin, tacrolimus does not stimulate production of TGFβ.

Pharmacokinetics

Tacrolimus is more water soluble than ciclosporin and undergoes more predictable, though poor, absorption from the gut. It is metabolised by the liver and has a highly variable half-life (4–41 h). Monitoring of the trough blood concentration of tacrolimus is essential for appropriate dose adjustment, especially early in treatment.

Unwanted effects

These are similar to those of ciclosporin except that tacrolimus causes less hypertension, hirsutism and gum hyperplasia. Effects that are more common with tacrolimus include:

■ pleural and pericardial effusions,
■ cardiomyopathy in children, who should be monitored by echocardiography.

MAMMALIAN TARGET OF RAPAMYCIN INHIBITORS

sirolimus

Mechanism of action and effects

Sirolimus (previously known as rapamycin) is a natural fungal fermentation product that inhibits T-cell proliferation by arresting the cell between the G_1 and S phases. It binds to intracellular FK-binding protein-12, and the complex inhibits the action of mammalian target of rapamycin (mTOR), a cytoplasmic kinase. mTOR is a key step in a series of intracellular Ca^{2+}-independent events that transduce signals from the cell surface IL-2 receptor and other growth factor receptors to cell-cycle regulators that promote DNA and protein synthesis and mitogenesis. The action of

sirolimus therefore differs from that of tacrolimus, despite binding to the same intracellular receptor.

Pharmacokinetics

Sirolimus is rapidly absorbed from the gut and the absorption is modulated by P-glycoproteins. It is metabolised by intestinal and hepatic cytochrome P450 and has a very long half-life (60 h).

Unwanted effects

■ Oedema, ascites, tachycardia, hypertension.
■ Abdominal pain, nausea, diarrhoea, stomatitis.
■ Anaemia, thrombocytopenia, neutropenia.
■ Hyperlipidaemia, hypokalaemia, hypophosphataemia.
■ Arthralgia, osteonecrosis.
■ Lymphocele (a complication of renal transplantation that is more common if sirolimus is used; it can cause ureteric compression).
■ Rash.
■ Drug interactions: rifampicin reduces plasma sirolimus concentrations by induction of CYP3A4; the antifungal agents itraconazole and ketoconazole increase plasma concentrations of sirolimus by enzyme inhibition.

ANTIPROLIFERATIVE AGENTS

Examples

azathioprine, cyclophosphamide, mycophenolate mofetil

Azathioprine

Mechanism of action

Azathioprine is widely used for immunosuppression. Most of the effects result from cleavage to 6-mercaptopurine in the intestine and liver and then to the active derivative thioinosinic acid, a purine analogue (Ch. 52). The antimetabolite action interferes with purine biosynthesis, thus impairing DNA synthesis in the S-phase of the cell cycle (Figs 52.1 and 52.2), and particularly affects fast-growing cells such as lymphocytes. The drug also blocks CD28 co-stimulation of T-cells. Both cell- and antibody-mediated immune reactions are suppressed (Figs 38.1 and 38.2), with impaired synthesis of immunoglobulins by B-cells, and inhibition of the infiltration and survival of mononuclear cells in inflamed tissue.

Pharmacokinetics

Oral absorption is almost complete. The half-lives of azathioprine and its 6-mercaptopurine metabolite are short (3–5 h). Azathioprine can be given by intravenous injection, but the solution is alkaline and very irritant.

Unwanted effects

■ Dose-dependent bone marrow suppression, especially leucopenia and thrombocytopenia. Regular monitoring of the full blood count (at least every 3 months) is essential.

- Hypersensitivity reactions, with malaise, dizziness, vomiting, diarrhoea, fever, myalgia, arthralgia, rash and hypotension. The drug should be stopped immediately if these arise.
- Increased susceptibility to infection, often with 'opportunistic' organisms.
- Alopecia.
- There is a small risk of carcinogenicity, especially lymphomas.
- Drug interactions: the most important interaction is with allopurinol (Ch. 31). Allopurinol inhibits xanthine oxidase, which is involved in the catabolism of 6-mercaptopurine, and the dose of azathioprine should be reduced by 75% if the drugs are used together.

Cyclophosphamide

Cyclophosphamide is an alkylating drug that is less commonly used as an immunosuppressant. It is discussed in detail in Ch. 52.

Mycophenolate mofetil and mycophenolic acid

Mechanism of action and effects

Mycophenolate mofetil is a prodrug of mycophenolic acid, which reduces purine synthesis by reversible non-competitive inhibition of inosine monophosphate (IMP) dehydrogenase and guanylyl synthase. These enzymes are involved in the conversion of IMP to xanthosine monophosphate, and then to the precursor of guanosine triphosphate that is involved in RNA, DNA and protein synthesis. Inhibition of these enzymes depletes the cell of guanine nucleotides and inhibits cellular DNA synthesis. T-cells, B-cells and monocytes rely on *de novo* purine nucleotide synthesis, unlike neutrophils and other cells, which can use preformed guanine released from the breakdown of pre-formed nucleic acids (the salvage pathway). Mycophenolate therefore is a selective inhibitor of lymphocyte function.

A further action of mycophenolate mofetil is inhibition of smooth muscle proliferation in arterial walls, which may also help to reduce graft rejection that arises from obliterative arteriopathy.

Pharmacokinetics

Mycophenolate mofetil is a prodrug ester which is almost completely absorbed from the gut and hydrolysed rapidly to mycophenolic acid. Elimination of mycophenolic acid is via hepatic metabolism and it has a long half-life (18 h) due to enterohepatic circulation. Mycophenolate mofetil and mycophenolic acid can also be given by intravenous infusion.

Unwanted effects

- Gastrointestinal upset is very common, including nausea, vomiting, diarrhoea, abdominal cramps and, occasionally, hepatitis or pancreatitis. Tolerance to the gastrointestinal symptoms often occurs.
- Hypertension, oedema, tachycardia, chest pain.
- Dyspnoea, cough.
- Dizziness, insomnia, headache, tremor, seizures.

- Bone marrow suppression resulting in leucopenia, thrombocytopenia and anaemia.
- Opportunistic infections may be increased, especially with cytomegalovirus, Herpes simplex, *Aspergillus* and *Candida*, as well as bacterial urinary tract infection and pneumonia.
- Lymphoproliferative disease and skin cancer.

FOLIC ACID ANTAGONIST

Example

methotrexate

Mechanism of action and uses

Methotrexate inhibits dihydrofolate reductase. This blocks purine and thymidylate synthesis and inhibits the synthesis of DNA, RNA and protein. It is specific for the S-phase of cell division and slows G_1- to S-phase (see Ch. 52). However, in inflammatory disease methotrexate may have a different action by inhibiting enzymes involved in purine metabolism, leading to accumulation of adenosine and its release from cells. Adenosine acts on specific cell surface receptors and suppresses the expression of adhesion molecules on T-cells and neutrophils, inhibiting their accumulation in inflamed tissues, and also reduces cytokine release from a variety of inflammatory cells.

Methotrexate is used by intermittent administration once a week in many conditions such as inflammatory joint disease, Crohn's disease and psoriasis (Chs 30, 34 and 49).

Pharmacokinetics

Methotrexate is well absorbed from the gut but can also be given intravenously, intramuscularly or subcutaneously. It is eliminated by renal excretion, but a small amount may be retained intracellularly for longer periods bound to dihydrofolate reductase and as polyglutamate conjugates.

Unwanted effects

- Toxicity to normal rapidly dividing tissues (especially the bone marrow).
- Hepatotoxicity can follow chronic therapy (as in psoriasis).

Toxicity is increased in the presence of reduced renal excretion and methotrexate should be avoided if there is significant renal impairment. Folic acid is frequently taken after methotrexate to reduce mucositis and myelosuppression. NSAIDs such as aspirin can reduce the renal excretion of methotrexate and increase its toxicity.

INTERLEUKIN-2 RECEPTOR ANTIBODIES

Examples

basiliximab

Basiliximab is a chimaeric monoclonal antibody with murine sequences in the hypervariable region. It binds to the IL-2 receptor on activated T-cells and prevents T-cell proliferation. It is used for initial induction therapy prior to transplantation or for treatment of acute transplant rejection.

Pharmacokinetics

Basiliximab is given by intravenous infusion immediately before and again 4 days after surgery. It has a very long half-life of over 1 week.

Unwanted effects

Hypersensitivity reactions occur rarely.

SELECTIVE CO-STIMULATION BLOCKER

belatacept

Belatacept is a fusion protein that binds to CD80 and CD86 molecules on APCs and blocks their co-stimulatory action with CD28 on T-cell activation. It is used to prevent rejection in adults undergoing renal transplantation who are seropositive for the Ebstein–Barr virus.

Pharmacokinetics

Belatacept is given by intravenous infusion and has a very long half-life (8–10 days).

Unwanted effects

- Hypersensitivity reactions occur rarely.
- lymphoproliferative disorder, especially in those with no prior exposure to Ebstein-Barr virus.

IMMUNOSUPPRESSION IN ORGAN TRANSPLANTATION

Immunosuppressant drugs block rejection at the steps of T-cell activation, T-cell proliferation and cytokine production (Figs 38.1 and 38.2). A major direction of current research is to find regimens that will induce immune tolerance and allow eventual withdrawal of immunosuppressant drugs.

Effective immunosuppression has improved the early survival of kidney, liver, heart, heart–lung, intestinal and haematopoietic stem cell transplants. However, suppression of acute rejection is more effective than prevention of chronic rejection, which responds poorly to immunosuppressant therapy. Regimens for immunosuppression vary among transplant units and according to the immunogenicity of the transplanted tissue. Combination therapy with a corticosteroid, calcineurin inhibitor and an antiproliferative agent is commonly used.

For kidney transplantation, induction therapy is given at the time of transplantation with either anti-CD3, which is inhibits T-cell activation in the thymus (anti-thymocyte immunoglobulin), or an IL-2 receptor antibody (basiliximab) to reduce initial acute rejection. Immunosuppression is then maintained with oral agents such as the corticosteroid prednisolone (Ch. 44) together with ciclosporin or tacrolimus, or with sirolimus or mycophenolate mofetil if the calcineurin inhibitors are poorly tolerated. Some units add azathioprine to this regimen. With such regimens, 90% of cadaveric kidney grafts will survive beyond 1 year. Only half of those that fail are lost due to rejection, and the rest from thrombosis of the graft blood supply. Progressive graft loss continues after the first year, with only 67% of grafts from 'brain death donors' surviving at 10 years. Grafts from living donors have better survival rates of 96% at 1 year and 78% at 10 years. Most of the late graft losses are as a result of chronic vascular rejection. If this occurs, increasing the dosages of the primary immunosuppressant drugs may help; however, there is continuing uncertainty about whether chronic rejection reflects nephrotoxicity from long-term use of calcineurin inhibitors or inadequate immunosuppression. It is possible that drugs such as sirolimus or mycophenolate mofetil may reduce the incidence of chronic rejection, but there are few long-term data on outcome. Late acute rejection is a less common problem. It can sometimes be overcome by high-dose corticosteroid or the use of polyclonal antilymphocytic globulin or monoclonal antilymphocytic antibody (although the use of these is associated with an increased risk of opportunistic infection and long-term malignancy). Tacrolimus or mycophenolate mofetil can also be used successfully as a rescue treatment during late episodes of acute rejection.

In contrast to renal transplants, pancreatic transplants are more immunogenic and quadruple immunosuppressant regimens are widely used. Induction treatment with antilymphocytic globulin is then followed by ciclosporin, azathioprine and a corticosteroid. Mycophenolate mofetil is sometimes substituted for azathioprine, or tacrolimus for ciclosporin. Despite these treatments, 5-year prancreatic graft survival is only about 60% and the risk of post-transplant infection is high.

Triple immunosuppressant therapy is used for heart (50% 10-year survival), heart–lung (30% 10-year survival), liver (70% 10-year survival) and intestinal (40–50% 3-year survival) transplants, often with initial use of an IL-2 receptor antibody (basiliximab). In addition to prednisolone, tacrolimus is often included in these regimens in place of ciclosporin. Mycophenolate mofetil as an alternative may reduce acute rejection rates but there is less evidence for an impact on chronic rejection.

With haematopoietic stem cell transplantation, graft-versus-host disease (GVHD) is the major barrier. This usually begins at least 3 months after the transplant and has three phases. The first phase involves damage to intestinal mucosa and the liver, with activation of host cells and release of inflammatory cytokines. These cytokines upregulate MHC proteins on the host cells, which are then recognised by the donor T-cells. The second phase involves activation and proliferation of donor T-cells, and the third phase includes tissue destruction by monocytes primed by inflammatory cytokines and lipopolysaccharide from T-cells and damaged intestinal mucosa. GVHD can be prevented by inhibition of phase 1, using a calcineurin inhibitor such as ciclosporin or tacrolimus, or possibly mycophenolate mofetil. Acute GVHD can be treated by a corticosteroid with ciclosporin.

IMMUNOSUPPRESSION IN OTHER DISORDERS

Immunosuppressant therapy is used for several diseases in which autoimmunity may contribute to the pathogenesis. These include many connective tissue diseases such as vasculitis and systemic lupus erythematosus, inflammatory arthritis, polymyalgia rheumatic, certain types of glomerulonephritis, autoimmune hepatitis, psoriasis, inflammatory bowel disease and some haematological disorders. Immunosuppressant drugs may be given alone or in combination. Those most widely used include corticosteroids, azathioprine, methotrexate and cyclophosphamide. Ciclosporin, tacrolimus and mycophenolate mofetil have also been used in disorders such as asthma, inflammatory bowel disease and psoriasis, with some success.

SELF-ASSESSMENT

True/false questions

1. Immunosuppression requires higher doses of methotrexate than used for cancer chemotherapy.
2. Ciclosporin and tacrolimus reduce interleukin (IL)-2 gene transcription in lymphocytes.
3. Ciclosporin causes bone marrow suppression.
4. Careful assessment of renal function is required with ciclosporin administration.
5. Azathioprine suppresses antibody-mediated immune responses.
6. Azathioprine interacts with allopurinol.
7. Sirolimus and tacrolimus share a common mechanism of action.
8. Corticosteroids have a narrow spectrum of immunosuppressant activity.
9. Mycophenolate is an alternative to azathioprine for preventing acute rejection.
10. Basiliximab is an antibody that blocks the IL-2 receptor.

Case-based questions

A 35-year-old woman was about to receive her second kidney transplant. The previous transplant had lasted 5 years but, despite immunosuppression with prednisolone and ciclosporin, it was eventually rejected.

A. How might the chances of acute rejection of the second transplant be reduced?

B. What could be the long-term risks of combination chemotherapy with corticosteroids, tacrolimus and azathioprine?

True/false answers

1. **False.** Immunosuppressant doses of drugs such as methotrexate, cyclophosphamide and azathioprine are lower than those used for cancer chemotherapy.
2. **True.** These calcineurin inhibitors reduce the transcriptional effects of NFAT on IL-2; the loss of IL-2 suppresses T-cell maturation and proliferation.
3. **False.** The calcineurin inhibitors are selective suppressors of lymphocyte proliferation.
4. **True.** Ciclosporin is nephrotoxic and renal monitoring is necessary.
5. **True.** Azathioprine has a cytotoxic action by inhibiting purine metabolism and the proliferation of lymphocytes and other immunocompetent cells is inhibited.
6. **True.** Allopurinol inhibits xanthine oxidase, which is involved in deactivating metabolites of azathioprine; doses of azathioprine should be reduced when given with allopurinol.
7. **False.** Sirolimus (rapamycin) binds to FK-binding protein-12, but the complex inhibits mammalian target of rapamycin (mTOR), a protein kinase involved in IL-2 signalling, unlike the calcineurin inhibitors that reduce IL-2 gene transcription.
8. **False.** Corticosteroids modulate the transcription of hundreds of immune and inflammatory genes encoding cytokines, mediators, adhesion molecules and apoptotic proteins.
9. **True.** Mycophenolate may have fewer toxic effects than azathioprine and is increasingly used in preventing acute rejection, but its place in preventing chronic rejection is less clear.
10. **True.** Basiliximab is a chimaeric monoclonal antibody that blocks the IL-2 receptor.

Case-based answers

A. Basiliximab given before and 4 days after renal transplant surgery reduces acute rejection by 35%. This is maintained typically with oral combination therapy of a corticosteroid (usually prednisolone) with a calcineurin or mTOR inhibitor (such as ciclosporin, tacrolimus or sirolimus), and an antiproliferative immunosuppressant (such as azathioprine or mycophenolate). When used in combination, lower doses of the drugs can be administered than when giving the drugs alone. Intensive monitoring of liver and renal functions is important.

B. Over-suppression of the immune response brings problems of opportunistic infections. Additional 'steroid effects' as described for iatrogenic Cushing-like syndrome may be also apparent (Ch. 44).

FURTHER READING

Ferrara JLM, Levine JE, Reddy P et al (2009) Graft-versus-host disease. *Lancet* 373, 1550–1561

Fishbein TM (2009) Current concepts: intestinal transplantation. *N Engl J Med* 361, 998–1008

Hirose R, Vincenti F (2006) Immunosuppression: today, tomorrow and withdrawal. *Semin Liver Dis* 26, 201–210

Jacobsohn DA, Vogelsang GB (2002) Novel pharmacotherapeutic approaches to prevention and treatment of GVHD. *Drugs* 62, 879–889

Jørgensen KA, Koefoed-Nielsen PB, Karamperis N (2002) Calcineurin phosphatase activity and immunosuppression. A review on the role of calcineurin phosphatase activity and the immunosuppressant effect of cyclosporin A and tacrolimus. *Scand J Immunol* 57, 93–98

Kobashigawa JA, Patel JK (2006) Immunosuppression for heart transplantation: where are we now? *Nat Clin Pract Cardiovasc Med* 3, 203–212

Mascarell L, Truffa-Bachi P (2003) New aspects of cyclosporin A mode of action: from gene silencing to gene upregulation. *Min Rev Med Chem* 3, 205–214

Snell GI, Westall GP (2007) Immunosuppression for lung transplantation: evidence to date. *Drugs* 67, 1531–1539

Thompson AW, Turnquist HR, Raimondi G (2009) Immunoregulatory functions of mTOR inhibition. *Nat Rev Immunol* 9, 324–337

Thiruchelvam PTR, Willicombe M, Hakim N et al (2011) Renal transplantation. *BMJ* 343:d7300

Webber SA, McCurry K, Keevi A (2006) Heart and lung transplantation in children. *Lancet* 368, 53–69

Compendium: immunosuppressant drugs

Drug	Kinetics (half-life)	Comment
Calcineurin inhibitors		
Ciclosporin	Oral bioavailability 40%; metabolised in liver and intestine, some active metabolites (10–40 h)	Lipid-soluble cyclic peptide; used in organ and tissue transplantation; oral or intravenous dosage
Tacrolimus	Oral bioavailability about 20%; extensive first-pass metabolism in the gut wall and liver (4–41 h)	Used for prophylaxis to prevent kidney and liver transplant rejection; oral or intravenous dosage
Mammalian target of rapamycin (mTOR) inhibitors		
Sirolimus	Low oral bioavailability (<30%), which is increased with fatty food; hepatic metabolism (60 h)	Potent non-calcineurin-inhibiting immunosuppressant; used for prophylaxis to prevent kidney transplant rejection; given orally as an oil solution
Antiproliferative agents		
Azathioprine	Good oral absorption; converted to active metabolites 6-mercaptopurine and thioinosinic acid (3–5 h); interacts with allopurinol	Used for transplant recipients, for autoimmune conditions and for rheumatoid arthritis; oral or intravenous dosage
Mycophenolate mofetil	Rapidly absorbed after oral dosage; hydrolysed within minutes to the active form, mycophenolic acid; hepatic metabolism (18 h)	Used for prophylaxis to prevent acute transplant rejection; oral or intravenous dosage
Mycophenolic acid	Active metabolite of mycophenolate mofetil	Used for prophylaxis to prevent acute transplant rejection; given orally as enteric-coated formulation
Interleukin-2 receptor antibodies		
Basiliximab	Binding to interleukin-2 receptor α-chain is maintained for 1–2 weeks after dosage	Monoclonal IL-2 receptor antibody that prevents T-lymphocyte proliferation; used to prevent acute kidney transplant rejection; given by intravenous infusion
Co-stimulation blocker		
Belatacept	Proteolysis (8–10 days)	Fusion protein that blocks CD80/CD86 co-stimulatory molecules; used to prevent renal transplant rejection in adults seropositive for Epstein–Barr virus; given by intravenous infusion

For the immunosuppressant activity of corticosteroids, see Ch. 44. See also the inflammatory arthritides (Ch. 30) and chemotherapy of malignancies (Ch. 52).

39 Antihistamines and allergic disease

ATOPY, ALLERGIC DISORDERS AND ANAPHYLAXIS

Allergic responses occur in atopic individuals who are pre-disposed to produce antigen-specific immunoglobulin E (IgE) when exposed to common, normally harmless environmental allergens such as house dust mite, grass pollen or animal dander. Immunological memory takes about 7 days to develop, and subsequent re-exposure to the allergen results in the antigen crosslinking IgE on mast cells and basophils and triggering an allergic response as explained below. Many atopic individuals have coexisting allergic diseases such as asthma, hay fever and eczema, although these are not invariably associated with atopy.

The control of antibody production in the immune response is shown in Figure 38.2. The key to the allergic reaction is that there is a preponderance of IgE production, rather than other classes of antibodies. This is because when atopic individuals are exposed to allergens they invoke a T-helper type 2 (Th2) lymphocyte response, rather than the usually dominant Th1-cell response (Ch. 38). The release of the Th2 profile of interleukins, including IL-4, IL-10 and IL-13, stimulates B-lymphocytes to produce IgE rather than IgG, a phenomenon known as class switching. Dominance of Th1 or Th2 response is partially programmed in early life, with exposure to microbial antigens thought to promote the normal Th1 dominance.

Most allergic reactions are predominantly of the type 1 (immediate) hypersensitivity category (see Ch. 38 for definitions). Immediate hypersensitivity to an allergen in a person with atopy produces a weal and flare reaction in the skin, or sneezing and a runny nose, or wheezing, within minutes. Pre-formed and newly synthesised mediators of the allergic response are released from mast cells and basophils after allergen crosslinks IgE that is bound to cell surface receptors. The pre-formed mediators include histamine and the newly synthesised mediators include platelet-activating factor, prostaglandin D₂ and the cysteinyl-leukotriene, LTC₄, which is converted to LTD₄ and LTE₄ extracellularly (Ch. 29). These mediators act at selective G-protein-coupled receptors on smooth muscle cells, endothelial cells, epithelial cells, mucus glands and leucocytes in various tissues. Tryptase is also released and stimulates protease-activated receptors (see Ch. 1).

Some allergic reactions, such as those that produce contact dermatitis, are driven by T-cell-mediated inflammatory processes. These reactions can result from involvement of Th1 or Th2 cells, or sometimes cytotoxic T-cells.

A prolonged inflammatory reaction (delayed-type hypersensitivity) may follow the initial allergic response, reaching a peak 6–9 h later. Depending on the site of the reaction, this produces an oedematous, red, indurated swelling in the skin, or a sustained blockage in the nose, or further wheezing. This delayed reaction is associated with tissue accumulation of eosinophils and neutrophils, followed by T-cells and basophils. Some delayed reactions arise without an immediate phase and may be triggered by primary activation of T-cells rather than mast cells. Chronic allergic inflammation is maintained by continuing release of several Th2-type cytokines which promote the production of mast cells and eosinophils, stimulate the expression of adhesion molecules and enhance the synthesis of IgE. Eosinophils release toxic basic proteins, cysteinyl-leukotrienes and platelet-activating factor. T-cells, mast cells and eosinophils also produce neurotrophins that release neuropeptides such as substance P, calcitonin gene-related peptide and neurokinin A from sensory neurons. These various mediators contribute to the inflammatory response by producing vasodilation with increased vascular permeability, and in the lung promote smooth muscle contraction and mucus secretion.

Allergic reactions to antigens vary in severity. At the most severe end of the spectrum is anaphylaxis, a systemic allergic reaction that is life-threatening because of upper airway swelling and obstruction and/or hypotension. Severe anaphylactic reactions can occur within minutes of exposure to the allergen. There are several causes of anaphylaxis (Box 39.1). If the allergen exposure is via systemic injection, then hypotension and shock will predominate.

> **Box 39.1** **Causes of anaphylaxis**
>
> Foods: especially peanuts, tree nuts, fish, shellfish,
>   eggs, milk
> Drugs: especially penicillin, intravenous anaesthetic agents,
>   aspirin and other non-steroidal anti-inflammatory drugs,
>   intravenous contrast media, morphine
> Bee and wasp stings
> Latex rubber

Foods are more likely to cause facial and laryngeal oedema with prominent respiratory problems.

Drugs can also act directly on mast cells to release mediators without the involvement of IgE. Such reactions are called anaphylactoid, and they present in the same way as true anaphylaxis.

HISTAMINE AS AN AUTACOID

Histamine is a heterocyclic amine that functions as a local hormone (autacoid). It is found in mast cells which are prominent in tissues that come into contact with the outside world, for example skin, lungs and gut, where they form part of the tissue defence mechanisms. Histamine is also present in circulating basophils, where it may also participate in tissue defence. Histamine has other roles in enterochromaffin-like cells in the stomach, where it participates in acid secretion (Ch. 33), and in the brain, where it acts as a neurotransmitter (Ch. 4).

Histamine is synthesised in mast cells and basophils by decarboxylation of dietary histidine and stored in intracellular granules. It is released by degranulation after activation of the cell either by a direct physical or chemical injury, by crosslinking of attached IgE molecules or by complement proteins. After release from these cells histamine is rapidly metabolised (see Ch. 4). Its effects are mediated by four distinct types of G-protein-coupled receptor, known as H_1, H_2, H_3 and H_4 (see the table of receptors at the end of Ch. 1). In general, H_1 receptors are involved in the 'defensive' actions of histamine and act through intracellular Ca^{2+} as a second messenger. Gastric acid secretion is mediated by H_2 receptors that generate cAMP as a second messenger (Ch. 33). These receptors are also involved in cardiac function (stimulation of rate and force of contraction) and are inhibitory postsynaptic receptors in the brain. There also H_3 and H_4 receptors in various locations (see Chs 1 and 4).

Allergic reactions involve the action of histamine at H_1 receptors. Histamine H_1 receptors are coupled to inositol phospholipid intracellular signalling pathways and activate the ubiquitous gene transcription factor nuclear factor κB (NF-κB; Ch. 30). NF-κB stimulates production of pro-inflammatory cytokines (particularly tumour necrosis factor α, IL-6 and IL-8) and expression of epithelial and endothelial adhesion molecules that attract inflammatory cells. The following are the major consequences of H_1 receptor stimulation.

- Capillary and venous dilation can produce marked hypotension. In the skin, histamine contributes to the weal and flare response; an axon reflex via H_1 receptors is responsible for the spread of vasodilation or flare from the oedematous weal.
- Increased capillary permeability can produce oedema. This can lead to urticaria, angioedema and laryngeal oedema. The consequent loss of fluid from the circulating blood volume contributes to hypotension.
- Smooth muscle contraction can occur, especially in bronchioles and the intestine.
- Skin itching can occur (produced by histamine in combination with kinins and prostaglandins).
- Pain may occur due to stimulation of nociceptors (Ch. 19).

HISTAMINE H_1 RECEPTOR ANTAGONISTS (ANTIHISTAMINES)

Examples

first-generation (sedating) antihistamines: chlorphenamine, clemastine, promethazine
second-generation (non-sedating) antihistamines: cetirizine, desloratidine, fexofenadine, levocetirizine, loratadine, mizolastine

MECHANISMS OF ACTION AND EFFECTS

The antihistamines are selective antagonists at histamine H_1 receptors; antagonists at other histamine receptors are traditionally not called antihistamines. Antihistamines are competitive inverse agonists (see Ch. 1) that reduce the basal level of spontaneous activity at histamine H_1 receptors as well as blocking the agonist effects of histamine. Useful actions of antihistamines include:

- suppression of many of the vascular effects of histamine,
- inhibition of inflammatory cell accumulation in tissues by second-generation antihistamines; this may result from downregulation of the activation of NF-κB in tissues at the site of an allergic response.

First-generation antihistamines have other actions that can be used therapeutically. They are lipophilic and cross the blood–brain barrier, producing sedation. They also have central antimuscarinic effects that may be clinically useful in suppressing nausea in motion sickness (e.g. cyclizine [no longer used as an antihistamine], promethazine; Ch. 32).

Second-generation (non-sedating) antihistamines such as cetirizine, fexofenadine, loratadine and mizolastine are either more hydrophilic or more ionised at physiological pH; they do not penetrate the blood–brain barrier well, and have little sedative effect. They also have little antimuscarinic action.

So-called 'third-generation' antihistamines, such as desloratadine, are active metabolites or optical isomers of second-generation drugs. They have similar efficacy to second-generation drugs but may have a different profile of unwanted effects.

PHARMACOKINETICS

Chlorphenamine is more slowly absorbed from the gut than promethazine; both undergo considerable first-pass hepatic metabolism to inactive compounds and have half-lives of 10–20 h. Formulations of chlorphenamine and promethazine are available for administration by intravenous or intramuscular injection in medical emergencies.

Most second-generation antihistamines are rapidly absorbed from the gut and metabolised in the liver to active compounds with half-lives ranging from 2 to 20 h. Cetirizine and fexofenadine undergo little metabolism and are mainly eliminated unchanged by the kidneys.

There are several topical formulations of antihistamines, including nasal sprays for allergic rhinitis, eye drops for allergic conjunctivitis and topical skin preparations for insect stings (although the latter are relatively ineffective).

UNWANTED EFFECTS

- Drowsiness or psychomotor impairment, especially with first-generation compounds, although paradoxical stimulation can occur in children and the elderly.
- Headache.
- Dry mouth, blurred vision, urinary retention and gastrointestinal upset from the antimuscarinic effects of first-generation compounds.
- Topical antihistamines for use on the skin can cause hypersensitivity reactions.

MANAGEMENT OF ALLERGIC DISORDERS

Most allergic reactions involve a complex series of chemical processes. However, the mainstay of treatment for many conditions is the use of antihistamines. Their efficacy indicates the importance of histamine as a mediator of allergic responses.

ANAPHYLAXIS

Anaphylaxis is a medical emergency and requires rapidly acting treatments. It most commonly arises as an allergic response to stings, nuts, penicillins, cephalosporins and muscle-relaxant drugs. The person should be laid flat with their feet raised if there is hypotension, and the airway secured. Adrenaline (epinephrine; Ch. 4) should be given intramuscularly and doses repeated every 10 min until the clinical state is stable. Adrenaline produces vasoconstriction by its action at α_1-adrenoceptors, reducing oedema, and bronchodilates via β_2-adrenoceptors. It also attenuates the release of mediators from mast cells by binding to cell surface β_2-adrenoceptors. People known to have allergies that cause anaphylaxis can carry a preloaded adrenaline syringe for emergencies, accompanied by detailed instructions on its appropriate use. Intravenous adrenaline should only be given if there is profound shock, and then in a very dilute solution with close cardiac monitoring. Intravenous use carries a risk of arrhythmias and intense vasoconstriction with myocardial ischaemic damage.

Once adrenaline has been given, late relapse can be prevented by intramuscular injection or slow intravenous injection of chlorphenamine and hydrocortisone (Ch. 44). Oxygen should be given in high concentration, and an inhaled β_2-adrenoceptor agonist such as salbutamol (Ch. 12) administered if there is marked bronchospasm. This can be particularly useful if a β-adrenoceptor antagonist has previously been taken, when adrenaline may be less effective on the airways. If there is persistent hypotension, intravenous fluid should be given rapidly, preferably a crystalloid such as isotonic saline.

SEASONAL AND PERENNIAL RHINITIS

Allergic inflammation of the lining of the nose produces symptoms of rhinitis including nasal obstruction, sneezing and itching. These result from increased glandular secretions producing nasal obstruction and mucous rhinorrhoea, as well as afferent nerve stimulation, which is responsible for itching and sneezing. Allergies can cause both perennial rhinitis (usually house dust mite) and seasonal rhinitis (pollens and moulds). The allergic response makes individuals more susceptible to the nasal irritant effects of other, non-allergenic stimuli, such as tobacco smoke and changes in temperature. Rhinitis also has several non-allergic causes, including acute infection and chronic sinus infection for which antibacterial treatment is indicated. Aspirin and other non-steroidal anti-inflammatory drugs can produce rhinitis (as well as asthma, see Ch. 12) in sensitive subjects, probably by enhancing cysteinyl-leukotriene generation. Less frequent causes include β-adrenoceptor antagonists (Ch. 5) and angiotensin-converting enzyme (ACE) inhibitors (Ch. 6).

Oral antihistamines are useful for reducing itching, sneezing and rhinorrhoea, but they are less effective for nasal obstruction. They can also suppress associated allergic conjunctivitis. Azelastine is an antihistamine used as a topical nasal spray. For more severe allergic rhinitis, a topical intranasal corticosteroid spray (Ch. 44) is the treatment of choice, providing relief from most symptoms. Topical sodium cromoglicate or nedocromil (Ch. 12) can be useful in atopic individuals, but they are less effective than antihistamines or topical corticosteroids and are no longer preferred treatments. An oral leukotriene receptor antagonist (montelukast) may be beneficial in allergic rhinitis with concomitant asthma. The antimuscarinic drug ipratropium bromide (Ch. 12) can be used topically for relief of non-allergic rhinorrhoea.

Topical nasal decongestants have a short-term role in treatment. These contain α_1-adrenoceptor agonists such as ephedrine or xylometazoline and produce local vasoconstriction. Prolonged use impairs ciliary activity in the nasal mucosa and can be associated with rebound nasal congestion during long-term use. Oral corticosteroids are reserved for the most severe symptoms.

If drugs fail the possibility of structural abnormalities such as nasal polyposis, hypertrophied inferior turbinates or a deviated nasal septum should be considered, since surgery may be helpful.

URTICARIA

Acute urticarial reactions often occur to the same allergens that cause anaphylaxis. Antihistamines are the treatment of choice, with an oral corticosteroid (Ch. 44) for more severe episodes.

Chronic urticaria can be provoked by physical factors such as cold, sun, scratching the skin or exercise, or it can be caused by urticarial vasculitis in association with connective tissue diseases such as systemic lupus erythematosus. In some cases, the cause may be autoimmune, caused by IgG autoantibodies to the IgE receptors on mast cells and basophils. Antihistamines can be useful to suppress the itch from urticaria, but often they have little effect on the weal. About 15% of the histamine receptors in the skin are H_2 receptors, and a histamine H_2 receptor blocker (Ch. 33) may be useful in addition to an antihistamine. Leukotriene receptor antagonists such as montelukast (Ch. 12) may be helpful for some people. Corticosteroids (Ch. 44) can be used in high dosage for severe symptoms, but long-term use should be avoided because of the unwanted effects. Immunosuppression with ciclosporin (Ch. 38) has been used successfully for some severe autoimmune urticarias.

ALLERGIC CONJUNCTIVITIS

Topical treatment with antihistamines, such as azelastine or levocabastine, or with sodium cromoglicate or nedocromil, is usually successful (see Ch. 50).

CONTACT AND ATOPIC ECZEMA

Contact and atopic eczemas are considered in Chapter 49.

ASTHMA

Although asthma often has an allergic component, antihistamines have little or no role. The management of asthma is considered in Chapter 12.

SELF-ASSESSMENT

True/false questions

1. Antihistamines do not reduce acid secretion from the gastric parietal cells.
2. Histamine is synthesised *de novo* when mast cell IgE receptors are crosslinked by allergen.
3. Loratadine is a non-sedating antihistamine.
4. Fexofenadine is associated with electrocardiographic (ECG) changes.
5. Fexofenadine reduces the release of histamine from mast cells.
6. Corticosteroids are effective for treating allergic rhinitis.
7. Histamine is the only mediator that causes symptoms in rhinitis.
8. Antihistamines have a well-defined place in the management of asthma.

One-best-answer (OBA) questions

1. Which *one* of the following contributes to an allergic response in an atopic individual?
   A. Increased production of cytokines from Th1-cells
   B. Increased production of IgM
   C. Stabilisation of mast cells
   D. Histamine release acting on both H_1 and H_2 receptors
   E. Reduction in leukotriene production from mast cells
2. Choose the *correct* statement below concerning antihistamines.
   A. Second-generation antihistamines readily cross the blood–brain barrier.
   B. Second-generation antihistamines have fewer antimuscarinic effects than first-generation antihistamines.
   C. First-generation antihistamines are the preferred first-line treatment for vomiting induced by cytotoxic drugs.
   D. Topical antihistamines are free from unwanted effects.
   E. Antihistamines cause vasodilation.

Case-based questions

A 10-year-old boy visited his doctor with his mother in the spring. His current symptoms of rhinorrhoea, nasal congestion, sneezing and itching eyes were interfering with his schoolwork. He gave a history of repeated episodes of recurrent otitis media, rhinorrhoea, nasal congestion, sneezing and itching eyes occurring over a 3-year period, but predominantly in the spring and autumn. He had had three episodes of otitis media over the previous 2 years, the last being 6 months before, which were treated with antibiotics because of prolonged residence of fluid in the middle ear. The boy had atopic dermatitis as an infant. He had no history of asthma; his mother had allergic rhinitis; they had two cats. Other than antibacterial drug treatment for his otitis media, he had taken no medication. Examination of the ears revealed healthy tympanic membranes with no current otitis media. He had no hearing loss and he was otherwise fit.

A. What was the likely diagnosis?
B. Were the boy's symptoms related to the history of otitis media?
C. Allergen skin testing showed him to be responsive to cat dander and house dust mite.
   What treatment would you give?

True/false answers

1. **True.** The term antihistamine is traditionally confined to H_1 receptor antagonists; these drugs do not block H_2 histamine receptors on the gastric parietal cells; selective histamine H_2 receptor antagonists include cimetidine and ranitidine.
2. **False.** Histamine is synthesised and stored in mast cell granules ready for release by IgE-dependent stimuli; in contrast, lipid mediators such as leukotrienes

and prostaglandins are synthesised *de novo* after stimulation.

3. **True.** Loratadine is a second-generation antihistamine, which lack the sedative action of first-generation antihistamines.
4. **False.** The parent drug of fexofenadine, terfenadine, was associated with ventricular arrhythmias in high doses and has been withdrawn; fexofenadine retains the antihistamine activity without the unwanted effects on the heart.
5. **False.** Fexofenadine blocks histamine activity only by blocking H_1 receptors.
6. **True.** Nasal corticosteroids are very effective in allergic rhinitis.
7. **False.** Mast cells also release prostaglandins and leukotrienes that contribute to nasal symptoms.
8. **False.** Antihistamines are not effective in asthma and have no place in asthma management guidelines.

OBA answers

1. **Answer D is correct.**
   A. Incorrect. In atopy there is a predominance of a Th2 response profile which is partially genetically determined and partly related to early life environment.
   B. Incorrect. The Th2 response leads to increased production of IgE.
   C. Incorrect. Mast cells degranulate following allergen crosslinking of IgE.
   D. **Correct.** Although the main effect of histamine in allergy is on the H_1 receptor, actions on H_2 receptors may also contribute to the allergic symptoms.
   E. Incorrect. Leukotriene synthesis in mast cells is increased and contributes to allergic responses.
2. **Answer B is correct.**
   A. Incorrect. Second-generation drugs are less able to cross the blood–brain barrier than first-generation drugs and cause less sedation.
   B. **Correct.** Second-generation antihistamines have less antagonist activity at muscarinic receptors.
   C. Incorrect. Antihistamines can be effective in motion sickness but not in vomiting caused by cancer chemotherapeutic agents.
   D. Incorrect. Topical antihistamines may cause hypersensitivity reactions.
   E. Incorrect. Antihistamines reduce vasodilation induced by the action of histamine at the H_1 receptor.

Case-based answers

A. The family history of atopy and the child's atopic dermatitis as an infant increase the likelihood that he would have had allergies. He is likely to have had seasonal allergic rhinitis but he may also have had sensitisation to cat and/or dust mite or other perennial allergens. His fitness and lack of current drug intake suggest that it is not non-allergic rhinitis, which may arise because of infections, drugs, etc.
B. Yes. As many as 50% of children older than 3 years with recurrent otitis media have confirmed allergic rhinitis.
C. It is important to carry out sensitivity testing, and sensitivity to cat dander and house dust mite was identified in this boy. Avoidance of exposure to allergens is advisable and should be actively pursued in the home and school environment. If pharmacological treatment is required, a non-sedating oral antihistamine should reduce rhinorrhoea, sneezing and itching but will have little effect on nasal congestion. A short course of nasal inhaled corticosteroids can be effective in controlling symptoms of allergic rhinitis, including congestion. Nasal sodium cromoglicate may also offer symptom relief but is not the preferred treatment.

FURTHER READING

Al Suleimani YM, Walker MJA (2007) Allergic rhinitis and its pharmacology. *Pharmacol Ther* 114, 233–260

Ardern-Jones MR, Friedmann PS (2010) Skin manifestations of drug allergy. *Br J Clin Pharmacol* 71, 672–683

De Groot H, Brand PLP, Fokkens WF et al. (2007) Allergic rhinoconjunctivitis in children. *BMJ* 335, 985–988

Greiner AN, Hellings PW, Rotiroti G et al. (2011) Allergic rhinitis. *Lancet* 378, 2112–2122

Kaplan AP (2002) Chronic urticaria and angioedema. *N Engl J Med* 346, 175–179

Kemp SF (2007) Office approach to anaphylaxis: sooner better than later. *Am J Med* 120, 664–668

Plaut M, Valentine MD (2005) Allergic rhinitis. *N Engl J Med* 353, 1934–1944

Saleh HA, Durham SR (2007) Perennial rhinitis. *BMJ* 335, 502–507

Compendium: antihistamines

Drug	Kinetics (half-life)	Comments
Non-sedating antihistamines		
All given orally, unless otherwise indicated, for symptomatic relief of allergic rhinitis and urticaria		
Acrivastine	Rapidly absorbed; high bioavailability; mainly renal excretion of unchanged drug (2 h)	
Azelastine	See Ch. 50	Used topically as nasal spray for allergic rhinitis and as eye drops for allergic conjunctivitis (Ch. 50)
Bilastine	Rapidly absorbed; bioavailability about 60%; eliminated unchanged in faeces and urine (14.5 h)	
Cetirizine	Complete oral bioavailability; eliminated by glomerular filtration and tubular secretion (6–10 h)	
Desloratadine	Hepatic metabolism, renal excretion (20–30 h)	The active metabolite of loratadine
Fexofenadine	Mostly eliminated in faeces (14 h)	The active metabolite of terfenadine (which is no longer used)
Levocetirizine	Rapidly absorbed; mostly excreted in urine unchanged (8–9 h)	The levo-isomer of cetirizine
Loratadine	Low oral bioavailability (about 10%) increased by food; prodrug metabolised to active desloratadine (8 h)	Prodrug of desloratadine
Mizolastine	Oral bioavailability about 70%; hepatic metabolism (15 h)	
Rupatadine	Hepatic metabolism; renal and faecal elimination (6 h)	May also block platelet-activating factor
Sedating antihistamines		
All drugs given orally unless otherwise indicated		
Alimemazine	Hepatic metabolism and renal excretion (4–7 h)	Used for urticaria and pruritus and as a premedication
Chlorphenamine (chlorpheniramine in USA)	Oral bioavailability about 50%; mainly renal excretion (22 h)	Used orally for symptomatic relief of hay fever and urticaria and by slow intravenous injection as an adjunct to adrenaline (epinephrine) for the emergency treatment of anaphylaxis and angioedema
Clemastine	Oral bioavailability 40%; hepatic metabolism, renal excretion (21 h)	Used for symptomatic relief of hay fever and urticaria
Cyproheptadine	Eliminated by hepatic metabolism (1–4 h); few kinetic data available	Used for symptomatic relief of hay fever and urticaria and in the treatment of migraine
Hydroxyzine	Rapidly absorbed; metabolised to cetirizine (20 h)	Used for pruritus and for the short-term treatment of anxiety
Ketotifen	Rapidly absorbed, 50% availability due to first-pass metabolism; hepatic metabolism (22 h)	Used for allergic conjunctivitis and allergic rhinitis
Promethazine	Low oral bioavailability (25%); hepatic metabolism and biliary excretion (10–14 h)	Used orally for symptomatic relief of hay fever and urticaria and by slow intravenous injection as an adjunct to adrenaline for the emergency treatment of anaphylaxis and angioedema; also used for motion sickness and as a premedication before anaesthesia; can also be given by deep intramuscular injection

Antihistamines are given orally, or topically in the eye (Ch. 50), nose and on the skin. Drugs with antihistamine actions which are not used to treat allergic conditions, such as cyclizine and meclozine, are used for the treatment of vestibular disorders and nausea and vomiting, especially motion sickness (see Ch. 32).

9

The endocrine system and metabolism

40

Diabetes mellitus

CONTROL OF BLOOD GLUCOSE

Glucose occupies a central position in metabolism as the predominant substrate for energy production. Cells receive their supply of glucose from blood, and control mechanisms ensure that the blood glucose concentration remains within narrow limits. Glucose enters the blood by absorption from the gut and from breakdown of stored glycogen or gluconeogenesis in the liver. At physiological concentrations, glucose is transferred from the blood into cells almost entirely by active transport. In most tissues this transfer is dependent on the action of the polypeptide hormone insulin.

Insulin is a protein that is secreted rapidly from the β-cells of the islets of Langerhans in the pancreas in response to a small rise in blood glucose, and its secretion is inhibited by a fall in blood glucose (Table 40.1). Insulin consists of two peptide chains, A and B, connected by two disulphide bridges. In the β-cell, insulin aggregates into hexamers with zinc, and after release from the cell it dissociates into dimers and eventually into the active monomeric form.

The presence of nutrients in the small intestine stimulates the release from gut endocrine cells of peptide hormones called incretins, which promote insulin secretion. The principal incretins are glucose-dependent insulinotropic peptide (GIP), secreted by the upper gut, and glucagon-like peptide-1 (GLP-1), which is released from the distal gut. Release is triggered by neural signals from the upper gut and direct interaction of nutrients with the secretory cells. GLP-1 has several actions that regulate glucose homeostasis:

- enhanced glucose-dependent insulin secretion; incretins are probably responsible for about 60% of the insulin that is secreted in response to a meal,
- inhibition of glucagon release,
- prolonged gastric emptying,
- promotion of satiety by an action on the hypothalamus (Ch. 37).

The actions of GLP-1 are brief as it has a very short plasma half-life of 1–2 min due to rapid degradation by dipeptidyl peptidase-4 (DPP-4).

Insulin is secreted into the blood under fasting conditions, with pulses every 10–14 min, and a slower cycle of release every 105–120 min. In response to a rise in plasma glucose (both the actual concentration and the rate of change) there is a superimposed biphasic pattern of insulin release.

- The *first phase* of release occurs within seconds, peaks at 3–5 min and lasts for about 10 min. This is achieved by the release of a small pool of insulin in secretory vesicles.
- The *second phase* of release is more gradual, rising to a lower peak than in phase 1, and is due to synthesis of new insulin.

Insulin secretion from pancreatic β-cells is modulated by K^+ channels in the cell membrane that are sensitive to ATP (K_{ATP} channels). The K_{ATP} channel has subunits known as sulfonylurea receptors (SURs), various isoforms of which act as regulatory proteins in the response to ATP in different tissues. First-phase insulin release is triggered when glucose enters the β-cell via the GLUT2 glucose transporter, and undergoes glycolysis with generation of intracellular ATP. Activation of the SUR1 receptor isoform by ATP closes the K_{ATP} channel, which reduces membrane K^+ efflux and depolarises the β-cell. Depolarisation opens

Table 40.1 Control of insulin release from pancreatic islets of Langerhans β-cells

Stimulants of insulin release	Inhibitors of insulin release
Parasympathetic stimulation (muscarinic receptors)	Sympathetic stimulation of α_2-adrenoceptors
Increased glucose	Decreased glucose
Amino acids	Somatostatin
Fatty acids	
Cortisol	
Gastrin	
Secretin	
Glucagon	
Incretins (GLP-1, GIP)	

GIP, glucose-dependent insulinotropic peptide; GLP-1, glucagon-like peptide.

Table 40.2 Metabolic effects of insulin

Site	Effect
Liver	Increased glucose storage as glycogen
	Decreased protein catabolism
	Increased protein synthesis
	Decreased gluconeogenesis
Muscle	Increased protein synthesis
	Increased glycogen synthesis
	Increased glucose uptake
	Increased amino acid uptake
Adipose tissue	Increased triglyceride storage
	Increased triglyceride synthesis
	Decreased lipolysis

voltage-gated L-type Ca^{2+} channels in the cell membrane, and an influx of Ca^{2+} ions into the cell triggers second messengers that lead to exocytosis of insulin granules. (See Fig. 5.4 for description of the K_{ATP} channel in vascular smooth muscle.) In addition to glucose, many other factors influence insulin secretion (Table 40.1).

Peripheral tissues express specific cell surface insulin receptors that are linked to a tyrosine kinase (insulin receptor kinase) (Ch. 1). Stimulation of these receptors leads to translocation of the GLUT4 glucose transporter to the cell surface, allowing glucose uptake, and activates pathways involved in glycogen synthesis, glycolysis and fatty acid synthesis. Metabolic effects of insulin include the following.

- Glucose metabolism: promotion of active transport of glucose into cells, particularly in skeletal muscle and adipose tissue, accompanied by K^+. Insulin enhances storage of glucose as glycogen in liver and muscle and inhibits the breakdown of glycogen (glycogenolysis). Insulin also inhibits gluconeogenesis from amino acids in the liver. The overall effect is to increase glycogen stores.
- Lipid metabolism: reduced plasma free fatty acids and increased adipocyte triglyceride storage. Insulin increases hydrolysis of circulating triglycerides from lipoproteins by enhancing the activity of lipoprotein lipase, and promotes fatty acid uptake by adipose cells. Glucose entry into adipocytes provides glycerol phosphate for esterification of fatty acids to triglycerides. In adipose tissue, insulin inhibits lipases and prevents triglyceride breakdown.
- Protein metabolism: inhibition of the catabolism of amino acids in the liver and increased amino acid transport into muscle with enhanced protein synthesis.

The effects of insulin on different tissues are summarised in Table 40.2.

Several hormones inhibit the anabolic actions of insulin, particularly on carbohydrate metabolism, although effects on protein metabolism vary. These include glucagon, growth hormone, cortisol and catecholamines. Most of these hormones are released in stressful situations that require the breakdown of glycogen reserves to provide energy.

DIABETES MELLITUS

Failure to secrete sufficient insulin to control the normal level of blood glucose results in diabetes mellitus. The condition is diagnosed when the fasting plasma glucose concentration exceeds 7 mmol·L^{-1}. The long-term consequences include increased risk of the development of vascular and neuropathic disease (Table 40.3). Two patterns of diabetes mellitus are recognised: type 1 and type 2. There is still dispute over whether they represent distinct entities, or different manifestations of the same disease process. There is a strong genetic predisposition for both conditions.

TYPE 1 DIABETES MELLITUS

Type 1 diabetes represents a severe deficiency of insulin production caused by autoimmune destruction of pancreatic β-cells, and usually presents in younger people. Type 1 diabetes typically presents with a short history of feeling tired and unwell, together with weight loss, polyuria and polydipsia. There is a high risk of ketoacidosis because of breakdown of fatty acids and amino acids in the liver to provide an energy source, which generates ketone bodies.

TYPE 2 DIABETES MELLITUS

Type 2 diabetes, which usually presents later in life, is the consequence of a relative deficiency of insulin. It accounts for 90% of cases of diabetes in the Western world. In established type 2 diabetes the first phase of insulin secretion is absent or attenuated, and the second phase is slowed.

People with type 2 diabetes are often overweight (the average body mass index at diagnosis is 30 kg·m^{-2}). This increases cellular resistance to insulin in the liver, muscles and adipose tissue so that less glucose is transported into cells. In addition to reduced tissue uptake of glucose,

Table 40.3 Complications of diabetes

Complication	Consequences
Microvascular	
Nephropathy	Microalbuminuria, macroalbuminuria, renal failure
Retinopathy	Background retinopathy, proliferative retinopathy leading to visual impairment
Peripheral neuropathy	Loss of peripheral sensation Pain, ulceration
Autonomic neuropathy	Impotence Gastrointestinal disturbance Orthostatic hypotension
Macrovascular	
Cardiovascular disease	Hypertension Ischaemic heart disease
Cerebrovascular disease	Stroke

glycogen in the liver is broken down and glucose is released into the circulation. In adipose tissue, triglycerides are broken down to free fatty acids which are released into the circulation.

In type 2 diabetes there is reduced or absent GLP-1 secretion in response to oral glucose, and a reduced sensitivity to the peptide at pancreatic β-cells. In addition, high circulating free fatty acids and the production of reactive oxygen species in response to a sustained high plasma glucose concentration reduce insulin secretion.

Insulin resistance characteristically precedes overt diabetes by several years, but for some time insulin secretion by the pancreas is sufficient to overcome cellular resistance. Eventually, β-cell dysfunction with loss of the first-phase insulin response to a glucose load results in loss of compensation for insulin resistance. In people with type 2 diabetes who are not obese the major defect is inadequate insulin secretion.

In type 2 diabetes, postprandial hyperglycaemia is the major defect in blood glucose control, with excess glucose outside the cells rather than a shortage inside. People with type 2 diabetes do not usually develop ketoacidosis, because sufficient glucose enters cells to permit adequate energy production for most situations. The ideal approach to treatment would be an intervention that restores the early phase of insulin secretion in response to a glucose load.

INSULINS AND INSULIN ANALOGUES

Normal insulin secretion from the pancreas is into the portal circulation and is strictly regulated to meet metabolic needs. Sixty per cent of the insulin that is released from the pancreas is extracted by the liver before it reaches the systemic circulation. In contrast, therapeutic delivery of insulin is to the systemic circulation, and the relationship to metabolic needs can only be approximated by the dosages used and their timing in relation to meals.

NATURAL INSULIN FORMULATIONS

Insulins for therapeutic administration were originally extracted from either bovine or porcine pancreas. Bovine insulin differs chemically from human insulin in three amino acid residues, and porcine in one, but their actions are very similar to human insulin. These insulins are now rarely used.

Human-sequence insulin is produced either by enzymatic modification of porcine insulin, or by recombinant DNA technology using bacteria or yeast. All current insulin preparations have a low impurity content, which has caused problems in the past, and have low immunogenic potential.

All insulins (and insulin analogues; see below) are formulated at a standard strength of 100 units·mL^{-1} to reduce confusion over doses. The choice of injection device, usually a form of prefilled syringe, is important to facilitate use.

Pharmacokinetics

Currently available insulins must be given parenterally, because insulin is a protein and would otherwise be digested in the gut. At present, subcutaneous injection is used for routine treatment, with intravenous infusion for emergency situations. Recommended subcutaneous injection sites include upper arms, thigh, buttocks and abdomen. Absorption is faster from the abdomen than from the limbs, although strenuous exercise can increase absorption from the limbs.

The half-life of insulin in plasma is very short (about 8–16 min), and to avoid the need for frequent injections during maintenance treatment the absorption of insulin from injection sites must be prolonged. Insulin is formulated either in a soluble preparation or complexed with a substance to delay absorption from the injection site (Table 40.4).

Soluble insulins aggregate to form hexamers, which delays their absorption from the injection site. After subcutaneous injection, the maximum plasma concentration of soluble insulin (also called neutral insulin) is achieved about 2 h later, compared with minutes after intravenous injection. To limit the increase in plasma glucose concentration generated by a meal, subcutaneous soluble insulin must be given 15–30 min before eating. The action of intravenous soluble insulin lasts less than an hour and is mainly terminated by degradation in the kidney. Continued absorption from a subcutaneous injection site prolongs the duration of action after injection to about 5 h.

To generate intermediate- or long-acting formulations, insulin is complexed with the following.

■ **Protamine**: to create an intermediate-acting complex *isophane insulin*. Isophane insulin can also be formulated together with a non-complexed solution of soluble insulin (*biphasic isophane insulin*). The ratio of soluble to isophane insulin in biphasic insulin varies from 10:90 through 20:80; 30:70 and 40:60 to 50:50.

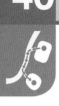

Table 40.4 Characteristics of insulins following subcutaneous administration

Type	Onset of action	Peak activity (h)	Duration (h)	
Insulin formulations				
Neutral (regular or soluble)	0.5 h	1–3	7	Short-acting
Isophane[a]	1 h	2–6	20	Intermediate-/long-acting
Zinc	2 h	6–14	22	Long-acting
Protamine–zinc	4 h	12–24	30	Long-acting
Insulin analogues				
Insulin lispro	10–20 min	0.5–0.75	2–5	Short-acting
Insulin aspart	10–20 min	0.6–0.7	2–4	Short-acting
Insulin glulisine	10–20 min	1	5	Short-acting
Insulin glargine	Plateau (4–24 h)		15–30	Long-acting
Insulin detemir	Plateau (7–24 h)		>20	Long-acting

[a]Sometimes called NPH (neutral protamine Hagedorn) insulin.

- **Zinc**: to create the intermediate-acting *insulin zinc* suspension or the long-acting *crystalline insulin zinc* suspension. Insulin molecules form hexamers which are stabilized by zinc, and the size of these molecular aggregates determines the rate of diffusion from the site of injection. Such complexes act as modified-release formulations for subcutaneous administration (Table 40.4).
- **Protamine and zinc**: to create the long-acting *protamine–zinc* insulin. This is only available as a bovine insulin and is now used rarely because it binds soluble insulin if given in the same syringe.

Unwanted effects

- The main problem is an excessive action producing hypoglycaemia. Neuroglycopenia with confusion and coma can occur. Treatment is with sugary foods or drinks, oral glucose or glucose gel (Hypostop®; 10–20 g) if the person is conscious. Intravenous injection of 20% glucose is used if the person is unconscious. Glucagon (see below) can be given intramuscularly if venous access is not available, followed by a sugary drink on waking. All people with diabetes who take insulin should carry a card with details of their treatment ('insulin passport'). Although most people experience warning symptoms of hypoglycaemia, some do not and are prone to sudden hypoglycaemia with loss of consciousness. Frequent hypoglycaemic attacks can reduce the awareness of the onset of symptoms.
- Rebound hyperglycaemia can occur after an episode of hypoglycaemia, especially at night (Somogyi effect). This results from the compensatory release of hormones such as adrenaline. It can produce ketonuria, leading to a mistaken belief that too little insulin has been given.
- Animal insulins produce circulating antibodies, although this is less common with current, highly purified preparations. These could diminish the activity of the insulin (insulin resistance) or produce local reactions (lipoatrophy) at injection sites.

- Insulins can cause local fat hypertrophy at the injection site, which can be minimized by rotating the site of injection.

INSULIN ANALOGUES

Examples

short-acting: insulin aspart, insulin glulisine, insulin lispro
long-acting: insulin detemir, insulin glargine

Mechanism of action and effects

The insulin analogues are recombinant chemical modifications of naturally occurring insulin. These changes have no effect on the binding of the molecule to cellular insulin receptors.

Short-acting insulin analogues

Unlike soluble insulins, these do not readily form dimers and hexamers, and therefore they are rapidly absorbed from an injection site with a faster onset and a shorter duration of action.

- Insulin aspart has one amino acid substitution of aspartic acid for proline at position B28.
- Insulin glulisine has two amino acid changes involving substitution with glutamic acid for lysine at B29 and lysine for asparagine at B3.
- Insulin lispro has the amino acids lysine and proline reversed at positions B28 and B29.

Insulin aspart and lispro are available complexed with protamine to give an intermediate duration of action, and in this form are combined with the short-acting formulations as ready mixed biphasic insulins.

Long-acting insulin analogues

- Insulin detemir has threonine at B30 omitted and a fatty acid chain added to the amino acid B29. This increases the formation of insulin complexes and enhances binding to albumin, which slows absorption from the injection site.

- Insulin glargine has two amino acid changes involving substitution of glycine for asparagine at A21 and addition of two arginines to the C-terminus of the B chain. This makes the molecule more soluble at acid pH, and less soluble at physiological pH. Insulin glargine precipitates after subcutaneous injection, slowly redissolves and is then absorbed.

Pharmacokinetics

Compared with standard soluble insulin, absorption of short-acting insulin analogues from a subcutaneous injection site occurs faster and leads to an early peak plasma concentration (Table 40.4). The duration of action is also shorter, at almost 3 h. They are usually given just before a meal, but can be mixed immediately after eating. They can be mixed with long-acting standard insulins, and are also available as biphasic formulations (insulin aspart with insulin aspart protamine in a 30:70 ratio; insulin lispro with insulin lispro protamine in a 25:75 or 50:50 ratio). Insulin analogues can be given by subcutaneous injection or infusion or by intravenous injection or infusion.

Long-acting insulin analogues are slowly and uniformly absorbed after subcutaneous injection, which avoids plasma insulin peaks.

Unwanted effects

- Unwanted effects are similar to those of other insulins. Despite the structural modifications, there is no reported excess of immunogenic reactions compared with standard insulin.
- There is a slightly reduced frequency of hypoglycaemia with insulin aspart or lispro compared with soluble insulin, because of the shorter duration of action.

THERAPEUTIC REGIMENS FOR INSULIN

The choice of regimen for insulin administration depends on the age, lifestyle, circumstances and preference of the individual. The general principle is to maintain a background (basal) level of insulin and then to give insulin boluses prior to meals to deal with the glucose load (basal-bolus regimens). Options include the following.

- **Single daily injections before breakfast or at bedtime**: used mainly for elderly people with type 2 diabetes who require insulin, and in whom the long-term complications of diabetes are less relevant. An intermediate- or long-acting insulin is used which can be combined with a short-acting insulin to improve control.
- **Twice-daily injections before breakfast and evening meal**: suitable for people who have a reasonably stable pattern of activity and eating habits. Short- and intermediate-acting insulins are combined, either in fixed ratios provided by the manufacturer (see above), or in varying ratios according to individual requirements.
- **Multiple injections before breakfast and evening meal and at bedtime** are increasingly used in younger,

active people who require more flexibility in their lifestyle. A number of tailored regimens can be employed using short- and intermediate-acting insulins. Examples include long-acting insulin at bedtime or intermediate-acting insulin at breakfast and at bedtime to ensure a 'background' level, and then short-acting insulin before breakfast and midday and evening meals.

There are also situations in which a basal-bolus regimen is not appropriate.

- **Continuous subcutaneous infusion** of short-acting insulin via a portable syringe pump and catheter is used if there is a problem with recurrent hypoglycaemia, unpredictable daily lives or hyperglycaemia before breakfast despite optimisation of a multiple-injection insulin regimen. The rate of infusion can be programmed, and boluses given before meals.
- **Intravenous infusion** is used for treatment of ketoacidotic crises, in labour, during and after surgery, or at other times when the person's usual routine cannot be adhered to. Short-acting insulin is infused in 5% glucose solution with added potassium chloride (unless there is hyperkalaemia).
- **Intraperitoneal infusion**: people with diabetes who are being treated for chronic renal failure by continuous ambulatory peritoneal dialysis can add their insulin to the dialysis fluid. Some implantable insulin pumps also use this route. This is the only therapeutic regimen in which insulin has direct access to the portal circulation.

OTHER PARENTERAL HYPOGLYCAEMIC DRUGS

SYNTHETIC INCRETIN MIMETICS

Examples

exenatide, liraglutide

Mechanism of action

Exenatide and liraglutide are peptides that share part of their amino acid sequences with the naturally occurring incretin, glucagon-like peptide-1 (GLP-1). They bind to and activate the GLP-1 receptor, leading to an increase in glucose-dependent synthesis of insulin and its secretion from β-cells. They restore the first-phase insulin response to an oral glucose load and, unlike insulin, promote weight loss. Unlike GLP-1 they are resistant to the enzymatic action of DPP-4.

Pharmacokinetics

Exenatide and liraglutide are given by subcutaneous injection. Exenatide is eliminated by the kidney and has a short half-life of about 2 h. Liraglutide is eliminated by proteolysis and has a half-life of 11–15 h.

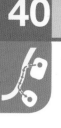

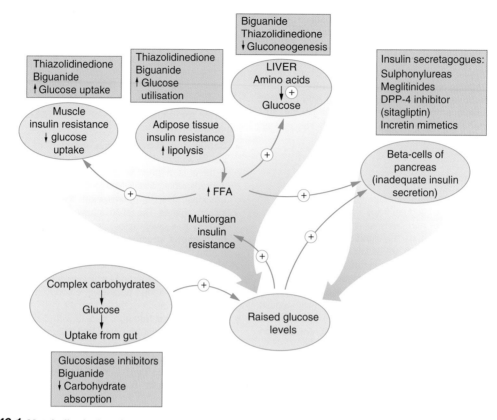

Fig. 40.1 Metabolic dysfunctions in type 2 diabetes and sites of drug action. The metabolic dysfunctions seen in type 2 diabetes result from inadequate insulin secretion and tissue resistance to the effects of insulin. Drug classes used to overcome the metabolic dysfunctions are 'insulin sensitisers' or increase insulin secretion and are shown with their main actions. DPP-4, dipeptidyl peptidase-4; FFA, free fatty acids.

Unwanted effects

- Nausea, vomiting, diarrhoea, abdominal pain, decreased appetite.
- Dizziness, headache, fatigue.
- Injection-site reactions.

ORAL HYPOGLYCAEMIC DRUGS

The main sites of action of oral hypoglycaemic drugs are shown in Figure 40.1.

SULFONYLUREAS

glibenclamide, gliclazide, glimepiride, glipizide, tolbutamide

Mechanism of action

Sulfonylureas act mainly by increasing the release of insulin from the pancreatic β-cells in response to stimulation by glucose (Fig. 40.1). They bind to the sulfonylurea (SUR1) receptor and close the K_{ATP} channel in the β-cell membrane. The resultant membrane depolarisation increases both first- and second-phase insulin secretion in response to glucose. Compounds with a short duration of action are usually preferred, to minimise the risk of hypoglycaemia. The long duration of action of glibenclamide carries a greater risk of hypoglycaemia and it is not recommended for treatment of the elderly.

Pharmacokinetics

Sulfonylureas are structurally related to sulphonamides. They are absorbed rapidly (although the rate of absorption is reduced when taken with food), are highly protein-bound and are metabolised by the liver. Tolbutamide, glipizide, glimepiride and gliclazide have half-lives of less than 10 h and short durations of action. Glibenclamide has a longer duration of action because of slow dissociation from the SUR1 receptor.

Unwanted effects

- Gastrointestinal disturbance, with nausea, vomiting, diarrhoea, constipation.
- Hypoglycaemia (particularly nocturnal) is most frequent with the longer-acting drugs or with excessive dosage since the drugs continue to work at low plasma glucose concentrations.
- Weight gain is almost inevitable unless dietary restrictions are observed.
- Hypersensitivity reactions (usually in the first 6–8 weeks of therapy) include skin rashes and, rarely, blood disorders.
- Glipizide and glimepiride can increase renal sensitivity to antidiuretic hormone and produce water retention with dilutional hyponatraemia.
- Sulfonylureas (except glipizide) should be avoided in people with acute porphyria.
- Concerns have been raised that sulfonylureas might increase cardiovascular mortality in type 2 diabetes, possibly as a result of binding to SUR2 receptors in the heart and inhibiting cardiac K_{ATP} channels. These channels have a cardioprotective role in ischaemic tissue, preventing cell depolarisation to conserve intracellular energy stores. Inhibition of the channels could lead to arrhythmias in people who have diabetes and ischaemic heart disease (see Ch. 5). However, recent clinical studies have failed to confirm the original concerns about cardiovascular mortality. Glimepiride and gliclazide bind less avidly than other sulfonylureas to cardiac SUR2 receptors.
- There is some evidence that sulfonylureas may accelerate the rate of pancreatic β-cell loss.

MEGLITINIDES

 Examples

nateglinide, repaglinide

Mechanism of action

The sulfonylurea moiety of glibenclamide is called meglitinide, and the currently available meglitinides are derived from this. Nateglinide binds to the SUR1 receptor on the β-cell, while repaglinide binds to a different nearby site. They stimulate insulin release in the same way as sulfonylureas. Nateglinide, unlike repaglinide, has a greater effect on insulin secretion when plasma glucose levels are rising and therefore produces little stimulation of insulin secretion in the fasting state. They have a rapid onset of action and a short duration of activity, and thus are taken shortly before main meals.

Pharmacokinetics

Both nateglinide and repaglinide are rapidly and well absorbed from the gut. They are metabolised in the liver and have short half-lives (1–2 h).

Unwanted effects

- Gastrointestinal upset, including nausea, vomiting, abdominal pain, diarrhoea or constipation, with repaglinide.
- Hypoglycaemia is much less frequent than with sulfonylureas due to the short duration of action. This also reduces the need to snack between meals, so weight gain is not usual.
- Hypersensitivity reactions with rashes and urticaria.

BIGUANIDE

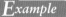 *Example*

metformin

Mechanism of action and effects

Metformin does not affect insulin secretion. Its molecular target is the protein kinase LKB1, which activates the hepatic enzyme 5′-AMP-activated protein kinase (AMPK). AMPK is a key regulator of the metabolism of fat and glucose. The major actions of metformin are as follows.

- Suppression of hepatic gluconeogenesis is the most important effect. Since some gluconeogenic activity remains, the risk of hypoglycaemia is minimal.
- Facilitation of glucose uptake in skeletal muscle and adipocytes. The full effect requires the presence of insulin. Metformin increases cell surface expression and activity of the membrane glucose transporter GLUT4.
- Decreased glucose absorption from the gut.
- Improvement in the adverse plasma lipid profile found in diabetes. Metformin increases fatty acid oxidation and reduces plasma triglycerides. It also raises plasma high-density lipoprotein (HDL) cholesterol (Ch. 48).

Metformin can suppress appetite and causes less weight gain than the sulfonylureas, which is useful in overweight people with diabetes.

Pharmacokinetics

Metformin is slowly and incompletely absorbed from the gut and excreted unchanged by the kidney.

Unwanted effects

- Gastrointestinal upset, including anorexia, nausea, abdominal discomfort and diarrhoea (usually transient).
- Metallic taste.
- Decreased vitamin B_{12} absorption.
- Inhibition of pyruvate metabolism encourages lactate accumulation. Lactic acidosis can result in situations that lead to an increase in anaerobic metabolism (e.g. shock with hypoxaemia), and metformin should be avoided in these situations. Lactic acidosis is more common in the presence of renal impairment, although the degree of renal impairment at which this becomes a significant risk is unclear.

THIAZOLIDINEDIONE

Example

pioglitazone

Mechanisms of action and effects

Pioglitazone has no effect on insulin secretion but is an insulin sensitiser. The effects are mediated through binding to peroxisome proliferator-activated receptor γ (PPAR-γ) in the cell nucleus. PPAR-γ associates as a heterodimer with the retinoid X receptor (RXR) (Ch. 1) in the cell nucleus and binds to PPAR-γ response elements in the promoter domains of target genes. In the absence of a ligand this heterodimer is further associated with a multiprotein co-repressor complex that has histone deacetylase activity and inhibits gene transcription. When a PPAR ligand binds to the PPAR–RXR heterodimer the co-repressor complex dissociates and a co-activator complex with histone acety-lase activity is recruited. In the case of PPAR-γ this results in the expression of genes that control adipocyte differentiation, and may increase the number of small adipocytes which are more insulin-sensitive.

The actions of pioglitazone include:

- enhanced insulin sensitivity and glucose utilisation in peripheral tissues, especially in adipocytes but also skeletal muscle and hepatocytes. Adipose tissue more readily takes up triglycerides from the blood. A secondary effect of the reduced availability of non-esterified fatty acids is improvement of insulin sensitivity in muscle cells. Other effects on adipocyte cell signalling may also influence tissue insulin sensitivity. These include reduced synthesis of pro-inflammatory cytokines that interfere with the insulin signalling cascade, such as tumour necrosis factor α and interleukin-6, and an increase in the insulin-sensitising and anti-inflammatory cytokine adiponectin,
- suppression of gluconeogenesis in the liver by inhibition of fructose-1,6-bisphosphatase,
- in addition to reducing the plasma glucose concentration, the effect on triglycerides also improves diabetic dyslipidaemia. Plasma HDL cholesterol concentration is increased, due to increased lipolysis of triglycerides in very-low-density lipoprotein (VLDL). The plasma low-density lipoprotein (LDL) fraction may also become larger and less dense, which may further reduce atherogenesis (Ch. 48). Overall, fat is redistributed from visceral to subcutaneous stores,
- a small reduction in blood pressure, possibly by improving endothelial function and reducing sympathetic nervous system activity. There is also a reduction in diabetic microalbuminuria.

Pharmacokinetics

Pioglitazone is well absorbed from the gut and is metabolised in the liver. The half-life (3–7 h) is not related to the duration of action. Since the mechanism of action involves gene transcription, the onset of the hypoglycaemic effect is gradual over 6–8 weeks.

Unwanted effects

- Gastrointestinal disturbances.
- Headache, dizziness, visual disturbances.
- Anaemia.
- Hypoglycaemia.
- Fluid retention leading to oedema, which can cause decompensation in heart failure.
- Weight gain because of fat-cell differentiation.
- Increased risk of fractures, especially in women.
- Liver dysfunction has been reported rarely, and liver function tests should be monitored during treatment.

DIPEPTIDYL PEPTIDASE-4 INHIBITORS

Examples

linagliptin, sitagliptin, saxagliptin, vildagliptin

Mechanism of action

The 'gliptins' are competitive inhibitors of DPP-4 and reduce the ability of the enzyme to inactivate the incretin hormones GLP-1 and GIP. As a consequence, insulin synthesis and secretion are increased and therefore blood glucose levels are decreased and β-cell function is improved.

Pharmacokinetics

DPP-4 inhibitors are rapidly absorbed from the gut. Sitagliptin is excreted by the kidney and linagliptin is excreted largely unchanged in faeces; they have half-lives of about 12 h. Saxagliptin is cleared mainly by P450 metabolism in the liver, whereas vildagliptin undergoes P450-independent hydrolysis in the liver and kidney; both have a half-life of about 3 h. The long duration of action of DPP-4 inhibitors is due to extended binding to the target enzyme.

Unwanted effects

- Nausea, vomiting, dyspepsia.
- Oedema.
- Headache, dizziness, fatigue, nasopharyngitis.

GLUCOSIDASE INHIBITOR

Example

acarbose

Mechanism of action and effects

Carbohydrate digestion in the intestine involves several enzymes that sequentially degrade complex polysaccharides such as starch into monosaccharides like glucose. Initial digestion of carbohydrates in the gut lumen is carried out by amylases from the saliva and pancreas. The final digestion of oligosaccharides is carried out by β-galactosidases (including lactase) and various α-glucosidase enzymes (such as maltase, isomaltase, glucoamylase and sucrase, which hydrolyse oligosaccharides) in the small-intestinal brush border. Acarbose competes with dietary oligosaccharides for α-glucosidase enzymes, and has a higher affinity for these enzymes. Binding to the enzymes is reversible, so that digestion and absorption of glucose after a meal is slower than usual but not prevented. As a result, the postprandial peak of blood glucose is reduced and blood glucose concentrations are more stable through the day. Acarbose has no effect on insulin secretion or its tissue action and is less effective for achieving glycaemic control than other oral hypoglycaemic agents. Its use is limited by the high incidence of unwanted effects.

Pharmacokinetics

Oral absorption of acarbose is very low, with only about 2% of the active parent drug reaching the circulation. Inactive metabolites are formed in the gut lumen by enzymic degradation.

Unwanted effects

Gastrointestinal effects include flatulence, abdominal distension and diarrhoea due to fermentation of unabsorbed carbohydrate in the bowel. These effects are dose-related and often transient.

INHIBITOR OF RENAL GLUCOSE TRANSPORT

dapagliflozin

Mechanism of action

Dapagliflozin is a competitive reversible inhibitor of the sodium-glucose co-transporter 2 (SGLT2) in the proximal convoluted tubule of the kidney. It reduces glucose absorption from the tubular filtrate and increases urinary glucose excretion. It does not predispose to hypoglycaemia, and its use is associated with modest weight loss. The place of dapagliflozin in therapy of type 2 diabetes is currently uncertain.

Pharmacokinetics

Dapagliflozin is well absorbed from the gut and metabolized in the liver. It has a half-life of 13 h.

Unwanted effects

- Increased risk of urinary tract and genital infections.
- Potential increased risk of hypovolaemia and electrolyte imbalance.
- A possible increased risk of bladder cancer cannot be excluded at present.

DRUGS TO INCREASE PLASMA GLUCOSE LEVELS

GLUCAGON

Mechanism of action and use

Glucagon is a polypeptide synthesised by the α-cells of the pancreatic islets of Langerhans. It binds to specific hepatocyte receptors and activates membrane-bound adenylyl cyclase. The consequent increase in intracellular cAMP leads to inhibition of glycogen synthase. This blocks the effect of insulin on hepatocytes and mobilises stored liver glycogen. Glucagon is used to raise blood glucose in severe acute insulin-induced hypoglycaemia.

Pharmacokinetics

Glucagon must be given by intramuscular, subcutaneous or intravenous injection, and acts within 10–20 min. It is degraded rapidly by enzymes in the plasma, liver and kidney.

Unwanted effects

These are not usually troublesome with a single injection but include nausea, vomiting and diarrhoea.

MANAGEMENT OF TYPE 1 DIABETES

The aim of treatment is to maintain a plasma glucose concentration as close to normal as possible. Maintenance treatment of type 1 diabetes should include an appropriate diet with a regulated carbohydrate intake distributed throughout the day. Excess dietary saturated fat should be avoided. The complications of type 1 diabetes can be reduced by close control of the blood glucose concentration using insulin, usually in a basal-bolus regimen (see above). The preferred regimens are those with multiple short-acting insulin doses before meals. Short-acting insulin analogues are used in place of soluble insulin for those who wish to inject shortly before or immediately after meals or when there are episodes of hypoglycaemia at night or between meals. Long-acting insulin analogues are recommended in place of isophane insulin if there is recurrent nocturnal hypoglycaemia or morning hyperglycaemia with difficult daytime control.

The success of the chosen approach can be monitored by measurement of the blood glucose concentrations, often carried out on a finger-prick blood specimen using a blood glucose reagent strip. If peak or trough blood glucose estimations are outside an acceptable range, the insulin regimen should be adjusted, although this should not be done more than once or twice a week. Long-term control of diabetes is usually assessed by the plasma concentration of glycosylated haemoglobin (HbA_{1c}). An HbA_{1c} level greater than 53 mmol·mol^{-1} (upper limit of normal is 42 mmol·mol^{-1})

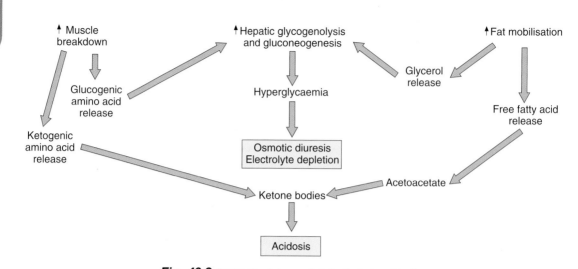

Fig. 40.2 Pathophysiology of diabetic ketoacidosis.

is associated with a higher risk of developing microvascular and neuropathic complications. Hyperglycaemia leads to the glycosylation of proteins which inhibits their function and may promote vascular and neurological damage. Several other mechanisms of vascular and neurological damage may also contribute to the complications of hyperglycaemia. In older people with type 1 diabetes, management of cardiovasular risk factors (see type 2 diabetes below) becomes increasingly important.

The most dramatic complication of untreated or poorly controlled type 1 diabetes is diabetic ketoacidosis (Fig. 40.2), which can lead to coma if it is severe. Systemic infection, dietary indiscretion or inappropriate insulin dose reduction or omission can precipitate ketoacidosis in a person with treated type 1 diabetes. Apart from the treatment of any precipitating cause, the management of ketoacidosis includes:

- restoration of extracellular volume: hyperglycaemia leads to an osmotic diuresis with excessive urinary salt and water loss. Replacement by isotonic (0.9%) saline is essential,
- potassium replacement: the osmotic diuresis results in excessive urinary potassium loss. Potassium is also shifted from within cells into extracellular fluid in exchange for hydrogen ions in the ketoacidotic state. Correction of the extracellular acidosis reverses this shift and can produce profound hypokalaemia. Once a good urine flow has been established, intravenous potassium supplements are usually required,
- intravenous insulin until the ketosis is abolished and the plasma glucose is below 15 mmol·L^{-1}. An intermediate-acting insulin should be continued subcutaneously during the infusion to maintain a basal blood insulin concentration. The metabolic acidosis will usually correct with treatment of the hyperglycaemia and fluid replacement. Intravenous sodium bicarbonate is occasionally required if the arterial pH is less than 7.0, but should be used with caution.

MANAGEMENT OF TYPE 1 DIABETES IN SPECIAL SITUATIONS

- Close attention to diabetic control is important before conception and during pregnancy because poor control will affect the fetus, leading to increased intra-uterine and perinatal mortality.
- At times of intercurrent illness, the dose of insulin will need to be increased, guided by blood glucose monitoring, to counteract the hyperglycaemic action of hormones released during stress reactions.
- During and after surgery, soluble insulin should be given in 10% glucose solution by intravenous infusion, dosage being guided by the blood glucose concentrations. Subcutaneous insulin can be restarted as soon as the person is able to eat and drink.

MANAGEMENT OF TYPE 2 DIABETES MELLITUS

The mainstays of treatment are lifestyle and dietary modifications. As for type 1 diabetes, close control of the blood glucose concentration in type 2 diabetes reduces the risk of microvascular complications, although the effect on macrovascular complications such as myocardial infarction is less convincing. The target HbA$_{1c}$ concentration is 48 mmol·mol^{-1}.

More than 75% of people with newly diagnosed type 2 diabetes are obese. Weight reduction not only improves blood glucose levels but also reduces other cardiovascular disease risk factors. Dietary advice should include:

- reducing energy intake if obese (an average weight loss of 18 kg is required to control blood glucose),
- eating small regular meals,

- ensuring that more than half the total energy intake is from carbohydrates, total fat contributing less than 35% of total energy intake,
- encouraging high-fibre foods and limiting sucrose and alcohol intake.

This should be combined with advice to exercise regularly and to stop smoking (because of the contribution to vascular disease) as appropriate. Lifestyle and dietary advice should initially be encouraged for obese people, with use of metformin if this fails. There is some evidence that metformin may reduce the risk of cardiovascular disease in obese people with type 2 diabetes. Combination therapy with a sulfonylurea and metformin can be useful if a single drug is insufficient to reduce the blood glucose concentration. By contrast, underweight people with type 2 diabetes often require early treatment with an oral hypoglycaemic agent, usually a sulfonylurea.

Pioglitazone should be considered if there is intolerance to combination therapy with metformin plus a sulfonylurea (replacing the drug to which there is intolerance). Failure of such combinations usually indicates declining insulin release and the need for exogenous insulin, although for some overweight people the combination of a sulfonylurea, metformin and pioglitazone may be helpful. The meglitinides are used alone for non-obese people with diabetes or when metformin is contraindicated. In other individuals meglitinides can be given in combination with metformin. A DPP-4 inhibitor such as sitagliptin can be considered when metformin alone is inadequate, but preferably in people without marked obesity. They can also be added to metformin with a sulfonylurea if insulin is not acceptable.

Within 3 years of diagnosis, 50% of individuals with type 2 diabetes will need combination therapy to achieve glycaemic control. Failure of oral treatment usually implies β-cell 'exhaustion' and up to 30% of those with type 2 diabetes require insulin with or without an oral hypoglycaemic drug. The most effective combination is a basal dose of intermediate-acting insulin at bedtime combined with metformin during the day. If the HbA_{1c} is greater than 75 mmol·mol^{-1} then biphasic insulin should be considered. A sulfonylurea can be used with insulin if metformin is contraindicated, but with a greater risk of hypoglycaemia and eventual loss of efficacy as β-cell exhaustion progresses. Combination therapy with insulin and a glitazone or a meglitinide has not been well studied. There is some evidence that insulin therapy is more likely to be successful if used early in type 2 diabetes to preserve β-cell function.

A GLP-1 mimetic, such as exenatide, is most appropriate for obese people for whom insulin is being considered. It can be added to metformin with a sulfonylurea, or used in combination with insulin. A GLP-1 mimetic is less likely to be effective if the diabetes has been present for many years, because β-cell exhaustion is often present.

Acarbose is of limited value when used alone or in combination with metformin. It may be most effective in early diabetes, when there is still sufficient insulin secretion for it to influence glycaemic control.

Intensive management of risk factors for cardiovascular disease is of crucial importance because the major complications of type 2 diabetes are vascular. In particular, control of raised blood pressure reduces both microvascular and macrovascular complications. There is little to choose between antihypertensive drugs for use in diabetes, except that thiazides and β-adrenoceptor antagonists may aggravate diabetes and should probably be avoided in the few people who are managed with dietary control alone. Use of an angiotensin-converting enzyme (ACE) inhibitor or an angiotensin II receptor antagonist reduces the risk of renal failure when there is evidence of diabetic nephropathy (either overt or with microalbuminuria) (Ch. 6). Treatment of the abnormal atherogenic plasma lipid profile that is common in type 2 diabetes is recommended for people over the age of 40 years (Ch. 48). Once a person with diabetes has developed coronary artery disease then management of all risk factors (Ch. 48) will reduce the risk of subsequent myocardial infarction or death to the same extent as for someone without diabetes.

SELF-ASSESSMENT

True/false questions

1. Oral hypoglycaemic drugs are only used in type 2 diabetes.
2. Glibenclamide is the drug of choice when there is no residual insulin secretion.
3. Sulfonylureas should be administered in conjunction with a dietary regimen in obese people.
4. Glibenclamide can cause hypoglycaemia, particularly in the elderly.
5. Metformin and the sulfonylurea gliclazide cannot be taken together.
6. The meglitinides are structurally related to glibenclamide.
7. Oral hypoglycaemics given to a pregnant mother can cause hypoglycaemia in the fetus.
8. Sulfonylureas should not be given together with the antibacterial trimethoprim.
9. Insulin lispro has a longer duration of action than isophane insulin.
10. Dipeptidyl peptidase-4 (DPP-4) synthesises incretin hormones.
11. Acarbose is completely absorbed from the gut after oral administration.
12. Glucagon mobilises glucose from glycogen in the liver.

One-best-answer (OBA) question

Ms JJ is a 55-year-old housewife with a body mass index (BMI) of 35 kg·m^{-2}. She was diagnosed with type 2 diabetes mellitus. Choose the *correct* statement below.

A. The mainstay of treatment is diet and exercise.
B. Diabetes presenting in this way is a medical emergency.
C. A sulfonylurea would be the drug of first choice.
D. Pioglitazone would be the drug of first choice.
E. Treatment with metformin may increase her risk of heart disease.

Case-based questions

A 25-year-old teacher, Mr JAH, was admitted to hospital as an emergency. He had developed a sore throat a week

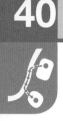

previously. His GP prescribed penicillin, but the soreness persisted and Mr JAH noticed profuse white spots on the back of his throat. He drank fluids copiously and passed more urine than usual. Two days before admission, he began to vomit, and on the day before admission he became drowsy and confused. He had lost approximately 12 kg in weight, despite eating more than usual. His great uncle had diabetes mellitus. Mr JAH was clinically dehydrated and ketones could be smelt on his breath. Results of blood tests indicated that he had diabetic ketoacidosis.

A. Which type of diabetes does Mr JAH have?
B. What was the significance of his sore throat?
C. Was it significant that his great uncle suffered from diabetes mellitus?
D. Explain his polydipsia and polyuria.
E. What treatments should have been instituted rapidly?
F. After he had recovered from the acute illness, what general advice should have been given about diet?
G. Mr JAH was a 'three-meals-a-day' man whose only exercise was walking a mile to work and back each day. Although insulin regimens vary widely, suggest a possible regimen and the types of insulin that could be given.
H. How long before meals should subcutaneous injection of soluble insulin have been given?
I. In addition to blood glucose levels, what other indicator could have been measured to signify good control in diabetes?

Mr JAH became more active, joined a health club and met a partner who liked to party. His eating became more irregular with hurried meals. His glycaemic control deteriorated.

J. What alterations to his insulin regimen could have been helpful?

True/false answers

1. **True.** Oral hypoglycaemic drugs (sulfonylureas, biguanides, meglitinides, thiazolidinediones, dipeptidyl peptidase-4 inhibitors) are only used in type 2 diabetes and act by different mechanisms to control glucose levels.
2. **False.** Glipizide is a sulfonylurea which stimulates insulin secretion from the islet β-cells and would be ineffective in the absence of any insulin-secreting ability.
3. **True.** Sulfonylureas cause weight gain partly by stimulating appetite; metformin might be a better choice.
4. **True.** Glibenclamide has a long duration of action and active metabolites can accumulate when renal function declines; hypoglycaemia is a greater problem in the elderly.
5. **False.** These drugs act in part by different mechanisms and can be combined. Unlike the sulfonylureas, metformin has a neutral or suppressive effect on appetite.
6. **True.** Meglitinides (glinides) chemically resemble the sulfonylurea moiety of glibenclamide.
7. **True.** Neonates born to mothers with diabetes who are taking oral hypoglycaemics in pregnancy have problems with hypoglycaemia; insulin is normally substituted in pregnancy.

8. **True.** Sulfonylureas have some structural similarities to the sulphonamides and trimethoprim and can produce severe hypoglycaemia when given together.
9. **False.** Isophane insulin is complexed with protamine and has a duration of action of 20 h, whereas synthetic insulin lispro is modified structurally and has a faster onset of action and shorter duration.
10. **False.** DPP-4 breaks down the incretin glucagon-like peptide-1 (GLP-1), so DPP-4 inhibitors such as sitagliptin enhance incretin activity on the islet β-cells.
11. **False.** Acarbose is very poorly absorbed and acts within the gut to reduce the digestion of glicose by α-glucosidases.
12. **True.** Glucagon reverses the effect of insulin on liver glycogen storage and is used to increase blood glucose in severe acute hypoglycaemia induced by insulin.

OBA answer

Answer A is correct.

A. **Correct.** Diet and exercise should be tried for 3 months before suggesting other treatments.
B. Incorrect. Treatment, support and advice should take place over many months.
C. Incorrect. Sulfonylureas can stimulate appetite by increasing insulin secretion and cause further weight gain.
D. Incorrect. The use of pioglitazone as second-line therapy added to either metformin or a sulfonylurea is not recommended, except for people who are unable to tolerate metformin and sulfonylurea combination therapy, or people in whom either drug is contraindicated; in such cases, the thiazolidinedione should replace the poorly tolerated or contraindicated drug.
E. Incorrect. Metformin has a cardioprotective effect which is not wholly explicable by its effects on glucose and may be due to improvements in the lipid profile.

Case-based answers

A. The ketoacidosis indicates that Mr JAH has type 1 diabetes mellitus.
B. An upper respiratory tract infection can be all that is necessary to precipitate ketoacidosis. Aggravating factors include the candidiasis in his throat, and over-breathing, causing dryness.
C. There is a strong familial tendency, but neither type 1 nor type 2 diabetes mellitus is a single-gene disorder, so there is no classic pattern of inheritance.
D. Once the tubular transport maximum for glucose reabsorption in the kidneys is exceeded the glucose in the distal tubules causes an osmotic diuresis, leading to polyuria and then to thirst.
E. Insulin, fluids and salts should be given to correct dehydration, glucose levels, ketoacidosis and electrolyte imbalances. Ketoacidosis can lead to coma.
F. A dietary regimen should be agreed to create a stable pattern of eating habits commensurate with his lifestyle. Diets low in animal fat and high in fibre are recommended, ideally with carbohydrate intake distributed throughout the day.

G. Initiate a stable pattern of eating habit and activity, and twice-daily subcutaneous insulin injections before breakfast and evening meal. The insulin regimen would contain a mixture of short- and long-acting insulins, the ratios of which vary depending upon his glucose levels. Insulins frequently used are soluble insulin and isophane insulin.

H. The time to onset of activity of neutral soluble insulin is 30 min, with peak activity at 1–3 h.

I. The amount of glycosylated haemoglobin (HbA_{1c}) can be measured. High concentrations indicate an increased risk of microvascular and neuropathic complications.

J. Rapid-acting monomeric insulin lispro may be helpful. This has a time to onset of only 15 min and a time to peak plasma levels of 0.5–0.75 h, so should be given immediately before a meal. Insulin lispro during the day with insulin isophane in the evening is a possible regimen, but education about eating and lifestyle would probably provide greater benefit than a change of insulin regimen.

FURTHER READING

Bailey CJ (2011) The challenge of managing coexistent type 2 diabetes and obesity. *BMJ* 342, d1996

Beckman JA, Creager MA, Libby P (2002) Diabetes and atherosclerosis. Epidemiology, pathophysiology, and management. *JAMA* 287, 2570–2581

Beigi FI (2012) Glycemic management of type 2 diabetes mellitus. *N Engl J Med* 366, 1319–1327

Bennett WL, Maruthur SS, Singh S et al. (2011) Comparative effectiveness and safety of medications for type 2 diabetes: update including new drugs and 2-drug combinations. *Ann Intern Med* 154, 602–613

Blood Pressure Lowering Treatment Trialists' Collaboration (2005) Effects of different blood pressure-lowering regimens on major cardiovascular events in individuals with and without diabetes mellitus. *Arch Intern Med* 165, 1410–1419

Daneman D (2006) Type 1 diabetes. *Lancet* 367, 847–858

De Witt DE, Hirsch IB (2003) Outpatient insulin therapy in type 1 and type 2 diabetes mellitus. *JAMA* 289, 2254–2264

Friedland SN, Leong A, Filion KB et al. (2012) The cardiovascular effects of peroxisome proliferator-activated receptor antagonists. *Am J Med* 125, 126–133

Gale EAM (2012) Newer insulins in type 2 diabetes. *BMJ* 345, e4611

Heine RJ, Diamant M, Mbanya J-C et al. (2006) Management of hyperglycaemia in type 2 diabetes. *BMJ* 333, 1200–1204

Kelly TN, Bazzano LA, Fonseca VA et al. (2009) Systematic review: glucose control and cardiovascular disease in type 2 diabetes. *Ann Intern Med* 151, 394–403

Metchick LN, Petit WA Jr, Inzucchi SE (2002) Inpatient management of diabetes mellitus. *Am J Med* 113, 317–323

Pickup JC (2012) Insulin-pump therapy for type 1 diabetes mellitus. *N Engl J Med* 366, 1616–1624

Plank J, Siebenhofer A, Berghold A et al. (2005) Systematic review and meta-analysis of short-acting insulin analogues in patients with diabetes mellitus. *Arch Intern Med* 165, 1337–1344

Selvin E, Bolen S, Yeh H-C et al. (2008) Cardiovascular outcomes in trials of oral diabetes medications: a systematic review. *JAMA* 168, 2070–2080

Snow V, Weiss KB, Mottur-Pilson C et al. (2003) Evidence for tight blood pressure control in type 2 diabetes mellitus. *Ann Intern Med* 138, 587–592

Stumvoll M, Goldstein BJ, van Haeften TW (2005) Type 2 diabetes: principles of pathogenesis and therapy. *Lancet* 365, 1333–1346

Tahrani AA, Bailey CJ, Del Prato S et al. (2011) Management of type 2 diabetes: new and future developments in treatment. *Lancet* 378, 182–197

Verspohl EJ (2009) Novel therapeutics for type 2 diabetes: incretin hormone mimetics (glucagon-like peptide-1 receptor agonists) and dipeptidyl peptidase-4 inhibitors. *Pharmacol Ther* 124, 113–138

Wilding JPH, Hardy K (2011) Glucagon-like peptide-1 analogues for type 2 diabetes. *BMJ* 342, d410

Compendium: drugs used in diabetes mellitus

Drug	Kinetics (half-life)	Comments
Treatment of hyperglycaemia		
Insulins		
Normally given by subcutaneous injection or subcutaneous infusion; onset and duration of action depend on the formulation used, many of which are combinations containing bovine, porcine or human insulin, e.g. insulin zinc suspension, isophane insulin, protamine–zinc insulin or recombinant human insulin analogues such as biphasic insulin aspart, biphasic insulin lispro and biphasic isophane insulin.		
Short-acting insulins		
Soluble insulin	See text and Table 40.4	A sterile solution of bovine, porcine or human insulin; may also be given by intramuscular or intravenous injection or by intravenous infusion, depending on requirements
Insulin aspart	See text and Table 40.4	A recombinant human insulin analogue; may also be given by intravenous injection or infusion, depending on requirements
Insulin glulisine	See text and Table 40.4	A recombinant human insulin analogue
Insulin lispro	See text and Table 40.4	A recombinant human insulin analogue; may also be given by intravenous injection or infusion, depending on requirements
Intermediate- and long-acting insulins		
Insulin detemir	See text and Table 40.4	A long-acting recombinant human insulin analogue
Insulin degludec	Duration of action over 40 h. Flat profile of action	Ultra-long acting human insulin analogue; less risk of nocturnal hypoglycaemia than with insulin glargine
Insulin glargine	See text and Table 40.4	A long-acting recombinant human insulin analogue with a longer duration of action than soluble insulin
Insulin complexes		
See text and Table 40.4.		
Sulfonylureas		
All are given orally for the treatment of type 2 diabetes mellitus.		
Glibenclamide	Complete oral bioavailability; hepatic metabolism to long-lived active metabolites (10 h)	Long-acting sulfonylurea; known as glyburide in the USA; used for people who are not overweight, or in whom metformin is contraindicated or not tolerated
Gliclazide	Variable absorption between individuals; hepatic metabolism (6–14 h)	Used for people who are not overweight, or in whom metformin is contraindicated or not tolerated
Glimepiride	Complete bioavailability; oxidised by P450 to active and inactive metabolites (5–9 h)	Used for people who are not overweight, or in whom metformin is contraindicated or not tolerated
Glipizide	Complete oral bioavailability; hepatic metabolism (2–4 h)	Used for people who are not overweight, or in whom metformin is contraindicated or not tolerated
Tolbutamide	Complete oral bioavailability; hepatic metabolism (4–6 h)	Used for people who are not overweight, or in whom metformin is contraindicated or not tolerated
Biguanide		
Given orally for the treatment of type 2 diabetes mellitus.		
Metformin	Oral bioavailability 50–60%; eliminated largely unchanged by renal tubular secretion (2–4 h)	Also available in combined formulations with pioglitazone, sitagliptin or vildagliptin
Meglitinides ('glinides')		
Given orally for the treatment of type 2 diabetes mellitus.		
Nateglinide	Oral bioavailability 70%; hepatic metabolism (1.5 h)	Given in combination with metformin when metformin alone is inadequate
Repaglinide	Oral bioavailability 60%; hepatic metabolism and faecal excretion (1 h)	Given alone, or in combination with metformin when metformin alone is inadequate

Compendium: drugs used in diabetes mellitus—cont'd

Drug	Kinetics (half-life)	Comments
Thiazolidinedione ('glitazone')		
Given orally for the treatment of type 2 diabetes mellitus.		
Pioglitazone	Rapidly absorbed; P450 metabolism (3–7 h) to long-lived active metabolites (16–24 h)	Used alone or in combination with metformin or a sulfonylurea or both
Other hypoglycaemics		
Acarbose	Negligible oral absorption (1–2%); absorbed fraction is renally excreted (3 h)	Glucosidase inhibitor, delays glucose absorption from gut; given orally for diabetes mellitus inadequately controlled by diet with or without other hypoglycaemic drugs
Dapagliflozin	Oral bioavailability 78%; hepatic metabolism to inactive products (13 h)	Inhibitor of sodium-glucose co-transporter 2 (SGLT2); reduces glucose reabsorption in renal tubule
Exenatide	Filtered in the glomerulus and metabolised in the kidney (2.4 h)	Synthetic incretin mimetic; given by subcutaneous injection with metformin or a sulfonylurea, or both, or with pioglitazone, or with both metformin and pioglitazone
Guar gum	Not absorbed	Given orally; acts in gut lumen to reduce glucose absorption
Linagliptin	Oral absorption 30%; mainly excreted unchanged in faeces (12 h)	DPP-4 inhibitor; given orally if metformin inappropiate, or with metformin, or with metformin and a sulfonylurea
Liraglutide	Subcutaneous bioavailability 55%; eliminated by proteolysis (11–15 h)	Synthetic incretin mimetic; given by subcutaneous injection; used with metformin or a sulfonylurea, or both, or with pioglitazone, or with both metformin and pioglitazone
Saxagliptin	Rapidly absorbed; hepatic P450 metabolism, with mainly renal elimination of parent drug and an active metabolite (2.5–3 h)	DPP-4 inhibitor; given orally with metformin or a sulfonylurea (if metformin inappropriate) or with pioglitazone
Sitagliptin	High oral bioavailability (87%); mostly excreted unchanged by renal tubular secretion (12 h)	DPP-4 inhibitor; given orally as monotherapy (if metformin inappropriate), or with metformin or a sulfonylurea, or with metformin and pioglitazone
Vildagliptin	Oral bioavailability 85%; hydrolysed in liver and kidney (3 h)	DPP-4 inhibitor; given orally with metformin or a sulfonylurea (if metformin inappropriate) or with pioglitazone
Treatment of hypoglycaemia		
Glucagon	Proteolysed rapidly by liver and kidneys (5–10 min)	Used for acute insulin-induced hypoglycaemia (*not* for chronic hypoglycaemia); given by subcutaneous, intramuscular or intravenous injection

DPP-4, dipeptidyl peptidase 4.

The thyroid and control of metabolic rate

THYROID FUNCTION

The main functions of thyroid hormones are the control of metabolism, growth and development. The term 'basal metabolism' refers to the energy-utilising biochemical processes of the body at rest. Basal metabolic rate is controlled by thyroid hormones, which stimulate tissue oxygen consumption and regulate energy and heat production, mainly through an increase in the metabolism of fats, carbohydrates and proteins. Most of these functions are a result of thyroid hormones acting in combination with other hormones such as insulin. Thyroid hormones have a thermogenic action on brown fat in infants, increasing synthesis of uncoupling proteins that divert the energy released during lipolysis into heat rather than high-energy phosphate synthesis. They also promote gluconeogenesis, obtaining the substrate for glucose formation from amino acids in tissues such as muscle and bone. Thyroid hormones facilitate the development of the nervous system, somatic growth (synergistically with growth hormone) and puberty. They also regulate the synthesis of proteins involved in hepatic, cardiac, neurological and muscular functions. Thyroid hormones increase the body's sensitivity to catecholamines, and therefore to sympathetic nervous system activation, in particular enhancing the effects of β-adrenoceptor stimulation (Ch. 4).

There are two thyroid hormones: triiodothyronine (T_3) and thyroxine (T_4). T_3 is mainly responsible for effects at a cellular level, while T_4 is now considered to be a prohormone. T_3 and T_4 are synthesised in the thyroid gland (Fig. 41.1), where inorganic iodide is trapped with great avidity by an enzyme-dependent process. The iodide is then oxidised to iodine by thyroid peroxidase. Iodine is very reactive and attaches to tyrosine (as tyrosyl residues of the glycoprotein thyroglobulin) to form mono-iodotyrosine and di-iodotyrosine residues. Two di-iodinated tyrosine molecules are conjugated to form T_4, and one di-iodinated molecule with one mono-iodinated tyrosine molecule conjugate to form T_3 (Fig. 41.1). Proteolytic enzymes from thyroid lysosomes then degrade thyroglobulin and release thyroid hormone into the circulation.

The synthesis and release of thyroid hormones are controlled by the anterior pituitary hormone thyrotropin (thyroid-stimulating hormone, TSH). This in turn is controlled by the hypothalamus, which secretes thyrotropin-releasing hormone (TRH). Circulating T_3 and T_4 exert negative feedback on both the hypothalamic and pituitary hormones (Fig. 41.2).

The thyroid secretes mainly T_4 and a small amount of T_3. Circulating thyroid hormones are highly protein-bound, mostly to thyroxine-binding globulin (TBG). Less than 0.03% of T_4 and less than 0.3% of T_3 circulate unbound and only this free fraction of hormone is available to bind to specific intracellular receptors. Most T_3 is derived from peripheral deiodination of T_4 by iodothyronine deiodinase, which is found in the liver, kidney, brain and brown adipose tissue. About 35% of T_4 is converted to T_3, while about 40% is converted to reverse T_3 (a metabolically inactive isomer of T_3). T_3 has a half-life in the circulation of about 1.5 days compared with about 7 days for T_4. Elimination of T_3 and T_4 is by conjugation, mainly in the liver.

Thyroid hormones cross cell membranes via active transporters and bind to intracellular thyroid hormone receptors (or TRs) (Ch. 1), which belong to the superfamily of nuclear receptors. Thyroid hormone receptors usually repress target genes but, following thyroid hormone binding, the complex recruits co-activators and regulates gene transcription via thyroid response elements. Thyroid hormone receptors are expressed in most tissues, but there are three isoforms which differ in their tissue distribution and may mediate different effects of thyroid hormones. T_3 also has non-genomic actions that include stimulation of cellular uptake of amino acids and glucose, and interactions with G-protein-coupled membrane receptors with activation of phosphatidylinositol 3-kinase and mitogen-activated protein kinase (MAPK) pathways.

HYPERTHYROIDISM

The commonest form of hyperthyroidism (often, and interchangeably, called thyrotoxicosis) is Graves' disease, an autoimmune condition in which thyroid-stimulating immunoglobulin binds to thyrotropin (TSH) receptors on thyroid cells and initiates signal transduction. This is often accompanied by an immunologically mediated inflammatory reaction in the extrinsic muscles and fat of the orbit, causing swelling and the characteristic exophthalmos. Toxic multinodular goitre, thyroid adenomas (toxic or 'hot' nodules) and various forms of thyroiditis are much less common causes of hyperthyroidism. Rarely, the condition arises from excess production of thyrotropin or it can be induced by

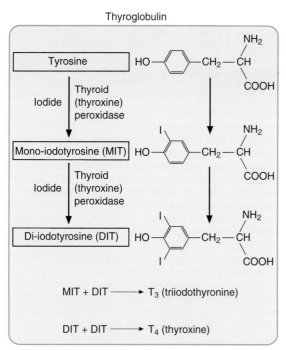

Thyroglobulin

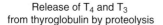

MIT + DIT ⟶ T₃ (triiodothyronine)

DIT + DIT ⟶ T₄ (thyroxine)

Release of T₄ and T₃
from thyroglobulin by proteolysis

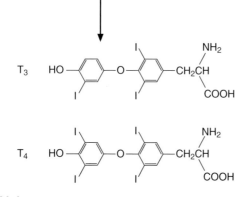

Fig. 41.1 **The synthesis of thyroid hormones.**
Iodide is oxidised to iodine by thyroid peroxidase and
incorporated into tyrosine residues of thyroglobulin, the
colloidal substance that fills the lumen of the thyroid
follicles. Conjugation of mono-iodotyrosine (MIT) and
di-iodotyrosine (DIT) residues into T3, or of two DIT
residues to form T4, is followed by the release of T3
and T4 when thyroglobulin is proteolysed.

treatment with amiodarone (Ch. 8). Symptoms of hyperthyroidism include weight loss, palpitation, sweating, fatigue,
nervousness, heat sensitivity and tremor. These are in part
mediated by the action of excess thyroid hormone, and
partly by excess sensitivity of tissues to β-adrenoceptor
stimulation. Signs are often less marked in the elderly, who
are more likely to present with atrial fibrillation that is resistant to treatment.

DRUGS FOR TREATMENT OF HYPERTHYROIDISM

Thionamides

Examples

carbimazole, propylthiouracil

Mechanism of action

Thionamides inhibit thyroid peroxidase and, therefore, the
synthesis of thyroid hormone (Fig. 41.2). The long half-life
of T₄ means that changes in the rate of synthesis take 4–6
weeks to lower circulating T₄ and T₃ concentrations to
within the normal range. These drugs also appear to have
an immunosuppressant effect in individuals with autoimmune thyroid disease. They reduce the levels of thyroid-
stimulating immunoglobulin, although the clinical importance
of this is uncertain. Large doses of propylthiouracil also
decrease peripheral conversion of T₄ to T₃.

Pharmacokinetics

Carbimazole is converted by first-pass metabolism to the
active derivative methimazole. Propylthiouracil has about
one-tenth of the activity of methimazole and a shorter half-
life; it is usually reserved for individuals intolerant to carbimazole. Both drugs accumulate in the thyroid, which
extends their duration of action.

Unwanted effects

- Gastrointestinal upset (especially nausea and epigastric
  discomfort), headache, arthralgia and pruritic rashes are
  common in the first 8 weeks of treatment.
- Allergic reactions, including vasculitis, a lupus-like syndrome, myopathy, cholestatic jaundice and nephritis.
  Some cross-sensitivity occurs between carbimazole and
  propylthiouracil.
- Bone marrow suppression, especially agranulocytosis,
  is an important unwanted effect and is more common
  with propylthiouracil than with carbimazole. A severe
  sore throat with fever is often the presenting complaint,
  and the occurrence of this, or any other infection, should
  be immediately reported to a doctor. The onset of agranulocytosis is sudden, and probably immunologically
  mediated, so that routine blood counts are unhelpful for
  monitoring. The blood count usually recovers about 3
  weeks after drug withdrawal.
- Placental transfer of the active metabolite of carbimazole can produce neonatal hypothyroidism, but propylthiouracil does not transfer in large enough quantities
  to cause problems. However, in Graves' disease the
  thyroid-stimulating antibody crosses the placenta and
  causes fetal thyrotoxicosis; therefore, carbimazole is the
  treatment of choice for maternal Graves' disease. Carbimazole is secreted in breast milk but rarely produces
  hypothyroidism in the infant.

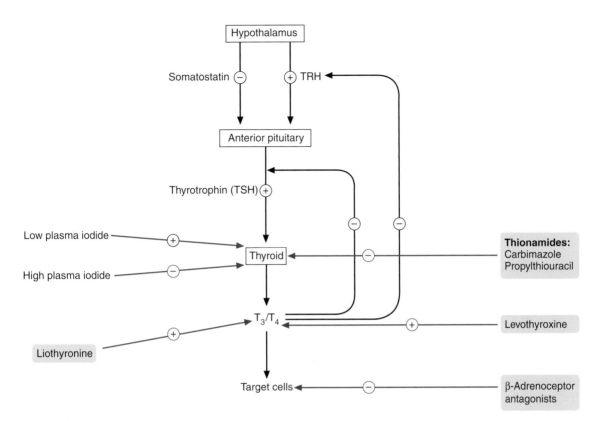

Fig. 41.2 **Control of thyroid hormone synthesis and release.** Thyrotropin (thyroid-stimulating hormone, TSH) and thyrotropin-releasing hormone (TRH) are inhibited by circulating levels of T_3 and T_4. The sites of action of drugs acting on thyroid pathways are also shown.

MANAGEMENT OF HYPERTHYROIDISM

Graves' disease

Carbimazole is the drug of choice for Graves' hyperthyroidism, and will usually decrease the thyroid hormone concentration to normal levels over 4–8 weeks. It is usual to start treatment with a high dosage unless the thyrotoxicosis is mild, when smaller initial doses may be more appropriate. Once the thyroid hormone concentration is normal, the dosage is then gradually reduced every 4–6 weeks to reach the lowest possible dose that controls the serum T_4. Initially treatment should be continued for 12–18 months, after which the dose can be tapered or treatment withdrawn. Occasionally, a block–replace regimen is used, giving a high dosage of carbimazole in conjunction with thyroxine replacement for 6–12 months. This maintains normal thyroid function regardless of the dose of carbimazole.

A β-adrenoceptor antagonist (especially propranolol because of its non-selective action; Ch. 5) is particularly useful for symptomatic relief from tremor, anxiety or palpitation during the early period of treatment with carbimazole. It has immediate effects on symptoms but does not alter the rate of thyroid hormone synthesis or secretion.

Exophthalmos associated with Graves' disease usually responds poorly to treatment with antithyroid drugs, since it is caused by TSH receptor antibody. Severe thyroid eye disease can be helped by treatment with oral prednisolone if antithyroid treatment is not improving the condition.

Approximately 50% of people with Graves' disease have a single episode that is cured by drug treatment (spontaneous remission). Those who relapse will usually do so within 6 months, and thereafter repeat relapses are common. Most are then offered definitive treatment by either a subtotal thyroidectomy (for a large goitre) or a therapeutic dose of radioactive iodine (^{131}I).

Radioiodine can be used as first-line treatment for Graves' disease or for relapse after antithyroid drug treatment. Radioiodine can make thyroid ophthalmopathy worse, but this can be prevented by treatment with a corticosteroid such as prednisolone for 2–3 months. Before radioiodine treatment it is often recommended that the thyrotoxicosis should be stabilised with carbimazole. This reduces the risk of exacerbation of hyperthyroidism from radiation thyroiditis immediately after isotope treatment. However, antithyroid drug treatment must be stopped 3–5 days before radioactive iodine is given or it will prevent uptake of the radioiodine by the thyroid cells. A β-adrenoceptor antagonist can be useful in this period to prevent symptomatic relapse. Carbimazole can be restarted 2–4 days after radioiodine, to cover the period of up to 8 weeks before radioiodine is fully effective. Between 10 and 20% of individuals will require a second dose of radioiodine to achieve euthyroid status. Permanent hypothyroidism can

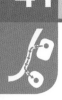

occur following radioiodine treatment. The incidence of hypothyroidism is related to the initial dose of radioactivity up to 1 year after treatment; thereafter, the risk is 2–3% annually. The theoretical increase in risk of cancer or leukaemia following radioiodine treatment has not been substantiated in clinical studies.

Surgery in Graves' disease is used if there is a poor response to antithyroid drugs, a very large goitre, for coexisting thyroid malignancy or if the person expresses a preference for this treatment. Before surgery, carbimazole is usually used to achieve a euthyroid state. If the thyrotoxicosis is drug-resistant then oral potassium iodide can be used for up to 2 weeks before surgery to inhibit thyroxine synthesis and release and to reduce the vascularity of the hyperplastic thyroid gland. Hypothyroidism, often delayed by several months or years, is common after surgery.

Toxic nodular goitre

Radioiodine is also used for toxic multinodular goitre. A solitary toxic thyroid nodule can be removed surgically, but radioactive iodine is extremely effective, because the isotope is taken up only by the abnormal tissue (the remainder is suppressed by the absence of thyrotropin in the circulation). Carbimazole is unsuitable as sole treatment for these conditions, since spontaneous remission does not occur. However, some elderly people may choose to continue treatment with carbimazole for life.

Amiodarone-induced thyrotoxicosis

Treatment of amiodarone-induced thyrotoxicosis (Ch. 8) depends on the clinical subtype. Type 1 is provoked in people with an underlying multinodular goitre by the iodide contained in the drug, and responds to antithyroid drug treatment. Type 2 is an inflammatory thyrotoxicosis that arises from a direct toxic effect of the drug on the gland, and responds well to treatment with a corticosteroid.

HYPOTHYROIDISM

Hypothyroidism is usually caused by primary thyroid failure, and the low circulating T_4 concentration is accompanied by a raised plasma thyrotropin (TSH) concentration. Autoimmune thyroiditis is the commonest cause, but hypothyroidism is occasionally congenital or can follow treatment for hyperthyroidism by surgery or radioiodine. Rarely, hypothyroidism can be secondary to pituitary or hypothalamic failure, when the circulating TSH concentrations will be low. Drug therapy with lithium (Ch. 22) or amiodarone (Ch. 8) can produce hypothyroidism.

Typical symptoms of hypothyroidism in an adult are non-specific and include lethargy, slowing of mental processes, cold intolerance, dry skin, hoarseness, weight gain, constipation and menorrhagia. Severe hypothyroidism (myxoedema) produces marked coarsening of the facial appearance and may ultimately lead to a hypothermic, comatose state. In children, hypothyroidism stunts mental and physical development, resulting in a condition known as cretinism.

MANAGEMENT OF HYPOTHYROIDISM

Standard treatment is with oral levothyroxine (T_4). Although its absorption is incomplete and variable, sufficient T_3 will be formed by peripheral deiodination of T_4. The proportion of circulating T_3 is usually lower than normal, so circulating levels of T_4 will often need to be higher than those in healthy individuals in order to obtain a satisfactory response. In some people, particularly those with ischaemic heart disease, a rapid increase in metabolic activity with levothyroxine replacement can cause excessive cardiac stimulation, and therefore levothyroxine should be introduced gradually in those at risk of cardiac complications. In others, the anticipated weight-related maintenance dose can be given from the start. Because of its long half-life, steady-state plasma concentrations of levothyroxine will not be achieved with constant dosage for 4–5 weeks. The adequacy of levothyroxine replacement therapy is best monitored by measurement of the serum TSH concentration 4–6 weeks after a change in levothyroxine dose. The TSH concentration should be in the lower third of the normal range, and then the plasma T_4 will usually be slightly high or in the upper part of the normal range. Once the dose of levothyroxine is correct an annual check of serum TSH is sufficient, unless there are symptoms suggesting hypo- or hyperthyroidism. When the hypothyroidism is caused by drug treatment the precipitating drug can be continued while levothyroxine is given. Problems with thyroid-replacement preparations are uncommon unless excessive doses are used, but allergic reactions have been reported, and transient scalp hair loss can occur in the first few weeks of treatment.

Some drugs interfere with the absorption of levothyroxine from the gut. These include iron, calcium carbonate, mineral supplements, colestyramine (Ch. 48) and sucralfate (Ch. 33). The metabolism of levothyroxine is accelerated by the concurrent use of the hepatic enzyme-inducing drugs phenobarbital, phenytoin, carbamazepine (Ch. 23) and rifampicin (Ch. 51). The therapeutic response to levothyroxine may be impaired in all of these situations.

Liothyronine (T_3) is usually reserved for intravenous use in severe hypothyroidism (myxoedema coma), when its potency, more rapid effect and shorter half-life allow more rapid attainment of a therapeutic blood concentration. However, even in this situation a large dose of levothyroxine has been successfully used, and may be associated with a lower mortality. An oral formulation of liothyronine is also available for rapid response in severe hypothyroid states.

SELF-ASSESSMENT

True/false questions

1. Secretion of triiodothyronine (T_3) and thyroxine (T_4) is controlled by anterior pituitary and hypothalamic hormones.
2. Circulating T_3 and T_4 are highly bound to plasma albumin.
3. T_4 has a long residence time in the body.
4. At target cells, T_4 is converted to T_3, which then binds to specific nuclear receptors.

5. Hyperthyroidism will be made worse by iodine administration.
6. Severe hypothyroidism causes cretinism in children.
7. Therapy with ^{131}I can cause hypothyroidism.
8. Propylthiouracil is the drug of choice for Graves' disease.
9. Hypothyroidism is treated with levothyroxine.
10. Liothyronine is used in myxoedema coma.

One-best-answer (OBA) questions

1. Choose the *incorrect* statement below about the treatment of thyrotoxicosis with carbimazole.
    A. Carbimazole takes several weeks to reduce circulating T_4 and T_3 to normal concentrations.
    B. Carbimazole is a prodrug.
    C. Carbimazole may cause bone marrow suppression.
    D. Carbimazole inhibits the stimulant action of thyrotropin on the thyroid.
    E. Carbimazole has a long duration of action.
2. Choose the *correct* statement below about hypothyroidism and its treatment.
    A. Low circulating T_4 levels in hypothyroidism are accompanied by low levels of thyrotropin.
    B. Hepatic enzyme-inducing drugs reduce the response to levothyroxine.
    C. During regular dosing, steady-state plasma levels of levothyroxine are reached within 7 days.
    D. No precautions are required when prescribing levothyroxine in a person with hypothyroidism who also has ischaemic heart disease.
    E. Oxygen consumption in metabolically active tissues is unaffected by levothyroxine.

Case-based questions

A 45-year-old man suffered from weight loss, palpitations, tremor, anxiety and sweating, plus eyelid retraction and orbital and ocular inflammation. Blood tests showed increased levels of free and bound T_3 and T_4 and suppressed TSH. A diagnosis of Graves' thyrotoxicosis was made. An electrocardiogram showed atrial fibrillation.

A. What is Graves' disease?
B. What other blood tests could be performed to confirm this diagnosis?
C. How could the symptoms be controlled?
D. What drug could be given to control the hyperthyroidism?
E. With treatment, he became euthyroid, but relapsed in the following year. A decision was made to treat him with ^{131}I.
    What treatment should be given before administering the ^{131}I and what are the reasons for this?
F. How long after treatment will benefit be seen?

True/false answers

1. **True.** T_3 and T_4 synthesis and release are controlled by thyrotropin-releasing hormone (TRH) and somatostatin from the hypothalamus, by thyrotropin (thyrotropin-stimulating hormone, TSH) from the anterior pituitary, and by plasma iodide.
2. **False.** T_3 and T_4 in the plasma are largely bound to thyroxine-binding globulin (TBG), which should not be confused with thyroglobulin in the thyroid gland.
3. **True.** Thyroxine has a half-life of about 7 days.
4. **True.** The complex of T_3 and thyroid hormone receptor (TR) activates gene transcription and protein synthesis.
5. **False.** Iodine is converted to iodide and inhibits T_3 and T_4 release.
6. **True.** Severe hypothyroidism causes myxoedema in adults and cretinism in children.
7. **True.** Permanent hypothyroidism can occur after radio-iodine treatment.
8. **False.** Propylthiouracil is usually reserved for people intolerant to carbimazole.
9. **True.** Oral levothyroxine is the standard treatment.
10. **True.** Liothyronine (T_3) is more potent and has a more rapid effect than levothyroxine, so is given intravenously in severe hypothyroidism (myxoedema coma)

OBA answers

1. **Answer D** is the incorrect statement.
    A. Correct. The long half-life of T_4 (about 7 days) means that carbimazole takes 5–6 weeks to reduce thyroid hormone levels to normal.
    B. Correct. The active metabolite of carbimazole is methimazole.
    C. Correct. Bone marrow suppression is a serious unwanted effect of carbimazole; it can be indicated by infection, especially fever and a severe sore throat.
    D. **Incorrect**. Carbimazole inhibits the liberation of iodine by thyroid peroxidase.
    E. Correct. Carbimazole accumulates in the thyroid and is given only once daily.
2. **Answer B** is correct.
    A. Incorrect. If T_4 levels were low, then thyrotropin levels would be raised, as the negative-feedback effect of T_4 on thyrotropin release would be reduced.
    B. **Correct**. Hepatic metabolism of levothyroxine is accelerated by cytochrome P450 inducers such as phenobarbitone and phenytoin.
    C. Incorrect. The half-life of levothyroxine is 6–7 days; therefore, the steady state would not be reached until 5–7 weeks of administration.
    D. Incorrect. Special care is required in ischaemic heart disease as a rapid increase in metabolic activity can cause excessive heart stimulation.
    E. Incorrect. Levothyroxine stimulates oxygen consumption in metabolically active tissues.

Case-based answers

A. Graves' disease is an autoimmune disease in which antibodies to TSH are generated which bind to and activate TSH receptors in the thyroid, promoting thyroid hormone release.

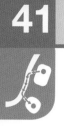

B. Thyrotropin (TSH) concentration could be measured. It will be low, due to the negative feedback effect of elevated T_3 and T_4.

C. Drugs of choice for controlling symptoms are β-adrenoceptor antagonists, although they do not improve fatigue and muscle weakness. Propranolol should also control a high ventricular rate due to the atrial fibrillation (Ch. 8) and anticoagulation with warfarin to prevent thromboembolism, which has an increased incidence in people with both atrial fibrillation and thyrotoxicosis.

D. Carbimazole is the drug of choice, given in a high dose, reducing over 4–6 weeks.

E. The clinical state should be stabilised with carbimazole and a β-adrenoceptor antagonist. Carbimazole is stopped 3–4 days before radioiodine is given, as it can prevent the uptake of iodine by thyroid cells.

F. It can take several months for the maximum benefit of ^{131}I to occur.

FURTHER READING

Brent GA (2008) Graves disease. *N Engl J Med* 358, 2594–2605

Pearce EN (2006) Diagnosis and management of thyrotoxicosis. *BMJ* 332, 1369–1373

Roberts CGP, Ladenson PW (2004) Hypothyroidism. *Lancet* 363, 793–803

Toft AD (2001) Subclinical hyperthyroidism. *N Engl J Med* 345, 512–516

Compendium: thyroid and antithyroid drugs

Drug	Kinetics (half-life)	Comments
Thyroid hormones		
Levothyroxine/thyroxine (T_4)	Oral bioavailability 50–80%; deiodinated in peripheral tissues to T_3 (6–7 days)	Treatment of choice for maintenance therapy; given orally
Liothyronine (L-triiodothyronine) (T_3)	Almost complete oral bioavailability; deiodination and hepatic conjugation (1–2 days)	More rapid onset of action than levothyroxine; given orally, or by slow intravenous injection for hypothyroid coma
Antithyroid drugs		
All drugs given orally once daily because of their long-duration effects on the thyroid. Beta-adrenoceptor antagonists such as propranolol (Ch. 5) can be used to treat the symptoms of thyrotoxicosis.		
Carbimazole	Complete absorption; presystemic metabolism to active methimazole; hepatic metabolism (3–5 h)	Thyroid peroxidase inhibitor; treatment of choice for Grave's hyperthyroidism
Iodine and potassium iodide	Complete oral absorption; incorporated into thyroid hormones; excreted largely in urine	Used as an adjunct to antithyroid drugs for 10–14 days before partial thyroidectomy, but should not be given for long-term treatment
Propylthiouracil	Bioavailability 50–75% due to poor absorption; hepatic glucuronidation (1–3 h)	Thyroid peroxidase inhibitor; used in people intolerant to carbimazole

42 Calcium metabolism and metabolic bone disease

REGULATION OF CALCIUM METABOLISM

Calcium ions play a part in a large number of cellular activities, including stimulus–response coupling in striated and smooth muscle, and in endocrine and exocrine glands. Calcium modulates the actions of intracellular cAMP and is a cofactor for numerous intracellular enzymes and for blood clotting. However, more than 98% of Ca^{2+} in the body is in the form of hydroxyapatite crystals deposited on the protein matrix of bone, which provides its mechanical strength.

Calcium circulates in plasma partly bound to protein (approximately 50%) and the rest in the free ionised (and therefore 'active') form. The free fraction in plasma is maintained precisely within narrow limits principally by the actions of parathyroid hormone (PTH) and 1,25-dihydroxyvitamin D_3 (calcitriol). Calcitonin secretion (see below) also reacts to changing plasma Ca^{2+} concentrations but it is less important in overall control of Ca^{2+} homeostasis. Calcium in plasma is in dynamic exchange with Ca^{2+} in the gut, renal tubules and bone. This is illustrated with the main controlling factors in Figure 42.1.

PTH is a polypeptide hormone which is the main physiological regulator of Ca^{2+} in blood. Its secretion from parathyroid chief cells is stimulated by a reduction of ionised Ca^{2+} in plasma. PTH secretion is inhibited when the plasma Ca^{2+} concentration rises.

The main actions of PTH relating to calcium homeostasis are:

- stimulation of the synthesis of the biologically active form of vitamin D (calcitriol) in the kidney by upregulation of the enzyme responsible for 1α-hydroxylation,
- enhanced reabsorption of Ca^{2+} from the kidney distal tubules and enhancement of urinary phosphate excretion. The rise in plasma Ca^{2+}/phosphate ratio also increases plasma free Ca^{2+},
- mobilisation of Ca^{2+} and phosphate from bone through stimulation of osteoclasts, which increases bone resorption. Osteoclasts do not have a receptor for PTH. PTH binds to osteoblasts and increases their expression of the surface molecule human receptor activator of nuclear factor-κB ligand (RANKL) and inhibits their expression of the surface receptor osteoprotegerin. Osteoprotegerin is the natural inhibitor of osteoclast activity by acting as a decoy receptor for binding RANKL. RANKL that is not bound to osteoprotegerin interacts with and activates RANK on osteoclasts and stimulates differentiation of osteoclast precursors to mature osteoclasts.

The effect of PTH on the kidney occurs within minutes of PTH release, whereas that on bone begins after 1–2 h.

Vitamin D (calciferol) is a group of compounds that have secosteroid nuclei (a steroid nucleus with one bond in the steroid ring broken). There are two precursors of active vitamin D. Ergocalciferol (vitamin D_2) is derived from food and absorbed from the gut. However, given adequate ultraviolet B sunlight, the major source of vitamin D is conversion of 7-dehydrocholesterol in the skin to cholecalciferol (vitamin D_3). Therefore, vitamin D is really a skin-derived hormone rather than a vitamin but this source was discovered after the dietary origins. Vitamins D_2 and D_3 are further metabolised in the liver to 25-hydroxyvitamin D_3 (calcidiol), and then in the kidney to 1,25-dihydroxyvitamin D_3 (calcitriol). 1α-Hydroxylation is an essential step for activation of vitamin D, and PTH stimulates 1α-hydroxylase activity in the kidney, increasing the formation of calcitriol. Calcitriol binds to specific vitamin D receptors in the target cell nucleus (Ch. 1) and the vitamin D–receptor complex acts as a transcription factor that increases the synthesis of Ca^{2+} transport proteins in the gut. The main effect of active forms of vitamin D is to increase the plasma concentration of Ca^{2+} by:

- facilitating absorption of Ca^{2+} from the small intestine,
- enhancing Ca^{2+} mobilisation from bone by increasing osteoclastic numbers and activity

In the kidney, vitamin D promotes phosphate retention, in contrast to the action of PTH. Therefore, vitamin D maintains the plasma Ca^{2+} and phosphate concentrations to allow normal osteoblast function. These actions of vitamin D affect Ca^{2+} turnover in bone over periods of days to weeks.

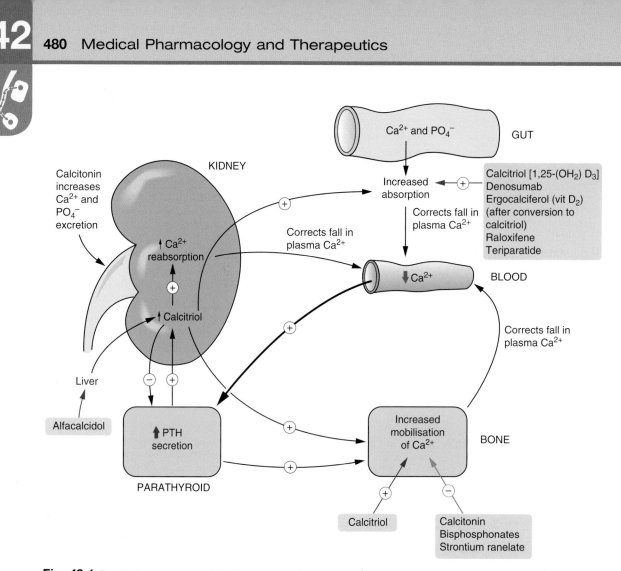

Fig. 42.1 Regulation of calcium metabolism. A fall in plasma Ca^{2+} leads to increased release of parathyroid hormone (PTH) from the parathyroid gland, which increases calcitriol [1,25-(OH_2)-D_3] formation in the kidney. This in turn increases gut absorption of Ca^{2+}. PTH further increases bone mobilisation of Ca^{2+} to return plasma Ca^{2+} to normal. An increase in plasma Ca^{2+}, conversely, decreases PTH secretion. Calcitonin, secreted by the thyroid, decreases Ca^{2+} reabsorption from the kidney and decreases bone turnover. Drugs used for hypercalcaemia are indicated by green arrows and drugs for hypocalcaemia by red arrows.

Calcitonin is a peptide secreted by the parafollicular cells of the thyroid when its calcium-sensing receptors detect a rise in plasma Ca^{2+}. The main target cell for calcitonin is the osteoclast, which it inhibits by stimulation of adenylyl cyclase, thus reducing bone turnover. Calcitonin also decreases Ca^{2+} and phosphate reabsorption by the kidney, thereby increasing their renal excretion.

PHYSIOLOGY OF BONE TURNOVER

Bone is constantly undergoing remodelling (bone turnover), which involves resorption and replacement of small areas of bone. Up to 10% of bone undergoes remodelling at any point in time, and trabecular bone (in the ends of long bones and in the vertebrae) undergoes greater turnover than cortical bone. Resorption leaves trenches on the bone surface and osteoclasts recruit osteoblasts to refill the trenches.

This process is essential for maintenance of Ca^{2+} homeostasis, replacement of apoptotic osteoclasts and repair of microfractures. There are many factors that regulate bone turnover, but the final pathway is via the balance between RANKL expressed by osteoblasts and activated T- and B-lymphocytes, and osteoprotegerin expressed by osteoblasts (see above). The balance between osteoblast and osteoclast activity and therefore the extent of bone remodelling is modulated by an interaction between various cells in the immune system (lymphocytes and dendritic cells), cytokines and circulating hormones.

HYPERCALCAEMIA

The main causes of hypercalcaemia are:

- increased resorption of Ca^{2+} from bone; for example, primary hyperparathyroidism, secretion of parathyroid-related hormone by cancer cells and bony metastases,

- increased absorption of Ca^{2+} from the gut through excessive use of vitamin D or in sarcoidosis,
- reduced renal excretion of Ca^{2+}; for example, as caused by thiazide diuretics (Ch. 14).

Hypercalcaemia occurs when the mobilisation of Ca^{2+} into the extracellular space exceeds the capacity to remove it. Chronic moderate hypercalcaemia leads to a progressive decline in renal function, formation of renal stones and ectopic calcification (e.g. cornea, blood vessels). Severe hypercalcaemia causes anorexia, nausea, vomiting, constipation, drowsiness and confusion, eventually leading to coma. Hypercalcaemia impairs the ability of the kidney to reabsorb salt and water which in conjunction with vomiting can lead to depletion of plasma volume and pre-renal failure. Urgent treatment is indicated when the plasma Ca^{2+} concentration rises above 3.5 mmol·L^{-1} (normal $<2.6 \text{ mmol·L}^{-1}$), since sudden death from cardiac arrest can occur.

ANTIRESORPTIVE DRUGS FOR HYPERCALCAEMIA

Bisphosphonates

 Examples

alendronic acid, disodium pamidronate, risedronate sodium, zoledronic acid

Mechanisms of action and effects

Bisphosphonates are pyrophosphate analogues that bind to hydroxyapatite crystals in bone matrix. They are preferentially deposited under osteoclasts, and are taken up by these cells and inhibit their resorptive action on bone. There are two different cellular actions of the drugs on osteoclasts, depending on the structure of the bisphosphonate.

- Amino-bisphosphonates (nitrogen-containing drugs: alendronic acid, disodium pamidronate, risedronate sodium, zoledronic acid) act by inhibition of the ATP-dependent enzyme farnesyl pyrophosphate synthase in the synthetic pathway from mevalonic acid to cholesterol; this reduces the production of lipids that are essential for signalling processes required for normal osteoclast function, and leads to impaired differentiation of osteoclast precursors, reduced ability of mature osteoclasts to reabsorb bone by altering the permeability of osteoclast membranes to small ions and, eventually, osteoclast apoptosis.
- Non-nitrogen-containing drugs (sodium clodronate, disodium etidronate) affect metabolism within the cell by forming a toxic analogue of ATP that induces osteoclast apoptosis. These drugs have a relatively weak antiresorptive action.

The actions of most bisphosphonates are relatively short-lived unless taken regularly, but zoledronic acid can suppress bone resorption for up to a year after a single dose.

Pharmacokinetics

Bisphosphonates are poorly absorbed from the gut, and oral formulations are best taken once weekly with the stomach empty to avoid binding by Ca^{2+} in food. Alendronic acid and risedronate sodium are only available in oral formulations while disodium pamidronate and zoledronic acid are only formulated for intravenous use. Removal of most bisphosphonates from blood via the kidney is rapid, but their effect is prolonged since a fraction remains tightly bound to Ca^{2+} in bone.

Unwanted effects

- Gastrointestinal disturbance, particularly nausea, abdominal pain, diarrhoea or constipation with the oral treatments.
- Headache, dizziness, musculoskeletal pain.
- Alendronic acid and risedronate sodium can cause severe oesophagitis and oesophageal strictures. To reduce the risk, the tablets should be swallowed intact with a full glass of water at least 30 min before food and followed by standing or sitting (but not lying down) for at least 30 min after ingestion. Once-weekly dosing also reduces the risk of oesophageal damage.
- Transient pyrexia and influenza-like symptoms after intravenous infusion.
- Osteonecrosis of the jaw, especially after intravenous use, and atypical femoral fractures.

Calcitonin

Mechanism of action and effects

The actions of calcitonin on bone and the kidney to reduce plasma Ca^{2+} concentrations have been discussed above. Calcitonin begins to act within a few hours of administration, with a maximum effect within 12–24 h. However, the hypocalcaemic effect produced by repeated administrations only lasts between 2 and 3 days. The loss of clinical response results from downregulation of calcitonin receptors on osteoclasts, leading to a rebound increase in bone resorption.

Pharmacokinetics

Salmon calcitonin (salcatonin) is usually given by intramuscular or subcutaneous injection, although intravenous infusion can be used. The half-life is very short (about 20 min) as it is degraded to inactive fragments in the plasma and the kidney.

Unwanted effects

- Facial flushing occurs in most people.
- Headache, dizziness.
- Nausea, vomiting, abdominal pain, diarrhoea.
- Taste disturbance.

TREATMENT OF HYPERCALCAEMIA

When possible, the primary cause should be corrected, for example removal of a parathyroid adenoma or treatment of myeloma. Oral Ca^{2+} supplements, vitamin D and thiazide diuretics should be discontinued. Additional measures may include correction of dehydration, enhancing renal excretion of Ca^{2+} and inhibiting bone resorption.

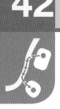

Most people with severe hypercalcaemia are fluid-depleted at presentation. Rehydration with intravenous isotonic saline is essential; this also promotes a sodium-linked Ca^{2+} diuresis in the proximal and distal renal tubules. Loop diuretics such as furosemide (Ch. 14) increase renal Ca^{2+} elimination but should only be given with high volumes of intravenous isotonic saline and intensive monitoring of fluid balance to avoid dehydration.

A bisphosphonate such as disodium pamidronate or zoledronic acid by intravenous infusion is the drug treatment of first choice for severe hypercalcaemia. Initial intravenous rehydration is essential to avoid precipitation of calcium bisphosphonate in the kidney. Oral bisphosphonate treatment may be sufficient for less severe hypercalcaemia. Following a single intravenous infusion of bisphosphonate the plasma Ca^{2+} concentration falls gradually after 2–4 days, with a maximum effect after 4–7 days and a response that persists for 1–4 weeks after treatment. Because of the delay in onset of action of the bisphosphonates, calcitonin can be given concurrently for an early effect. Corticosteroids such as prednisolone (Ch. 44) are effective for lowering plasma Ca^{2+} when vitamin D excess is an important factor, for example in sarcoidosis and for acute treatment of vitamin D overdose, or for hypercalcaemia associated with haematological malignancy such as myeloma or lymphoma. Corticosteroids probably act by reducing the effect of vitamin D on intestinal Ca^{2+} transport, but can take several days to work.

HYPOCALCAEMIA

There are two major underlying causes of hypocalcaemia:

- deficiency of PTH; for example, idiopathic hypoparathyroidism, after surgical parathyroid removal,
- deficiency of vitamin D; for example, dietary deficiency, limited exposure to sunlight, renal failure (failure of 1α-hydroxylation).

Hypocalcaemia produces neuromuscular irritability with paraesthesiae of the extremities or around the mouth, muscle cramps and tetany. When severe, it can produce seizures. Chronic hypocalcaemia, especially in congenital hypoparathyroidism, is associated with mental deficiency, seizures, intracranial calcification (e.g. choroid plexus) and ocular cataracts.

DRUGS FOR HYPOCALCAEMIA

Vitamin D compounds

alfacalcidol (1α-hydroxycholecalciferol), calcitriol (1,25-dihydroxyvitamin D_3 or 1,25-dihydroxycholecalciferol), ergocalciferol (vitamin D_2), paricalcitol

Mechanism of action

This is discussed above. A dose-related increase in Ca^{2+} and phosphate absorption from the gut occurs at lower concentrations of vitamin D than those which stimulate bone resorption. Ergocalciferol is inactive and can only be used if 1α-hydroxylation by the kidney is intact. In renal impairment, the hydroxylated active forms alfacalcidol or calcitriol should be used. Paricalcitol is a synthetic vitamin D analogue used in chronic renal failure; it binds to the vitamin D receptor and inhibits PTH synthesis and secretion, but has less effect than natural vitamin D on the plasma Ca^{2+} concentration.

Pharmacokinetics

The fat-soluble D vitamins are well absorbed orally in the presence of bile. They can also be given intravenously. Both alfacalcidol and calcitriol are active forms of vitamin D; they have short half-lives (about 3 h) and are metabolised and excreted mainly in the bile. Paricalcitol requires intravenous injection.

Unwanted effects

- Excessive dosing will produce hypercalcaemia.
- Excretion of vitamin D supplements in breast milk can cause hypercalcaemia in a suckling infant.

TREATMENT OF HYPOCALCAEMIA

Mild hypocalcaemia can be treated with oral Ca^{2+} supplements, taken between meals to avoid binding to dietary phosphate and oxalate which forms salts that are poorly absorbed. In the absence of reversible pathology such as malabsorption due to coeliac disease, the mainstay of treatment for more severe hypocalcaemia is vitamin D supplements. The few individuals who have vitamin D deficiency from inadequate diet or lack of exposure to sunlight (such as may be found in Asian women in the UK) will respond to small doses of vitamin D. Most causes of hypocalcaemia, however, require much larger doses (usually given as ergocalciferol) to maintain normocalcaemia. Oral Ca^{2+} supplements (as carbonate or citrate salts) are often used with vitamin D for the treatment of chronic hypocalcaemia.

For treatment of hypoparathyroidism, alfacalcidol is given; PTH is not used for replacement therapy (although PTH and a synthetic PTH fragment, teriparatide, are now licensed for treatment of osteoporosis; see below). Large doses of ergocalciferol could be used, but carry a risk of hypercalcaemia. The action of vitamin D begins after 2–4 weeks of treatment, because there is deficient renal hydroxylation of vitamin D in hypoparathyroidism; the action of calcitriol is much more rapid, beginning after 1–2 days, but it is rarely required unless a very rapid onset of action is necessary.

Acute severe hypocalcaemia (sometimes occurring after parathyroidectomy) must be treated with intravenous Ca^{2+} (as gluconate, gluceptate or chloride salt).

METABOLIC BONE DISEASE

OSTEOMALACIA

Osteomalacia is the bone disease resulting from failure of adequate bone mineralisation due to lack of vitamin D.

Bone pain is prominent and low plasma concentrations of Ca^{2+} and phosphate produce proximal muscle weakness. In developing children the bones become distorted (rickets). Treatment is with vitamin D (ergocalciferol) supplements, but it will take at least a year to achieve a normal bone structure.

SCREENING FOR VITAMIN D DEFICIENCY

Vitamin D deficiency is most common in people with pigmented skin. In adults there is an additional risk in the elderly who have less exposure to sunlight, obese people, those with malabsorption or renal disease, or those who take anticonvulsants, rifampicin or highly active antiretroviral drugs. The rising incidence of vitamin D deficiency in infants has led to a recommendation that vitamin D supplements should be routinely given to children under 5 years old. In adults who are at risk, deficiency of vitamin D is usually suspected from bone pain affecting the ribs, hips and pelvis together with proximal muscle weakness.

RENAL BONE DISEASE

Chronic renal disease is associated with deficient activation of vitamin D and hypocalcaemia. At the same time, reduced renal phosphate excretion leads to hyperphosphataemia. The low serum Ca^{2+} stimulates PTH secretion (secondary hyperparathyroidism) in an attempt to maintain the plasma Ca^{2+} concentration. The result is demineralisation of bone (renal bone disease) and soft tissue calcification from the increased plasma calcium–phosphorus product. Vascular calcification is associated with increased cardiovascular disease and mortality.

Treatment of renal bone disease requires a 1α-hydroxylated vitamin D derivative (such as alfacalcidol or calcitriol), which will increase plasma Ca^{2+} but does not affect the plasma phosphate. An oral non-Ca^{2+}-containing phosphate binder such as aluminium hydroxide is necessary to reduce the plasma phosphate concentration if this is raised to avoid tissue calcification. People who are undergoing haemodialysis or ambulatory peritoneal dialysis cannot readily excrete absorbed aluminium, and an alternative phosphate binder such as sevelamer or lanthanum is used. Despite the symptomatic benefit of vitamin D in renal disease there is little evidence for any improvement in long-term mortality.

OSTEOPOROSIS

Osteoporosis is the loss of bone mass due to reduced organic bone matrix and, consequently, mineral content, which decreases the mechanical strength of bone. It results from an imbalance between bone resorption and formation, and affects trabecular bone more than cortical bone. It is a natural and inevitable part of the ageing process (beginning from age 30–35 years), and in females a marked increase in bone loss occurs after the menopause. Other predisposing factors include smoking, heavy alcohol intake, malnutrition, malabsorption and lack of exercise. Osteoporosis in younger people is associated with trabecular bone loss and predisposes to spontaneous vertebral fractures. In older people, cortical bone is also lost, increasing the risk of low-impact traumatic fracture, particularly of the neck of the femur. Sometimes osteoporosis is secondary to other conditions such as myeloma or thyrotoxicosis or occurs as a result of prolonged corticosteroid therapy (Ch. 44).

The diagnosis of osteoporosis is usually made by estimating bone mineral density from dual-energy X-ray absorptiometry (DEXA) scanning. Bone mineral density is then compared to mean bone density in a young adult reference population, and a T-score calculated (standard deviations of bone mineral density from the mean of the reference population):

- T-score −1.0 or above is normal,
- T-score between −1.0 and −2.5 means 'low bone mass' (osteopenia),
- T-score −2.5 or below indicates osteoporosis.

Once established, osteoporosis is difficult to reverse, and emphasis should be placed on prevention where possible. Management of osteoporosis includes:

- non-pharmacological approaches, removing factors that increase the risk of demineralisation,
- the use of either antiresorptive therapies (with an associated decrease in markers of bone formation and bone resorption: bisphosphonates, raloxifene, oestrogen, denosumab) or,
- anabolic therapies that lay down new bone (with increases in markers of bone formation and bone resorption: calcitonin, teriparatide),
- supplementary vitamin D which increases the laying down of hydroxyapatite on bone collagen organic matrix,
- strontium ranelate, which does not conform to any of the above patterns of effect on bone metabolism (see below).

Prevention of osteoporosis

Preventive strategies are important in those identified as being at high risk of osteoporosis. Use of a prediction tool for calculating the risk of future fractures can help to target treatment. Early use of preventive treatments is important if prolonged corticosteroid treatment is planned (Ch. 44).

- **Oral calcium supplements** increase bone mineral density in the spine in postmenopausal women, but with an uncertain effect on the risk of vertebral fractures. The addition of vitamin D (ergocalciferol) confers greater benefit, with a reduction in the risk of non-vertebral fractures. Recently, concern has been raised that high-dose Ca^{2+} supplements may increase the risk of myocardial infarction, but any increase in risk is modest.
- **Oral bisphosphonates** (see above) are the treatment of choice for prevention of postmenopausal osteoporosis and corticosteroid-induced osteoporosis.
- **Hormone-replacement therapy (HRT)** with oestrogen (Ch. 45) in peri- and postmenopausal women was once the mainstay of preventative treatment for osteoporosis. However, 5–10 years of oestrogen therapy may be required and long-term use of HRT increases the risk of breast cancer and thromboembolic events. As a consequence, the use of HRT for this indication has declined.

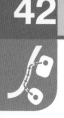

Treatments for established osteoporosis

The choice of treatment depends on the clinical circumstances. Pain relief is important if there are fractures, and salmon calcitonin given subcutaneously can aid pain relief when used for up to 3 months after a vertebral fracture. Drug treatment to prevent bone loss can reduce the risk of further fractures by up to 50%. Options include the following.

- **Oral bisphosphonates** increase bone density, with the best evidence in postmenopausal women. Alendronic acid and risedronate sodium have been shown to reduce hip, vertebral and wrist fractures. Bisphosphonates are also first-line treatment for the management of corticosteroid-induced osteoporosis. If there has been a good response in bone mineral density after 5 years then treatment is usually stopped for 3–5 years while monitoring markers of bone turnover. Such a strategy does not increase the risk of subsequent fractures. Intravenous bisphosphonates such as zoledronic acid once a year or ibandronic acid every 3 months are used when oral treatment is poorly tolerated.
- **Raloxifene** is a selective oestrogen receptor (ER) modulator. It binds to both types of oestrogen receptor (ERα and ERβ; Ch. 45) and is a partial agonist of ERα (which acts as a gene activator) but also an antagonist of ERβ by recruiting co-repressor molecules (which suppresses genes). The distribution of the two receptors may explain the tissue specificity of raloxifene, which has oestrogen receptor agonist effects on bone and lipids (reducing low-density lipoprotein [LDL] cholesterol) but acts as an anti-oestrogen on the breast and endometrium (Ch. 45). Raloxifene reduces the risk of oestrogen receptor-positive breast cancer in postmenopausal women by 75%, but its effects on pre-existing breast cancer are unknown. It does not affect menopausal vasomotor symptoms. Raloxifene reduces the risk of vertebral fractures by 40%, but has no effect on non-vertebral fractures, which may reflect the tissue distribution of oestrogen receptor subtypes. It is recommended for women who have had a vertebral fragility fracture who cannot take a bisphosphonate, or who have a fragility fracture after at least 1 year of treatment with a bisphosphonate. Unwanted effects include hot flushes and leg cramps. In addition, raloxifene doubles the risk of venous thromboembolism, particularly during the first 4 months of treatment.
- **Teriparatide** is a synthetic recombinant fraction of PTH (amino acids 1–34) that is used for the treatment of postmenopausal osteoporosis. It is given daily by subcutaneous injection. The most common unwanted effects are nausea, oesophageal reflux, postural hypotension, dyspnoea, depression and dizziness. It is recommended for postmenopausal women who cannot tolerate a bisphosphonate. There is also evidence that it is effective for osteoporosis treatment in men, and corticosteroid-induced osteoporosis. Human recombinant PTH can also be given by subcutaneous injection.
- **Strontium ranelate** is preferentially taken up by trabecular bone and incorporated into bone in the same way as Ca^{2+}. It stimulates osteoblast activity and inhibits osteoclast differentiation and resorptive activity. Strontium ranelate reduces the risk of both hip and vertebral fractures. The pattern of bone remodelling, with increases in markers of bone formation and a decrease in bone resorption, differs from that seen with both antiresorptive and anabolic therapies. Unwanted effects include nausea, diarrhoea, headache and rashes. Strontium ranelate is recommended for use in postmenopausal women who cannot tolerate a bisphosphonate, and may be the first-choice treatment for women older than 80 years.
- **Denosumab** is a human monoclonal antibody which binds specifically to RANKL and prevents activation of the RANK receptor found on osteoclasts and their precursors. As a result, formation of osteoclasts is reduced, their function is inhibited and their survival reduced. Resorption of both cortical and trabecular bone is decreased, and denosumab reduces both vertebral and non-vertebral fractures with a greater efficacy than oral bisphosphonates in postmenopausal women. Denosumab is also effective for treatment of osteoporosis in men taking androgen-depletion therapy for prostate cancer. Denosumab has a very long half-life of about 26 days and is given subcutaneously twice a year. Unwanted effects include diarrhoea, constipation, dyspnoea, increased frequency of urinary tract and upper respiratory tract infections, limb pains, sciatica, hypocalcaemia, hypophosphataemia, rash, sweating and cataracts.
- **Calcitriol** is used when bisphosphonates are unsuitable, and is given for postmenopausal and corticosteroid-induced osteoporosis.
- **Testosterone** (Ch. 46) is sometimes used for prophylaxis and treatment of corticosteroid-induced osteoporosis in men.

PAGET'S DISEASE OF BONE

Paget's disease of bone is a disturbance of bone remodelling characterised by both excessive bone reabsorption by osteoclasts and an increase in formation of poor-quality bone. The new bone matrix is non-lamellar woven bone (haphazard organization of the collagen matrix due to rapid bone formation) with areas of osteosclerosis, leaving bone that is structurally weakened. Paget's disease mainly affects the skull and long bones. The aetiology is unknown but there is a genetic predisposition and a slow virus infection may initiate the disease.

About a third of pagetic bone lesions are asymptomatic, but the remainder can produce bone pain and deformity, nerve entrapment and pathological fractures. Active treatment should be given if symptoms are present or a risk of complications is identified. Apart from symptomatic measures such as analgesics, two main treatments are used, as follows.

- **Bisphosphonates** are effective by inhibiting bone resorption. They can relieve pain to a greater extent than analgesics but may not reduce bone deformity or decrease the risk of fractures. Oral treatment is usually sufficient, with intravenous treatment reserved for severe disease.

■ **Calcitonin**, by reducing osteoclastic bone resorption, can reduce pain and then improve the structural abnormalities in pagetic bone. Pain relief usually begins within 2 weeks, but treatment may be necessary for several months to improve bone remodelling. Approximately 50% of people will relapse on stopping treatment. Calcitonin is often used for initial treatment while awaiting a response to a bisphosphonate.

SELF-ASSESSMENT

True/false questions

1. Hypocalcaemia develops when there is a deficiency in parathyroid hormone (PTH) or vitamin D activity.
2. Vitamin D deficiency can lead to hypoparathyroidism.
3. Calcitonin decreases Ca^{2+} resorption in the kidney.
4. Bisphosphonates lower blood Ca^{2+} levels rapidly.
5. Oestrogens maintain bone density by directly enhancing Ca^{2+} absorption from the intestine.
6. Raloxifene stimulates oestrogen receptors on bone, breast and uterine tissue.
7. Denosumab binds to RANK ligand and reduces osteoclast activity.
8. Teriparatide is used in the treatment of postmenopausal osteoporosis.

One-best-answer (OBA) questions

1. Identify the *inaccurate* statement below concerning osteoporosis.
   A. High doses of oral prednisolone increase the risk of osteoporosis.
   B. Raloxifene has oestrogenic activity at all oestrogen receptors.
   C. Oral bisphosphonates reduce Ca^{2+} mobilisation in bone.
   D. Raloxifene causes hot flushes in some women.
   E. Lack of exercise increases the risk of osteoporosis.
2. Identify the *inaccurate* statement below concerning osteomalacia and rickets.
   A. Lack of sunlight can contribute to osteomalacia.
   B. Renal failure may reduce the effectiveness of ergocalciferol treatment in osteomalacia.
   C. Intestinal absorption of Ca^{2+} is decreased in osteomalacia.
   D. Vitamin D promotes bone mineralisation.
   E. Osteomalacia results in low levels of PTH.

True/false answers

1. **True.** Deficiencies in the production of PTH or vitamin D or in the responsiveness of their target tissues cause hypocalcaemia.
2. **False.** Vitamin D deficiency leads to hyperparathyroidism, which may assist in reducing the worst excesses of vitamin D deficiency. PTH increases calcitriol formation and calcitriol has a negative feedback effect on PTH.
3. **True.** Calcitonin reduces Ca^{2+} resorption and inhibits bone turnover.
4. **False.** Bisphosphonates inhibit bone dissolution and their effects occur slowly; plasma Ca^{2+} concentrations fall slowly with a maximum effect after about a week.
5. **False.** Oestrogens inhibit the cytokines that recruit the bone-resorbing osteoclasts. Oestrogens also inhibit the actions of PTH.
6. **False.** Raloxifene has been licensed to increase bone density in postmenopausal women. It is an oestrogen receptor agonist selective for its actions on oestrogen receptors in bone and without stimulant effects on oestrogen receptors in breast and uterus.
7. **True.** Denosumab prevents activation of RANK receptors on osteoclasts by RANK ligand (RANKL), and reduces osteoclast proliferation, function and survival.
8. **True.** Teriparatide is a recombinant version of amino acids 1–34 of PTH and is given daily by subcutaneous injection for postmenopausal osteoporosis.

OBA answers

1. **Answer B** is the inaccurate statement.
   A. Correct. Corticosteroids can reduce the number of bone-forming cellular units (osteoclasts/osteoblasts), decrease Ca^{2+} absorption, increase renal Ca^{2+} excretion and increase bone resorption.
   B. **Incorrect**. Raloxifene is oestrogenic on bone but anti-oestrogenic on receptors in the breast and uterus.
   C. Correct. Bisphosphonates reduce bone Ca^{2+} mobilisation and are particularly useful in corticosteroid-induced osteoporosis.
   D. Correct. The anti-oestrogenic effects of raloxifene can result in hot flushes and thromboembolism in some women.
   E. Correct. Load-bearing exercises increase bone turnover.
2. **Answer E** is the inaccurate statement.
   A. Correct. Sunlight is involved in the formation of cholecalciferol in the skin, which is then converted to active vitamin D compounds in the liver and kidneys.
   B. Correct. Ergocalciferol is hydroxylated in the kidney to calcitriol before it can exert its biological activity. In renal failure, if 1α-hydroxylase activity is defective, alfacalcidol or calcitriol may have to be substituted.
   C. Correct. Because of the lack of active vitamin D formed in the kidney, less Ca^{2+} and phosphate will be absorbed from the gut.
   D. Correct. Vitamin D promotes bone mineralisation by promoting the laying down of hydroxyapatite on the collagen organic matrix.
   E. **Incorrect**. Low levels of Ca^{2+} and lack of vitamin D may result in higher levels of PTH (secondary hyperparathyroidism).

FURTHER READING

Andress DL, Coyne DW, Kalantar-Zadeh K et al. (2008) Management of secondary hyperparathyroidism in stages 3 and 4 chronic kidney disease. *Endocr Pract* 14, 18–27

Canalis E, Giustina A, Bilezikian JP (2007) Mechanisms of anabolic therapies for osteoporosis. *N Engl J Med* 357, 905–916

Cooper MS, Gittoes NJL (2008) Diagnosis and management of hypocalcaemia. *BMJ* 336, 1298–1302

Favus MJ (2010) Bisphosphonates for osteoporosis. *N Engl J Med* 363, 2027–2035

Holick MF (2007) Vitamin D deficiency. *N Engl J Med* 357, 266–281

Laroche M (2008) Treatment of osteoporosis: all the questions we still cannot answer. *Am J Med* 121, 744–747

MacLean C, Newberry S, Maglione M et al. (2008) Systematic review: comparative effectiveness of treatments to prevent fractures in men and women with low bone density or osteoporosis. *Ann Intern Med* 148, 197–213

Mallick S, Kanthety R, Rahman M (2009) Vitamin D: bone and beyond, rationale and recommendations for supplementation. *Am J Med* 122, 793–802

Marcocci C, Cetani F (2011) Primary hyperparathyroidism. *N Engl J Med* 365, 2389–2397

Mazziotti G, Canalis E, Giustina A (2010) Drug-induced osteoporosis: mechanisms and clinical implications. *Am J Med* 123, 877–884

Pallan S, Omair Rahman M, Khan AA (2012) Diagnosis and management of primary hyperparathyroidism. *BMJ* 344, e1013

Palmer SC, McGregor DO, Macaskill P et al. (2007) Meta-analysis: vitamin D compounds in chronic kidney disease. *Ann Intern Med* 147, 840–853

Poole KES, Compston JE (2006) Osteoporosis and its management. *BMJ* 333, 1251–1256

Rachner TD, Khosla S, Hofbauer LC (2011) Osteoporosis: now and the future. *Lancet* 377, 1276–1287

Ralston SH, Langston AL, Reid IR (2008) Pathogenesis and management of Paget's disease of bone. *Lancet* 372, 155–163

Rosen CJ (2005) Postmenopausal osteoporosis. *N Engl J Med* 353, 595–603

Rosen CJ (2011) Vitamin D insufficiency. *N Engl J Med* 364, 248–254

Shoback D (2008) Hypoparathyroidism. *N Engl J Med* 359, 391–403

Sitges-Serra A, Bergenfelz A (2007) Clinical update: sporadic primary hyperparathyroidism. *Lancet* 370, 468–470

Stewart AF (2005) Hypercalcemia associated with cancer. *N Engl J Med* 352, 373–379

Whyte MP (2006) Paget's disease of bone. *N Engl J Med* 355, 593–600

Compendium: drugs used to regulate calcium metabolism and in metabolic bone disease

Drug	Kinetics (half-life)	Comments
Calcitonin and parathyroid hormone		
Calcitonin (salmon)/ salcatonin	Rapidly metabolised by the kidney (12–21 min), but biological effects persist for hours or days	Involved with parathyroid hormone in regulation of bone turnover; used to lower plasma Ca^{2+} in hypercalcaemia and for treatment of Paget's disease; given intranasally, by subcutaneous or intramuscular injection or by slow intravenous infusion
Parathyroid hormone	Bioavailability 55% after subcutaneous injection; proteolysed in the liver and kiney (1.5 h)	Human recombinant parathyroid hormone; given by subcutaneous injection for the treatment of postmenopausal osteoporosis
Teriparatide	Eliminated by hepatic and extrahepatic metabolism after subcutaneous injection (1h)	A recombinant fragment (amino acids 1–34) of parathyroid hormone used for postmenopausal and corticosteroid-induced osteoporosis; given by subcutaneous injection
Bisphosphonates		
All these drugs are used for osteoporosis. They are adsorbed onto hydroxyapatite crystals and reduce bone turnover; there is an extremely long half-life of release from bone. They are poorly absorbed from the gut after oral administration.		
Alendronic acid (alendronate)	Very low oral bioavailability (<1%); some of the absorbed fraction is eliminated renally; the fraction bound to bone is eliminated very slowly (11 years)	First-line option for the prevention and treatment of osteoporosis; given orally
Clodronate (sodium)	Very low bioavailability (1–2%); renal elimination (2 h) but fraction bound to bone is eliminated very slowly (years)	Used for hypercalcaemia of malignancy; given orally or by slow intravenous infusion
Etidronate (disodium)	Low absorption (1–9%); some eliminated rapidly within 24 h; fraction retained in bone is eliminated very slowly (years)	Used for prevention and treatment of osteoporosis; given orally

Compendium: drugs used to regulate calcium metabolism and in metabolic bone disease—cont'd

Drug	Kinetics (half-life)	Comments
Ibandronic acid	Renal elimination (10–60 h) but fraction bound to bone is eliminated very slowly (years)	Potent bisphosphonate used for osteoporosis (given every 3 months) and for hypercalcaemia of malignancy
Pamidronate (disodium)	Renally eliminated (0.5 h) but fraction bound to bone is eliminated very slowly (2 years)	Used for hypercalcaemia of malignancy and Paget's disease; given by slow intravenous infusion
Risedronate sodium	Lipophilic moiety improves oral bioavailability (about 60%); renal elimination (10 days) but fraction bound to bone is eliminated very slowly (years)	Potent bisphosphonate which is used for the prevention and treatment of osteoporosis and Paget's disease; given orally
Zoledronic acid	Renal elimination (7 days) but fraction bound to bone is eliminated very slowly	Used for hypercalcaemia of malignancy and prevention and treatment of osteoporosis; given by intravenous infusion only; used once a year for osteoporosis

Vitamin D

Because vitamin D requires metabolic activation in the kidneys, alfacalcidol or calcitriol should be used in cases of severe renal impairment.

Alfacalcidol	High oral bioavailability; oxidised by a 25-hydroxylase to active calcitriol (3 h)	1α-Hydroxycholecalciferol; given orally or by intravenous injection
Calcitriol	Completely absorbed; oxidised to inactive metabolites (3–6 h)	$1\alpha,25$-Dihydroxycholecalciferol; given orally or by intravenous injection
Colecalciferol (vitamin D_3)	High oral bioavailability; oxidised to 25-hydroxycholecalciferol (calcidiol) then to active 1,25-dihydroxyvitamin D_3 (calcitriol) in kidney	Given orally or by intravenous injection
Dihydrotachysterol	High oral bioavailability; few kinetic data available	Synthetic analogue of vitamin D_2; given orally
Ergocalciferol (calciferol; vitamin D_2)	High oral bioavailability; metabolised to cholecalciferol, then to active 1,25-dihydroxyvitamin D_3 (calcitriol) in liver and kidney (19–24 h)	Given orally or by intravenous injection
Paricalcitol	Hepatic metabolism (4–6 h)	19-Nor-1α-25-dihydroxyvitamin D_2; binds to vitamin D receptor and inhibits parathyroid hormone synthesis; used for secondary hyper-parathyroidism in chronic renal failure; given by slow intravenous injection

Other drugs affecting bone metabolism

Denosumab	Subcutaneous bioavailability 78%; eliminated by proteolysis (26 days)	Human monoclonal antibody that blocks RANKL–RANK interaction; given subcutaneously twice yearly
Raloxifene	Rapidly absorbed; extensive first-pass hepatic glucuronidation and enterohepatic cycling (28 h)	Used for the treatment and prevention of postmenopausal osteoporosis; does not affect menopausal vasomotor symptoms; given orally
Strontium ranelate	Bioavailability 25%; binds avidly to bone; renal and faecal elimination (60 h)	Used for postmenopausal osteoporosis in women over 75 years if bisphosphonates are poorly tolerated; given orally

43 Pituitary and hypothalamic hormones

ANTERIOR PITUITARY AND HYPOTHALAMIC HORMONES

Thyrotropin and thyrotropin-releasing hormone are considered in Chapter 41.

GROWTH HORMONE

Growth hormone (GH), or somatotropin, is a 191-amino acid peptide that is synthesised in specific cells in the anterior pituitary. Its secretion is controlled by the hypothalamus by a balance between growth hormone-releasing hormone (GHRH) via specific receptors and somatostatin (SST; also called growth hormone release-inhibiting hormone, GHRIH) via specific somatostatin receptors (or SSTRs) (Fig. 43.1). Many other factors modulate this balance such as the stimulant effects of ghrelin, sex hormones, sleep and exercise or the inhibitory effects of plasma GH, glucose and glucocorticoids.

GH is released in pulses repeatedly throughout the day and night. Like other peptide hormones, GH binds to cell surface receptors and activates adenylyl cyclase, and has direct metabolic effects on several tissues. In addition it produces other effects via the production of insulin-like growth factor 1 (IGF-1, a somatomedin). IGF-1 is synthesised by the liver in response to GH stimulation, and is highly protein bound in plasma.

The effects of GH are anabolic in relation to protein metabolism, especially in skeletal muscle leading to increased muscle mass, and in epiphyseal cartilage, where the proliferating effects stimulate bone growth. These actions are mediated by IGF-1. IGF-1 also has effects on the liver via the insulin receptor, and promotes hepatic gluconeogenesis. However, GH has an opposing direct effect on carbohydrate metabolism, reducing glucose uptake by skeletal muscle and adipose tissue, creating an insulin-resistant state (Box 43.1).

The effect of GH on fat is catabolic, with a direct action on adipocytes that promotes lipolysis and reduces lipogenesis.

Growth hormone for therapeutic use

Example

somatropin (synthetic human GH)

Somatropin has several therapeutic uses in children, which include:

- to improve linear growth in children with proven GH deficiency (who usually lack GHRH; pituitary dwarfism),
- chronic renal insufficiency before puberty,
- Turner's syndrome,
- Prader–Willi syndrome.

To be effective, the hormone must be given before the closure of the epiphyses in long bones. Treatment should be stopped if growth velocity does not increase by at least 50% from baseline.

Adult GH deficiency may warrant treatment with somatropin if all the following criteria are fulfilled:

- severe GH deficiency,
- impaired quality of life,
- already receiving treatment for another pituitary hormone deficiency.

Pharmacokinetics

Somatropin is usually given by subcutaneous injection, although the intramuscular route can be used. Plasma concentrations fluctuate widely following both routes, although the latter gives more stable levels because of slower uptake into the circulation. Somatropin has a very short half-life (0.5 h), but the plasma concentration of IGF-1 is much more constant due to its high protein binding. As a consequence, three doses of somatropin per week give good clinical results, although daily dosing is often used.

Unwanted effects

- Headache, occasionally associated with visual problems, nausea and vomiting, and papilloedema from benign intracranial hypertension.
- Fluid retention with peripheral oedema.

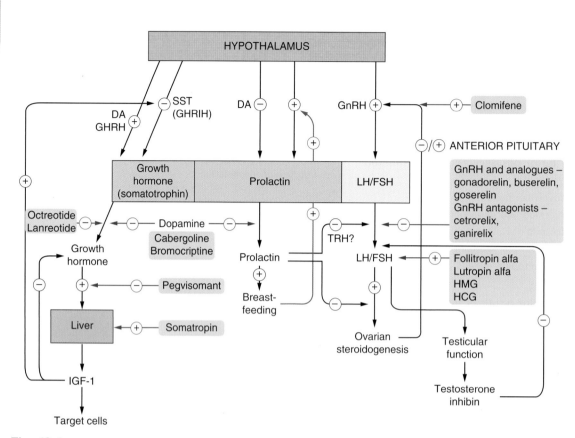

Fig. 43.1 Control mechanisms for the release of growth hormone, gonadotropins and prolactin from the anterior pituitary. For control of other hormones, see Ch. 41 (thyroid) and Ch. 44 (adrenocorticotropic hormones). Oestrogen effects on gonadotropin-releasing hormone (GnRH) are shown as both positive and negative because oestrogen suppresses luteinizing hormone (LH) secretion in the early follicular phase but enhances secretion around ovulation (Ch. 45). The actions of drugs are shown by red arrows. Gonadorelin is a synthetic GnRH and buserelin and goserelin are GnRH analogues. Pulsatile administration of GnRH or its analogues enhances LH/follicle-stimulating hormone (FSH). On continuous administration, they downregulate the GnRH receptors, inhibiting LH/FSH release, an effect produced more rapidly by GnRH antagonists (cetrorelix, ganirelix). Somatropin is synthetic growth hormone, and octreotide and lanreotide are somatostatin analogues that suppress growth hormone release. For details of dopamine (DA) agonists, see Ch. 24. GHRH, growth hormone-releasing hormone; HMG, human menopausal gonadotropins (menotrophin); HCG, human chorionic gonadotropin; IGF-1 insulin-like growth factor 1; SST, somatostatin (also called GHRIH, growth hormone release-inhibiting hormone); ? = regulating hormone not yet established. Note: dopamine stimulates growth hormone release in healthy individuals, but paradoxically in acromegaly it inhibits release.

Box 43.1 **Effects of growth hormone**

Anabolic effects on protein synthesis in muscle
Increases bone growth, mineralisation and Ca^{2+} retention
Increases fat catabolism
Stimulates growth of most internal organs
Reduces liver uptake of glucose and promotes
    gluconeogenesis
Stimulates the immune system

- Arthralgia, myalgia, carpal tunnel syndrome.
- A transient insulin-like action occasionally produces hypoglycaemia.
- If excessive doses are used (as may happen during illicit use by athletes to build muscle mass) there is a risk of diabetes mellitus in predisposed individuals.
- Pain at the injection site.

Acromegaly

Acromegaly results from excessive production of GH, almost always by an adenoma in the anterior pituitary which also secretes prolactin in one-third of cases (Fig. 43.1). The most common clinical features arise from excessive growth of bone and soft tissue. Complex metabolic consequences include insulin resistance with diabetes mellitus and hypertension.

The morbidity and mortality of acromegaly vary according to its severity. Untreated acromegalic individuals have a life expectancy approximately half that of people without acromegaly, due to an excess incidence of cardiovascular and respiratory disease and of carcinoma of the colon. Acromegaly is therefore usually treated actively.

Drugs for acromegaly

Somatostatin analogues

lanreotide, octreotide

Mechanisms of action and uses

The synthetic derivatives of SST are both more potent and longer-acting inhibitors of GH secretion than the native compound. They are selective for the SST receptor subtypes that are highly expressed on GH-secreting adenomas. Like SST, they also inhibit the release of gastro-entero-pancreatic peptide hormones, such as insulin, glucagon, cholecystokinin, gastrin and vasoactive intestinal peptide (VIP), via intestinal SST receptors, which generate intracellular cAMP and modulate Ca^{2+} influx into the cell. These actions make SST analogues useful also for the treatment of a variety of conditions associated with excess secretion of gut hormones.

Uses of SST analogues include:

- management of acromegaly,
- management of other endocrine tumours, for example carcinoid tumours (to reduce flushing and diarrhoea), VIPoma (to reduce diarrhoea) and glucagonoma (to improve the characteristic necrolytic rash),
- management of medullary thyroid tumours (lanreotide) and prevention of complications following pancreatic surgery (octreotide),
- octreotide is sometimes used to stop bleeding from oesophageal varices (Ch. 36).

Pharmacokinetics

Octreotide is given by subcutaneous injection. It has a short half-life (1–2 h) but suppresses GH secretion for up to 8 h so it is used three times daily. A depot preparation is available in which octreotide is adsorbed onto microspheres; given by deep intramuscular injection it has a duration of action of about 4 weeks. The depot is used once control has been achieved by the use of the conventional formulation. Lanreotide also has a short half-life (1–2 h) and is formulated as a sustained-release preparation given by subcutaneous or intramuscular injection every 1–4 weeks.

Unwanted effects

- Gastrointestinal upset is common, especially anorexia, nausea, vomiting, abdominal pain, bloating and diarrhoea. It usually resolves with continued treatment.
- Impaired glucose tolerance.
- Gallstones, due to suppression of cholecystokinin secretion with decreased gallbladder motility. In addition, an increase in bowel transit time alters colonic flora and makes bile salts more lithogenic.
- Pain at the injection site.

Growth hormone receptor antagonist

pegvisomant

Mechanism of action

Pegvisomant is a pegylated synthetic analogue of GH that acts as a highly selective GH receptor antagonist.

Pharmacokinetics

Pegvisomant is given by subcutaneous injection. The mechanism of its clearance is unknown; the half-life is very long (6 days).

Unwanted effects

- Nausea, vomiting, dyspepsia, abdominal distension, diarrhoea, constipation.
- Hypertension.
- Headache, dizziness, fatigue, drowsiness, tremor, sleep disturbance.
- Influenza-like symptoms, arthralgia, myalgia.
- Weight gain, hypo- or hyperglycaemia.

Dopamine receptor agonists

In healthy people, dopaminergic receptor stimulation increases the secretion of GH, but in acromegaly there is a paradoxical decrease. Bromocriptine was originally used to treat acromegaly, but the clinical response was unpredictable and control of plasma IGF-1 was achieved in only about 20% of cases. It has been superseded by better-tolerated drugs such as cabergoline, which adequately suppress IGF-1 concentrations in about 40% of people with acromegaly. Further details of these drugs can be found in Ch. 24.

Treatment of acromegaly

Surgery by the trans-sphenoidal route is the usual treatment of choice, sometimes followed by external radiotherapy if the tumour is large.

Three groups may be suitable for drug treatment:

- those in whom an excess of GH persists despite surgery and radiotherapy; after radiotherapy the plasma GH concentration can take 1–2 years to fall,
- those with mild acromegaly,
- the elderly.

SST analogues are the first-line treatment, with pegvisomant used when there is intolerance or failure to respond. Cabergoline is sometimes used with a SST analogue when there is resistance to other treatments. The effectiveness of treatment is monitored by the plasma concentration of IGF-1.

ADRENOCORTICOTROPIC HORMONE

Adrenocorticotropic hormone (ACTH; corticotropin) is a single-chain polypeptide with 39 amino acids, of which the

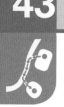

24 that form the N-terminal region are essential for full biological activity. It promotes steroidogenesis in adrenocortical cells by occupying cell surface receptors and stimulating adenylyl cyclase. Release of ACTH occurs in response to the hypothalamic peptide corticotropin-releasing hormone (CRH). CRH secretion is pulsatile and has a diurnal rhythm, with maximal release in the morning around the time of waking (see further detail in Ch. 44). The release of CRH is affected by other factors, including chemical (e.g. antidiuretic hormone, opioid peptides), physical (e.g. heat, cold, injury) and psychological influences. The main inhibitory influence on ACTH release is negative feedback control by circulating glucocorticoids. This occurs at both hypothalamic and pituitary levels. Adrenal androgens, although stimulated by ACTH, play no part in feedback control.

ACTH for therapeutic use

tetracosactide

ACTH preparations of animal origin have been replaced by a less allergenic synthetic peptide analogue, tetracosactide, which consists of the active N-terminal amino acids 1–24 of the ACTH molecule.

Pharmacokinetics

There are two formulations of tetracosactide:

- a rapid-acting form that increases steroidogenesis for about an hour and is suitable for tests of adrenocortical function. In adrenal insufficiency there is a subnormal or no rise of plasma cortisol 30 min after intramuscular or intravenous injection of tetracosactide,
- a depot form that is absorbed slowly into the circulation over several hours and can be used as an alternative to exogenous corticosteroid therapy. However, the unpredictable corticosteroid response means that the therapeutic value of this form is limited.

Once absorbed into the circulation, tetracosactide is metabolised rapidly with a very short half-life (0.2 h).

Unwanted effects

Prolonged use will produce all the features of corticosteroid excess (Ch. 44).

PROLACTIN

Prolactin is a glycoprotein similar in structure to GH but secreted by distinct cells in the anterior pituitary (Fig. 43.1). The major hypothalamic control mechanism is inhibition by dopamine via D_2 receptors on the prolactin-secreting cells of the anterior pituitary (Ch. 45). Thyrotropin-releasing hormone (or TRH) is involved in stimulating prolactin release, and oestrogen increases prolactin production. The main target tissue for prolactin is the breast, which secretes milk in response to prolactin if the mammary glands have been primed by ovarian and other hormones. At delivery, the maternal plasma prolactin concentration is high. Release of further prolactin continues as long as suckling continues. A high plasma concentration of prolactin suppresses follicle-stimulating hormone (FSH) release from the pituitary and leads to a failure of ovarian follicle growth. This may explain the relative subfertility of women who are breastfeeding.

Prolactin has other functions, including producing sexual gratification after intercourse and contributing to maturation of the fetal lung and proliferation of oligodendrocytes that form the neural myelin sheath.

Hyperprolactinaemia

Persistent hyperprolactinaemia is usually caused by a microadenoma of the anterior pituitary or by the action of dopamine receptor antagonist drugs such as phenothiazines (Ch. 21). In younger women hyperprolactinaemia can produce amenorrhoea, infertility and signs and symptoms of oestrogen deficiency (e.g. vaginal dryness and dyspareunia, galactorrhoea and osteoporosis). In men it may cause hypogonadism. Withdrawal of a provoking drug should be considered. For a microadenoma, a dopamine D_2 receptor agonist such as cabergoline (Ch. 24) can be used to suppress prolactin secretion. Pituitary surgery may be considered for treatment failure.

GONADOTROPIN-RELEASING HORMONE

Gonadotropin-releasing hormone (GnRH) is a decapeptide that is synthesised in the hypothalamus and is transported by neuronal axons to the pituitary. It is then released in pulses into the capillaries of the pituitary-portal circulation and positively controls the synthesis and release of both luteinizing hormone (LH) and FSH from the anterior pituitary (Fig. 43.1). The cell surface receptors for GnRH are G-protein-linked and are found widely in the body, although their role is poorly understood, as well as on the gonadotropic cells in the anterior pituitary. These receptors are upregulated by repeated stimulation with GnRH, but pulsatile exposure is essential to maintain responsiveness. Low-frequency pulses stimulate FSH release, and high-frequency pulses stimulate LH release. In males, pulse frequency remains constant, whereas in females it varies through the menstrual cycle with a surge just before ovulation (see Ch. 45).

There is rapid tolerance to constant-rate infusions of GnRH because of downregulation of cell surface receptors. Therapeutic administration of GnRH can mimic pulsatile stimulation or produce receptor downregulation, and these have different clinical uses, as described below. There is negative feedback control of GnRH release via neural pathways and sex steroids (Fig. 43.1).

GnRH-related products for therapeutic use

Synthetic GnRH (gonadorelin)

Synthetic GnRH is available for assessing hypothalamic-pituitary function and is given as a subcutaneous or intravenous injection. Unwanted effects are unusual, but include nausea, headaches and abdominal pain.

Gonadorelin analogues

buserelin, goserelin

Mechanism of action

Structurally similar to the natural hormone, gonadorelin analogues (Ch. 52) initially stimulate GnRH receptors, but rapidly promote receptor downregulation, which then inhibits further gonadotropin production. The result is reduced production of oestrogen or androgen. This latter action underlies their clinical uses.

Clinical uses of gonadorelin analogues

- The main use is to reduce testosterone secretion to castration levels in men with prostatic cancer. An initial rise in testosterone from receptor stimulation can produce tumour 'flare' in the first 1–2 weeks of treatment (Ch. 52). An anti-androgen such as cyproterone acetate (Ch. 46) is usually given to counteract this effect.
- Treatment of endometriosis by reducing oestrogen secretion (for up to 6 months only).
- Treatment of advanced breast cancer in women, by reducing oestrogen secretion.
- To reduce endometrial thickness for 3–4 months prior to intra-uterine surgery.
- Preparation of women for assisted conception by methods such as in vitro fertilisation (IVF) (see below).
- Suppression of precocious puberty.
- 'Hormonal castration' of males with severe sexual deviation.

Pharmacokinetics

Buserelin can be given by either subcutaneous injection or intranasal spray and has a short half-life (1–1.5 h). Goserelin, which has a half-life of 4 h, must be given by subcutaneous injection and is available as an oily depot preparation. Depot formulations inhibit gonadotropin production for up to 4 weeks after a single injection.

Unwanted effects

- Menopause-like symptoms in women, with hot flushes, sweating, vaginal dryness and loss of libido.
- Orchidectomy-like effects in men, with loss of libido, gynaecomastia and vasomotor instability.
- Headache.
- Hypersensitivity reactions, including skin rashes, asthma and anaphylaxis.
- Osteoporosis with prolonged use.
- Local reactions at injection sites, or intranasally with spray.

GnRH antagonists

cetrorelix, ganirelix

Mechanism of action and uses

These drugs are competitive GnRH receptor antagonists that produce immediate, reversible suppression of gonadotropin secretion. They are used in assisted reproduction techniques in the management of female infertility (IVF; see below). They have advantages compared with gonadorelin analogues in this role, since there is no initial surge of LH release (which can lead to cancellation of the IVF in about 20% of cycles).

Pharmacokinetics

Both cetrorelix and ganirelix are given by subcutaneous injection, and inactivated by hepatic metabolism. They have long half-lives (>12 h).

Unwanted effects

- Nausea.
- Headache.
- Injection-site reactions.

GONADOTROPINS

LH and FSH are glycoproteins that are released from the anterior pituitary when it is stimulated by pulsatile exposure to GnRH. Negative feedback by inhibin, a hormone produced by the gonads, selectively inhibits FSH secretion. In addition, both gonadotropins are subject to negative feedback from gonadal steroids, including progesterone (Ch. 45).

In males, LH acts on specific receptors on the surface of the Leydig cells in the testes and stimulates adenylyl cyclase, leading to the production of testosterone. FSH acts in a similar way on the Sertoli cells of the seminiferous tubules, stimulating the formation of a specific androgen-binding protein.

In females, receptors for FSH and LH are found in granulosa cells of ovarian follicles. FSH is responsible for follicular development. The rising oestradiol concentration in the late follicular phase has a positive-feedback effect on secretion of LH, and produces a short-lived surge of LH release. This triggers rupture of the follicle, release of the ovum and formation of the corpus luteum (Ch. 45). Both FSH and LH, like human chorionic gonadotropin (HCG), are also produced in large quantities by the placenta during pregnancy.

Gonadotropins for therapeutic use

- Human menopausal gonadotropins (HMGs) are FSH and LH (in a 1:1 ratio, also known as menotrophin) extracted from urine obtained from postmenopausal women.
- HCG contains large quantities of LH with little FSH. It is secreted by the placenta and extracted from the urine of pregnant women. An alternative preparation is human choriogonadotropin alfa (recombinant human chorionic gonadotropin).
- Follitropin alfa and beta (recombinant human FSH) (Fig. 43.1) and corifollitropin alfa (modified recombinant FSH).
- Lutropin alfa (recombinant human LH) (Fig. 43.1).

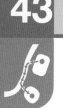

Gonadotropins are given by intramuscular or subcutaneous injection.

Unwanted effects

- Nausea and vomiting.
- Breast, abdominal and pelvic pain.
- Headache.
- In women the most serious problem is ovarian hyperstimulation syndrome, in which the ovaries can become grossly enlarged as a result of multiple follicle stimulation, leading to considerable abdominal pain, ascites and even pleural effusions.
- In men the commonest problem is gynaecomastia or oedema with prolonged use.

Clinical uses of gonadotropins

- Treatment of infertility in women with hypopituitarism.
- Treatment of infertility in women after failure of clomifene treatment (see below).
- For superovulation treatment for assisted conception (such as IVF).
- In men with hypogonadotropic hypogonadism and oligospermia. This requires long courses of gonadotropin injections, initially to achieve external sexual maturation and then to maintain satisfactory sperm production. Spermatozoa take 70–80 days to mature, and a year or more of treatment may be needed to achieve optimal response. A combination of HMG and HCG is usually given.

INFERTILITY

Infertility is said to be present after 1 year of unprotected intercourse without conception. It has several causes, which need full evaluation of both partners before treatment is given or IVF is considered.

Clomifene

Mechanism of action and use

Clomifene is an agent with both oestrogenic and antioestrogenic properties. The latter are related to its ability to block pituitary oestrogen receptors and increase gonadotropin secretion. It is used to stimulate ovulation in anovulatory infertility.

Pharmacokinetics

Clomifene is well absorbed from the gut. It is metabolised in the liver and has a very long half-life (5 days).

Unwanted effects

- Reversible ovarian enlargement and cyst formation.
- Hot flushes.
- Abdominal or pelvic pain.
- Nausea, vomiting.
- Breast tenderness, weight gain.

Drug treatment of female infertility

If there is hyperprolactinaemia then a dopamine agonist such as cabergoline should suppress prolactin levels and permit ovulation in 70–80% of women. The management of polycystic ovary syndrome is considered below.

When deficiency of gonadal stimulation by gonadotropin is the limiting factor, FSH (follitropin) can be given with LH (HMG), or in combination as HCG to encourage the development of a single mature ovarian follicle (see Ch. 45). Ovarian hyperstimulation can be a problem.

If the hypothalamic–pituitary axis is normal, the anti-oestrogen clomifene blocks oestrogen receptors in the pituitary, which decreases the negative feedback on FSH (Fig. 43.1), giving increased FSH concentrations that stimulate follicle growth. There is a small risk of ovarian hyperstimulation, and multiple fetuses develop in about 11% of those who become pregnant.

Preparation for assisted conception (*in vitro* fertilisation)

Ovulation is targeted on a particular date, and initial inhalation of a gonadorelin analogue or use of a GnRH antagonist will 'switch off' natural cyclical menstrual activity. Ovarian stimulation treatment is then begun to achieve maturation of oocytes at the time chosen for egg recovery prior to IVF. This involves giving large doses of HCG or HMG to stimulate the maturation of several follicles (superovulation treatment). These ova are then 'harvested' by aspiration of the follicles.

Polycystic ovary syndrome

This is a common cause of infertility, affecting 5–10% of women of reproductive age. It is characterised by abnormal ovarian function with hyperandrogenism. Other complaints include menstrual disturbance, hirsutism and acne. Polycystic ovary syndrome is often associated with obesity and insulin resistance in adipose and muscle tissue, conferring an increased risk of diabetes mellitus and cardiovascular disease in later life. Increased insulin secretion is also a factor in stimulating ovarian androgen production. Assessment and treatment of cardiovascular risk is an important component of management.

Weight loss (especially if the body mass index is greater than 29 $kg \cdot m^{-2}$) may restore ovulatory cycles if infertility is the main concern. Metformin (Ch. 40) can be used if this is inadequate, and the resulting improvement in insulin sensitivity reduces androgen concentrations. This leads to weight loss, reduction of the consequences of hyperandrogenisation, and improved fertility. Clomifene can be added if fertility is not restored. Because of the absence of good safety data metformin is usually stopped during pregnancy.

Alternative approaches to treatment include a combined oral hormonal contraceptive for management of amenorrhoea or oligomenorrhoea (Ch. 45) or anti-androgen therapy with cyproterone acetate (often used in combination with an oestrogen) for hirsutism (Ch. 46). Topical therapies are available for managing hirsutism associated with polycystic ovary syndrome. These include minoxidil cream (Ch. 6) to reverse male-pattern hair loss, and eflornithine cream (an ornithine decarboxylase inhibitor) to slow facial hair growth by inhibiting cell division in hair follicles.

POSTERIOR PITUITARY HORMONES

VASOPRESSIN (ANTIDIURETIC HORMONE)

Vasopressin is a nonapeptide, sometimes referred to as arginine-vasopressin (AVP) because human vasopressin has an arginine residue in position 8. It is also known as antidiuretic hormone (ADH). Vasopressin is released from neurosecretory cells of the hypothalamus and transported down the axons of the nerve cells that form the pituitary stalk. It is stored in the nerve endings in the posterior pituitary and released in response to stimulation of the hypothalamus via osmoreceptors, sodium receptors and volume receptors in response to reduced plasma volume or increased plasma osmolality. Vasopressin has two main target tissues.

- Stimulation of vascular smooth muscle via V1 receptors leads to Ca^{2+} influx and vasoconstriction. Vasoconstriction sufficient to raise blood pressure only occurs at high plasma vasopressin concentrations.
- At the collecting ducts of the kidney nephron, stimulation of V2 receptors increases intracellular cAMP production which leads to expression of aquaporin-2 channels that allow water reabsorption down an osmotic gradient to produce more concentrated urine. Expression of urea transporters in the collecting duct is also enhanced with consequent urea reabsorption from the renal filtrate.

Vasopressin is metabolised in many tissues, including the liver and kidney, and has a very short half-life of about 10 min. It is given therapeutically by subcutaneous or intramuscular injection or by intravenous infusion.

Vasopressin analogues

Examples

desmopressin, terlipressin

Vasopressin has a short duration of action. Desmopressin (DDAVP, des-amino-D-arginine-vasopressin) has an increased antidiuretic potency and reduced pressor activity compared with vasopressin. It is absorbed through the nasal mucosa and is most conveniently administered by a metered-dose nasal spray or sublingually. It can also be given by subcutaneous, intramuscular or intravenous injection. An additional action of parenteral desmopressin is to increase clotting factor VIII concentration in blood (Ch. 11).

Terlipressin is also a vasopressin analogue that is used to treat bleeding oesophageal varices. It is discussed in Chapter 36.

Pharmacokinetics

Like vasopressin, desmopressin is metabolised in the liver and kidney, but it has a longer half-life (0.5–2 h). Terlipressin is a prodrug hydrolysed to active lysine-vasopressin, which has a formation rate-limited half-life of 0.5 h.

Unwanted effects

- Excessive water retention, producing dilutional hyponatraemia.
- Headache.
- Nausea, vomiting and abdominal pain.

Clinical uses of vasopressin and its analogues

- Vasopressin can be given acutely for treatment of cranial diabetes insipidus (see below), using the longer-acting derivative desmopressin for maintenance treatment.
- Desmopressin can be given sublingually for primary nocturnal enuresis.
- Terlipressin will control bleeding from oesophageal varices in portal hypertension (Ch. 36). Vasopressin is sometimes used for this indication.
- Desmopressin by injection is used to boost factor VIII concentration and reduce bleeding in mild to moderate haemophilia.
- Desmopressin can be given to test for urine-concentrating ability in suspected diabetes insipidus (see below).
- Vasopressin is given for its pressor activity in the treatment of shock associated with hypotension, when it also increases vascular sensitivity to noradrenaline.

Diabetes insipidus

Diabetes insipidus is usually caused by a failure of secretion of vasopressin in the hypothalamus ('cranial' diabetes insipidus). Tumours, inflammatory conditions, granulomatous conditions such as sarcoidosis, and trauma to the hypothalamus are the main causes. A distinct condition known as nephrogenic diabetes insipidus occurs when the kidney is unresponsive to vasopressin. It can result from a hereditary deficiency of renal vasopressin receptors, or from drug therapy, particularly with lithium (Ch. 22) or the tetracycline demeclocycline (Ch. 51). Diabetes insipidus presents clinically with thirst, polyuria and a tendency to high plasma osmolality together with an inappropriately low urine osmolality.

Vasopressin produces concentrated urine in people with cranial diabetes insipidus; desmopressin is used for long-term treatment. Treatment of nephrogenic diabetes insipidus is more difficult, because the kidney does not respond to vasopressin. Paradoxically, thiazide diuretics (Ch. 14) can reduce the polyuria. This may be due to initial contraction in extracellular volume, with subsequent increase in proximal tubular salt and water retention. Carbamazepine (Ch. 23) is also effective, by sensitising the renal tubule to the effect of vasopressin.

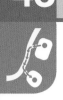

Syndrome of inappropriate antidiuresis

This is a condition caused by inappropriately high secretion of vasopressin, resulting in excess water retention and a dilutional hyponatraemia. There are many causes, including malignant tumours that secrete vasopressin, pulmonary disorders (including infection) and various disorders of the central nervous system. Drugs such as antidepressants (Ch. 22), carbamazepine (Ch. 23) and various cytotoxic agents can also produce the syndrome.

Vasopressin V2 receptor antagonist

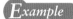

tolvaptan

Mechanism of action and uses

Tolvaptan is a competitive antagonist at vasopressin V2 receptors. Its major action is in the renal collecting ducts to reduce water reabsorption and produce aquaresis without sodium loss, thus increasing free water clearance, and correcting dilutional hyponatraemia. In the UK, tolvaptan is currently licensed for the treatment of hyponatraemia secondary to inappropriate ADH secretion. However, it is also effective for correction of hyponatraemia in cirrhosis and in heart failure when it arises from diuretic use. Tolvaptan is not suitable for urgent treatment of severe hyponatraemia, when there is a risk of significant neurological complications. When initiating treatment, it is important to monitor the rise in serum sodium to avoid rapid correction and precipitation of osmotic demyelination syndrome.

Pharmacokinetics

Tolvaptan is fairly well absorbed from the gut and eliminated by hepatic metabolism with a half-life of about 12 h.

Unwanted effects

- Thirst, dry mouth, polyuria.
- Hypotension.
- Hypernatraemia.
- Hypoglycaemia.

Treatment of syndrome of inappropriate antidiuresis

Severe hyponatraemia can cause confusion, seizures and coma. Slow correction of the serum Na$^+$ concentration with intravenous saline 0.9% is the mainstay of treatment. Rapid correction can disturb the osmotic balance across neurons and cause irreversible damage known as central pontine myelinolysis, which produces dysarthria, spastic quadriparesis and pseudobulbar palsy.

Less severe hyponatraemia may respond to fluid restriction. Demeclocycline, a tetracycline antimicrobial agent that reduces the sensitivity of the collecting ducts to vasopressin, can also be used. The vasopressin V2 receptor antagonist tolvaptan is sometimes used, but not for urgent treatment due to the risk of neurological complications.

OXYTOCIN

Oxytocin is discussed in Chapter 45.

HYPOPITUITARISM

Pituitary insufficiency can arise from traumatic brain injury and subarachnoid haemorrhage, when a single hormonal axis is often affected. Pituitary irradiation or surgery, by contrast, often affects multiple axes. Less common causes include both pituitary and non-pituitary intracranial tumours, and ischaemic damage.

Replacement of a deficiency of glucocorticoid (Ch. 44) and thyroid (Ch. 41) hormonal function is essential and urgent. Female sex hormone (Ch. 45) or testosterone (Ch. 46) replacement can be important at a later stage to restore libido and bone mass. In some individuals deficiency of GH or vasopressin may also require replacement.

SELF-ASSESSMENT

True/false questions

1. The release of growth hormone (GH, somatotropin) is reduced by somatostatin.
2. Somatostatin is only produced by the hypothalamus.
3. Octreotide is a useful drug for the treatment of acromegaly.
4. Pegmisovant is a pegylated GH analogue that stimulates GH receptors.
5. Prolactin suppresses ovarian steroidogenesis.
6. Cabergoline reduces prolactin secretion.
7. Continuous administration of gonadorelin analogues stimulates sex steroid synthesis.
8. The gonadorelin analogue buserelin stimulates gonadotropin-releasing hormone (GnRH) receptors and is used for the treatment of endometriosis, but has no clinical use in males.
9. Cetrorelix and ganirelix are GnRH receptor antagonists used in female infertility.
10. Follitropin alfa is a recombinant follicle-stimulating hormone (FSH) analogue used in preparation for *in vitro* fertilisation.
11. The production of vasopressin is impaired in nephrogenic diabetes insipidus.
12. Vasopressin increases expression of aquaporin channels.
13. Desmopressin is administered by intranasal spray in cranial diabetes insipidus.
14. Tolvaptan is used in the urgent treatment of severe hyponatraemia.
15. In nephrogenic diabetes insipidus, thiazide diuretics increase the polyuria.

One-best-answer (OBA) question

Identify the *inaccurate* statement below about GH.

A. The release of GH is constant over a 24 h period.
B. GH acts by stimulation of insulin-like growth factor 1 (IGF-1) release.

C. In acromegaly, cabergoline reduces IGF-1 levels.
D. IGF-1 has a negative feedback effect on GH release.
E. Somatropin is used for GH deficiency in children.

Case-based questions

An assessment of a 10-year-old girl with short stature showed that she had abnormally low levels of growth hormone-releasing hormone (GHRH) and GH.

A. Was this girl too old to benefit from treatment?
B. What treatment should be recommended and how should it be administered?
C. What unwanted effects might occur?

True/false answers

1. **True.** Somatostatin is also known as growth hormone release-inhibiting hormone (GHRIH).
2. **False.** Somatostatin is also produced from intestinal and pancreatic cells.
3. **True.** Octreotide is a long-acting analogue of somatostatin and therefore inhibits GH release.
4. **False.** Pegvisomant is a pegylated GH analogue but it selectively blocks GH receptors; it is used when somatostatin analogues such as octreotide are poorly tolerated or ineffective.
5. **True.** Prolactin inhibits FSH release and suppresses ovarian follicle growth and steroidogenesis.
6. **True.** Cabergoline is a dopamine receptor agonist and inhibits prolactin release from the anterior pituitary; it can be used to improve fertility in women with hyperprolactinaemia.
7. **False.** Although brief administration of gonadorelin analogues stimulates sex steroid synthesis, on continued administration gonadotropin receptors are rapidly downregulated and sex steroid synthesis declines.
8. **False.** Gonadorelin analogues downregulate GnRH receptors and are used to inhibit testosterone synthesis in prostate cancer, as well as reducing synthesis of ovarian hormones in endometriosis.
9. **True.** GnRH receptor antagonists produce immediate suppression of gonadotropin secretion without the initial surge in LH caused by gonadorelin analogues.
10. **True.** Follitropin alfa is a synthetic FSH analogue and promotes follicle growth.

11. **False.** In nephrogenic diabetes insipidus the kidney is unresponsive to vasopressin; vasopressin secretion is impaired in cranial diabetes insipidus.
12. **True.** Vasopressin (antidiuretic hormone) acting at V2 receptors enhances water reabsorption by increasing aquaporin channels in the renal collecting duct.
13. **True.** Desmopressin is a modified vasopressin with a longer duration of action and selectivity for V2 receptors in the kidney.
14. **False.** The vasopressin V2 antagonist tolvaptan is licensed for maintenance treatment of hyponatraemia caused by excessive ADH secretion, but if used for acute treatment of severe hyponatraemia it can cause neurological complications.
15. **False.** Paradoxically, in diabetes insipidus, the response to thiazide diuretics is a beneficial reduction in polyuria.

OBA answer

Answer A is the inaccurate statement.

A. **Incorrect.** GH is released in a pulsatile manner and is higher during deep sleep, particularly in children.
B. Correct. GH stimulates IGF-1 release from the liver, which then acts on receptors in many tissues and in concert with other hormones.
C. Correct. In normal individuals dopamine receptor agonists such as cabergoline stimulate GH release, but in acromegaly they paradoxically inhibit GH release.
D. Correct. IGF-1 inhibits GH release and also stimulates somatostatin release from the hypothalamus, which further inhibits GH release.
E. Correct. Somatropin is a recombinant GH.

Case-based answers

A. Epiphyseal closure occurs much later than 10 years of age, so treatment of this girl with short stature can increase her growth.
B. Low levels of GHRH and GH suggest pituitary dwarfism and therefore synthetic GH (somatropin) would be appropriate. Although somatropin has a half-life of only 25 min, it generates IGF-1 which is highly protein-bound, so three subcutaneous injections of somatropin a week are sufficient to maintain IGF-1 levels.
C. Transient insulin-like effects of somatropin can produce hypoglycaemia and there may be pain at the site of injection. Headache and oedema can also occur.

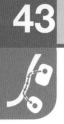

FURTHER READING

Balen AH, Rutherford AJ (2007) Management of infertility. *BMJ* 335, 608–611

Balen AH, Rutherford AJ (2007) Managing anovulatory infertility and polycystic ovary syndrome. *BMJ* 335, 663–666

Danzig J (2007) Acromegaly. *BMJ* 335, 824–825

Dattani M, Preece M (2004) Growth hormone deficiency and related disorders: insights into causation, diagnosis, and treatment. *Lancet* 363, 1977–1987

Ehrmann DA (2005) Polycystic ovary syndrome. *N Engl J Med* 352, 1223–1236

Ellison DH, Beri T (2007) The syndrome of inappropriate antidiuresis. *N Engl J Med* 356, 2064–2072

Khanna A (2006) Acquired nephrogenic diabetes insipidus. *Semin Nephrol* 26, 244–248

Melmed S (2006) Acromegaly. *N Engl J Med* 355, 2558–2573

Norman RJ, Dewailly D, Legro RS et al. (2007) Polycystic ovary syndrome. *Lancet* 370, 685–697

Olive DL (2008) Gonadotropin–releasing hormone agonists for endometriosis. *N Engl J Med* 359, 1136–1142

Sands JM, Bichet DG (2006) Nephrogenic diabetes insipidus. *Ann Intern Med* 144, 186–194

Schneider HJ, Almaretti G, Kreitschmann-Andermahr I et al. (2007) Hypopituitarism. *Lancet* 369, 1461–1470

Setji TJ, Brown AJ (2007) Polycystic ovary syndrome: diagnosis and treatment. *Am J Med* 120, 128–132

Van Voorhis BJ (2007) In vitro fertilization. *N Engl J Med* 356, 379–388

Compendium: pituitary and hypothalamic hormones

Drug	Kinetics (half-life)	Comments
Hypothalamic hormones and antagonists		
GnRH		
Gonadorelin	Very short half-life (4 min) due to tissue uptake and intracellular metabolism	Synthetic preparation identical to GnRH; used for endometriosis (Ch. 45) and breast and prostate cancer (Ch. 52); given by subcutaneous or intravenous injection
Gonadorelin analogues		
Buserelin	See Ch. 52	Used for prostate cancer (Ch. 52)
Goserelin	See Ch. 52	Used for prostate cancer (Ch. 52)
Leuprorelin acetate	See Ch. 52	Used for prostate cancer (Ch. 52)
Nafarelin	See Ch. 45	Used for endometriosis (Ch. 45)
Triptorelin	See Ch. 52	Used for prostate cancer (Ch. 52)
GnRH antagonists		
Inhibit the release of gonadotropins (LH and FSH); used to inhibit premature LH surges in the treatment of female infertility (under specialist supervision).		
Cetrorelix	Metabolised by peptidases; some is eliminated unchanged in urine and bile (20–60 h)	Synthetic decapeptide given by subcutaneous injection
Ganirelix	Metabolised by peptidases; some is eliminated unchanged in urine and bile (16 h)	Synthetic decapeptide given by subcutaneous injection
Drugs that interfere with gonadotropin release (anti-oestrogens)		
Anti-oestrogens used in the treatment of female infertility due to oligomenorrhoea or secondary amenorrhoea; they reduce negative feedback and induce gonadotropin release.		
Clomifene	Biliary excretion and enterohepatic circulation (5 days)	Given orally
Tamoxifen	See Ch. 52	Main use is in breast cancer (Ch. 52)
GHRIH (somatostatin) analogues		
Lanreotide	Eliminated by renal excretion and probably by tissue uptake and metabolism (1.3 h)	Used for acromegaly and for neuroendocrine and thyroid tumours; given by intramuscular or deep subcutaneous injection
Octreotide	Eliminated by renal excretion (about 40%) and probably by tissue uptake and metabolism (1.7 h)	Used for acromegaly and neuroendocrine tumours, and for reducing vomiting in palliative care and stopping oesophageal variceal bleeds; given by subcutaneous injection or by intravenous injection if a more rapid response is required
Anterior pituitary hormones and antagonists		
Corticotrophins		
Tetracosactide	Metabolised by endopeptidases in serum (0.2 h)	ACTH analogue; used largely as a test of adrenocortical function; given by intramuscular or intravenous injection
Gonadotropins (FSH, LH and HCG) and analogues		
Follitropin alfa and beta (FSH)	Slow release from injection site; mostly eliminated by metabolism (24–40 h)	Recombinant human FSH; given by subcutaneous or intramuscular injection
Lutropin alfa (LH)	About 50% absorbed from the injection site as active drug (14 h)	Recombinant human LH; given by subcutaneous injection
Human menopausal gonadotropins (menotrophin)	Metabolites eliminated in urine (FSH 7–10 h; LH 3 h)	Contains 1:1 mixture of FSH and LH; given by deep intramuscular or subcutaneous injection
Human chorionic gonadotropin (HCG	Slow release from the site of injection; hepatic metabolism (30–35 h)	Mainly LH activity; extracted from urine of pregnant women; given by subcutaneous or intramuscular injection

Compendium: pituitary and hypothalamic hormones—cont'd

Drug	Kinetics (half-life)	Comments
Choriogonadotropin alfa	Metabolic routes not defined; about 10% is excreted in urine (29 h)	Recombinant HCG; given by subcutaneous injection
Corifollitropin alfa	Slow release from injection site; renal elimination (59–79 h)	Synthetic FSH (modified); given by subcutaneous injection
Growth hormone		
Somatropin	Slow release from injection site; proteolytic degradation (4 h)	Synthetic form of growth hormone (somatotropin); given by subcutaneous or intramuscular injection
Growth hormone receptor antagonists		
Pegvisomant	Route of elimination not defined (6 days)	Pegylated synthetic antagonist of growth hormone receptors; given by subcutaneous injection
Prolactin antagonists		
Used to suppress lactation.		
Bromocriptine	See Ch. 24	D_2 receptor agonist; given orally (Ch. 24)
Cabergoline	See Ch. 24	D_2 receptor agonist; better tolerated than bromocriptine; given orally (Ch. 24)
Quinagolide	Well absorbed; hepatic metabolism; renal and faecal excretion (17 h)	Non-ergot D_2 receptor agonist; better tolerated than bromocriptine; given orally
TSH		
Thyrotropin alfa	Mainly renal elimination (22 h)	Recombinant TSH; used to detect thyroid remnants post-thyroidectomy; given by intramuscular injection
Posterior pituitary hormones and antagonists		
Demeclocycline	Oral bioavailability 66%; renal and biliary elimination (10–15 h)	Tetracycline antibiotic with anti-ADH action in renal tubule; used for treatment of hyponatraemia resulting from inappropriate secretion of ADH; given orally
Desmopressin	Poor oral bioavailability due to presystemic metabolism; metabolised by liver, kidney and plasma (0.5–2 h)	Vasopressin analogue; used for treatment of cranial diabetes insipidus; given orally, intranasally, or by subcutaneous, intramuscular or intravenous injection
Terlipressin	Prodrug hydrolysed to active lysine-vasopressin (which has half-life of 0.5 h)	Used for treatment of oesophageal varices; given by intravenous injection
Tolvaptan	Oral bioavailability 56%; hepatic metabolism (8 h)	Antagonist of vasopressin V2 receptors in renal collecting ducts; used for treating hyponatraemia resulting from inappropriate secretion of ADH; given orally
Vasopressin (ADH)	Rapidly metabolised in kidney, liver, brain and placenta (5–15 min)	Used for treatment of cranial diabetes insipidus and bleeding oesophageal varices; given by subcutaneous or intramuscular injection or by intravenous infusion

ACTH, adrenocorticotropic hormone; ADH, antidiuretic hormone; FSH, follicle-stimulating hormone; GHRIH, growth hormone-release inhibiting hormone; GnRH, gonadotropin-releasing hormone; HCG, human chorionic gonadotropin; LH, luteinizing hormone; TSH, thyroid-stimulating hormone.

STRUCTURE AND SYNTHESIS OF STEROID HORMONES

Steroid hormones comprise several compounds synthesised mainly in the adrenal cortex and the gonads. They are derived from cholesterol and share a distinctive core structure of four conjoined rings (Fig. 44.1). The pathways of steroid hormone synthesis are shown in Figure 44.2. The steroid hormones responsible for phenotypic gender differences are known as the sex hormones; these compounds are considered in Chapters 45 and 46.

This chapter considers steroid hormones derived predominantly from the adrenal cortex that are known as adrenal corticosteroids. They have two distinct classes of action (see below and Table 44.1):

■ glucocorticoid activity, which affects carbohydrate and protein metabolism,
■ mineralocorticoid activity, which affects water and electrolyte balance.

The natural glucocorticoid is cortisol (also known as hydrocortisone), which has a hydroxyl grouping at position 17 and approximately equal affinity for glucocorticoid and mineralocorticoid receptors (but see below). The natural mineralocorticoid is aldosterone, which has an aldehyde grouping at position 18 and has little glucocorticoid activity. Synthetic corticosteroids that have been modified structur-

ally to enhance either the glucocorticoid or mineralocorticoid activity are widely used therapeutically.

Although hydrocortisone and various synthetic derivatives are used for their glucocorticoid activity, they are frequently referred to as 'corticosteroids' or much less accurately as 'steroids'. In this chapter, the distinction between glucocorticoid and mineralocorticoid is emphasised. In the rest of the book drugs with mainly glucocorticoid activity are usually referred to as corticosteroids.

Cortisol (hydrocortisone) is released from the zona fasciculata of the adrenal cortex, and its secretion is controlled by the hypothalamo–pituitary–adrenal axis (Fig. 44.3). An increase in the plasma glucocorticoid concentration feeds back negatively to the hypothalamus and pituitary to reduce the release of corticotropin-releasing hormone (CRH) and adrenocorticotropic hormone (ACTH; corticotropin). Glucocorticoid receptors are found in most tissues, giving cortisol a wide range of actions.

Aldosterone is secreted from the zona glomerulosa of the adrenal cortex. Aldosterone secretion is regulated by several factors, of which angiotensin II (Ch. 6), low plasma Na^+ and high plasma K^+ are the most important. Angiotensin II acts via specific AT_1 receptors (see Chs 1 and 6) to induce aldosterone release. ACTH has a modest stimulatory effect on aldosterone secretion. Mineralocorticoid receptors are found in several tissues including the kidney, colon and heart. Important target cells are in the distal renal tubule and cortical collecting duct, where aldosterone increases the permeability of the luminal tubular membrane to Na^+ by increasing the number of epithelial Na^+ channels. It also stimulates the Na^+/K^+-ATPase pump in the basolateral membrane, which leads to active Na^+ reabsorption and loss of K^+ into tubular urine (Ch. 14). Water is passively reabsorbed with Na^+, so that extracellular fluid volume and blood pressure are both increased. Target cells for aldosterone, especially in the renal tubule, contain 11β-hydroxysteroid dehydrogenase which metabolises cortisol to cortisone. Cortisone has very low affinity for the mineralocorticoid receptor and this ensures that most aldosterone-responsive tissues are not stimulated by endogenous glucocorticoid.

MODE OF ACTION OF STEROID HORMONES

All steroid hormones have similar intracellular receptor mechanisms, but there are distinct receptors for the different structural variants (Ch. 1). The distribution of the various receptors among tissues gives tissue specificity to each type of steroid hormone and defines its activity. In the circulation, steroid hormones are bound to specific

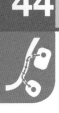

globulins, including transcortin and sex hormone-binding globulin. Steroids are highly lipophilic and cross cell membranes by diffusion and bind to a specific cytoplasmic receptor (Ch. 1). In the absence of a steroid molecule, the receptor is retained in the cytoplasm and prevented from migrating to the cell nucleus because it is associated with a heat-shock protein (HSP). Binding of the steroid to the

receptor dissociates the complex from the HSP, and the steroid–receptor complex then enters the nucleus and binds to a steroid-response element in the promoter region of the target genes (see Fig. 1.8). The binding usually involves the presence of other proteins, called chaperone proteins, and can lead to either increased or decreased transcription of proteins, depending on the target cell. Some genes are activated by simple interaction of the steroid receptor with the steroid-response element, but the rate of gene transcription is modulated by recruitment of various intranuclear co-regulator proteins and complexes.

The corticosteroid receptor only interacts with the steroid-response element for a matter of seconds before dissociating, and appears to have a 'hit-and-run' effect on gene transcription. When corticosteroids are given for a therapeutic effect, the response is delayed by many hours due to the time taken for modulation of protein synthesis. However, some actions of glucocorticoids are relatively rapid in onset and do not require gene transcription (non-genomic signalling pathways). They may produce direct activation of various kinases in the cell cytoplasm through a ligand-activated glucocorticoid receptor or through G-protein-coupled receptors, leading to effects such as vasodilation and regulation of cell growth.

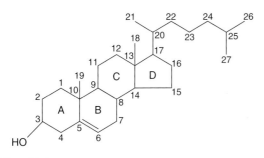

Fig. 44.1 **The core structure of steroid hormones is derived from the cholesterol molecule shown.** The four rings are each identified by a letter A–D, and each carbon atom by a number.

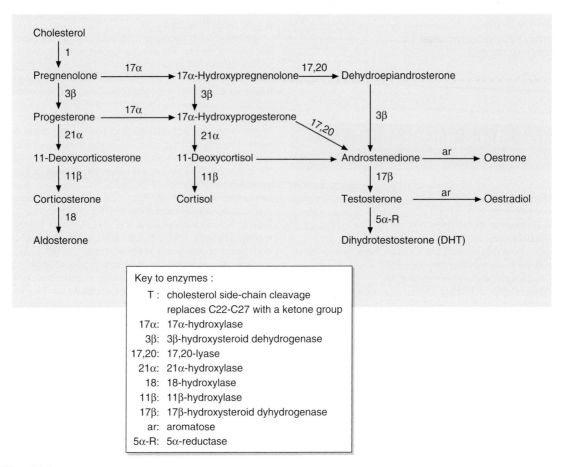

Fig. 44.2 Pathways of biosynthesis of steroid hormones, including progestogens, oestrogens, androgens, mineralocorticoids and glucocorticoids.

Table 44.1 Relative glucocorticoid and mineralocorticoid activities of some natural and synthetic corticosteroid hormones

	Glucocorticoid	Mineralocorticoid
Cortisol (hydrocortisone)	1	1
Prednisolone	4	0.8
Dexamethasone	30	Negligible
Betamethasone	30	Negligible
Aldosterone	0	80
Fludrocortisone	10	125

All potencies are relative to the glucocorticoid and mineralocorticoid activities of cortisol, each assigned an arbitrary value of 1. Due to intracellular metabolism by 11β-hydroxysteroid dehydrogenase in aldosterone-sensitive cells, cortisol has about one-thousandth of the mineralocorticoid activity of aldosterone *in vivo*.

GLUCOCORTICOIDS

Examples

betamethasone, dexamethasone, hydrocortisone, prednisolone

ACTIONS OF GLUCOCORTICOIDS

Immunosuppressant and anti-inflammatory actions

Glucocorticoids have important immunomodulatory actions that underpin many of their therapeutic uses. A major action of glucocorticoids is to silence pro-inflammatory genes (gene transrepression). These genes are activated by pro-inflammatory transcription factors such as nuclear factor κB (NF-κB) and activator protein 1 (AP-1) produced in response to inflammatory cytokines. NF-κB and AP-1 attach to the promoter region of pro-inflammatory genes and recruit co-activator molecules such as cAMP response element-binding protein (CBP) that have histone acetyltransferase activity. CBP acetylates core histones at the transcription complex which in turn activates pro-inflammatory gene transcription.

When glucocorticoid receptors are activated they bind to CBP at the glucocorticoid response element of inflammatory genes and inhibit histone acetyltransferase activity by recruiting co-repressor molecules. The glucocorticoid receptors also recruit histone deacetylase to suppress the pro-inflammatory genes. As a consequence, glucocorticoids inhibit the synthesis of many inflammatory cytokines, chemokines, adhesion molecules, inflammatory enzymes and receptors for inflammatory mediators.

Glucocorticoids also activate anti-inflammatory genes (gene transactivation). This is achieved by stimulation of core histone acetylation at the promoter regions of anti-inflammatory genes.

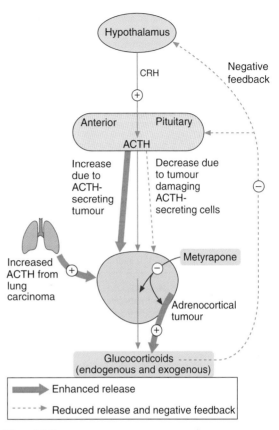

Fig. 44.3 Control of secretion of glucocorticoids. Corticotropin-releasing hormone (CRH) from the hypothalamus stimulates adrenocorticotropic hormone (ACTH; corticotropin) from the anterior pituitary, which increases the release of glucocorticoids from the adrenal cortex. The level of glucocorticoids in the blood feeds back negatively to control the release of CRH and ACTH. Synthetic glucocorticoids have the same suppressive action on the hypothalamo–pituitary axis. In conditions in which excess glucocorticoids are released, for example in ACTH-secreting tumours or adrenocortical tumours, glucocorticoid synthesis and release can be reduced by metyrapone (red arrows). In people with tumours that result in hormone-induced reduction in glucocorticoids, synthetic glucocorticoids can be administered.

Anti-inflammatory effects

As a result of the above actions, glucocorticoids:

- reduce T-lymphocyte proliferation and increase T-cell apoptosis, which impairs cell-mediated immunity (Ch. 38). They also inhibit humoral immunity by reducing T-cell activation, B-lymphocyte proliferation and immunoglobulin production, particularly IgG (Ch. 38),
- inhibit mononuclear cell and neutrophil leucocyte migration and their adhesion to inflamed capillary endothelium. The ability of these inflammatory cells to phagocytose and destroy micro-organisms and to release oxygen free radicals is also reduced through downregulation of their surface receptors (Ch. 38),

- reduce the synthesis of inflammatory prostaglandins by inhibition of phospholipase A_2 activity (via induction of annexin-1) and by suppression of cyclo-oxygenase expression (Ch. 29),
- impair fibroblast activity with reduced collagen synthesis and inhibition of matrix metalloproteinases, which impairs wound repair,
- decrease capillary permeability, which has a protective effect on blood volume and raises blood pressure. The sensitivity of vascular walls to the vasoconstrictor actions of catecholamines and angiotensin II is also enhanced.

Metabolic effects

- Gluconeogenesis is increased, particularly in the liver, using amino acids and glycerol from triglycerides. Storage of glycogen in the liver and, to a lesser extent, in muscle is increased, and uptake and utilisation of glucose in muscle and adipose tissue are impaired. These actions promote hyperglycaemia.
- Protein is degraded, particularly in muscle, to release amino acids for synthesis of glucose while protein synthesis is inhibited. As a result there is an overall negative nitrogen balance.
- Fat is redistributed from the glucocorticoid-sensitive fat stores in the limbs to the glucocorticoid-resistant stores in the face, neck and trunk. This action results from enhancement of the lipolytic response to catecholamines, and releases glycerol for glucose synthesis.

Effects on bone metabolism

- Osteoblast formation is decreased, and apoptosis of mature osteoblasts is increased. The function of mature osteoblasts is inhibited by reducing production of osteocalcin, a key extracellular matrix protein in bone that promotes bone mineralisation. Osteocyte apoptosis is increased which reduces bone strength. By contrast, survival of osteoclasts is prolonged. These actions lead to bone resorption and demineralisation.
- Inhibition of the proliferation and differentiation of chondrocytes at the epiphyseal end of the growth plate of long bones reduces bone growth in children.

Central nervous system effects

Plasma cortisol concentrations rise to a peak at the time of awakening and are lowest during sleep. In general, high circulating concentrations of cortisol are associated with alertness, but severe disturbances of mood may occur with abnormally high levels of glucocorticoid. Low concentrations produce a feeling of lethargy.

Mineralocorticoid effects

Natural glucocorticoids also have mineralocorticoid activity, although this has minimal impact at physiological doses (see above). Synthetic glucocorticoid compounds are altered structurally to minimise the amount of mineralocorticoid activity (Table 44.1).

PHARMACOKINETICS OF GLUCOCORTICOIDS

Both hydrocortisone and synthetic glucocorticoids are used in clinical practice. They are readily absorbed from the gut. Hydrocortisone binds to corticosteroid-binding globulin (transcortin) and to albumin in the blood, and is extensively metabolised in the gut wall and liver. Synthetic glucocorticoids are more potent than hydrocortisone and bind to albumin but not to transcortin. They are more slowly metabolised in the liver, giving them a longer duration of action. Of the many synthetic glucocorticoids, dexamethasone is the most potent and has the least mineralocorticoid activity.

Most glucocorticoids are available in formulations for parenteral use. This does not appreciably shorten the time to onset of action, since most effects are delayed by up to 8 h while protein synthesis is modulated intracellularly. Some glucocorticoids are available in formulations for topical use (e.g. beclometasone, budesonide and fluticasone by inhaler for asthma). This reduces their systemic actions although systemic unwanted effects can still occur, particularly with high doses (see also Chs 12 and 34).

The plasma half-lives of glucocorticoids vary, but, because their mechanism of action depend on gene transcription and changes in protein synthesis, their biological (i.e. effective) half-lives are long (varying from 8 h for hydrocortisone to 2 days for dexamethasone).

CLINICAL USES OF SYSTEMICALLY ADMINISTERED GLUCOCORTICOIDS

The anti-inflammatory and immunosuppressant effects of glucocorticoids are used for control of various inflammatory diseases (especially those which are immunologically mediated) and treatment of neoplastic conditions, particularly when they involve lymphoid tissue (Box 44.1). Powerful glucocorticoids with little mineralocorticoid activity, such as prednisolone, are usually chosen. Dexamethasone is used to reduce oedema around malignant tumours in the brain and those compressing the spinal cord. It is also used in some anti-emetic regimens during cancer chemotherapy (Ch. 32).

Resistance to the anti-inflammatory and immunosuppressant effects of glucocorticoids occurs in some individuals. The mechanisms are complex, and arise from a variety of excessively activated intracellular inflammatory pathways. There are no reliable strategies to overcome glucocorticoid resistance, and alternative immunosuppressant drugs may need to be used (Ch. 38).

Physiological replacement therapy for corticosteroid deficiency

Hydrocortisone or an equivalent synthetic glucocorticoid is given orally twice or three times daily in doses as close as possible to the amount normally secreted by the adrenal

Box 44.1 **Examples of diseases for which systemic glucocorticoid therapy is useful**

Replacement therapy in corticosteroid deficiency
Acute inflammatory disease:
    Bronchial asthma
    Anaphylaxis and angioedema
    Acute fibrosing alveolitis

Chronic inflammatory disease:
    Connective tissue disorders, e.g. systemic lupus
       erythematosus, polymyositis, vasculitis
    Renal disorders, e.g. glomerulonephritis
    Hepatic disorders, e.g. chronic active hepatitis
    Bowel disorders, e.g. inflammatory bowel disease
    Eye disorders, e.g. posterior uveitis

Neoplastic disease:
Myeloma
    Lymphomas
    Lymphocytic leukaemias

Miscellaneous disorders:
Bell's palsy
    Sarcoidosis
    Organ transplantation
    Anti-emetic therapy (for cytotoxic chemotherapy)

Box 44.2 **Causes of glucocorticoid excess (Cushing's syndrome) and corticosteroid deficiency**

Causes of Cushing's syndrome

- Excessive secretion of ACTH by the anterior pituitary (pituitary adenoma) (Cushing's disease)
- Excessive secretion of ACTH from an ectopic source (most commonly carcinoma of the bronchus)
- A tumour of the adrenal cortex secreting predominantly cortisol
- Iatrogenic: administration of glucocorticoid or ACTH in pharmacological doses

Causes of corticosteroid deficiency

- Primary adrenal insufficiency (Addison's disease):
  - Autoimmune adrenalitis
  - Infections, e.g. tuberculosis, various fungi, opportunistic infections in AIDS
  - Metastatic carcinoma
- Secondary adrenocortical failure (deficient ACTH from the anterior pituitary):
  - Pituitary tumour
  - Sarcoidosis
  - Suppression of the hypothalamo–pituitary–adrenal axis by prolonged glucocorticoid treatment at pharmacological doses
- Various enzyme defects in cortisol synthesis (congenital adrenal hyperplasia)

Table 44.2 Examples of topical corticosteroid administration

Disease	Mode of administration	Chapter in this book
Asthma	Aerosol	12
Vasomotor rhinitis	Aerosol	39
Eczema	Ointment or cream	49
Superficial ocular inflammation	Aqueous solution	50
Ulcerative colitis	Aqueous solution or foam enema	34
Proctitis	Suppository	34
Arthritis	Aqueous solution by intra-articular injection	30

CLINICAL USES OF TOPICALLY ADMINISTERED GLUCOCORTICOIDS

Topical use of glucocorticoids can deliver high concentrations to a target site and reduce systemic unwanted effects. However, significant absorption into the blood occurs at higher doses. Examples of the clinical uses of topical glucocorticoids are given in Table 44.2.

UNWANTED EFFECTS OF GLUCOCORTICOIDS

Pharmacological doses of systemic glucocorticoids given over long periods will produce the typical features of adrenocortical overactivity (Cushing's syndrome). Unwanted glucocorticoid actions are shown in Box 44.3. These effects do not occur when physiological replacement doses of a glucocorticoid are used.

CUSHING'S SYNDROME

Cushing's syndrome is characterised by excessive glucocorticoid effects (Box 44.3). There are four possible causes (Box 44.2).

Surgery is the definitive treatment for excessive pituitary secretion of ACTH (usually from an adenoma) and for unilateral adrenal tumours, with subsequent radiotherapy for some pituitary tumours.

Drug treatment to reduce glucocorticoid secretion is desirable for several weeks before surgery, in order to reverse the excessive tissue catabolism and correct the metabolic disturbances. This is usually achieved with metyrapone, which reduces glucocorticoid biosynthesis by competitive inhibition of 11β-hydroxylase (Fig. 44.2). Metyrapone also inhibits cytochrome P450 in the liver, which can produce important drug interactions. Gastrointestinal upset is the main unwanted effect. The antifungal agent ketoconazole (Ch. 51) also reduces cortisol synthesis by inhibition of 11β-hydroxylase, but its onset of action is slower than that of metyrapone. In addition, it inhibits sex steroid production and therefore often causes gynaecomastia and decreased libido in males and hirsutism in

cortex. The dose must be doubled or tripled in stressful situations, for example intercurrent infection. Acute adrenal insufficiency requires immediate treatment with high-dose intravenous hydrocortisone. Conditions that can give rise to glucocorticoid deficiency are shown in Box 44.2.

For uses of ACTH and its analogues, see Chapter 43.

- Central obesity with 'buffalo hump', moon face and abdominal striae
- Loss of supporting tissue in skin with skin atrophy, bruising and poor wound healing; local atrophy can be marked at the site of topical corticosteroid application
- Osteoporosis due to catabolism of protein matrix in the bone and defective mineralisation
- Proximal (i.e. shoulder and hip girdle) muscle wasting and weakness
- Hyperglycaemia, which may lead to overt diabetes mellitus (Ch. 40)
- Peptic ulceration due to inhibition of gastrointestinal prostaglandin (Ch. 33)
- Mood changes, including euphoria and occasionally psychosis
- Posterior capsular cataracts in the eye, and exacerbation of glaucoma
- Increased susceptibility to infection with bacteria, viruses or fungi; activation of latent infections such as tuberculosis can also occur
- Growth retardation in children, with reduced linear bone growth and premature epiphyseal closure
- After long-term treatment, sudden withdrawal can produce an acute adrenal crisis due to suppression of the hypothalamic–pituitary–adrenal axis and adrenal atrophy. Recovery of adrenal responsiveness can take several months. Basal cortisol secretion is restored before maximal responses, leaving patients at risk during stress and intercurrent infection.
- Mineralocorticoid effects (which vary between the different drugs)

females. Ketoconazole can be used alone or in combination with metyrapone. All these drugs have relatively short-lived benefit, with rapid loss of control (escape) when increased ACTH secretion is the cause of the syndrome.

Mitotane is a chemotherapeutic drug (Ch. 52) that causes more profound suppression of glucocorticoid synthesis with no escape. It can be used for long-term control of symptoms for people who are unwilling or too unfit to undergo surgery. Glucocorticoid-replacement therapy is usually necessary during treatment with mitotane.

Ectopic ACTH secretion is not usually amenable to surgical cure, but palliative drug treatment can be helpful (Fig. 44.3).

MINERALOCORTICOIDS

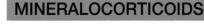

fludrocortisone

FLUDROCORTISONE

Pharmacokinetics

Aldosterone is almost completely inactivated on its first passage through the liver and is therefore unsuitable for oral use. Fludrocortisone (9α-fluorohydrocortisone) is a synthetic alternative but only about 10% escapes first-pass metabolism. Its half-life is short (0.5 h) due to rapid hepatic metabolism.

Clinical uses

- Fludrocortisone is given as replacement therapy for defective aldosterone production. This is usually the result of primary adrenal pathology with destruction of all three zones of the adrenal cortex (Addison's disease).
- Expansion of blood volume by fludrocortisone can be used to raise blood pressure in postural hypotension resulting from autonomic neuropathy. However, it often produces supine hypertension without fully eliminating the postural fall in blood pressure.

Unwanted effects

Excessive Na⁺ retention and K⁺ loss can occur with pharmacological doses of fludrocortisone. Hypertension can result, but the expansion of blood volume stimulates cardiac stretch receptors, leading to secretion of natriuretic peptides. This results in an 'escape' natriuresis which establishes a new equilibrium between Na⁺ intake and excretion at a higher blood volume. Consequently, oedema does not usually occur.

PRIMARY HYPERALDOSTERONISM (CONN'S SYNDROME)

Autonomous oversecretion of aldosterone causes hypertension and a hypokalaemic alkalosis. Some cases are caused by an adenoma in the zona glomerulosa of the adrenal cortex and are treated surgically. The majority are caused by hyperplasia of both zonae glomerulosa. This usually causes less marked clinical consequences, and a potassium-sparing diuretic (usually spironolactone) is the treatment of choice to preserve the plasma K⁺ concentration and reduce blood pressure (Ch. 14).

SELF-ASSESSMENT

True/false questions

1. Glucocorticoids take many hours to produce their clinical effects.
2. Inhaled glucocorticoids do not cause systemic unwanted effects.
3. Oral fludrocortisone is a useful anti-inflammatory corticosteroid in severe asthma.
4. Fluticasone is not used orally.
5. Metyrapone inhibits glucocorticoid synthesis.
6. Hypoglycaemia is common during glucocorticoid administration.
7. If prolonged administration of prednisolone results in unwanted effects, it should be withdrawn immediately.
8. Mineralocorticoid secretion is decreased in Addison's disease.

9. Aldosterone secretion is inhibited by angiotensin II.
10. Glucocorticoids do not affect inflammatory responses provoked by infection.
11. Dexamethasone causes vomiting.
12. Glucocorticoids delay wound healing.

Case-based questions

Case 1

A 35-year-old woman showed signs of cortisol excess, including centripetal obesity, muscle weakness, easy bruising and amenorrhoea.

A. What were the possible causes?
B. She was not taking corticosteroids, eliminating an iatrogenic cause. The cortisol level in a 24-h urine sample was elevated, and the plasma adrenocorticotropic hormone (ACTH) level was also high.
   What did these results indicate?
C. A single high dose of dexamethasone was administered and resulted in only marginal suppression of plasma cortisol.
   What did this result indicate?
D. A computed tomography scan and other tests showed an inoperable carcinoma of the bronchus.
   What treatment could be given?

Case 2

Mr BFG, a 69-year-old man, had late-onset asthma, which was poorly controlled by β_2-adrenoceptor agonists. His GP prescribed a low-dose inhaled corticosteroid that helped him initially.

A. Which glucocorticoids could have been given by aerosol inhaler?
B. What were the possible unwanted effects of the low-dose inhaled glucocorticoid?
C. Mr BFG then had a particularly severe attack (acute severe asthma or status asthmaticus) which led to his admission to hospital as an emergency.
   Among the drugs he was given was an intravenous corticosteroid. Which drug was likely to have been given and what was the objective of its use?
D. Mr BFG's status asthmaticus resolved and he was then prescribed a course of oral corticosteroid while in hospital and subsequently sent home with high-dose inhaled corticosteroid.
   Which corticosteroid could have been used for oral therapy?
E. Mr BFG's asthma was poorly controlled by a higher dose of inhaled corticosteroid and it was decided to recommence oral therapy.
   Why might oral therapy be better than inhaled therapy in severe chronic asthma?
F. How would you have determined the dose to be used and monitor its appropriateness?
G. After many months of this therapy, Mr BFG started to complain of apparently unrelated problems, including: recurrent minor infections, minor epigastric discomfort, especially on an empty stomach, weight gain and increased appetite, a tendency to bruise easily and severe back pain after a minor fall. Examination revealed a cushingoid appearance, and investigation showed a raised plasma glucose level and a decreased plasma level of cortisol and ACTH. Discuss the reasons for Mr BFG's symptoms.

True/false answers

1. **True.** Glucocorticoids act principally by modulating gene transcription so most of their clinical effects are not seen for several hours.
2. **False.** In maximum recommended doses, inhaled glucocorticoids can cause systemic effects.
3. **False.** Fludrocortisone is a synthetic mineralocorticoid with weak anti-inflammatory effects; glucocorticoids such as prednisolone are used orally in severe asthma.
4. **True.** Inhaled fluticasone is used for topical effects on the airways in the treatment of asthma.
5. **True.** Metyrapone inhibits synthesis of cortisol, and to a lesser extent that of aldosterone, by inhibiting steroid 11β-hydroxylase.
6. **False.** Corticosteroids cause hyperglycaemia by reducing tissue uptake of glucose and increased gluconeogenesis ('steroid-induced diabetes').
7. **False.** Prolonged administration of a systemic glucocorticoid may suppress the hypothalamo–pituitary–adrenal axis. The drug should be withdrawn slowly to allow the adrenals to recover their normal cortisol secretion and avoid corticosteroid deficiency.
8. **True.** Addison's disease can be caused by autoimmune disease or drugs such as ketoconazole.
9. **False.** Angiotensin II is produced by the action of renin, which is secreted when plasma sodium concentrations are low; angiotensin II then stimulates aldosterone release from the adrenal cortex and this increases Na^+ reabsorption in the renal tubule.
10. **False.** Glucocorticoids suppress all inflammatory responses including those produced by infection.
11. **False.** Dexamethasone can inhibit vomiting and will add to the anti-emetic actions of agents such as ondansetron used in cancer chemotherapy.
12. **True.** Glucocorticoids delay wound healing because of their catabolic effect on proteins.

Case-based answers

Case 1

A. Possible causes include a tumour of the adrenal cortex secreting cortisol; excess secretion of adrenocorticotropic hormone (ACTH) by a pituitary tumour, or by a non-pituitary tumour (commonly small-cell carcinoma of the lung, medullary or thyroid carcinoma); or therapeutic administration of glucocorticoids or ACTH (iatrogenic).
B. The cause could not be a primary cortisol-secreting adrenocortical tumour or glucocorticoid administration, as the plasma ACTH level would then be low due to negative feedback of glucocorticoid on the anterior

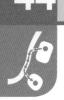
pituitary and hypothalamus. The possibilities are an ACTH-secreting pituitary or non-pituitary tumour.

C. Dexamethasone suppresses ACTH of pituitary origin but not from ectopic ACTH-producing tumours or adrenocortical tumours. The result might therefore exclude a tumour of pituitary origin.

D. Metyrapone, an inhibitor of adrenal corticosteroid synthesis, could be given. She would probably also show signs of excess mineralocorticoid activity, which should be treated concomitantly with spironolactone.

Case 2

A. Inhaled glucocorticoids include beclometasone, budesonide and fluticasone (see Ch. 12).

B. Systemic unwanted effects are unlikely at low doses of inhaled glucocorticoids. Local problems such as oral candidiasis could be managed with a spacer device and good oral hygiene.

C. Intravenous hydrocortisone is likely to have been used to reduce airway inflammation in this acute exacerbation of asthma, although its onset of action would be delayed by several hours.

D. A short course (5 days) of oral prednisolone could have been used.

E. A high concentration of glucocorticoid is needed at inflammatory cells in the airways, and poor inhaler technique or airway obstruction by inflammation and mucus might prevent inhaled drugs reaching their target. Systemic prednisolone reaches airway inflammatory leucocytes more effectively than after inhalation in these circumstances, and may also reduce bone marrow proliferation and airway recruitment of eosinophils.

F. The lowest possible doses of glucocorticoid should be used in chronic asthma management, using peak expiratory flow measurements and a symptom diary at home to monitor asthma control and to step the dosages up or down as appropriate.

G. Glucocorticoids have a wide range of metabolic effects in addition to their anti-inflammatory and immunomodulatory actions. The cushingoid symptoms described can all be attributed to actions on carbohydrate, protein and lipid metabolism and suppression of the hypothalamo–pituitary–adrenal axis.

FURTHER READING

Barnes PJ, Adcock IM (2009) Glucocorticoid resistance in inflammatory disease. *Lancet* 373, 1905–1917

Feldman RD, Gros R (2011) Unravelling the mechanisms underlying the rapid vascular effects of steroids: sorting out the receptors and the pathways. *Br J Pharmacol* 163, 1163–1169

Lipworth BS (1999) Systemic adverse effects of inhaled corticosteroid therapy. *Arch Intern Med* 159, 941–955

Lovas K, Husebye ES (2003) Replacement therapy in Addison's disease. *Expert Opin Pharmacother* 4, 2145–2149

Newell-Price J, Bertagna X, Grossman AB et al. (2006) Cushing's syndrome. *Lancet* 367, 1605–1617

Nieman LK, Ilias I (2005) Evaluation and treatment of Cushing's syndrome. *Am J Med* 118, 1340–1346

Rhen T, Cidlowski JA (2005) Antiinflammatory effects of glucocorticoids–new mechanisms for old drugs. *N Engl J Med* 353, 1711–1723

Weinstein RS (2011) Glucocorticoid-induced bone disease. *N Engl J Med* 365, 62–70

Young WF Jr (2003) Minireview: primary aldosteronism – changing concepts in diagnosis and treatment. *Endocrinology* 144, 2208–2213

Compendium: corticosteroids

Drug	Kinetics (half-life)	Comments
Glucocorticoids		
The durations of action (biological half-lives) of glucocorticoids greatly exceed their chemical half-lives because of their mechanism of action.		
Betamethasone	Ester prodrugs are hydrolysed to betamethasone; betamethasone is rapidly absorbed if given orally; hepatic metabolism (35–55 h)	Used for suppression of inflammatory and allergic disorders, congenital adrenal hyperplasia and cerebral oedema; given orally, topically, by intramuscular or slow intravenous injection, or by intravenous infusion; phosphate ester prodrug used for injections
Cortisone acetate	Oral bioavailability 20–90%; rapidly converted to cortisol (hydrocortisone)	Formerly used for replacement therapy; given orally
Deflazacort	Rapidly hydrolysed to active 21-desacetyl metabolite; mainly renal excretion (1–2 h)	Used for suppression of inflammatory and allergic disorders; given orally
Dexamethasone	High but variable oral bioavailability; hepatic metabolism (2–4 h)	Used for suppression of inflammatory and allergic disorders, congenital adrenal hyperplasia and cerebral oedema, and diagnosis of Cushing's disease; given orally, by intramuscular or slow intravenous injection, or by intravenous infusion; anti-emetic; phosphate ester prodrug is used for injections
Hydrocortisone (cortisol)	Variable absorption (30–90%) due to first-pass metabolism; metabolised to cortisone and to dihydro- and tetrahydrocortisol (1–2 h)	Numerous anti-inflammatory and anti-allergic uses; given orally, by intramuscular or slow intravenous injection, or by intravenous infusion; phosphate ester prodrug is used for injections
Methylprednisolone	High oral bioavailability (80–90%); esters are rapidly hydrolysed; metabolised in liver and kidney (1–3 h)	Used for suppression of inflammatory and allergic disorders, cerebral oedema and connective tissue disease; given orally, by intramuscular or slow intravenous injection, or by intravenous infusion; injectable forms are lipid-soluble esters in solvents
Prednisolone	High oral bioavailability (70–80%); hepatic metabolism (2–4 h)	Used for suppression of numerous inflammatory and allergic disorders; given orally, topically and by intramuscular injection; injectable form is the acetate ester as an aqueous suspension
Triamcinolone	Hepatic metabolism (2–5 h)	Used for suppression of inflammatory and allergic disorders; given by deep intramuscular injection as an aqueous suspension
Mineralocorticoids		
The durations of action (biological half-lives) of mineralocorticosteroids greatly exceed their chemical half-lives because of their mechanism of action.		
Fludrocortisone acetate	Low bioavailability (10%) due to first-pass metabolism; hydrolysed to fludrocortisol (0.5 h)	Mineralocorticoid used in combination with hydrocortisone for adrenocortical insufficiency; given orally
Inhibitor of steroid metabolism		
Metyrapone	Rapid oral absorption; metabolised to active metabolite (metyrapol) (2 h)	Competitive inhibitor of 11β-hydroxylation in the adrenal cortex; used to control the symptoms of Cushing's syndrome, especially prior to surgery; given orally

Additional corticosteroids used for specific purposes are covered in other chapters (see Table 44.2).

45 Female reproduction

PHYSIOLOGY OF THE MENSTRUAL CYCLE

The endocrine function of the hypothalamo–pituitary–ovarian axis acts through a series of feedback loops to control the reproductive processes of the menstrual cycle (Fig. 45.1). The menstrual cycle begins with the uterus shedding its lining (*menstrual phase*: usually days 1 to 3–5 of the menstrual cycle). Following the shedding of the endometrium, a group of five to seven follicles in the ovary that have been growing for up to a year start to mature. This occurs under the influence of the gonadotropic hormone follicle-stimulating hormone (FSH) secreted from the anterior pituitary (*follicular phase*: approximately days 5–13 of the menstrual cycle). The secretion of FSH starts during the menstrual phase and continues during the early follicular phase, and is a result of the low circulating concentration of oestrogen. Release of the gonadotropic hormones FSH and luteinizing hormone (LH) is controlled by pulsatile secretion of gonadotropin-releasing hormone (GnRH) from the hypothalamus (see also Ch. 43). The small follicles produce gonadotropin surge-attenuating factor (GnSAF) that acts on the hypothalamus to inhibit GnRH release and prevent a rise in LH. The follicles also produce inhibin, which reduces FSH release. A single dominant ovarian follicle (or occasionally two) is selected and matures in preparation for ovulation at the expense of the remaining follicles. Regression of the other follicles is probably due to a lack of receptors for FSH.

FSH drives the developing ovarian follicle to convert androgens produced by its thecal cells into oestradiol (Fig. 44.2) within its granulosa cells. Oestradiol secretion from the follicle slowly rises as the follicle matures. In the window of time between the early to mid-follicular phase of the menstrual cycle the modest amount of oestrogen secreted by the follicle exerts negative feedback on both the hypothalamus and pituitary to keep gonadotropin secretion low (Fig. 43.1). The low plasma concentration of progesterone also weakly suppresses gonadotropin secretion in the early follicular phase.

In the late follicular phase a cohort of granulosa cells in the maturing ovarian follicle differentiates under the influence of FSH and starts to express LH receptors. These granulosa cells can then be stimulated by LH to secrete progesterone and are destined to become the corpus luteum after ovulation. In the mid- to late follicular phase the circulating oestradiol concentration rises dramatically as the follicle secretes more of the hormone under the influence of FSH. Eventually the plasma oestradiol reaches a critical concentration of about 200 pg · mL^{-1} for 48 h. The rapid rise and sustained high concentration of oestradiol triggers a switch from negative feedback to positive

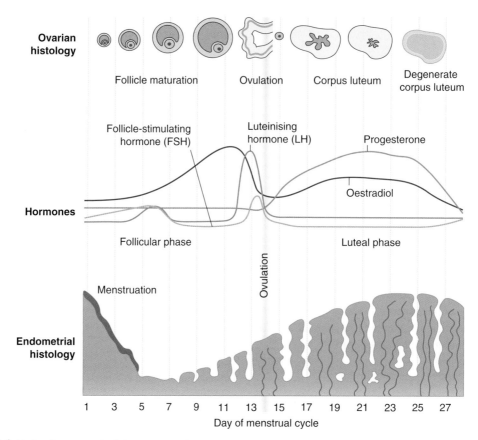

Fig. 45.1 Endocrine control of the menstrual cycle.

feedback of oestradiol upon the pituitary and hypothalamus, causing pulsatile release of GnRH. As a result there is an acute mid-cycle surge of LH for about 48 h, which is essential for ovulation. Ovulation involves release of the secondary oocyte from the follicle, which rapidly matures into an ovum.

Following *ovulation* (about day 14 of the menstrual cycle) the residual follicle transforms into the corpus luteum under the influence of the pituitary gonadotropins. The plasma LH concentration falls rapidly and remains low throughout the *secretory (luteal) phase* (days 15–26 of the menstrual cycle). The reason for this is that granulosa cells expressing LH receptors proliferate in the corpus luteum and produce increasing amounts of progesterone. Progesterone suppresses LH and FSH production by negative feedback on the hypothalamus and pituitary. If implantation of a fertilised ovum does not occur the corpus luteum regresses after about 10 days, since it requires gonadotropins to maintain itself.

From day 5 to late in the menstrual cycle the gradually increasing plasma concentrations of oestrogens, and subsequently progesterone, which are produced as the menstrual cycle progresses, result in proliferation and vascularisation of endometrial cells that are able to secrete a variety of fluids and nutrients aimed at making the endometrium receptive for implantation. The temporal

precision of the change in receptivity is critical if successful implantation of a fertilised oocyte is to occur. Oestrogen and progesterone cause the endometrium to become oedematous, and its glands secrete increasing quantities of amino acids, sugars and glycoproteins in a viscous liquid. At the end of the menstrual cycle the circulating concentrations of progesterone and oestrogen eventually fall to levels that no longer support the endometrium. Deprived of hormonal support, the endometrial spiral arteries go into spasm and the endometrial cells die, producing digestive enzymes (*ischaemic phase*: days 27–28 of the menstrual cycle). As a consequence of this and other changes the endometrium is shed during menstruation.

The cervical mucus is also influenced by oestrogen and progesterone concentrations. Under the dominant influence of progesterone cervical mucus is viscid and less penetrable by sperm, whereas at ovulation the high plasma oestradiol concentration results in thinner and more elastic mucus that is easily penetrable by sperm. Progesterone also inhibits the motility of the fallopian tube, altering the transport of sperm, and the fertilised or unfertilised oocyte. Excess progesterone may alter the chance of fertilisation occurring or the embryo may reach the uterine cavity when the endometrium is not receptive to implantation. Oestrogens have the opposite action, increasing tubal motility, and may accelerate the transport of the ovum into the uterine cavity.

PHYSIOLOGY OF PREGNANCY

Pregnancy is accompanied by considerable hormonal changes. When a fertilised ovum implants in the uterine lining the corpus luteum becomes essential for the production of progesterone and maintenance of pregnancy during the first 6–8 weeks. After this placental production of hormones takes over and the combined feto-placental unit produces progressively greater quantities of oestrogen and progesterone which reach the maternal circulation. The dividing cells of the implanted ovum start to secrete human chorionic gonadotropin (HCG) from about 9 days after fertilisation (Ch. 43). HCG stimulates the corpus luteum to continue to secrete progesterone. Eventually, the placenta takes over the production of HCG, progesterone and oestrogen. The placenta also produces human placental lactogen as pregnancy advances, resulting in the development of duct and milk-secreting cells in the mother's breasts. The precise balance of sex steroids also contributes to quiescence of the uterus during pregnancy and the onset of labour at term.

MECHANISM OF ACTION OF OESTROGENS AND PROGESTOGENS

In common with other steroid hormones, both oestrogens and progestogens act by influencing gene transcription (see also Ch. 44). They passively diffuse into the cell and bind to specific receptors in either the cytoplasm or cell nucleus (see Fig. 1.8). The receptors are associated with heat-shock protein (HSP) when in their unbound state in the cytosol. HSP dissociates when the hormone binds to the receptor, and the receptor forms dimers that are translocated by active transport to the cell nucleus. The steroid–receptor complex associates with hormone-response elements of numerous oestrogen- or progesterone-responsive genes. This leads to recruitment of co-activator molecules to the complex, and produces gene transcription (co-activation). Oestrogen binds to two specific cytoplasmic receptors (ERα and ERβ), which have different tissue distributions. Progesterone also has two specific receptors (PR-A and PR-B) that regulate progesterone-responsive genes. Oestrogen increases and progesterone decreases the expression of the progesterone receptors.

STEROIDAL CONTRACEPTIVES

Oral hormonal contraceptives ('the pill') are the most widely used form of contraception and contain either a combination of a synthetic oestrogen with a synthetic progestogen (a C19 synthetic progesterone derivative) or a progestogen alone.

MECHANISMS OF HORMONAL CONTRACEPTION

Elevated circulating concentrations of synthetic oestrogen and progestogen prevent the precise cyclic pattern of hormone-related events seen in the normal menstrual cycle (Fig. 45.2), and can be used for contraception.

- The combination of oestrogen and progestogen exerts its contraceptive effect mainly through suppression of FSH release, which prevents development of the follicles

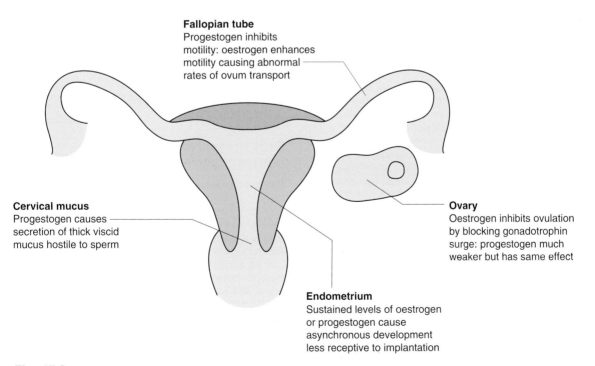

Fallopian tube
Progestogen inhibits motility: oestrogen enhances motility causing abnormal rates of ovum transport

Cervical mucus
Progestogen causes secretion of thick viscid mucus hostile to sperm

Ovary
Oestrogen inhibits ovulation by blocking gonadotrophin surge: progestogen much weaker but has same effect

Endometrium
Sustained levels of oestrogen or progestogen cause asynchronous development less receptive to implantation

Fig. 45.2 **The main contraceptive actions of the synthetic oestrogens and progestogens in the combined hormonal contraceptive pill.** FSH, follicle-stimulating hormone; LH, luteinizing hormone.

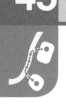
in the ovary. The lack of a dominant follicle means that production of oestradiol is impaired. The failure of plasma oestradiol to rise, combined with negative feedback from the progestogen, prevents the mid-cycle LH surge that is essential for ovulation to occur.

- Progestogen produces asynchronous development of the endometrium with stromal thinning, which makes it less receptive to implantation of the fertilised ovum. Fallopian tube motility is increased by oestrogens and decreased by progestogens; this may affect fertility by altering the rate of transport of the ovum.
- Progestogen alters cervical mucus, making it thicker and less copious, thereby creating an environment more hostile to sperm penetration.

Progestogens can be used alone for contraception, when the mechanism depends on the dose of progestogen. Low-dose progestogen inhibits ovulation in only about 50% of cycles, and contraception relies upon the other actions of the hormone. With higher doses, inhibition of follicular development and ovulation becomes more important.

THE 'COMBINED' HORMONAL CONTRACEPTIVE

Combined hormonal contraceptives (often called the combined oral contraceptive pill, or COCP) contain both a synthetic oestrogen and progestogen. The oestrogen component is usually ethinylestradiol (an oestrogen that is alkylated at C17 to slow its metabolism) but in some combinations is mestranol, a compound that is metabolised in the liver to ethinylestradiol. Over the years since the combined oral hormonal contraceptive was introduced, the dose of the oestrogen component has been reduced to minimise unwanted effects. 'Second-generation' combined hormonal contraceptives have a lower oestrogen concentration than 'first-generation' combined hormonal contraceptives, which are no longer used. The lowest dose of oestrogen that gives good menstrual cycle control (absence of breakthrough bleeding; see below) is preferred.

The progestogen component of the second-generation combined oral hormonal contraceptives is either levonorgestrel (the active isomer of norgestrel) or norethisterone; these compounds are testosterone analogues that also possess residual androgenic activity. 'Third-generation' oral combined hormonal contraceptives contain modified progestogens that have less androgenic activity – desogestrel, gestodene, norgestimate (which are all derivatives of norgestrel) – or anti-androgenic activity – dienogest, drospirenone (a derivative of the aldosterone antagonist spironolactone with some anti-mineralocorticoid activity). Modified progestogens are used if there are unacceptable unwanted effects with the second-generation progestogens.

Other differences and similarities between second- and third-generation combined hormonal contraceptives are discussed below.

Monophasic preparations

Monophasic preparations contain fixed amounts of oestrogen and progestogen. They are taken daily for the first 21 days of the menstrual cycle followed by seven contraceptive-free days with tablets containing an inactive substance, such as lactose. The oestrogen concentration should be the lowest that maintains good cycle control and produces minimal unwanted effects. There is a choice of:

- low-strength preparations that contain 20 µg ethinylestradiol,
- standard-strength preparations that contain 30 or 35 µg ethinylestradiol, or 50 µg mestranol.

The monophasic oral combined hormonal contraceptive contains one of several progestogens. In some women it may be necessary to change the formulation to reduce minor unwanted effects, such as breakthrough bleeding or weight gain during the menstrual cycle. The degree of androgenic activity possessed by different progestogens (see combined hormonal contraceptive section above) may influence the suitability of an individual preparation for a particular woman.

A transdermal patch formulation of low-strength ethinylestradiol with the third-generation progestogen norelgestromin is also available; this is applied weekly for 3 weeks followed by a 7-day patch-free interval. There is also a vaginal contraceptive ring that contains ethinylestradiol with the progestogen etonorgestrel.

Biphasic and triphasic preparations

Biphasic and triphasic preparations are designed to mimic more closely the changes in sex hormone concentrations that occur during the natural menstrual cycle. The total sex hormone intake through the cycle is no less than with monophasic preparations. Several preparations are available, all of which contain ethinylestradiol in combination with levonorgestrel, norethisterone or gestodene. The dose of ethinylestradiol is either kept constant throughout, as in the monophasic pills, or increased during days 7–12. Progestogen doses are increased once (biphasic) or twice (triphasic) as the menstrual cycle proceeds.

PROGESTOGEN-ONLY CONTRACEPTIVES

Oral progestogen-only contraceptives

The oral progestogen-only contraceptive ('progestogen-only pill', or POP) is particularly useful for women in whom the administration of oestrogen is considered to be undesirable, for example if there is a history of thromboembolic disorders (see below). Pregnancy rates are slightly higher than with a low-dose combined oral hormonal contraceptive. Various progestogens are used, such as desogestrel, etynodiol diacetate, gestodene, levonorgestrel or norethisterone. The progestogen-only contraceptive must be taken daily, without a break, and within 3 h of the usual time every day (see efficacy below). Because the dose of progestogen is low, bleeding does occur at monthly intervals but may be irregular. Breakthrough bleeding occurs in up to 40% of women; this is much higher than with the combined hormonal contraceptive. Some women become amenorrhoeic while using progestogen-only contraception.

Parenteral progestogen-only contraceptives

Intramuscular injection of a progestogen, either medroxyprogesterone acetate or norethisterone, can provide contraception for up to 8–12 weeks. The higher dose of progestogen compared with the oral preparations reliably inhibits ovulation, and therefore there is a low incidence of ectopic pregnancy. The contraceptive effect is fully reversible, but there is a high incidence of amenorrhoea when its effect wears off. Prolonged use of medroxyprogesterone acetate can reduce bone mineral density and cause osteoporosis. The loss of bone mineral density occurs over the first 2–3 years of use and then stabilises. Prolonged use of medroxyprogesterone acetate beyond 2 years, or its use in adolescents or people with other risk factors for osteoporosis, is discouraged.

A subcutaneous implant of etonogestrel provides contraception for up to 3 years, after which time it should be replaced. The progestogen is released from a flexible rod inserted subdermally on the lower surface of the upper arm. Local irritation is experienced by some women. The implants are radio-opaque so they can be easily located by radiography. Unwanted effects are similar to those experienced with the oral progestogen-only contraceptive, but lower doses of progestogen are needed because first-pass metabolism in the gut and liver is avoided.

Intra-uterine progestogen-only device

A plastic intra-uterine contraceptive system (IUS) with a levonorgestrel-releasing system from a silicone reservoir provides effective contraception with reduced menstrual blood loss compared with copper intra-uterine contraceptive devices (IUCDs) that do not contain a progestogen, and carries less risk of pelvic inflammatory disease. The progestogen is released from the device for a period of 5 years. The device is also used to control menstrual bleeding in women with primary menorrhagia by preventing endometrial proliferation.

EFFICACY OF HORMONAL CONTRACEPTION

When taken according to the recommended schedule, the failure rate for the combined hormonal contraceptive is 0.2%. With the combined oral hormonal preparations, contraceptive protection is reduced if there is a delay of more than 24 h in taking the daily dose. In such circumstances the missed dose should be taken as soon as possible. If two doses are missed then additional contraceptive measures should be used for 7 days.

Failure of the progestogen-only oral contraceptive is age-related and is up to 5% in young women, falling with decreasing fertility to about 0.3% at the age of 40 years. With the oral progestogen-only contraceptive, other contraceptive precautions should be taken for 2 days if there is a delay of only 3 h or more after the normal time of taking the daily dose.

EMERGENCY CONTRACEPTION

This can be carried out with the progestogen levonorgestrel, the progesterone receptor modulator ulipristal acetate, or a copper-containing IUCD. A single large dose of levonorgestrel is taken within 72 h after unprotected intercourse, and preferably within 12 h. Levonorgestrel inhibits ovulation, but only if taken before the LH surge. The treatment is successful in up to 99% of cases, but the efficacy is greatly reduced if used between 72 and 120 h after unprotected intercourse. Nausea is a frequent unwanted effect, occurring in up to 22% of women, and an anti-emetic (e.g. domperidone; Ch. 32) may be needed. Absorption takes 2 h and vomiting after this time will not affect the efficacy of treatment. A larger dose may be required if drugs that induce drug-metabolising enzymes in the liver are being taken. In the UK, levonorgestrel can be purchased without prescription by women over the age of 16 years.

The progesterone receptor modulator ulipristal acetate suppresses the mature follicle up to and including the time of the LH surge, so can be effective when taken up to 120 h after unprotected intercourse. Insertion of a copper IUCD up to 5 days after unprotected sexual intercourse is more effective as emergency contraception than levonorgestrel, but it is not known whether it is more effective than ulipristal acetate.

PHARMACOKINETICS OF CONTRACEPTIVE STEROIDS

The synthetic oestrogens, like the naturally occurring oestradiol-17β (oestradiol), and progestogens are highly lipid-soluble molecules that are rapidly and completely absorbed from the gut lumen after oral administration. Synthetic drugs are metabolised more slowly, including less first-pass metabolism, than the natural hormones oestradiol (half-life 1–2 h) and progesterone (half-life 5–20 min), so they have greater oral bioavailability and longer half-lives. For example, ethinylestradiol undergoes some first-pass metabolism (about 20%) but this is low compared with oestradiol (90–95%), and its half-life is longer (8–24 h). Some synthetic drugs are prodrugs that undergo first-pass metabolism to the active entity. Oestrogens and progestogens are eliminated by hepatic metabolism, often involving CYP3A4-mediated oxidation and/or conjugation with glucuronic acid and/or sulphate. The conjugates may undergo enterohepatic cycling. Enterohepatic cycling of ethinylestradiol is responsible for maintaining effective plasma concentrations with low-dose formulations. There is considerable inter-individual variation in plasma levels of oestrogens and progestogens after ingestion of the combined hormonal contraceptive.

The kinetics of oestrogens and progestogens can be affected by the administration of other drugs. Contraceptive failure may occur if there is concomitant treatment with drugs that induce liver cytochrome P450 enzymes (Table 2.7), such as anticonvulsants (e.g. barbiturates, carbamazepine or phenytoin), antiretroviral drugs (e.g. nelfinavir, nevirapine or ritonavir) or antibacterials (e.g. rifampicin and rifabutin) (Ch. 51). A higher dose of ethinylestradiol (using multiple tablets) should be used during and for 4

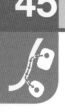
weeks after stopping these drugs. Alternatively, a form of contraception unaffected by enzyme-inducing drugs should be used (such as an IUCD or parenteral progestogen).

The pharmacokinetics of individual synthetic oestrogens and progestogens vary widely and details are given in the drug compendium at the end of this chapter.

BENEFICIAL AND UNWANTED EFFECTS OF CONTRACEPTIVE STEROIDS

Beneficial effects

- Cancer: there is a 40% reduction in the risk of ovarian cancer after 5 years of use and persisting for up to 15 years after stopping. Endometrial cancer is reduced by 50%, with a similar duration of protection.
- Acne can be treated with combined oral hormonal contraceptives, since they reduce the concentration of free testosterone (Ch. 49). A combination of ethinylestradiol with cyproterone acetate, a weak progestogen with antiandrogenic activity (Ch. 46), is sometimes used for this purpose.
- Dysfunctional uterine bleeding, for example menorrhagia, is reduced by the combined oral hormonal contraceptive or an intra-uterine progestogen-only device.

Unwanted effects

Both oestrogens and progestogens have a number of minor and major unwanted effects, but the incidence of the major effects, although important, is relatively low.

- Thromboembolism: the incidence of venous thromboembolic disease is increased in some subgroups of women taking the combined hormonal contraceptive. The mechanisms are complex but include procoagulant activity from increased production of clotting factors X and II and decreased production of anticoagulant antithrombin (Ch. 11). Fibrinolysis is impaired, while reduced prostacyclin generation enhances platelet aggregation (Ch. 11). The risk of thromboembolism increases with age, and is greater in women who smoke (because smoking increases the risk of thrombogenesis) or who are obese and in those with a thrombophilic tendency, such as deficiency of protein C or protein S or the presence of factor V Leiden. The baseline risk of venous thromboembolism in women of reproductive age not taking the combined oral hormonal contraceptive is about 5 per 100 000 per year. The risk in women taking second-generation preparations (containing levonorgestrel) is about 15 per 100 000 per year and in those taking third-generation preparations containing desogestrel or gestodene (and possibly drospirenone) is about 25 per 100 000 per year. It is important that these risks are put into context; for example the risk of venous thromboembolism in pregnancy is 60 per 100 000 pregnancies.
- Ischaemic heart disease and ischaemic stroke: there is an increased risk of myocardial infarction and stroke in women taking the combined hormonal contraceptive who smoke or who are hypertensive, particularly in those over the age of 35 years. The added risk in those

over 40 years is 20 per 100 000 for smokers and 29 per 100 000 for women with hypertension. It has been suggested that enhanced thrombogenesis rather than premature atherogenesis is responsible for the excess cardiovascular risk with the combined hormonal contraceptive. The lowest possible dose of oestrogen should be given to older women who use the combined hormonal contraceptive.

- Increase in blood pressure: a small increase in blood pressure, typically 5/3 mmHg, is common during use of the combined hormonal contraceptive, but not of progestogen-only contraceptives. A significant rise can occur in about 5% of women with previously normal blood pressure and in up to 15% of women with preexisting hypertension. The mechanism is probably an increase in plasma renin substrate (Ch. 6) produced by oestrogen and, to a lesser extent, progestogen. Blood pressure may remain elevated for some months after the combined hormonal contraceptive has been stopped. Regular monitoring of blood pressure is advisable during use of the combined hormonal contraceptive, and it should be stopped if the blood pressure rises above 160 mmHg systolic or 95 mmHg diastolic.
- Cancer: there is a small excess risk of breast cancer, but it is uncertain whether this relates to earlier diagnosis. The rate of diagnosis remains higher for 10 years after the combined hormonal contraceptive is stopped. The incidence of cervical cancer is slightly increased by combined hormonal contraceptives after 5 years of use.
- Nausea, mastalgia, depression, headache, weight gain and provocation of migraine may be minimised by prescribing preparations with low oestrogen content, or by changing the progestogen to desogestrel, drospirenone or gestodene. Women who have migraine with aura are at increased risk of stroke if they take a combined hormonal contraceptive.
- Breakthrough bleeding occurs frequently in some women, whereas in others withdrawal bleeding fails to occur. Gestodene-containing pills or triphasic preparations probably give the best cycle control. Amenorrhoea after stopping the combined hormonal contraceptive can last beyond a few months in about 5% of women, and a small number can experience amenorrhoea for more than a year. A history of irregular periods before taking the combined hormonal contraceptive increases the chance of prolonged amenorrhoea.
- Metabolic effects: oestrogens alone increase protective plasma high-density lipoprotein (HDL) cholesterol, decrease low-density lipoprotein (LDL) cholesterol and increase plasma triglycerides (see also Ch. 48). When used in combination with the second-generation progestogens, HDL cholesterol is reduced. Oestrogens increase vascular prostacyclin and nitric oxide synthesis, inhibit platelet adhesion and suppress smooth muscle cell proliferation. Some progestogens such as norethisterone and medroxyprogesterone acetate may oppose the beneficial effects of oestrogens on the arterial wall. The third-generation combined hormonal contraceptives containing gestodene and desogestrel increase plasma triglycerides but, unlike the progestogens in the second-generation pills, they increase HDL cholesterol. The clinical relevance of these small changes is uncertain.

- Increased skin pigmentation can occur in some women who take oestrogens. The androgenic progestogens can sometimes cause or aggravate hirsutism and acne or produce weight gain. In women with hyperandrogenaemia (such as occurs with polycystic ovary syndrome) a third-generation combined hormonal contraceptive would be preferred, as gestodene and desogestrel have little androgenic activity.
- Effects on the liver are occasionally seen. Cholestatic jaundice can be produced by progestogens, and oestrogens increase the risk of gallstones.
- Drug interactions: drugs that increase the metabolism of oestrogen may cause a reduction in the efficacy of the combined hormonal contraceptive, which may result in breakthrough bleeding and contraceptive failure (see above).

NON-CONTRACEPTIVE USES OF STEROIDAL CONTRACEPTIVES

The combined hormonal contraceptive can be used:

- to reduce excessive blood loss from menorrhagia,
- to reduce the pain of dysmenorrhoea,
- to treat premenstrual tension,
- to treat endometriosis,
- to treat acne in women.

Menorrhagia

Excessive menstrual blood loss is a common gynaecological problem. Menstrual loss can be reduced to a variable extent by non-steroidal anti-inflammatory drugs (NSAIDs; Ch. 29), and numerous different NSAIDs have been used. They are taken only during the time of menstruation. The combined hormonal contraceptives and the progestogen-only contraceptives can also reduce excessive menstrual loss. To be useful the progestogen-only contraceptive has to be taken for 3 weeks at a fairly high dose. A more effective way of giving the progestogen is from an intra-uterine progestogen system (IUS), which reduces blood loss by up to 90%.

The antifibrinolytic agent tranexamic acid (Ch. 11) can also reduce menstrual blood loss by up to 50%. Its effect is rapid in onset and therapy is only required during the time of menstruation.

Dysmenorrhoea

The cause of primary dysmenorrhoea (pain associated with menstruation) is unknown. Many explanations have been proposed, including uterine hyperactivity, excessive prostaglandin or leukotriene generation and excessive production of vasopressin. Various NSAIDs (Ch. 29) have been used for the relief of dysmenorrhoea, with approximately 70% of women being relieved of their symptoms. There are differences in efficacy among the NSAIDs that are poorly understood and do not seem to be simply related to their analgesic or anti-inflammatory activity. NSAIDs with a licence for this indication in the UK include ibuprofen, mefenamic acid and naproxen.

The combined hormonal contraceptive and the progestogen-only contraceptive are effective in reducing symptoms of dysmenorrhoea.

Premenstrual disorders

Many women experience a variety of symptoms precipitated by ovulation that may continue up to the end of menstruation. The term premenstrual syndrome is used to describe the symptom complex if a woman has at least one week free of symptoms every cycle. Physical symptoms include joint and muscle pains, breast tenderness, abdominal bloating, headaches, weight gain and oedema of the hands or feet. These are often accompanied by increased appetite, fatigue, mood swings, irritability and sleep disturbance. Second-generation combined hormonal contraceptives can produce similar symptoms to premenstrual syndrome.

Treatment is varied, and includes cognitive behavioural therapy and aerobic exercise. If symptoms are more severe, the diuretic spironolactone (Ch. 14) can reduce abdominal bloating, breast discomfort and mood disturbance. Selective serotonin reuptake inhibitors, such as citalopram (Ch. 22), are effective when used for 2 weeks prior to menstruation at lower doses than required to treat depression. A combined hormonal contraceptive containing drospirenone is helpful if fertility is not an issue, or ovulation can be suppressed with a gonadorelin agonist analogue such as goserelin (Ch. 43) or use of the 'impeded' androgen danazol (Ch. 46) in the luteal phase.

Endometriosis

Endometriosis is the presence and proliferation of endometrial tissue outside the uterine cavity. It may arise from retrograde menstrual flow through the fallopian tubes. The main consequences are pelvic pain, dysmenorrhoea, dyspareunia and infertility. Treatment is either medical or surgical.

Medical treatment can be given to suppress ovarian activity and create a hypo-oestrogenic anovulatory state, but does not restore fertility. Symptoms often improve in pregnancy, and the combined hormonal contraceptive or a progestogen-only contraceptive are often effective treatments. Alternative strategies include induction of a pseudo-postmenopausal state with the use of danazol (Ch. 46) or gonadotropin-releasing hormone (GnRH) analogues (Ch. 43). Treatment is usually necessary for at least 6 months, but up to 50% of women have recurrence of painful symptoms in the 2 years after it is stopped.

If fertility is the major problem, then treatment involves surgery or *in vitro* fertilisation techniques (Ch. 43).

HORMONE-REPLACEMENT THERAPY

The menopausal transition from regular periods to amenorrhoea begins at a median age of 51 years and takes place over about 4 years. It arises because there is a natural depletion of ovarian follicles and as a result the plasma oestrogen concentration falls, with a consequent rise in plasma FSH. After the menopause, the ovaries do not produce oestrogen or progesterone, but continue to produce testosterone. Some oestrogen is still produced by conversion of adrenal corticosteroids to oestradiol in peripheral adipose tissue. The consequences of oestrogen deficiency during and after the menopause include the following.

■ Symptoms such as vasomotor instability (hot flushes and night sweats), and altered sexual and urinary function. Vasomotor instability results from resetting of the hypothalamic temperature set-point so that it perceives that the body is warmer than it is. Vasodilation and sweating represent an attempt to disperse heat. The mechanism is uncertain but may be due to either reduced oestrogen or increased FSH leading to a reduction in noradrenergic or serotonergic neurotransmission in the hypothalamus. Loss of connective tissue in the vagina and trigone of the bladder, and a less acidic vaginal pH underlie many of the other problems. These include vaginal dryness, discomfort and itching, dyspareunia, and urinary urgency, frequency and incontinence. Breast atrophy and thinning of the skin also occur. Other postmenopausal symptoms such as irritability and depression are less clearly related to oestrogen deficiency.

■ Bone loss leading to osteoporosis (Ch. 42) and an increased susceptibility to fragility fracture occur after the menopause. The ERβ receptor is present in higher concentrations in developing cancellous bone (such as vertebrae), and the ERα receptor in developing cortical bone (such as the hip). Oestrogen deficiency increases bone turnover, with bone resorption increasing more than formation.

■ Cardiovascular disease and cerebrovascular disease are more common. The cause is uncertain. Unfavourable changes in lipids may be part of the explanation, due to a reduced HDL_2 cholesterol subfraction and increased LDL cholesterol (see Ch. 48). However, an independent effect of oestrogen in reducing plasma fibrinogen (a factor in thrombogenesis) may be more important. Oestrogen receptors are found on the cells of the arterial wall, and stimulation decreases arterial resistance and increases vessel compliance, which may also be relevant.

Treatment with oestrogens during the peri- and postmenopausal period is often advocated to try to reverse the effects of oestrogen deficiency, but recent evidence of both lack of efficacy and potential harm has limited their use (see benefits and risks below).

ORAL HORMONE-REPLACEMENT THERAPY AND OTHER DRUGS USED FOR POSTMENOPAUSAL CONDITIONS

Examples

estradiol, raloxifene, tibolone

Oral oestrogens and progestogens

For hormone-replacement therapy (HRT), oestrogens are given at much lower doses than are used for contraception. However, if oestrogen is given alone for more than a few weeks to a woman who has a uterus then cystic hyperplasia of the endometrium can occur. Progestogen is given concurrently to avoid this, and is used for 12 days each calendar month or continuously if withdrawal bleeding is to be avoided. Oestrogen can be used alone if the woman has had a hysterectomy.

The majority of oral HRT preparations contain the natural estradiol as the oestrogen, although preparations with conjugated equine oestrogens are also available. Synthetic progestogens are used: dydrogesterone, medroxyprogesterone, norethisterone, levonorgestrel or drospirenone.

Oral oestrogen replacement will reduce the symptoms of postmenopausal oestrogen deficiency, although relief may take up to 3 months. Treatment for symptom relief probably should be given for at least 6 months to perimenopausal women, after which withdrawal can be attempted to see whether symptoms have resolved spontaneously.

Tibolone

Tibolone is a synthetic compound with combined weak oestrogenic, progestogenic and androgenic properties. Its effects are predominantly oestrogenic, although in breast tissue it inhibits the enzyme responsible for activation of its metabolites, giving a low incidence of breast tenderness. In the endometrium it activates progesterone and androgen receptors, and the effects are mainly progestogenic, without stimulation of the endometrium or producing bleeding. Tibolone reduces postmenopausal symptoms and prevents postmenopausal bone loss. Vaginal bleeding can occur in women who still produce some endogenous oestrogen, and therefore tibolone is not usually given to women who are within 12 months of their last period.

Pharmacokinetics

Tibolone is a prodrug that is well absorbed from the gut and is metabolised in the liver to active metabolites, which have half-lives of about 8 h.

Unwanted effects

■ Hot flushes.
■ Leg cramps.
■ Increased risk of stroke.
■ Increased risk of breast cancer and endometrial cancer, but to a lesser extent than combined hormonal HRT.

Raloxifene

Raloxifene is a selective oestrogen receptor modulator which has oestrogenic effects on bone but anti-oestrogenic actions on breast and uterine receptors. It increases bone mineral density in postmenopausal osteoporosis, but does not treat menopausal symptoms. More details on raloxifene and osteoporosis are given in Chapter 42.

VAGINAL OESTROGEN

Oestrogen cream (usually estradiol) or pessaries can be used to treat vaginal atrophy and dyspareunia and can relieve perimenopausal urinary symptoms such as frequency and dysuria. Considerable systemic absorption occurs with some formulations, and an oral progestogen may be needed to prevent endometrial hyperplasia. Creams or pessaries are used daily for 2–3 weeks initially and then applied twice weekly for as long as required.

SUBCUTANEOUS OESTROGEN IMPLANTS

Estradiol can be implanted surgically as pellets that release drug for up to 6 months. The major use for this option is when tolerance of oral oestrogen is poor, perhaps because of nausea. Oral progestogen must also be taken for 10–12 days each month if the woman has a uterus, and continued for up to 2 years after stopping oestrogen, to prevent vaginal bleeding from persistently high oestrogen levels.

TRANSDERMAL OESTROGEN WITH PROGESTOGEN

A variety of transdermal patches that deliver sex steroids are available. In some preparations, oestrogen alone is delivered by patches applied twice weekly for 2 weeks, followed by patches delivering oestrogen plus progestogen for 2 weeks. In other regimens, progestogen is taken orally for at least 12 days of the cycle while continuing with the patch-delivered oestrogen. Patches delivering continuous oestrogen plus progestogen (levonorgestrel or norethisterone) are also available. A lower dose of progestogen can be used because the transdermal route avoids first-pass metabolism, and this might reduce unwanted effects. Estradiol gels applied twice daily are also available and require co-administration of oral progestogen for 12 days per month in women with a uterus. It is recommended that patches are applied below the waistline, and not close to the breasts.

BENEFITS AND RISKS OF HORMONE-REPLACEMENT THERAPY

The benefits and risks of oestrogen-based HRT are highly individual for the patient. For most women it is recommended that HRT is reserved for short-term alleviation of menopausal symptoms. Any treatment should be reviewed at least annually. Tibolone (see above) or alternative approaches to the treatment of menopausal symptoms (see below) should be considered. Atrophic vaginitis may respond to a short course of topical oestrogen.

HRT reduces the risk of vertebral and non-vertebral osteoporotic fractures. However, because of the potential risks of treatment, HRT is not considered to be first-line treatment except for women with early natural or surgical menopause before the age of 45 years, in whom it is not recommended that treatment should continue beyond the age of 50 years.

UNWANTED EFFECTS OF HORMONE-REPLACEMENT THERAPY

- Breakthrough bleeding can be troublesome, and regular withdrawal bleeds during the cycle are common unless continuous progestogen is used. These may be preceded by symptoms of premenstrual tension.
- Breast pain and abdominal or leg cramps.
- Nausea and vomiting.
- Headache, dizziness.
- Depression, irritability, loss of energy and poor concentration due to progestogen.
- Transdermal delivery can cause contact sensitisation.
- Increased risk of venous thromboembolism, especially in the first year and in those with other risk factors (obesity, smoking, immobility, previous thromboembolic disease). The risk after 5 years of use is increased by about 40% for combined HRT (added risk is 4 cases per 1000 for combined HRT, and 1 case per 1000 for oestrogen-only HRT over 5 years if aged 50–59 years; the excess risk is more than doubled between 60 and 69 years). Transdermal oestrogen replacement may not increase the risk of venous thromboembolism.
- Increased risk of stroke (excess risk is 1 case per 1000 for combined HRT and 2 cases per 1000 for oestrogen-only HRT over 5 years if aged 50–59 years; this excess risk is tripled between 60 and 69 years).
- HRT does not prevent coronary heart disease, and may increase the risk in the first year of treatment.
- Increased risk of breast cancer within 1–2 years of starting use, increasing further with duration of use. The excess risk is lost 5 years after stopping HRT. Taking combined HRT for 10 years leads to a 40% increase in the risk of developing breast cancer in women aged 50–64 years (excess risk is 6 cases per 1000). Oestrogen-only HRT carries about one-quarter of this excess risk.
- The risk of endometrial cancer is increased by oestrogen-only HRT, which should be avoided in women who have a uterus.
- The risk of cholecystitis is increased by oral but not transdermal oestrogen.

ALTERNATIVE TREATMENTS FOR MENOPAUSAL SYMPTOMS

Oestrogens are by far the most effective treatment for menopausal symptoms. Vasomotor symptoms may be alleviated by the use of high doses of progestogens but unwanted effects are common. There is limited evidence for the use of antidepressants that modulate monoaminergic neurotransmission, such as selective serotonin reuptake inhibitors (SSRIs) and serotonin and noradrenaline reuptake inhibitors (SNRIs) (Ch. 22). The anticonvulsant gabapentin (Ch. 23) is effective for treating hot flushes.

THE ONSET AND INDUCTION OF LABOUR

The aetiology of the induction of labour is still uncertain (Fig. 45.3). The actual onset may be multifactorial in nature

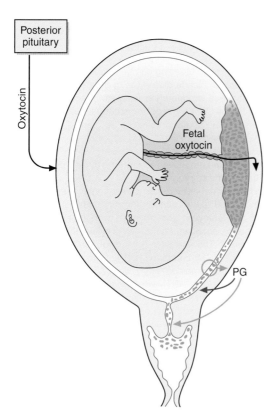

Fig. 45.3 **Induction of labour.** The mechanisms involved in the onset of labour in humans are uncertain but likely to be multifactorial. Prostaglandins (PG) are synthesised by the amnion and decidua and they stimulate the uterus and soften the cervix. Fetal and maternal oxytocin and prostaglandins may be involved in the processes of labour; their role in the initiation of labour is uncertain.

and it is probable that prostaglandins, oxytocin, progesterone, oestrogen and corticosteroids are among the agents involved. Lack of knowledge about the mechanisms that underpin the onset of labour is directly reflected in a poor ability to prevent preterm labour, where at best parturition can be delayed for only short periods of time (see below).

CORTICOTROPIN-RELEASING HORMONE

The critical factor in the timing of birth in humans is development of the placenta, and particularly expression of the gene for corticotropin-releasing hormone (CRH; also known as corticotropin-releasing factor) by the placenta. Placental CRH production increases dramatically at the end of pregnancy. Prior to this, its production is suppressed by progesterone, but it is stimulated by a rise in glucocorticoid production and catecholamine release prior to parturition. The increase in CRH drives the fetal hypothalamo–pituitary–adrenal axis to produce corticosteroids and dehydroepiandrosterone (Ch. 43). In the fetus, CRH and cortisol stimulate

the fetal lung to produce surfactant protein A (Ch. 13), which enters amniotic fluid and then the amnion, where it stimulates synthesis of prostaglandin E_2 (PGE_2). In the mother, the formation of myometrial $PGF_{2\alpha}$ is also increased.

PROSTAGLANDINS

$PGF_{2\alpha}$ and PGE_2 are synthesised by the cells of the amnion and decidua and have many actions that could contribute to labour. Uterine contractile sensitivity to prostaglandins is approximately 10-fold higher at term than in earlier pregnancy. The contractility of the uterus during labour commences at the utero-tubular junction and progresses through the body of the uterus to the cervix, thus promoting efficient labour. This type of synchronous contractile pattern, which does not occur in early pregnancy, is caused by prostaglandins and oestrogens promoting the synthesis of 'contraction-associated proteins' and increasing connectivity between myometrial cells. Gap junctions are specialised connections between the smooth muscle cells that allow excitatory impulses to pass between cells. The type of uterine contractions that result in efficient progress of labour can only occur in uterine muscle cells that are rich in gap junctions. The progesterone-dominated uterus has few gap junctions. Prostaglandins also increase the release of Ca^{2+} from intracellular stores in myometrial cells, which promotes muscle contraction.

PGE_2 softens the cervix, an essential prerequisite for the smooth passage of labour. Prostaglandins also increase the synthesis of oxytocin from the posterior pituitary.

OXYTOCIN

Oxytocin is a peptide produced by the posterior pituitary (Ch. 43). There is a marked increase in the expression of uterine oxytocin receptors from about 35 weeks of pregnancy onwards, so that oxytocin has a marked uterotonic action at term but is much less effective earlier in pregnancy. Oxytocin acts synergistically with prostaglandins to release Ca^{2+} from intracellular stores in the myometrial cells and promote muscle contraction. The oxytocin concentration in the maternal circulation does not increase until the second stage of labour.

SEX STEROID HORMONES

Oestrogens and progesterone both increase during pregnancy. Overall, the actions of oestradiol promote uterine contractility while progesterone decreases contractility. Production of dehydroepiandrosterone is also increased just before parturition.

- **Progesterone:** decreases gap junctions, diminishes uterine pacemaker activity and decreases the sensitivity of the uterus to oxytocin and prostaglandins. At the onset of labour there is reduced responsiveness of progesterone receptors which blocks the cellular action of the hormone.
- **Oestradiol:** increases the number of uterine oxytocin receptors and increases oxytocin release from the posterior pituitary. It increases gap junctions, and fundal dominance of uterine contractility is increased by an

effect on the functional pacemaker at the utero-tubular junction. Oestradiol increases the synthesis of prostaglandins and increases the sensitivity of the uterus to their effects and has a softening effect on the cervix.

- **Dehydroepiandrosterone**: this has high activity at oestrogen ERβ receptors that contributes to fetal lung maturation. It also enhances the production of oestrogen by the placenta, which may be important in the timing of the onset of labour.

DRUGS USED FOR INDUCING LABOUR

Oxytocin and prostaglandins are the only drugs currently used to induce labour.

Oxytocin

Oxytocin is given by slow intravenous infusion for the induction of labour and to augment contractions in inadequate labour. The concentration given depends upon the response: the aim is to produce regular coordinated contractions at intervals of approximately 1.5–2 min with complete relaxation between contractions. Oxytocin is an effective uterine stimulant in women at term, and labour will usually proceed well if the cervix is partially dilated and softened prior to its use. Inappropriately high concentrations of oxytocin can cause uterine hypertonus, in which the uterus does not relax between contractions, and fetal distress can occur. As labour progresses and the woman's 'endogenous' induction mechanisms come into play, the concentration of oxytocin may need to be reduced. Following delivery, oxytocin can also be useful to reduce postpartum haemorrhage (see below). Oxytocin, unlike prostaglandins, does not soften the cervix and is now often used after intravaginal prostaglandin (usually dinoprostone) has been given for this purpose (see below). Oxytocin in high doses has a weak antidiuretic activity as it is related to vasopressin and large doses can cause fluid retention (Ch. 43).

Dinoprostone

Dinoprostone (the name for exogenous PGE_2) causes contractions of both the non-pregnant and the pregnant uterus. The sensitivity of the uterus to prostaglandins is higher than to oxytocin prior to term. Like oxytocin, correct doses of prostaglandins can produce contractions that are indistinguishable from spontaneous labour. Prostaglandins have the added advantage of softening ('ripening') the cervix, so they can be used for induction of labour before term. Dinoprostone is given as vaginal tablets, pessaries or gels for induction of labour or for priming of the uterus prior to rupture of membranes and induction by oxytocin. In some women dinoprostone will result only in ripening of the cervix, whereas others will go into labour. Dinoprostone is rarely used intravenously for the induction of labour, as it produces more unwanted effects.

Unwanted effects

- Gastrointestinal disturbances, particularly nausea, vomiting and diarrhoea.
- Uterine hypertonus, amniotic fluid embolism, abruptio placenta.
- Maternal hypertension.
- Bronchospasm.

INDUCTION OF ABORTION

Prostaglandin derivatives

Prostaglandins are widely used for the induction of abortion. In the second trimester their use results in fewer complications than surgical abortion. Gemeprost (a PGE_1 analogue), given as an intravaginal pessary, is used for the medical induction of first- or second-trimester therapeutic abortion or management of intra-uterine death. Misoprostol is an alternative that can be given orally or vaginally. Both drugs produce prolonged uterine contraction. Mifepristone pretreatment (see below) is used before vaginal administration of a prostaglandin.

Gemeprost is also given as a pessary to ripen and soften the cervix prior to early surgical abortion.

Mifepristone

Mechanism of action and uses

Mifepristone is a potent progesterone receptor antagonist. It is given orally and sensitises the uterus to prostaglandin-induced contractions and softens the cervix. For medical termination of pregnancy up to 24 weeks' gestation or following spontaneous fetal death, mifepristone is given as a single oral dose followed 36 h later by either oral gemeprost, or oral or vaginal misoprostol (Ch. 33). It can also be given alone to soften the cervix 36 h before surgical termination of early pregnancy.

Pharmacokinetics

Mifepristone is well absorbed from the gut and is metabolised slowly in the liver (half-life 18 h), partially to an active metabolite.

Unwanted effects

- Abdominal cramps.
- Vaginal bleeding.
- Uterine pain, which can be severe.

POSTPARTUM HAEMORRHAGE

Bleeding can arise after incomplete abortion or after a normal delivery. In the latter situation, preventative treatment is routinely given to avoid excessive blood loss.

Ergometrine maleate

Ergometrine causes hypertonic contractions of the uterus and is therefore not used for induction of labour as it would result in fetal distress and poor progress in labour. After placental separation, uterine hypertonus produced by ergometrine squeezes the uterine blood vessels and reduces blood loss. It also causes vasoconstriction by α-adrenoceptor stimulation (see ergotamine Ch. 26), which further limits haemorrhage.

Pharmacokinetics

Ergometrine is given intramuscularly and works within 2–7 min.

Unwanted effects

- Nausea, vomiting, abdominal pain.
- Headache, dizziness, tinnitus.
- Chest pain, peripheral vasoconstriction, hypertension, dyspnoea.

Management of postpartum haemorrhage

To minimise bleeding after delivery, ergometrine should be given together with oxytocin by intramuscular injection on delivery of the anterior shoulder. Following delivery of the baby, postpartum haemorrhage can also be reduced by increasing the concentrations of intravenous oxytocin being administered. This causes hypertonic contraction of the uterus and compresses intra-uterine blood vessels. If bleeding continues, the prostaglandin carboprost (15-methyl-$PGF_{2\alpha}$, a compound related to dinoprostone) is given by intramuscular injection.

MYOMETRIAL RELAXANTS (TOCOLYTICS) AND PRETERM LABOUR

Preterm birth is a delivery that occurs before 37 weeks of gestation, and affects more than 10% of pregnancies. It is possible that preterm labour has multifactorial origins, such as myometrial and fetal membrane overdistension (as may occur with multiple fetuses), early fetal endocrine activation, decidual haemorrhage and intra-uterine infection or inflammation.

Prematurity is the largest cause of neonatal morbidity and mortality, but relatively poor pharmacological tools are available currently to prevent it. Therapeutic strategies have concentrated on inhibition of myometrial contractions (tocolysis) between 24 and 33 weeks gestation. Tocolytics have not been shown to improve fetal morbidity or mortality, but they provide a limited time for treatment with a corticosteroid to enhance lung maturation (Ch. 13), or for transfer of the mother to a specialist unit. Prophylactic treatment with antibacterials may improve outcome in particular at-risk groups but has not been widely adopted.

Atosiban

Mechanism of action

Atosiban is a peptide analogue of oxytocin that is an antagonist at oxytocin receptors in the decidua and myometrium, reducing the release of intracellular Ca^{2+}.

Pharmacokinetics

Atosiban is given by intravenous injection or infusion. It is metabolised to an active derivative, and has a very short half-life (about 15 min).

Unwanted effects

- Nausea, vomiting.
- Headache, dizziness.
- Tachycardia, hypotension, hot flushes.
- Hyperglycaemia.

Beta₂-adrenoceptor agonists

Examples

salbutamol, terbutaline

β_2-Adrenoceptor agonists inhibit uterine contractility by increasing the intracellular concentration of cAMP. Salbutamol and terbutaline are given intravenously or orally for up to 48 h following the start of preterm labour, after which the risks to the mother increase with no benefit to the fetus. Unwanted effects include nausea, vomiting, flushing and maternal and fetal tachycardia with hypotension (see also Ch. 12).

Calcium channel blockers

Nifedipine (Ch. 5) is used orally and is as effective as other tocolytics, with fewer unwanted effects than β_2-adrenoceptor agonists. The use of nifedipine may improve fetal outcome.

Other agents for preterm labour

Magnesium sulphate has been widely used in the USA for treating women in preterm labour. Recent evidence indicates that it may be no better than placebo, and may be associated with worse fetal outcomes. Intravenous or transdermal glyceryl trinitrate (Ch. 5) may be effective through nitric oxide generation in smooth muscle, but is not widely used.

The NSAID indometacin (Ch. 29) can be successful for delaying delivery, but there are concerns about transient neonatal renal impairment and premature closure of the ductus arteriosus.

SELF-ASSESSMENT

True/false questions

1. Oestrogen has a negative feedback effect on luteinizing hormone (LH) and follicle-stimulating hormone (FSH) secretion from the anterior pituitary throughout the follicular phase of the menstrual cycle.
2. In the luteal phase, the elevated level of progesterone is controlled by gonadotropins.
3. Progesterone causes cervical mucus to be viscous and hostile to the passage of sperm.
4. The oral progestogen-only contraceptive reliably inhibits ovulation.
5. Both oestrogen and progesterone inhibit the motility of the fallopian tube.

6. The functioning corpus luteum maintains pregnancy for the first 6–8 weeks after implantation.
7. Progestogens used in combined hormonal contraceptives do not differ in their androgenic activity.
8. Biphasic and triphasic formulations of combined hormonal contraceptives result in lower overall dosages of oestrogen and progestogen than monophasic formulations.
9. Effective protection is lost if there is a delay of more than 3 h in taking the daily oral dose of an oral combined hormonal contraceptive.
10. Emergency contraception with ulipristal acetate is effective taken up to 120 h after unprotected intercourse.
11. An etonogestrel implant beneath the skin of the upper arm provides effective contraception for 5 years.
12. Antiepileptic drugs such as carbamazepine can reduce the plasma concentrations of oestrogens and progestogens.
13. Mortality from venous thromboembolism is increased in women using the oral combined hormonal contraceptive who smoke, particularly those over the age of 35 years.
14. The combined hormonal contraceptive significantly increases blood pressure in most women.
15. Oestrogen used on its own as hormone-replacement therapy (HRT) may cause endometrial hyperplasia.
16. Postmenopausal women taking continuous HRT with both oestrogen and progestogens do not experience breakthrough bleeding.
17. Oestrogens and progestogens can be given transdermally.
18. Raloxifene blocks oestrogen receptors in bone.
19. Tibolone reduces bone loss in postmenopausal women.
20. Oxytocin is preferred to prostaglandins for the induction of labour at 34 weeks of gestation.
21. Progesterone increases the number of gap junctions in the uterus.
22. Ergometrine can be used for the induction of labour.
23. Atosiban is a tocolytic drug that acts by blocking oxytocin receptors.
24. Non-steroidal anti-inflammatory drugs (NSAIDs) are used in treating dysmenorrhoea.

One-best-answer (OBA) questions

1. Identify the *incorrect* statement below concerning drugs used during labour and abortion.
   A. Mifepristone is a progesterone receptor antagonist used to induce abortion.
   B. Prostaglandin E$_2$ (PGE$_2$) is preferred to oxytocin for induction of labour at 35 weeks of gestation.
   C. Oxytocin is less likely than prostaglandins to cause uterine hypertonus.
   D. β$_2$-Adrenoceptor agonists do not reduce mortality in children born preterm.
   E. Ergometrine reduces postpartum haemorrhage by constricting uterine blood vessels.
2. Identify the *most accurate* statement below concerning the contraceptive options for a 35-year-old woman who smokes 40 cigarettes a day, but who, despite treatment, has not been able to stop smoking.

A. The oral combined hormonal contraceptive would be suitable for her contraception.
B. The oral combined hormonal contraceptive would increase her risk of endometrial cancer.
C. The oral combined hormonal contraceptive would have a lower failure rate than an intra-uterine contraceptive device (IUCD).
D. The oral progestogen-only contraceptive would provide adequate contraception without increasing the risk of venous thromboembolism.
E. An intramuscular injection of medroxyprogesterone acetate would give contraceptive protection for at least 6 months.

True/false answers

1. **False.** The negative feedback in the early part of the follicular phase switches to positive feedback at an oestradiol level of approximately 200 pg·mL^{-1}, resulting in the mid-cycle surge in LH and FSH.
2. **True.** The LH levels fall precipitously after the mid-cycle surge, but they are high enough to support the secretion of progesterone in the luteal phase.
3. **True.** The effect on cervical mucus is an important action of the oral progestogen-only contraceptive.
4. **False.** Ovulation occurs in up to 50% of women with the oral progestogen-only contraceptive, as other effects are responsible for its contraceptive action. Ovulation is reliably inhibited in women using parenteral progestogens.
5. **False.** Progesterone inhibits fallopian tube motility, and oestrogens enhance it. An imbalance may alter oocyte transport and the probability of fertilisation and implantation.
6. **True.** After 6–8 weeks of pregnancy maintained by the corpus luteum, the placenta takes over production of sex steroids under the influence of HCG.
7. **False.** Progestogens in second-generation combined hormonal contraceptives (such as levonorgestrel and norethisterone) have variable androgenic activity, but gestodene and desogestrel used in third-generation combined contraceptives have little or no androgenic activity.
8. **False.** Biphasic and triphasic formulations mimic more closely the steroidal changes in the menstrual cycle, but they do not reduce the overall administered load of sex steroids.
9. **False.** Protection is reduced if there is a delay of more than 12 h in taking a daily dose of the combined hormonal contraceptive, but this can occur with a delay of only 3 h in taking oral progesterone-only contraceptives.
10. **True.** The progesterone receptor modulator ulipristal acetate suppresses the follicle until the time of the LH surge and is effective up to 120 h after unprotected intercourse.
11. **False.** Etonogestrel implants must be replaced every 3 years.
12. **True.** By inducing liver microsomal enzymes, the effective concentrations of oestrogens and progestogens may be reduced as their metabolism is enhanced.

13. **True.** The excess risk of thromboembolic disease in women taking the combined hormonal contraceptive is significantly greater in smokers over the age of 35 years.

14. **False.** A small increase in blood pressure is commonly seen with the combined contraceptive, but a significant rise occurs in only 5% of previously normotensive women.

15. **True.** The risk of endometrial hyperplasia with oestrogen is reduced by giving progestogens concurrently; oestrogens can be used alone in women who have had a hysterectomy.

16. **False.** Breakthrough bleeding frequently occurs, particularly in the first 6 months of treatment.

17. **True.** Both oestrogens and progestogens undergo first-pass metabolism and this can be avoided by transdermal absorption from patches.

18. **False.** Raloxifene is a selective oestrogen receptor modulator; it stimulates oestrogen receptors in bone but not in breast or uterine tissue.

19. **True.** Tibolone has weak oestrogenic and progestogenic activity and reduces bone loss.

20. **False.** Oxytocin is less effective in earlier pregnancy compared with full term. An intravaginal pessary of prostaglandin would increase uterine contractility and also soften the cervix.

21. **False.** Oestrogens increase uterine gap junctions in the uterus, facilitating uterine contractility, while progesterone opposes this action of oestrogens.

22. **False.** Ergometrine is given alone or together with oxytocin at the time of delivery and produces hypertonic uterine activity to reduce postpartum haemorrhage; it should not be given for labour induction.

23. **True.** Antagonism of oxytocin receptors by atosiban reduces uterine contractility in preterm labour; other tocolytic drugs include β_2-adrenoceptor agonists and calcium channel blockers.

24. **True.** NSAIDs relieve dysmenorrhoea in approximately 70% of women; the combined and progestogen-only hormonal contraceptives may also be effective.

OBA answers

1. **Answer C** is the incorrect statement.
   A. Correct. Blockade of the actions of progesterone by mifepristone results in abortion, although the precise mechanisms are uncertain.
   B. Correct. Women should be given intravaginal prostaglandins to soften the cervix prior to rupture of the membranes, and then intravenous oxytocin if required.
   C. **Incorrect.** Both oxytocin and prostaglandins can cause uterine hypertonus and fetal distress if given in inappropriate amounts.
   D. Correct. β_2-Adrenoceptor agonists may delay labour for 48 h, but they have not been shown to decrease morbidity or mortality in the preterm newborn child.
   E. Correct. Ergometrine constricts uterine blood vessels via α_1-adrenoceptors and uterine hypertonus further compresses blood vessels, reducing postpartum blood loss.

2. **Answer D** is the most accurate statement.
   A. Incorrect. In a 35-year-old woman who smokes, the oral combined hormonal contraceptive is not a good choice due to an increased risk of cardiovascular complications.
   B. Incorrect. The oral combined hormonal contraceptive reduces the risk of endometrial cancer.
   C. Incorrect. The IUCD is as effective as the combined hormonal contraceptive.
   D. **Correct.** The risk of thromboembolic complications is related to the oestrogen content of the combined hormonal contraceptive.
   E. Incorrect. Intramuscular medroxyprogesterone acetate is effective for 8–12 weeks.

FURTHER READING

Boulvain M, Kelly A, Irion O (2008) Intracervical prostaglandins for induction of labour. *Cochrane Database Syst Rev* 1, CD006971

Farquhar C (2007) Endometriosis. *BMJ* 334, 249–253

Grady D (2006) Management of the menopause. *N Engl J Med* 355, 2338–2347

Gruber CJ, Tschuggel W, Schneeberger C et al. (2002) Production and actions of estrogens. *N Engl J Med* 346, 340–352

Hickey M, Davis SR, Sturdee DW (2005) Treatment of menopausal symptoms: what shall we do now? *Lancet* 366, 409–421

Hickey M, Elliott J, Davison SL (2012) Hormone replacement therapy. *BMJ* 344, e763

Kaunitz AM (2008) Hormonal contraception in women of older reproductive age. *N Engl J Med* 358, 1262–1270

Norwitz ER, Robinson JN, Shallis JRG (1999) The control of labor. *N Engl J Med* 341, 660–666

O'Brien S, Rapkin A, Dennerstein L et al. (2011) Diagnosis and management of premenstrual disorders. *BMJ* 342, d2994

Peterson HB, Curtis KM (2005) Long-acting methods of contraception. *N Engl J Med* 353, 2169–2175

Petitti DB (2003) Combination estrogen–progestin oral contraceptives. *N Engl J Med* 349, 1443–1450

Prabakar I, Webb A (2012) Emergency contraception. *BMJ* 344, e1492

Prentice A (1999) Medical management of menorrhagia. *BMJ* 319, 1343–1345

Riggs BL, Hartmann LC (2003) Selective estrogen-receptor modulators. Mechanisms of action and application to clinical practice. *N Engl J Med* 348, 618–629

Sanchez-Ramos L (2005) Induction of labor. *Obstet Gynecol Clin North Am* 32, 181–200

Simhan HN, Caritis SN (2007) Prevention of preterm delivery. *N Engl J Med* 357, 477–487

Stearns V, Ullmer L, Lopez JF et al. (2002) Hot flushes. *Lancet* 360, 1851–1861

Stubblefield PG, Carr-Ellis S, Borgatta L (2004) Methods for induced abortion. *Obstet Gynecol* 104, 174–185

Compendium: drugs acting on the female reproductive system

Drug	Kinetics (half-life)	Comments
Oestrogens		
Components of oral contraceptives and for HRT; all compounds are lipid-soluble and rapidly absorbed after oral dosage; other uses are specified. Some oestrogens, progestogens and oestrogen receptor antagonists are used for the treatment of malignant disease (see Ch. 52).		
Conjugated oestrogen (equine)	Components are absorbed both intact and after hydrolysis; excreted as sulphate conjugates	Given as sulphate conjugates of >10 equine oestrogens; used as a component of oral HRT
Estradiol	Rapidly absorbed; first-pass hepatic metabolism to estrone and estriol (1–2 h)	
Estradiol valerate	Assumed to be a prodrug for estradiol	
Ethinylestradiol	Oral bioavailability 83%; hepatic oxidisation and conjugation (8–24 h)	Component of oral combined hormonal contraceptive; replaced by other oestrogens for treatment of menopausal symptoms; also used in hereditary haemorrhagic telangiectasia
Mestranol	More than 50% converted to ethinylestradiol, in part during first-pass metabolism (8–24 h)	
Progestogens		
Components of oral contraceptives and for HRT; other uses are specified.		
Desogestrel	Prodrug undergoes rapid P450-mediated oxidation in gut wall and liver to etonogestrel (30 h)	Third-generation progestogen; component of oral hormonal contraceptives
Drospirenone	Oral bioavailability about 80%; hepatic metabolism (36–42 h)	Third-generation progestogen with anti-mineralocorticoid and anti-androgen activity; component of oral hormonal contraceptives
Dydrogesterone	Metabolised to active product (5–7 h) with longer half-life (14 h)	Progesterone analogue used in endometriosis, infertility, recurrent miscarriage, premenstrual syndrome, amenorrhoea and dysmenorrhoea
Etonogestrel	Slow release from implant; P450 hepatic metabolism (29 h)	Etonogestrel-releasing implant can be inserted subdermally to give prolonged contraception
Etynodiol (ethynodiol)	Rapidly absorbed; complete hepatic first-pass metabolism to active norethindrone (half-life 5–14 h)	Used in progestogen-only oral contraceptives
Gestodene	Metabolism by CYP3A4 results in irreversible inhibition of the enzyme (18 h)	Third-generation progestogen; component of oral hormonal contraceptives
Levonorgestrel	Bioavailability 100%; hepatic metabolism (8–30 h)	Component of oral combined hormonal contraceptive; effective emergency contraception up to 72 h after unprotected intercourse; also used in an intra-uterine device for contraception and primary menorrhagia
Medroxyprogesterone acetate	Hepatic metabolism (30 days)	Long-acting progestogen; given as aqueous suspension by deep intramuscular injection
Norelgestromin	Transdermal patch gives sustained blood levels; hepatic metabolism (28 h)	Progestogen; used as a once-weekly transdermal patch with ethinylestradiol; applied for 3 weeks in every four
Norethisterone	Hepatic metabolism; eliminated in urine and bile (5–12 h)	Testosterone analogue used for endometriosis, premenstrual syndrome, dysmenorrhoea and postponement of menstruation; component of oral hormonal contraceptives
Norethisterone acetate	Hydrolysed to norethisterone	Component of oral hormonal contraceptives
Norethisterone enantate	Hydrolysed to norethisterone	Long-acting progestogen; given as an oil solution by very slow deep intramuscular injection

Compendium: drugs acting on the female reproductive system—cont'd

Drug	Kinetics (half-life)	Comments
Norgestimate	Prodrug converted to active metabolites including norelgestromin and levonorgestrel (half-lives 8–30 h)	Component of oral hormonal contraceptives
Norgestrel	Hepatic metabolism (20 h)	Component of oral hormonal contraceptives
Progesterone	Metabolised in liver to pregnanediol then glucuronidated (5–20 min)	Given as rectal or vaginal pessaries for infertility, premenstrual syndrome and postnatal depression, or by injection for dysmenorrhoea
Ulipristal acetete	Oral bioavailability 99%; hepatic metabolism, faecal excretion (32 h)	Progesterone receptor modulator; effective emergency contraception up to 120 h after unprotected intercourse; given orally

Drugs used primarily for endometriosis

Other uses are specified.

Danazol	Hepatic metabolism (4–5 h)	Anti-gonadotrophic drug with androgenic, anti-oestrogenic and anti-progestogenic effects; also used for severe pain in benign fibrocystic breast disease and hereditary angioedema; given orally
Gestrinone	Hepatic metabolism (27 h)	Actions similar to danazol; given orally
Gonadorelin	See Ch. 43	Gonadotropin-releasing hormone (see Ch. 43); given by intravenous injection for assessment of pituitary function

Gonadorelin analogues

Downregulate gonadotropin-releasing hormone (GnRH) receptors and thereby reduce the release of gonadotropins; used for endometriosis and infertility, and before intra-uterine surgery; other uses are specified.

Buserelin	Metabolism plus urinary excretion (1–1.5 h)	Used for prostate cancer (see Ch. 52); given nasally for endometriosis and by subcutaneous injection
Goserelin	Metabolised by cell peptidases (4 h)	Used for prostate cancer and early and advanced breast cancer (see Ch. 52); given by subcutaneous implant
Leuprorelin acetate	Metabolised by cell peptidases (3 h)	Used for prostate cancer (see Ch. 52); given by subcutaneous or intramuscular injection
Nafarelin	Slow hydrolysis (3–4 h)	Used for endometriosis; given as a nasal spray
Triptorelin	Routes of elimination unknown (3 h)	Used for prostate cancer (see Ch. 52); given by intramuscular injection

Drugs used for menopausal symptoms and/or osteoporosis

Given orally.

Raloxifene	Rapidly absorbed; extensive first-pass glucuronidation and enterohepatic cycling (28 h)	Used in treatment of postmenopausal osteoporosis (Ch. 42)
Tibolone	Rapidly converted to active metabolites with oestrogenic activity (half-lives 4–14 h)	Oestrogenic, progestogenic and weak androgenic activities; used for the short-term treatment and prevention of menopausal vasomotor symptoms and postmenopausal osteoporosis

Anti-oestrogens

Induce gonadotropin release by suppressing negative feedback by oestrogen

Clomifene	See Ch. 43	Used for the treatment of female infertility associated with oligomenorrhoea or secondary amenorrhoea; given orally
Tamoxifen	See Ch. 52	Main use is in breast cancer (Ch. 52)

Compendium: drugs acting on the female reproductive system—cont'd

Drug	Kinetics (half-life)	Comments
Drugs used to treat mastalgia		
Bromocriptine	–	See Chs 24 and 43
Danazol	–	See above
Tamoxifen	–	See Ch. 52
Prostaglandins, oxytocics and drugs used to reduce postpartum haemorrhage		
Carbetocin	Metabolic routes not defined (40 min)	Oxytocin receptor agonist; used for uterine atony and postpartum haemorrhage after caesarean section; given by intravenous injection
Carboprost	Slower metabolism than $PGF_{2\alpha}$ (8 min)	15-Methyl derivative of $PGF_{2\alpha}$; used for severe postpartum haemorrhage due to uterine atony; given by deep intramuscular injection
Dinoprostone (PGE_2)	Metabolised by dehydrogenation (30 s)	Used for induction of labour; given intravaginally (or rarely by intravenous injection)
Ergometrine (ergonovine)	Hepatic metabolism (2 h)	Used to prevent and treat postpartum haemorrhage; given by intramuscular injection
Gemeprost	Rapidly hydrolysed locally (minutes); absorbed fraction (12–28%) mostly eliminated in urine	Used to soften the cervix in labour induction and to induce abortion; given intravaginally
Oxytocin	Rapid metabolism (2–10 min)	Used for induction of labour; given by slow intravenous injection or infusion
Drugs used for effects on ductus arteriosus		
Alprostadil (PGE_1)	Metabolised by dehydrogenation (30 s)	Used to maintain patency of the ductus arteriosus in neonates with congenital heart defects; given as an intravenous infusion
Indometacin	See Ch. 29	Used to close the ductus arteriosus in premature babies; given by intravenous injection
Drugs used primarily for therapeutic abortions		
Gemeprost	See above.	PGE_1 analogue; used for the medical induction of late therapeutic abortion; given as an intravaginal pessary
Mifepristone	Hepatic metabolism and enterohepatic cycling (18 h)	Given orally or vaginally prior to therapeutic abortion to sensitise uterus to actions of prostaglandins
Misoprostol	Rapidly absorbed; eliminated as urinary metabolites (20–40 min)	Used for the induction of second trimester abortion; given orally or vaginally
Myometrial relaxant drugs		
Atosiban	Metabolised to active derivative (15 min)	Oxytocin receptor antagonist used for inhibition of uncomplicated premature labour at 24–33 weeks of gestation; given by intravenous injection or infusion
Nifedipine	See Ch. 5	Calcium channel blocker (Ch. 5); given orally
Salbutamol	See Ch. 12	β_2-Adrenoceptor agonist used for inhibition of uncomplicated premature labour at 24–33 weeks of gestation; given by intravenous infusion and then orally
Terbutaline	See Ch. 12	β_2-Adrenoceptor agonist used for inhibition of uncomplicated premature labour at 24–33 weeks of gestation; given orally, subcutaneously or by intravenous infusion

HRT, hormone-replacement therapy; PG, prostaglandin.

Androgens, anti-androgens and anabolic steroids

ANDROGENS

Naturally occurring androgens are 19-carbon steroid hormones that are synthesised in the adrenal cortex and gonads (see Fig. 44.2). They have characteristic actions on the reproductive tract and other tissues as well as an anabolic effect on metabolism. A number of synthetic androgenic steroids have been developed. The term 'anabolic steroid' is used when the predominant action of the compound is anabolic rather than reproductive. There are a few medical uses for anabolic steroids, but they have achieved notoriety because of their abuse by athletes to enhance muscle development.

Testosterone is secreted by the Leydig cells of the testis, and its synthesis and release are stimulated by the gonadotropin luteinizing hormone (LH). In many tissues testosterone is aromatized to form oestradiol, which accelerates closure of bony epiphyses and contributes to brain development. It is oestradiol rather than testosterone that inhibits the release of gonadotropin-releasing hormone (GnRH) from the hypothalamus and LH via a negative-feedback loop (Ch. 43). Androgens are also released from the adrenal cortex, in response to stimulation by adrenocorticotropic hormone (ACTH; corticotropin); these are mainly dehydroepiandrosterone and androstenedione (see Fig. 44.2). Men produce large amounts of androgens and small amounts of oestrogens, while the reverse is the case in women.

The actions of testosterone are in part due to its metabolite dihydrotestosterone (DHT). This is produced from testosterone in the prostate, skin and reproductive tissues by the enzymatic action of 5α-reductase (Fig. 44.2). DHT has a higher affinity than testosterone for the androgen receptor, and is five times more potent as an androgen. DHT is mainly responsible for the development of secondary sexual characteristics in men.

The cellular mechanism of action of steroid hormones is discussed in Chapters 1 and 44. Androgens act mainly through genomic effects on protein synthesis via the cytoplasmic androgen receptor (AR), which is then translocated to the cell nucleus. The androgen receptor also produces rapid-onset, non-genomic actions in the cytoplasm by affecting signal transduction and ion transport. This is responsible for effects such as vasodilation (see also Ch. 44).

Circulating androgens are bound largely to a specific transport protein, sex hormone-binding globulin (SHBG), which has a greater affinity for androgens than for oestrogen.

MALE SEX HORMONES

Examples

mesterolone (methyltestosterone), testosterone

Actions of testosterone

Actions of androgens include the following:

- sexual differentiation in the fetus,
- sexual development of the male testis, penis, epididymis, seminal vesicles and prostate at puberty, and maintenance of these tissues in adults,
- spermatogenesis in adults,
- stimulation and maintenance of sexual function and behaviour,
- metabolic actions. Testosterone is a powerful anabolic agent producing a positive nitrogen balance with an increase in the bulk of tissues such as muscle and bone. In the skin, sebum production is increased, which can provoke acne. Growth of axillary, pubic, facial and chest hair is stimulated. In the liver, testosterone increases the synthesis of several proteins, including clotting factors, but decreases high-density lipoprotein (HDL) synthesis (Ch. 48). Testosterone also induces several liver enzymes, including steroid hydroxylases,
- haematological actions. Testosterone stimulates the production of erythropoietin by the kidneys, leading to higher haemoglobin concentrations in men than in women.

Pharmacokinetics

- Oral preparations. Testosterone is well absorbed from the gut but is almost completely degraded by first-pass metabolism in the gut wall and liver. Oral absorption can be enhanced by esterification of testosterone to create hydrophobic compounds, such as testosterone undecanoate, which are absorbed via lacteals into the lymphatic system, thus avoiding hepatic metabolism. Mesterolone is a synthetic testosterone derivative that has a greater oral bioavailability than testosterone, but less androgenic activity.

- Depot injection. The most popular form of therapy for hypogonadism in men is an intramuscular injection of a testosterone ester, usually in oily solution, given at intervals from 2–3 weeks up to 10–14 weeks depending on the formulation. Testosterone is absorbed gradually after ester hydrolysis at the site of injection. Examples are testosterone enantate, propionate and undecanoate.
- Transdermal delivery. A transdermal delivery patch containing testosterone can be applied to the back, abdomen, upper arm or thigh, rotating the site daily to avoid skin irritation. Testosterone gel is an alternative way to deliver the drug transdermally.
- Buccal delivery. Testosterone can be delivered via a buccal tablet which softens to a gel and adheres to the mucosa. This provides sustained release of testosterone, and avoids hepatic first-pass metabolism.
- Subcutaneous implant. A pellet of pure crystalline testosterone provides a reservoir for gradual absorption into the systemic circulation for 4–5 months. A minor surgical procedure is necessary, and therefore this method of delivery is rarely used.

Testosterone is metabolised in the liver to androstenedione, and then to inactive compounds. Some testosterone undergoes conversion in specific organs to dihydrotestosterone, and a small amount undergoes aromatisation to oestradiol (see above). Mesterolone is not metabolised to oestrogenic compounds.

Unwanted effects

- Prostate cancer.
- In hypogonadal adolescents, initial nitrogen retention and a spurt in linear growth is followed by premature epiphyseal closure and short stature. A short course of testosterone can be used for the treatment of delayed puberty without inducing epiphyseal closure.
- Headache.
- Anxiety, depression.
- Nausea, vomiting, gastrointestinal bleeding.
- Sodium retention with oedema and hypertension.
- Hirsutism, male-pattern baldness, acne. Virilisation occurs in women given testosterone.
- Conversion to oestrogens by aromatase can produce gynaecomastia (see Fig. 44.2). This is less likely to occur with mesterolone.
- Suppression of gonadotropin release with diminished testicular size and reduced spermatogenesis. Hypogonadal men will not regain fertility while taking androgens.
- Cholestatic jaundice. Liver tumours are a rare complication.
- Local irritation from topical formulations.

Clinical uses of testosterone

- The main clinical use is as hormone-replacement therapy for primary hypogonadism in adult males. Late-onset

hypogonadism may present with erectile dysfunction, fatigue, depression, hot flushes, muscle weakness and reduced body hair. Testosterone replacement can improve quality of life in this situation.

- It can be used briefly in constitutionally delayed puberty, even in the absence of hypogonadism.
- Androgens are occasionally beneficial for promoting erythropoiesis in some forms of aplastic anaemia.

DANAZOL

Mechanism of action

Danazol is an androgen derivative described as an 'impeded' androgen, which is weakly androgenic on peripheral tissues. It has no oestrogenic activity as, unlike testosterone, it is not converted into an oestrogen by aromatases. Its main action is feedback inhibition of gonadotropin and gonadotropin-releasing hormone (GnRH) secretion. It therefore has anti-oestrogenic and anti-progestogenic actions.

Pharmacokinetics

Danazol is well absorbed orally, metabolised in the liver and has a short half-life (3 h).

Unwanted effects

- Nausea, epigastric pain.
- Acne, hirsutism, oedema, hair loss or deepening of voice, due to androgenic effects.
- Depression, anxiety.
- Dizziness, headache.
- Vaginal dryness, reduction in breast size, changes in libido, amenorrhoea, hot flushes.

Clinical uses of danazol

- Treatment of endometriosis (Ch. 45).
- Treatment of menorrhagia (Ch. 45).
- Management of gynaecomastia (Ch. 45).
- Long-term management of hereditary angioedema.

ANABOLIC STEROIDS

Examples

nandrolone, oxymetholone

Anabolic steroids are most frequently encountered as drugs of abuse to improve athletic performance (doping). In medical practice there are few indications for these compounds and there is little evidence for efficacy in many conditions where their use has been advocated.

Pharmacokinetics

Nandrolone is given as a decanoate ester depot formulation by intramuscular injection every 3 weeks. Oxymetholone is available as an oral formulation from specialist suppliers.

Unwanted effects

Androgenic effects may be troublesome in women.

Clinical uses

- Promotion of erythropoiesis in aplastic anaemias.
- Itching associated with chronic biliary obstruction in palliative care.

Abuse of anabolic steroids

The ability of androgens to promote an increase in muscle mass has led to their abuse to improve physical performance by athletes, weightlifters and bodybuilders. Often, several different androgens are used for prolonged periods, perhaps with a brief 'drug-free' period. Abused compounds include testosterone, nandrolone and oxymetholone and many others that are licensed only for veterinary use. The consequences of abuse include:

- weight gain from muscle hypertrophy and fluid retention,
- acne in adolescent and young men,
- decreased testicular size and reduced sperm count,
- hepatotoxicity with cholestasis, hepatitis or, occasionally, hepatocellular tumours,
- atherogenic changes in the plasma lipids with a rise in plasma LDL cholesterol and a fall in HDL cholesterol (Ch. 48); these changes may predispose to premature vascular disease,
- psychological disturbance, including changes in libido, increased aggression and psychotic symptoms.

ANTI-ANDROGENS

BICALUTAMIDE AND FLUTAMIDE

Mechanism of action

Bicalutamide and flutamide are non-steroidal, relatively pure anti-androgens. They bind to androgen receptors in the cell cytoplasm, either to the hormone binding site or to an adjacent site producing distortion of the co-activator binding site, so that the receptor cannot initiate gene transcription.

Pharmacokinetics

Bicalutamide and flutamide are well absorbed orally, and are metabolised in the liver. Bicalutamide has a very long half-life of 7–10 days, while that of flutamide is 8 h.

Unwanted effects

- Anti-androgenic effects, for example gynaecomastia, hot flushes, impotence, decreased libido and inhibition of spermatogenesis.
- Nausea, vomiting, diarrhoea, weight gain.
- Cholestatic jaundice.

CYPROTERONE ACETATE

Mechanism of action

Cyproterone acetate, a 21-carbon steroid, is a progestogen and a weak glucocorticoid (Ch. 44). Its progestational activity produces feedback inhibition of gonadotrophin (LH) secretion (Ch. 45). At high doses cyproterone inhibits androgen binding to its receptors.

Pharmacokinetics

Cyproterone acetate is well absorbed orally and metabolised in the liver, and has a very long half-life of 2 days.

Unwanted effects

- Anti-androgenic effects, for example gynaecomastia, hot flushes, impotence, decreased libido and inhibition of spermatogenesis.
- Fatigue.
- Hepatotoxicity with long-term use, causing hepatitis and, occasionally, hepatic failure.

CLINICAL USES OF ANTI-ANDROGENS

- The main use of anti-androgens is in the treatment of carcinoma of the prostate (Ch. 52), usually in conjunction with a gonadorelin analogue (Ch. 43).
- Cyproterone acetate is used in male sexual offenders as 'chemical castration'.
- Cyproterone acetate can be given for manifestations of hyper-androgenisation in females, such as acne and hirsutism, in conjunction with ethinylestradiol in an oral combined hormonal contraceptive (Ch. 45).

5α-REDUCTASE INHIBITORS

Examples

dutasteride, finasteride

Mechanism of action and effects

Dutasteride and finasteride reduce the formation of dihydrotestosterone by inhibiting 5α-reductase, rather than acting as an antagonist at androgen receptors. In the adult male finasteride and dutasteride can produce regression of benign prostatic hypertrophy and improve the symptoms of prostatism. More details are found in Ch. 15.

SELF-ASSESSMENT

True/false questions

1. Androgen deficiency in adult men may cause decreased libido.
2. Testosterone cannot be given orally.
3. Testosterone alone is used to stimulate spermatogenesis.
4. Nandrolone causes less virilisation in women than testosterone.
5. Cyproterone acetate is used as an adjunct to the treatment of prostate cancer.
6. Anti-androgens can cause gynaecomastia.

One-best-answer (OBA) question

Choose the *most accurate* statement concerning drugs that affect androgenic and anabolic activities.

A. 5α-Reductase inactivates dihydrotestosterone.
B. Cyproterone acetate promotes spermatogenesis.
C. Nandrolone reduces muscle mass.
D. Danazol is used in the treatment of endometriosis.
E. Testosterone has marked anti-anabolic activity.

True/false answers

1. **True.** Androgen deficiency may also cause impotence, reduced muscle mass, loss of body hair and other effects.
2. **True.** Testosterone is ineffective when given orally as it undergoes very extensive first-pass metabolism; it is given as testosterone ester formulations or in transdermal patches.
3. **False.** Other treatments are required, including human chorionic gonadotropin (HCG) and other gonadotropins.
4. **True.** Nandrolone has fewer androgenic effects than testosterone, but has many other unwanted effects.
5. **True.** Cyproterone acetate is an anti-androgen used with a gonadorelin analogue in prostate cancer.
6. **True.** Anti-androgens can cause gynaecomastia, inhibition of spermatogenesis and other unwanted effects.

OBA answer

Answer D is correct.

A. Incorrect. 5α-Reductase converts testosterone to active dihydrotestosterone.
B. Incorrect. Cyproterone is an anti-androgen; it inhibits spermatogenesis.
C. Incorrect. Nandrolone is an androgen and causes an increase in muscle mass.
D. **Correct.** Danazol has anti-androgen, anti-oestrogen and anti-progesterone activity and is used in the treatment of endometriosis.
E. Incorrect. Testosterone is markedly anabolic, increasing turnover and growth in many tissues and cells.

FURTHER READING

Di Luigi L, Romanelli F, Lenzi A (2005) Androgenic-anabolic steroids abuse in males. *J Endocrinol Invest* 28 (suppl 3), 81–84

Kazi M, Geraci SA, Koch CA (2007) Considerations for the diagnosis and treatment of testosterone deficiency in elderly men. *Am J Med* 120, 835–840

Rhoden EL, Morgentaler A (2004) Risks of testosterone-replacement therapy and recommendations for monitoring. *N Engl J Med* 350, 482–492

Schneider HPG (2003) Androgens and antiandrogens. *Ann NY Acad Sci* 997, 292–306

Traish AM, Miner MM, Morgentaler A et al. (2011) Testosterone deficiency. *Am J Med* 124, 578–587

Compendium: drugs acting on the male reproductive system and anabolic agents

Drug	Kinetics (half-life)	Comment
Androgens		
Danazol	See Ch. 45	Inhibits pituitary gonadotropins; used for endometriosis (Ch. 45)
Mesterolone (methyltestosterone)	Almost completely absorbed; hepatic metabolism (12–13 h)	Used for androgen deficiency and male infertility associated with hypogonadism; given orally
Testosterone and testosterone esters	Testosterone has low oral bioavailability due to extensive first-pass metabolism; slow release from esters, depot formulations, implants or patches; rapidly cleared from blood (2–4 h)	Used for androgen deficiency and for breast cancer in women; given orally (as undecanoate), by intramuscular injection (as enantate or propionate), or as an implant (as testosterone) or as patches (as testosterone)
Anabolic steroids		
Nandrolone decanoate	Slow release from depot injection; hydrolysed (5–17 h)	Not used for effects on male reproductive system; used for aplastic anaemia; given as deep intramuscular injection
Oxymetholone	Oral bioavailability 95%; hepatic metabolism, renal excretion (9 h)	Given for 3–6 months for aplastic anaemia (see Ch. 47); given orally
Gonadorelin analogues		
Given for advanced prostate cancer (see Ch. 52) and for actions on the female reproductive system (see Ch. 45).		
Buserelin	See Ch. 45	Given by subcutaneous injection followed by intranasal dosage
Goserelin	See Ch. 45	Given by subcutaneous implant
Leuprorelin acetate	See Ch. 45	Given by subcutaneous or intramuscular injection
Triptorelin	See Ch. 45	Given by subcutaneous or intramuscular injection
Anti-androgens		
Abiraterone acetate	Prodrug of abiraterone; hepatic metabolism and faecal excretion (12 h)	17α-Hydroxylase inhibitor that reduces androgen synthesis; used for metastatic castration-resistant prostate cancer; given orally
Bicalutamide	Oxidised and conjugated products excreted in urine and bile (7–10 days)	Used for advanced prostate cancer; given orally
Cyproterone acetate	Hepatic metabolism (2 days)	Used as an adjunct for prostate cancer, for hirsutism and acne in women, and for severe hypersexuality and sexual deviation in men; given orally
Flutamide	Essentially complete oral bioavailability; rapid hepatic oxidation to active 2-hydroxy-flutamide (8 h)	Used for advanced prostate cancer; acts by inhibition of the uptake and/or nuclear binding of testosterone and dihydrotestosterone by prostatic tissue; given orally
5α-Reductase inhibitors		
Inhibit 5α-reductase, the enzyme that converts testosterone to 5α-dihydrotestosterone (DHT), the primary androgen that stimulates the development of prostatic tissue.		
Dutasteride	Oral bioavailability 60%; accumulates over 6 months due to long half-life (5 weeks)	Used for benign prostatic hyperplasia; inhibitor of type I and type II 5α-reductase; given orally
Finasteride	Hepatic metabolism (5–6 h)	Used for benign prostatic hyperplasia and male-pattern baldness in men; selective inhibitor of type II 5α-reductase; given orally

47 Anaemia and haematopoietic colony-stimulating factors

ANAEMIA

The definition of anaemia is rather arbitrary and the absolute normal ranges for haemoglobin concentration in blood vary among laboratories. In adults, anaemia equates to a blood concentration of haemoglobin in males below about 130 g·L^{-1} (normal is about 130–170 g·L^{-1}) or in non-pregnant females below about 120 g·L^{-1} (normal is about 120–150 g·L^{-1}). Many individuals, however, have concentrations below these ranges without apparent detriment. Lower concentrations can be normal in children and during pregnancy. Anaemia can cause many symptoms, including shortness of breath and fatigue. There are many causes of anaemia (Box 47.1), the forms of which are classified by red cell size and haemoglobin content (Box 47.2).

There are three key dietary factors that are required for normal red cell synthesis, referred to as haematinics:

- iron,
- folic acid,
- vitamin B$_{12}$.

IRON

Dietary iron is absorbed from the duodenum and upper jejunum. In an omnivorous diet most iron is absorbed from meat, in which it is present as haem. Haem is the ferrous form of iron (Fe^{2+}) complexed with a porphyrin ring. Haem is readily absorbed from the gut, but non-haem iron in a vegetarian diet, which is mainly in the ferric state (Fe^{3+}), is inefficiently absorbed. Absorption of ferric iron is facilitated by several factors:

- gastric acid, which increases its solubility,
- conversion to ferrous iron by ferric reductase on the brush border of enterocytes, which is enhanced by dietary reducing agents such as ascorbic acid, fructose and some amino acids,
- intestinal absorption mediated by the divalent metal transporter (DMT-1), mainly in the duodenum. Expression of DMT-1 is increased in iron deficiency and in hereditary haemochromatosis.

Within enterocytes, iron is oxidized to the ferric state and transported to the circulation by the protein ferroportin. In the blood, ferric iron is bound to the globulin transferrin and transported to the bone marrow and iron stores. Cellular iron uptake occurs via transferrin receptors, and in most cells iron is stored as ferritin (a complex of iron with the apoferritin protein). In some tissues iron is also found as relatively insoluble aggregates of degraded forms of ferritin, known as haemosiderin. Two-thirds of the iron in the body is present in circulating red cells, and about half of the remainder is found in macrophages, reticuloendothelial cells and hepatocytes. The rest is present in myoglobin in muscle cells or associated with various intracellular enzymes.

When ageing red cells are broken down by the reticuloendothelial system, most of the released iron is recycled via macrophages for further erythropoiesis. Iron loss from the body is normally low, and occurs through shedding of mucosal cells containing ferritin; there is negligible renal loss of iron.

Iron deficiency

The main cause of iron deficiency in the UK is abnormal loss of blood, particularly from the gut or from exaggerated menstrual loss. Iron malabsorption can result from disease of the upper small intestine, for example coeliac disease, or following partial gastrectomy. Dietary deficiency is rarely a major cause in Western societies, although worldwide a vegetarian diet low in absorbable forms of iron is the commonest contributory cause of iron deficiency.

Therapeutic iron preparations

Oral iron

Oral iron supplements are preferred and are given as ferrous salts; for example, ferrous sulphate, fumarate or gluconate. Tablets are normally used, but some people find that a syrup is more palatable. In the presence of iron deficiency, a daily oral dose equivalent to 100–200 mg of elemental iron produces the maximum rate of rise of haemoglobin (200 mg ferrous sulphate contains 65 mg iron). About one-third of this dose will be absorbed. Some oral iron preparations contain vitamin C, but the therapeutic advantage is minimal compared to the ferrous salt alone.

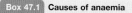

Unwanted effects

- Gastrointestinal intolerance is common, especially nausea and dyspepsia. The prevalence of these effects depends both on the dose of elemental iron and on psychological factors, rather than on the iron salt used. They can be minimised by taking iron supplements with food or by reducing the dose. Modified-release iron formulations have been developed to improve tolerability, but much of the iron is released beyond the duodenum, the site where it is best absorbed. These formulations should only be used when other methods for improving iron tolerance are ineffective. Diarrhoea or constipation also occur, but are not dose-related.
- Oral iron turns stools black.

Parenteral iron

Iron can be given by slow intravenous injection or infusion, or less commonly by deep intramuscular injection. Formulations involve complexing ferric hydroxide to a carrier to form iron sucrose, iron dextran (the only formulation for intramuscular use), ferric carboxymaltose or iron isomaltoside 1000. The iron in these formulations is not bound to transferrin in plasma but accumulates in reticuloendothelial cells. When calculating the amount of iron to give, the approximate total body iron deficit (haemoglobin and body stores) is estimated from the person's size and haemoglobin concentration.

Unwanted effects

- Nausea, vomiting, diarrhoea, abdominal pain.
- Flushing, fever.
- Headache, dizziness.
- Chest pains, arthralgia, myalgia.
- Urticaria.
- Anaphylactoid/anaphylactic reactions, including cardiovascular collapse; facilities for resuscitation should always be available.

Therapeutic use of iron

The cause of iron deficiency should always be sought when starting symptomatic treatment with iron. If this is not done, then serious disorders such as gastrointestinal malignancy can be overlooked. Oral iron supplements are adequate for most mild or moderate iron-deficiency anaemias. After an initial delay of a few days while new red cells are formed, oral iron supplements should raise the blood haemoglobin concentration by about 20 g·L^{-1} over the first 3–4 weeks, and about 10 g·L^{-1} per week thereafter. Oral iron supplements should be continued for 3 months after the haemoglobin concentration has been restored, in order to replenish tissue iron stores.

Failure to respond to oral iron can be caused by several factors:

- incorrect diagnosis, for example anaemia of chronic disorder, thalassaemia,
- poor adherence to oral iron therapy,
- inadequate iron dosage, for example in some modified-release formulations,
- continuing excessive blood loss,
- malabsorption,
- concurrent deficiency of other substances necessary for haemoglobin synthesis.

Parenteral iron preparations are used if there are intractable unwanted effects from oral preparations, if there is severe uncorrectable malabsorption or continuing heavy blood loss and when adherence to oral treatment is poor. Parenteral iron does not raise the haemoglobin concentration any faster than oral iron, except during haemodialysis for severe renal failure.

Oral iron supplements are occasionally given for prophylaxis against iron deficiency at times of high demand for iron, for example pregnancy, menorrhagia or if there is a poor dietary intake. The reduced iron absorption after subtotal or total gastrectomy can also be overcome by long-term iron supplements.

FOLIC ACID

Folate is required for a number of cellular biochemical processes, including DNA synthesis, and is essential for cell replication, including the formation of red cells. Folic acid (pteroylglutamic acid) is ingested as conjugated folate polyglutamates, found mainly in fresh leaf vegetables (in which it is heat-labile) and in liver (where it is more heat-stable). Before absorption, the polyglutamates are deconjugated to the monoglutamate. Folate monoglutamate is absorbed principally in the duodenum and jejunum, and is methylated

Box 47.3   Causes of folate deficiency

- Poor diet: folate stores are adequate for a few weeks only. Lack of folate is uncommon in Western diets, but may be more common in the diet of elderly people or in alcoholism.
- Increased requirements: e.g. pregnancy, malignancies, haemolytic anaemias, exfoliative dermatitis.
- Malabsorption: e.g. coeliac disease, tropical sprue.
- Drugs that interfere with folate metabolism: anticonvulsants (especially phenytoin; Ch. 23), methotrexate (Ch. 52), pyrimethamine (Ch. 51).

and reduced to 5-methyltetrahydrofolate by dihydrofolate reductase during absorption. Methyltetrahydrofolate enters cells, where it is demethylated and converted back to folate polyglutamates. These are coenzymes in the synthesis of pyrimidines and purines and hence of DNA (see also Ch. 52).

Folate deficiency

The most obvious consequence of folate deficiency is a macrocytic anaemia with the presence of megaloblasts in the marrow, a feature it shares with vitamin B_{12} deficiency. Folate deficiency can arise for a number of reasons (Box 47.3). Unlike iron, folate cannot be recycled from old red cells that are removed from the circulation.

Therapeutic use of folic acid

Folate deficiency almost always responds to oral folic acid supplements. Folic acid is a poor substrate for dihydrofolate reductase, and is largely absorbed unchanged and then converted to tetrahydrofolic acid in the plasma and liver. Most causes of folate deficiency are self-limiting, and folic acid treatment is usually given for 4 months to correct the anaemia and replace folate stores.

Folic acid is given prophylactically in pregnancy. It is given in higher doses if there is an increased risk of conceiving a child with a neural tube defect. Those at higher risk include a partner with a neural tube defect, history of neural tube defect in a previous pregnancy, or if the woman has coeliac disease, diabetes mellitus, sickle-cell anaemia or is taking antiepileptic drugs (Ch. 23). Folic acid is also given prophylactically to premature infants, during renal dialysis, and for chronic haemolytic anaemia.

Treatment of deficiencies of both vitamin B_{12} and folate using only folic acid may correct the anaemia, but irreversible neurological damage can be precipitated (see below). Therefore, vitamin B_{12} deficiency must be excluded before folic acid is used, or both vitamin B_{12} and folic acid should be given if there is a possibility of vitamin B_{12} deficiency.

For folate deficiency produced by drugs that inhibit dihydrofolate reductase (e.g. methotrexate; Ch. 52 and Fig. 51.4) it is necessary to 'bypass' this enzyme blockade by giving the synthetic tetrahydrofolic acid, folinic acid (5-formyl tetrahydrofolic acid). This is the basis of 'folinic acid rescue' to reduce the toxic effects on healthy tissues of high-dose methotrexate used for treatment of

malignancy (Ch. 52). Folinic acid is formulated as a salt and given orally, usually as calcium folinate. When low-dose methotrexate is used in a once-a-week regimen for immunosuppression folic acid can be given on a separate day to reduce toxicity.

VITAMIN B_{12}

Vitamin B_{12} has many roles in the body, including participation in DNA synthesis and fatty acid synthesis. The term vitamin B_{12} refers to a group of cobalt-containing compounds, also known as cobalamins. Bacteria are the only organisms that can synthesise cobalamins *de novo*. Humans obtain vitamin B_{12} from meat (particularly liver), from animal products (milk, cheese, eggs, etc.) or from vegetables contaminated by bacteria. Absorption is by an unusual mechanism: dietary vitamin B_{12} binds in the stomach to a glycoprotein called intrinsic factor that is produced by gastric parietal cells. This complex is absorbed principally from the terminal ileum after binding to receptors on the luminal membranes of ileal cells.

Most vitamin B_{12} in plasma is bound to a glycoprotein, transcobalamin I, from which it is rapidly taken up by the tissues, especially the liver, which stores about 50% of the body content of vitamin B_{12}. A second protein, transcobalamin II, is mainly responsible for rapid transport of vitamin B_{12} to tissues, and for enhancing its uptake by the bone marrow via specific receptors. Vitamin B_{12} is essential as a coenzyme in nucleic acid synthesis, and in other metabolic pathways in conjunction with folate. Many functions of vitamin B_{12} can be performed by folic acid, but there are two enzyme families that only vitamin B_{12} can facilitate. These are responsible for isomerisation of methylmalonyl coenzyme A to succinyl coenzyme A, isomerisation of α-leucine to β-leucine, and methylation of homocysteine to methionine (a reaction that results in demethylation of methyltetrahydrofolate).

Vitamin B_{12} deficiency

Impairment of vitamin B_{12}-dependent enzyme reactions affects DNA synthesis. The major organs affected by vitamin B_{12} deficiency are those with a rapid cell turnover, particularly the bone marrow and the gastrointestinal tract.

Vitamin B_{12} deficiency presents with a macrocytic anaemia and a megaloblastic bone marrow. The tongue becomes smooth, and changes to the lining of the small bowel can lead to malabsorption. Damage to the posterior and lateral neuronal tracts in the spinal cord can also occur, leading to a condition known as subacute combined degeneration of the cord. The biochemical basis for the neurological damage is poorly understood, and it may not be fully reversible after correction of vitamin B_{12} deficiency.

Causes of vitamin B_{12} deficiency include:

- diet: strict vegetarians (vegans) only,
- intestinal malabsorption due to damage to the terminal ileum; for example, Crohn's disease, lymphoma,
- deficiency of intrinsic factor: pernicious anaemia (destruction of gastric parietal cells with achlorhydria and failure of intrinsic factor production), total and subtotal gastrectomy.

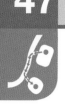

Therapeutic use of vitamin B$_{12}$

Most people with vitamin B$_{12}$ deficiency have problems absorbing it from the gut, and treatment is usually by intramuscular injection of vitamin B$_{12}$ in aqueous solution. Hydroxocobalamin, the form of vitamin B$_{12}$ produced by bacteria, is used for treatment of deficiency. Following initial injections on alternate days for 2 weeks to replenish stores, maintenance injections every 3 months for life are adequate. In the rare dietary causes of vitamin B$_{12}$ deficiency, oral cyanocobalamin supplements can be given, but otherwise oral treatment is never indicated.

ERYTHROPOIETIN

darbepoetin, epoetin

Erythropoietin is a glycosylated protein hormone produced mainly by the kidney. It regulates red cell production by reducing apoptosis and stimulating differentiation and proliferation of erythroid progenitor cells. Erythropoietin binds to its receptor, which is found in high concentration on erythroid precursors, and enables the receptor to activate several intracellular signalling pathways. Deficiency of erythropoietin in end-stage renal disease contributes to the anaemia that characterises this disorder. Interestingly, the hormone has also been found to have a protective effect on ischaemic neurons in the brain. Human erythropoietin has been synthesised using recombinant DNA technology (epoetin): it is produced in four forms – alfa, beta, theta and zeta – which have similar clinical effects. Erythropoietin is also available as two longer-acting derivatives: a hyperglycosylated derivative, darbepoetin alfa, and methoxy polyethylene glycol-epoetin beta.

Pharmacokinetics

Epoetin can be given intravenously or, more conveniently, subcutaneously, when a 25–50% lower dose can be used. The red cell response is more rapid after intravenous use, but ultimately greater after subcutaneous injection. Epoetin has a half-life of about 4–6 h, and is normally given two or three times a week. Darbepoetin has a longer half-life and is given once a week, and methoxy polyethylene glycol-epoetin beta is given every 2–4 weeks. The route of elimination of epoetin is uncertain, but may be largely by receptor-mediated uptake in the bone marrow and subsequent intracellular degradation.

Unwanted effects

- Nausea, vomiting, diarrhoea.
- Headache.
- Influenza-like symptoms early in treatment.
- Hypertension, which is dose-dependent and can be severe, leading to encephalopathy with seizures.
- Thrombosis of arteriovenous shunts.
- Pure red cell aplasia (not affecting white cells or platelets) occurs rarely during subcutaneous administration

in renal failure; this is usually associated with formation of antibodies to epoetin, and treatment must be discontinued if this occurs.

Therapeutic uses of epoetin

- Anaemia of end-stage renal disease. Other causes of anaemia should be excluded. Adequate iron stores are essential, since erythropoiesis demands large amounts of iron, and iron supplements (often intravenously) may be needed to maximise the response. Anaemia can be corrected in more than 90% of those treated, and treatment improves quality of life. Epoetin also modulates lipid metabolism, creating a less atherogenic plasma lipid profile, which may reduce the high cardiovascular mortality in renal failure. However, recent evidence suggests that cardiovascular mortality and morbidity may be increased if the haemoglobin concentration is raised above 120 g·L^{-1}.
- To increase red cell production prior to surgery. Autologous blood transfusion is becoming more popular to reduce the use of banked blood. Epoetin given twice weekly for 3 weeks before surgery can increase the number of units of blood that can be obtained.
- Anaemia associated with human immunodeficiency virus (HIV) infection or acquired immunodeficiency syndrome (AIDS).
- Anaemia associated with cytotoxic chemotherapy of non-myeloid malignant disease (Ch. 52).
- Epoetin is sometimes abused by athletes to increase haematocrit and improve performance. This abuse is associated with an increased risk of arterial and venous thromboses.

DRUG TREATMENT IN OTHER ANAEMIAS

Certain other anaemias require specific drug therapy.

Aplastic anaemia

Failure of haematopoietic stem cell production has many causes, including certain drugs (Box 47.4). Drugs do not

---

Box 47.4   Causes of aplastic anaemia

Drugs:
- Cytotoxic agents
- Chloramphenicol
- Sulphonamides
- Non-steroidal anti-inflammatory drugs
- Gold salts
- Carbimazole
- Phenytoin
- Carbamazepine
- Phenothiazines
- Chlorpropamide

Radiation
Infections, e.g. hepatitis, Epstein–Barr virus
Inherited, e.g. Fanconi anaemia
Malignant, e.g. myelodysplastic syndrome

have a major role in treatment of aplastic anaemia. The anabolic steroid oxymetholone (Ch. 46; available in the UK only on a named-patient basis) is sometimes used, but its effectiveness is unpredictable. Antilymphocyte globulin is helpful in some acquired aplastic anaemias, and is sometimes used in combination with ciclosporin (Ch. 38).

Sideroblastic anaemia

This can also be caused by drugs (Box 47.5). It is characterised by accumulation of iron in the mitochondria of erythroblasts, which lie in a ring around the nucleus. Staining for iron reveals the characteristic ring sideroblasts. Pyridoxine supplements can increase the haemoglobin concentration in idiopathic acquired and hereditary forms of the disorder. They can also be useful for reversible sideroblastic anaemia associated with pregnancy, haemolysis, alcohol dependence or during treatment with the antituberculous drug isoniazid (Ch. 51).

Autoimmune haemolytic anaemia

This can respond to immunosuppression with corticosteroids (Ch. 44).

Beta-thalassaemia major

This is a genetic disorder of haemoglobin synthesis with a hyperplastic bone marrow and refractory anaemia. Blood transfusions or excessive iron supplements lead to iron overload, with damage to the liver, heart and pancreas. Iron overload can be prevented with infusions of desferrioxamine mesilate (Ch. 53) together with vitamin C, which enhances iron excretion. The oral iron chelators, deferiprone or deferasirox, are used when desferrioxamine is poorly tolerated or contraindicated.

Sickle cell anaemia

This inherited disorder occurs when more than 80% of the haemoglobin is HbS; fetal haemoglobin (HbF) forms the remainder. Hydroxycarbamide (see Ch. 52) reduces the frequency and severity of sickle cell crises. It raises the HbF concentration and also reduces the number of young red cells, which are those most likely to adhere to endothelium and occlude blood vessels.

DRUGS AS A CAUSE OF ANAEMIA

- Iron deficiency: especially drugs causing bleeding from the upper gut, for example non-steroidal anti-inflammatory drugs (NSAIDs).
- Aplastic anaemia: see Box 47.4.
- Sideroblastic anaemia: see Box 47.5.
- Haemolysis in glucose-6-phosphate dehydrogenase (G6PD) deficiency: see Box 47.6. G6PD is involved in generating reduced glutathione, which protects red cells against oxidative stresses. Oxidant drugs produce haemolysis in GP6D-deficient individuals, who are usually male (Ch. 53).

NEUTROPENIA

Leucocytes are part of the first line of defence against pathogens. They include phagocytic cells (neutrophils, monocytes and eosinophils) and non-phagocytic cells (lymphocytes and basophils). In addition to their role in acute inflammation, all these cells participate in regulation of cellular and humoral immunity through the production of cytokines (Ch. 38). A reduction in the number of circulating neutrophils (neutropenia) in particular increases the risk of serious infection. There are several causes of neutropenia (Box 47.7). Neutropenia does not give rise to symptoms, but predisposes to infection, especially if the neutrophil count falls below 0.5×10^9 L^{-1}.

Box 47.6 **Drugs causing haemolysis in glucose-6-phosphate dehydrogenase deficiency**

Antimalarials
- Primaquine
- Pamaquine

Analgesics
- Aspirin (high dose)

Others
- Sulphonamides
- Nalidixic acid
- Dapsone

Box 47.7 **Causes of neutropenia**

Inherited
Congenital agranulocytosis
Cyclical neutropenia

Acquired
Viral infection, e.g. hepatitis, influenza, rubella, infectious mononucleosis
Bacterial infection
Radiotherapy
Drugs, especially cytotoxic drugs, carbimazole
Autoimmune neutropenia
Hypersplenism
Marrow infiltration

Box 47.5 **More common causes of sideroblastic anaemia**

Congenital
Acquired
- Myelodysplastic syndrome
- Drugs and toxins:
  - Isoniazid
  - Chloramphenicol
  - Alcoholism
  - Lead poisoning

DRUGS FOR NEUTROPENIA

Granulocyte colony-stimulating factors

Granulocyte colony-stimulating factors are produced by many cells, such as endothelial cells, monocytes and fibroblasts, and stimulate the maturation of pluripotent stem cells in the bone marrow. Granulocyte colony-stimulating factor (G-CSF) is produced by recombinant DNA technology. Therapeutic agents include:

- filgrastim (recombinant human G-CSF),
- lenograstim (glycosylated recombinant human G-CSF),
- pegfilgrastim (pegylated filgrastim).

G-CSF is glycosylated in its natural state, but this does not seem to be a prerequisite for effectiveness. A transient fall in circulating neutrophils occurs within minutes of the injection, followed a few hours later by a substantial rise.

Pharmacokinetics

Granulocyte colony-stimulating factors are given by prolonged intravenous infusion or subcutaneous infusion or injection. Daily injections of filgrastim or lenograstim are given until there is an adequate neutrophil response. Pegfilgrastim has a longer duration of action than filgrastim, and is only given once after chemotherapy. Filgrastim and lenograstim are eliminated both by the kidney and by neutrophil uptake. Pegfilgrastim is not eliminated by the kidney, and has a prolonged effect in neutropenia, since few neutrophils are available to contribute to its elimination.

Unwanted effects

- Musculoskeletal or bone pain.
- Headache.
- Fever.
- Fatigue.
- Anorexia, nausea, vomiting, diarrhoea.
- Myeloproliferative disorders with long-term treatment.
- Osteoporosis with long-term treatment.

THERAPEUTIC USE OF COLONY-STIMULATING FACTORS

The use of these drugs remains controversial in many indications.

Congenital neutropenia

Survival is prolonged by G-CSF which reduces life-threatening infection, but 10% of people develop acute myeloid leukaemia as a result of treatment.

Chemotherapy-induced neutropenia

The duration of neutropenia may be reduced, with a limitation of associated sepsis. However, with many chemotherapy regimens there is no evidence that long-term survival is improved by G-CSF, and with some regimens the risk of acute myeloid leukaemia may be increased. G-CSF treatment is therefore reserved for those regimens that have greater than 20% historical risk of febrile neutropenia. It is also used when chemotherapy has previously been associated with a febrile neutropenic episode and the drug dosage cannot be reduced for subsequent courses.

Mobilisation of progenitor cells into peripheral blood for harvesting prior to bone marrow transplantation

The white blood cell count rises 7–12 days after treatment and is accompanied by an increase in haematopoietic stem cells, which are collected via a cell-separation machine. G-CSF use can be followed by the chemokine receptor antagonist plerixafor, which mobilises haematopoietic stem cells into peripheral blood.

SELF-ASSESSMENT

True/false questions

1. Dietary iron is transported in the blood mostly bound to ferritin.
2. Pernicious anaemia is caused by reduced vitamin B_{12} absorption.
3. In vitamin B_{12} deficiency treatment is rarely required for more than 3 months.
4. The blood film in pernicious anaemia shows microcytosis.
5. Both vitamin B_{12} and folate are essential for DNA synthesis.
6. Folic acid cannot be given orally.
7. Phenytoin can cause folate deficiency.
8. Erythropoietin reduces apoptosis of red blood cell progenitors.
9. Filgrastim is a recombinant form of erythropoietin.
10. Plerixafor is a chemokine antagonist.

One-best-answer (OBA) questions

1. Identify the *correct* statement below concerning the properties of erythropoietin.
   A. Erythropoietin is mainly synthesised by the adrenal glands.
   B. Erythropoietin can correct anaemia in end-stage renal disease.
   C. Erythropoietin is an effective anaemia treatment even if iron levels are low.
   D. Erythropoietin impairs athletic performance by increasing hamatocrit.
   E. Erythropoietin can be given orally.
2. Identify the *incorrect* statement below concerning the usage and properties of folic acid and its metabolites.
   A. Tetrahydrofolate is involved in the synthesis of the nucleotide bases in DNA.
   B. Folic acid is often given with hydroxocobalamin.
   C. Folate is absorbed in the stomach.

D. Tetrahydrofolic acid is given rather than folic acid to correct the folate deficiency caused by methotrexate.
E. Folic acid in pregnancy reduces the risk of neural tube defects.

Case-based questions

A 40-year-old woman complained to her GP of fatigue and heavy menstrual periods lasting 7 days and occurring every 28 days. Her GP noted that she was pallid; her haemoglobin level was 67 $g \cdot L^{-1}$ and mean cell volume (MCV) was 61 fL (normal 76–96). Other blood measurements of platelets and white cell counts were unremarkable.

A. How would you interpret these data and what were the possible reasons?
B. What biochemical tests could have helped the diagnosis?
C. The tests confirmed iron-deficiency anaemia.
  What pharmaceutical preparation should have been given?
D. Several iron formulations were tried, as the woman felt unwell taking ferrous sulphate.
  What unwanted effects might she have experienced?
E. Where was the iron absorbed?
F. After 2 months of oral iron therapy, the haemoglobin value was 80 $g \cdot L^{-1}$.
  Was this a sufficient response?
G. The woman was intolerant of oral iron.
  What could have been the reasons for the poor response?
H. What alternative treatment could have been administered?

With the new treatment regimen her haemoglobin rose to 115 $g \cdot L^{-1}$ over 2–3 weeks.

True/false answers

1. **False.** Iron is transported in the blood bound to transferrin and stored in tissues as ferritin and haemosiderin.
2. **True.** Autoimmune loss of gastric parietal cells reduces production of intrinsic factor, which is needed for vitamin B_{12} absorption in the distal ileum.
3. **False.** In pernicious anaemia vitamin B_{12} is given (as hydroxocobalamin) by intramuscular injection every 2–3 months for life.
4. **False.** Macrocytes (enlarged red cells) are found in the blood in pernicious anaemia.
5. **True.** Folate is necessary for synthesis of purines and pyrimidines, and vitamin B_{12} is a cofactor in their synthesis.
6. **False.** Folic acid is given orally each day for up to 4 months to replenish stores.
7. **True.** Phenytoin and a number of other drugs interfere with folate metabolism.
8. **True.** Erythropoietin increases survival of erythroid progenitor cells in the bone marrow.
9. **False.** Filgrastim is a recombinant form of granulocyte colony-stimulating factor (G-CSF), which promotes

formation of neutrophils and other granulocytes in the bone marrow.
10. **True.** Plerixafor is an antagonist of the CXCR4 chemokine receptor and is used with a recombinant G-CSF to mobilise stem cells for harvesting.

OBA answers

1. **Answer B** is correct.
  A. Incorrect. The kidneys are the main site of erythropoietin production.
  B. **Correct**. Anaemia due to renal disease is commonly treated with erythropoietin.
  C. Incorrect. Adequate iron stores are necessary for erythropoietin to be successful.
  D. Incorrect. Erythropoietin may enhance performance by increasing haematocrit, but with an increased risk of thrombosis.
  E. Incorrect. It is a glycoprotein given by intravenous or subcutaneous routes.
2. **Answer C** is the incorrect statement.
  A. Correct. Tetrahydrofolate is a folic acid metabolite utilised in the synthesis of the purine and pyrimidine bases in DNA.
  B. Correct. Neurological damage can be caused if folic acid is given alone when both folate and vitamin B_{12} are deficient.
  C. **Incorrect.** Folate is absorbed in the proximal jejunum, and absorption is deficient in coeliac disease.
  D. Correct. Methotrexate inhibits the synthesis of tetrahydrofolate by dihydrofolate reductase. Synthetic tetrahydrofolate (folinic acid) bypasses this block.
  E. Correct. Folic acid is given prophylactically in pregnancy, and in higher amounts if there is a history of a neural tube defect in a previous pregnancy.

Case-based answers

A. The haemoglobin concentration (67 $g \cdot L^{-1}$) is below normal for a non-pregnant woman (115 $g \cdot L^{-1}$), indicating anaemia. The MCV (61 fL) is also low. A common cause of low MCV is iron-deficiency anaemia, which is common in menstruating women. Another cause is gastrointestinal bleeding, including haemorrhoids.
B. Serum ferritin would be low and total iron-binding capacity elevated.
C. Oral ferrous salts (e.g. ferrous sulphate, the form most easily absorbed).
D. Gastrointestinal distension and loose bowel movements are common.
E. Iron is absorbed from the duodenum and upper jejunum.
F. The rise in haemoglobin was insufficient: it should be about 10 $g \cdot L^{-1}$ each week.
G. Poor response could be due to poor adherence to treatment, continued bleeding or malabsorption.
H. Alternative treatment could have been slow intravenous injection or infusion of iron sucrose or iron dextran.

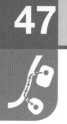

FURTHER READING

Cappellini MD, Fiorelli G (2008) Glucose-6-phosphate dehydrogenase deficiency. *N Engl J Med* 371, 64–74

Crawford J, Dale DC, Lyman GH (2004) Chemotherapy-induced neutropenia: risks, consequences and new directions for its management. *Cancer* 100, 228–237

Frewin R, Henson A, Provan D (1997) Iron deficiency anaemia. *BMJ* 314, 360–363

Henry DH, Bowers P, Romano MT et al. (2004) Epoetin alpha. Clinical evolution of a pleiotropic cytokine. *Arch Intern Med* 164, 262–276

Hoffbrand V, Provan D (1997) Macrocytic anaemias. *BMJ* 314, 430–433

Hubell K, Engert A (2003) Clinical applications of granulocyte colony-stimulating factor: an update and summary. *Ann Haematol* 82, 207–213

Kaushansky K (2006) Lineage-specific hematopoietic growth factors. *N Engl J Med* 354, 2034–2046

Lyman GH, Shayne M (2007) Granulocyte colony-stimulating factors: finding the right indication. *Curr Opin Oncol* 19, 299–307

Macdougall IC, Eckardt K-U (2006) Novel strategies for stimulating erythropoiesis and potential new treatments for anaemia. *Lancet* 368, 947–953

Provan D, Weatherall D (2000) Red cells II: acquired anaemias and polycythaemias. *Lancet* 355, 1260–1268

Umbreit J (2005) Iron deficiency: a concise review. *Am J Haematol* 78, 225–231

Weatherall D, Provan D (2000) Red cells I: inherited anaemias. *Lancet* 355, 1169–1175

Compendium: drugs used to treat anaemias and neutropenia

Drug	Kinetics (half-life)	Comments
Drugs used in iron-deficiency anaemia		
Iron		
Oral formulations		
Ferrous sulphate Ferrous fumarate Ferrous gluconate Polysaccharide–iron complex Sodium feredetate	—	Often given as co-formulations with folic acid; extent of absorption depends on form, the presence of food, and iron status; water-soluble forms are the sulphate and gluconate, the fumarate is only sparingly soluble
Parenteral formulations		
Iron carboxymaltose	Uptake by bone marrow, liver and spleen	Ferric hydroxide core stabilized by a carbohydrate shell; given by slow intravenous injection or infusion
Iron dextran	Extensive uptake by macrophage-rich spleen	A complex of ferric hydroxide with dextran containing 5% iron; given by slow intravenous injection or infusion
Iron isomaltoside 1000	Uptake by reticuloendothelial cells (21-24 h)	Ferric hydroxide complexed with carbohydrate; given by slow intravenous injection or infusion
Iron sucrose	Extensive uptake by macrophage-rich spleen	A complex of ferric hydroxide with sucrose containing 2% iron; given by slow intravenous injection or infusion
Drugs used in megaloblastic anaemias		
Hydroxocobalamin has replaced cyanocobalamin as the drug of choice in the UK.		
Cyanocobalamin	Dose-dependent absorption and renal elimination (6 days); metabolism to cobalamin, incorporated into vitamin B_{12}	Given orally or by intramuscular injection
Folic acid	Absorption 70–80%; metabolised to tetrahydrofolate; dose-dependent renal excretion	Folate deficiency responds to a short course of treatment; given orally, often with hydroxocobalamin
Hydroxocobalamin	Dose-dependent renal elimination and metabolism (2–6 h)	Given by intramuscular injection
Drugs used in hypoplastic, haemolytic and renal anaemias		
Darbepoetin alfa	Eliminated largely by undefined metabolism (20 h); half-life longer after subcutaneous dosage (30–90 h)	Long-acting recombinant form of renal erythropoietin; used for anaemia associated with chronic renal disease and anaemia in adults receiving chemotherapy for non-myeloid malignancies; given by intravenous or subcutaneous injection
Epoetin alfa, beta, theta and zeta	Probably catabolised by target cells after internalisation (4–6 h)	Used for anaemia associated with chronic renal disease, to increase autologous blood in healthy people and for anaemia in adults receiving chemotherapy for malignancies; given by intravenous or subcutaneous injection
Methoxy polyethylene glycol-epoetin beta	Slow subcutaneous absorption; bioavailability 50–60%; probably catabolised by target cells after internalisation (140 h)	Long-acting, pegylated version of epoetin beta; used for anaemia associated with chronic renal disease; given by intravenous or subcutaneous injection
Oxymetholone	Oral bioavailability 95%; hepatic metabolism, renal excretion (9 h)	Used for 3–6 months for treatment of aplastic anaemia; given orally
Treatment of iron overload		
Deferasirox	Eliminated by glucuronidation and biliary excretion (8–16 h)	Used for iron overload in thalassaemia major, for people requiring frequent blood transfusions and those intolerant to desferrioxamine; given orally
Deferiprone	Mainly renal excretion (1.5 h)	Used for iron overload in thalassaemia major and for people intolerant to desferrioxamine; given orally

Compendium: drugs used to treat anaemias and neutropenia—cont'd

Drug	Kinetics (half-life)	Comments
Desferrioxamine mesilate (deferoxamine mesilate)	Eliminated unchanged in urine (15–65%) and by metabolism (6 h)	Chelating agent used for iron overload in thalassaemia major (or aluminium overload in people undergoing dialysis), and for haemochromatosis in people in whom repeated venesection is contraindicated; given by subcutaneous infusion

Drugs used in neutropenia

All drugs are recombinant colony-stimulating factors given parenterally; for specialist use only.

Filgrastim	Mainly renal elimination (3.5 h)	Unglycosylated recombinant human G-CSF; used for neutropenia, following cytotoxic chemotherapy of malignancy, and for severe congenital neutropenia; given by subcutaneous injection or infusion or by intravenous infusion
Lenograstim	Pathways of metabolism not defined (1–3 h)	Glycosylated recombinant human G-CSF; used for reduction in the duration of neutropenia, for example following cytotoxic chemotherapy of malignancy; given by subcutaneous injection or intravenous infusion
Pegfilgrastim	Clearance by neutrophil uptake (15–80 h)	Long-acting pegylated derivative of filgrastim; used for neutropenia, for example following cytotoxic chemotherapy of malignancy; given by subcutaneous injection
Plerixafor	Renal excretion (3–5 h)	Chemokine receptor (CXCR4) antagonist; used with G-CSF to improve mobilisation and yield of stem cells for transplantation; given by subcutaneous injection

G-CSF, granulocyte colony-stimulating factor.

48

Lipid disorders

LIPIDS AND LIPOPROTEINS

Lipid and lipoprotein metabolism is complex and the following account is a very brief summary, sufficient to establish the mechanism of action of drugs used to correct lipid abnormalities.

CHOLESTEROL AND TRIGLYCERIDES

Cholesterol is a sterol that is a vital structural component of cell membranes and a precursor of many steroids, including bile salts and steroid hormones. About 20–25% of daily production of cholesterol is by the liver; the rest is synthesised in the intestines, adrenal glands and reproductive organs or ingested in the diet from eggs, cheese, meat or fish. The synthesis of cholesterol involves several enzymes, but the rate-limiting step is catalysed by β-hydroxy-β-methylglutaryl-coenzyme A (HMG-CoA) reductase. Intracellular cholesterol is sensed by the cell and produces negative feedback on HMG-CoA reductase to reduce further cholesterol synthesis.

Cholesterol leaves hepatocytes either by transport into the circulation (see below) or by secretion into the bile after incorporation into bile salt micelles (Figs 48.1 and 48.2). Virtually all of the cholesterol secreted in bile is reabsorbed and taken up by the liver, which also retains about 50% of cholesterol that is not incorporated into bile salts.

Triglycerides (fatty acids esterified with glycerol) are the major dietary fat, and can also be synthesised from intermediary metabolites formed in the liver from excess carbohydrate in the diet. Triglycerides are stored in adipose tissue, from where they can be mobilised as non-esterified free fatty acids to act as an energy substrate during periods of fasting.

THE BASIS OF LIPOPROTEIN METABOLISM

Lipids (triglycerides and esters of cholesterol) have low water solubility. They circulate in plasma encased in a coat of apolipoproteins within a phospholipid monolayer, creating lipoproteins that are water soluble and which make the triglycerides and cholesterol esters transportable. The lipoproteins can be differentiated according to the triglyceride/cholesterol ratio they carry, their apolipoprotein constituent and their density (Table 48.1). They are usually classified according to their density into very-low-density (VLDL), low-density (LDL), intermediate-density (IDL) and high-density (HDL) lipoproteins. There are specific cell-surface receptors for processing different apolipoproteins and these determine where and how particular fractions of circulating cholesterol and triglyceride will be handled (Table 48.1). In healthy individuals, about 70% of plasma cholesterol is carried by LDL and 20% by HDL. The least-dense and largest-diameter particles, known as chylomicrons, are exclusively concerned with the transport of dietary lipid from the intestine to the liver. Their low density and large size reflect their high content of triglycerides (Table 48.1), and they are almost completely removed from blood after a 12 h fast. VLDL carries about 60% of plasma triglyceride in the fasting state. The ratio of cholesterol to triglyceride carried is greatest in the HDL fraction.

PROCESSING OF LIPIDS ABSORBED FROM THE GUT

Cholesterol and free fatty acids are solubilised by bile acids in the gut lumen to facilitate absorption into enterocytes (see Fig. 48.1). Soluble cholesterol is transported into the enterocyte from the intestinal lumen by a specific lipid transmembrane transporter called Nieman-Pick C1-like 1 protein (NPC1L1). Triglyceride absorption does not require a specific transporter. Cholesterol and triglycerides are then incorporated into chylomicrons within the enterocytes (see Table 48.1). Chylomicrons pass into the lymphatic system and then into the circulation. Hydrolysis of triglycerides to free fatty acids in the chylomicrons is carried out by a lipoprotein lipase attached to the endothelium of capillaries in muscle and adipose tissue, and requires the chylomicron-associated apolipoprotein C (subtype C2) as a cofactor (Table 48.1). Free fatty acids are utilised by muscle and liver as an energy source or stored as triglycerides in adipose tissue. After removal of triglycerides from the chylomicrons, the remaining surface lipoprotein and lipid fractions leave the particles to enter the HDL pool as 'nascent HDL' (Fig. 48.1). The chylomicron remnants are taken into hepatocytes

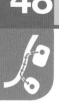

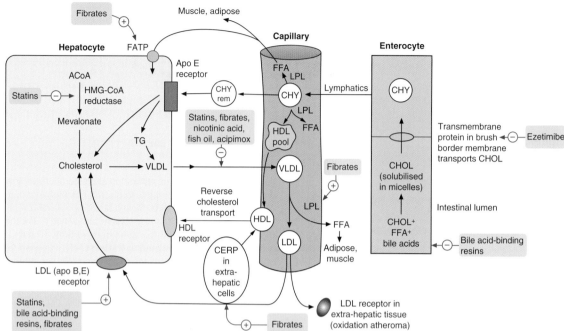

Fig. 48.1 Major pathways in lipoprotein formation and metabolism. Dietary lipids including cholesterol (CHOL) and free fatty acids (FFA) in the gut are emulsified by bile acids and transported within chylomicrons (CHY) to the liver. They are then circulated as cholesterol and triglycerides (TG) to tissues in very-low-density lipoproteins (VLDL), where endothelial lipoprotein lipase (LPL) liberates FFA in adipose and muscle for storage or metabolism. The resulting low-density lipoproteins (LDL) are returned to hepatocytes via LDL receptors, or taken up by LDL receptors in extrahepatic tissues where they are oxidised and contribute to atherogenesis. The high-density lipoprotein (HDL) pool (nascent HDL) is derived from the chylomicrons following the action of LPL, and the reverse cholesterol pathway returns HDL to the liver via HDL receptors. Lipid-lowering drugs and their principal targets are shown with red arrows. ACoA, acetyl coenzyme A; Apo, apolipoprotein; CERP, cholesterol efflux regulatory protein; CHY rem, chylomicron remnant; FATP, fatty acid transport protein; HMG-CoA reductase, β-hydroxyl-β-methylglutaryl-coenzyme A reductase.

by specific chylomicron remnant (apolipoprotein E, or apo E) receptors.

PLASMA TRANSPORT AND LIVER PROCESSING OF LIPIDS

Cholesterol is transported to tissues in chylomicrons, VLDL and LDL; it is transported from tissues to the liver by HDL. A high plasma concentration of LDL is associated with atheromatous disease.

Liver cholesterol (as esters) and any triglycerides in the liver that are surplus to synthetic and oxidative requirements are released into the circulation complexed to VLDL. Peripheral lipoprotein lipase acts on VLDL to release free fatty acids, leaving IDL (not shown in Fig. 48.1); triglycerides in IDL are also hydrolysed by hepatic lipase to release free fatty acids, which generates LDL. LDL therefore contains a higher concentration of cholesterol and a lower concentration of triglyceride compared with VLDL (Table 48.1). LDL is removed from the circulation by uptake into liver cells (75%) and peripheral tissues (25%). Some 70% of this uptake is by

specific receptors for the apolipoproteins type B and E (Fig. 48.1), while the rest is by non-receptor-mediated pathways. The circulating concentration of LDL rises if there is either excess production of LDL or deficient LDL receptor numbers. When plasma LDL rises, non-receptor-mediated uptake of cholesterol in peripheral tissues such as arterial walls will increase. Within arterial walls, LDL cholesterol undergoes oxidation which leads to formation of lipid-rich deposits and atheromatous plaques (see below).

HDL carries cholesterol mobilised from peripheral tissues (and particularly oxidized cholesterol derivatives), and transports it to the liver (reverse cholesterol transport). The efflux of cholesterol from peripheral cells is facilitated by cholesterol efflux regulatory protein (CERP). This cholesterol is bound to nascent HDL, and then the cholesterol is esterified by the circulating enzyme lecithin-cholesterol acyltransferase (LCAT) to create mature HDL. HDL is believed to protect against atheroma by this reverse cholesterol transport from peripheral tissues to the liver. The enzyme cholesterol ester transfer protein (CETP) can transfer cholesterol from HDL to VLDL in exchange for triglycerides. The extent of this exchange depends on the concentration of circulating triglycerides.

HYPERCHOLESTEROLAEMIA AND ATHEROMA

Abnormalities of plasma lipoprotein metabolism produce excessive concentrations of circulating cholesterol and/or triglyceride. Their clinical importance lies in their relationship to the production of atheroma (mainly raised plasma LDL cholesterol with a contribution from triglycerides) and pancreatitis (plasma triglycerides >12 mmol·L^{-1}). Atheroma is focal thickening of the intima of arteries, produced by a combination of cells, elements of connective tissue, lipids and debris.

Excess LDL accumulates in the arterial wall, where its cholesterol undergoes enzymatic and free radical oxidation to produce a cytotoxic and chemotactic lipid that can activate the endothelium. Activated endothelium (a state which is also initiated by other atherogenic factors such as

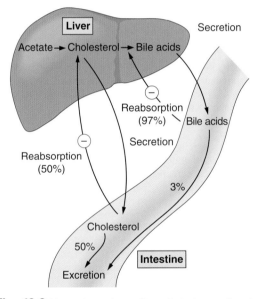

Fig. 48.2 Enterohepatic cycling of cholesterol and bile acids. Bile acids are secreted via the bile duct into the duodenum, where they aid in dietary lipid absorption, and are then returned to the liver by the portal circulation. A circled minus sign indicates a negative-feedback effect. Percentages are in relation to the amount excreted in bile.

smoking, diabetes or hypertension) expresses adhesion molecules that attract platelets, monocytes and some T-lymphocytes. These cells migrate into the sub-endothelial space, where the monocytes differentiate into macrophages under the influence of endothelial cytokines. The macrophages take up oxidised LDL cholesterol via scavenger receptors, and the cholesterol accumulates as droplets in the cytosol, creating lipid-rich foam cells. Foam cells initiate fatty streaks that are the precursor of atheroma. T-cells in the developing atheromatous lesion recognise lipid antigens and release various cytokines that attract further inflammatory cells and initiate a T-helper cell type 1 inflammatory response (Ch. 38). These processes also result in formation of a cap of smooth muscle cells and collagen-rich matrix over the lesion. The extent of the inflammatory response determines whether the cap becomes fibrous and stable, or is destabilised by infiltration of inflammatory cells that make the cap prone to rupture or surface erosion. Plaque destabilisation underlies the development of acute coronary syndromes and many cases of ischaemic stroke (see Chs 5 and 9).

Atherogenic patterns of lipoproteins can result from the following:

- high dietary intake of saturated fat,
- primary (inherited) disorders of enzymes or receptors involved in lipid metabolism. Most inherited hyperlipidaemias are polygenic, but an important inherited defect is familial hypercholesterolaemia, a single recessive gene disorder that affects 1 in 500 of the population, who have reduced synthesis of LDL receptors,
- secondary lipid disorders, when hyperlipidaemia results from diseases that affect lipid metabolism; for example liver disease, nephrotic syndrome, hypothyroidism.

A classification for the various phenotypic patterns of primary hyperlipidaemia adopted by the World Health Organization is shown in Table 48.2.

DRUGS FOR HYPERLIPIDAEMIAS

HMG-CoA reductase inhibitors ('statins')

Examples

atorvastatin, pravastatin, rosuvastatin, simvastatin

Table 48.1 Apolipoprotein and lipid composition of major lipoproteins and their sources

Lipoprotein	Major associated apolipoproteins[a]	Cholesterol (%)	Triglycerides (%)	Source
Chylomicrons	Apo A/apo B/apo B$_{48}$/apo C/apo E	3	90	Intestine
VLDL	Apo C/apo B$_{100}$/apo E	20	50	Liver
LDL	Apo B$_{100}$	50	7	VLDL
HDL	Apo A	40	6	Chylomicrons, VLDL, liver, intestine

[a]The apolipoproteins supply structural integrity and also have roles in controlling lipoprotein metabolism and as receptor ligands.
HDL, high-density lipoproteins; LDL, low-density lipoproteins; VLDL, very-low-density lipoproteins.

Table 48.2 The Fredrickson classification of dyslipidaemias

Type	Triglyceride	Total cholesterol	LDL cholesterol	Raised lipoprotein	Atheroma risk
I	+++	+	N	Chylomicrons	N
IIa	N	++	++	LDL	+++
IIb	++	++	++	LDL/VLDL	+++
III	++	+	N	VLDL and chylomicron remnants	++
IV	++	N/+	N	VLDL	++
V	+++	+	N	VLDL/chylomicrons	N

N, normal; +, slightly raised; ++, moderately raised; +++, extremely raised.

Box 48.1 **Non-lipid effects of statins[a]**

- Improved function of vascular endothelium damaged by hypercholesterolaemia, either by a direct effect or as a consequence of reduction in plasma LDL cholesterol
- Stabilisation of atherosclerotic plaques by altered smooth muscle proliferation and migration
- Changes in haemostasis: decreased plasma fibrinogen and enhanced fibrinolysis
- Reduction of inflammatory cell infiltration into atherosclerotic plaques
- Reduced plasma C-reactive protein (CRP), reflecting anti-inflammatory action

[a]Statins vary in these non-lipid effects.

Mechanism of action and effects

HMG-CoA reductase inhibitors competitively inhibit the enzyme that catalyses the rate-limiting step in the synthesis of cholesterol (Fig. 48.1). Their most important action is in the liver, where the fall in hepatic cholesterol levels produces a compensatory upregulation in the number of LDL receptors on hepatocytes, with increased clearance of circulating LDL cholesterol. In the liver, the cholesterol is reprocessed to form bile salts. The extent of the reduction in plasma LDL cholesterol depends on the specific drug and the dose of the drug ranges from 25 to 50%. Short-acting statins, such as simvastatin, are most effective when taken at night, which is the time when most cholesterol synthesis occurs. Statins also reduce the circulating concentration of VLDL by stimulating lipoprotein lipase, and therefore reduce circulating triglycerides. A modest increase in HDL cholesterol is usually seen, due to increased synthesis of the constituent apolipoprotein A1. This is due to activation of peroxisome proliferator-activated receptor α (PPAR-α) (see also fibrates, below).

Statins have several other actions, which may be distinct from their ability to reduce plasma lipids (Box 48.1). There is increasing evidence that some of these may contribute significantly to the beneficial actions of statins in reducing clinical events in people with atherothrombotic disease.

Pharmacokinetics

The statins are well absorbed from the gut. Simvastatin is a prodrug (Ch. 2) that is activated in first-pass metabolism in the liver by cytochrome P450 (CYP3A4). Further metabolism inactivates the drug and only 5% of the active compound reaches the circulation. Atorvastatin undergoes first-pass metabolism, in part to active derivatives, and has a very long half-life. Pravastatin is a hydrophilic drug that is eliminated mainly by the kidneys; its half-life is 1–2 h. Rosuvastatin has a low oral bioavailability and is eliminated mainly in the bile, with a half-life of 20 h.

Unwanted effects

- Gastrointestinal upset, including nausea, vomiting, abdominal pain, flatulence and diarrhoea.
- Central nervous system effects, such as dizziness, blurred vision and headache.
- Transient disturbance of liver function tests and, rarely, hepatitis.
- Myalgia (muscle pain) or myositis (muscle inflammation) and rarely rhabdomyolysis. In some people there is a raised serum creatine kinase concentration suggesting muscle damage, but no muscle symptoms. The mechanism of the myopathy remains uncertain but it is likely that some people have minor metabolic abnormalities in their striated muscle that makes the muscle more susceptible to reduction of its fat substrate. There is an increased risk when a statin is used in combination with a fibrate, nicotinic acid, fusidic acid, ciclosporin and several other drugs (Ch. 38).

Specific cholesterol absorption inhibitors

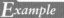

Example

ezetimibe

Mechanism of action

Ezetimibe acts at the brush border of the small intestinal mucosa to specifically inhibit the NPC1L1 transporter and reduces cholesterol absorption by about 50%. It has no effect on the absorption of triglycerides, bile acids or fat-soluble vitamins. Given alone, ezetimibe reduces plasma total cholesterol by about 15% and LDL cholesterol by about 20%. When taken with a low dose of statin the combination is as effective as three doublings of the statin dose in reducing plasma total cholesterol.

Pharmacokinetics

Ezetimibe is rapidly but incompletely absorbed from the gut, and metabolised in the gut wall and the liver. It undergoes enterohepatic circulation, which gives it a long half-life (about 22 h), and about 80% is excreted in the faeces.

Unwanted effects

- Diarrhoea, abdominal pain.
- Headache.
- Angioedema.

Bile acid-binding (anion-exchange) resins

colesevelam, colestipol, colestyramine

Mechanism of action

Bile acids are synthesised from cholesterol in the liver, and are secreted into the duodenum to aid absorption of dietary fat. They are then reabsorbed in the terminal ileum and returned to the liver in the portal circulation (Fig. 48.2). Bile acid-binding resins are insoluble, non-absorbable polymers that bind bile salts in the gut and prevent enterohepatic circulation of bile acids.

When reabsorption of bile acids is impaired by binding to the resin, bile acid synthesis is increased from cholesterol in the liver. This reduces intrahepatic cholesterol, and there is compensatory upregulation of hepatic LDL receptors in order to replenish liver cholesterol. LDL cholesterol is cleared more rapidly from plasma, with a fall in circulating levels of 15–20%. Stimulation of VLDL synthesis produces a small rise in plasma triglycerides. There is a small rise in HDL cholesterol, but the mechanism for this is unclear.

Unwanted effects

- Unpalatability. Sachets containing several grams of powder have to be taken, usually mixed with food. The taste and texture limit acceptability and for this reason resins are no longer widely used.
- Constipation or, occasionally, diarrhoea.
- Interference with the absorption of certain acidic drugs, for example digoxin (Ch. 7), warfarin (Ch. 11) and levothyroxine (Ch. 41). These drugs should be given at least 1 h before or 4 h after taking a resin.

Fibrates

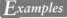

bezafibrate, ciprofibrate, fenofibrate, gemfibrozil

Mechanism of action

The main mechanism of fibrate drugs is activation of gene transcription factors known as PPARs, particularly PPAR-α, which regulate the expression of genes that control lipoprotein metabolism. Fibrates are related to thiazolidinediones and their PPAR-mediated actions are described in Chapter 40. PPAR-α is expressed in several tissues, including the liver, heart and kidney. There are several consequences of PPAR-α activation:

- increased free fatty acid uptake by the liver due to induction of the fatty acid transporter protein in the cell membrane. In the liver, fatty acid conversion to acyl-coenzyme A is enhanced as a result of increased acyl-CoA synthetase activity. The esterified fatty acids are less available for hepatic triglyceride synthesis,
- increased lipoprotein lipase activity, which enhances the clearance of triglycerides from lipoproteins in the plasma (Fig. 48.1),
- formation of LDL with increased affinity for its receptors, thus removing it more readily from the circulation,
- increased plasma HDL because of enhanced apolipoprotein A1 and A2 production in the liver.

Pharmacokinetics

Fibrates are well absorbed from the gut and highly protein bound in the plasma. Fenofibrate is an ester prodrug that undergoes complete first-pass metabolism to the active form. Excretion is primarily by the kidney, although some metabolism occurs in the liver. The half-lives of bezafibrate and gemfibrozil are short, and other fibrates have longer half-lives.

Unwanted effects

- Gastrointestinal upset.
- Rash or pruritus.
- Dizziness, headache.
- Increased lithogenicity of bile theoretically increases the risk of gallstones, but this has not been a problem with the clinical uses of these drugs.
- Myalgia and myositis are uncommon, unless there is impaired renal function or the fibrate is used in combination with a statin (especially gemfibrozil with simvastatin).
- Drug interactions include inhibition of the effect of warfarin (Ch. 11).

Nicotinic acid and derivatives

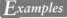

nicotinic acid (niacin), acipimox

Mechanism of action

Nicotinic acid is a B vitamin which has effects on lipids at pharmacological doses. It inhibits hepatic diacylglycerol acyltransferase-2, which is a key enzyme for triglyceride synthesis. As a result, hepatic apo B degradation is enhanced and the hepatic secretion of VLDL and LDL is reduced. The action of nicotinic acid at a specific niacin receptor on adipocytes, skin and immune cells appears to be less important in lipid regulation. However, activation of the receptor may contribute to an anti-atherogenic action and the flushing caused by the drug. Nicotinic acid reduces circulating triglycerides by up to 35% and LDL cholesterol modestly by up to 15%. HDL cholesterol is increased by up to 25% as a result of reduced hepatic uptake of the HDL molecule. A decrease in the activity of hepatic lipase also shifts the distribution of HDL subfractions, with a predominant elevation of HDL_2, which has greater protective effect than HDL_3.

Pharmacokinetics

Nicotinic acid is well absorbed from the gut. Hepatic metabolism occurs via two pathways. Oxidation is a high-affinity, low-capacity pathway that generates metabolites which are thought to be responsible for the hepatotoxicity that can occur with high doses of nicotinic acid. The other pathway is a low-affinity, high-capacity conjugation pathway. Large doses of nicotinic acid are excreted unchanged in the urine. Acipimox is a synthetic derivative of nicotinic acid that is longer-acting but less effective for lowering LDL cholesterol.

Unwanted effects

Nicotinic acid is often poorly tolerated, but unwanted effects can be reduced by gradual dosage increases. A modified-release formulation that minimises the risk of flushing, and acipimox, are better tolerated.

- Cutaneous vasodilation is particularly troublesome and causes flushing and itching. The action of nicotinic acid on specific G-protein-coupled receptors in the skin increases the production of prostaglandin (PG) D_2 and PGE_2, which cause the flushing. The flushing can be reduced by taking a small dose of aspirin 30 min before nicotinic acid, by taking the drug with food, or by using a modified-release formulation.
- Gastrointestinal upset and peptic ulceration.
- Headache, dizziness.
- Glucose intolerance with high doses of nicotinic acid (not with acipimox).
- Exacerbation of gout.
- Hepatotoxicity, which is less common with a modified-release formulation of niacin.

Omega-3 fatty acids

Omega-3 fatty acids are long-chain polyunsaturated acids such as α-linolenic acid, which is found in plants, and eicosapentaenoic acid (EPA) and docosahexaenoic acid (DHA), which are found in high quantities in oily fish such as mackerel and sardines. They have several potential cardioprotective effects:

- because they are poor substrates for the enzymes that synthesise triglycerides, they lead to the production of triglyceride-poor LDL and reduce triglycerides in plasma, although total cholesterol is increased. They also increase conversion of VLDL to LDL, and increase circulating HDL cholesterol,
- reduction of plasma fibrinogen, decreasing thrombogenesis,
- they substitute for arachidonic acid in platelet phospholipids, which results in increased production of the prostanoid thromboxane A_3 in platelets. This has a lower

ability to induce platelet aggregation compared with the thromboxane A_2 usually formed (Ch. 11),
- retardation of growth of atherosclerotic plaques by reduced expression of endothelial adhesion molecules and an anti-inflammatory action,
- promotion of nitric oxide-mediated vasodilation,
- membrane stabilisation in heart muscle, with reduced susceptibility to ventricular arrhythmias and sudden cardiac death.

Unwanted effects

- Gastrointestinal upset with nausea, belching, diarrhoea or constipation.
- Prolonged bleeding time.

MANAGEMENT OF HYPERLIPIDAEMIAS

Cardiovascular disease is the major risk associated with raised plasma LDL cholesterol. The relationship with raised LDL cholesterol is strongest for coronary atherosclerosis and peripheral vascular atherosclerosis, and to a lesser extent for cerebrovascular disease and atherothrombotic stroke. HDL cholesterol is protective against atherosclerosis and a low HDL cholesterol (<1.0 mmol·L^{-1}) is associated with the highest risk of disease. The ratio of total cholesterol to HDL cholesterol provides a much more sensitive indicator of the relative risk of developing cardiovascular disease than total cholesterol alone.

While a high ratio of total cholesterol to HDL cholesterol predicts the relative risk of cardiovascular disease, the absolute risk (i.e. the overall number of individuals in the population who will develop disease in a particular time period) will be determined by the coexistence of other risk factors (see below).

Raised plasma triglycerides are an independent predictor of the risk of atherosclerosis, but less so than raised plasma cholesterol. Nevertheless, when raised triglycerides coexist with an atherogenic cholesterol profile, the overall risk is enhanced. A markedly raised plasma triglyceride concentration (>12 mmol·L^{-1}) confers an increased risk of acute pancreatitis. Isolated hypertriglyceridaemia should be treated intensively for this reason alone.

Secondary cause of hyperlipidaemia, such as diabetes, hypothyroidism and nephrotic syndrome, should be excluded or treated before embarking on other aspects of management.

Primary prevention of cardiovascular disease

Atherothrombotic disease has a multifactorial aetiology, and any strategy for primary prevention must consider all relevant treatable factors. Drug treatment of hyperlipidaemia with drugs for primary prevention should only be considered if there is a sufficiently high absolute risk of disease, and should not be based on the cholesterol level alone. Important factors to consider in risk management include the following.

- Smoking: smoking doubles the risk of coronary artery disease. Stopping smoking reduces the risk close to that of a non-smoker in 3–5 years (see Ch. 5).

- Physical activity: a physically active lifestyle reduces the risk of myocardial infarction by up to 50% compared with a sedentary lifestyle.
- Maintaining ideal body weight: obesity (see Ch. 37) increases the risk of myocardial infarction by up to 50%.
- Mild-to-moderate alcohol consumption: a modest alcohol intake (see Ch. 54) can reduce the risk of myocardial infarction by about one-third. A high alcohol intake increases blood pressure, and thus increases cardiovascular risk.
- Treating hypertension (see Ch. 6): although this is more effective for the prevention of stroke, it also reduces the risk of myocardial infarction, especially in older people.
- Control of diabetes: there is conflicting evidence on whether close control of plasma glucose reduces vascular events. However, since the risk of ischaemic heart disease in diabetes is at least twice that of people without diabetes, intensive management of coexistent risk factors should be undertaken.
- Modifying the diet: dietary management should be advised for all people with hypercholesterolaemia, with a reduction in saturated fat intake (saturated fat decreases hepatic LDL receptors) and an increase in monounsaturated fats (which increases hepatic LDL cholesterol receptors). Eating a diet containing fresh fruit and vegetables reduces oxidation of LDL cholesterol and therefore makes it less atherogenic.
- Treating raised LDL cholesterol: this is a powerful predictor of future cardiovascular disease, especially in young people. The greatest risk is present when there is familial hypercholesterolaemia (FH), a dominantly inherited genetic defect that predisposes to premature coronary heart disease even in the absence of other risk factors. Heterozygous FH is associated with reduced LDL receptors on liver cells, and the total serum cholesterol is usually greater than 7.5 mmol·L^{-1} in adult life. Lipid-lowering therapy in FH, usually with a statin, should normally begin before the age of 10 years with the goal of reducing plasma LDL cholesterol by 50%.

For other forms of multigenic and acquired hypercholesterolaemia, the risk of cardiovascular disease should first be estimated using risk tables that assess the contribution of the total cholesterol/HDL ratio, systolic blood pressure, smoking, family history and other risk factors such as rheumatoid arthritis and socioeconomic deprivation. The question exercising the minds of health economists is not whether treatment is effective, but when it becomes cost-effective. As part of a multiple risk factor intervention strategy, drug therapy for raised LDL cholesterol has a role for those at higher absolute risk, usually because several other risk factors coexist or there is a history of premature coronary artery disease in a first-degree relative. In the UK, lipid-lowering drugs are recommended if the predicted 10-year cardiovascular disease risk (a combination of coronary heart disease and stroke risk) is greater than 20%. There is no target cholesterol recommendation for primary prevention, except for those with FH for whom a 50% reduction in LDL cholesterol is recommended. For other people, using a dose of statin that has been shown to reduce cardiovascular events is recommended, regardless of the achieved reduction in plasma LDL cholesterol.

The ability of cholesterol-lowering drugs (and particularly statins) to prevent ischaemic heart disease has been demonstrated in many trials. Reducing plasma total cholesterol by 25–30% (with a reduction in LDL cholesterol of 30–35%) with a statin reduces the subsequent risk of myocardial infarction or vascular death by about 30%.

Secondary prevention of cardiovascular disease

Once cardiovascular disease is clinically apparent the subsequent risk of death from vascular events is increased. People with clinical evidence of vascular disease are at much greater absolute risk of a further event than are those without clinical coronary artery disease but who have similar, or even higher, plasma cholesterol concentrations. A recent myocardial infarction or an episode of unstable angina confers the highest risk. At slightly lower absolute risk are those with stable angina pectoris, peripheral vascular disease or ischaemic stroke. Reduction of even 'normal' plasma cholesterol concentrations (to as low as 4.0 mmol·L^{-1}) in people with established vascular disease reduces the subsequent risk of both fatal and non-fatal cardiovascular events.

Current evidence supports the use of statins as first-line therapy. Trials with fibrates have shown less marked benefit unless the major lipid abnormality is low HDL cholesterol (see also Ch. 5). The target cholesterol concentration is total cholesterol below 4.0 mmol·L^{-1} (LDL cholesterol <2 mmol·L^{-1}). When this is not achieved with a statin alone, then combinations of drugs, such as a statin with ezetimibe or a fibrate, may be used, although there is little evidence of improved clinical outcomes. The use of omega-3 fatty acids after myocardial infarction has a cardioprotective effect, which may not entirely relate to their effects on plasma lipids.

Lowering plasma cholesterol for secondary prevention of coronary artery disease should be only one aspect of a comprehensive strategy for improving prognosis (see Ch. 5).

Mechanisms of prevention of coronary events by lipid-lowering drugs

There is a close relationship between the degree of LDL cholesterol reduction and the reduced risk of coronary events, especially when it is achieved with a statin. Overall there is a 2–3% reduction in risk for every 1% reduction in plasma total cholesterol concentration. Reducing plasma cholesterol probably stabilises existing atheromatous plaques by preventing lipid accumulation in their core and therefore reduces the risk of plaque rupture. Statins prevent the growth of existing coronary artery plaques and reduce the formation of new plaques. High doses of a statin may even produce some regression of existing plaque. An antiinflammatory effect of statins may be important, measured by a reduction in plasma high-sensitivity C-reactive protein. Other actions of statins, such as reduction in thrombogenicity of blood and inhibition of smooth muscle proliferation in atheromatous plaques, may contribute to the clinical benefit, but their roles remain speculative.

There is uncertainty whether lipid-lowering drugs other than statins have the same ability to reduce cardiovascular events. Although it is widely accepted that lowering LDL cholesterol should provide some protection against atheroma, however it is achieved, there is little evidence to confirm this.

Management of hypertriglyceridaemia

When triglycerides are markedly raised, control of diabetes, weight loss and reduction of alcohol intake should be considered when appropriate. When drug therapy is necessary, modest hypertriglyceridaemia in association with hypercholesterolaemia will usually respond to a statin. Extremely high plasma triglyceride concentrations usually respond well to a fibrate or to nicotinic acid. Combination therapy with a statin and a fibrate may be necessary in some high-risk individuals to achieve an acceptable lipid profile.

SELF-ASSESSMENT

True/false questions

1. The risk of coronary disease is strongly related to the plasma triglyceride concentration.
2. Genetic factors contribute to the development of hypercholesterolaemia.
3. Anion-exchange resins enhance the absorption of bile acids from the gut.
4. Statins inhibit β-hydroxy-β-methylglutaryl-coenzyme A (HMG-CoA) reductase activity.
5. Decreased hepatic cholesterol synthesis results in increased numbers of high-density lipoprotein (HDL) receptors.
6. Pravastatin lowers plasma low-density lipoprotein (LDL) cholesterol by about 10%.
7. Co-administration of statins and fibrates has no greater effect than giving each drug separately.
8. Ezetimibe blocks cholesterol absorption in the intestinal mucosa.
9. Gemfibrozil inhibits lipoprotein lipase by activating peroxisome proliferator-activated receptor α (PPAR-α).
10. Nicotinic acid reduces triglyceride synthesis in the liver.
11. Skin flushing is a common unwanted effect of nicotinic acid.
12. Arachidonic acid is an omega-3 fatty acid.

One-best-answer (OBA) questions

1. Identify the *most accurate* statement below concerning lipids and cardiovascular disease.
   A. A high total plasma cholesterol/HDL cholesterol ratio reduces cardiovascular risk.
   B. Very-low-density lipoprotein (VLDL) has a greater percentage of cholesterol than HDL.
   C. The outer coat of lipoproteins is a phospholipid bilayer.
   D. Reducing dietary saturated fat reduces coronary disease risk.

E. Even moderate alcohol consumption increases the risk of myocardial infarction.

2. Identify the *inaccurate* statement below concerning the actions of statins.
   A. Statins alter smooth muscle proliferation in atherosclerotic plaques.
   B. Statins may cause myalgia.
   C. Statins reduce plasma C-reactive protein (CRP).
   D. Statins suppress lipoprotein lipase activity.
   E. Statins decrease plasma HDL concentrations.

Case-based questions

A 58-year-old man recovered from an anterior myocardial infarction. His fasting plasma cholesterol was 7.8 mmol·L^{-1}. You want to reduce his risk of a further myocardial infarction by lowering his cholesterol.

A. What advice should be offered?
B. What drug should be recommended and why?
C. What reduction in plasma cholesterol should be aimed for and when should a response be expected?
D. What unwanted effects should be looked out for?

True/false answers

1. **False.** Cardiovascular risk is mostly associated with high low-density lipoprotein (LDL) cholesterol, which leads to lipid peroxidation and formation of foam cells in atheromatous plaque.
2. **True.** The best understood genetic risk is familial hypercholesterolaemia, in which a recessive gene disorder predisposes to premature coronary disease.
3. **False.** The anion-exchange resins sequester bile acids in the gut, decreasing the absorption of dietary cholesterol. They also increase incorporation of hepatic cholesterol into bile acids, leading to further loss of cholesterol in bile secretions into the gut.
4. **True.** HMG-CoA reductase is the rate-limiting enzyme for cholesterol synthesis in the liver.
5. **False.** Reducing cholesterol synthesis in the liver results in increased LDL receptors and hence increased LDL clearance from the plasma.
6. **False.** Statins reduce plama LDL cholesterol by 25–50%.
7. **False.** Statins and fibrates act mainly by different mechanisms, and their co-administration can help achieve target plasma cholesterol concentrations, although the additional benefit on clinical outcomes is unclear.
8. **True.** Ezetimibe reduces cholesterol absorption by blocking the intestinal NPC1L1 cholesterol transporter.
9. **False.** Fibrates activate PPAR-α but this increases lipoprotein lipase activity and clears triglycerides from the plasma.
10. **True.** Nicotinic acid inhibits triglyceride synthesis by diacylglycerol acyltransferase-2 in the liver, hence reducing production of VLDL and LDL.
11. **True.** Nicotinic acid may cause skin flushing by stimulating prostaglandin synthesis and it can be reduced by a non-steroidal anti-inflammatory drug (NSAID).
12. **False.** Arachidonic acid is an omega-6 fatty acid and the precursor of prothrombotic thromboxane A$_2$. Omega-3 fatty acids include eicosapentaenoic acid

(EPA) and docosahexaenoic acid (DHA) found in fish oils, which may have cardioprotective effects.

OBA answers

1. **Answer D** is correct.
    A. Incorrect. A low ratio of total cholesterol to HDL cholesterol is associated with lower cardiovascular risk.
    B. Incorrect. VLDL carries a greater load of triglycerides, so the proportion of cholesterol is lower in VLDL (20%) than in HDL (40%).
    C. Incorrect. The lipoprotein coat is a phospholipid monolayer, in which apolipoproteins are embedded, and provides a lipophilic interior for the transport of triglycerides.
    D. **Correct.** High dietary intake of saturated fat is associated with coronary disease.
    E. Incorrect. Moderate alcohol consumption reduces myocardial infarction risk by 30–40%.
2. **Answer E** is the inaccurate statement.

    A. Correct. The effect on smooth muscle proliferation may improve plaque stability.
    B. Correct. Statins can cause muscle pain and, rarely, rhabdomyolysis.
    C. Correct. The reduced plasma CRP reflects an anti-inflammatory action of statins.

D. Correct. This action on lipoprotein lipase reduces plasma triglycerides.
E. **Incorrect**. Statins increase plasma HDL concentration by 5–15%.

Case-based answers

A. General advice would include a low-fat diet, exercise and stopping smoking. Concomitant risk factors including obesity, diabetes and hypertension should be investigated.
B. A statin would be recommended as first-choice drug in preventing cardiovascular events. Statins are of proven benefit based on data from many studies and they are well tolerated.
C. The response would depend upon the chosen statin, its dosage and additional lifestyle changes, but the recommended targets are a total cholesterol concentration less than 4 mmol·L^{-1} and LDL cholesterol less than 2 mmol·L^{-1}. Several weeks of treatment may be required.
D. Gastrointestinal upsets are common. Use of statins is not recommended in people with hypothyroidism or liver disease. Thyroid and liver function tests should be performed. He should be advised to report unexplained muscle pain.

FURTHER READING

Afilalo J, Majdan AA, Eisenberg MJ (2007) Intensive statin therapy in acute coronary syndromes and stable coronary heart disease: a comparative meta-analysis of randomised controlled trials. *Heart* 93, 914–921

Almuti K, Rimawi R, Spevack D et al. (2006) Effects of statins beyond lipid lowering: potential for clinical benefits. *Int J Cardiol* 109, 7–15

Armitage J (2007) Safety of statins in clinical practice. *Lancet* 370, 1781–1790

Baber U, Toto RD, de Lemos J (2007) Statins and cardiovascular risk reduction in patients with chronic kidney disease and end-stage renal failure. *Am Heart J* 153, 471–477

Cholesterol Treatment Trialists' Collaborators (2005) Efficacy and safety of cholesterol-lowering treatment: prospective meta-analysis of data from 90 056 participants in 14 randomised trials of statins. *Lancet* 366, 1267–1278

Cholesterol Treatment Trialists' Collaborators (2008) Efficacy of cholesterol-lowering therapy in 18 686 people with diabetes in 14 randomised trials of statins: a meta-analysis. *Lancet* 371, 117–125

Durrington P (2003) Dyslipidaemia. *Lancet* 362, 717–731

Gami AS, Montori VM, Erwin PJ et al. (2003) Systematic review of lipid lowering for primary prevention of coronary heart disease in diabetes. *BMJ* 326, 528–529

Gutierrez J, Ramirez G, Rundek T et al. (2012) Statin therapy in the prevention of recurrent cardiovascular events: a sex-based meta-analysis. *Arch Intern Med* 172, 909–919

Hachem SB, Mooradian AD (2006) Familial dyslipidaemias. An overview of genetics, pathophysiology and management. *Drugs* 66, 1949–1969

Joy TR, Hegele RA (2009) Narrative review: statin-related myopathy. *Ann Intern Med* 150, 858–868

Kwak SM, Nyung S-K, Lee YJ et al. (2012) Efficacy of omega-3 fatty acid supplements (eicosapentaenoic acid and docasahexaenoic acids) in the secondary prevention of cardiovascular disease: a meta-analysis of randomized, double-blind, placebo-controlled trials. *Arch Intern Med* 172, 686–694

Lee C-H, Olson P, Evans RM (2003) Minireview: lipid metabolism, metabolic diseases, and peroxisome proliferator-activated receptors. *Endocrinolog y* 144, 2201–2207

Minder CM, Blaha MJ, Horne A et al. (2012) Evidence-based use of statins for primary prevention of cardiovascular disease. *Am J Med* 125, 440–446

Nicholls SJ, Tuczu EM, Sipahi I et al. (2007) Statins, high-density lipoprotein cholesterol, and regression of coronary atherosclerosis. *JAMA* 297, 499–508

Nissen SE, Tuzcu EM, Schoenhagen P et al. (2005) Statin therapy, LDL cholesterol, C-reactive protein, and coronary artery disease. *N Engl J Med* 352, 29–38

Rallidis LS, Lekakis, J, Kremastinos DT (2007) Current questions regarding the use of statins in patients with coronary heart disease. *Int J Cardiol* 122, 188–194

Saravanan P, Davidson NC, Schmidt EB et al. (2010) Cardiovascular effects of marine omega-3 fatty acids. *Lancet* 376, 540–550

Sathasivam S, Lecky B (2008) Statin induced myopathy. *BMJ* 337, a2286

Schillinger M, Exner M, Mlekusch W et al. (2004) Statin therapy improves cardiovascular outcome of patients with peripheral vascular disease. *Eur Heart J* 25, 742–748

Walsh JME, Pignone M (2004) Drug treatment of hyperlipidaemia in women. *JAMA* 291, 2243–2253

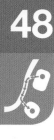

Compendium: drugs used to treat hyperlipidaemias

Drug	Kinetics (half-life)	Comments
HMG-CoA reductase inhibitors ('statins')		
Statins are first-line drugs for lowering LDL cholesterol; used in symptomatic cardiovascular disease and in asymptomatic patients at increased cardiovascular risk.		
Atorvastatin	Low bioavailability (14%); P450 oxidation to active metabolites with long half-lives (32–36 h)	Used for primary hypercholesterolaemia, heterozygous familial hypercholesterolaemia or mixed hyperlipidaemia
Fluvastatin	Bioavailability 24%; hepatic metabolism (2–3 h)	Used as adjunct to diet in primary hypercholesterolaemia and mixed hyperlipidaemias and for prophylaxis of coronary atherosclerosis
Pravastatin	Low oral bioavailability (17%), partly due to first-pass metabolism; renal excretion (1–2 h)	Used as adjunct to diet in primary hypercholesterolaemia and for prophylaxis of coronary atherosclerosis
Rosuvastatin	Bioavailability 20%; limited P450 metabolism, mainly eliminated in bile (20 h)	Used in primary hypercholesterolaemia, mixed dyslipidaemia and homozygous familial hypercholesterolaemia
Simvastatin	Prodrug extensively first-pass metabolised by hepatic P450 to active hydroxyacid analogue	Used as an adjunct to diet in primary hypercholesterolaemia and mixed hyperlipidaemias, and for prophylaxis of coronary atherosclerosis
Drugs binding bile acids or inhibiting cholesterol absorption		
Bile acid sequestrants reduce LDL cholesterol but can aggravate hypertriglyceridaemia.		
Colesevelam	Not absorbed	A lipid-lowering polymer used for primary hypercholesterolaemia as an adjunct to dietary measures, given alone or with a statin; improves glycaemic control in type 2 diabetes in adults
Colestipol	Not absorbed	Anion-exchange resin that binds bile acids; used for hyperlipidaemias in people not responding to diet and other measures
Colestyramine	Not absorbed	Anion-exchange resin that binds bile acids; used for hyperlipidaemias, and for primary hypercholesterolaemia in men aged 35–59, and to treat pruritus associated with biliary obstruction
Ezetimibe	Rapidly absorbed and metabolised to a glucuronide conjugate, which undergoes biliary excretion and hydrolysis to the active drug in the lower bowel, the site of cholesterol reabsorption (22 h)	Inhibits intestinal cholesterol transporter; used as adjunct to dietary measures and a statin in primary and homozygous familial hypercholesterolaemia
Fibrates		
Act mainly by reducing serum triglycerides, with variable effects on LDL cholesterol; used as first-line treatment for hypertriglyceridaemia, or in people intolerant of statins.		
Bezafibrate	Complete oral bioavailability; eliminated equally by renal excretion and metabolism (1–2 h)	
Ciprofibrate	Complete oral bioavailability; hepatic conjugation; long half-life (38–86 h)	Not used in type V hyperlipidaemia
Fenofibrate	Prodrug of fenofibric acid, which is glucuronidated and renally excreted (20 h)	Ester prodrug of fenofibric acid
Gemfibrozil	Complete oral bioavailability; half is excreted unchanged and remainder by hepatic metabolism (1–2 h)	Should not be combined with statins

Compendium: drugs used to treat hyperlipidaemias—cont'd

Drug	Kinetics (half-life)	Comments
Nicotinic acid and derivatives		
Used in combination with statins or as monotherapy in patients intolerant to statins.		
Acipimox	Complete oral bioavailability; mostly eliminated unchanged in urine (1–2 h)	Less effective for hypertriglyceridaemias than nicotinic acid, but fewer unwanted effects
Nicotinic acid (niacin)	Completely absorbed; hepatic metabolism and renal excretion (0.3–0.8 h)	Reduces both cholesterol and triglycerides, but limited by prostaglandin-mediated vasodilation
Other treatments		
Ispaghula	Not relevant	Soluble fibre which probably reduces reabsorption of bile acids; acts as a bulk laxative (see Ch. 35)
Omega-3 acid ethyl esters	Incorporated in lipoproteins; metabolised as dietary fatty acids	Used as adjunct for treating hypertriglyceridaemia
Omega-3 marine triglycerides	Incorporated in lipoproteins; metabolised as dietary fatty acids	Used as adjunct for treating hypertriglyceridaemia

All drugs given orally unless otherwise stated.
HMG-CoA reductase, β-hydroxyl-β-methylglutaryl-coenzyme A reductase; LDL, low-density lipoprotein.

10

The skin and eyes

Skin disorders

VEHICLES FOR TOPICAL SKIN APPLICATIONS

Topical preparations for the treatment of skin disorders usually have two components: a vehicle or base, and the active ingredient such as a corticosteroid or an antifungal agent. Five types of base are used:

- ointments, which are greases such as white or yellow soft paraffin. They are more occlusive on the skin than creams, and this keeps the skin hydrated,
- pastes, which are suspensions of fine powder in an ointment and will stay where they are placed on the skin. Their main use is to apply noxious chemicals that should be confined to one area of the skin,
- creams, which are emulsions of water with a grease. They are less greasy than ointments, are absorbed more quickly into the skin and are often used as a vehicle for active ingredients,
- lotions, which are any kind of liquid. They are less messy for use on wet surfaces and hairy areas and their main advantage is a cooling effect,
- gels, which can be hydrophilic or hydrophobic and have a high water content. They are combined with an active ingredient, particularly for use on the face or scalp.

ATOPIC AND CONTACT DERMATITIS

Dermatitis is a term used to describe eczematous inflammation of the skin. It has significant underlying genetic influences, but is triggered by external factors.

ATOPIC DERMATITIS (ECZEMA)

The pathogenesis of atopic dermatitis is determined by a combination of genetic, environmental, pharmacological and immunological factors. There are two forms of atopic dermatitis. The extrinsic type (70–80% of cases) is associated with a food or aero-allergen. There is an association with other atopic disorders such as asthma and hay fever. It is associated with IgE-mediated sensitisation, with eosinophilia in the peripheral blood and with a raised plasma IgE concentration. In atopic individuals, circulating mononuclear cells have a reduced ability to produce interferon γ, which normally inhibits both IgE production and the proliferation of T-helper type 2 (Th2) lymphocytes. The function of regulatory T-cells is also abnormal. Keratinocytes produce cytokines that stimulate eosinophil activation and adhesion to vascular walls. The intrinsic form of atopic dermatitis also involves immune dysregulation, but there is no IgE excess or eosinophilia.

As a result of the changes in immune regulation in atopic individuals, Th2-cells proliferate. Dominance of either a Th1 or Th2 response is partially programmed in early life, with exposure to microbial antigens promoting the normal Th1 dominance. Th1-cell responses are induced by infections, and suppress the development of Th2-cells. It is possible that the increasing use of antibacterial drugs in childhood may partially explain the rise in atopic dermatitis (Chs 38 and 39).

Affected skin is red, scaly and extremely dry, often affecting the flexures. The dryness is a consequence of the inflammation, but the permeability barrier function of the skin is also impaired, resulting in increased transepidermal water loss. There may be vesicles and weeping with crusting over the skin surface. Scratching produces excoriation and thickening of the skin. The affected skin is infiltrated with activated T-cells, with selective recruitment of Th2-cells, and eosinophils. Increased carriage of *Staphylococcus aureus* on the affected skin may also maintain inflammation by activating T-cells and macrophages.

CONTACT DERMATITIS

There are two main triggers:

- an external agent producing direct irritation,
- immunological sensitisation involving a delayed hypersensitivity response (Ch. 39). Once the skin has been sensitised, the potential for further reaction persists indefinitely. Sensitisation can arise in response to topical application of drugs.

OTHER TYPES OF DERMATITIS

These include nummular (discoid) eczema, photosensitive dermatitis and seborrhoeic dermatitis.

TREATMENT OF ATOPIC DERMATITIS

- Emollients (substances that soften the skin) are helpful as hydrophobic agents that seal the surface of the skin and reduce water loss. Paraffin derivatives are most effective but are greasy and not well accepted by most people. Alternatives, such as aqueous creams, are more cosmetically acceptable.
- Avoidance of irritants, such as soaps, detergents, alcohols and astringents. Wet dressings may help to prevent skin fissuring and reduce scratching.
- Identification of allergens by patch tests and their subsequent elimination.
- Topical corticosteroid ointment (Ch. 44) is effective, but a low-potency corticosteroid should be chosen if there is continuous use, to minimise unwanted effects. The anti-inflammatory effect of these drugs makes them the mainstay of treatment, but diminished effectiveness with prolonged use (tachyphylaxis) limits their long-term value. Tachyphylaxis may be delayed by twice-weekly application of a more potent corticosteroid.
- Topical calcineurin inhibitors, such as tacrolimus (Ch. 38), directly or indirectly reduce activation of many of the inflammatory cells involved in the pathogenesis of the dermatitic lesions, including T-cells, dendritic cells, mast cells and keratinocytes. Local burning is the major unwanted effect, and skin malignancy has been reported. Tacrolimus is more effective than a potent corticosteroid for moderate to severe eczema.
- Sedative antihistamines (Ch. 39) at night assist sleep, although they have little effect on itching. A topical formulation of the tricyclic antidepressant doxepin (see Ch. 22) is available to treat itch. It is uncertain whether its antihistamine activity is the major mode of action.
- Immunosuppressant therapy with azathioprine, ciclosporin or mycophenolate mofetil (Ch. 38) can be tried for treatment-resistant dermatitis. Apart from unwanted effects the main problem is rapid relapse when treatment is stopped.
- Phototherapy with natural sunlight is helpful, but sweating can increase pruritus. Narrow-band ultraviolet B (UVB) radiation is a useful alternative.
- Tar bandages on the limbs are messy, but have anti-inflammatory and anti-pruritic effects.
- Systemic antibacterial drugs are given for secondary infection. Anti-staphylococcal agents are often helpful if the skin lesions are poorly controlled.

TREATMENT OF CONTACT DERMATITIS

- Provision of a barrier to an irritant; for example wearing gloves or removing an allergen may be sufficient.
- Dilute topical corticosteroid ointment (Ch. 44).
- Potassium permanganate soaks can help to dry up exudative lesions.

PSORIASIS

Psoriatic skin lesions are produced by a very rapid proliferation of epidermal cells. Cell turnover time is decreased from about 28 days to 3–4 days, which prevents adequate maturation. Instead of producing a normal keratinous surface layer, the skin thickens, forming a silvery scale with dilated upper dermal blood vessels. Psoriatic plaques (psoriasis vulgaris, accounting for 90% of cases) are usually found on the elbows, knees, lower back, buttocks and scalp. Various subtypes of psoriasis present with different clinical manifestations. An inflammatory arthritis occurs in up to 25% of people with psoriasis (see Ch. 30).

There is a genetic component to psoriasis, which interacts with unknown environmental factors to produce an immune reaction in the dermis. Antigen-presenting cells in the dermis mature after contact with the antigen, migrate to regional lymph nodes and activate T-cells. T-cells then proliferate and enter the circulation and extravasate into the skin at sites of inflammation, assisted by local chemokine production. In the dermis, interaction with the initiating antigen results in Th1 immune responses, with secretion of cytokines such as interferon γ, interleukin (IL)-12 and IL-23 and tumour necrosis factor α (TNFα). The cytokines stimulate cell proliferation and impair maturation of keratinocytes, and produce vascular changes in the skin.

Psoriasis can be provoked or exacerbated by several drugs, including lithium, chloroquine, hydroxychloroquine, β-adrenoceptor antagonists, non-steroidal anti-inflammatory drugs and angiotensin-converting enzyme inhibitors.

There are several treatments for the skin lesions, both topical and systemic, but none produce long-term remission. Increasingly, combinations of treatments have been found to be more effective than one agent alone.

TOPICAL THERAPY

Emollients

These reduce scaling and itching and may be sufficient in mild psoriasis (see atopic dermatitis, above). They can also be used with a keratolytic.

Keratolytics

Keratolytics such as salicylic acid break down keratin and soften skin, which improves penetration of other treatments. Salicylic acid ointment is most frequently used.

Vitamin D analogues

Vitamin D regulates epidermal proliferation and differentiation. It also has immunosuppressant properties. Vitamin D analogues (e.g. calcipotriol, calcitriol) are clean and simple to apply and are particularly useful for chronic plaque psoriasis, although complete clearing of the plaques is unusual. Ointment has a greater emollient effect than has cream, but is messy to apply. Calcipotriol should not usually be used on the face, where it often causes irritation; calcitriol may be better tolerated on this site, although it is less effective elsewhere. Excessive use of vitamin D analogues can lead to hypercalcaemia, but this is not a problem at recommended dosages. The ease of use of these compounds makes them a popular choice if a keratolytic is insufficient.

Topical retinoids

Retinoids are discussed more fully under systemic treatments. Tazarotene gel can be applied to plaque psoriasis and has minimal systemic absorption. Unlike other retinoids, tazarotene is selective for retinoic acid receptor (RAR) proteins, with no affinity for retinoid X receptors (RXR) (see below). This may reduce unwanted effects, which are mainly local irritation of healthy skin with pruritus. Tazarotene should be avoided for 1 month before conception, because of potential teratogenic effects.

Dithranol

This anthraquinone decreases cell division and is effective for healing psoriatic plaques. In hospital it is applied in a stiff paste to the plaque so that the dithranol does not burn normal skin, and is left in contact with the plaque for 24 h. At home, dithranol is used as a cream that is applied to the plaque for 30 min and then washed off. The oxidation products of dithranol stain the skin brown, leaving discoloration of healed areas for a few days. They also stain clothes and bedding a mauve colour that will not wash out. Since dithranol irritates normal skin, it should not be used in flexures.

Coal tar preparations

Crude coal tar is a mixture of a large number of hydrocarbons that have a cytostatic action. It enhances the healing effect of UVB radiation on psoriatic lesions. The main disadvantage is messiness, and its efficacy when used alone is modest. More refined tar preparations have greater acceptability, but are even less effective.

Phototherapy

Ultraviolet light produces improvement by inhibiting DNA synthesis and depleting intra-epidermal T-cells. It should not be used on individuals with very fair skin who burn in the sun. Broad-band UVB ('sunburn' wavelength 270–350 nm) has largely been replaced by the more effective narrow-band UVB (311–313 nm). Long-wavelength UVA (320–400 nm) requires more specialised equipment and prior administration of an oral psoralen as a photosensitising drug (a process called photochemotherapy or PUVA therapy). Psoralen probably intercalates between pyrimidine base pairs in the DNA helix and inhibits cell replication. PUVA is usually reserved for severe, resistant psoriasis and is more effective than treatment with UVB. Psoralen can produce nausea and headache acutely. The long-term risks of PUVA include accelerated skin ageing and an increased incidence of skin cancer, and systemic treatments are increasingly preferred.

Topical corticosteroid preparations

These should be used sparingly on limited areas, since unwanted effects can be troublesome (Ch. 44). Withdrawal of a high-potency corticosteroid can produce a rebound exacerbation and even generalised pustular psoriasis.

SYSTEMIC TREATMENTS

Apart from emollients and corticosteroids, which are most useful for chronic plaque psoriasis, topical treatments should be avoided in more inflammatory forms of the condition because they can cause troublesome skin irritation. Systemic treatment is used for the more severe forms of disease.

Methotrexate

This is a very effective treatment at low dosages for resistant and widespread psoriasis. Its main actions are cytostatic and immunosuppressant (see Chs 38 and 52). Oral or intramuscular dosing is commonly used once a week. Bone marrow depression and hepatotoxicity with liver fibrosis are the main complications; blood counts and serum procollagen III, to identify liver toxicity, must be checked every 3 months.

Retinoids

This term covers vitamin A (retinol) and therapeutically useful synthetic vitamin A derivatives, such as acitretin, the active metabolite of etretinate (which is no longer used). Given orally, they are anti-inflammatory and cytostatic. Vitamin A, and its metabolites all-*trans*-retinoic acid and 9-*cis*-retinoic acid, are involved in epithelial cell growth and differentiation. Retinoids enter cells by endocytosis and interact with two forms of retinoic acid nuclear receptor, retinoic acid receptors (RARs) and retinoid X receptors (RXRs), which are related to steroid/thyroid hormone receptors (Ch. 1). The retinoid–receptor complex initiates gene transcription and may affect cell growth and differentiation by modulation of growth factors and their receptors. Response of psoriatic lesions is delayed by up to 2 months. Elimination of retinoids is by hepatic metabolism. Unwanted effects are almost universal and include dry lips and nasal mucosa, dryness of the skin with localised peeling over the digits, and transient thinning of hair. These effects are dose-dependent and reversible. Longer-term problems include ossification of ligaments, increased plasma triglycerides and, to a lesser extent, increased plasma cholesterol. There is a high risk of teratogenesis and women must use adequate contraception during treatment, and stop treatment for 3 years before conception.

Ciclosporin or tacrolimus

These immunosuppressants (Ch. 38) are effective in psoriasis at lower doses than those required for prevention of allograft rejection. However, remissions induced by these drugs are usually short-lived.

Biologic agents

Etanercept, infliximab and adalimumab (Chs 30 and 34) are intravenous therapies that block TNFα and are highly effective in treatment-resistant psoriasis. They inhibit the production of chemokines and endothelial adhesion molecules that attract activated lymphocytes into the skin. Infliximab produces a more rapid response than etanercept. Ustekinumab, an inhibitor of IL-12 and IL-23, is effective for plaque psoriasis that has not responded to at least two standard systemic therapies. IL-12 and IL-23 are products of dendritic cells and macrophages which activate T-cells involved in the inflammatory response in psoriasis.

Fumaric acid esters

This is an oral unlicensed treatment for severe psoriasis that probably works by promoting a Th2-cell response in place of the Th1-dominant response found in psoriasis. This results from inhibition of nuclear factor κB (NF-κB), enhancing T-cell apoptosis. Fumaric acid is poorly absorbed from the gut and is therefore given as an ester that is rapidly hydrolysed to monomethylfumarate, the active compound. Unwanted effects include gastrointestinal upset in more than two-thirds of people, and flushing in one-third.

ACNE

Acne most commonly arises in adolescence and often regresses in the late teens or early twenties. Acne affects areas of skin with large numbers of sebaceous glands, especially the face, back and chest. There is increased production of sebum, which distends the pilosebaceous duct, producing a small closed papule (comedo) called a whitehead. Hyperkeratosis at the mouth of the hair follicle blocks the duct. If the duct then opens, compacted follicular cells at the tip give comedones the appearance of a blackhead. A resident anaerobic bacterium, *Propionibacterium acnes*, degrades triglycerides in sebum to free fatty acids and glycerol. It also produces chemotactic factors and inflammatory mediators. These mediators together with the irritant free fatty acids produce inflamed lesions of pustules and nodules, which can coalesce to form multilocular cysts. The inflammatory lesions can scar, leaving permanent disfigurement.

Acne has a genetic background, which determines the rate of sebum production, particularly in response to androgens. Androgens are produced at puberty and induce hypertrophy of sebaceous glands, and the excess secretion rate in predisposed individuals triggers the acne. Acne can also be produced by systemic corticosteroids or anabolic steroids (Ch. 46). In women, it can be a manifestation of polycystic ovary syndrome (Ch. 43).

TREATMENT OF ACNE

There are several effective treatments for acne. The choice will depend on the nature of the lesions and their severity. Topical treatments do not influence the rate of production of sebum.

Topical treatments

- **Benzoyl peroxide** has antibacterial activity against *P. acnes* and a keratolytic action, both of which reduce the numbers of comedones. It produces scaling and skin irritation, which may limit its use to short treatment periods.
- **Topical antibacterials**, for example clindamycin and erythromycin (Ch. 51), are less effective than oral antibacterials but have fewer unwanted effects. Their efficacy is similar to that of benzoyl peroxide, but they produce less skin irritation. Combination therapy with benzoyl peroxide reduces the problem of bacterial resistance. Topical antibacterials are used for mild to moderate acne, and are particularly useful in pregnant women since there is no systemic absorption.
- **Isotretinoin** (13-*cis*-retinoic acid) is a vitamin A derivative with a keratolytic action that unblocks the pilosebaceous follicles and allows flow of sebum to extrude the plug. The mechanism of action within the cell is similar to that of acitretin (see under psoriasis). It also reduces sebum production by up to 90% by decreasing sebocyte proliferation; this action is probably independent of effects on nuclear retinoid receptors. Topically, isotretinoin produces erythema and scaling, which can be minimised by starting with a low concentration. Adapalene is an extensively modified retinoid that has a faster onset of action and produces less skin irritation.
- **Azelaic acid** is an aliphatic dicarboxylic acid that has an antibacterial action against propionibacteria and is effective against bacteria that have become resistant to erythromycin and tetracycline. It also inhibits the division of keratinocytes, which may reduce follicular plugging and prevent the development of comedones. The most frequent unwanted effects are local burning, scaling or itching, although hypopigmentation can also be a problem. Azelaic acid is most effective for mild to moderate non-inflammatory comedonal acne, especially of the face.
- **Nicotinamide** gel has equivalent efficacy to topical antibacterials. It has an anti-inflammatory action by inhibiting production of lipids in sebaceous secretions (Ch. 48). Unwanted effects include dryness, pruritus and burning of the skin.

Systemic treatments

- Oral antibacterials that are active against *P. acnes* are used for inflammatory acne (papules/pustules). Penetration into sebaceous follicles is poor, but they produce some improvement after 2–3 months, requiring 4–6 months of treatment for maximal benefit. Treatment should be given for extended periods, since relapse is common if it is stopped. Among the more useful antibacterial agents are tetracyclines, for example oxytetracycline and doxycycline. Alternatives include ciprofloxacin and trimethoprim (Ch. 51). Widespread resistance to erythromycin makes it a less suitable choice.

- The anti-androgen cyproterone acetate (Ch. 46) is useful in women with moderate or severe acne and is usually given in combination with ethinylestradiol as a combined oral hormonal contraceptive (Ch. 45). The combination reduces sebum flow by 40%. Alternatively, oestrogen can be given with a non-androgenic progestogen such as norgestimate or desogestrel. Improvement can take 2–4 months.
- Isotretinoin is used orally in severe acne and gives an almost 100% probability of complete remission. High doses can produce prolonged remission. Unwanted effects include dry lips, nose and eyes, increased plasma triglycerides and, less commonly, myalgia. Teratogenesis is a major problem and, although the half-life of the metabolites is less than 2 days, conception should be avoided during treatment and for 1 month after stopping treatment.

CHOICE OF TREATMENT FOR ACNE

Initially, management of non-inflammatory comedones is by topical treatment such as azelaic acid or retinoids. For early inflammatory lesions a topical antibacterial or benzoyl peroxide can be considered, alone or in combination. More severe inflammatory acne usually requires topical or systemic antibacterials with topical retinoid. Systemic treatment with isotretinoin is used for severe unresponsive acne. Oestrogen and anti-androgen therapy are alternatives for women, and combined oral hormonal contraceptives can be of benefit. Overall, the most common reason for treatment failure is probably non-adherence to the recommended regimen.

SELF-ASSESSMENT

True/false questions

1. Atopic dermatitis is the most common form of dermatitis.
2. Oral corticosteroids are the mainstay of treatment of atopic dermatitis.
3. Oral antihistamines reduce itching in atopic dermatitis.
4. Th2-lymphocytes are the dominant immune cells in psoriasis.
5. Immunosuppressant drugs are contraindicated in severe psoriasis.
6. Retinoids reduce cell growth and differentiation.
7. Severe inflammatory acne should be treated with topical or systemic antibacterials.
8. Antibacterial drug resistance in *Propionibacterium acnes* is rare.

One-best-answer (OBA) question

Choose the *accurate* statement below about psoriasis and its treatment.

A. Psoriasis may be improved by atenolol.
B. Psoriasis may be exacerbated by exposure to sunshine.
C. Methotrexate has few unwanted effects in the treatment of psoriasis.
D. Calcipotriol is a vitamin D analogue applied topically for psoriasis.
E. Ustekinumab is a monoclonal antibody against tumour necrosis factor α (TNFα).

Case-based questions

A 7-year-old girl with a history of atopic asthma developed a red, scaly and dry rash in her knee and elbow flexures and on her arms and cheeks. The rash was extremely itchy and she was scratching the affected areas, causing excoriation and weeping. Her mother had had atopic dermatitis when she was young.

A. What was the possible diagnosis?
B. What treatments should be tried initially?
C. What other factors should be considered?

True/false answers

1. **True.** Atopic dermatitis is an inflammatory condition with a familial tendency.
2. **False.** Corticosteroids are used topically in atopic dermatitis for up to 4 weeks.
3. **True.** A sedative antihistamine (e.g. promethazine) may be of value, although direct effects on itching are limited.
4. **False.** Psoriasis is thought to be driven mainly by Th1-lymphocytes, with production of tumour necrosis factor α (TNFα), interleukin (IL)-12 and IL-23.
5. **False.** The immunosuppressants ciclosporin or methotrexate can be used in severe psoriasis resistant to other drugs.
6. **True.** Oral retinoids such as vitamin A and its derivatives reduce cell growth and can be used in psoriasis, but may be teratogenic. Oral and topical retinoids are also useful in acne.
7. **True.** A topical retinoid is used together with oral or topical antibacterials; suitable topical antibacterials are erythromycin and clindamycin.
8. **False.** Resistance of *P. acnes* to antibacterials is increasing, including cross-resistance to erythromycin and clindamycin; when possible, drugs with an antibacterial action should be used, such as benzoyl peroxide or azelaic acid.

OBA answer

Answer D is correct.

A. Incorrect. Beta-adrenoceptor antagonists can exacerbate psoriasis.

B. Incorrect. Regular short exposures to sunlight or ultraviolet light benefit psoriasis by increasing production of vitamin D and slowing skin cell proliferation.

C. Incorrect. Methotrexate can produce bone marrow depression and hepatoxicity and regular monitoring is required.

D. **Correct**. Calcipotriol is a topical vitamin D analogue with beneficial actions in psoriasis including inhibition of T-cell proliferation and cytokine release.

E. Incorrect. Ustekinumab is an inhibitor of IL-12 and IL-23 and is used in drug-resistant psoriasis; modulators of TNFα (e.g. infliximab, etanercept) are also used.

Case-based answers

A. Atopic dermatitis is possible because of the appearance of the rash, the child's atopy, and her mother's history of the condition.

B. Initial management approaches should include good skin hygiene with regular bathing (but avoiding soaps), and the use of emollients in bath water and applied topically to moisturise the skin. Drug treatments should include short courses of topical hydrocortisone, and a topical antihistamine or oral sedative antihistamine if the itch is severe, although there is no consensus that antihistamines are beneficial. Topical doxepin may also help reduce itch.

C. Contributory factors such as allergies to food and other allergens, psychological factors and removal of irritants and allergens should be assessed. Severe acute exacerbations may require rigorous topical measures and antibacterial treatment.

FURTHER READING

Bieber T (2008) Atopic dermatitis. *N Engl J Med* 358, 1483–1494

Brown S, Reynolds NJ (2006) Atopic and non-atopic eczema. *BMJ* 332, 584–588

Haider A, Shaw JC (2004) Treatment of acne vulgaris. *JAMA* 292, 726–735

Menter A, Griffiths CEM (2007) Psoriasis 2. Current and future management of psoriasis. *Lancet* 370, 272–284

Naldi L, Rebora A (2009) Seborrheic dermatitis. *N Engl J Med* 360, 387–396

Purdy S, de Berker D (2006) Acne. *BMJ* 333, 949–953

Reynolds NJ, Al-Daraji WI (2002) Calcineurin inhibitors and sirolimus: mechanisms of action and application in dermatology. *Clin Exp Dermatol* 27, 555–561

Schön MP, Boehncke WH (2005) Psoriasis. *N Engl J Med* 352, 1899–1912

Smith CH, Barker JNWN (2006) Psoriasis and its management. *BMJ* 333, 380–384

Wasserbauer N, Ballow M (2009) Atopic dermatitis. *Am J Med* 122, 121–125

Weger W (2010) Current status and new developments in the treatment of psoriasis and psoriatic arthritis with biological agents. *Br J Pharamcol* 160, 810–820

Williams HC (2005) Atopic dermatitis. *N Engl J Med* 352, 2314–2324

Compendium: drugs used in the treatment of skin disorders

Drug	Kinetics (half-life)	Comments
Absorption of topical formulations is slow and limited and their duration of action is not related to the systemic half-life.		
Corticosteroids		
Given topically for inflammatory skin conditions.		
Alclometasone dipropionate	About 3% of applied dose is absorbed across the skin over 8 h	Synthetic corticosteroid
Beclometasone dipropionate	Poorly absorbed; metabolised to active monopropionate (0.5 h)	Use restricted to severe conditions, such as eczema unresponsive to less potent drugs
Betamethasone esters	Poor absorption, particularly from forearm but higher absorption from the forehead, scrotum, eyelids and inflamed skin; skin hydration increases absorption	Use restricted to severe conditions, such as eczema unresponsive to less potent drugs
Clobetasol propionate	Very poor absorption (see betamethasone esters)	Use restricted to short-term treatment of severe resistant conditions, such as eczema unresponsive to less potent drugs; suppression of adrenocortical function possible in people with psoriasis
Clobetasone butyrate	Poorly absorbed (see betamethasone esters)	Used for eczema and dermatitis of all types
Diflucortolone valerate	Absorption probably similar to betamethasone esters	Use restricted to severe conditions, such as eczema unresponsive to less potent drugs, and for psoriasis
Fludroxycortide	No kinetic data available	
Fluocinolone acetonide	Poorly absorbed (see betamethasone esters); hepatic metabolism	
Fluocinonide	Poorly absorbed (see betamethasone esters)	Use restricted to severe conditions, such as eczema unresponsive to less potent drugs, and for psoriasis
Fluocortolone	Few data available after topical dosing (1.5 h)	Use restricted to severe conditions, such as eczema unresponsive to less potent drugs, and for psoriasis
Fluticasone propionate	Poorly absorbed transdermally (see betamethasone esters)	Use restricted to severe conditions, such as eczema unresponsive to less potent drugs, and for psoriasis
Hydrocortisone	Poorly absorbed transdermally (see betamethasone esters); probably metabolised within skin (1.5 h)	Low potency; can be used for perioral inflammatory lesions
Hydrocortisone butyrate	Poorly absorbed transdermally (see betamethasone esters); hydrolysed in skin to hydrocortisone	Use of the butyrate ester is restricted to severe conditions, such as eczema unresponsive to less potent drugs
Mometasone furoate	Very poor absorption (see betamethasone esters); hepatic metabolism (5 h)	Use restricted to severe conditions, such as eczema unresponsive to less potent drugs, and for psoriasis
Triamcinolone acetonide	Poorly absorbed from the skin (see betamethasone esters); rapidly eliminated (2–5 h)	Use restricted to severe conditions, such as eczema unresponsive to less potent drugs, and for psoriasis
Drugs for eczema and/or seborrhoeic dermatitis		
Topical corticosteroids may also be given.		
Ichthammol	—	A sulphonated shale oil; used as an ointment or cream
Pimecrolimus	Very limited absorption across the skin hepatic metabolism (30–40 h)	Calcineurin inhibitor; used for mild to moderate atopic eczema
Tacrolimus	Limited absorption across the skin (see Ch. 38)	Calcineurin inhibitor; applied topically for moderate to severe atopic eczema unresponsive to other treatment
Drugs for psoriasis		
Acitretin	Oral bioavailability 60%; slow hepatic metabolism (50 h)	Retinoid used for severe extensive and resistant psoriasis; teratogenic risk; given orally

Compendium: drugs used in the treatment of skin disorders—cont'd

Drug	Kinetics (half-life)	Comments
Calcipotriol (calcipotriene)	About 5% absorbed after topical application; hepatic metabolism (5–6 h)	Vitamin D analogue used for plaque psoriasis; applied topically
Calcitriol	Metabolised by hydroxylation and conjugation (3–6 h)	Vitamin D analogue used for mild to moderate plaque psoriasis; applied topically; see Ch. 42
Ciclosporin	Oral bioavailability about 30%; metabolised in gut and liver (27 h) (see Ch. 38)	Used for short-term treatment of severe atopic dermatitis and severe psoriasis; given orally
Coal tar	High transdermal absorption; activated by P450 oxidation	Contains polycyclic aromatic hydrocarbons; used for chronic atopic eczema; applied topically
Dithranol (anthralin)	Poorly absorbed; metabolised within the skin	Used for subacute and chronic psoriasis; applied topically
Fumaric acid esters	Ester prodrugs rapidly hydrolysed to active monomethylfumarate, which has half-life of about 36 h.	Used for severe psoriasis; given orally; not licensed in UK
Methotrexate	Oral absorption 20–95%; metabolised to active polyglutamates and by oxidation (8–10 h)	Folate antagonist used in the treatment of severe uncontrolled psoriasis, rheumatoid arthritis (Ch. 30) and malignant disease (Ch. 52); given orally or by intravenous or intramuscular injection
Salicylic acid	See Ch. 29	Used with coal tar and dithranol preparations as a keratolytic in scaly psoriasis; applied as a paste containing zinc oxide
Tacalcitol	Negligible absorption across skin	Vitamin D_3 analogue (1,24-dihydroxy-vit D_3) used for plaque psoriasis; applied topically as ointment
Tazarotene	Poorly absorbed; hydrolysed in skin to active tazarotenic acid, which has half-life 18 h	Retinoid used for mild to moderate plaque psoriasis; applied topically
Ustekinumab	Kinetics unclear (15–32 days)	Antibody directed at IL-12, IL-23; used for moderate to severe psoriasis resistant to other therapy; given by subcutaneous injection

Drugs for acne and rosacea

In addition to topical preparations below, antibiotics such as clindamycin, doxycycline, erythromycin, minocycline, oxytetracycline, tetracycline and trimethoprim (see Ch. 51) can be used in the treatment of acne.

Drug	Kinetics (half-life)	Comments
Adapalene	Very low topical absorption; eliminated in bile	Retinoid-like drug; binds to nuclear but not cytosolic retinoid receptors; applied topically
Azelaic acid	Low absorption (about 4%); eliminated unchanged in urine (1–2 h)	Antimicrobial and anticomedonal actions; applied topically
Benzoyl peroxide	Absorption about 5%; reduced to benzoic acid	Powerful oxidising agent; applied topically
Co-cyprindiol		Coformulation of cyproterone acetate (Ch. 46) and ethinylestradiol (Ch. 45); used for the treatment of severe acne unresponsive to antibiotics and for hirsutism in women
Isotretinoin	Metabolised by oxidation and glucuronidation (10–20 h); isomerises to all-*trans*-retinoic acid (a teratogen)	Retinoid (13-*cis*-retinoic acid); applied topically; may be given orally but known to be teratogenic
Tretinoin	Metabolised by oxidation and glucuronidation (1–2 h)	Retinoid (all-*trans*-retinoic acid); applied topically

Drugs used to assist wound healing

Drug	Kinetics (half-life)	Comments
Becaplermin	Not absorbed	Recombinant human platelet-derived growth factor; enhances formation of granulation tissue; applied topically

Compendium: drugs used in the treatment of skin disorders—cont'd

Drug	Kinetics (half-life)	Comments
Preparations for warts and calluses		
Preparations not suitable for application to face or anogenital areas		
All compounds used topically to produce localised tissue destruction.		
Formaldehyde	—	Used for warts, particularly plantar warts
Glutaraldehyde	—	Used for warts, particularly plantar warts
Salicylic acid	—	Used for plantar and mosaic warts, corns, verrucas and calluses
Silver nitrate	—	Used for warts, verrucas, umbilical granulomas and over-granulation tissue
Preparations suitable for application to anogenital areas		
Both compounds used topically for soft non-keratinised external warts; risk of severe systemic toxicity.		
Imiquimod	Slow absorption from skin extends systemic half-life (20–30 h)	Left on treated area for a maximum of 8–10 h; also used for superficial basal cell carcinoma
Podophyllum (podophyllotoxin)	—	Left on treated area for a maximum of 6 h

50

The eye

Vision depends upon the eye converting light that falls on the retina into an electrical signal to be carried to the brain through the optic nerve. The eye must focus objects sharply on the retina, a process called accommodation. To adjust the innate focus to achieve this, the ciliary muscle alters the shape of the lens, allowing the eye to accommodate to objects at different distances. The iris determines the size of the pupil and the amount of light entering the eye. The autonomic nervous system innervates the ciliary muscles and the iris.

Accommodation

The ciliary muscle is a circular (constrictor) smooth muscle that is attached to the lens by suspensory ligaments. The ciliary muscle only has a parasympathetic nerve supply (mediated by acetylcholine acting through muscarinic receptors; Ch. 4) and contracts in response to parasympathetic stimulation. This reduces tension on the suspensory ligaments and the capsule of the lens is relaxed, so that the lens becomes shorter and fatter and accommodates for viewing near objects. Drugs that are agonists at muscarinic receptors produce ciliary muscle contraction and fix the lens for viewing near objects, blurring far vision.

In the absence of parasympathetic stimulation the ciliary muscle is relaxed and tension in the suspensory ligaments increases. This pulls on the lens capsule, which flattens the lens and adjusts visual acuity for distant vision. Drugs that are antagonists at muscarinic receptors prevent ciliary muscle contraction and fix the lens for viewing far objects, with blurring of near vision. This state is called cycloplegia (Fig. 50.1).

Pupil size

(ciliary muscle)

This is determined by the relative tone in the two smooth muscle layers of the iris. The circular (constrictor) muscle is the more powerful and receives parasympathetic nervous innervation, producing muscle contraction that is mediated by acetylcholine acting on muscarinic receptors. The radial (dilator) muscle is sympathetically innervated, and contraction of the muscle is mediated by noradrenaline acting on α_1-adrenoceptors.

The light reflex is the primary determinant of pupil size with increased light causing the pupil to constrict and reduce the amount of light that reaches the retina. Pupillary constriction is known as miosis and also accompanies accommodation for near vision, a response mediated by the parasympathetic nervous system. Miosis can be produced by drugs that stimulate muscarinic receptors and contract the circular muscle of the iris. Dilation of the pupil is called mydriasis and is caused by contraction of the radial muscle. Mydriasis can be produced by drugs that are antagonists at muscarinic receptors in the circular muscle (leaving unopposed action of the radial muscle) or by drugs that stimulate α_1-adrenoceptors in the radial muscle.

Dilation of the pupil also has the effect of moving the iris towards the cornea and narrowing the anterior angle between the iris and the cornea. This can reduce aqueous humour outflow through the canal of Schlemm. *→ by antimuscarinic!*

Drainage of aqueous humour

The space between the cornea, at the front of the eye (Fig. 50.1), and the iris is the anterior chamber and is filled with a clear liquid known as aqueous humour. Aqueous humour is constantly secreted by the ciliary body. Most aqueous humour flows through the pupil to the anterior chamber, and leaves the eye via the trabecular meshwork that drains to the episcleral veins through the canal of Schlemm (Fig. 50.1). Some aqueous humour drains through the sclera (uveoscleral outflow). Production of aqueous humour is influenced by innervation from the autonomic nervous system. Alpha$_2$-adrenoceptor stimulation of the ciliary body reduces the production of aqueous humour, while β_1-adrenoceptor stimulation increases its production. Outflow

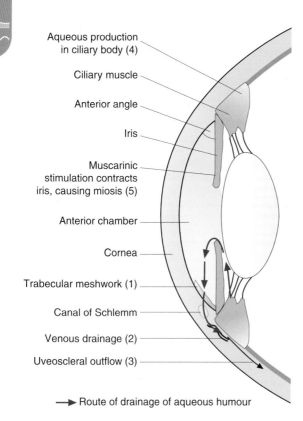

Aqueous production in ciliary body (4)

Ciliary muscle

Anterior angle

Iris

Muscarinic stimulation contracts iris, causing miosis (5)

Anterior chamber

Cornea

Trabecular meshwork (1)

Canal of Schlemm

Venous drainage (2)

Uveoscleral outflow (3)

→ Route of drainage of aqueous humour

Fig. 50.1 **The route of drainage of aqueous humour from the eye and the sites of action of drugs used in the treatment of glaucoma.** The mechanisms by which some drugs benefit glaucoma are still uncertain but are thought to include the following:

- in angle-closure glaucoma, muscarinic agonists, e.g. pilocarpine, facilitate aqueous humour drainage (1, 2) by constricting the iris circular constrictor pupillae (5), which widens the anterior angle,
- carbonic anhydrase inhibitors, e.g. acetazolamide, decrease aqueous humour production (4),
- beta-adrenoceptor antagonists, e.g. timolol, reduce aqueous humour production (4) and increase outflow (1),
- selective α_2-adrenoceptor agonists, e.g. brimonidine, decrease aqueous humour production (4),
- prostaglandin analogues selective for stimulating the prostaglandin $F_{2\alpha}$ receptor, e.g. latanoprost, enhance aqueous humour outflow (1, 2, 3) and may improve ocular blood flow.

of aqueous humour is also influenced by innervation from the autonomic nervous system, and by prostaglandins. Contraction of the ciliary muscle aids drainage of aqueous humour through the trabecular meshwork into the episcleral veins. Pressure in the eye is maintained by a balance between the production of aqueous humour and its drainage. The intraocular pressure rises if drainage of the aqueous humour is impaired. High intraocular pressure can damage retinal ganglion cells, and is one of the factors that leads to progressive loss of vision in the disease known as glaucoma. If the anterior chamber of the eye is abnormally

shallow, there will be a narrow anterior-chamber angle between the iris and cornea (iridocorneal angle) (Fig. 50.1).

Dilation of the pupil can narrow the angle further to an extent where it impedes drainage of aqueous humour through the trabecular meshwork. This can produce an acute rise in pressure in the eye (Fig. 50.1). Conversely, constriction of the circular muscle of the iris makes the pupil smaller and moves the iris away from the trabecular meshwork, widening the anterior angle and facilitating aqueous humour drainage through the canal of Schlemm.

TOPICAL APPLICATION OF DRUGS TO THE EYE

Drugs applied in solution to the anterior surface of the eye can penetrate to the anterior chamber and the ciliary muscle, principally via the cornea. The high water content of the cornea makes lipid solubility less important for adequate penetration of a drug than is the case for transdermal drug delivery, but formulation of the carrier is important to avoid irritation of the conjunctiva. There is little diffusion to the more posterior structures of the eye.

Systemic absorption of drug following topical application to the surface of the eye can occur either via conjunctival vessels or from the nasal mucosa after drainage of excess drug through the tear ducts. Topical administration of drugs to the eye can therefore produce systemic effects. Drainage can be reduced by shutting the eyes for at least 1 min after putting in the drops and by compressing the nasolacrimal duct at the medial corner of the eye with a finger. Both eye drops and ointments are usually administered into the pocket that can be formed by gently pulling the lower eyelid downwards (the lower fornix).

Microbial contamination is a potential problem once eye preparations have been opened. Multiple-application containers have preservative added to reduce the risk, but it is not advisable to use any eye preparation more than a month after it has been opened.

GLAUCOMA

Glaucoma is a group of disorders characterised by loss of retinal ganglion cells and is a form of optic neuropathy. In some cases the intraocular pressure is raised, and ischaemia of the optic nerve head may be the cause. In many cases, however, the pressure in the anterior chamber of the eye is normal and a genetic susceptibility to retinal ganglion cell apoptosis is responsible. The diagnosis requires both structural and functional changes in the eye. There is evidence of optic disc damage with deepening and widening of the depression or cup of the optic disc. Progressive visual defects occur, initially as scotomas (blind spots) in the peripheral visual field. These scotomas enlarge, resulting in tunnel vision and finally total blindness. Glaucoma is the second most common cause of blindness in the UK.

Open-angle glaucoma is caused by obstruction to outflow through the trabecular meshwork, caused by injury or death of cells. It can be associated with raised intraocular pressure, but in other cases the pressure in the eye is normal and retinal cell loss is related to the ability of the optic nerve head to withstand stress imposed by the pressure in the eye.

Angle-closure glaucoma is less common, and results from the iris blocking the drainage angle and preventing drainage through the trabecular meshwork. This usually arises when there is a shallow anterior chamber, such as occurs in long-sighted individuals. The condition is usually chronic and asymptomatic, with a risk of acute attacks of high intraocular pressure with pain and sudden visual loss.

DRUGS FOR GLAUCOMA

Beta-adrenoceptor antagonists

Examples

betaxolol, timolol

Beta-adrenoceptor antagonists reduce the formation of aqueous humour by the ciliary body. They have no effect on accommodation or pupil size. Systemic absorption can produce the typical unwanted effects associated with these compounds, particularly bronchospasm, bradycardia and worsening of uncontrolled heart failure (Ch. 5). The contraindications for topical use in the eye are the same as those for oral use. Timolol is a non-selective β-adrenoceptor antagonist whereas betaxolol is 'cardioselective', but they have similar efficacy in the eye.

Sympathomimetics

Example

brimonidine

Brimonidine is a selective α_2-adrenoceptor agonist that reduces aqueous humour production. It can cause dry mouth, gastrointestinal disturbances, taste disturbances and headache.

Carbonic anhydrase inhibitors

Examples

acetazolamide, brinzolamide, dorzolamide

The intracellular mechanism of action of carbonic anhydrase inhibitors is discussed in Ch. 14. Carbonic anhydrase in the eye plays a key role in controlling aqueous humour production. It is responsible for secreting about 70% of the Na^+ that enters the anterior chamber, which is accompanied by water to maintain isotonicity. Therefore, inhibition of the enzyme reduces aqueous humour production.

Acetazolamide is taken orally. Dorzolamide and brinzolamide are topical preparations for the eye, with fewer systemic unwanted effects; their duration of action in the eye is 6–12 h, but they have extremely long plasma half-lives (≥2 weeks) due to retention within erythrocytes.

Prostaglandin analogues

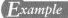
Example

latanoprost, travoprost

These drugs are analogues of prostaglandin $F_{2\alpha}$. Their precise mechanism of action in glaucoma remains uncertain, but they increase uveoscleral outflow of aqueous humour. This may result in part from an increase in extracellular matrix metalloproteinases in ciliary smooth muscle cells, and from remodelling of the uveal meshwork. Prostaglandin analogues also increase blood flow to the optic nerve, and this may contribute to neuroprotection in the retina. The reduction in intraocular pressure is greater than that achieved by β-adrenoceptor antagonists. The major disadvantage of prostaglandin analogues is an increase in brown pigmentation of the iris and growth of eyelashes. A rare complication in people who have no lens in the eye (aphakia) is the development of cystoid macular oedema, which responds to treatment with non-steroidal anti-inflammatory drugs. The prostaglandin analogues have a long duration of action of 1–2 days that is not a reflection of their half-lives.

Miotic drugs (muscarinic agonists)

Example

pilocarpine

Pilocarpine is usually given for angle-closure glaucoma to contract the circular sphincter muscle of the iris to produce miosis and open up the drainage channels in the anterior chamber of the eye (see also Ch. 4). The miotic effect lasts for about 4 h, but more prolonged miosis can be achieved by the use of a gel delivery system. It is not widely used since ciliary muscle spasm is an undesirable consequence and produces blurred vision and an ache over the eye (especially in younger people).

TREATMENT OF GLAUCOMA

In open-angle glaucoma, reducing intraocular pressure can slow the rate of disease progression sufficiently to prevent significant visual impairment. A target pressure reduction of at least 30% below the presenting pressure is usually set. Treatment of ocular hypertension without evidence of visual loss may prevent the onset of glaucoma.

In primary open-angle glaucoma, a topical β-adrenoceptor antagonist or a prostaglandin analogue is the treatment of choice, because of their relative lack of ocular unwanted effects. If either treatment alone is insufficient, then a combination can give an additive effect. If these agents cannot be used then the choice of a second-line drug lies between a topical carbonic anhydrase inhibitor or a sympathomimetic. Surgery may also be considered at this point. Laser burns applied to the trabecular meshwork can produce a temporary increase in aqueous humour outflow, but drug treatment may still be required. Drainage surgery is the alternative and can often bring about long-term pressure control. The therapeutic challenge is to develop neuroprotective drugs to retard neuronal apoptosis in the retina.

Angle-closure glaucoma is treated by laser peripheral iridotomy or surgical peripheral iridectomy to provide a channel for aqueous humour to flow through the iris. If drug therapy is required after surgery then topical treatment with a prostaglandin analogue or a β-adrenoceptor antagonist can be used.

MYDRIATIC AND CYCLOPLEGIC DRUGS

ANTIMUSCARINICS

 Examples

atropine, cyclopentolate, homatropine, tropicamide

Antimuscarinic drugs (see also Ch. 4) are both mydriatic (dilating the pupil) and cycloplegic (paralysing the ciliary muscle). Tropicamide is weak and short-acting (about 3 h), which makes it useful for dilating the pupil for fundal examination. Cyclopentolate is longer-acting (up to 24 h) and has a rapid onset of action. Homatropine and atropine have actions up to 3 and 7 days, respectively. The longer-acting compounds are used to prevent adhesions (posterior synechiae) in anterior uveitis (often in combination with phenylephrine). Dark irises are more resistant to pupillary dilation with these drugs, as the pigments adsorb the applied drug.

The degree of cycloplegia will depend on the dose of drug; small doses produce pupil dilation and diffusion is insufficient to reach the ciliary muscle and has little effect on accommodation. UK law does not specifically prohibit driving after pupil dilation, but many people find that their vision is impaired for several hours. Care must be taken when using these drugs in individuals predisposed to acute angle-closure glaucoma. Local irritation in the eye is the most common unwanted effect, but systemic effects occasionally occur in children or the elderly (see Ch. 4).

SYMPATHOMIMETICS

 Example

phenylephrine

Phenylephrine is a relatively selective α_1-adrenoceptor agonist that stimulates the radial muscle of the iris and produces mydriasis. It does not affect the ciliary muscle, and therefore does not affect accommodation. It is a vasoconstrictor, and can decrease vascular congestion of the conjunctiva and oedema of the eyelid in allergic conjunctivitis. In this role it is often combined with an antihistamine in over-the-counter preparations. Local irritation is the most common unwanted effect, although systemic vasoconstriction with hypertension or coronary artery spasm can occur occasionally. It is often given together with muscarinic receptor-blocking drugs to produce pupil dilation for procedures such as cataract operations.

OTHER TOPICAL APPLICATIONS FOR THE EYE

Several other drugs are used topically in the eye.

ANTIBACTERIAL AGENTS

These are given for local infections such as blepharitis, conjunctivitis or trachoma (caused by chlamydial infection) (see also Ch. 51). Aqueous solutions are diluted rapidly or flushed away by lacrimation and should initially be used every 1–2 h; ointments are often given for longer action, for example at night. Examples of broad-spectrum antibacterial agents are gentamicin, chloramphenicol, ciprofloxacin, fusidic acid, neomycin and (for trachoma) chlortetracycline.

ANTIVIRAL AGENTS

These are mainly used for herpes simplex infection, which causes dendritic corneal ulcers (see also Ch. 51). Aciclovir is most frequently used.

CORTICOSTEROIDS

Local inflammatory conditions of the anterior part of the eye, such as uveitis and scleritis, are treated with corticosteroids, for example dexamethasone or prednisolone (Ch. 44). Care must be taken to exclude a viral dendritic ulcer and glaucoma before using them, since these conditions can be exacerbated by corticosteroids. Prolonged use of corticosteroids can lead to thinning of the sclera or cornea, or formation of a 'steroid cataract'.

ANTIALLERGIC AGENTS

Topical antihistamines such as antazoline (usually given in combination with the sympathomimetic xylometazoline) or levocabastine (Ch. 39) can be given for allergic conjunctivitis. Topical sodium cromoglicate or nedocromil (Ch. 12) are generally less effective than antihistamines.

LOCAL ANAESTHETICS

Oxybuprocaine or lidocaine eye drops provide surface anaesthesia (Ch. 18) for tonometry (measurements of pressure in the anterior chamber). For minor surgical procedures, such as removal of cataracts, tetracaine gives more profound anaesthesia and may be combined with injection of a small amount of lidocaine into the anterior chamber.

NON-STEROIDAL ANTI-INFLAMMATORY DRUGS

Diclofenac, flurbiprofen and ketorolac (Ch. 29) can be applied topically for pain following surgery or laser treatment in the eye.

ARTIFICIAL TEARS

Hypromellose (hydroxypropyl-methylcellulose) is most commonly used to treat dry eyes, such as occurs in Sjögren's syndrome. It may need to be reapplied every hour. The surface mucin in the eye is often abnormal when there is tear deficiency, and the mucolytic agent acetylcysteine is often added to hypromellose. Carbomers, synthetic high-molecular-weight polymers of acrylic acid, cling better to the surface of the eye than hypromellose and need less frequent application.

AGE-RELATED MACULAR DEGENERATION

Age-related macular degeneration (ARMD) is the main cause of irreversible visual loss in the Western world. Damage to the macula, the central part of the retina, leads to partial or complete loss of central vision. There are two clinical types:

- dry (non-exudative) ARMD that involves hypertrophic changes in the retinal pigment epithelium under the macula, with formation of yellow deposits called drusen,
- wet (exudative) ARMD with development of new blood vessels (choroidal neovascularisation) under the macula, with leakage of blood and fluid.

Dry maculopathy is common (85–90% of all macular pathology) and is associated with minor visual disturbance. By contrast, wet ARMD produces severe visual loss in 70% of eyes within 2 years. The dry form of ARMD can progress to the wet form.

TREATMENT OF AGE-RELATED MACULAR DEGENERATION

Treatment is only available for wet ARMD. Options include:

- high-dose antioxidants,
- laser photocoagulation of neovascular tissue,
- photodynamic therapy using the photosensitising agent verteporfin. Verteporfin is infused intravenously and activated in the eye by non-thermal red light, producing cytotoxic derivatives,
- intravitreal injection of a vascular endothelial growth factor (VEGF) inhibitor such as the monoclonal antibodies ranibizumab or bevacizumab (Ch. 52). VEGF is a protein that induces angiogenesis and increases vascular permeability

Treatment of exudative ARMD slows the loss of visual acuity in 20–30% of eyes compared to no treatment.

SELF-ASSESSMENT

True/false questions

1. The production of aqueous humour is not altered in glaucoma.
2. Brimonidine reduces aqueous humour secretion and causes mydriasis.
3. Stimulation of β-adrenoceptors in the ciliary body reduces aqueous humour production.
4. Tropicamide should be avoided in people with glaucoma.
5. Accommodation of the lens is controlled by the sympathetic autonomic nervous system.
6. Cocaine causes mydriasis when administered topically to the eye.
7. Cyclopentolate is a short-acting mydriatic drug used for fundal examination.
8. Pilocarpine causes accommodation for near vision.
9. Dry (non-exudative) age-related macular degeneration (AMRD) produces severe visual loss.
10. Bevacizumab may be given by intravitreal injection in wet AMRD.

Extended-matching-item questions

Match each statement 1–4 below with the appropriate drug from options A–F.

A. Pilocarpine
B. Phenylephrine
C. Tetracaine
D. Tropicamide
E. Timolol
F. Atropine

1. An antagonist of receptors in the ciliary body that will reduce aqueous production in glaucoma but with no effect on pupil size.
2. A drug that dilates the pupil without affecting accommodation or production of aqueous humour.
3. A relatively short-acting drug that will dilate the pupil and is weakly cycloplegic.
4. A long-acting and strongly cycloplegic drug that can be used to prevent adhesions (posterior synechiae) in anterior uveitis.

Case-based questions

During a routine eye examination, the optician noted a raised intraocular pressure with optic nerve changes in a 56-year-old woman. Further tests revealed she had open-angle (simple) glaucoma.

A. What is the most common cause of open-angle glaucoma?
B. What drugs could be used for this condition?
C. What precautions should be taken when using these drugs?

True/false answers

1. **True.** Glaucoma is due to reduced outflow of aqueous humour, resulting from obstruction of the trabecular meshwork or closure of the anterior angle.
2. **False.** The selective action of brimonidine on α_2-adrenoceptors reduces aqueous humour production in the ciliary body but does not cause mydriasis or reduce the anterior angle.
3. **False.** Aqueous humour production in the ciliary body is reduced by antagonists of β-adrenoceptors, such as timolol.
4. **True.** Tropicamide blocks muscarinic receptors in the circular muscle of the iris, causing mydriasis, which narrows the anterior angle and may reduce aqueous drainage in angle-closure glaucoma.
5. **False.** The ciliary muscle of the lens is innervated only by parasympathetic autonomic nerves.
6. **True.** Formerly used as a local anaesthetic, cocaine causes mydriasis by preventing reuptake of released noradrenaline, which contracts the iris radial muscle.
7. **False.** Cyclopentolate acts for 12–24 h; tropicamide acts for about 3 h and is therefore more useful for fundal examination.
8. **True.** Pilocarpine is a muscarinic receptor agonist; it contracts the ciliary muscle, causing the lens to accommodate for near vision, and the iris circular muscle, causing miosis.
9. **False.** Dry AMRD causes only minor visual disturbance. Wet (exudative) ARMD produces severe visual loss in 70% of eyes within 2 years.
10. **True.** Bevacizumab is a vascular endothelial growth factor (VEGF) inhibitor that reduces angiogenesis in wet AMRD.

Extended-matching-item answers

1. **Answer E**. Timolol is a β-adrenoceptor antagonist and reduces aqueous production but does not affect the pupil size, which is controlled by muscarinic and α_1-adrenergic receptors on the iris circular and radial muscles, respectively.
2. **Answer B**. Phenylephrine will dilate the pupil by α_1-adrenoceptor stimulation of the iris, but not the ciliary muscle (muscarinic receptors).
3. **Answer D**. Tropicamide is a relatively short-acting muscarinic antagonist with only a relatively weak blocking action on muscarinic receptors on the ciliary muscle.
4. **Answer F**. Atropine is a long-acting mydriatic that can be used to prevent adhesions but strongly blocks accommodation for near vision (cycloplegia).

Case-based answers

A. Reduced drainage of aqueous humour through the trabecular meshwork into the canal of Schlemm and the episcleral veins.
B. Beta-adrenoceptor antagonists or prostaglandin analogues are the drugs of first choice for open-angle glaucoma. Alpha$_2$-adrenoceptor agonists, carbonic anhydrase inhibitors or muscarinic agonists could also be used.
C. Beta-adrenoceptor antagonists: avoid in asthma, bradycardia, heart block, heart failure. Prostaglandin analogues: avoid in pregnancy and asthma. Alpha$_2$-adrenoceptor agonists: avoid in severe cardiovascular disease. Carbonic anhydrase inhibitors: avoid in pregnancy; they can cause hypokalaemia and electrolyte imbalance. Muscarinic agonists: avoid in conjunctival or corneal damage, cardiac disease, asthma.

FURTHER READING

Bielory L (2002) Ocular allergy guidelines. *Drugs* 62, 1611–1634

Chakravarthy U, Evans J, Rosenfeld PJ (2010) Age related macular degeneration. *BMJ* 340, c981

Ghate D, Edelhauser HF (2008) Barriers to glaucoma drug delivery. *J Glaucoma* 17, 147–156

Hylton C, Robin AL (2003) Update on prostaglandin analogs. *Curr Opin Ophthalmol* 14, 65–69

Ishida N, Odani-Kawabata N, Shimazaki A et al. (2006) Prostanoids in the therapy of glaucoma. *Cardiovasc Drug Rev* 24, 1–10

Jager RD, Mieler WF, Miller JW (2008) Age-related macular degeneration. *N Engl J Med* 358, 2606–2617

Quigley HA (2011) Glaucoma. *Lancet* 377, 1362–1377

Saw S-M, Gazzard G, Friedman DS (2003) Interventions for angle-closure glaucoma. An evidence-based update. *Ophthalmology* 110, 1869–1879

Singh A (2005) Medical therapy of glaucoma. *Ophthalmol Clin North Am* 18, 397–408

Takeda AL, Colquitt J, Clegg AJ et al. (2007) Pegaptanib and ranibizumab for neovascular age-related macular degeneration: a systematic review. *Br J Ophthalmol* 91, 1177–1182

Compendium: drugs used in the eye

Drug	Kinetics (half-life)[a]	Comments
Treatment of infections		
Antibacterials		
Systemic treatment may be necessary in some cases (see Ch. 51).		
Azithromycin	No detectable systemic absorption after topical use	Macrolide; used for purulent bacterial conjunctivitis and trachomatous conjunctivitis
Chloramphenicol	Eliminated mainly by glucuronidation (2–12 h)	Broad-spectrum, used for a wide range of infections; drug of choice for superficial eye infections
Ciprofloxacin	Renal elimination, some metabolism (3–4 h)	Quinolone; broad-spectrum, used for a wide range of infections, including *Pseudomonas aeruginosa*; used for corneal ulcers
Fusidic acid	Hepatic metabolism, biliary excretion (9 h)	Used for staphylococcal infections
Gentamicin	Renal elimination (1–4 h)	Aminoglycoside; broad-spectrum, used for a wide range of infections, including *Pseudomonas aeruginosa*
Levofloxacin	Almost 90% excreted unchanged in urine (6–8 h)	Quinolone; active against Gram-positive and especially Gram-negative organisms
Moxifloxacin	Minimal systemic bioavailability after topical use	Quinolone; broad-spectrum, used for a wide range of infections
Neomycin	Renal elimination (2 h)	Aminoglycoside; broad-spectrum, used for a wide range of infections
Ofloxacin	Limited metabolism, mainly renal elimination (6–7 h)	Quinolone; broad-spectrum, used for a wide range of infections, including *Pseudomonas aeruginosa*
Polymyxin B	Renal elimination (4–6 h); elimination prolonged in renal impairment	Used for Gram-negative organisms
Propamidine isetionate	No kinetic data available	Principal use is treatment of the rare but devastating condition *Acanthamoeba* keratitis
Tobramycin	Renal elimination (2 h)	Aminoglycoside; broad-spectrum, used for a wide range of infections, including *Pseudomonas aeruginosa*
Antivirals		
Aciclovir	Renal elimination, some metabolism to inactive products (3 h)	Used for local treatment of herpes simplex infections (see Ch. 51)
Ganciclovir	Renal elimination (4 h)	Used as slow-release implants inserted surgically for sight-threatening cytomegalovirus retinitis (see Ch. 51)
Treatment of inflammation		
Corticosteroids		
The drugs shown below are used locally for short-term treatment of inflammation. Oral corticosteroids (see. Ch. 44) are given for anterior segment inflammation.		
Betamethasone sodium phosphate	Hydrolysed to betamethasone, then inactivated by metabolism (35–55 h)	Available in coformulations with neomycin
Dexamethasone	Hepatic oxidation (2–4 h)	Also given as intravitreal implant for treatment of macular oedema following branch retinal vein occlusion
Fluorometholone	Some metabolism locally in the eye	Only used topically
Hydrocortisone acetate	Metabolised to cortisone and other products (1–2 h)	
Loteprednol etabonate	Negligible systemic absorption	Only used topically
Prednisolone	Extensively metabolised (2–4 h)	
Rimexolone	Hepatic metabolism, faecal excretion (1–2 h)	Only used topically

Compendium: drugs used in the eye—cont'd

Drug	Kinetics (half-life)[a]	Comments
Other anti-inflammatory preparations		
Many are histamine H_1 receptor antagonists (see also Ch. 39).		
Antazoline	No kinetic data available	Histamine H_1 receptor antagonist; used for allergic conjunctivitis
Azelastine	Hepatic metabolism to active desmethyl metabolite (17 h)	Histamine H_1 receptor antagonist; used for allergic conjunctivitis
Emedastine	Oxidised; eliminated in urine (3–4 h)	Histamine H_1 receptor antagonist; used for seasonal allergic conjunctivitis
Epinastine	Mainly eliminated unchanged in urine and faeces (12 h)	Histamine H_1 receptor antagonist; used for seasonal allergic conjunctivitis
Ketotifen	Metabolised by glucuronidation (22 h)	Used for seasonal allergic conjunctivitis; antihistamine and mast cell stabiliser; rapid onset of action after application to the eye and negligible systemic exposure
Lodoxamide	Eliminated largely in the urine as the parent drug (8 h)	Mast cell stabiliser; used for allergic conjunctivitis
Nedocromil	Slow absorption; renal elimination (2 h)	Mast cell stabiliser; used for allergic conjunctivitis
Olopatadine	Minimal systemic absorption; renal elimination (8–12 h)	Antihistamine and mast cell stabiliser; used for seasonal allergic conjunctivitis
Sodium cromoglicate	Limited absorption; renal elimination (1–1.5 h)	Mast cell stabiliser; used for allergic conjunctivitis
Mydriatics and cycloplegics		
Atropine	Extensive hepatic metabolism (2–5 h)	Long-acting antimuscarinic; used for refraction procedures in children and for anterior uveitis
Cyclopentolate	Rapidly absorbed; elimination routes not defined	Long-acting antimuscarinic; used for refraction procedures in children
Homatropine	Probably well absorbed; no kinetic data available	Antimuscarinic; used for treatment of anterior segment inflammation
Phenylephrine	Eliminated in metabolites and parent compound (2–3 h)	Sympathomimetic α_1-selective adrenoceptor agonist
Tropicamide	Rapidly absorbed and eliminated (0.3 h)	Short-acting antimuscarinic; used to facilitate examination of the fundus
Local anaesthetics		
See Chapter 18.		
Lidocaine	Dealkylated and hydrolysed (2 h)	
Oxybuprocaine (benoxinate)	Few kinetic data available (<3 h)	Widely used
Proxymetacaine	Few kinetic data available	Causes less initial stinging and is useful for children
Tetracaine	Rapidly hydrolysed by plasma cholinesterase	Widely used; produces more profound anaesthesia and is suitable for minor procedures
Treatment of glaucoma		
Beta-adrenoceptor antagonists		
Effective in primary open-angle glaucoma.		
Betaxolol	Oxidised in liver, renal elimination (13–24 h)	Selective β_1-adrenoceptor antagonist
Carteolol	Mostly eliminated in urine unchanged (3–7 h)	Non-selective β-adrenoceptor antagonist
Levobunolol	Extensive metabolism, renal elimination (5–8 h)	Non-selective β-adrenoceptor antagonist

Compendium: drugs used in the eye—cont'd

Drug	Kinetics (half-life)[a]	Comments
Timolol	Eliminated by metabolism and renal excretion (2–5 h)	Non-selective β-adrenoceptor antagonist
Miotic		
Pilocarpine	Limited systemic absorption; oxidation (1 h)	Muscarinic agonist; ocular effects persist for 4–14 h
Sympathomimetics		
Apraclonidine	Some systemic absorption (8 h)	α_2-Adrenoceptor agonist; used short term before or after surgery
Brimonidine	Limited systemic absorption; binds to melanin; hepatic oxidation; rapid urinary elimination (3 h)	α_2-Adrenoceptor agonist; used alone or with a β-adrenoceptor antagonist for ocular hypertension, and alone for open-angle glaucoma if β-adrenoceptor antagonists are ineffective or inappropriate
Carbonic anhydrase inhibitors		
Acetazolamide	Renal elimination (6–9 h)	Used for open-angle, and secondary and preoperative angle-closure glaucoma; given orally or by intravenous injection as an adjunct to other treatments; not recommended for long-term use
Brinzolamide	Distributes into erythrocytes, where it has a very long half-life (11 days)	Used topically alone or in combination with a β-adrenoceptor antagonist for ocular hypertension and open-angle glaucoma if β-adrenoceptor antagonists are ineffective or inappropriate
Dorzolamide	Negligible systemic bioavailability	Used topically alone or in combination with a β-adrenoceptor antagonist for ocular hypertension, and open-angle and pseudo-exfoliative glaucoma if β-adrenoceptor antagonists are ineffective or inappropriate
Prostaglandin analogues		
Used to reduce pressure in ocular hypertension and open-angle glaucoma.		
Bimatoprost	Rapid absorption; metabolised by oxidation and conjugation (45 min)	Prostamide analogue of $PGF_{2\alpha}$; used alone or as adjunctive therapy
Latanoprost	Rapid absorption; active metabolite has half-life of 0.3 h	Synthetic analogue of $PGF_{2\alpha}$; also available as coformulation with timolol
Tafluprost	Hydrolysed to tafluprost acid	Fluorinated analogue of $PGF_{2\alpha}$; preservative-free to reduce irritation
Travoprost	Prodrug hydrolysed by esterases in the eye to active travoprost acid	Synthetic analogue of $PGF_{2\alpha}$

[a]The half-life data are systemic data following absorption into the general circulation; the duration of local action will depend on the rate of uptake by, and removal from, the eye. Drugs are usually given topically to reduce unwanted systemic effects.
PG, prostaglandin.

11

Chemotherapy

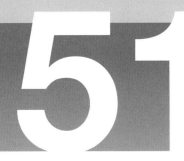

Chemotherapy of infections

Antimicrobial drugs are natural or synthetic chemical substances that suppress the growth of, or destroy, micro-organisms including bacteria, fungi, helminths, protozoa and viruses. The term antibiotic is widely used, but strictly should be reserved for those antimicrobial drugs that are derived from micro-organisms. The term antimicrobial or the more restrictive terms antibacterial, antifungal, antihelminthic, antiprotozoal and antiviral are used in this book.

Effective antimicrobial drugs have certain key attributes. In order to minimise unwanted effects in humans, most are designed to act on processes that are unique to the target pathogen. They must also be able to penetrate human tissues to reach the site of infection. Micro-organisms can acquire resistance to various antimicrobial drugs and will then no longer be affected by the drug, so there is a continuing effort to discover and develop antimicrobial drugs that avoid or overcome the evolving mechanisms of resistance.

BACTERIAL INFECTIONS

CLASSIFICATION OF ANTIBACTERIAL DRUGS

Antibacterial drugs can be classified in several overlapping ways.

Firstly, they can be **bacteriostatic** or **bactericidal**. This categorisation depends largely on the concentration of drug that can be achieved safely in plasma without causing significant toxicity in the person who takes the drug. Bacteriostatic antibacterials inhibit bacterial growth but do not destroy the bacteria at concentrations in plasma that are safe for humans; following inhibition of growth, the natural immune mechanisms of the body are able to eliminate the bacteria. Such drugs will be less effective in immunocompromised individuals or when the bacteria are dormant and not dividing. At plasma concentrations that are safe for humans, bactericidal antibacterials kill bacteria but, even then, immune mechanisms will play a role in the final elimination of the bacteria. Some bactericidal drugs are more effective when bacterial cells are actively dividing, and may therefore be less effective if taken together with a bacteriostatic drug. For antibacterials to be bactericidal they must be present at adequate concentration; too low a concentration may render them bacteriostatic.

Secondly, antibacterials can be grouped according to their **mechanisms of action** (Fig. 51.1):

- inhibition of the synthesis of bacterial cell wall peptidoglycans or activation of enzymes that disrupt the cell wall (e.g. β-lactams),
- increased permeability of the bacterial cell phospholipid membrane, leading to leakage of intracellular contents (e.g. polymyxins),
- impaired bacterial ribosome function, producing a reversible inhibition of protein synthesis (e.g. aminoglycosides, macrolides). Such drugs can show selectivity because bacterial 70S ribosomes differ structurally from the 80S ribosomes in humans,
- selective block of bacterial metabolic pathways (e.g. trimethoprim),
- interference with replication of bacterial DNA or RNA (e.g. quinolones).

Thirdly, antibacterials may be classified according to whether their **spectrum of activity** against bacteria is limited (narrow-spectrum) or extensive (broad-spectrum).

Finally, they can be classified by **chemical structure**. In the following text, the antimicrobial drugs are grouped according to their mechanism of action and then by their

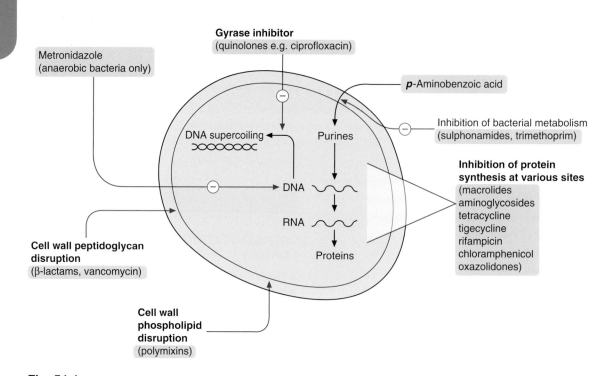

Fig. 51.1 The sites of action of the main classes of antibacterial drugs.

chemical structure. Cross-referencing to other methods of classification may be necessary. The drug compendium at the end of the chapter is organised to accord with the *British National Formulary*.

ANTIMICROBIAL RESISTANCE

When an antibacterial is ineffective against a bacterium, the organism is said to be resistant to the antibacterial drug. Resistance to antibacterial drugs can be intrinsic to the bacterium (innate resistance) or can be acquired by modification of its genetic structure (acquired resistance).

Resistance is a major problem in treating infections with bacteria, and also for many protozoa (e.g. malaria) and viruses (e.g. HIV), but is less significant in fungal infections (unless the person has immunodeficiency).

ANTIBACTERIAL DRUG RESISTANCE

There are four general processes by which a bacterium can acquire resistance to antibacterial drugs (Fig. 51.2):

- modification of the bacterium such that it produces enzymes that inactivate the drug; examples are β-lactamase enzymes, which inactivate some penicillins, and acetylating enzymes, which can inactivate aminoglycosides,
- modification of the bacterium so that penetration of the drug is reduced; an example is the absence of the membrane protein D2 porin in resistant *Pseudomonas aeruginosa*, which prevents penetration of the β-lactam antibacterial imipenem,

- acquisition of efflux pumps that remove the antibacterial drug from the cell faster than it can enter; an example is quinolone efflux pumps in *Staphylococcus aureus*,
- structural change in the target molecule for the antibacterial drug; examples are mutated penicillin-binding proteins in resistant enterococci that have a low affinity for binding of cephalosporins, and mutated dihydrofolate reductase that is not inhibited by trimethoprim (see Fig. 51.4, below).

The major mechanisms by which bacteria acquire resistance to antibacterial drugs are spontaneous mutation, conjugation, transduction and transformation.

Spontaneous mutation

In this process, a single-step genetic mutation in a bacterial population leads to resistant organisms that selectively survive and grow while sensitive bacteria are killed by an antibacterial drug. This is termed *vertical evolution*.

The other three mechanisms involve acquisition from other resistant organisms of genetic material that confers resistance. This is termed *horizontal evolution*.

Conjugation

Direct cell-to-cell contact is a way of exchanging genetic material that confers antibacterial resistance. It usually involves transfer of self-replicating circular fragments of DNA (plasmids), which can contain multiple resistance genes. A transposon (a DNA sequence that can change its relative position within the genome) may facilitate transfer of sections of DNA from one organism to another by

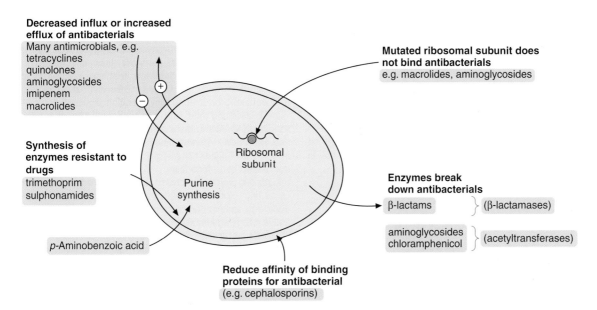

Decreased influx or increased efflux of antibacterials
Many antimicrobials, e.g.
tetracyclines
quinolones
aminoglycosides
imipenem
macrolides

Mutated ribosomal subunit does not bind antibacterials
e.g. macrolides, aminoglycosides

Ribosomal subunit

Synthesis of enzymes resistant to drugs
trimethoprim
sulphonamides

Purine synthesis

Enzymes break down antibacterials
β-lactams } (β-lactamases)

aminoglycosides
chloramphenicol } (acetyltransferases)

p-Aminobenzoic acid

Reduce affinity of binding proteins for antibacterial
(e.g. cephalosporins)

Fig. 51.2 Mechanisms of bacterial resistance to antibacterial drugs.

jumping to plasmid DNA. Transfer of the plasmid occurs via a connecting structure called a pilus. The plasmid can remain outside the genome of the bacterium or can be incorporated into it, when it is more stable but less transmissible. Conjugation is by far the most important source of extrinsic DNA transfer between bacteria.

Transduction

Bacteria are susceptible to infection by viruses known as bacteriophages. During replication of the bacteriophages, the host bacterial cell's DNA (containing resistance genes) may be replicated along with bacteriophage DNA and taken into the virus. The phage carrying the resistance genes can then infect other bacterial cells and spread resistance. This method of acquired resistance is rare.

Transformation

Uptake of DNA from dead bacteria by live bacteria can spread resistance genes.

ANTIBACTERIAL DRUGS

The antibacterial drugs in this section are grouped by their mechanism of action and then by their chemical structure.

Drugs affecting the cell wall: β-lactam antibacterials

The drugs in this class all have a β-lactam ring which must be intact for them to be active (Fig. 51.3). The β-lactam antibacterials include penicillins, cephalosporins and cephamycins, monobactams and carbapenems. Some are susceptible to attack by bacterial enzymes (β-lactamases, also known as penicillinases) that split the β-lactam ring,

but others have structural modifications that confer resistance to β-lactamase inactivation.

Mechanism of action of β-lactam antibacterials

Beta-lactam antibacterials bind to several penicillin-binding proteins in bacteria. Some of these proteins are transpeptidases that are required for crosslinking of the peptidoglycan layer of the cell wall which surrounds certain bacteria and is essential for their survival. Inhibition of transpeptidase activity by β-lactam antibacterials prevents the bacterium synthesising an intact cell wall when it divides. The transmembrane osmotic gradient then leads to swelling, rupture and death of the bacterium.

Some bacterial cells also contain enzymes that cause cell lysis when activated. The binding of β-lactam antibacterials to other specific penicillin-binding proteins within bacteria reduces the production of natural inhibitors of lysis-inducing enzymes, promoting lysis of the bacterial cell wall.

Penicillins

penicillins: benzylpenicillin, phenoxymethylpenicillin
aminopenicillins: amoxicillin, ampicillin, flucloxacillin
ureidopenicillins: piperacillin
amidinopenicillin: pivmecillinam
carboxypenicillin: ticarcillin

Spectrum of activity

Penicillins consist of a thiazolidine ring connected to a β-lactam ring, to which is in turn attached a side-chain (Fig. 51.3). The side-chain determines many of the antibacterial and pharmacological characteristics of particular penicillins (Table 51.1).

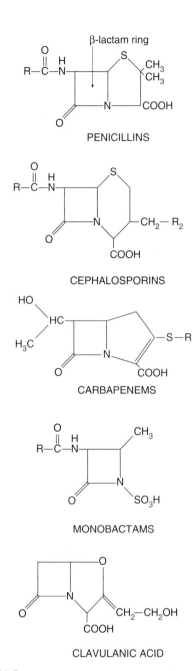

Fig. 51.3 **The structural backbones of β-lactam antibacterial drugs.** Also shown is the β-lactamase inhibitor, clavulanic acid.

Benzylpenicillin (penicillin G) and phenoxymethylpenicillin (penicillin V) are active against many aerobic Gram-positive bacteria, a more limited range of Gram-negative bacteria, for example cocci (e.g. gonococci and meningococci), and many anaerobic micro-organisms. Gram-negative bacilli are not sensitive to these drugs. Benzylpenicillin and phenoxymethylpenicillin are only effective against organisms that do not produce β-lactamases (see below).

Flucloxacillin has an acyl side chain attached to the β-lactam ring which prevents access of β-lactamase to the ring and makes the drug resistant to inactivation by the enzyme. Flucloxacillin is generally less effective than benzylpenicillin against bacteria that do not produce β-lactamase, and is usually reserved for treating β-lactamase-producing staphylococci.

Ampicillin and amoxicillin are aminopenicillins that have an extended spectrum of activity to include many Gram-negative bacilli. However, they are less effective than benzylpenicillin against Gram-positive cocci. Both drugs are inactivated by β-lactamase.

Other extended-spectrum penicillins include ureidopenicillins (e.g. piperacillin), which are active against *P. aeruginosa*, and amidinopenicillins (e.g. pivmecillinam), which are active mainly against Gram-negative bacteria. Carboxypenicillins (e.g. ticarcillin) are not widely used, but have activity against *Pseudomonas* species, *Proteus* species and *Bacteroides fragilis*.

Clavulanic acid is a potent inhibitor of several β-lactamases. It is structurally related to the β-lactam antibiotics, although it has little intrinsic antibacterial activity (Fig. 51.3). It is available in combined formulations with penicillins that are destroyed by β-lactamase, such as amoxicillin (as co-amoxiclav) or ticarcillin (Table 51.1); the combination drugs can be used to treat infections caused by some β-lactamase-producing organisms that would otherwise be resistant to the antibacterial. Tazobactam has similar properties to clavulanic acid and is used in combination with piperacillin.

Resistance

Resistance to penicillins is most often due to the production of β-lactamases which hydrolyse the β-lactam ring (Fig. 51.3). There are hundreds of β-lactamases, many of which are closely related to penicillin-binding proteins, but some are structurally different metalloenzymes. The β-lactamases produced by various organisms have widely differing spectra of activity. Some bacteria release extracellular β-lactamases, particularly *S. aureus*. In Gram-negative bacteria the β-lactamases are located between the inner and outer cell membranes in the periplasmic space. Extended-spectrum β-lactamases (ESBLs) are β-lactamases that also hydrolyse extended-spectrum 'third-generation' cephalosporins, such as cefotaxime and ceftriaxone, and monobactams such as aztreonam (see below). ESBLs are most often produced by enterobacteria. The genetic information for β-lactamase production is often encoded in a plasmid and this may be transferred to other bacteria by conjugation. By contrast, the broader-spectrum β-lactamases are often encoded by chromosomal genes.

An alternative type of penicillin resistance occurs in gonococci and in meticillin-resistant *S. aureus* (MRSA), which develop mutated penicillin-binding proteins that do not bind β-lactam antibacterials. Meticillin has now been discontinued, but the name MRSA is still used.

Pharmacokinetics

Only about one-third of an oral dose of benzylpenicillin (penicillin G) is absorbed; the rest is destroyed by acid in the stomach. Benzylpenicillin is therefore restricted to intramuscular or intravenous administration. The phenoxymethyl

Table 51.1 Examples of penicillins and their properties

	Streptococci	Staphylococcus aureus		Enterobacteriaceae (coliforms)	Pseudomonas aeruginosa	Bacteroides fragilis
		GRAM-POSITIVE STAINING		GRAM-NEGATIVE STAINING		
		β-Lactamase negative	β-Lactamase positive			
Benzylpenicillin/ phenoxymethylpenicillin	+	+	0	0	0	++
Broader spectrum						
Amoxicillin/ampicillin	+	+	0[a]	++	0	0
Beta-lactamase-resistant						
Flucloxacillin	+	+	+[b]	0	0	0
Antipseudomonal						
Ticarcillin	+	+	0[c]	+	+	+/0
Piperacillin	+	+	0[c]	+	+	+/0

+, Active; +/0, variable activity; 0, inactive or poor activity.
[a]Can be used combined with a β-lactamase inhibitor, e.g. amoxicillin plus clavulanic acid (co-amoxiclav).
[b]Resistance is increasing.
[c]Ticarcillin only available with clavulanic acid. Piperacillin is combined with the β-lactamase inhibitor tazobactam.

derivative (penicillin V) is more acid-stable and better absorbed from the gut; it has a similar spectrum of activity as benzylpenicillin but is generally less active. Penicillins are widely distributed through the body, although transport across the meninges is poor unless they are acutely inflamed (e.g. in meningitis). The half-lives of benzylpenicillin and phenoxymethylpenicillin, in common with most penicillins, are short (about 1 h) because they are rapidly eliminated by the kidney, mainly by active secretion at the proximal tubule. Flucloxacillin and amoxicillin are rapidly and almost completely absorbed from the gut, but ampicillin is incompletely absorbed. These drugs can also be given intramuscularly or intravenously. They are eliminated by the kidney in a similar way to benzylpenicillin. The amidinopenicillin pivmecillinam is a prodrug for oral use which is hydrolysed to mecillinam. The carboxypenicillin ticarcillin is only available in combination with clavulanic acid for intravenous use. The ureidopenicillin piperacillin is given intravenously in combination with the β-lactamase inhibitor tazobactam.

Unwanted effects

Penicillins are normally well tolerated and have a high therapeutic index.

- Nausea, vomiting.
- Allergic reactions in 1–10% of exposed individuals. Penicillins and their breakdown products bind to proteins and act as haptens, stimulating the production of antibodies that mediate the allergic response (Chs 38 and 53). Manifestations of allergy to penicillins include fever, vasculitis, serum sickness, exfoliative dermatitis, Stevens–Johnson syndrome and anaphylactic shock. Cross-allergenicity is widespread among various penicillins and to a lesser extent with cephalosporins.
- Aminopenicillins (e.g. amoxicillin) frequently produce a non-allergic maculopapular rash in people with glandular fever. This does not recur if another type of penicillin is given.
- Reversible neutropenia and eosinophilia with prolonged high doses.
- Encephalopathy with excessively high cerebrospinal fluid (CSF) concentrations of penicillin. This occurs in severe renal failure or after inadvertent intrathecal injection (which should never be given).
- Diarrhoea or *Clostridium difficile*-related colitis as a result of disturbance of normal colonic flora, especially with broad-spectrum penicillins.
- Cholestatic jaundice, especially with flucloxacillin or clavulanic acid.

Cephalosporins

first generation: cefadroxil, cefalexin
second generation: cefaclor, cefuroxime
third generation: cefotaxime, cefixime, ceftazidime, ceftriaxone

Spectrum of activity

Cephalosporins, like penicillins, have a β-lactam ring, to which is fused a dihydrothiazine ring, which makes them more resistant to hydrolysis by β-lactamases (Fig. 51.3). Cephalosporins are often classified by 'generations', the members within each generation sharing similar antibacterial activity. Successive generations tend to have increased activity against Gram-negative bacilli, usually at the expense of Gram-positive activity, and an increased ability to cross the blood–brain barrier (Table 51.2).

Table 51.2 Examples of β-lactams other than penicillins and their spectra of activity

	Staphylococcus aureus	Haemophilus influenzae	Enterobacteriaceae (coliforms)	Pseudomonas aeruginosa	Bacteroides fragilis	Ability to cross blood–brain barrier	Resistance to β-lactamase
Cephalosporins							
First generation							
Cefadroxil/cefradine (oral)	+	0	+/0	0	0	+/0	+
Cefalexin (oral)	+	0	+/0	0	0	+/0	+
Second generation							
Cefuroxime axetil (oral)	+	+	+	0	+	+	+
Cefuroxime (parenteral)	+	+	+	0	+	+	+
Third generation							
Cefixime (oral)	0	+	+	0	0	+	+
Cefotaxime (parenteral)	+	+	+	0	+	+	+
Ceftazidime (parenteral)	0	0	+	+	0	+/0[a]	+
Monobactams (aztreonam)	0	+	0	+	+	+	+/0
Carbapenems (imipenem)	+	+	+	+	+	+	+

This table is a general guide to selected drugs and susceptibilities of organisms can vary widely.
Staphylococcus aureus is a Gram-positive staining organism. Other illustrative bacteria are Gram-negative staining.
[a]Some cephalosporins penetrate better into the CNS in the presence of inflamed meninges.

■ First-generation cephalosporins (e.g. cefadroxil or cefalexin) have activity against staphylococci and most streptococci, but not enterococci.

■ Second-generation cephalosporins (e.g. cefuroxime) have additional activity against some Gram-negative bacteria such as *Haemophilus influenzae* and *Neisseria gonorrhoeae*. They are able to penetrate the blood–brain barrier.

■ Third-generation cephalosporins have improved β-lactamase stability and are able to penetrate the CSF in useful quantities. They also have greater Gram-negative activity than the other two generations. Cefixime adds *Proteus* and *Klebsiella* species to its spectrum, but it has no activity against staphylococci (Table 51.2). Ceftazidime has good activity against *Pseudomonas* species.

Resistance

The later generations are more resistant to β-lactamase-mediated enzymatic hydrolysis of the β-lactam ring than are the earlier generations (Table 51.2). However, ESBLs can be acquired by *Escherichia coli* and and other enterobacteria, which confers resistance to third-generation cephalosporins.

Pharmacokinetics

First-generation oral cephalosporins are well absorbed from the gut. Several second- and third-generation drugs, for example cefuroxime and cefotaxime, are acid-labile and must be given by a parenteral route. Cefuroxime has been formulated as a prodrug for oral use (cefuroxime axetil), which is hydrolysed to cefuroxime at first pass through the liver. Most cephalosporins are excreted primarily by the kidney and have short half-lives (less than 3 h), but cefixime is mainly eliminated by biliary excretion. Ceftriaxone has a longer half-life (6–9 h), probably as a result of extensive plasma protein binding.

Unwanted effects

■ Nausea, vomiting, abdominal discomfort.

■ Headache.

■ Rashes, including erythema multiforme and toxic epidermal necrolysis.

■ Cephalosporins can produce allergic reactions similar to those observed with the penicillins. Fewer than 10% of people who are allergic to penicillins show cross-allergy to cephalosporins, but a history of a serious reaction to penicillins precludes the use of cephalosporins.

■ Diarrhoea or *C. difficile*-related colitis can be caused by disturbance of normal bowel flora. This is more common with oral cephalosporins, and is more frequent than with many other antimicrobials.

Monobactams

Example

aztreonam

Aztreonam is a β-lactam antibacterial related to the penicillins but with a single ring structure ('monocyclic β-lactam')

(Fig. 51.3). It has little cross-allergenicity with the penicillins and has been successfully given to people with proven penicillin allergy. Its spectrum of activity is limited to Gram-negative bacteria, including *P. aeruginosa*, *Neisseria meningitidis*, *N. gonorrhoeae* and *H. influenzae*, with no activity against Gram-positive bacteria or anaerobes. Aztreonam is given intramuscularly or intravenously and is resistant to most β-lactamases. However, ESBLs can be acquired by *E. coli* and other enterobacteria, which confer resistance to aztreonam. Aztreonam is excreted by the kidney and has a half-life of about 2 h. Unwanted effects are similar to those of other β-lactam antibacterials.

Carbapenems

Examples

ertapenem, imipenem, meropenem

Imipenem is a β-lactam drug that has an extremely broad spectrum of bactericidal activity. It has potent activity against Gram-positive cocci, including some β-lactamase-producing pneumococci (Table 51.2), Gram-negative bacilli, including *P. aeruginosa*, *Neisseria suppurans* and *Bacteroides* species, and also many anaerobic bacteria. Imipenem can penetrate the blood–brain barrier and is resistant to β-lactamases. Narrow-spectrum resistance to imipenem in *P. aeruginosa* occurs from a mutation that results in loss of a specific cell membrane uptake pathway.

Meropenem and ertapenem are structurally related and have broad spectra of activity against Gram-positive and Gram-negative bacteria, but ertapenem is inactive against *Pseudomonas* species. Imipenem, meropenem and ertapenem are given intravenously; imipenem can also be given by deep intramuscular injection. Imipenem is rapidly hydrolysed by dihydropeptidases in the kidney and so is given in combination with the dihydropeptidase inhibitor cilastatin. Meropenem and ertapenem are not inactivated by the renal dihydropeptidase and can be given alone.

These drugs are mainly excreted by the kidney and have short half-lives (1–5 h). Unwanted effects are similar to those of other β-lactam antibacterials, except for neurotoxicity with seizures, which is more common with imipenem than with other carbapenems.

Other drugs affecting the cell wall

Glycopeptides

Examples

teicoplanin, vancomycin

Mechanism of action

Vancomycin and teicoplanin are high-molecular-weight glycopeptide compounds that inhibit bacterial cell wall synthesis by preventing the linking of peptidoglycan constituents (Fig. 51.1). Glycopeptides are bactericidal.

Spectrum of activity

Vancomycin and teicoplanin are active only against Gram-positive bacteria, particularly meticillin-resistant staphylococci. They do not penetrate the cell wall of Gram-negative bacteria. Both are usually reserved for treatment of serious Gram-positive bacterial infection or for bacterial endocarditis that is not responding to other treatments. Vancomycin given orally is also effective against *C. difficile*, which colonises the colon when the normal gut flora is disturbed by antibacterial drugs, causing diarrhoea and colitis. Metronidazole (see below) is preferred for this indication, but resistance to metronidazole is increasingly common.

Resistance

Acquired resistance to vancomycin is uncommon. In *S. aureus* it arises as a result of a multi-step genetic acquisition of a thickened peptidoglycan cell wall. This traps the drug and prevents it reaching its target on the cytoplasmic membrane. For other bacteria, plasmid-mediated resistance involves incorporation of D-lactate into the cell wall in place of D-alanine. This modification prevents binding of the glycopeptide.

Pharmacokinetics

Both vancomycin and teicoplanin are poorly absorbed orally and are given by intravenous infusion for systemic infection. Teicoplanin can also be given by intramuscular injection. Oral vancomycin is only used for treating *C. difficile*-related colitis. Both drugs are excreted by the kidney; vancomycin has a shorter half-life (5–11 h) than teicoplanin (32–176 h). Plasma concentration monitoring of vancomycin is used to minimise the risk of toxicity.

Unwanted effects

Dose adjustment based on monitoring of the trough plasma concentration of vancomycin may reduce the risk of toxic effects.

- Nephrotoxicity, which may be enhanced if used in combination with an aminoglycoside.
- Thrombophlebitis at the site of infusion.
- Rashes, including Stevens–Johnson syndrome and toxic epidermal necrolysis. Rapid intravenous injection of vancomycin produces upper body flushing, the 'red man' syndrome.
- Blood disorders, including neutropenia, thrombocytopenia.
- Ototoxicity is uncommon. It usually starts with tinnitus.
- Nausea.

Daptomycin
Mechanism of action

Daptomycin is a lipopeptide antibacterial with a unique mode of action. It binds to the cell wall of Gram-positive bacteria, and creates transmembrane channels that allow leakage of intracellular ions, destroying the membrane potential across the cell.

Spectrum of activity

Daptomycin does not penetrate the membrane of Gram-negative bacteria. It is bactericidal against a similar spectrum of organisms as vancomycin and is used to treat complicated skin and soft tissue infections.

Resistance

Resistance occurs when the bacterial membrane structure changes to prevent binding of the drug.

Pharmacokinetics

Daptomycin is given intravenously and eliminated unchanged by the kidneys, with a half-life of about 8 h.

Unwanted effects

- Gastrointestinal upset.
- Injection-site reactions.

Polymyxins

Example

colistimethate sodium

Mechanism of action

Polymyxins bind to membrane phospholipids in susceptible bacteria and alter the permeability of the membrane to K^+ and Na^+ ions. The cell's osmotic barrier is lost and the bacteria are killed by lysis (Fig. 51.1).

Spectrum of activity

Polymyxins have bactericidal action against Gram-negative bacteria, including *Pseudomonas* species, but are inactive against Gram-positive bacteria.

Resistance

Acquired resistance is rare.

Pharmacokinetics

Colistimethate sodium is very poorly absorbed from the gut and is usually given by inhalation or topically to the skin. Penetration into joint spaces and CSF is poor. It is excreted unchanged by the kidney and has a half-life of 4–8 h. It is occasionally given by mouth for bowel sterilisation.

Unwanted effects

Substantial toxicity limits the systemic administration of polymyxins.

- Nephrotoxicity with dose-related reversible renal impairment.
- Neurotoxicity produces dizziness, circumoral and peripheral paraesthesiae, and confusion. Rarely, neuromuscular blockade produces respiratory paralysis with apnoea.
- Bronchospasm or sore throat after inhalation.

Drugs affecting bacterial DNA

Quinolones (fluoroquinolones)

Examples

ciprofloxacin, moxifloxacin, norfloxacin

Mechanism of action

Quinolones inhibit replication of bacterial DNA. They block the activity of bacterial DNA gyrase and DNA topoisomerase, the enzymes that form DNA supercoils and are essential for DNA replication and repair (Fig. 51.1). The effect is bactericidal.

Spectrum of activity

Ciprofloxacin has a broad spectrum of activity and is active against many micro-organisms resistant to penicillins, cephalosporins and aminoglycosides. Its spectrum includes Gram-positive bacteria, but with only moderate activity against *Streptococcus pneumoniae* and *Enterococcus faecalis*. It is active against most Gram-negative bacteria, including *H. influenzae*, *P. aeruginosa*, *N. gonorrhoeae*, and *Enterobacter* and *Campylobacter* species. Its spectrum extends to chlamydia and some mycobacteria, but not anaerobes.

Moxifloxacin has a broad spectrum of activity against Gram-positive and Gram-negative bacteria, but is inactive against *P. aeruginosa*. It has greater activity than ciprofloxacin against pneumococci. Norfloxacin is mainly useful for urinary tract pathogens.

Resistance

Resistance to quinolones is relatively uncommon but can be produced by a mutation that results in a DNA gyrase that is less susceptible to the drug's action, or by increased active drug efflux from the cell (Fig. 51.2).

Pharmacokinetics

Oral absorption of ciprofloxacin is variable but adequate. Intravenous formulations of some quinolones are available, including ciprofloxacin and moxifloxacin. Ciprofloxacin is widely distributed but CSF penetration is poor unless there is meningeal inflammation. Ciprofloxacin and norfloxacin are eliminated mainly by the kidney and have short half-lives (3–4 h). Moxifloxacin is well absorbed from the gut, is metabolised in the liver and has a longer half-life (12 h).

Unwanted effects

- Nausea, vomiting, abdominal pain, diarrhoea.
- Central nervous system (CNS) effects: dizziness, headache, tremor, seizures (especially in those with a history of epilepsy).
- Rashes.
- Pain and inflammation in tendons, occasionally with tendon rupture (especially in the elderly or with concomitant use of corticosteroids).
- Moxifloxacin prolongs the Q–T interval on the electrocardiogram (ECG) and predisposes to ventricular arrhythmias. The risk is greater if used in combination with other proarrhythmic drugs (Ch. 8).
- Drug interactions: inhibition of hepatic cytochrome P450 by ciprofloxacin and norfloxacin increases the plasma concentrations of theophylline (Ch. 12), warfarin (Ch. 11) and ciclosporin (Ch. 38), which can produce toxicity. The absorption of quinolones from the gut is decreased by oral iron salts.

Metronidazole and tinidazole

Mechanism of action

Metronidazole and tinidazole are bactericidal only after they have been converted to an intermediate transient toxic metabolite, which inhibits bacterial DNA synthesis and breaks down existing DNA. Only some anaerobes and some protozoa contain the oxidoreductase enzyme that converts these drugs to their antibacterial derivatives. The intermediate metabolite is not produced in human cells, or in aerobic bacteria. These drugs are equally active against dividing and non-dividing cells.

Spectrum of activity

Metronidazole and tinidazole are mainly active against anaerobic bacteria and protozoa, including *B. fragilis*, *Clostridium* species, *Gardnerella vaginalis* and *Giardia lamblia*. Metronidazole is an important drug for treating *C. difficile*-related colitis caused by broad-spectrum antimicrobial use. Metronidazole or tinidazole are important constituents of the triple or quadruple therapy utilised for the elimination of *Helicobacter pylori* (Ch. 33). They are also amoebicidal, with activity against *Entamoeba histolytica*.

Resistance

Acquired resistance is becoming more common. For example, in some countries a significant percentage of strains of *H. pylori* are resistant to metronidazole, as are some strains of *C. difficile*. Resistance can result from the development of oxidoreductases that do not act on metronidazole, or from the induction of oxidative stress mechanisms that inhibit the action of the drug. Resistance to tinidazole is less common.

Pharmacokinetics

Metronidazole is well absorbed orally and can also be given intravenously or by rectal suppositories. Metronidazole penetrates well into body fluids, including vaginal, pleural and cerebrospinal fluids, and can cross the placenta. Metronidazole and tinidazole are eliminated mainly by metabolism in the liver and have half-lives of 6–9 h and 12–14 h, respectively.

Unwanted effects

- Nausea, vomiting, metallic taste.
- Intolerance to alcohol can occur by a mechanism similar to the disulfiram reaction (Ch. 54).
- Rash.

Nitrofurantoin

Mechanism of action

Nitrofurantoin is activated inside bacteria by reduction via the flavoprotein nitrofurantoin reductase to unstable metabolites, which disrupt ribosomal RNA, DNA and other intracellular components. It is bactericidal, especially to bacteria present in acid urine.

Spectrum of activity

Nitrofurantoin is active against most Gram-positive cocci and *E. coli*. *Pseudomonas* species are naturally resistant, as are many *Proteus* species. Its use is confined to infections of the lower urinary tract.

Resistance

Chromosomal resistance is uncommon, and due to inhibition of nitrofurantoin reductase.

Pharmacokinetics

Nitrofurantoin is well absorbed from the gut. Its half-life in plasma is very short (<1 h) and therapeutic plasma concentrations are not achieved. It is excreted largely unchanged in the urine, giving urinary concentrations high enough to treat lower urinary tract infections, but the low tissue concentrations are inadequate for the treatment of acute pyelonephritis.

Unwanted effects

- Gastrointestinal upset is common, including anorexia, nausea and vomiting.
- Pulmonary toxicity with long-term use produces acute allergic pneumonitis or chronic interstitial fibrosis.
- Peripheral neuropathy.

Drugs affecting bacterial protein synthesis

Macrolides

azithromycin, clarithromycin, erythromycin, telithromycin

Mechanism of action

Macrolides interfere with bacterial protein synthesis by binding reversibly to the 50S subunit of the bacterial ribosome. This causes dissociation of the aminoacyl-transfer RNA (tRNA) from its translocation site. The action is primarily bacteriostatic (Fig. 51.1).

Spectrum of activity

Erythromycin has a similar spectrum of activity to broad-spectrum penicillins and is often used for treating individuals who are allergic to penicillin. It is effective against Gram-positive bacteria and gut anaerobes, but has poor activity against *H. influenzae*. It is also used for infections by *Legionella*, *Mycoplasma*, *Chlamydia*, *Mycobacterium* and *Campylobacter* species and for *Bordetella pertussis*. Although erythromycin is primarily bacteriostatic, it is bactericidal at high concentrations for some Gram-positive species, such as group A streptococci and pneumococci.

Azithromycin has less activity than erythromycin against Gram-positive bacteria, but enhanced activity against *H. influenzae*. Clarithromycin has slightly greater activity than erythromycin and is also used as part of the multidrug treatment of *H. pylori* (Ch. 33). Telithromycin is a derivative of erythromycin active against penicillin- and erythromycin-resistant *S. pneumoniae*.

Resistance

Bacteria become resistant to macrolides by activation of an efflux mechanism. A less common mechanism is a mutation in the gene encoding a methyltransferase that modifies the drug target site on the ribosome.

Pharmacokinetics

Erythromycin is destroyed at acid pH and is therefore given as an enteric-coated tablet or as an acid-stable ester prodrug (erythromycin ethyl succinate). It can also be administered intravenously. Clarithromycin is acid-stable and well absorbed from the gut, but undergoes first-pass metabolism in the liver. Erythromycin and clarithromycin are metabolised in the liver and have short half-lives (1–3 h). Azithromycin is poorly absorbed from the gut. It is widely distributed and released slowly from the tissues, and then excreted unchanged in the bile. It has a long half-life of about 2 days. Telithromycin is well absorbed from the gut, is metabolised in the liver and has a half-life of 10 h.

Unwanted effects

- Epigastric discomfort, nausea, vomiting and diarrhoea are common with the oral preparation of erythromycin. Other macrolides are better tolerated.
- Rashes.
- Cholestatic jaundice with erythromycin, usually if treatment is continued for more than 2 weeks.
- Prolongation of the Q–T interval on the ECG, with a predisposition to ventricular arrhythmias (Ch. 8).
- Drug interactions: erythromycin and clarithromycin inhibit P450 drug-metabolising enzymes (CYP1A2, CYP3A4) and can increase the plasma concentration of other drugs metabolised by these enzymes, including carbamazepine (Ch. 23) and ciclosporin (Ch. 38).

Aminoglycosides

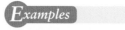

gentamicin, netilmicin, streptomycin, tobramycin

Mechanism of action

The aminoglycosides have similar properties, but with some important differences that can be exploited in particular clinical circumstances, as illustrated below. Aminoglycosides inhibit protein synthesis in bacteria by binding irreversibly to the 30S ribosomal subunit (Fig. 51.1). This inhibits transfer of aminoacyl-tRNA to the peptidyl site, causing premature termination of the peptide chain, and also increases the frequency of misreading of mRNA. Aminoglycosides may also damage bacterial cell membranes, causing leak of intracellular contents. They are bactericidal.

Spectrum of activity

Aminoglycosides are active against many Gram-negative bacteria (including *Pseudomonas* species) and some Gram-positive bacteria. They are inactive against anaerobes, which are unable to take up the aminoglycosides. Aminoglycosides are particularly useful for serious Gram-negative infections, when they have a synergistic action with drugs that disrupt cell wall synthesis (e.g. penicillins). Gentamicin is the most widely used aminoglycoside. Streptomycin is used rarely, but is occasionally used as a component of the drug regimen to treat *Mycobacterium tuberculosis* (see below).

Resistance

Resistance to aminoglycosides is transferred by plasmids and is an increasing problem. It can occur by several mechanisms, the most frequent being production of enzymes that acetylate, phosphorylate or adenylyl aminoglycosides in the bacterial periplasmic space, with poor uptake of the modified drug (Fig. 51.2). Resistance resulting from reduced penetration of the drug can be overcome by co-administration of antibacterials that disrupt cell wall synthesis, such as penicillins. Netilmicin is less susceptible to these enzymes and is effective against many gentamicin-resistant bacteria. Changes in the ribosomal proteins in bacteria can also reduce drug binding and antibacterial effectiveness, particularly for streptomycin.

Pharmacokinetics

Aminoglycosides are poorly absorbed from the gut and are given parenterally. They are rapidly excreted by the kidney and have short half-lives (1–4 h). They do not cross the blood–brain barrier, but they cross the placenta. Blood concentrations should always be measured to guide dosing. With multiple daily doses the peak plasma concentration (measured 1 h after dosing) and the trough concentration immediately before the next dose are important, both to ensure bactericidal efficacy and to minimise the risk of toxic effects. Once-daily dosage regimens for aminoglycosides are increasingly used and are no more toxic than multiple daily dosages.

Tobramycin is also available in a preservative-free solution for administration by nebuliser for the management of people with bronchiectasis (including cystic fibrosis) whose respiratory tracts are colonised by *P. aeruginosa*.

Unwanted effects

Most unwanted effects of aminoglycosides are dose-related and many are reversible; they are most closely related to high trough concentrations of the drug.

- Ototoxicity can lead to both vestibular and auditory dysfunction. Prolonged treatment or high plasma drug concentrations lead to accumulation of the aminoglycoside in the inner ear, resulting in disturbances of balance or deafness that are often irreversible. Mutations in the human gene encoding mitochondrial 12S ribosomal RNA predispose to ototoxicity. Netilmicin causes less ototoxicity than the other aminoglycosides.
- Renal damage occurs through retention of aminoglycosides in the proximal tubular cells of the kidney. It is usually reversible and is manifest initially by a defect in the concentrating ability of the kidney, with mild proteinuria followed by a reduction in the glomerular filtration rate.
- Acute neuromuscular blockade can occur, usually if the aminoglycoside is used with anaesthetic drugs (Ch. 17), and aminoglycosides can enhance the effects of other neuromuscular-blocking drugs (Ch. 27). This action is the result of inhibition of pre-junctional acetylcholine release and also reduced postsynaptic sensitivity. It is reversed by intravenous Ca^{2+} salts.

Tetracyclines

doxycycline, minocycline, oxytetracycline

Mechanism of action

Tetracyclines enter bacteria mainly by an active uptake mechanism that is not found in human cells. They are bacteriostatic and inhibit bacterial protein synthesis by binding reversibly to the 30S subunit of ribosomes, inhibiting the binding of aminoacyl-tRNAs.

Spectrum of activity

Tetracyclines have a broad spectrum of activity against many Gram-positive and Gram-negative bacteria and in infections caused by rickettsiae, amoebae, *Chlamydia psittaci*, *Chlamydia trachomatis*, *Coxiella burnetii*, *Vibrio cholerae* and *Mycoplasma*, *Legionella* and *Brucella* species. They are useful in acne (Ch. 49). Minocycline is active against *N. meningitidis*, unlike other tetracyclines.

Resistance

Resistance is carried by plasmids and is usually due to increased transport of the drug out of the bacterium (Fig. 51.2). An alternative mechanism is decreased binding of tetracyclines to bacterial ribosomes. Resistance to the tetracyclines develops slowly, but in the UK is now widespread among most Gram-positive and several Gram-negative bacteria. Micro-organisms that have developed resistance to one tetracycline frequently display resistance to the others.

Pharmacokinetics

Tetracyclines are incompletely absorbed from the gut, particularly if taken with food. Absorption of oxytetracycline is further impaired by milk, antacids (Ch. 33), iron and increased intestinal pH; tetracyclines bind to divalent and trivalent cations, forming inactive chelates (Ch. 56).

The tetracyclines diffuse reasonably well into sputum, urine, and peritoneal and pleural fluid, and cross the placenta, but penetrate the CSF poorly. Tetracyclines are concentrated in the liver and some is excreted via the bile into the small intestine, from where it is partially reabsorbed. Drug concentrations in the bile may be three to five times higher than in the plasma.

Tetracyclines are mainly eliminated unchanged in the urine, with the exception of doxycycline, which is largely eliminated in the bile. All of the tetracyclines have half-lives within the range 8–22 h.

Unwanted effects

- Nausea, vomiting, epigastric discomfort and diarrhoea.
- In children, tetracyclines produce permanent yellow–brown discoloration of growing teeth by chelating with Ca^{2+}, and can also cause dental hypoplasia. Tetracyclines should be avoided during the latter half of pregnancy and in children during the first 12 years of life.
- Anti-anabolic effects can occur in human cells from inhibition of protein synthesis (not seen with doxycycline or minocycline). If there is pre-existing impairment of renal function it can lead to uraemia.
- Idiopathic intracranial hypertension, with headache and visual disturbances.

Tigecycline
Mechanism of action

Tigecycline has structural similarities to the tetracyclines and also binds to the 30S ribosomal subunit of bacteria.

Spectrum of activity

Tigecycline has a broad spectrum of activity against Gram-positive and Gram-negative bacteria, including some anaerobes. It is used for complicated skin and soft tissue infections, and for complicated abdominal infections caused by resistant bacteria. Tigecycline is active against MRSA, vancomycin-resistant enterococci, *Proteus* species and *P. aeruginosa*.

Resistance

Many strains of *Proteus* species and *P. aeruginosa* are resistant, usually as a result of possessing a drug-efflux pump.

Pharmacokinetics

Tigecycline is given intravenously and is excreted largely unchanged in the bile and urine; it has a long half-life (about 27 h).

Unwanted effects

The most common unwanted effects are similar to those of tetracyclines.

Chloramphenicol
Mechanism of action

Chloramphenicol inhibits protein synthesis in bacteria by binding reversibly to the 50S subunit of bacterial ribosomes (Fig. 51.1), where it blocks peptide chain elongation by inhibiting peptidyl transferase activity. The effect is mainly bacteriostatic, but can be bactericidal in some bacteria.

Spectrum of activity

Chloramphenicol is a broad-spectrum antibacterial, active against many Gram-positive cocci (both aerobic and anaerobic) and Gram-negative bacteria. The sensitivities of all these bacteria are variable, but it has a bactericidal effect on *E. coli*, *S. pneumoniae*, *H. influenzae*, *N. meningitidis*, *B. pertussis*, *V. cholerae*, and *Salmonella*, *Shigella* and *Bacteroides* species. It is bacteriostatic for some streptococci and staphylococci.

Because of its toxicity, chloramphenicol is reserved for life-threatening infections, particularly with *H. influenzae* or *Salmonella typhi*. It is used topically for conjunctivitis (Ch. 50).

Resistance

Resistance is transferred by plasmids and involves the production of an acetyltransferase that inactivates the drug by acetylation, preventing it from binding to the ribosome. The acetyltransferase is produced by many Gram-negative bacteria but can also be induced in Gram-positive bacteria. Resistant bacteria may also show reduced uptake of the drug.

Pharmacokinetics

Chloramphenicol is well absorbed orally and can also be given intravenously. It is widely distributed, including into CSF and the biliary tree; it crosses the placenta and is present in breast milk. Chloramphenicol is metabolised in the liver and has a half-life of 2–12 h.

Unwanted effects

- The most important unwanted effect is bone marrow toxicity. Reversible anaemia, thrombocytopenia or neutropenia can occur, particularly in those receiving high or prolonged dosing. Aplastic anaemia is rare, but usually fatal.
- Peripheral neuritis, optic neuritis, headache.
- Rashes.
- Premature infants and babies less than 2 weeks old have immature glucuronyl transferase and reduced drug elimination. Chloramphenicol can accumulate in neonates, causing the 'grey baby syndrome'. Initial symptoms include vomiting and cyanosis, followed by hypothermia, vasomotor collapse and an ashen grey discoloration of the skin. There is a high mortality.

Lincosamides

clindamycin

Mechanism of action

Clindamycin inhibits bacterial protein synthesis in a similar manner to the macrolide antibacterials.

Spectrum of activity

Clindamycin is used for staphylococcal bone infection such as osteomyelitis and sometimes for soft tissue infections.

Resistance

Resistance develops by modification of the 50S ribosomal binding site.

Pharmacokinetics

Clindamycin is well absorbed orally. It is eliminated largely by hepatic metabolism and has a half-life of 2.5 h.

Unwanted effects

- Nausea, vomiting, abdominal discomfort, diarrhoea and, rarely, *C. difficile*-related colitis.
- Rashes.
- Jaundice and abnormal liver function tests.
- Neutropenia, thrombocytopenia.

Fusidic acid

Mechanism of action

Fusidic acid is a steroid compound that inhibits bacterial protein synthesis. It forms a complex with the ribosome and inhibits elongation of the peptide chain.

Spectrum of activity

Fusidic acid is a narrow-spectrum antibacterial, mainly active against Gram-positive bacteria. It is most commonly used for treatment of penicillin-resistant *S. aureus*, especially in the treatment of osteomyelitis. It is bactericidal.

Resistance

Resistance occurs usually transferred by plasmids, and involves an altered ribosomal binding site for the drug. Resistance develops rapidly when fusidic acid is used alone, so it is usually given in combination with another drug.

Pharmacokinetics

Oral absorption is complete, but an intravenous formulation is available. Distribution into synovial fluid and soft tissues is good, and the drug concentrates in bone. Fusidic acid is metabolised in the liver and has a half-life of 9 h.

Unwanted effects

- Thrombophlebitis with intravenous infusions.
- Cholestatic jaundice.
- Nausea, vomiting.

Oxazolidinones

Linezolid

Mechanism of action

The oxazolidinones are active against non-replicating bacteria. They have a unique mechanism of action, binding to the ribosomal 50S subunit and preventing initiation of protein synthesis, unlike many other antibacterials which inhibit chain elongation.

Spectrum of activity

Linezolid is active against a range of Gram-positive organisms, including MRSA and also vancomycin-resistant *Enterococcus faecium*.

Resistance

Resistance is due to mutation, leading to modification of the ribosomal target for the drug. This can develop with prolonged treatment, or with inadequate doses.

Pharmacokinetics

Linezolid is well absorbed orally. It is mainly metabolised in the liver; it has a half-life of 5 h.

Unwanted effects

- Headache.
- Nausea, vomiting, taste disturbances, diarrhoea.
- Myelosuppression with anaemia, neutropenia and thrombocytopenia.
- Optic neuropathy with prolonged use (over 28 days).
- Linezolid is a weak non-selective monoamine oxidase inhibitor, and dietary restriction of tyramine is advisable (see Ch. 22).

Drugs affecting bacterial metabolism

Sulphonamides

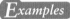

sulfadiazine, sulfamethoxazole

The therapeutic importance of the sulphonamides has diminished because of the spread of resistance and there are now only a few situations (nonetheless important) in which they are first-choice drugs. Sulfamethoxazole is only used in combination with trimethoprim, as co-trimoxazole (see below).

Mechanism of action

Folate is a nutrient essential for cell growth and is used to manufacture purines and thymidine for incorporation into DNA. Unlike humans, who obtain folate from the diet, bacteria cannot utilise pre-formed folate and must synthesise it from *p*-aminobenzoic acid (PABA). Sulphonamides are structurally similar to PABA and inhibit dihydropteroate synthetase in the synthetic pathway for folic acid (Fig. 51.4).

Spectrum of activity

Sulphonamides have a bacteriostatic action against a wide range of Gram-positive and Gram-negative bacteria and are also active against *Toxoplasma*, *Chlamydia* and *Nocardia* species. Because of the frequency of resistance in many of these micro-organisms, sulphonamides are given as sole therapy only for the treatment of nocardiosis or toxoplasmosis.

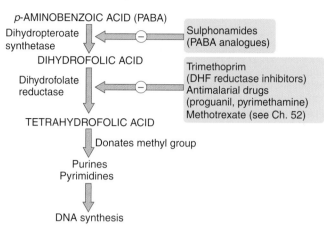

The Folic Acid Pathway:

Fig. 51.4 **Sites of action of sulphonamides and dihydrofolate (DHF) reductase inhibitors in the folic acid pathway.** Selective inhibitors of bacterial, plasmodial and human DHF reductase isozymes are used respectively as antibacterial (trimethoprim), antimalarial (proguanil, pyrimethamine) and anti-cancer (methotrexate) drugs.

Resistance

Resistance is common and occurs through the production of a mutated dihydropteroate synthetase with reduced affinity for sulphonamide binding (Figs 51.2 and 51.4). Resistance is transmitted among Gram-negative bacteria by plasmids. Resistance in *S. aureus* occurs as a result of excessive synthesis of PABA. Some resistant bacteria have reduced uptake of sulphonamides.

Pharmacokinetics

Sulphonamides are well absorbed orally, and a parenteral preparation of sulfadiazine is available. They are widely distributed and cross the blood–brain barrier and placenta.

Sulphonamides are metabolised in the liver, initially by acetylation, which shows genetic polymorphism (Ch. 2). The acetylated products have no antibacterial action but retain a risk of toxicity. The parent drugs and their N-acetyl metabolites are excreted by the kidney. Most sulphonamides have half-lives of about 12 h.

Unwanted effects

- Nausea and vomiting.
- Rashes, including toxic epidermal necrolysis and Stevens–Johnson syndrome.
- Haemolysis in individuals with glucose-6-phosphate dehydrogenase deficiency (Chs 47 and 53).
- Neutropenia, thrombocytopenia.
- Sulphonamides should not be used in the last trimester of pregnancy or in neonates, because the drug competes for bilirubin-binding sites on albumin; this can raise the concentration of unconjugated bilirubin and increases the risk of kernicterus.

Trimethoprim

Trimethoprim can be used alone or, less commonly, combined with the sulphonamide sulfamethoxazole as co-trimoxazole.

Mechanism of action

Trimethoprim inhibits dihydrofolate reductase, which converts dihydrofolate to tetrahydrofolate (Fig. 51.4). The bacterial enzyme is inhibited at much lower concentrations of trimethoprim than its mammalian counterpart. The combination of trimethoprim with sulfamethoxazole (co-trimoxazole) acts synergistically to prevent folate synthesis by bacteria. However, resistance to the sulfamethoxazole component and the incidence of unwanted effects limit the value of this combination.

Spectrum of activity

Trimethoprim has broad-spectrum bacteriostatic activity against Gram-positive and Gram-negative bacteria. In many urinary and respiratory tract infections trimethoprim alone gives results similar to the combination with sulfamethoxazole. Co-trimoxazole is effective against the protozoan *Pneumocystis jirovecii*, which causes pneumonia in people with AIDS or other immunodeficiencies, and this is now its major indication (see below).

Resistance

Resistance to trimethoprim occurs in a variety of ways, including the production of mutated dihydrofolate reductase that is insensitive to trimethoprim.

Pharmacokinetics

Trimethoprim is well absorbed from the gut and most is eliminated unchanged by the kidney; it has a half-life of 9–17 h. Both trimethoprim and co-trimoxazole are available for intravenous use.

Unwanted effects

- Nausea, vomiting and diarrhoea, which are usually mild.
- Rashes.
- Bone marrow depression.
- Folate deficiency, leading to megaloblastic changes in the bone marrow, is rare except in people with depleted folate stores.

Drugs used for tuberculosis

Tuberculosis is usually treated with a multidrug regimen because of the rapid development of resistance. Some drugs used to treat mycobacterial infections also have other clinical uses.

Rifamycins

rifabutin, rifampicin, rifaximin

Mechanism of action and spectrum of activity

Rifamycins act by inhibition of bacterial DNA-dependent RNA polymerase and inhibit mRNA transcription. They have a bactericidal action. Rifampicin (rifampin) has a broad spectrum of activity and is used in combination with other drugs for the treatment of mycobacterial infections (*M. tuberculosis* and *M. leprae*), brucellosis, *Legionella* infections, serious staphylococcal infections and endocarditis. In the UK, rifampicin is considered an essential drug for treatment of tuberculosis. Rifampicin is also used for prophylaxis against meningococcal meningitis and *H. influenzae* type b infection. Rifabutin is used for treatment of tuberculosis and for prophylaxis against *Mycobacterium avium* complex infection (which most commonly occurs in people who are infected with HIV) and other mycobacterial infections. Rifaximin is a non-absorbable rifamycin used to treat traveller's diarrhoea (Ch. 35).

Resistance

Resistance develops rapidly, which limits the wider use of rifampicin as an antibacterial drug, other than as part of combination treatment for tuberculosis. It is acquired by a one-step genetic mutation of the bacterial DNA-dependent RNA polymerase.

Pharmacokinetics

Oral absorption of rifampicin and rifabutin is good and an intravenous formulation of rifampicin is also available. The bioavailability of rifabutin is low (20%) compared with rifampicin. Rifampicin and rifabutin are metabolised in the liver and have half-lives of 1–6 h and 35–40 h, respectively.

Unwanted effects

- Nausea and anorexia.
- Diarrhoea and antibiotic-associated colitis with rifampicin.
- Hepatotoxicity, usually only producing a transient rise in plasma transaminases but occasionally more severe; regular monitoring is recommended.
- Orange coloration of tears, sweat, urine.
- Leucopenia, thrombocytopenia or anaemia with rifabutin.
- Various symptoms with intermittent use of rifampicin, which include influenza-like symptoms, respiratory symptoms, renal failure, shock, disseminated intravascular coagulation and acute haemolytic anaemia.
- Drug interactions of rifamycins: induction of drug-metabolising enzymes in the liver (Ch. 2) can reduce

plasma concentrations of oestrogen in those taking oral contraceptives (Ch. 45) and of several other drugs including phenytoin (Ch. 23), warfarin (Ch. 11) and sulfonylureas (Ch. 40).

Isoniazid
Mechanism of action

Isoniazid is an important and specific drug for the treatment of *M. tuberculosis*. It is a prodrug activated by catalase–peroxidase activity within the mycobacteria. The activated drug acts on enzymes in the cell to inhibit the synthesis of long-chain mycolic acids, which are unique to the cell wall of mycobacteria. It is bactericidal against dividing organisms, but bacteriostatic on resting organisms. In the UK it is considered an essential drug for treatment of tuberculosis along with rifampicin.

Resistance

Resistance occurs rapidly if isoniazid is used alone and may be due to mutations in the enzymes responsible for the synthesis of mycolic acids, making them less susceptible to the drug. Resistance is currently uncommon in developed countries, but can be troublesome in developing countries.

Pharmacokinetics

Oral absorption of isoniazid is good but reduced by food. It is metabolised by acetylation in the liver, which is subject to genetic polymorphism. Rapid acetylators show extensive first-pass metabolism and plasma isoniazid concentrations are half of those in slow acetylators. The half-life is 0.5–2 h in rapid acetylators and 2–6.5 h in slow acetylators.

Unwanted effects

- Nausea, vomiting, constipation, dry mouth.
- Peripheral neuropathy with high doses. This can be prevented by prophylactic use of oral pyridoxine supplements in people at high risk, for example those with diabetes, alcoholism, chronic renal failure, malnutrition or HIV infection. Neuropathy is more common in slow acetylators.
- Hepatitis is rare, but regular monitoring with liver function tests is recommended.
- Systemic lupus erythematosus-like syndrome. Positive antinuclear antibodies are found in 20% of people during long-term treatment, but fewer develop symptoms.

Pyrazinamide
Mechanism of action

Pyrazinamide is a prodrug that acts through metabolites formed by pyrazinamidase, an enzyme found in *M. tuberculosis*. The product pyrazinoic acid lowers intracellular pH, inactivates a vital enzyme in fatty acid synthesis and destroys the bacterium. It is bactericidal to dividing cells.

Resistance

Resistance results from a point mutation in the gene which codes for pyrazinamidase. It develops rapidly if pyrazinamide is used as a sole treatment for tuberculosis.

Pharmacokinetics

Oral absorption of pyrazinamide is good and metabolism occurs in the liver; it has a long half-life (10–24 h).

Unwanted effects

- Hepatotoxicity: a rise in plasma bilirubin usually requires cessation of treatment; regular monitoring is recommended.
- Nausea and vomiting.
- Arthralgia.
- Sideroblastic anaemia.

Ethambutol

Mechanism of action

Ethambutol probably functions as an arabinose analogue and inhibits arabinosyl transferase, resulting in impaired synthesis of the cell wall of mycobacteria. Ethambutol is primarily bacteriostatic. It is effective against *M. tuberculosis* and several other mycobacteria, including *M. avium* complex.

Resistance

Resistance may be due to gene mutations that inhibit the binding of ethambutol to its target enzyme. It develops slowly, but is common during prolonged treatment of tuberculosis if ethambutol is used alone.

Pharmacokinetics

Oral absorption is good. It is mainly eliminated unchanged by the kidney. The half-life is long (10–15 h).

Unwanted effects

- Optic neuritis produces initial red/green colour blindness, then reduced visual acuity; it is dose-related but usually reversible.
- Peripheral neuritis.

Other drugs used in the treatment of tuberculosis

Other drugs can be used as second-line treatments in multidrug-resistant tuberculosis. These include cycloserine, capreomycin, amikacin, ciprofloxacin, moxifloxacin, azithromycin, clarithromycin, streptomycin and *p*-aminosalicylic acid. Drugs used in countries other than the UK include thiacetazone and protionamide.

Drugs used for leprosy

The drugs recommended for treatment of leprosy, which is caused by *Mycobacterium leprae*, are rifampicin (see above), dapsone and clofazimine.

Dapsone

Mechanism of action and use

Dapsone is similar to the sulphonamides and acts by inhibition of folate synthesis. It is the most active drug against *M. leprae*. Dapsone is also used to treat pneumocystis pneumonia and dermatitis herpetiformis.

Resistance

Resistance can develop as for sulphonamides (see above).

Pharmacokinetics

Dapsone is well absorbed from the gut. It is metabolised in the liver and undergoes enterohepatic cycling. It has a long half-life (27 h).

Unwanted effects

- Blood disorders: haemolysis and methaemoglobinaemia (Ch. 53), although these are rare at the doses used for treatment of leprosy.
- Neuropathy.
- Anorexia, nausea, vomiting.
- Allergic dermatitis.

Clofazimine

Mechanism of action and use

Clofazimine is a dye that interferes with DNA replication and is used as a second-line drug in the event of dapsone intolerance in people with leprosy. It is given orally.

Pharmacokinetics

Clofazimine has a variable oral bioavailability and is eliminated slowly in the bile. It has a long half-life (10 days) and can accumulate in the body.

Unwanted effects

- Gastrointestinal upset.
- Brownish-black discoloration of the skin.
- Acne.

PRINCIPLES OF ANTIBACTERIAL THERAPY

Antibacterial therapy is widely misused, which encourages selection of resistant organisms. In particular, use of antibacterials for viral illnesses such as the common cold or sore throats is to be discouraged. The following guidelines outline the principles that should be considered in the choice of a safe and effective antibacterial therapy.

Empirical treatment

Most antibacterial therapy is started without prior identification of the organism and its antibacterial drug sensitivities. Such treatment should be guided by the clinical diagnosis and knowledge of the most common pathogenic bacteria responsible for the infection to be treated. Local information about patterns of antibacterial resistance is an important consideration.

Spectrum of antibacterial activity

A drug with a narrow spectrum of activity should be used in preference to a broad-spectrum drug whenever possible. The unnecessary use of broad-spectrum antibacterials encourages the development of resistant bacteria. This can present problems for the person treated, due to the selection of resistant pathogens or colonisation by resistant bacteria from the environment. For the community, the selection of resistant pathogens can create problems by rendering standard antibacterial therapy less reliable. Broad-spectrum antibacterial cover is sometimes appropriate, for example in a seriously ill person when the infecting bacterium is unknown and a variety of bacteria could be causing the condition being treated.

Combination therapy

Treatment with more than one antibacterial drug should not be used routinely. It may, however, be valuable to provide broad-spectrum cover in serious illness when the organism is unknown, for example the combination of cefotaxime and metronidazole to cover aerobic and anaerobic organisms in suspected Gram-negative septicaemia. When resistance is likely to develop readily to the first-choice drug during prolonged treatment, the use of combination therapy can minimise that risk, for example in the treatment of infective endocarditis or tuberculosis.

Bactericidal versus bacteriostatic drugs

In some situations, bactericidal drugs are preferred to bacteriostatic drugs, for example for the treatment of infective endocarditis (when bacteria divide infrequently) or when the person being treated is immunocompromised (and host defences are ineffective for assisting eradication). In most other situations the choice is not important.

Site of infection

This may determine the choice of drug; for example, some antibacterials only achieve low concentrations in the biliary tree, urine, bone or cerebrospinal fluid.

Mode of administration

Oral therapy is usually preferred to parenteral treatment. Exceptions include the treatment of serious infections for which reliable plasma drug concentrations are essential, when the drug is only available in parenteral formulation, or when gastrointestinal absorption may be unreliable, for example after abdominal surgery.

Duration of therapy

This should be as short as is compatible with adequate treatment of the infection. The decision is often arbitrary, for example 7–10 days in many infections. Some infections can be effectively treated over much shorter periods; for example, courses of 1–3 days are usually adequate for uncomplicated lower urinary tract infections in women. There is evidence that the conventional longer courses of treatment for many other infections may be unnecessary. For a few infections, long periods of treatment may be essential to eliminate semi-dormant organisms or those in 'privileged sites' to which antibacterial drug penetration is poor. Examples include infective endocarditis, osteomyelitis and tuberculosis. Some antibacterials produce a 'post-antibiotic effect', in which there is delayed regrowth of surviving bacteria following exposure to the drug. This is most marked with aminoglycosides such as gentamicin, but also occurs with other drugs, including β-lactam antibacterials.

Chemoprophylaxis

The use of chemoprophylaxis to prevent infection is important in many situations. Common examples include prevention of meningococcal meningitis, H. influenzae type b infection or pertussis in close contacts of an infected person, and pre-operative prophylaxis before many surgical procedures. More prolonged prophylaxis is used to prevent pneumococcal infection after splenectomy or in people with sickle cell disease.

TREATMENT OF SELECTED BACTERIAL INFECTIONS

This section is not intended to be comprehensive. It will outline the approach to antibacterial therapy in several common bacterial infections. The choice of antibacterial drug for these infections will depend on factors such as local patterns of bacterial resistance or the risk of C. difficile infection, which make universal recommendations impossible.

Upper respiratory tract infections

Most upper respiratory tract infections are caused by viruses, producing symptoms of the common cold. Symptomatic treatment is all that should be offered, with an antihistamine (e.g. chlorphenamine; Ch. 39) or an antimuscarinic spray (e.g. ipratropium; Ch. 12) to reduce rhinorrhoea and sneezing. An α-adrenoceptor agonist given orally or nasally (e.g. xylometazoline) can reduce nasal congestion, but prolonged use can provoke a rebound effect (rhinitis medicamentosa) (Ch. 39). A non-steroidal anti-inflammatory drug (NSAID; Ch. 29) can be used to reduce associated headache and malaise. Antibacterial drugs are widely prescribed for upper respiratory tract symptoms but have no benefit.

Sinusitis and otitis media

Sinusitis and otitis media accompany catarrhal conditions in childhood and frequently follow an upper respiratory tract infection. Sinusitis produces headache, facial pain, fever and purulent rhinorrhoea. A nasal decongestant such as an α-adrenoceptor agonist can be helpful, in conjunction with an analgesic. An antibacterial is often not beneficial in acute sinusitis unless there is marked facial swelling and pain, or failure to resolve after 7 days. The most common infecting organisms are H. influenzae (which often produces β-lactamase), S. pneumoniae and Moraxella catarrhalis. Suitable antibacterial drugs include amoxicillin (or amoxicillin plus clavulanic acid if there is no improvement after 48 h), doxycycline and clarithromycin. Chronic sinusitis usually requires correction of an anatomical obstruction in the nose.

Otitis media is very common in childhood. When associated with an effusion in the middle ear, increased pressure causes pain and perforation of the eardrum. The organisms responsible are similar to those causing acute sinusitis. In more than 80% of affected children the condition is self-limiting over 2–3 days without treatment. An antibacterial such as amoxicillin or clarithromycin should be used if symptoms have not resolved after 72 h, or if there are systemic symptoms. Surgery is occasionally necessary for recurrent infections.

Lower respiratory tract infections

Acute bronchitis

This is characterised by new-onset, often productive cough without evidence of pneumonia. It is usually caused by a viral infection and the cough often takes 2–4 weeks to resolve without treatment. Antibacterial treatment is inappropriate and does not alter the course of the illness. Even if there is underlying chronic obstructive airways disease, the evidence for benefit from antibacterial drugs is small, although they may slightly shorten the duration of symptoms. In such cases *S. pneumoniae* (pneumococcus), *H. influenzae* or *M. catarrhalis* are commonly found in the sputum, but these micro-organisms are often isolated in remissions as well. If an antibacterial drug is used then 5 days' treatment with amoxicillin, doxycycline or clarithromycin will be effective against the most likely pathogens. Co-amoxiclav (amoxicillin with clavulanic acid) can be used for resistant *H. influenzae*.

Pneumonia

Primary community-acquired pneumonia is most commonly caused by *S. pneumoniae*, and less commonly by *H. influenzae* and staphylococci. 'Atypical' micro-organisms can also cause pneumonia, such as *Legionella* species, *Mycoplasma pneumoniae* or *Chlamydia pneumoniae*. Appropriate antibacterial treatment will be dictated by the most likely infecting agent.

Amoxicillin is the treatment of choice if pneumococcus is suspected. For people who are penicillin-allergic, clarithromycin will cover most likely micro-organisms, including 'atypical' ones. Oral amoxicillin combined with clarithromycin is often used for community-acquired pneumonia requiring admission of the person to hospital. Doxycycline is increasingly used as an alternative oral treatment because of a lower risk of *C. difficile*-related colitis. Severe community-acquired pneumonia (defined by the CURB-65 score; Table 51.3) is usually treated with intravenous therapy comprising benzylpenicillin with intravenous clarithromycin or doxycycline. Co-amoxiclav is often used in place of benzylpenicillin for life-threatening pneumonia, or when Gram-negative organisms are suspected, to cover β-lactamase-producing organisms. A quinolone with activity against pneumococci, such as moxifloxacin, would be an alternative choice. Adjunctive treatment of pneumonia may include supplemental oxygen via a facemask, pain relief for pleurisy and ensuring adequate hydration.

Table 51.3 CURB-65 score for predicting mortality in community-acquired pneumonia

Confusion of new onset (abbreviated mental test score ≤8/10)
Serum **u**rea >7 mmol·L⁻¹
Respiratory rate ≥30 breaths·min⁻¹
Blood pressure: systolic <90 mmHg or diastolic ≤60 mmHg
Age ≥**65** years

Each risk factor above scores one point.
Total score: 0–1 points, mortality 1.5%; 2 points, mortality 9.2%; ≥3 points, mortality 22%.

Secondary pneumonias occur in patients with other concurrent diseases, often during a stay in hospital (nosocomial or hospital-acquired pneumonia). A wide range of pathogens may be involved and parenteral drug treatment is usually necessary. A cephalosporin (e.g. cefuroxime) or co-amoxiclav are often used for early-onset infections, or an antipseudomonal penicillin (e.g. piperacillin with tazobactam) or ciprofloxacin for late-onset infection. An aminoglycoside such as gentamicin can be added for severe infection where *P. aeruginosa* infection is suspected.

Chronic lung sepsis

This encompasses lung abscess, empyema and bronchiectasis. The pathogens in lung abscesses vary according to the immune status of the individual. Ideally, the antibacterial treatment should be directed by isolation and sensitivity testing of the bacteria. Empyema requires drainage and then specific antibacterial therapy directed at the cultured pathogen. Bronchiectasis is most frequently associated with colonisation by *H. influenzae*, and less often *Pseudomonas* species or *S. pneumoniae*. A quinolone such as moxifloxacin or a macrolide such as azithromycin are suitable empirical treatment choices. Increasing use is being made of inhaled nebulised antibacterial drugs, such as tobramycin, to treat frequent exacerbations. Adjunctive treatment with bronchodilators, mucolytics and physiotherapy may be useful (see also cystic fibrosis, Ch. 13).

Urinary tract infections

Urinary tract infections are more common in women than men, because of their shorter urethra. Infections can occur in structurally normal urinary tracts or in association with a structural genitourinary abnormality that impairs drainage of urine or acts as a focus for infection, such as a stone in the kidney or bladder. An indwelling urinary catheter is often associated with bacterial colonisation of the urine that is almost impossible to eradicate, but often does not cause any symptoms.

The most frequent bacterial cause of urinary tract infection is *E. coli*. Hospital-acquired infections are often caused by *Klebsiella*, *Enterobacter* and *Serratia* species or by *P. aeruginosa*, because these organisms can be selected as resistant bacteria following antibacterial usage. *Proteus mirabilis* is often found if there are stones in the urinary tract. Less commonly, staphylococci, especially *Staphylococcus saprophyticus*, are responsible.

Uncomplicated urinary tract infection is confined to the bladder (cystitis) and in women can be treated by a short course (3 days) of an aminopenicillin such as amoxicillin. Alternative drugs include a first-generation cephalosporin (e.g. cefalexin), trimethoprim and nitrofurantoin. A quinolone such as ciprofloxacin can be useful for *P. aeruginosa* infections. Men should be treated for longer (usually 7 days).

Complicated urinary tract infections also involve the kidney (pyelonephritis), or the prostate in males, and require longer courses of treatment. For pyelonephritis, initial intravenous therapy is usually started with broad-spectrum drugs such as aztreonam, ciprofloxacin or cefuroxime, sometimes with an initial dose of gentamicin; treatment is usually continued for 10–14 days. For acute prostatitis, oral treatment with trimethoprim or ciprofloxacin for at least 4 weeks is recommended.

Treatment of infection with an indwelling urinary catheter is only recommended if there are systemic symptoms of infection such as fever or rigors.

Long-term antibacterial prophylaxis against urinary tract infections may be necessary to prevent recurrent infection if there are underlying urinary tract abnormalities. Suitable drugs, usually given at low dosage, include trimethoprim, nitrofurantoin and cefalexin.

Gastrointestinal infection

In the UK, infectious diarrhoea is usually caused by viruses and is self-limiting. However, gastroenteritis (a syndrome that includes nausea, vomiting, diarrhoea and abdominal discomfort) can result from ingestion of bacterial pathogens.

'Food poisoning' of bacterial origin can occur from ingestion of a pre-formed bacterial toxin (e.g. from *Clostridium botulinum* or *S. aureus*), with onset of symptoms usually within hours, or it can be caused by ingested bacteria infecting the bowel. Severe bacterial infection of the large intestine can cause dysentery, an inflammatory disorder often associated with fever, abdominal pain, and blood and pus in the faeces. The most common cause of bacterial diarrhoea (especially in children in developing countries) is *E. coli*, which produces powerful enterotoxins. In other circumstances, *Salmonella* species, *Campylobacter* species, *V. cholerae*, *Shigella* species or various other organisms are responsible.

If diarrhoea is severe, fluid replacement is often necessary. Antibacterial treatment is not usually recommended even if bacterial infection is suspected, unless there are systemic symptoms such as fever, rigors and hypotension. Ciprofloxacin and clarithromycin are effective for *Campylobacter* enteritis and shigellosis. Salmonella infections can be treated with ciprofloxacin, unless *S. typhi* is suspected, when cefotaxime is preferred.

Antibacterial drugs can cause diarrhoea due to alteration of bowel flora, which usually resolves rapidly when the drug is withdrawn. However, if it is complicated by colonisation with *C. difficile* then oral metronidazole or oral vancomycin will be necessary to eliminate the pathogen.

Biliary tract infection

Acute cholecystitis and cholangitis are often caused by *E. coli* and most often occur if there is biliary obstruction. Supportive treatment with fluid and electrolyte replacement is usually required. Antibacterial therapy with a cephalosporin, ciprofloxacin or gentamicin is usually effective. Combination therapy is recommended if the infection is severe; alternatively, a ureidopenicillin such as piperacillin with tazobactam can be given alone. Treatment is usually given for 7–10 days.

Osteomyelitis

Infection of bone produces necrotic tissue and generates an avascular privileged site for bacteria that antibacterial drugs penetrate to only a limited extent. Organisms involved include *S. aureus*, which adheres readily to bone matrix, various streptococci, *Serratia* species, *P. aeruginosa* and enteric Gram-negative rods.

Early antibacterial treatment is essential and surgical intervention may be necessary to remove necrotic tissue. The choice of drug depends on the suspected organisms. First-line treatment is often with flucloxacillin or clindamycin, combined with fusidic acid or rifampicin for the first 2 weeks if a prosthesis is present or the infection is severe. Amoxicillin or cefuroxime is usually used if *H. influenzae* is identified, or vancomycin for MRSA. Acute infections are treated with intravenous antimicrobials for 6 weeks, but chronic infections are treated for at least 12 weeks. If long-term therapy is necessary for chronic refractory osteomyelitis an oral quinolone such as ciprofloxacin can be substituted.

Septic arthritis

The most common organism is *S. aureus*, or less frequently streptococci. The standard treatment is with flucloxacillin or clindamycin for individuals who are penicillin-allergic. Vancomycin is used for MRSA. Treatment should be continued for 4–6 weeks.

Cellulitis

This usually complicates a wound, ulcer or dermatosis. In most cases the infecting organisms are *S. aureus* or streptococci. Treatment is usually with a β-lactam antibacterial that is active against β-lactamase-producing *S. aureus*. Flucloxacillin is normally used. Clarithromycin or clindamycin is used for individuals who are penicillin-allergic.

Septicaemia

Septicaemia is a bacterial infection involving the bloodstream and can present with fever or, if more severe, result in circulatory collapse from vasodilation, capillary leak and impaired myocardial contractility. Gram-positive organisms are a more frequent cause than Gram-negative organisms, with about 60% of infections arising from respiratory, intra-abdominal and urinary tract sources. Septicaemia is a medical emergency requiring intensive fluid replacement, plasma volume expansion and electrolyte correction. Noradrenaline (norepinephrine) or other vasopressors may be used to support the blood pressure (Ch. 4). There have been many advances in our understanding of the pathogenesis of sepsis and the associated immune activation, but little improvement in our ability to manage the complications of sepsis. Adrenal insufficiency is common in severe sepsis and treatment with low-dose hydrocortisone may reduce the duration of shock.

If the source of the infection is not clinically apparent then empirical antibacterial therapy is given to cover as wide a range of potential infecting organisms as possible. The prognosis is much worse if first-line drugs are ineffective. Suitable treatment would be with an antipseudomonal penicillin such as piperacillin with tazobactam or a broad-spectrum cephalosporin (e.g. cefotaxime, or ceftazidime if pseudomonal infection is suspected). A carbapenem such as meropenem or imipenem (with cilastatin) can be used if the infection was hospital-acquired. Metronidazole is added if anaerobic infection is suspected, or vancomycin if MRSA is suspected.

Immunocompromised and neutropenic individuals are at particularly high risk from septicaemia. A combination of gentamicin with a broad-spectrum penicillin, cephalosporin, piperacillin with tazobactam or meropenem can be given. Metronidazole is usually added if anaerobic infection is suspected; flucloxacillin or vancomycin is added if Gram-positive infection is suspected. Failure to respond to such triple therapy within 48 h may indicate a fungal infection, for which amphotericin can be added (see below).

Infective endocarditis

The majority of cases of infective endocarditis are caused by bacterial pathogens, most commonly oral streptococci, followed by enterococci, S. aureus and coagulase-negative staphylococci. Endocarditis usually arises on the endothelial surface of a pre-existing heart defect (e.g. valvular heart defect, ventricular septal defect) or on a prosthetic heart valve. It arises when micro-organisms enter the bloodstream and become established on the endocardium, where they may adhere to pre-existing fibrin–platelet vegetations. Bacteria enter the blood during dental procedures, vigorous teeth cleaning or some surgical procedures.

Untreated infection can destroy the infected heart valve and produce severe haemodynamic disturbance. Systemic complications can also arise from embolisation of vegetation from the valve, from bacteraemia, or through immune complexes that form in response to the infection.

When infection is suspected, blood cultures must be taken and empirical antimicrobial treatment started. Prior to identification of the organism, treatment is usually started with intravenous flucloxacillin or benzylpenicillin combined with low-dose gentamicin. If the organism is sensitive to penicillin, then the benzylpenicillin is continued for 4 weeks and the gentamicin stopped after 2 weeks. Vancomycin and rifampicin are substituted for the penicillin in people with penicillin allergy when there is infection on a prosthetic heart valve or if MRSA is suspected.

Antibacterial prophylaxis is no longer recommended prior to procedures such as dental treatment, since there is no good evidence that it prevents endocarditis.

Table 51.4 Organisms causing bacterial meningitis

Age	Organism
<1 month	Group B streptococci
1 month–4 years	Haemophilus influenzae
>4 years to young adult	Neisseria meningitidis (meningococcus)
Older adults	Streptococcus pneumoniae (pneumococcus)

Meningitis

Bacterial meningitis is a medical emergency. The most likely organism depends on the age of the person (Table 51.4). Empirical selection of therapy is usually necessary and treatment should be started at the first suspicion of bacterial meningitis. A single dose of benzylpenicillin can be given if the person is outside hospital, but cefotaxime (with the addition of amoxicillin for those over 50 years old) is the preferred treatment in hospital. Chloramphenicol is an option for those who have an allergy to both penicillin and cephalosporins. Treatment is given for 7 days for meningococcus, and 10 days for H. influenzae or pneumococcus. Rifampicin is given for 2–4 days before hospital discharge if the meningitis was caused by meningococcus or H. influenzae. Close contacts of people with meningococcal or H. influenzae type b meningitis are usually given rifampicin as prophylaxis against infection.

Dexamethasone should be considered immediately, and no later than 12 h after starting the antibacterial. This reduces the frequency of neurological complications.

Tuberculosis

M. tuberculosis readily develops resistance to single-drug therapy. Three or four drugs are used for the first 2 months ('initial phase') to rapidly reduce the bacterial population prior to information on bacterial sensitivities becoming available, following which treatment is continued with two drugs for a further 4 months ('continuation phase') to achieve a cure. In some cases, more prolonged treatment may be necessary, especially for tuberculous meningitis or for resistant mycobacteria.

A standard regimen in the UK includes rifampicin, isoniazid, ethambutol and pyrazinamide for the initial phase (or until bacterial sensitivities are known), followed by rifampicin and isoniazid (preferably in a combination preparation) for a further 4 months. More prolonged treatment is sometimes necessary for cavitating lung disease or slow clearance of bacteria from the sputum. Ethambutol is not used for treatment of young children because of difficulty in monitoring for eye toxicity.

Streptomycin is used in some countries in the initial phase of treatment or if resistance to isoniazid is known. Thiacetazone is often used with isoniazid and initially streptomycin in countries that cannot afford rifampicin. Adherence to the treatment regimen can be a major problem in the treatment of tuberculosis, and combination tablets are often used to maximise this. In developed countries, directly observed treatment (or DOT) has been instituted to improve adherence. This can result in major improvements in eradication rates.

Multidrug-resistant tuberculosis (with resistance to at least rifampicin and isoniazid) is becoming more common, and new treatment strategies are needed to deal with emerging strains of *M. tuberculosis*. There are also increasing problems with the treatment of tuberculosis in people with HIV infection. This reflects the propensity for interactions among the antiretroviral drugs and antituberculous therapy, and overlapping unwanted effects.

FUNGAL INFECTIONS

Fungi (including yeasts) usually infect skin or superficial mucous membranes, but can more rarely involve internal organs. Most fungal infections occur because of an underlying defect in host resistance. Fungi grow more readily in immunosuppressed individuals or following the suppression of normal flora with antibacterials. Good hygiene and the avoidance of sources of infection are important complementary approaches to the use of antifungal drugs.

Compared with antibacterial drugs, fewer drugs have been developed that have activity against fungi, and many of these are toxic to humans. A simplified outline of the ways in which antifungal drugs work is shown in Figure 51.5.

ANTIFUNGAL DRUGS

Drugs that impair membrane barrier function

Polyenes

 Examples

amphotericin, nystatin

Mechanism of action

Polyenes bind to ergosterol in the cell wall of fungi and form aqueous pores that promote leakage of intracellular ions and disruption of active transport mechanisms in the membrane. They can be fungistatic or fungicidal.

Spectrum of activity

Nystatin is particularly effective for infections with *Candida* species. Amphotericin is active against all common fungi that cause systemic infection (*Candida*, *Aspergillus*, *Mucor* and *Cryptococcus* species).

Resistance

Acquired resistance is rare but can occur in immunosuppressed people. Fungi develop a mutation that permits synthesis of the cell membrane without using ergosterol.

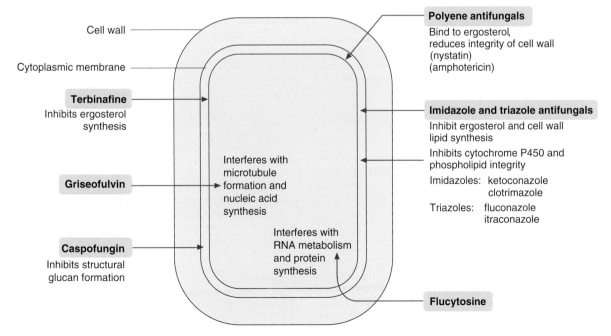

Fig. 51.5 Sites of action of antifungal drugs.

Pharmacokinetics

Nystatin is too toxic for systemic use and is not absorbed from the gastrointestinal tract. It is therefore used topically for *Candida albicans* infections, for example as cream for skin infection, as vaginal pessaries or orally for buccal and bowel infections.

Amphotericin is poorly absorbed from the gut and is usually given intravenously for treatment of serious systemic fungal infections. An oral formulation is used for buccal and intestinal candidal infections. Amphotericin can also be given intrathecally for fungal meningitis. Amphotericin binds to steroid molecules in human tissue, and is released slowly and eliminated via the biliary tract and kidney. It has a very long half-life (about 2 days).

Lipid delivery vehicles for amphotericin have been developed to reduce its nephrotoxicity. These formulations alter drug distribution and help to concentrate the drug at the site of infection. Formulations include liposomal spheres (in which the drug is dissolved in phospholipid membrane vesicles), lipid complexes (in which the lipid exists in ribbons interspersed with amphotericin) and a colloidal dispersion of lipid discs that incorporate the drug. The lipid component is probably cleared from the blood by mononuclear phagocytes.

Unwanted effects

Nystatin is virtually free of both toxic and allergic unwanted effects when used topically. Used orally for intestinal infection, it can cause gastrointestinal upset. Host toxicity with amphotericin is due to binding to cholesterol rather than ergosterol. Intravenous infusion of amphotericin is commonly associated with the following:

- fever and rigors during the first week of therapy,
- anorexia, nausea, vomiting, diarrhoea,
- headache, muscle and joint pain,
- anaphylaxis, which makes a test dose advisable,
- dose-related nephrotoxicity, which is the major limiting factor in treatment. It presents with reduced glomerular filtration rate and produces hypokalaemia and hypomagnesaemia through tubular leakage of K^+ and Mg^{2+}. Lipid formulations substantially reduce the risk of nephrotoxicity and are particularly useful to treat people with pre-existing renal impairment,
- arrhythmias,
- hearing loss, diplopia, convulsions, peripheral neuropathy.

Drugs that inhibit cell wall synthesis

Imidazoles

clotrimazole, ketoconazole, miconazole

Mechanism of action

The imidazoles alter fungal cell membrane fluidity by inhibiting lanosterol 14α-demethylase, a form of cytochrome P450 that participates in the conversion of lanosterol to ergosterol. Reduced ergosterol synthesis alters fungal cell membrane fluidity, reduces the activity of membrane-associated enzymes and increases cell wall permeability. Accumulation of ergosterol precursors in the cell causes growth arrest. Although the equivalent human enzyme is much less sensitive to the effects of the drug, inhibition of cytochrome P450 isoenzymes can occur in human tissues, especially with ketoconazole (Ch. 2).

Spectrum of activity

The imidazoles are active against a wide variety of filamentous fungi including many *Candida* species. They are less active against *Candida krusei*. Clotrimazole is used for vaginal candidiasis and for dermatophyte infections, such as ringworm (tinea), the causative fungi of which vary geographically, but which generally are *Trichophyton*, *Microsporon* or *Epidermophyton* species. Ketoconazole can be used for systemic mycoses, resistant mucocutaneous candidiasis, resistant vaginal candidiasis and resistant dermatophyte infections.

Resistance

The development of resistance is rare, except during long-term use in people with AIDS. The mechanism involves a point mutation in the target enzyme, lanosterol 14α-demethylase, or development of an active pump that removes drug from the cell, especially in *Candida* species.

Pharmacokinetics

Absorption of imidazoles from the gastrointestinal tract is poor, but oral ketoconazole achieves plasma concentrations high enough to treat systemic infection. Clotrimazole is only used in topical formulations for superficial infections, for example skin and vagina. The imidazoles are metabolised in the liver. Ketoconazole has a half-life of about 6–10 h.

Unwanted effects

These are unusual with topical formulations, although oral miconazole can cause gastrointestinal upset. Oral ketoconazole can cause the following:

- nausea, vomiting, abdominal pain,
- rash, urticaria, pruritus,
- hepatitis: asymptomatic elevation of liver enzymes is common; more severe hepatic reactions are unusual but can be fatal. Liver function must be monitored during systemic use of ketoconazole,
- high doses of ketoconazole suppress androgen production and in males can cause oligospermia or gynaecomastia,
- drug interactions: ketoconazole can inhibit metabolism of drugs that are eliminated by cytochrome P450; examples of drugs affected include ciclosporin, tacrolimus (Ch. 38) and warfarin (Ch. 11).

Triazoles

Examples

fluconazole, itraconazole, voriconazole

Mechanism of action and spectrum of activity

The triazoles have a similar mechanism of action and spectrum of activity to the imidazoles (see above). Fluconazole is used for candidiasis and for cryptococcal infection. Itraconazole is used for mucocutaneous candidiasis and for dermatophyte infections, such as pityriasis versicolor (caused by an organism known as *Malassezia furfur* or *Pityosporum orbiculare*) and tinea corporis or pedis (ringworms). Voriconazole is an 'extended-spectrum' triazole used for invasive aspergillosis, and serious infections caused by *Scedosporium* species, *Fusarium* species, or invasive fluconazole-resistant *C. krusei* and *Candida glabrata.*

Resistance

As with imidazoles, the development of resistance is rare, except during long-term use in people with AIDS. The mechanism involves development of an active pump that removes drug from the cell, especially in *Candida* species.

Pharmacokinetics

Oral absorption of triazoles is good. Formulations are also available for intravenous (fluconazole, voriconazole) and topical (itraconazole) use. The triazoles are metabolised in the liver and have long half-lives (6–30 h). Fluconazole penetrates well into cerebrospinal fluid, which is useful for treatment of cryptococcal meningitis.

Unwanted effects

- Nausea, abdominal pain and diarrhoea.
- Headache, dizziness.
- Abnormalities of liver function and, occasionally, hepatitis or cholestasis. These are more common during prolonged treatment with itraconazole. Monitoring of liver function during systemic treatment is essential.
- Increased risk of heart failure with itraconazole. The mechanism of its negative inotropic effect is not known.
- Rashes, including Stevens–Johnson syndrome.

Terbinafine
Mechanism of action and use

Terbinafine is an allylamine that inhibits squalene epoxidase, the enzyme that converts squalene to ergosterol in the cell wall. It impairs fungal cell wall synthesis, and the intracellular accumulation of squalene is probably cytotoxic (Fig. 51.5). It is used topically for treatment of dermatophyte infections of the nails, and systemically for ringworm infections.

Resistance

Resistance is rare, but similar to that for imidazole antifungals.

Pharmacokinetics

Terbinafine penetrates well into the stratum corneum and hair follicles after topical use. After oral administration it is metabolised in the liver and has a long half-life (11–17 h).

Unwanted effects

These are unlikely with topical use of the drug, but include:

- nausea, taste disturbance, abdominal discomfort and diarrhoea,
- headache,
- rashes, which are occasionally severe.

Echinocandins

Example

caspofungin

Mechanism of action

Caspofungin inhibits fungal cell wall synthesis, targeting the glucans that are found in fungal cell walls but not in human cells (Fig. 51.5). It inhibits the enzyme $\beta(1,3)$-D-glucan synthase, and prevents production of the main structural polymer in the fungal cell wall. Caspofungin is used to treat invasive aspergillosis as a second-line drug, and invasive candidiasis.

Resistance

This is uncommon at present, but can occur from a point gene mutation coding for a structural change in the target enzyme, which no longer binds the drug.

Pharmacokinetics

Caspofungin is only given by intravenous infusion. It is metabolised in the liver and has a very long half-life (40–50 h).

Unwanted effects

- Nausea, vomiting, abdominal pain, diarrhoea.
- Dyspnoea.
- Flushing, fever.
- Headache.
- Rashes.
- Hypokalaemia, hypomagnesaemia.

Drugs that inhibit macromolecule synthesis

Flucytosine
Mechanism of action and use

Flucytosine is converted to 5-fluorouracil (5-FU) selectively in fungal cells by cytosine deaminase. 5-FU is an antimetabolite that competes with uracil for incorporation into fungal RNA, and is metabolised to compounds that inhibit enzymes involved in DNA synthesis (Fig. 51.5).

Flucytosine is only active against yeasts such as *Candida*, *Aspergillus* and *Cryptococcus* species and is used for systemic infections.

Resistance

Resistance occurs readily and arises through a mutation that produces a deficiency of cytosine deaminase or through excessive synthesis of uracil, which competes with the antimetabolite. For this reason, flucytosine is only used in combination with amphotericin or fluconazole.

Pharmacokinetics

Flucytosine is only available for intravenous use. It is mainly eliminated unchanged in the urine and has a short half-life (3 h).

Unwanted effects

- Nausea, abdominal pain, diarrhoea.
- Rashes.

Drugs that interact with microtubules

Griseofulvin

Mechanism of action and use

Griseofulvin inhibits dermatophyte mitosis by impairing the polymerisation of microtubule protein (Fig. 51.5). It is active against dermatophytes such as *Microsporum*, *Epidermophyton* and *Trichophyton* species.

Resistance

Resistance has not been shown.

Pharmacokinetics

Griseofulvin shows variable absorption from the gut. It is selectively concentrated in skin and nail beds; only low concentrations are found in plasma. Elimination is by hepatic metabolism and the half-life is long (10–21 h).

Unwanted effects

- Nausea, vomiting, diarrhoea.
- Headache.

TREATMENT OF SPECIFIC FUNGAL INFECTIONS

Aspergillus

Aspergillus species can cause an invasive fungal infection that most commonly affects the lung. However, in immunocompromised individuals it can invade more widely and infect the heart, brain, sinuses and skin. The treatment of choice is voriconazole, which is more effective and less toxic than amphotericin. If this fails then itraconazole can be used. Caspofungin is reserved for infections that have failed to respond to standard treatments, or for those people who cannot tolerate the other drugs.

Candida

Amphotericin or nystatin is often used for oral candidiasis. If there is oropharyngeal disease that is refractory to topical treatment, then an absorbed drug such as fluconazole or itraconazole is used orally. Vulvovaginal infection is treated with cream and pessaries, and imidazole drugs such as clotrimazole are usually the first choice. Nystatin is an alternative for vulvovaginal candidiasis, but stains clothing yellow. For recurrent vulvovaginal infections, oral fluconazole or itraconazole should be taken once a week for 6 months. Superficial candidal infections of the skin are treated topically with cream, usually containing an imidazole. Terbinafine or nystatin can also be used topically.

Invasive candidiasis mainly occurs as a hospital-acquired infection, particularly in people who have had abdominal surgery, parenteral nutrition, multiple antibacterial drugs or central vascular lines. *C. albicans* is still the single most common organism, but *C. krusei*, *C. glabrata* and *Candida parapsilosis* are increasingly common. Amphotericin is the treatment of choice, sometimes combined with fluconazole. Caspofungin is an alternative.

Cryptococcus

Infection with *Cryptococcus* species usually occurs in people who are immunocompromised. It can cause life-threatening meningitis and is treated with intravenous amphotericin with flucytosine. Fluconazole is an alternative and can be given orally for prophylaxis against relapse.

Skin and nail infections

Topical therapy is usually suitable for infections with most dermatophytes. Fungal infection of the scalp (tinea capitis), body (tinea corporis), groin (tinea cruris), hand (tinea manuum), foot (tinea pedis) or nail (tinea unguium) will respond to most azoles. Griseofulvin is usually reserved for treatment of scalp infections. Nail infection usually requires systemic treatment with terbinafine or itraconazole.

Pityriasis versicolor can be treated topically or orally with itraconazole, or with oral fluconazole.

Prophylaxis in immunocompromised individuals

Individuals who are immunocompromised are at greater risk of fungal infection. Prophylaxis is often given with oral fluconazole, since this has better oral absorption than most azoles, and is less toxic than ketoconazole.

VIRAL INFECTIONS

Viruses are small infective particles consisting of either DNA or RNA inside a protein coating (capsule), which in some viruses may be further surrounded by a lipoprotein coating. The proteins can have antigenic properties. Viruses lack any inherent metabolic machinery and must use the host's metabolic processes to replicate. Viruses access host cells after binding to recognition sites that are endogenous receptors for normal cellular constituents; for example, adrenoceptors, cytokine receptors, glycoproteins, etc. (Fig. 51.6). Drugs that interfere with host cell membrane cytokine receptors, such as CCR5 (see below), and surface glycoproteins will inhibit viral entry and interrupt virus replication.

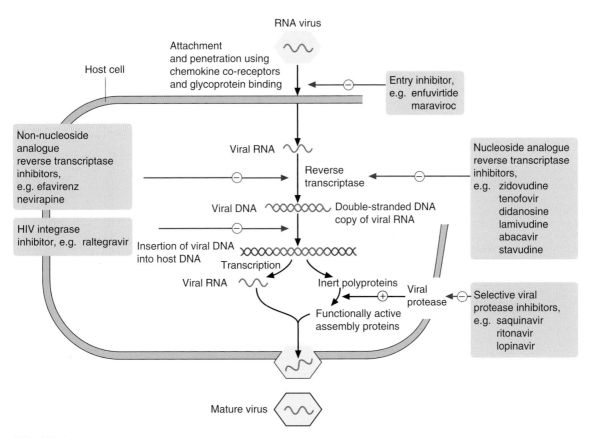

Fig. 51.6 **Principles of RNA virus replication and sites of action of antiviral drugs.**

The host will normally eliminate the virus by killing the infected cell. Cytotoxic T-lymphocytes recognise the viral surface proteins that are expressed by infected cells. The host can also produce antibodies that bind to and inactivate virus particles extracellularly. Vaccination is designed to generate this response.

Viruses utilise the host's metabolic processes and this makes it difficult to damage the virus without damaging the host. Importantly, antiviral drugs are only effective while the virus is replicating, so the earlier they are given in the course of the infection the more likely they are to work. An outline of the replication of RNA and DNA viruses is shown in Figures 51.6 and 51.7. Since the replicative mechanisms involved may be distinctive to one type of virus, some antiviral drugs are specific for a particular class of virus.

New antiviral drugs are being introduced into clinical practice at an increasing rate. Drugs are available to treat infection by RNA viruses (e.g. HIV, hepatitis C and influenza viruses) and DNA viruses (e.g. herpesviruses, cytomegalovirus and hepatitis B virus). Most of these drugs work by disturbing various steps in the replicative pathways of the virus. Because of the development of resistance and the variability in viral sensitivity to drugs it is sometimes necessary to use concurrently drugs that target different processes in the virus replication.

Resistance to antiviral drugs occurs readily. This relates to the high rate of natural occurrence of mutations in the viral genome and production of quasi-species of the virus.

Viral polymerases have a high inherent error rate (especially RNA viruses) and viruses tolerate a large number of nucleoside mutations without losing their infectivity. Normally the large variety of viral quasi-species will be dominated by the variant most selected for survival and therefore use of an antiviral drug will select for growth of resistant variants.

ANTIVIRAL DRUGS

Drugs active against HIV

Nucleoside analogue HIV reverse transcriptase inhibitors

Examples

abacavir, emtricitabine, lamivudine, tenofovir disoproxil, zidovudine

Mechanism of action

Reverse transcriptase inhibitors are active against human immunodeficiency virus (HIV), an RNA virus. These drugs inhibit RNA virus replication by reversible inhibition of the viral enzyme HIV reverse transcriptase, which reverse transcribes viral RNA into viral DNA for insertion into the host DNA sequence. The nucleoside analogue reverse

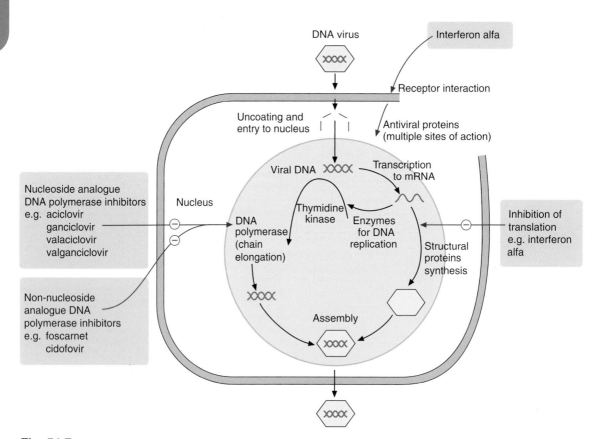

Fig. 51.7 Principles of DNA virus replication and sites of actions of antiviral drugs.

transcriptase inhibitor drugs (Fig. 51.6) are activated by phosphorylation inside the virus to the 5′-triphosphate form. Inhibition of viral replication is achieved by competitive binding of the activated drug to the enzyme–template–primer complex in place of the natural 5′-deoxynucleoside triphosphates, thus terminating further DNA chain elongation.

The nucleoside reverse transcriptase inhibitors are analogues of precursors of the natural purines and pyrimidines involved in DNA transcription initiated by the virus. Zidovudine is an analogue of thymidine, emtricitabine and lamivudine are analogues of cytidine, abacavir is an analogue of deoxyguanosine and tenofovir is an analogue of adenosine.

Resistance

Resistant quasi-species emerge within weeks or months by mutation of the drug-binding site on reverse transcriptase, resulting in an increase in the affinity for the natural substrate compared with the drug. Because of the rapid development of resistance, multiple drug therapy is used for treatment of HIV infection.

Pharmacokinetics

These drugs are almost completely absorbed from the gut. Elimination of abacavir and zidovudine is mainly by hepatic metabolism and the half-lives are short (1–2 h). Emtricitabine, lamivudine and tenofovir (the metabolite of tenofovir disoproxil) are mainly eliminated unchanged by the kidney, with half-lives in the range 1–17 h.

Unwanted effects

These are often so severe that they lead to withdrawal of therapy. They are probably related to inhibition of host mitochondrial enzymes, with impaired generation of intracellular ATP.

- Neutropenia and anaemia are the most frequent unwanted effects (usually occurring in individuals with advanced AIDS).
- Nausea, vomiting, diarrhoea, abdominal pain.
- Headache, insomnia.
- Myalgia or myositis, especially with high doses.
- Severe, potentially life-threatening, hepatomegaly with steatosis and lactic acidosis.
- Pancreatitis.
- Lipodystrophy syndrome with fat redistribution (loss of subcutaneous fat, buffalo hump, breast enlargement), insulin resistance and dyslipidaemia; this may be due to inhibition of regulatory proteins in adipocytes.

Non-nucleoside HIV reverse transcriptase inhibitors

Examples

efavirenz, nevirapine, rilpivirine

Mechanism of action and resistance

The non-nucleoside drugs inhibit HIV reverse transcriptase by binding remotely from the enzyme active site to produce a conformational change that prevents substrate binding. They have greater antiviral activity than nucleoside analogue inhibitors and are better tolerated. Resistance still emerges rapidly by single point mutations, unless they are used in combination with at least two other antiretroviral drugs.

Pharmacokinetics

Oral absorption of nevirapine and rilpivirine is good, while that of efavirenz is variable and incomplete. They are metabolised by hepatic CYP3A4, and also induce the enzyme. They have very long half-lives of about 2 days.

Unwanted effects

- Rash (severe in 10%), especially with nevirapine and efavirenz.
- Nausea, vomiting, abdominal pain, diarrhoea.
- Headache, drowsiness, fatigue.
- Depression with efavirenz and rilpivirine.
- Hepatotoxicity with nevirapine, which can cause potentially fatal fulminant hepatitis.
- Drug interactions with drugs metabolised by hepatic cytochrome P450.

HIV protease inhibitors

 Examples

atazanavir, darunavir, fosamprenavir, lopinavir, ritonavir

Mechanism of action

In HIV infection there are some steps in viral replication that differ from the RNA translation processes in host cells. In the virus, RNA is translated into inert polyproteins rather than the functional proteins that are the products of host cells. Proteases found only in the virus cleave these polyproteins to the functionally active proteins required by the virus for its continued existence (Fig. 51.6). Protease inhibitors are specific for the enzymes found in HIV. They block the infectivity of the virus but do not affect virus activity in host cells that are already infected.

Resistance

Resistance occurs by mutation in the amino acid sequence of the HIV proteases that form the targets for the drug. Multiple mutations are required for high-level resistance, but over one-third of the amino acid residues in HIV protein can be changed without altering viral function. High plasma drug concentrations delay the onset of resistance, as does the combination of a protease inhibitor with two reverse transcriptase inhibitors. Sequential use of more than one protease inhibitor encourages high-level resistance.

Pharmacokinetics

Oral absorption varies between the protease inhibitors. All are metabolised by, and inhibit, CYP3A4 in the liver. They have half-lives in the range 2–10 h.

Unwanted effects

- Nausea, vomiting, abdominal pain, diarrhoea.
- Lipodystrophy syndrome (see nucleoside analogue HIV reverse transcriptase inhibitors).
- Hepatic dysfunction.
- Pancreatitis.
- Circumoral and peripheral paraesthesiae with ritonavir.
- Drug interactions (Ch. 56): inhibition of the P450 enzyme CYP3A4 can enhance the unwanted effects of protease inhibitors; the concurrent use of inducers of CYP3A4 can lower plasma concentrations of the protease inhibitor and encourage viral resistance. Inhibition of CYP3A4 by a low dose of ritonavir can increase the clinical effect of other protease inhibitors (boosted protease inhibition), a useful action that allows less frequent dosing with the other drug. Ritonavir also inhibits the metabolism of drugs such as warfarin (Ch. 11) and carbamazepine (Ch. 23). The use of protease inhibitors with simvastatin (Ch. 48) should be avoided because of an increased risk of myopathy.

HIV binding–fusion–entry inhibitors

 Example

enfuvirtide

Mechanism of action

To enter a host cell, HIV fuses with the host cell membrane. This fusion is facilitated by a conformational change in a viral glycoprotein, gp41, in the viral cell membrane. Enfuvirtide is a 36-amino-acid peptidomimetic that binds to the gp41 glycoprotein and prevents the conformational change, blocking HIV entry into host cells. Enfuvirtide is used when there is resistance or intolerance to other antiretroviral drugs.

Resistance

This occurs by gene mutation that modifies the gp41 glycoprotein target of the drug.

Pharmacokinetics

Enfuvirtide is given by subcutaneous injection. It is metabolised by hydrolysis to its constituent amino acids, and has a half-life of 4 h.

Unwanted effects

- Injection-site reactions.
- Pancreatitis, gastro-oesophageal reflux disease, anorexia, weight loss.
- Peripheral neuropathy, tremor, anxiety, nightmares, vertigo.
- Diabetes mellitus.

CCR5 co-receptor antagonists

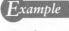 *Example*

maraviroc

Mechanism of action

Chemokine (C-C motif) receptor 5 (CCR5) is a receptor for several chemokines, including RANTES (regulated upon activation, normal T-cell expressed and secreted) and macrophage inflammatory proteins MIP-1α and MIP-1β. It is expressed on many cells, including T-cells, macrophages, dendritic cells and microglia. CCR5 acts as a viral co-receptor that facilitates entry of HIV into the cell. Some HIV strains use other chemokine receptors such as CCR4, or both CCR4 and CCR5, to access cells. HIV strains which use CCR5 are predominant early in the infection. Maraviroc selectively binds to CCR5 and prevents interaction with CCR5-tropic strains of HIV, inhibiting their entry into the cell. It has no effect on viruses that use CCR4 or are dual-tropic for CCR4 and CCR5. Maraviroc is used in combination with other antiretroviral drugs for individuals who have already received other antiretroviral treatment.

Pharmacokinetics

Maraviroc is only partially absorbed from the gut. It is metabolised in the liver and has a long half-life (14–18 h).

Unwanted effects

- Nausea, diarrhoea, abdominal pain, anorexia.
- Malaise.
- Rash.
- Depression, insomnia, headache.

HIV integrase inhibitors

raltegravir

Mechanism of action

Once inside a host cell, HIV integrates its DNA into the host genome. This requires the action of a specific viral integrase. Raltegravir inhibits the integrase and prevents DNA strand transfer from the viral genome. Raltegravir is used when there is resistance to other antiretroviral drugs.

Resistance

This occurs when there is amino acid substitution in the viral integrase.

Pharmacokinetics

Raltegravir is well absorbed from the gut, and is excreted in the bile after glucuronide conjugation and unchanged in the urine. It has a half-life of 9 h.

Unwanted effects

- Nausea, vomiting, diarrhea, abdominal pain.
- Headache, dizziness, insomnia.
- Rashes, sometimes with fever, arthralgia, myalgia, angioedema and hepatitis.

Drugs for herpesvirus and cytomegalovirus infections

Nucleoside analogue inhibitors of viral DNA polymerase

aciclovir, ganciclovir, valaciclovir, valganciclovir

Mechanism of action

Aciclovir and the other drugs in this class are guanosine analogues that are active against many DNA viruses and inhibit the synthesis of viral DNA (Fig. 51.7). Before they can exert their antiviral activity they all require phosphorylation by viral enzymes that are not present in uninfected host cells. However, the phosphorylating enzymes are not present in all DNA viruses. This dependency on viral enzymes prevents cytotoxic effects in human tissue.

Aciclovir and ganciclovir are activated by phosphorylation to a monophosphate by viral thymidine kinase. The monophosphate is then converted to a triphosphate derivative by other intracellular enzymes. The triphosphate derivatives are potent inhibitors of viral DNA polymerase. This terminates viral DNA synthesis and thus inhibits viral replication (Fig. 51.7).

Spectrum of activity

Aciclovir is most active against herpesviruses (both simplex and zoster). It is only active against cytomegalovirus (CMV) at high doses. Ganciclovir is also active against herpesviruses and has much greater activity than aciclovir against CMV, possibly because it is a better substrate for the CMV protein kinase which activates it.

Resistance

Viral mutants are selected that are unable to phosphorylate the drugs. Thymidine kinase-deficient mutants of herpesvirus usually develop in immunocompromised individuals, for example those with AIDS or after bone marrow transplantation, when resistance rates average 5–10%.

Pharmacokinetics

Aciclovir can be given orally, intravenously or topically to the skin or eye. Absorption from the gut is poor. The drug is widely distributed, but concentrations in the cerebrospinal fluid are low compared with those in plasma. Most is eliminated by the kidney, and the half-life is 3 h. Valaciclovir is an ester of aciclovir with higher oral bioavailability.

Ganciclovir is given intravenously for acute infections since it is poorly absorbed from the gut; it penetrates into CSF moderately well. It is eliminated by the kidney and has a half-life of 4 h. Valganciclovir is an oral prodrug of ganciclovir with better absorption.

Unwanted effects

Most unwanted effects occur with intravenous use, and are much more frequent with ganciclovir than with aciclovir.

- Severe local phlebitis at an infusion site.
- Nausea, vomiting, abdominal pain, diarrhoea.

- Rashes, including photosensitivity.
- Headache, dizziness, confusion, convulsions.
- Nephrotoxicity is caused by crystallisation of aciclovir in the kidney. It can be limited by a high fluid intake.
- Bone marrow suppression is the most frequent serious unwanted effect with ganciclovir, with neutropenia occurring in up to 40% of people, and thrombocytopenia less frequently.

Non-nucleoside analogue inhibitors of viral DNA polymerase

cidofovir, foscarnet sodium

Mechanism of action

Foscarnet is an inorganic pyrophosphate compound that binds to the pyrophosphate-binding sites of viral DNA polymerase, preventing DNA chain elongation. Affinity for the viral DNA polymerase is a hundred times greater than for the host cell DNA polymerase. Cidofovir is similar in structure to aciclovir but contains a phosphate moiety. Its action is similar to that of foscarnet. Foscarnet and cidofovir do not rely on intracellular activation for their antiviral activities (Fig. 51.7). These drugs are reversible inhibitors of CMV and herpes simplex replication.

Pharmacokinetics

Because both foscarnet and cidofovir are highly polar molecules, they are only given intravenously. Foscarnet and cidofovir are eliminated by the kidney and have half-lives of about 5 h and 3 h, respectively. Cidofovir is given with probenecid (and adequate hydration), which inhibits renal tubular secretion of cidofovir and minimises its nephrotoxicity.

Unwanted effects

- Nausea, vomiting, diarrhoea.
- Neutropenia.
- Headache, tremor, dizziness, mood disturbances with foscarnet.
- Both drugs are highly nephrotoxic, causing a rise in plasma creatinine; good hydration reduces kidney damage.
- Iritis or uveitis with cidofovir.

Drugs for treating hepatitis viruses

The nucleoside analogues entecavir, lamivudine, ribavirin and tenofovir disoproxil, and the protease inhibitors bocepravir and telaprevir as well as interferon alfa are used in the treatment of infections with hepatitis B and C viruses. Ribavirin is also used to treat respiratory syncytial virus (RSV). These drugs are discussed in Chapter 36.

Drugs for treating influenza virus

M₂ ion channel inhibitors

amantadine

Amantadine is active only against influenza A and inhibits the transmembrane M_2 ion channel that permits H^+ entry into the viral particle. This is required for uncoating of the virus once it has penetrated the host cell, so viral replication is inhibited. Amantadine is discussed in Chapter 24.

Neuraminidase inhibitors

oseltamivir, zanamivir

Mechanism of action

Influenza viruses carry two surface glycoproteins, a haemagglutinin and a neuraminidase. The haemagglutinin mediates entry of the virus into the host cell. Neuraminidase cleaves cellular-receptor sialic acid residues to which newly formed viruses are attached as they bud from the infected cell. The released virions can then infect new cells. Neuraminidase inhibitors inhibit the neuraminidases of both influenza A and B, and are effective against isolates resistant to amantadine.

Pharmacokinetics

Zanamivir is administered by inhalation; only 2% of the inhaled drug is absorbed, and then excreted unchanged. Oseltamivir is a more lipophilic molecule that is taken orally, and is converted by hepatic esterases to the active oseltamivir carboxylate, which is excreted by the kidneys and has a half-life of 6–10 h.

Unwanted effects

- Gastrointestinal disturbance with oseltamivir.
- Headache, fatigue, insomnia, dizziness with oseltamivir.
- Bronchospasm with inhaled zanamivir.

Immunomodulators

Interferon alfa

Interferon alfa is most often used in the treatment of chronic hepatitis B infection and is discussed in Chapter 36. Other clinical uses of interferon alfa include the treatment of:

- condylomata acuminata,
- AIDS-related Kaposi's sarcoma,
- hairy cell leukaemia,
- recurrent or metastatic renal cell carcinoma (Ch. 52).

Palivizumab

Mechanism of action and use

Palivizumab is a humanised monoclonal antibody produced by recombinant DNA technology. It has potent neutralising and fusion-inhibiting activity against RSV. It reduces the ability of RSV to replicate and infect cells by binding to an antigenic site on the surface of RSV. RSV is a common cause of mild respiratory illness in infants but can produce more severe illness in premature infants or those with congenital heart disease or bronchopulmonary dysplasia. Palivizumab can be given to at-risk children under the age of 2 years prior to commencement of the RSV season (October to April in the northern hemisphere) and monthly thereafter.

Pharmacokinetics

Palivizumab is given intramuscularly into the anterolateral aspect of the thigh. The routes of elimination are unknown; it has a long half-life of about 20 days.

Unwanted effects

- Fever.
- Injection-site reactions.

TREATMENT OF SPECIFIC VIRAL INFECTIONS

HIV infection

Multiple drug therapy is essential for HIV infection because of the rapid emergence of resistant strains. The most frequently used treatment regimens include two nucleoside analogue reverse transcriptase inhibitors (e.g. tenofovir with emtricitabine, or abacavir with lamivudine) combined with either a protease inhibitor (e.g. atazanavir, darunavir or raltegravir) or a non-nucleoside reverse transcriptase inhibitor (e.g. efavirenz). A low dose of ritonavir is often added to the protease inhibitor (boosted protease therapy) to prolong its action and simplify the dosing regimen. Such combinations are referred to as highly active antiretroviral therapy (HAART). HAART involves complex regimens that require adherence by the individual and careful assessment of the progress of viral suppression. Key principles include the following.

- Combination drug treatment should be started before substantial immunodeficiency is present. The goal is to suppress the virus before resistant mutants emerge or irreversible immune damage occurs. The optimal time to start treatment is not known, but should definitely be started when the CD4+ T-lymphocyte count falls below 200×10^6 L^{-1}. If this stage is missed, then treatment is given when symptoms arise as a result of HIV infection.
- When resistance occurs, modification in drug therapy should involve the addition or change of at least two drugs. Resistance of the HIV virus persists indefinitely. However, if toxicity limits the tolerability of one drug, a single substitution of a similar drug is a reasonable option.

- Optimal treatment should reduce the viral load to below detectable limits and achieve a rise in CD4+ lymphocyte count. This may take 6 months of optimal therapy.
- Failure to achieve full suppression of viral load should prompt a change in therapy if adherence is believed to be good. Poor adherence with therapy is likely to encourage the development of drug resistance (see above) and thus treatment failure. Drug therapy is ideally guided by patterns of resistance in the virus.
- The optimal duration of treatment is unclear, but withdrawal even when the CD4+ T-cell count rises is probably associated with less favourable long-term outcomes.

Prophylaxis after accidental exposure to HIV may be required. The regimen depends on the level of risk: two drugs are often used for moderate-risk exposures, or three drugs if the risk is high.

Varicella–zoster virus infections

Varicella–zoster virus (VZV) is a herpesvirus responsible for both chickenpox and shingles (herpes zoster). Shingles arises from reactivation of the virus, which lies dormant in a dorsal root ganglion after the primary chickenpox infection. Chickenpox is rarely treated with antiviral therapy, although the use of oral aciclovir reduces lesion formation and results in quicker healing.

Herpes zoster is most commonly found in the elderly and in immunosuppressed people. The rash is often preceded by pain for 1–4 days. Complications of infection occur in 15–20% of people who develop herpes zoster and include meningoencephalitis, motor nerve paralysis, ocular complications and postherpetic neuralgia. Oral antiviral drug therapy reduces pain and accelerates healing. It must be given while the virus is still replicating, and therefore started within 72 h of the onset of the rash. Oral aciclovir or valaciclovir are often used and are particularly indicated for those over 50 years (who are at greater risk of complications), for ophthalmic infections or in immunosuppressed people. The use of aciclovir has little effect on the risk of developing postherpetic neuralgia but does reduce the risk of motor nerve damage. Corticosteroids such as prednisolone as an adjunctive treatment to antiviral therapy reduce pain and produce more rapid healing of lesions, but do not prevent the development of post-herpetic neuralgia. Analgesics are often required in the early phases of zoster, and postherpetic neuralgia may require specific therapy (Ch. 19).

Herpes simplex virus infections

Herpes simplex virus exists in two forms: type 1 produces either oral or genital ulceration, and type 2 produces genital ulceration. Oral herpes simplex infection will respond to early topical application of aciclovir. Primary genital herpes produces multiple painful lesions and responds to oral aciclovir or valaciclovir given for 7–10 days. Recurrent lesions occur from reactivation of latent virus in the dorsal root ganglia, producing symptoms that are usually less severe than with primary episodes. After initial therapy with aciclovir or valaciclovir for up to 3 days, continuous suppressive therapy can be given to prevent further relapses.

Cytomegalovirus infection

CMV infection is common and usually produces mild symptoms. However, it can be devastating in immunosuppressed individuals. Troublesome complications in this group include retinitis (which can threaten sight), gastrointestinal manifestations (including oesophagitis, gastritis, cholecystitis or colitis), pneumonia and CNS involvement.

Intravenous ganciclovir is the treatment of choice for severe manifestations of CMV infection. Foscarnet can be used as an alternative to ganciclovir, or cidofovir if both are contraindicated. For CMV retinitis, oral valganciclovir is used both for treatment and to prevent relapse. Oral valganciclovir or valaciclovir are given for the prevention of CMV infection, especially in renal transplant and bone marrow transplant recipients in whom CMV pneumonia is a major potential complication. Combined therapy with ganciclovir and CMV immunoglobulin may be more effective than ganciclovir alone for treatment of pneumonia in this situation.

Influenza

The use of a neuraminidase inhibitor, such as zanamivir or oseltamivir, reduces the duration of uncomplicated influenza by about 1 day. Treatment must be started within 48 h of the onset of an influenza-like illness. People who are at greater risk of complications of influenza include those with chronic respiratory disease, significant cardiovascular disease, chronic renal disease, diabetes mellitus or those who are immunocompromised. However there is little evidence that these drugs prevent the complications of influenza. Neuraminidase inhibitors are also effective for the prevention of influenza during an epidemic, reducing the likelihood of developing the illness by 70–90%. They should be considered for high-risk individuals who have not been vaccinated and who can be treated within 48 h of contact with someone who has an influenza-like illness. Such prophylaxis is not a substitute for an effective vaccination campaign.

Viral hepatitis

This is discussed in Ch. 36.

Respiratory syncytial virus

RSV most commonly causes respiratory infections in children under 2 years old. It causes bronchiolitis and increased airway reactivity with wheezing. Treatment is usually symptomatic, but severe infection is sometimes treated with ribavirin. Palivizumab is given to prevent serious lower respiratory tract disease from RSV in children under 2 years old who are at high risk of complications.

PROTOZOAL INFECTIONS

MALARIA

Five species of the protozoan *Plasmodium* produce malaria in humans: *Plasmodium vivax*, *Plasmodium ovale* (two subspecies), *Plasmodium knowlesi*, *Plasmodium malariae* and *Plasmodium falciparum.* The motile infective form of the parasite, sporozoites, are formed by repeated division of oocysts in the body of the infected female *Anopheles* mosquito (the vector) and transferred in the mosquito's saliva into the host circulation during a blood meal (only female mosquitoes feed on blood). The parasite is rapidly sequestered in the liver and matures to tissue schizonts which divide asexually to form merozoites (Fig. 51.8). When the pre-erythrocytic (liver) cycle is complete after 5–16 days, 20 000–40 000 merozoites escape into the blood and invade erythrocytes. *P. vivax* and *P. ovale* may continue to multiply in the liver, but *P. malariae*, *P. knowlesi* and *P. falciparum* do not.

Merozoites released from the liver then undergo the erythrocytic cycle, multiplying asexually in erythrocytes and using haemoglobin as the main source of nutrition. Infected erythrocytes rupture (haemolyse) and release merozoites to invade other erythrocytes. Some merozoites in the plasma differentiate into male and female gametocytes. A mosquito biting an infected individual ingests gametocytes, which then go through a sexual development cycle in the mosquito to form sporozoites.

Release of merozoites from erythrocytes every 2 or 3 days causes repeated bouts of tertian or quartan fever in humans. Premonitory clinical symptoms of malaria include chills, and nausea, vomiting and headache are common. A fever follows, and the attack concludes with sweating. *P. falciparum* produces the most severe symptoms (malignant tertian malaria) because high levels of parasitaemia cause agglutination of red cells, which produces capillary thrombosis, especially in the brain, leading to cerebral malaria.

Because *P. vivax* and *P. ovale* continue to multiply in the liver as hypnozoites, they form a reservoir of parasites that are difficult to eradicate and can emerge to give relapses months or years after the initial infection. Drugs that treat only the erythrocytic phase will not produce a radical cure (elimination of all parasites), and relapsing infection can occur. Although *P. falciparum*, *P. malariae* and *P. knowlesi* do not have persistent liver forms, disease can recrudesce if parasites are not completely eliminated from the blood.

Antimalarial drugs

Chloroquine

Mechanism of action

Erythrocytes infected by malaria parasites concentrate chloroquine more than 100-fold compared to uninfected erythrocytes, since it binds to a breakdown product of haemoglobin (haemin) induced by the parasite.

- Chloroquine is then ingested by the erythrocyte-resident parasite and this raises lysosomal pH, which reduces the ability of the parasite to digest haemoglobin and thereby inhibits its growth.
- Chloroquine interacts with haemin (ferriprotoporphyrin IX) formed during digestion of haemoglobin, an action that prevents further degradation by the parasite.

Chloroquine (and its close relative hydroxychloroquine) also possess slow-onset anti-inflammatory activity, which is useful in the treatment of rheumatoid arthritis (Ch. 30).

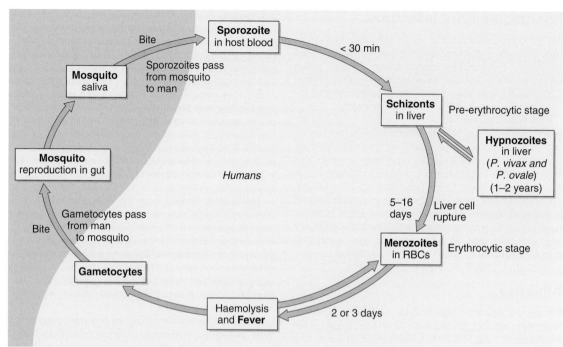

Fig. 51.8 **Life-cycle of the malarial parasite.** Most antimalarial drugs kill the *Plasmodium* parasites that cause repeated cycles of red blood cell (RBC) lysis and fever (erythrocytic stage). Primaquine kills parasites of *P. vivax* and *P. ovale* (hypnozoites) dormant in the liver (pre-erythrocytic stage).

Pharmacokinetics

Chloroquine is completely absorbed from the gut or can be given intravenously. It has a very high volume of distribution because of selective concentration in melanin-containing tissues, for example the retina of the eye, and in the liver, spleen and kidney. Approximately half is converted in the liver to active metabolites and the rest is excreted unchanged by the kidney. The half-life is very long during chronic dosing; an initial half-life of up to 6 days is followed by a second slow phase of tissue elimination with a half-life of greater than 1 month.

Unwanted effects

- Nausea, vomiting, diarrhoea and abdominal pain.
- Cardiovascular depression after intravenous use, with hypotension and heart block.
- Seizures.
- Retinopathy with cumulative doses, producing retinal pigmentation and visual field defects. Visual function should be monitored.
- Rashes and pruritus, hair loss and skin depigmentation.

Mefloquine
Mechanism of action

Mefloquine has a similar mode of action to that of chloroquine.

Pharmacokinetics

Mefloquine is well absorbed from the gut and has a high affinity for lung, liver and lymphoid tissue. Extensive metabolism occurs in the liver, but the elimination half-life is extremely long (2–4 weeks).

Unwanted effects

- CNS effects: dizziness, vertigo, headache, sleep disorders. Less commonly, severe psychiatric disturbance can occur, and mefloquine should not be given to people with a previous history of psychiatric disorder.
- Gastrointestinal effects occur that are similar to those seen with chloroquine.
- Myalgia, arthralgia.
- Chest pain, tachycardia, hypotension.

Primaquine
Mechanism of action

Unlike the structurally related drugs chloroquine and mefloquine, primaquine only affects the exoerythrocytic parasite. It enters the parasite in the liver and may inhibit mitochondrial respiration. It is used after treatment with chloroquine, to eradicate *P. vivax* or *P. ovale* from the liver (a radical cure).

Pharmacokinetics

Primaquine is completely absorbed from the gut and rapidly metabolised in the liver, producing active compounds. The half-life is 4–10 h.

Unwanted effects

- Intravascular haemolysis in people with glucose-6-phosphate dehydrogenase (G6PD) deficiency (Ch. 47). G6PD activity in erythrocytes produces NADPH, which keeps glutathione in the reduced state, thereby maintaining cell wall integrity and preventing haemolysis (see Ch. 53). G6PD activity should be checked before initiating treatment.
- Gastrointestinal effects are similar to those seen with chloroquine.

Quinine
Mechanism of action

Quinine is similar to chloroquine in its action.

Pharmacokinetics

Quinine is well absorbed from the gut but can also be given by intravenous infusion. Metabolism in the liver is extensive and the half-life is about 6 h in healthy people, becoming much longer in severe malaria.

Unwanted effects

- 'Cinchonism': tinnitus, headache, nausea, flushing, visual disturbances with vertigo, and, if severe, hearing loss.
- Stimulation of insulin secretion, producing hypoglycaemia.
- Bradycardias, heart block or ventricular tachycardia, most often with intravenous loading doses.

Pyrimethamine with sulfadoxine
Mechanism of action

Selective inhibition of dihydrofolate reductase in the malaria parasite by pyrimethamine reduces folic acid synthesis (Fig. 51.4). Pyrimethamine should only be given in combination with the sulphonamide sulfadoxine because of the widespread emergence of resistance.

Pharmacokinetics

Pyrimethamine is well absorbed from the gut and undergoes extensive hepatic metabolism. The half-life is approximately 2–6 days.

Unwanted effects

Pyrimethamine is usually well tolerated; occasional effects are:
- Photosensitive rashes.
- Insomnia.
- Megaloblastic anaemia due to inhibition of human folate metabolism (with high doses).

Proguanil
Mechanism of action

Proguanil inhibits plasmodial dihydrofolate reductase (Fig. 51.4), mainly through its active metabolite, cycloguanil, which inhibits folate production in both pre-erythrocytic and erythrocytic parasites. It is often used for malaria

prophylaxis in combination with chloroquine. It can also be used in the prophylaxis and treatment of *P. falciparum* in combination with atovaquone (see below).

Pharmacokinetics

Absorption of proguanil from the gut is good and extensive metabolism occurs in the liver to cycloguanil, its potent active derivative. Cycloguanil has a short half-life (2 h) but its plasma profile reflects its slow formation from proguanil (12–24 h).

Unwanted effects

- Mouth ulcers.
- Epigastric discomfort, diarrhoea.

Artemether with lumefantrine
Mechanism of action

Artemether is a herb extract that is activated by complexing with iron in the haem ingested by the malarial parasite. The resulting compound produces reactive oxygen species that disrupt Ca^{2+} transporter function in the parasite. It is used with lumefantrine, which may work by inhibiting the production of β-haematin in the erythrocyte. The combination reduces the emergence of resistance.

Pharmacokinetics

Artemether is well absorbed from the gut and rapidly hydrolysed to an active metabolite that has a short half-life of 2–3 h.

Unwanted effects

- Abdominal pain, nausea, anorexia, diarrhoea.
- Headache, dizziness, sleep disturbance, fatigue.

Treatment of malaria

Chemotherapy of malaria falls into three categories:

- rapid-acting blood schizonticides (to kill schizonts in acute malaria): chloroquine, mefloquine, quinine, artemether with lumefantrine,
- slow-acting blood schizonticides (to suppress blood infections): pyrimethamine with sulfadoxine, proguanil,
- tissue schizonticide (to eliminate liver parasites): primaquine.

The recommended drug to use within each category depends on the type of parasite and the pattern of resistance where the infection was acquired. If the infecting organism is unknown, it is assumed to be *P. falciparum*, which carries the greatest risk. The latest drug recommendations should be obtained from tropical disease advisory centres.

Examples are given for current recommended treatments for acute attacks of high- and low-risk malaria.

For *P. falciparum*, chloroquine and mefloquine resistance is common. Oral quinine (or intravenous quinine for serious infections) for 5–7 days is followed by pyrimethamine with sulfadoxine for 7 days or by doxycycline or clindamycin (see antibacterials, above) if the plasmodia are resistant to sulfadoxine. Alternatively, proguanil with atovaquone or artemether with lumefantrine are used for 3 days.

For benign malaria, chloroquine is taken for 3 days. For *P. vivax* and *P. ovale* primaquine is then taken for 14 days to destroy hepatic parasites.

Prophylaxis against malaria

The recommendations for prophylaxis depend on patterns of resistance in the area to be visited. Chloroquine or proguanil is often recommended for areas where resistance is low. For many areas a combination of both drugs is desirable. Mefloquine, doxycycline, or proguanil with atovaquone are recommended in some areas where there is a high risk of chloroquine-resistant malaria. Prophylaxis must also take into account the unwanted effects of the drugs and other factors such as pregnancy and renal or hepatic impairment. Prophylaxis must be started 1 week before travel (2–3 weeks for mefloquine; 1–2 days for proguanil with atovaquone, or for doxycycline) and continued for 4 weeks after leaving a malarial area (7 days for proguanil with atovaquone), to protect against infection acquired immediately prior to departure.

OTHER PROTOZOAL INFECTIONS

Details of the natural history of other protozoal infections are not given in this book. Important drugs available in the UK for these conditions are discussed below. An outline of therapeutic uses is given in Table 51.5.

Atovaquone

Mechanism of action and uses

Atovaquone interferes with DNA synthesis by inhibiting pyrimidine synthesis. It is selective for protozoa that cannot utilise pre-formed pyrimidines. It affects mitochondrial electron transport and ATP synthesis.

Atovaquone is used as a second-line drug for treatment of *P. jirovecii* infections and for treating *Toxoplasma gondii* infection. It is also active against *Plasmodium* species, *E. histolytica* and *Trichomonas vaginalis*.

Pharmacokinetics

Oral absorption of atovaquone is poor. The absorbed fraction is excreted in the urine and bile, which results in enterohepatic cycling giving it a very long half-life of about 3 days.

Unwanted effects

- Diarrhoea, nausea, vomiting.
- Rash.
- Headache, insomnia.
- Neutropenia.

Pentamidine

Mechanism of action and uses

Pentamidine undergoes active uptake into the cell, where it probably inhibits DNA synthesis and ribosomal synthesis of protein and phospholipid.

Pentamidine is used in pneumocystis pneumonia, leishmaniasis and trypanosomiasis. It is cytotoxic to *P. jirovecii* in the non-replicating state, but because of its toxicity it is usually reserved for people who are intolerant of co-trimoxazole.

Pharmacokinetics

Pentamidine is given intravenously or inhaled as an aerosol for pneumocystis pneumonia. It can be given by deep intramuscular injection for leishmaniasis or trypanosomiasis. Pentamidine is metabolised in the liver and has a very long half-life (13 days).

Unwanted effects

- Inhaled pentamidine produces bronchial irritation with cough and bronchospasm.

Table 51.5 Selected protozoan infections and antiprotozoal drugs

Protozoa	Disease	Drug examples
Plasmodium species	Malaria	Chloroquine, mefloquine, primaquine, quinine, proguanil, pyrimethamine with sulfadoxine, atovaquone, artemether with lumefantrine
Entamoeba histolytica	Amoebic dysentery	Metronidazole, tinidazole, diloxanide
Trichomonas vaginalis	Vaginitis	Metronidazole, tinidazole
Giardia lamblia	Gastrointestinal dysfunction	Metronidazole, tinidazole, mepacrine
Leishmania species	Cutaneous or visceral (kala-azar) leishmaniasis	Stibogluconate, pentamidine
Trypanosoma species	Trypanosomiasis, Chagas' disease, sleeping sickness	Suramin[a], nifurtimox[a], benznidazole[a], eflornithine, pentamidine, melarsoprol[a]
Toxoplasma gondii	Encephalomyelitis, toxoplasmosis	Pyrimethamine plus sulfadiazine, trimetrexate[a]
Pneumocystis jirovecii	Pneumocystis pneumonia	Co-trimoxazole, pentamidine, atovaquone, trimetrexate[a]

[a]Not available or used in the UK for protozoal infection.

■ Intravenous pentamidine is nephrotoxic, and can produce irreversible hypoglycaemia and life-threatening arrhythmias such as ventricular tachycardia.

Sodium stibogluconate

Mechanism of action and use

Sodium stibogluconate is an organic antimony derivative that may act by binding to thiol groups in the parasite and inhibiting the formation of high-energy phosphates. Sodium stibogluconate is used to treat visceral leishmaniasis.

Pharmacokinetics

Sodium stibogluconate must be given parenterally, either by intramuscular injection or slow intravenous infusion. It has a half-life of 6 h and is eliminated by the kidney.

Unwanted effects

■ Anorexia, nausea, vomiting, abdominal pain, diarrhoea.
■ Headache.
■ Lethargy.
■ Myalgia, arthralgia.
■ Cough and substernal pain during intravenous infusion.

Diloxanide furoate

Mechanism of action and use

The mechanism of action is unknown. Diloxanide is used to treat chronic amoebiasis in asymptomatic individuals who are excreting cysts of *E. histolytica* in the stool. Acute infection is treated with metronidazole or tinidazole (Table 51.5).

Pharmacokinetics

It is given orally and hydrolysed in the gut to diloxanide and furoic acid; 90% of the diloxanide is then absorbed and rapidly conjugated in the liver. There is little information about its fate in the body. The unabsorbed fraction of diloxanide may contribute to the drug's effectiveness in amoebic dysentery.

Unwanted effects

■ Flatulence, anorexia, nausea and diarrhoea.
■ Urticaria, pruritus.

HELMINTHIC INFECTIONS

Details of the natural history of helminth infections are not given here, but an outline of the more commonly encountered conditions and drug treatments is given in Table 51.6. Drugs specifically for helminth infections are discussed below.

ANTIHELMINTHIC DRUGS

Ivermectin

Mechanism of action and use

Ivermectin is used to treat filariasis (especially onchocerciasis, for which it is the drug of choice), hookworm and *Strongyloides stercoralis* infection. Treatment with a single dose reduces microfilarial levels for several months and can be repeated every 6–12 months if necessary. It is available in the UK on a 'named-patient' basis.

Ivermectin produces an influx of Cl^- ions via an action on glutamate-gated membrane ion channels, generating muscle hyperpolarisation and paralysis of the filariae.

Pharmacokinetics

Ivermectin is well absorbed from the gut and excreted mainly in the faeces. It undergoes some hepatic metabolism and has a long half-life (12 h).

Unwanted effects

■ Itching.
■ Rash.

Diethylcarbamazine

Mechanism of action and use

Diethylcarbamazine is a first-line treatment for filariasis. Its mechanism of action is not well understood. It may inhibit arachidonic acid metabolism in the filariae. It also triggers exposure of antigens on the surface coat, leading to antibody-mediated phagocytosis. Treatment is usually required for 2–3 weeks to eliminate the microfilariae. Diethylcarbamazine is not marketed in the UK.

Table 51.6 Helminth infections

Helminth	Common name	Drug examples
Enterobius vermicularis	Threadworm	Mebendazole, piperazine
Ascaris lumbricoides	Roundworm	Mebendazole, piperazine, levamisole
Toxocara canis	Dog roundworm	Tiabendazole, diethylcarbamazine
Taenia species	Tapeworm	Niclosamide, praziquantel
Ancylostoma species, *Necator* species	Hookworm	Mebendazole, ivermectin, albendazole
Microfilariae (e.g. *Loa loa, Wuchereria bancrofti, Brugia malayi*)		Diethylcarbamazine, ivermectin
Strongyloides stercoralis		Tiabendazole, albendazole, ivermectin
Echinococcus granulosa	Hydatid disease	Albendazole

Pharmacokinetics

Oral absorption is good, and approximately half the drug is metabolised in the liver; the rest is excreted unchanged by the kidney. The half-life is not well established.

Unwanted effects

Most problems are caused by release of antigens from dying filariae. The onset is about 2 h after dosing and is almost diagnostic of the disease. The reaction is occasionally severe and life-threatening. The reaction includes:

- fever,
- headache,
- nausea,
- muscle and joint pains,
- itching,
- postural hypotension.

Benzimidazoles

albendazole, mebendazole, tiabendazole

Mechanism of action and uses

The benzimidazoles bind to tubulin, preventing its polymerisation into the cytoskeletal microtubules. The effect is selective for parasitic tubulin and the drugs are active against the adults, larvae and eggs. Tiabendazole and albendazole are available in the UK on a 'named-patient' basis.

Uses include (see also Table 51.6):

- mebendazole: threadworm, roundworm, hookworm,
- tiabendazole: *S. stercoralis*, hookworm (cutaneous larva migrans),
- albendazole: hydatid cysts, *S. stercoralis*, hookworm (including cutaneous larva migrans).

Pharmacokinetics

Oral absorption of tiabendazole is almost complete; metabolism in the liver is extensive and the half-life is very short (about 1 h). The oral absorption of mebendazole and albendazole are very poor; these drugs act principally within the gut.

Unwanted effects

- Gastrointestinal effects are common with tiabendazole and include anorexia, nausea, vomiting and diarrhoea; they are less severe with the other drugs.
- Dizziness and drowsiness can occur with tiabendazole.

Piperazine

Mechanism of action and uses

Piperazine is given orally to treat threadworm and roundworm infections. It competitively inhibits the effect of acetylcholine on the smooth muscle of the worm, producing a reversible flaccid paralysis.

Pharmacokinetics

Absorption of piperazine is rapid from the gut; up to 30% of the dose is eliminated unchanged in urine but little is known about the fate of the remainder.

Unwanted effects

Gastrointestinal upset can occur.

Niclosamide

Mechanism of action and use

Niclosamide is given orally to treat tapeworm infection. It inhibits generation of ATP by preventing phosphorylation of ADP in mitochondria. It is ineffective against larval worms. Purgatives are usually given after niclosamide to remove viable ova from the gut. Niclosamide is available in the UK on a 'named-patient' basis.

Pharmacokinetics

Some oral absorption (up to 20%) occurs, with subsequent liver metabolism.

Unwanted effects

- Gastrointestinal upset, nausea, abdominal pain.
- Lightheadedness.
- Pruritus.

Praziquantel

Mechanism of action and uses

Praziquantel is given orally to treat tapeworm infection and schistosomiasis. It is not well understood how praziquantel acts; it is known to increase the permeability of the cell membrane of sensitive helminths to Ca^{2+}, causing muscular contraction and paralysis. It may also reduce cellular transport of adenosine, which cannot be synthesised by the parasites. Praziquantel is available in the UK on a 'named-patient' basis.

Pharmacokinetics

Praziquantel is well absorbed from the gut and penetrates most tissues well; it is extensively metabolised by the liver and has a plasma half-life of 2 h.

Unwanted effects

- Dizziness, headache, lassitude.
- Gastrointestinal upset.

SELF-ASSESSMENT

True/false questions

1. Resistance to antibacterials may be due to mutations in bacterial ribosomes.
2. Benzylpenicillin has a short half-life as it is rapidly excreted by the kidneys.

3. Broad-spectrum penicillins do not disturb normal colonic flora.
4. Penicillins are bactericidal by binding to bacterial ribosomal sites.
5. The antipseudomonal penicillin ticarcillin is resistant to β-lactamase.
6. Cefotaxime is a third-generation cephalosporin.
7. Individuals who are allergic to penicillins cannot be given cephalosporins.
8. Imipenem is rapidly metabolised in the kidney.
9. Imipenem has only bacteriostatic activity.
10. Ciprofloxacin is ineffective for *Pseudomonas aeruginosa* infections in cystic fibrosis.
11. Ciprofloxacin interacts with theophylline used in asthma management.
12. Erythromycin commonly causes gastrointestinal disturbances.
13. Gentamicin has a low incidence of unwanted effects.
14. Gentamicin is not active when given orally.
15. Metronidazole can be used for eradicating *Helicobacter pylori*.
16. Antibacterials are effective for the majority of people with sore throat.
17. Tetracyclines should be avoided during pregnancy and in young children.
18. Vancomycin is active against β-lactamase-producing Gram-positive bacteria.
19. Rifampicin is an important drug for the treatment of tuberculosis.
20. Isoniazid is active against a wide range of bacteria.
21. Co-trimoxazole is the drug of choice for hospital-acquired acute urinary tract infection.
22. Trimethoprim administration can result in folate deficiency.
23. Imidazoles and triazoles have the same mechanism of antifungal action.
24. Griseofulvin inhibits squalene epoxidase.
25. Amphotericin can be given in liposomal formulations.

One-best-answer (OBA) questions

1. Choose the *most accurate* statement about HIV:
   A. Binding of HIV to the chemokine receptor CCR5 in the host cell membrane inhibits entry of the virus.
   B. Low doses of ritonavir reduce the activity of other protease inhibitors.
   C. Once resistance of HIV has developed, it persists indefinitely.
   D. Zidovudine acts in HIV by preventing viral entry to the host cells.
   E. The non-nucleoside reverse transcriptase inhibitors treat HIV by preventing insertion of the viral DNA into the host genome.
2. Identify the *least accurate* statement regarding the treatment of malaria:
   A. Primaquine kills parasites in the liver (hypnozoites) in *Plasmodium falciparum* infections.
   B. Chloroquine concentrates in erythrocytes and prevents the erythrocytic stage of malarial parasite reproduction.
   C. In many areas prophylaxis against malaria requires administration of two drugs.

D. Primaquine can induce haemolysis in people with glucose-6-phosphate dehydrogenase (G6PD) deficiency.
E. Proguanil acts to inhibit malarial parasite folate production.

Case-based questions

Case 1

Mr JW, age 40 years, lives at home and was previously healthy, but saw his GP in August, 5 days after returning from a conference abroad, where he had stayed in a large hotel and indulged his passion for frequent whirlpool baths. He had characteristic symptoms of pneumonia, including pleuritic chest pain and sudden development of fever and cough, producing yellow sputum. He was disorientated. Physical examinations and chest radiograph supported the diagnosis.

A. Before the results of the microbiological test were available, what treatment would you have commenced and by what route of administration?
B. How do the drugs that you are proposing to give work?

Case 2

Mr RH, age 80 years, had influenza and was admitted to hospital when he developed symptoms similar to Mr JW (see above) and became seriously ill. A chest radiograph showed multiple abscesses.

A. What treatment would you have commenced before microbiological results were available?
B. What antibacterial could be used if the organism was not treatable by β-lactamase-resistant penicillins?

Case 3

A 31-year-old man suffering from AIDS was admitted with shortness of breath, cough and generalised chest discomfort. Chest radiograph revealed diffuse bilateral opacities and a blood gas analysis demonstrated an arterial partial oxygen pressure (P_aO_2) of 8.0 kPa (normal range 11.0–14.0 kPa). Sputum culture was uninformative. A bronchoalveolar lavage was performed and transbronchial biopsies taken.

A. What was the likely clinical diagnosis?
B. What microscopic investigation could have been useful and what might it have shown?
C. How could this man have been managed and what factors needed to be considered?
D. What drug treatment unrelated to the infection could have further exposed him to the increased risk of opportunistic infection?
E. What prophylactic treatment could be commenced?

Case 4

Twenty-four hours after attending a convention, a 36-year-old man became ill with a temperature, abdominal pain, vomiting and diarrhoea. Faeces were collected and inoculated onto culture plates with several different types of culture medium. Pale-coloured colonies that were non-lactose fermenting were identified.

A. What organisms might have been causing this infection?
B. *Salmonella enteritidis* phage type 4 was eventually identified. How should this man be managed?
C. What was most likely to have caused this infection?

True/false answers

1. **True.** Mutations in bacterial ribosomes can reduce binding of many antibacterials that inhibit protein synthesis.
2. **True.** Benzylpenicillin is actively secreted into the proximal tubule by the organic acid transporter (Ch 2). This can be inhibited by probenecid or by other drugs that use the same secretory mechanism, such as aspirin.
3. **False.** Broad-spectrum penicillins in particular may alter the balance of gut flora, allowing overgrowth of pathogenic bacteria such as *Clostridium difficile*.
4. **False.** Penicillins disrupt cell membrane peptidoglycans.
5. **False.** Ticarcillin is broken down by β-lactamase.
6. **True.** Cefotaxime is a third-generation cephalosporin that penetrates the CNS and is resistant to β-lactamases.
7. **False.** Cephalosporins can be given, but with caution, as 8–16% of penicillin-allergic people will also have allergy to cephalosporins.
8. **True.** Imipenem (but not other carbapenems) is rapidly metabolised by renal dihydropeptidase and is always given in combination with cilastatin, a dihyhdropeptidase inhibitor.
9. **False.** Like all β-lactam antibacterials given in correct doses, imipenem is bactericidal.
10. **False.** The quinolones have good activity against *Pseudomonas* species.
11. **True.** Ciprofloxacin inhibits hepatic metabolism of theophylline and increases its toxicity.
12. **True.** Erythromycin often causes nausea and diarrhoea. Azithromycin is better tolerated.
13. **False.** Gentamicin is nephrotoxic and ototoxic, and its plasma levels should be monitored.
14. **True.** Gentamicin is poorly absorbed from the gastrointestinal tract and is given parenterally.
15. **True.** Metronidazole can be used with a proton pump inhibitor and other antibacterials to eliminate *H. pylori*.
16. **False.** Most sore throats are caused by viruses; those with bacterial causes usually resolve without antibacterials.
17. **True.** Tetracyclines can chelate with Ca^{2+} and form permanent yellow–brown deposits on developing teeth.
18. **True.** Vancomycin is reserved for meticillin-resistant *Staphylococcus aureus* (MRSA) and metronidazole-resistant *C. difficile*, which causes colitis.
19. **True.** Rifampicin is a broad-spectrum antibacterial also used in some serious diseases caused by Gram-negative bacteria such as *Legionella* and mycobacteria, and for MRSA.

20. **False.** Isoniazid is a highly selective inhibitor of the production of mycolic acids, which are unique to the cell wall of *Mycobacterium* species.
21. **False.** Trimethroprim alone is usually preferred to co-trimoxazole in urinary tract infections due to the lower risk of severe side effects compared to the combination drug.
22. **True.** Trimethroprim inhibits the role of folate in the synthesis of nucleotides; folate deficiency can result in megaloblastic anaemia, preventable during long-term treatment by giving folinic acid.
23. **True.** Imidazoles and triazoles suppress ergosterol synthesis by inhibiting lanosterol 14α-demethylase and they also share a similar spectrum of antifungal activity.
24. **False.** Griseofulvin inhibits dermatophyte mitosis by impairing microtubule formation.
25. **True.** Liposomes and other lipid delivery vehicles reduce the nephrotoxicity of amphotericin.

OBA answers

1. **Answer C** is the most accurate.
   A. Incorrect. The virus binds to a number of cell surface molecules including CCR5 receptors and glycoproteins to facilitate entry.
   B. Incorrect. Ritonavir inhibits breakdown of other protease inhibitors by CYP3A4 enzymes and is used to enhance their activity.
   C. **Correct.** Resistance of HIV persists indefinitely and drug treatment should be modified.
   D. Incorrect. Zidovudine is an RNA reverse transcriptase inhibitor and prevents the formation of viral DNA from viral RNA.
   E. Incorrect. See answer D.
2. **Answer A** is the least accurate.
   A. **Incorrect.** Only infections by *Plasmodium vivax* and *Plasmodium ovale* result in schizonts that remain in the liver as hypnozoites, and they require primaquine for their eradication.
   B. Correct. Chloroquine concentrates 100-fold in red cells and interferes with the ability of the parasite to digest haemoglobin.
   C. Correct. Resistance is a problem in many areas, where prophylaxis with chloroquine plus proguanil or atovaquone plus one of mefloquine, doxycycline or proguanil is recommended.
   D. Correct. Toxic metabolites of primaquine can induce haemolysis in people with G6PD deficiency.
   E. Correct. Proguanil inhibits dihydrofolate (DHF) reductase.

Case-based answers

Case 1

A. The most common cause of community-acquired infection is *Streptococcus pneumoniae*, but other 'atypical' organisms could be involved. In Mr JW, who was previously well, a recent stay in a hotel abroad might indicate the involvement of *Legionella* species, which multiply in warm water, for example in the tanks of air-conditioning systems. The incubation time is 5–10 days. Co-amoxiclav (amoxicillin and clavulanic acid) plus erythromycin or another macrolide should be given orally before the diagnosis is confirmed. If his condition is severe, rifampicin should also be given. The treatment should be reviewed immediately the microbiology sensitivities are known.

B. Amoxicillin is bactericidal and acts by interfering with bacterial cell wall peptidoglycan synthesis. It also allows greater activity of enzymes that lyse bacterial cells. Clavulanic acid inhibits β-lactamase, thus extending the spectrum of activity of amoxicillin. Erythromycin inhibits bacterial protein synthesis by acting on the bacterial ribosome. Rifampicin, perhaps better known for its role in treating tuberculosis, inhibits DNA-dependent RNA polymerase in many Gram-positive and Gram-negative bacteria.

Case 2

A. *Staphylococcus aureus* is a likely cause of acute pneumonia following an attack of influenza. Although the treatment must be guided by the sensitivity tests, most *S. aureus* strains are sensitive to flucloxacillin and this is the most appropriate antibiotic to start with. In the circumstances, it may be combined with fusidic acid or gentamicin. *S. aureus* commonly produces abscesses in the lungs. Pulmonary infection with *S. aureus* may also occur in people with cystic fibrosis. A Gram stain of the sputum would demonstrate Gram-positive cocci in clusters, typical of staphylococci. The production of coagulase and DNase would identify the organism as *S. aureus*. Many different species of coagulase-negative staphylococci exist and are found as part of the normal skin flora. The coagulase-negative staphylococci are typical causes of prosthetic valve endocarditis, joint prostheses and infected venous catheters. Of concern is the large number of meticillin-resistant staphylococci (MRSA), which pose a threat to people who are frail or immunocompromised.

B. A range of other second-choice antibacterials effective against β-lactamase-producing *S. aureus* might be useful. For example, fusidic acid, gentamicin, a cephalosporin, a quinolone or erythromycin may be effective. There are increasing concerns about MRSA. Vancomycin, a bactericidal glycopeptide that inhibits cell wall synthesis, is effective against some MRSA, or linezolid may be used if the glycopeptide is unsuitable.

Case 3

A. Clinically, the man is likely to have *Pneumocystis jirovecii* pneumonia (PCP), which is the predominant respiratory illness in people with AIDS. The causative organism, which is a protozoan, is believed to be acquired at a young age and reactivates with waning immunity. The organism is endemic in the community and multiplies within the lungs and causes symptoms. There is often a seasonal prevalence of PCP. Symptoms can be scant and, if present, consist of breathlessness and cough. Induced sputum or bronchoalveolar lavage specimens should be sent to laboratory for detection of PCP and routine culture.

B. PCP can be detected in sputum or lavage by staining with methenamine silver stain for typical casts. It can also be detected by use of the polymerase chain reaction, and on lung biopsy.

C. The treatment of choice is high-dose co-trimoxazole. Many people with AIDS have hypersensitivity reactions to sulphonamides and are taking multiple drug combinations. Alternative treatments for PCP are aerosolised or parenteral pentamidine, dapsone and trimethoprim, primaquine, etc.

D. Long-term treatment with corticosteroids or other immunosuppressants.

E. After an attack of PCP, a prophylactic regimen should be taken, for example nebulised pentamidine or oral trimethoprim 3 days per week.

Case 4

A. *Salmonella*, *Shigella*, *Proteus* and *Pseudomonas* species are non-lactose fermenting and produce pale-coloured colonies on this medium. All were contenders.

B. Antibacterials have no role to play in the management of the majority of cases of *Salmonella* gastroenteritis. Exceptions are when the gastroenteritis occurs in an individual who is immunocompromised or if there is evidence of systemic invasion. Ciprofloxacin would be the antibacterial of choice; it can be given orally and is cheaper than intravenous preparations. Dehydration and electrolyte imbalance should be corrected by fluid replacement. Control of the diarrhoea by antidiarrhoeal drugs is contraindicated because of the risk of inducing paralytic ileus and causing septicaemia.

C. Food poisoning, as this case would seem to be from the history, is a notifiable condition and should be reported to the consultant in Communicable Disease Control. Because the man has attended a convention, it is possible that this is part of an outbreak and all persons attending the convention should be contacted to find out if they have been symptomatic and to collect faecal specimens for culture. Specimens of food, if still available, should also be collected for culture.

FURTHER READING

Antibacterial drugs

Bartlet JG (2002) Antibiotic-associated diarrhoea. *N Engl J Med* 346, 334–339

Calhoun JH, Manring MM (2005) Adult osteomyelitis. *Infect Dis Clin North Am* 19, 765–786

Durrington HJ, Summers C (2008) Recent changes in the management of community acquired pneumonia. *BMJ* 336, 1429–1433

Fihn SD (2003) Acute uncomplicated urinary tract infection in women. *N Engl J Med* 349, 259–266

Fitch MT, Abrahamian FM, Moran GJ et al. (2008) Emergency department management of meningitis and encephalitis. *Infect Dis Clin North Am* 22, 33–52

Grant A, Gothard P, Thwaites G (2008) Managing drug resistant tuberculosis. *BMJ* 337, 564–569

Gruchella RS, Pirmohamed M (2006) Antibiotic allergy. *N Engl J Med* 354, 601–609

Hawkwy PM, Livermore DM (2012) Carbapenem antibiotics for serious infections. *BMJ* 344, e3236

Hirschmann JV (2002) Antibiotics for common respiratory tract infections in adults. *Arch Intern Med* 162, 256–264

Jacoby GA, Munoz-Price LS (2005) The new β-lactamases. *N Engl J Med* 352, 380–391

Lawn SD, Zumia AI (2011) Tuberculosis. *Lancet* 378, 57–72

Mathews CJ, Weston VC, Jones A et al. (2010) Bacterial septic arthritis in adults. *Lancet* 375, 846–855

Mackenzie I, Lever A (2007) Management of sepsis. *BMJ* 335, 929–932

Mansharamani NG, Koziel H (2003) Chronic lung sepsis: lung abscess, bronchiectasis and empyema. *Curr Opin Pulm Med* 9, 181–185

Moreillon P, Que Y-A (2004) Infective endocarditis. *Lancet* 363, 139–149

Niederman MS (2007) Recent advances in community-acquired pneumonia: inpatient and outpatient. *Chest* 131, 1205–1215

Phoenix G, Das S, Joshi M (2012) Diagnosis and management of cellulitis. *BMJ* 345, e4955

Picazo JJ (2004) Management of the febrile neutropenic patient: a consensus conference. *Clin Infect Dis* 15 (suppl 1), S1–S6

Rovers MM, Schilder AGM, Zielhuis GA et al. (2004) Otitis media. *Lancet* 363, 465–473

ten Hacken NHT, Wijkstra PJ, Kerstjens HAM (2007) Treatment of bronchiectasis in adults. *BMJ* 335, 1089–1093

Tenover FC (2006) Mechanisms of antimicrobial resistance in bacteria. *Am J Med* 119 (suppl 1), S3–S10

Thuny F, Grisoli D, Collart F et al. (2012) Infective endocarditis. *Lancet* 379, 965–975

Turnidge J (2001) Responsible prescribing for upper respiratory tract infections. *Drugs* 61, 2065–2077

Westphal J-F, Brogard J-M (1999) Biliary tract infections. *Drugs* 57, 81–91

Antifungal drugs

Moriarty B, Hay R, Morris-Jones R (2012) The diagnosis and management of tinea. *BMJ* 345, e4380

Patterson TF (2005) Advances and challenges in management of invasive mycoses. *Lancet* 366, 1013–1025

Pfaller MA (2012) Antifungal drug resistance mechanisms, epidemiology, and consequences for treatment. *Am J Med* 125 (suppl), S3–S13

Sobel JD (2003) Management of patients with recurrent vulvovaginal candidiasis. *Drugs* 63, 1059–1066

Antiviral drugs

Clavel F, Hance AJ (2004) HIV drug resistance. *N Engl J Med* 350, 1023–1035

Esté JA, Telenti A (2007) HIV entry inhibitors. *Lancet* 370, 81–88

Glezen WP (2008) Prevention and treatment of seasonal influenza. *N Engl J Med* 359, 2579–2585

Gupta R, Warren T, Wald A (2007) Genital herpes. *Lancet* 370, 2127–2137

Moscana A (2005) Neuraminidase inhibitors for influenza. *N Engl J Med* 353, 1363–1373

Volberding PA, Deeks SG (2010) Antiretroviral therapy and management of HIV infection. *Lancet* 376, 49–62

Wareham DW, Breuer J (2007) Herpes zoster. *BMJ* 334, 1211–1215

Antiprotozoal drugs

Davies AP, Chalmers RM (2009) Cryptosporidiosis. *BMJ* 339, b4168

Freedman DO (2008) Malaria prevention in short-term travellers. *N Engl J Med* 359, 603–612

Kremsner PG, Krishna S (2004) Antimalarial combinations. *Lancet* 364, 285–294

Lalloo DG, Hill DR (2008) Preventing malaria in travellers. *BMJ* 336, 1362–1366

Montoya JG, Liessenfeld O (2004) Toxoplasmosis. *Lancet* 363, 1965–1977

Stanley SL Jr (2003) Amoebiasis. *Lancet* 361, 1025–1034

Whitty CJM, Lalloo D, Ustianowski A (2006) Malaria: an update on treatment of adults in non-endemic countries. *BMJ* 333, 241–245

Antihelminthic drugs

de Silva N, Guyatt H, Bundy D (1997) Antihelminthics. *Drugs* 53, 769–788

Gray DJ, Ross AG, Li Y-S et al. (2011) Diagnosis and management of schistosomiasis. *BMJ* 342, d2651

McManus DP, Gray DJ, Zhang W et al. (2012) Diagnosis, treatment and management of echinococcus. *BMJ* 344, e3866

Compendium: drugs used for infections

Drug	Kinetics (half-life)	Comments
Antibacterial drugs		
Penicillins		
Amoxicillin	Oral bioavailability (90%) not influenced by food; rapid renal excretion (1 h)	Broad-spectrum penicillin; used for urinary tract infections, otitis media, sinusitis, bronchitis, uncomplicated community-acquired pneumonia, *Haemophilus influenzae* infections, invasive salmonellosis and listerial meningitis; given orally, by intramuscular injection, or by intravenous injection or infusion; also given with clavulanic acid as co-amoxiclav
Ampicillin	Low oral bioavailability, reduced if taken with food; eliminated largely by renal clearance (1–2 h)	Broad-spectrum penicillin; see amoxicillin for uses; given orally, by intramuscular injection, or by intravenous injection or infusion
Benzylpenicillin (penicillin G)	Unreliable oral absorption due to hydrolysis by gastric acid; rapidly eliminated by renal excretion (0.5–1 h)	Used for throat infection, otitis media, streptococcal endocarditis, meningococcal disease, pneumonia and anthrax; given by intramuscular injection, slow intravenous injection or infusion
Flucloxacillin (floxacillin)	Oral bioavailability 80%; cleared largely by the kidneys (0.8–1.2 h)	Beta-lactamase-resistant penicillin; used for infections caused by β-lactamase-producing staphylococci; given orally, by intramuscular injection, or by intravenous injection or infusion; also given combined with ampicillin as co-fluampicil
Phenoxymethyl penicillin (penicillin V)	Bioavailability 60%; eliminated unchanged by renal excretion and as penicilloic acid metabolite (0.5 h)	Used for tonsillitis, otitis media, erysipelas, rheumatic fever and pneumococcal infection prophylaxis; given orally
Piperacillin	Poorly absorbed from gut, so not given orally; excreted largely unchanged in urine and bile (0.7–1.2 h)	Antipseudomonal penicillin used for infections of lower respiratory tract, urinary tract, abdomen and skin; given by intravenous infusion; only available in combination with tazobactam (β-lactamase inhibitor)
Pivmecillinam	Prodrug rapidly hydrolysed to mecillinam, which has a half-life of 1–2 h	Antipseudomonal penicillin; also active against many Gram-negative bacteria; used for urinary tract infections; given orally
Temocillin	Eliminated largely unchanged in urine (4–5 h)	Beta-lactamase-resistant penicillin; used for infections caused by Gram-negative bacteria; given by intramuscular or intravenous injection or by intravenous infusion
Ticarcillin	Excreted largely unchanged in urine (1 h)	Antipseudomonal penicillin active also against *Proteus* species; given by intravenous infusion in combination with clavulanic acid
Cephalosporins, carbapenems and other β-lactams		
Aztreonam	Eliminated unchanged by kidney (1.7 h)	Monobactam; active only against Gram-negative bacteria and used for infections by *Pseudomonas aeruginosa*, *H. influenzae* and *Neisseria meningitides;* given by deep intramuscular injection, or by intravenous injection or infusion
Cefaclor	Extensively absorbed; mostly renal elimination, plus limited metabolism (0.5–1 h)	Second-generation cephalosporin; used for sensitive Gram-negative or Gram-positive infections of urinary tract (unresponsive to other drugs), respiratory tract and soft tissues, and for otitis media and sinusitis; given orally
Cefadroxil	Completely absorbed (not affected by food); eliminated mostly unchanged in urine (1–2 h)	First-generation cephalosporin; For uses, see under cefaclor; given orally
Cefalexin	Rapidly and completely absorbed; eliminated in urine unchanged (1 h)	First-generation cephalosporin; for uses, see under cefaclor; given orally
Cefixime	Incomplete absorption (50%); renal and biliary excretion (2.5–3.8 h)	Third-generation cephalosporin; for uses, see under cefaclor (but acute infections only), also used for gonorrhoea; given orally

Compendium: drugs used for infections—cont'd

Drug	Kinetics (half-life)	Comments
Cefotaxime	Renal elimination with some metabolism (0.9–1.3 h)	Third-generation cephalosporin; for uses, see under cefaclor; also used for gonorrhoea, surgical prophylaxis, *Haemophilus epiglottitis* and meningitis; given by deep intramuscular injection, or by intravenous injection (over 3–5 min) or infusion
Cefpodoxime	Proxetil prodrug hydrolysed to active cefpodoxime, which is renally eliminated (1.9–3.2 h)	Third-generation cephalosporin; used for upper and lower respiratory tract infections, skin and soft tissue infections, uncomplicated urinary tract infections and uncomplicated gonorrhoea; given orally as the proxetil derivative prodrug
Cefradine	Completely absorbed but rate affected by food; eliminated unchanged in urine (1.3 h)	First-generation cephalosporin; for uses, see under cefaclor; also used for surgical prophylaxis; given orally, by deep intramuscular injection, or by intravenous injection (over 3–5 min) or infusion
Ceftaroline fosamil	Fosamil prodrug converted by phosphatases to ceftaroline, which is mostly excreted in urine (2.5 h)	Fifth-generation cephalosporin; similar to cefotaxime but extended activity against Gram-positive bacteria including MRSA; used for community-acquired pneumonia and complicated skin and soft-tissue infections; given by intravenous infusion
Ceftazidime	Eliminated unchanged by glomerular filtration (1.8–2.2 h)	Third-generation cephalosporin; for uses, see under cefaclor; also used for surgical prophylaxis; given by deep intramuscular injection, or by intravenous injection or infusion
Ceftriaxone	Extensive plasma protein binding; eliminated unchanged in urine (6–9 h)	Third-generation cephalosporin; for uses, see under cefaclor; also used for surgical prophylaxis and prophylaxis of meningococcal meningitis; given by deep intramuscular injection, or by intravenous injection or infusion
Cefuroxime	Axetil prodrug hydrolysed to cefuroxime; absorbed better if taken after food; eliminated by renal filtration and secretion (1.2 h)	Second-generation cephalosporin; for uses, see under cefaclor; also used for surgical prophylaxis; given orally (as cefuroxime axetil), by deep intramuscular injection, or by intravenous injection or infusion
Doripenem	Eliminated largely unchanged in urine (1 h)	Carbapenem; broad-spectrum activity against both Gram-negative and Gram-positive organisms; used for hospital-acquired pneumonias and for complicated intra-abdominal and urinary tract infections; given by intravenous infusion
Ertapenem	Eliminated in urine as parent drug and as an inactive metabolite (4.5 h)	Carbapenem; broad-spectrum activity against both Gram-negative and Gram-positive organisms; used for abdominal and acute gynaecological infections and for community-acquired pneumonia; given by intravenous infusion
Imipenem (with cilastatin)	Hydrolysed by renal dihydropeptidase and also eliminated unchanged in urine (1 h); always given with cilastatin (dihydropeptidase inhibitor)	Carbapenem; active against aerobic and anaerobic Gram-negative and Gram-positive organisms; used for hospital-acquired septicaemia and for surgical prophylaxis; given with cilastatin by deep intramuscular injection or intravenous infusion
Meropenem	Eliminated mainly by kidneys with some hepatic metabolism (1 h)	Carbapenem; used for aerobic and anaerobic Gram-negative and Gram-positive infections; given by intravenous injection or intravenous infusion

Beta-lactamase inhibitors

Given with some β-lactam antibacterial agents susceptible to hydrolysis by β-lactamase (penicillinase).

Clavulanic acid	Extensive metabolism and glomerular filtration (1 h)	Given in combination with amoxicillin or ticarcillin
Tazobactam	Eliminated by the kidney (0.7–1.5 h)	Given in combination with piperacillin

Compendium: drugs used for infections—cont'd

Drug	Kinetics (half-life)	Comments
Quinolones		
Ciprofloxacin	Bioavailability 50–80%; eliminated renally plus biliary excretion and metabolism (3–4 h)	Active against Gram-positive and especially Gram-negative organisms, including *Salmonella*, *Shigella*, *Campylobacter*, *Neisseria* and *Pseudomonas* species; used for respiratory (not pneumococcal pneumonia), urinary and gastrointestinal tract infections, chronic prostatitis, gonorrhoea and septicaemia; given orally or by intravenous infusion
Levofloxacin	Complete bioavailability, unaffected by food; eliminated largely unchanged in urine (6–8 h)	Similar activity to ciprofloxacin, but more active against pneumococci; used for bronchitis, community-acquired pneumonia, and infections of urinary tract, skin and soft tissues; given orally or as an intravenous infusion
Moxifloxacin	Bioavailability 90%; hepatic metabolism (12 h)	Similar activity to ciprofloxacin but more active against pneumococci and inactive against *P. aeruginosa* or MRSA; used for bronchitis, community-acquired pneumonia and sinusitis; given orally
Nalidixic acid	Essentially complete bioavailability; hepatic metabolism (1.5 h)	Used in uncomplicated urinary tract infections; given orally
Norfloxacin	Absorption reduced if taken with food; eliminated mainly by kidneys, with some metabolism (3 h)	Used in uncomplicated urinary tract infections; given orally
Ofloxacin	Complete oral absorption; eliminated by kidneys plus limited metabolism (6–7 h)	Used for infections of urinary tract and lower respiratory tract, and for gonorrhoea, non-gonococcal urethritis and cervicitis; given orally or as intravenous infusion
Macrolides		
Antibacterial spectrum similar to penicillins and used as alternatives in penicillin-allergic patients.		
Azithromycin	Low bioavailability (37%), reduced by food; eliminated largely unchanged in bile (40–60 h)	Used for respiratory tract infections, otitis media, skin and soft tissue infections, uncomplicated chlamydial infections, non-gonococcal urethritis, and moderate typhoid due to multiple antibacterial-resistant organisms; given orally
Clarithromycin	Oral bioavailability 55%; eliminated by metabolism and renal excretion; half-life (3 h) increases at high doses (9 h)	Used for respiratory tract infections, otitis media, mild to moderate skin and soft tissue infections, and for *Helicobacter pylori* eradication; given orally or by intravenous infusion
Erythromycin	Oral formulations are enteric coated or ester prodrugs that are rapidly hydrolysed; eliminated largely by liver (1–1.5 h)	Used for campylobacter enteritis, pneumonia, Legionnaires' disease, syphilis, non-gonococcal urethritis, chronic prostatitis, diphtheria and whooping cough prophylaxis, and for acne vulgaris and rosacea; given orally or by intravenous infusion
Spiramycin	Renal and biliary elimination (6–8 h)	Used on a 'named-patient' basis for toxoplasmosis
Telithromycin	Oral bioavailability 60%; hepatic metabolism (10 h)	Used for community-acquired pneumonia, bronchitis, sinusitis, β-haemolytic streptococcal pharyngitis, or tonsillitis when β-lactams are inappropriate; given orally
Aminoglycosides		
Bactericidal drugs active against Gram-negative and Gram-positive organisms; gentamicin is the aminoglycoside of choice in the UK and is used for serious infections.		
Amikacin	Eliminated by glomerular filtration (2 h)	Used for serious Gram-negative infections resistant to gentamicin; given by intramuscular injection, slow intravenous injection or intravenous infusion
Gentamicin	Eliminated by glomerular filtration (1–4 h)	Used for septicaemia and neonatal sepsis, CNS infections (including meningitis), biliary tract infections, acute pyelonephritis and prostatitis, endocarditis, pneumonia in hospital and as adjunct in listerial meningitis; given by intramuscular injection, slow intravenous injection, intravenous infusion or by intrathecal injection

Compendium: drugs used for infections—cont'd

Drug	Kinetics (half-life)	Comments
Neomycin	Absorption <5%; renal elimination (2 h)	Toxicity restricts use to skin infections and for bowel sterilisation before surgery; given orally
Tobramycin	Eliminated by glomerular filtration (2–3 h)	For uses, see gentamicin; given by intramuscular injection, slow intravenous injection or intravenous infusion

Tetracyclines

Broad-spectrum antibacterials; increasing resistance but they remain drugs of choice for infections caused by *Chlamydia*, *Rickettsia* or *Brucella* species, and for Lyme disease; all are given orally; no parenteral formulations available.

Drug	Kinetics (half-life)	Comments
Demeclocycline	Oral bioavailability 66%; excreted unchanged in urine and bile (10–15 h)	Main uses given above
Doxycycline	Oral bioavailability >90%; eliminated in bile and urine (18–22 h)	Main uses given above; also for chronic prostatitis, sinusitis, syphilis, pelvic inflammatory disease, anthrax, malaria, rosacea and acne vulgaris; also used with quinine in the treatment of malaria
Lymecycline	Degraded in gastrointestinal tract into tetracycline, lysine and formaldehyde (8–10 h)	Main uses given above
Minocycline	Oral bioavailability >90%; mainly biliary elimination (12–16 h)	Main uses given above; also for meningococcal carrier state and acne vulgaris
Oxytetracycline	Variable absorption (up to 60%); renal and biliary elimination (9 h)	Main uses given above; also for acne vulgaris and rosacea
Tetracycline	Incomplete absorption; eliminated in bile and urine, with some metabolism (9 h)	Main uses given above; also for acne vulgaris and rosacea
Tigecycline	Mainly eliminated unchanged in bile and urine (27 h)	Glycylcycline structurally related to tetracyclines, with similar unwanted effects; used for complicated intra-abdominal, skin or soft tissue infections; given by intravenous infusion

Sulphonamides

Importance of sulphonamides has decreased due to increasing resistance and the availability of better alternatives.

Drug	Kinetics (half-life)	Comments
Sulfadiazine	Oral bioavailability 60–90%; parent drug and acetyl metabolite eliminated by kidney (7–12 h)	Used for prevention of rheumatic fever recurrence; given orally or by intravenous infusion; silver sulfadiazine cream is available for topical use
Sulfamethoxazole	Rapidly absorbed; eliminated mainly by acetylation (6–20 h)	Used only in combination with trimethoprim (as co-trimoxazole) for *Pneumocystis jirovecii* (where it is the drug of choice), toxoplasmosis, nocardiasis and for other susceptible acute infections; given orally or by intravenous infusion
Trimethoprim	Complete bioavailability; eliminated largely by kidneys, with some metabolism (9–17 h)	Used with sulfamethoxazole and alone for urinary tract infections and bronchitis (when it is given orally)

Other antibacterial drugs

Drug	Kinetics (half-life)	Comments
Chloramphenicol	Oral bioavailability 80–90%; mainly hepatic elimination (2–12 h)	Bacteriostatic antibiotic; potent but toxic broad-spectrum activity; use limited to life-threatening infections, especially *H. influenzae* and typhoid fever; given orally or by intravenous injection or infusion
Clindamycin	Extensive oral absorption; mostly eliminated by hepatic metabolism (2.5 h)	Lincosamide; use limited by toxicity to staphylococcal bone and joint infections and for peritonitis; given orally, by deep intramuscular injection or by intravenous infusion
Colistin (colistimethate sodium)	Not absorbed orally; renal elimination (4–8 h)	Polymyxin; used for infections by Gram-negative organisms, including *P. aeruginosa*; given orally (for bowel sterilisation only), by intravenous injection or infusion, or by inhalation (nebuliser)

Compendium: drugs used for infections—cont'd

Drug	Kinetics (half-life)	Comments
Daptomycin	Mostly excreted unchanged in urine (8–9 h)	Lipopeptide; used for complicated skin and soft tissue infections by Gram-positive bacteria; given by intravenous infusion
Fidaxomicin	Very low oral absorption; parent drug and main metabolite excreted in faeces	Macrocyclic drug; used for *Clostridium difficile* infection; given orally
Fusidic acid (sodium fusidate)	Complete oral bioavailability; hepatic metabolism and biliary excretion (9 h)	Narrow-spectrum steroid antibacterial; use restricted to penicillin-resistant staphylococcal infections; given orally or by intravenous infusion
Linezolid	Eliminated unchanged in urine and by oxidative metabolism (5 h)	Oxazolidinone; used for pneumonia and complicated skin and soft tissue infections caused by Gram-positive organisms; given orally or by intravenous infusion
Methenamine	Degraded by acid to formaldehyde and ammonia, so given as enteric-coated formulation; mainly urinary excretion (4 h)	Used for prophylaxis and long-term treatment of lower urinary tract infections; given orally for urinary tract infections
Metronidazole	Complete oral bioavailability; metabolites eliminated in urine (6–9 h)	Active against anaerobic bacteria; used for surgical and gynaecological sepsis, antibiotic-associated colitis and eradication of *H. pylori*; given orally, rectally or by intravenous infusion
Nitrofurantoin	Complete oral bioavailability; eliminated unchanged in urine and by metabolism (0.3–1 h)	Used for urinary tract infections, when it is given orally
Rifaximin	Oral absorption <1%	Non-absorbable rifamycin compound; used for uncomplicated traveller's diarrhoea; given orally
Teicoplanin	High plasma protein binding (90%); eliminated mostly unchanged in urine (32–176 h)	Glycopeptide; used for Gram-positive infections, including endocarditis, peritonitis and for prophylaxis in orthopaedic surgery; given by intramuscular injection, intravenous injection or infusion
Tinidazole	Complete oral bioavailability; parent drug and metabolites eliminated in urine and bile (12–14 h)	Actions and uses similar to metronidazole; given orally
Vancomycin	Negligible absorption from gut; eliminated by glomerular filtration (5–11 h)	Glycopeptide; used for prophylaxis and treatment of endocarditis and other serious Gram-positive cocci infections and for *C. difficile*-related colitis; given orally (for colitis) or by intravenous infusion
Antituberculous drugs		
Capreomycin	Few data available; about 50% eliminated by renal excretion	Used in combination with other drugs when resistance to first-line drugs occurs; given by deep intramuscular injection
Cycloserine	Oral bioavailability >90%; mostly excreted in urine, with some metabolism (4–30 h)	Used in combination with other drugs when resistance to first-line drugs occurs; given orally
Ethambutol	Oral bioavailability 80%; mainly renal elimination, with some metabolism (10–15 h)	First-line drug (initial phase only) included in regimen if resistance to isoniazid is suspected; given orally
Isoniazid	High oral bioavailability; prodrug activated within cells; eliminated largely by acetylation; half-life 0.5–2 h in rapid acetylators and 2–6.5 h in slow acetylators	First-line drug; given orally or by intramuscular or intravenous injection
Pyrazinamide	High oral bioavailability; prodrug activated by hydrolysis to pyrazinoic acid, which undergoes renal elimination (10–24 h)	First-line drug (initial phase only), particularly useful in tuberculous meningitis; given orally

Compendium: drugs used for infections—cont'd

Drug	Kinetics (half-life)	Comments
Rifabutin	Bioavailability 12–20%; accumulates intracellularly; hepatic metabolism, renal excretion (35–40 h)	Rifamycin compound; used for prophylaxis against *Mycobacterium avium* complex infections and for treatment of non-tuberculous mycobacterial disease and pulmonary tuberculosis; given orally
Rifampicin (rifampin)	High oral bioavailability; hepatic metabolism; multiple elimination routes (1–6 h)	Rifamycin compound, key first-line drug; also used for brucellosis, Legionnaires' disease and serious staphylococcal infections; given orally or by intravenous infusion
Streptomycin	About 50–60% eliminated by kidney (2–3 h)	Aminoglycoside; use is mainly restricted to resistant organisms (also used as adjunct in treatment of brucellosis); given by deep intramuscular injection

Drugs used in leprosy

Drug	Kinetics (half-life)	Comments
Clofazimine	Bioavailability 20–85%, enhanced by food; eliminated unchanged in bile (10 days)	Given orally
Dapsone	Bioavailability >90%; hepatic metabolism and about 10% eliminated in urine unchanged (27 h)	Given orally
Rifampicin	–	See above

Antifungal agents

Drug	Kinetics (half-life)	Comments
Amorolfine	Limited transdermal absorption; accumulates in skin	Alkylamine; used for fungal infections of skin and nails; applied as a cream or nail lacquer
Amphotericin	Negligible oral absorption; slow renal excretion (1–14 days)	Polyene; active against most fungi; given orally (for intestinal candidiasis) or by intravenous infusion for systemic infections
Caspofungin	Hepatic metabolism, biliary elimination (40–50 h)	Echinocandin; used for invasive aspergillosis unresponsive to amphotericin or itraconazole and for invasive candidiasis; given by intravenous infusion
Clotrimazole	Negligible absorption across the skin; 5–10% absorption after vaginal use and fungicidal concentrations are maintained locally for up to 3 days	Imidazole; used for fungal skin infections and vaginal candidiasis; applied as a cream, powder or spray
Econazole	Negligible absorption across the skin	Imidazole; used for fungal skin infections and vaginal candidiasis; applied as a cream
Fluconazole	Oral bioavailability 90%; mainly renal excretion, some metabolism (30 h)	Triazole; used for local and systemic fungal infections; penetrates blood–brain barrier so useful for fungal meningitis; given orally or by intravenous infusion
Flucytosine	Partly converted to 5-fluorouracil; mostly eliminated unchanged by glomerular filtration (3 h)	Antimetabolite; used for systemic fungal infections; used in combination with amphotericin or fluconazole; given by intravenous infusion
Griseofulvin	Variable absorption, increased by fatty foods; hepatic metabolism (10–21 h)	Microtubule inhibitor; used for widespread or intractable dermatophyte infections of the skin, scalp and nails where topical treatment has been ineffective; given orally
Itraconazole	Oral bioavailability 55%; hepatic metabolism, biliary excretion (20 h)	Triazole; used for numerous local and systemic fungal infections; given orally
Ketoconazole	Hepatic metabolism, biliary excretion (6–10 h)	Imidazole; used for systemic mycoses and for a range of serious and resistant infections; given orally or topically
Miconazole	Poorly absorbed from the gut; extensive metabolism (20–25 h)	Imidazole; used for oral and intestinal infections; given orally
Nystatin	Not absorbed from gut or intact skin	Polyene; principally used for *Candida albicans* infections of skin and mucous membranes; given topically (for oral, vaginal and skin infections)

Compendium: drugs used for infections—cont'd

Drug	Kinetics (half-life)	Comments
Posaconazole	Incomplete absorption, enhanced by food; renal, biliary and faecal excretion (35 h)	Triazole; used in infections unresponsive to amphotericin or other suitable treatments; given orally
Terbinafine	Oral bioavailability about 80%; numerous pathways of metabolism (11–17 h)	Allylamine; drug of choice for fungal nail infections (also used for ringworm infection); given orally or topically
Tioconazole	Negligible systemic absorption after topical treatment	Imidazole; used for fungal nail infections; applied as a solution
Voriconazole	Oral bioavailability 96%; variable hepatic metabolism (6 h)	Triazole; used for invasive aspergillosis and other serious infections; given orally or by intravenous infusion

Antiviral agents

Reverse transcriptase inhibitors

Drugs below are used for treatment of HIV infection in combination with other antiretroviral drugs; any other indications are listed under individual drugs.

Drug	Kinetics (half-life)	Comments
Abacavir	Oral bioavailability 80%; hepatic metabolism (1.5 h)	Nucleoside drug; given orally
Didanosine	Absorption 20–40%; eliminated unchanged in urine and by metabolism (0.6–1.4 h)	Nucleoside drug; given orally
Efavirenz	Variable absorption; induces own hepatic metabolism (40–70 h)	Non-nucleoside drug; given orally
Emtricitabine	Completely absorbed; eliminated largely by renal secretion and hepatic metabolism (10 h); intracellular active triphosphate has longer half-life (about 40 h)	Nucleoside drug; given orally
Etravirine	Hepatic metabolism, faecal excretion (30–40 h)	Non-nucleoside drug; given orally
Lamivudine	Absorption 90%; eliminated largely unchanged in urine (5–7 h); intracellular triphosphate has longer half-life (11–16 h)	Nucleoside drug; also used for chronic hepatitis B with evidence of viral replication; given orally
Nevirapine	Bioavailability 90%; eliminated by hepatic metabolism (25–30 h)	Non-nucleoside drug; used in advanced disease in combination with at least two other drugs; given orally
Rilpivirine	Hepatic metabolism, mainly faecal excretion (45 h)	Non-nucleoside drug; given orally
Stavudine	Oral bioavailability >80%; eliminated unchanged in urine and by metabolism (1–1.6 h)	Nucleoside drug; given orally
Tenofovir disoproxil	Converted to tenofovir within gut, giving bioavailability of 25%; forms active intracellular diphosphate; eliminated by kidney (17 h)	Nucleoside drug; given orally
Zidovudine	Oral bioavailability about 65%; mainly hepatic metabolism, some excreted unchanged in urine (1 h)	Nucleoside drug; also used for prevention of maternal–fetal HIV transmission; given orally or by intravenous infusion

HIV protease inhibitors

Drugs below are used for treatment of HIV infection in combination with other antiretroviral drugs; any other indications are listed under individual drugs.

Drug	Kinetics (half-life)	Comments
Atazanavir	Oral bioavailability 70%; hepatic metabolism (7 h)	Used in individuals treated previously with other antiretroviral drugs; given orally
Darunavir	Oral bioavailability 37%; hepatic metabolism (15 h)	Given orally

Compendium: drugs used for infections—cont'd

Drug	Kinetics (half-life)	Comments
Fosamprenavir	Phosphate ester prodrug completely hydrolysed to amprenavir in gut mucosa	Used in individuals treated previously with other antiretroviral drugs; given orally
Indinavir	Oral bioavailability 18–20%; metabolised in gut and liver, faecal excretion (2 h)	Used in combination with nucleoside reverse transcriptase inhibitors; given orally
Lopinavir (with ritonavir)	Absorption increased markedly by fatty food; hepatic metabolism (5–6 h)	Given orally
Nelfinavir	Hepatic metabolism; biliary excretion of parent drug and active metabolite (3.5–5 h)	Given orally
Ritonavir	Oral bioavailability >70% in animals; hepatic metabolism by CYP3A4 and potently inhibits the enzyme, parent drug and an active metabolite eliminated in faeces (3–5 h)	Low doses increase effects of several other protease inhibitors by blocking their metabolism by CYP3A4; used for progressive and advanced HIV infection in combination with nucleoside reverse transcriptase inhibitors and protease inhibitors; given orally
Saquinavir	Oral bioavailability 1–30%, influenced by food; hepatic metabolism, faecal elimination (5–7 h)	Given orally
Tipranavir	Absorption enhanced by food; hepatic metabolism (6 h)	Used for HIV infection resistant to other protease inhibitors and in those treated previously with other antiretroviral drugs; given orally

Viral DNA polymerase inhibitors

Drug	Kinetics (half-life)	Comments
Aciclovir	Oral bioavailability 10–20%; mainly renal elimination, some metabolism (3 h)	Used for herpes simplex and varicella-zoster infections; given orally, topically or by intravenous infusion
Cidofovir	Undergoes intracellular phosphorylation to mono-, di- and triphosphates, which have longer half-lives; renal elimination (3 h)	Used for CMV in people with AIDS; phosphorylated analogue of aciclovir; given by intravenous infusion
Famciclovir	Prodrug converted to penciclovir which is renally eliminated (2 h); intracellular active triphosphate has a longer half-life	Used for treatment of herpes zoster, acute genital herpes simplex and suppression of recurrent genital herpes infections; given orally
Foscarnet	Highly polar compound; renal elimination (3–7 h)	Used for CMV retinitis in people with AIDS and for mucocutaneous herpes simplex infections unresponsive to aciclovir in immunocompromised people; given by intravenous infusion
Ganciclovir	Mainly renal elimination (4 h)	Used for life-threatening or sight-threatening CMV infections in immunocompromised people only; given by intravenous infusion
Penciclovir	Not absorbed from skin	Used as a cream for herpes simplex labialis
Valaciclovir	Bioavailability 55%; rapidly metabolised to aciclovir	Uses similar to aciclovir; given orally
Valganciclovir	Ester prodrug converted by intestinal and hepatic esterases to ganciclovir	Used for CMV retinitis in people with AIDS and for prevention of CMV infection following transplantation from an infected donor; given orally

Other antivirals

Drug	Kinetics (half-life)	Comments
Adefovir dipivoxil	Diester prodrug converted to adefovir, which is renally eliminated (8 h)	Used for chronic hepatitis B infection with either compensated liver disease and evidence of viral replication or decompensated liver disease; given orally
Amantadine	Completely absorbed from the gut; renally eliminated (10–15 h)	M_2 ion channel inhibitor; used for herpes zoster and influenza A; given orally

Compendium: drugs used for infections—cont'd

Drug	Kinetics (half-life)	Comments
Enfuvirtide	Peptide probably undergoes hepatic hydrolysis (4 h)	HIV entry inhibitor; used with other antiretroviral drugs for resistant HIV infection or in people intolerant to other drugs; given by subcutaneous injection
Idoxuridine	Phosphorylated metabolite incorporated into viral DNA and impairs transcription; few kinetic data available	Used as 5% solution in dimethyl sulfoxide (DMSO) for topical infections with herpes simplex and herpes zoster; rarely used and of little value
Inosine pranobex	Few data available; complex decomposes to generate inosine (<1 h)	Used for mucocutaneous herpes simplex, genital warts and subacute sclerosing panencephalitis; given orally
Maraviroc	Partially absorbed from gut; hepatic metabolism (14–18 h)	Chemokine co-receptor CCR5 antagonist; used with other antiretroviral drugs for treatment of resistant HIV infection; given orally
Oseltamivir	Complete first-pass metabolism to active carboxylic acid analogue (1–3 h), which is renally excreted (6–10 h)	Neuraminidase inhibitor; used to treat influenza in at-risk people if started within 48 h of onset of symptoms; given orally
Palivizumab	Few data available; probably eliminated by peptide hydrolysis (≈20 days)	Humanised monoclonal antibody against RSV antigen; used for prevention of serious lower respiratory tract infection by RSV in neonates and children under 2 years; given by intramuscular injection
Raltegravir	Good oral absorption; eliminated by conjugation and excretion unchanged in urine (9 h)	HIV integrase inhibitor; used for the treatment of HIV infection resistant to other antiretroviral drugs; given orally
Ribavirin (tribavirin)	Oral bioavailability 50%; metabolised by hydrolysis, renal excretion; slowly cleared from tissues (7–21 days)	Used for severe RSV bronchiolitis in infants and children, and with interferon alfa or peginterferon alfa for chronic hepatitis C infection; given orally or by inhalation
Zanamivir	Eliminated in urine (2–5 h)	Neuraminidase inhibitor; used to treat influenza in at-risk subjects if started within 48 h of onset of symptoms; given by inhalation for influenza

Antiprotozoal drugs

Antimalarials

Drug	Kinetics (half-life)	Comments
Artemether with lumefantrine	Artemether rapidly demethylated to active metabolite (2–3 h); lumefantrine slowly metabolised (2–6 days); faecal elimination	Used for the treatment of acute uncomplicated falciparum malaria; given orally
Atovaquone	Variable absorption influenced by food; most eliminated unabsorbed in faeces (3 days)	Given orally with proguanil for the treatment of acute uncomplicated falciparum malaria and for prophylaxis of falciparum malaria; also used for mild to moderate pneumocystis pneumonia
Chloroquine	Complete oral bioavailability; accumulates in infected erythrocytes and other tissue sites; mostly renal elimination (30–60 days)	Used for chemoprophylaxis and treatment of malaria and also used for rheumatoid arthritis and lupus erythematosus; given orally or by intravenous infusion
Mefloquine	Bioavailability 80%; accumulates in infected erythrocytes; metabolised by hydrolysis, metabolites eliminated in bile and urine (15–33 days)	Used for chemoprophylaxis and treatment of uncomplicated falciparum and chloroquine-resistant vivax malaria; given orally
Primaquine	Almost complete bioavailability; metabolised to active carboxyprimaquine (4–10 h)	Used for eradication of liver stages of vivax and ovale malaria; given orally
Proguanil	High oral bioavailability; prodrug of cycloguanil, which has shorter half-life (2 h) than parent drug (12–24 h)	Folate inhibitor; used for chemoprophylaxis of malaria; given orally (alone or with atovaquone)
Pyrimethamine	Well absorbed; numerous metabolites eliminated mainly in faeces (2–6 days)	Folate inhibitor; used for malaria only in combination with sulfadoxine; given orally

Compendium: drugs used for infections—cont'd

Drug	Kinetics (half-life)	Comments
Quinine	Oral bioavailability 80–90%; eliminated largely by metabolism (6–47 h)	Used for treatment but not prophylaxis of falciparum malaria, or when the infection is either mixed or not known; given orally or by intravenous infusion
Sulfadoxine	Metabolised by acetylation (10 days)	Sulphonamide; used for malaria only in combination with pyrimethamine; given orally
Other antiprotozoals		
Diloxanide furoate	Completely hydrolysed in gut to diloxanide; absorbed diloxanide is rapidly conjugated with glucuronic acid; mainly renal excretion	Used for amoebiasis and drug of choice for asymptomatic *Entamoeba histolytica* infections; given orally
Eflornithine	Renal elimination (8 h)	Ornithine decarboxylase inhibitor; given intravenously for trypanosomiasis (sleeping sickness); also used topically for hirsutism
Mepacrine	Few data available; slowly eliminated by metabolism	Used for giardiasis and discoid lupus erythematosus; given orally
Metronidazole	Complete oral bioavailability; metabolites eliminated in urine (6–9 h)	Antibacterial; used for intestinal and extra-intestinal amoebiasis and for urogenital trichomoniasis and giardiasis; given orally
Pentamidine	Hepatic metabolism, renal excretion (10–14 days)	Used for pneumocystis pneumonia, leishmaniasis and trypanosomiasis; given by inhalation (nebuliser), by deep intramuscular injection or by intravenous infusion
Stibogluconate	Pentavalent antimony is eliminated in urine (6 h)	Pentavalent antimony compound; used for leishmaniasis; given by intramuscular injection or slow intravenous infusion
Tinidazole	Complete oral bioavailability; parent drug and metabolites eliminated in urine and bile (12–14 h)	Antibacterial; uses as antiprotozoal are similar to metronidazole; given orally
Antihelminthic drugs		
Albendazole	Low oral bioavailability; parent compound and sulphoxide metabolite are active (8–12 h)	Used on a 'named-patient' basis either alone or as an adjunct to surgery for echinococcal infections and for cutaneous hookworm larval infections; given orally
Diethylcarbamazine	Good oral absorption; eliminated by hepatic metabolism and renal excretion	First line drug for use against filariae (not approved in UK); given orally
Ivermectin	Well absorbed; eliminated as metabolites in faeces (12 h)	Used on a 'named-patient' basis as the drug of choice for onchocerciasis; also used for cutaneous hookworm larval infections and for chronic *Strongyloides* infections; given orally
Levamisole	Bioavailability 60–70%; hepatic metabolism (4–6 h)	Used on a 'named-patient' basis as the drug of choice for *Ascaris lumbricoides* infection; given orally
Mebendazole	Bioavailability <20%; metabolites excreted in urine (3–9 h)	Used for threadworm, roundworm, whipworm and hookworm infections; given orally
Niclosamide	Some oral absorption (up to 20%), with subsequent liver metabolism	Used on a 'named-patient' basis for tapeworm infections; given orally; not used in the USA
Piperazine	About 5–30% of oral dose is excreted in urine unchanged within 24 h	Used for threadworm and roundworm infections; given orally
Praziquantel	Probably extensive first-pass metabolism; rapidly metabolised and excreted (2 h)	Used on a 'named-patient' basis for tapeworm infections and bilharziasis; given orally
Tiabendazole	Extensively absorbed; hepatic metabolism (1.2 h)	Used on a 'named-patient' basis as the drug of choice for *Strongyloides* infection; also for cutaneous hookworm larval infections; given orally

CMV, cytomegalovirus; MRSA, meticillin-resistant *Staphylococcus aureus;* RSV, respiratory syncytial virus.

52

Chemotherapy of malignancy

Approximately 20–25% of people in the Western world die from cancer. Surgery and radiotherapy are valuable for treating localised cancers but are less effective in prolonging life once the tumour has spread to produce metastases. However, the introduction of cytotoxic chemotherapy to kill rapidly proliferating neoplastic cells has had a major impact on the treatment of malignant disease, especially diffuse tumours. The successful treatment of cancer frequently involves a multidisciplinary approach, which also includes psychological and social support.

A wide range of different drugs to treat cancer has been introduced into clinical practice since the 1970s with a variety of mechanisms and sites of action within cancer cells. Although the drugs differ in their specific cellular targets, the majority rely on the rapid rate of growth and division of cancer cells to provide a degree of selectivity between normal and malignant tissue. Recent developments in molecular biology are resulting in the discovery of new potential targets for drug action and a resurgence of cytotoxic drug development. The ability of molecular biological approaches to define the mechanisms of cell–cell communication, apoptosis and angiogenesis will undoubtedly prove a major stimulus for the production of new drugs with greater selectivity for cancer cells. In addition, there is growing understanding of the potential for immunotherapy in the treatment of cancer.

There are a number of *in vivo* animal tests for detecting antineoplastic activity, but these frequently over-predict the likely effectiveness of a compound in clinical use because the animal tumours used as models have a much higher growth fraction. A placebo-controlled clinical trial of a new antineoplastic drug given as sole treatment is now unethical if an effective drug is already available. Therefore, the efficacy of any new drug is usually assessed by adding it to the best available current therapy. A successful new drug would have to show a clinically significant benefit above that of the optimal current treatment. As a result, many recent advances in cancer chemotherapy have arisen from the more effective use of existing drugs, by optimising drug combinations and regimens, and by minimising toxicity, rather than the introduction of novel compounds.

Cytotoxic drugs share a number of generic properties and characteristics, both beneficial and adverse, which will be discussed first. The major classes of drug will then be discussed with information on mechanisms of action and general toxic effects.

MOLECULAR ORIGINS OF CANCER

Most cancers probably arise from multiple genetic mutations in a cell, with sequential gene defects resulting in progressive

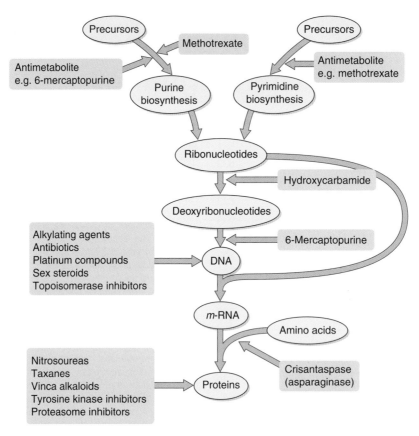

Fig. 52.1 Sites of action of the main groups of anti-cancer drugs.

changes through initial metaplastic and dysplastic phases, and then to invasive and ultimately metastatic cancer. Normal cells are regulated by numerous external factors that control their growth and death. These include growth factors, cytokines and hormones that activate or suppress the genes controlling cell division. Cancers develop as a result of abnormalities in the control of cell function.

About 85% of cancers arise from exposure to environmental factors such as viruses and chemicals, with inherited genetic mutations accounting for the remainder. The environmental factors produce DNA damage, which in the normal cell can be repaired before the cell completes its cycle of division. A second protective mechanism is apoptosis (programmed cell death) of severely damaged cells. Cancer may arise by various mechanisms that influence gene expression and cell cycle control:

- **inactivation of tumour suppressor genes** or changes in microRNA genes (encoding RNA molecules which regulate gene expression) will promote unregulated cell proliferation,
- **inactivation of genes that repair DNA**,
- **activation of proto-oncogenes to growth-promoting oncogenes**: proto-oncogenes are normal gene sequences that control cell proliferation and differentiation. They are capable of being activated to oncogenes, the expression of which leads to tumour development. Oncogene activation occurs as a result of chromosomal

rearrangement, gene mutations or gene amplification. Products of oncogene activation include transcription factors, chromatin remodellers, growth factors, altered growth factor receptors, intracellular signal transducers and apoptosis regulators. Gene mutations that activate oncogenes allow cell growth in the absence of stimulation by an external regulator,

- **suppression of apoptosis:** cells with damaged genetic material fail to undergo programmed cell death if oncogenes are activated and tumour suppressor genes are not functional. Defective function of the tumour suppressor protein p53 may be a factor in reducing apoptosis and permitting cell proliferation.

Activation of telomerase may also be important. Telomeres are found at the ends of chromosomes and their progressive shortening as healthy cells divide ultimately arrests further division. In cancer cells, telomerase activation extends the telomeres and promotes cell growth and division. Defective function of the tumour suppressor protein p53 may be a factor in reducing apoptosis and permitting cell proliferation. Growth factors secreted by cancer cells promote angiogenesis and increase blood supply to the tumour. Other secreted factors can impede the host's immune response to the cancer cells. Genetic changes in cancer cells can give rise to metabolic changes or expression of transporters such as P-glycoprotein that confer resistance to chemotherapy (Ch. 2).

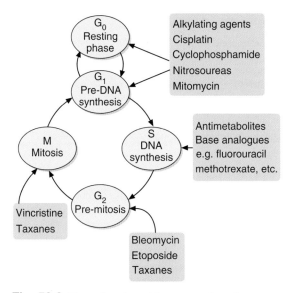

Fig. 52.2 Sites of action of key examples of cell-cycle-specific anti-cancer drugs.

ANTINEOPLASTIC DRUGS

MECHANISMS OF ACTION

The majority of antineoplastic drugs act on the process of DNA synthesis within the cancer cell, as summarised in Figure 52.1. Selectivity of these drugs for cancer cells compared with normal tissues is determined by the rate of DNA synthesis and cell division. Resting cells in the G_0 phase (Fig. 52.2) are resistant to many antineoplastic drugs. *Cell cycle-specific antineoplastic drugs*, such as the antimetabolites (Fig. 52.2), work effectively only when the cells are in the appropriate phase of the cell cycle at the time of treatment. *Non-cell cycle-specific antineoplastic drugs*, such as the alkylating drugs, nitrosoureas and cisplatin, have a 'hit-and-run' action on DNA, and it is not critical when the cell is exposed because the drug effect becomes apparent when the cells attempt to divide.

The sensitivity of a cancer to treatment depends on its growth fraction, which is the fraction of cells undergoing mitosis at any time. For example, in Burkitt's lymphoma almost 100% of neoplastic cells are undergoing division simultaneously and are they are very sensitive to chemotherapy, showing a dramatic response to a single dose of cyclophosphamide. In contrast, the growth fraction in a carcinoma of the colon is less than 5% of cells, resulting in its relative resistance to chemotherapy. However, metastases from colonic carcinoma deposited in the liver and elsewhere initially have a high growth fraction and are more sensitive to anti-cancer drugs.

Using *in vitro* cancer cell lines, it has been shown that:

- antineoplastic drugs produce a proportional cell kill; in other words, a proportion such as 95% of the cells present may be eliminated during a single course of treatment; consequently, multiple treatments may be necessary to eradicate the cancer, with successive treatments producing an exponential decrease in the number of residual viable cancer cells,
- essentially complete eradication of tumour cells is necessary to prevent regrowth,
- efficacy of chemotherapy *in vitro* is increased if treatment with cell cycle-specific drugs is timed to coincide with the appropriate phase of cell division within the cell population.

In vivo, the immune system probably contributes to the final removal of residual malignant cells; however, most antineoplastic drugs compromise immunoresponsiveness, which will reduce this removal process. The periodicity of doses is probably less critical *in vivo* because cancer cell cycles are not synchronised within the target cell population between treatments. In clinical practice, dose intervals are often established to allow recovery of healthy cells from toxic effects of the treatment. Therefore, while these concepts apply to *in vivo* cancer treatment, risk–benefit considerations may change with successive treatments and preclude complete eradication of the tumour.

RESISTANCE

Resistance to chemotherapeutic drugs may develop in a number of ways. These are explained later in the text for individual drugs, but include:

- reduced drug uptake into cancer cells, e.g. methotrexate enters cells by the high-affinity transport system (the reduced folate carrier) for tetrahydrofolic acid, and downregulation of the transporter limits the uptake of methotrexate and confers resistance to the drug,
- use of alternative metabolic pathways and salvage mechanisms to circumvent a blocked biochemical process; such mechanisms are usually drug-specific, e.g. induction of asparagine synthesis in cells exposed to crisantaspase (asparaginase),
- alteration of intracellular drug targets, e.g. production of topoisomerase II with reduced sensitivity to the inhibitory effects of anthracyclines,
- increased inactivation of the compound within the cancer cell, e.g. high intracellular levels of glutathione S-transferase isozymes inactivate cisplatin and alkylating drugs,
- reduced activation of prodrugs, e.g. low intracellular levels of deoxycytidine kinase reduces activation of cytarabine (cytosine arabinoside); increased activity of thiopurine S-methyltransferase increases the metabolism of mercaptopurine and tioguanine,
- increased removal of the drug from the cancer cell. This involves the possibility of increased transcription of the gene for proteins which act as carriers for the elimination from the cell of complex foreign chemicals (Fig. 2.1), including a number of cytotoxic compounds. There are several such proteins (see Table 2.1), including P-glycoprotein and the multidrug resistance-related proteins (MRPs). Increased production of the carrier protein confers multidrug resistance to a number of structurally unrelated natural compounds or their derivatives, including vinca alkaloids, etoposide, taxanes, anthracyclines, dactinomycin (actinomycin D), mitomycin C and mitoxantrone. The carrier can be inhibited by calcium channel blockers, such as nifedipine or verapamil, by ciclosporin,

or by tamoxifen. These drugs may be added to cytotoxic drug regimens to prevent resistance.

UNWANTED EFFECTS

Cytotoxic antineoplastic drugs are among the most toxic compounds given to humans. Many have a therapeutic index of approximately 1, as the therapeutic dose is essentially the same as the toxic dose. Because drug action is usually greater in tissues with a high growth fraction, a number of normal, rapidly dividing non-malignant tissues are also affected. In addition to effects that occur in all rapidly dividing tissues, many chemotherapeutic drugs also have specific toxic effects on other tissues. Dosage regimens are usually designed so that normal tissues, especially bone marrow and gut, can recover between doses (Fig. 52.3).

Gastrointestinal tract

Mucosal cells have a rapid turnover. Toxicity can produce anorexia, mucosal ulceration or diarrhoea. A sore mouth is most common with fluorouracil, methotrexate and the anthracyclines. Nausea and vomiting are common, especially with alkylating drugs and cisplatin, and this may limit an individual's ability to tolerate an optimal dosage regimen (see Ch. 32).

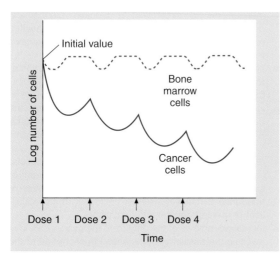

Fig. 52.3 Hypothetical dosing schedule of anti-cancer drugs to allow recovery of normal tissues. At least 10^9 tumour cells are usually present when tumours are first detectable. The malignant cells show a greater proportional kill than normal cells because a larger fraction is in division at any time. Theoretically, the response of the malignant cells to dose 2 would be greater than for dose 1 if cell cycles became synchronised and dose 2 was given during the correct phase of the growth cycle. A typical dose interval is 3–4 weeks.

Bone marrow

Myelosuppression is a serious consequence of treatment and can lead to severe neutropenia, thrombocytopenia and sometimes anaemia. It often occurs 7–10 days after a cycle of chemotherapy, but is delayed with drugs such as melphalan and lomustine. These haematological consequences may limit the drug dosage that the person is able to tolerate. There is a high risk of both infection (neutropenic sepsis) and haemorrhage following cytotoxic chemotherapy.

Hair follicle cells

Partial or complete alopecia may occur, but this is usually temporary.

Reproductive organs

Both sexes are affected and sterility can result, particularly after therapy with cyclophosphamide or cytarabine. Because of the mechanisms of action of cytotoxic drugs, most have teratogenic activity. Pregnant women should not be exposed to cytotoxic drugs for treatment or as members of the healthcare team. Alkylating agents or procarbazine can cause permanent male infertility. Drugs that mimic or affect the activity of sex hormones are frequently used for the treatment of breast or prostate cancer, and these inevitably produce adverse effects on sexual function.

Growing tissues in children

Of particular concern in children is the possibility that intensive cytotoxic chemotherapy can impair growth. Children treated with cytotoxic drugs for malignancy also have an increased risk of the subsequent development of a second malignancy (about 10%), which is often leukaemia.

Extravasation of intravenous drug

If anti-cancer drugs leak from a vein into the surrounding tissues, they can cause severe local tissue necrosis.

Tumour lysis syndrome

Rapid breakdown of malignant cells can produce hyperuricaemia, hyperkalaemia, hypophosphataemia, hypocalcaemia with consequent renal damage or arrhythmias. The syndrome is most common with treatment of non-Hodgkin's lymphoma, Burkitt's lymphoma and acute leukaemias. Tumour lysis syndrome can be ameliorated by good hydration and the prophylactic use of allopurinol (Ch. 31).

DRUG COMBINATIONS

It is common practice to treat many cancers with a combination of different antineoplastic drugs simultaneously. Potential combinations of drugs are investigated using in vitro and in vivo experiments before they are subjected to clinical evaluation in humans. The most successful combinations are those that show synergism in their actions on cancer cells, rather than a simple additive effect, while showing no increase in their systemic toxicity. Criteria for selecting ideal combinations are:

- each drug should be an active antineoplastic drug in its own right; a second drug would not be given simply to increase the formation of an active metabolite of the first, although sometimes drugs are given to reduce the development of toxicity or resistance to another drug,
- each drug should have a different mechanism of action and target site within the cancer cell; this will increase efficacy while reducing the likelihood of resistance,
- each drug should have a different site for any organ-specific toxicity; some common toxicity is almost inevitable because nearly all drugs affect tissues with a high growth fraction.

SPECIFIC ANTINEOPLASTIC DRUGS

The drug compendium at the end of this chapter outlines the licensed uses of individual drugs and notes any unusual or limiting toxicity.

DRUGS AFFECTING NUCLEIC ACID FUNCTION

Alkylating drugs

Examples

busulfan, chlorambucil, cyclophosphamide, melphalan

Mechanism of action and uses

The nitrogen mustards were developed from the sulphur mustard gases used as chemical warfare agents in World War I. These gases caused bone marrow suppression in addition to the respiratory toxicity for which they were developed. Replacement of the divalent sulphur atom by trivalent nitrogen allowed the introduction of a complex side chain, which resulted in a range of more stable nonvolatile drugs that could be given therapeutically under controlled conditions. Alkylating drugs contain side chains which undergo a metabolic activation step that involves loss of part of the molecule (for example the Cl is lost from – CH_2CH_2Cl) and yields a highly reactive product which binds to DNA or proteins. Many alkylating drugs are bifunctional (i.e. have two reactive groups). The reactive alkylating group(s) in the molecule may be:

- nitrogen mustard $N–CH_2CH_2Cl$ (with Cl being the leaving group), e.g. carmustine (BCNU), chlorambucil, cyclophosphamide, ifosfamide, lomustine (CCNU), melphalan,
- sulphonate ester $–CH_2OSO_2CH_3$ (with SO_2CH_3 being the leaving group), e.g. busulfan, treosulfan,
- nitrosourea $–NNO$, e.g. carmustine, lomustine,
- cyclic nitrogen derivative (ethylenimines, e.g. thiotepa).

The mechanism of action is by covalent binding to DNA (nitrogen mustards, sulphonate esters and cyclic nitrogen compounds), which prevents DNA and RNA synthesis, or by covalent binding to proteins (nitrosoureas), which blocks DNA repair processes.

When alkylating drugs bind to DNA nucleotides, such as to guanine, the alkylated nucleotide may either be repaired in which case the cell survives, or it may interfere with DNA replication by:

- being misread,
- undergoing further metabolism via ring opening,
- crosslinking to another guanine molecule via a second reactive group (with bifunctional drugs).

Because of the covalent nature of the product, these effects are not cell cycle-specific (Fig. 52.2). Alkylating agents are used to treat a wide variety of leukaemias, lymphomas and solid tumours.

Pharmacokinetics

The pharmacokinetic characteristics of the alkylating drugs depend on the nature of the reactive group(s) and the third non-reactive substituent on the N atom. Cyclophosphamide is an orally active prodrug that undergoes metabolic activation to produce two toxic metabolites, acrolein and phosphoramide mustard. Ifosfamide metabolism is similar to that of cyclophosphamide, and toxic metabolites of both cyclophosphamide and ifosfamide are excreted in the urine. Melphalan and chlorambucil, which have an aromatic substituent, undergo rapid metabolism. Most alkylating agents have half-lives of less than 6 h, but the duration of action on DNA is very long.

Unwanted effects

- Alkylating drugs are highly cytotoxic and cause bone marrow suppression and neutropenia. Amifostine is a compound used to reduce the severity of neutropenia induced by cyclophosphamide or cisplatin (see cisplatin below). It is a prodrug that is metabolised in neutrophils by alkaline phosphatase to a free thiol metabolite that binds to the reactive metabolites of these cytotoxic drugs.
- Fertility is reduced through impaired gametogenesis.
- A particular problem with the long-term use of alkylating drugs is the development of acute myeloid leukaemia, especially if combined with radiotherapy.
- Busulfan, carmustine and treosulfan can cause pulmonary fibrosis.
- Busulfan and treosulfan commonly cause skin pigmentation.
- Cyclophosphamide and ifosfamide cause bladder toxicity with haemorrhagic cystitis due to formation of acrolein; it can be prevented by prior treatment with mesna (mercaptoethane sulphonic acid; Ch. 53), which provides free thiol groups in the urinary bladder to detoxify acrolein. Bladder cancer can develop years after cyclophosphamide therapy.

Cytotoxic antibiotics

Examples

anthracyclines: doxorubicin, epirubicin
other antibiotics: bleomycin, dactinomycin, mitomycin,
    mitoxantrone

Mechanisms of action and uses

The cytotoxic antibiotics have diverse chemical structures.

- The anthracyclines are all quinone-containing planar four-ringed structures that contain an amino sugar group.
- Mitoxantrone has a three-ringed planar quinone structure with amino-containing side chains (an anthracycline derivative), and mitomycin is a non-planar tricyclic quinone.
- Bleomycin and dactinomycin are complex peptide or glycopeptide derivatives.

Cytotoxic antibiotics have several possible mechanisms of action.

- Intercalation: this is shown particularly by the anthracyclines, with the planar ring system intercalating between DNA bases and the amino sugar part binding to the deoxyribose phosphate groups. Intercalation blocks reading of the DNA template and also inhibits repair of DNA double-strand breaks by topoisomerase II.
- Free radical attack: the metabolism of the drugs gives rise to superoxide and hydroxyl radicals and hydrogen peroxide, which cause DNA damage and cytotoxicity.
- Membrane effects: interference with membrane function can occur either directly or via oxidative damage.

In general, the mechanisms of action are not cell cycle-specific, although some members of the class show greatest activity at certain phases of the cycle, for example S phase (doxorubicin, mitoxantrone), G_1 and early S phase (mitomycin), and G_2 phase and mitosis (bleomycin).

Cytotoxic antibiotics have a wide spectrum of activity and are used for treatment of several leukaemias and lymphomas, as well as some solid tumours.

Pharmacokinetics

The cytotoxic antibiotics are poorly absorbed from the gut and are given intravenously. They are eliminated by metabolism and some have very long half-lives (mostly 12 h or longer).

Unwanted effects

Many of these drugs have radiomimetic properties. They should not be used at the same time as radiotherapy, since toxicity can be greatly increased.

- General cytotoxicity.
- Doxorubicin, epirubicin and mitoxantrone produce dose-related irreversible myocardial damage leading to cardiomyopathy through free radical release and oxidative stress, as well as nuclear cytotoxicity. The cardiomyopathy may not become apparent until several years after treatment. Liposomal formulations of doxorubicin and longer infusion times may reduce the cardiac toxicity, as does concurrent infusion of the iron chelator dexrazoxane.
- Painful skin eruptions with liposomal doxorubicin.
- Bleomycin often causes skin pigmentation.
- Bleomycin and mitomycin produce dose-related pulmonary fibrosis.
- Tissue extravasation during infusion of anthracyclines produces severe necrosis, which can be minimised by subsequent intravenous infusion of dexrazoxane.

PLATINUM COMPOUNDS

Examples

carboplatin, cisplatin, oxaliplatin

Mechanism of action and uses

The platinum drugs enter cells and generate a reactive complex that crosslink guanine units in DNA. The result is similar to the effect of alkylating drugs by breaking the DNA chain. Cisplatin and carboplatin are used for ovarian and lung tumours. Cisplatin is also used for several other solid tumours. Oxaliplatin is used for advanced colorectal cancer.

Pharmacokinetics

These drugs are given by intravenous infusion and are mainly excreted by the kidney as platinum compounds. Cisplatin and oxaliplatin have long half-lives (24–60 h), largely owing to extensive protein binding.

Unwanted effects

- Severe nausea and vomiting.
- Nephrotoxicity with irreversible renal impairment; hydration is important to minimise the risk.
- Hypomagnesaemia.
- Ototoxicity with hearing loss and tinnitus.
- Peripheral neuropathy (especially with oxaliplatin).
- Myelosuppression (more marked for carboplatin).

Most effects are more marked for cisplatin than for carboplatin. Amifostine (see above) is used to reduce the severity of cisplatin-induced neutropenia in advanced ovarian cancer. It also reduces the nephrotoxicity of cisplatin.

ANTIMETABOLITES

Folic acid antagonists

Example

methotrexate

Mechanism of action and uses

An astute clinical observation that the administration of folic acid to children with leukaemia exacerbated their condition led to the development of a folate antagonist, methotrexate. This represented an important landmark in cancer chemotherapy.

Folic acid in its reduced form (tetrahydrofolic acid, THF) is an important biochemical intermediate. It is essential for synthetic reactions that involve the addition of a single carbon atom during a biochemical reaction, such as the introduction of the methyl group into thymidylate and the synthesis of the purine ring system. During such reactions, THF is oxidised to dihydrofolic acid (DHF), which has to be reduced by dihydrofolate reductase back to THF before it can accept a further one-carbon group and be reused.

Methotrexate has a very high affinity for mammalian dihydrofolate reductase and inhibits its active site. This blocks purine and thymidylate synthesis and inhibits the synthesis of DNA, RNA and protein. It may show selectivity for cancer cells because these rely more on *de novo* synthesis of purines and pyrimidines, whereas normal tissues use salvage pathways that reutilise preformed purines and pyrimidines to a greater extent. Methotrexate is specific for S phase and slows G_1 to S phase.

Methotrexate is given for acute lymphoblastic leukaemia, non-Hodgkin's lymphomas and various solid tumours. It is also used an immunosuppressant at lower doses in non-malignant conditions such as inflammatory joint diseases and psoriasis. The mechanism of its immunosuppressant effect is different to its anti-cancer actions (Ch. 38).

Pharmacokinetics

Methotrexate is well absorbed from the gut but can also be given intravenously or intrathecally. It is eliminated by renal excretion, but a small amount may be retained for longer periods both strongly bound to dihydrofolate reductase and intracellularly as polyglutamate conjugates.

Unwanted effects

- Toxicity to normal rapidly dividing tissues, especially the bone marrow.
- Hepatotoxicity can follow chronic therapy as an immunosuppressant (see Ch.38).

Toxicity is increased in the presence of reduced renal excretion, and methotrexate should be avoided if there is significant renal impairment. Folinic acid (leucovorin) is frequently administered shortly after high-dose methotrexate to reduce mucositis and myelosuppression. Non-steroidal anti-inflammatory drugs such as aspirin can reduce the renal excretion of methotrexate and increase its toxicity.

Base analogue antimetabolites

Examples

purine antagonists: fludarabine, gemcitabine, mercaptopurine, tioguanine
pyrimidine antagonists: capecitabine, cytarabine, fluorouracil, raltitrexed, tegafur

Mechanism of action and uses

A number of useful chemotherapeutic drugs have been produced by simple modifications to the structures of normal purine and pyrimidine bases (Fig. 52.4). These act in a number of ways to interfere with DNA synthesis, typically following intracellular phosphorylation and the incorporation of the triphosphate product into DNA or RNA. Detailed mechanisms are given for each drug in the Compendium at the end of the chapter. Base analogue antimetabolites are used for a wide variety of leukaemias, lymphomas and solid tumours.

Pharmacokinetics

Base analogues are mainly absorbed and metabolised by the pathways involved in absorption and metabolism of the corresponding unmodified base. Oral absorption is often erratic and most are given intravenously. The urine is a minor route of elimination (up to 1% of the parent drug) and most half-lives are in the range 1–8 h. Tegafur is a prodrug of fluorouracil and is given in combination with uracil, or with gimeracil and oteracil, which inhibit the breakdown of fluorouracil.

Unwanted effects

- Typical cytotoxic effects are common; myelosuppression, in particular, can be severe and prolonged after cladribine, cytarabine, fludarabine and tioguanine.

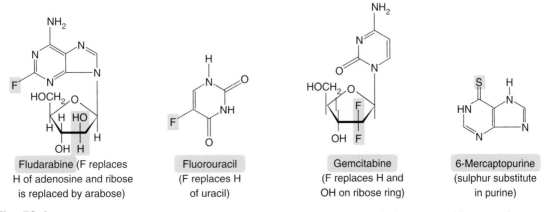

Fludarabine (F replaces H of adenosine and ribose is replaced by arabose)

Fluorouracil (F replaces H of uracil)

Gemcitabine (F replaces H and OH on ribose ring)

6-Mercaptopurine (sulphur substitute in purine)

Fig. 52.4 **The structures of some antimetabolite drugs, illustrating their similarity to normal bases and nucleotides.** The structural changes are highlighted.

- Drug interaction: allopurinol (Ch. 31) interferes with the metabolism of 6-mercaptopurine, and the dose should be reduced if these drugs are used concurrently.

MITOTIC INHIBITORS

Vinca alkaloids

Examples

vinblastine, vincristine, vindesine, vinorelbine

Mechanism of action and uses

The vinca alkaloids are complex natural chemicals isolated from the periwinkle plant (*Vinca rosea*). Vinca alkaloids bind to tubulin and inhibit polymerisation and therefore assembly of microtubules, thus producing M-phase arrest of mitosis. They are therefore cycle-specific. Microtubules are essential for numerous cellular functions, including maintenance of cell shape, motility, transport between organelles and cell division.

The vinca alkaloids are used for various lymphomas and for acute leukaemia. They are also effective in some solid tumours.

Pharmacokinetics

Vinca alkaloids are usually given intravenously. Elimination is largely by metabolism with little renal excretion. They have very long half-lives.

Unwanted effects

The spectrum of unwanted effects differs between various drugs, despite their close structural similarities.

- General cytotoxicity. Myelosuppression is dose-limiting for vinblastine, vindesine and vinorelbine, but unusual with vincristine.
- Neurotoxicity, usually a sensory neuropathy, is dose-limiting with vincristine. It causes peripheral paraesthesiae, loss of tendon reflexes, abdominal pain and constipation. Motor weakness occasionally accompanies the sensory neuropathy.
- Severe tissue damage if the drugs extravasate from the infusion site.

Camptothecin analogues (topoisomerase I inhibitors)

Examples

irinotecan, topotecan

Mechanism of action and uses

These drugs are semi-synthetic derivatives of a cytotoxic alkaloid isolated from the Chinese tree *Camptotheca acuminata*. The drugs inhibit topoisomerase I, which is important in DNA transcription and translation. The enzyme relieves the torsional strain in DNA by producing single-strand breaks that, under normal cell conditions, are then re-ligated. The drugs bind to the DNA–topoisomerase I complex and prevent re-ligation. Although this binding is readily reversible, the consequences are irreversible, because cell death occurs when a double-strand break is produced at the DNA replication fork during S phase. Inhibition of DNA repair increases the sensitivity of the cell to ionising radiation.

Irinotecan is given as second-line treatment for metastatic colorectal cancer. Topotecan is used for lung, cervical or ovarian cancer.

Pharmacokinetics

They are large complex molecules that are given by intravenous infusion and eliminated mainly by hepatic metabolism.

Unwanted effects

- General cytotoxicity, with dose-limiting myelosuppression.
- Diarrhoea; cholinergic stimulation produces early diarrhoea, but other toxicity can result in delayed onset of diarrhoea.

Epipodophyllotoxins (topoisomerase II inhibitors)

Example

etoposide

Mechanism of action and uses

Etoposide is a synthetic derivative of a compound extracted from the mandrake root (*Podophyllum peltatum*). It is active during the G_2 phase and binds to the complex of DNA and topoisomerase II (an enzyme involved in the breaking and rejoining of DNA strands during cell division). The etoposide-bound complex prevents DNA replication by preventing re-ligation of DNA, and leads to cell apoptosis.

Etoposide is used for small cell lung carcinoma, lymphomas and testicular cancer.

Pharmacokinetics

Etoposide can be given orally or intravenously. Elimination is largely by metabolism.

Unwanted effects

- General cytotoxicity.
- Severe tissue damage if the drug extravasates from the infusion site.

Taxanes

Examples

docetaxel, paclitaxel

Mechanism of action and uses

The clinically used drugs are produced from taxane, a diterpenoid extracted from the bark of the Pacific yew tree (*Taxus brevifolia*). Taxanes promote the assembly of microtubules and inhibit their depolymerisation, leading to the formation of stable and non-functional microtubular bundles in the cell. They bind to a different site to that targeted by vinca alkaloids. The cell is inhibited during the G_2 and M phases of the cell cycle. Taxanes are also radiosensitisers, since cells in the G_2 and M phases are more sensitive to radiation.

Taxanes are used for ovarian, breast and prostate cancer and a variety of other solid tumours.

Pharmacokinetics

These drugs are given intravenously because of poor oral absorption. They are extensively metabolised in the liver and have half-lives of 10–20 h.

Unwanted effects

- General cytotoxicity.
- Severe hypersensitivity reactions can occur, with hypotension, angioedema and bronchospasm. Routine premedication with histamine (H_1 and H_2) receptor antagonists (Chs 33 and 39) combined with a corticosteroid (Ch. 44) is recommended for paclitaxel, and premedication with a corticosteroid for docetaxel.
- Neutropenia is dose-limiting.
- Arthralgia/myalgia syndrome.
- Paclitaxel causes peripheral sensory neuropathy, with motor neuropathy at high dosages.
- Docetaxel causes persistent leg oedema due to fluid retention.

DRUGS AFFECTING TYROSINE KINASE FUNCTION

The products of activated oncogenes include various cell surface receptors that activate a range of intracellular tyrosine kinases which autophosphorylate the receptor (see Ch. 1). There are about 20 families of receptors, including vascular endothelial growth factor receptors (VEGFRs; of which there are three types), the human epidermal growth factor (EGF) receptors HER1 (often called EGFR), HER2, HER3 and HER4, and platelet-derived growth factor receptors (PDGFRs). Autophosphorylation of the receptor triggers a series of intracellular pathways that stimulate cancer cell proliferation and block apoptosis.

Drugs acting on these processes can be subdivided into monoclonal antibodies that inhibit the cell surface receptor and small organic molecules that act intracellularly on the tyrosine kinase enzyme.

Tyrosine kinase receptor inhibitors

bevacizumab, cetuximab, trastuzumab

Mechanism of action and uses

Bevacizumab is a monoclonal antibody that inhibits VEGFR and reduces tumour angiogenesis. It is given by intravenous infusion as part of the first-line treatment of metastatic colorectal cancer, lung cancer and renal cell carcinoma. Unwanted effects include mucocutaneous bleeding, gastrointestinal perforation and impaired wound healing.

Cetuximab is a monoclonal antibody that binds to the extracellular domain of the EGFR (HER1) and blocks ligand-induced activation of tyrosine kinase. It is given by intravenous infusion in cases of colorectal tumour expressing EGFR and in combination with radiotherapy for locally advanced squamous cell cancer of the head and neck. Unwanted effects may occur with the infusion, including chills, fever and hypersensitivity reactions. Severe keratitis leading to blindness has also been reported.

Trastuzumab is a monoclonal antibody used for metastatic breast cancer when the tumour overexpresses HER2. It binds to HER2 and prevents activation of tyrosine kinase. Unwanted effects may occur with the infusion, including chills, fever and hypersensitivity reactions. Cardiotoxicity occurs if trastuzumab is used with anthracyclines, leading to heart failure.

Tyrosine kinase inhibitors

dasatinib, erlotinib, imatinib, sorafenib, sunitinib

These drugs block tyrosine kinase enzyme activity intracellularly, preventing transduction of signals from a variety of tyrosine kinase-linked cell surface receptors, and inhibiting cell growth and enhancing apoptosis. The drugs compete with ATP for binding to the enzyme and inhibit autophosphorylation of the receptor (see Ch. 1).

- Dasatinib inhibits multiple tyrosine kinases, including those associated with VEGFR and PDGFR families and with Bcr-Abl (a fusion protein found in leukaemias associated with Philadelphia chromosome). Dasatinib is used for chronic myeloid leukaemia and acute lymphoblastic leukaemia.
- Erlotinib inhibits signals from the EGFR (HER1). It is used for lung and pancreatic cancers.
- Imatinib inhibits signals from the PDGFR family and Bcr-Abl. It is used for chronic myeloid leukaemia, acute lymphoblastic leukaemia and a variety of rare tumours.
- Sunitinib and sorafenib inhibit signals from several receptors, including VEGFR and PDGFR families. They are used for renal cell carcinoma; sunitinib is also used for gastrointestinal stromal tumours and sorafenib also for hepatocellular cancer.

Pharmacokinetics

These drugs are well absorbed from the gut. They are metabolised in the liver, sometimes to active metabolites. The half-lives are typically about 1–5 days (except 3–5 h for dasatinib).

Unwanted effects

- Cytotoxic effects.
- Gastrointestinal upset.
- Dizziness, headache, insomnia.
- Oedema with dasatinib and imatinib.

PROTEASOME INHIBITORS

bortezomib

Mechanism of action

Proteasomes are large protein complexes that degrade ubiquitinated proteins (proteins conjugated to ubiquitin, which directs them to parts of the cell for destruction). Inhibition of the 26S proteasome by bortezomib interferes with degradation of pro-apoptotic proteins, leading to cell death.

Pharmacokinetics

Bortezomib is given intravenously. It is metabolised in the liver and has a half-life of 9–15 h.

Unwanted effects

- Cytotoxic effects.
- Peripheral neuropathy, fatigue.
- Gastrointestinal disturbances.
- Pyrexia.
- Postural hypotension.

HORMONAL AGENTS

Some drugs used in cancer therapy suppress cell division by actions at intracellular steroid receptors or by influencing the metabolism of steroidal hormones; examples include corticosteroids and drugs that control the division of cells sensitive to sex hormones. Cancers that arise from cell lines possessing steroid receptors that promote their growth and cell division are frequently susceptible to inhibitory steroids.

Glucocorticoids

Glucocorticoids (Ch. 44) suppress lymphocyte mitosis and are used in leukaemia and lymphoma; they are also helpful in reducing oedema around a tumour.

Oestrogens

Oestrogens such as ethinylestradiol (Ch. 45) suppress prostate cancer cells, both locally and in metastases, and provide symptomatic improvement; gynaecomastia is a common unwanted effect.

Progestogens

Progestogens such as hydroxyprogesterone acetate (Ch. 45) suppress endometrial cancer cells and kidney cancer metastases.

Oestrogen receptor antagonists

Breast cancer can be suppressed by oestrogen receptor antagonists such as tamoxifen. Tamoxifen is active orally and binds competitively to oestrogen receptors. It shows both oestrogenic effects (on bone) and anti-oestrogenic effects (on breast tissue). Tamoxifen inhibits oestrogen-regulated genes and reduces the secretion of growth factors by tumour cells. Tumour cells are affected mainly in the G_2 phase of the cell cycle. Tamoxifen is extensively metabolised in the liver and has active metabolites with long half-lives, so several weeks of treatment are necessary to achieve steady-state concentrations. Unwanted effects include hot flushes and amenorrhoea in premenopausal women and vaginal bleeding in postmenopausal women. Tamoxifen inhibits CYP3A4 and, therefore, reduces the metabolism of other substrates, such as warfarin.

Androgen receptor antagonists

These drugs (e.g. flutamide; Ch. 46) suppress prostate cancer cells.

Gonadorelin analogues

Gonadorelin is synthetic gonadotrophin-releasing hormone (GnRH) (see Ch. 43). Gonaldorelin analogues (e.g. buserelin) suppress prostate cancer cells.

Aromatase inhibitors

Aromatase is the enzyme that converts androgens to oestrogens. Inhibitors of aromatase (e.g. anastrazole and letrozole, which are non-steroidal, or exemestane, which is a steroid) reduce oestrogen production in postmenopausal women, who produce oestrogen mainly from androstenedione and testosterone in many tissues such as adipose tissue, skin, muscle and liver. Aromatase is also present in the cells of two-thirds of breast cancers. Aromatase inhibitors are used in post-menopausal women to treat breast cancers that are oestrogen-dependent.

MISCELLANEOUS ANTI-CANCER DRUGS

There are many individual anti-cancer drugs with a variety of mechanisms of action. Further details (including therapeutic uses and adverse effects) are given in the drug compendium at the end of this chapter.

Mechanisms of action and uses

Most potential biochemical sites within cells have been investigated as targets for anti-cancer drugs. Actions of different drugs include the following:

- removal of asparagine required for protein synthesis (crisantaspase),
- inhibition of incorporation of thymidine and adenine into DNA (procarbazine),
- inhibition of adenosine deaminase, which causes a build-up of deoxyadenosine triphosphate (dATP) that inhibits the formation of other deoxyribonucleotide triphosphates (pentostatin),
- inhibition of reduction of ribonucleotides to deoxyribonucleotides (hydroxycarbamide),
- intercalation between DNA base pairs (amsacrine),
- alkylating action, especially on thiol groups, to inhibit DNA repair (dacarbazine and temozolomide),
- superoxide production causing DNA backbone cleavage and cell apoptosis (trabectedin),
- increased cell differentiation and inhibition of proliferation by action on retinoid receptors (retinoic acid receptors, RARs, and retinoid X receptors, RXRs) (bexarotene, tretinoin) (Ch. 49),
- photodynamic activation in superficial tumours by laser light to produce cytotoxic oxygen free radicals (porfimer sodium, temoporfin),
- immunomodulation (by inhibition of tumour necrosis factor α and several other pro-inflammatory chemokines) and inhibition of angiogenesis (lenalidomide and thalidomide),
- activation of cytotoxic killer cells (Ch. 38); interleukin-2 (aldesleukin) is a cytokine produced by T-lymphocytes that is made by recombinant DNA technology,
- monoclonal antibodies: several monoclonal antibodies have been developed that have anti-cancer activity; for example:
  - alemtuzumab (which produces lysis of B-lymphocytes in treatment-resistant or rapidly relapsing chronic lymphocytic leukaemia),
  - rituximab (which produces lysis of B-lymphocytes in chemotherapy-resistant advanced follicular lymphoma) (see also Ch. 49),
  - catumaxomab (a trifunctional molecule that binds to the epithelial cell adhesion molecule (EpCAM), lymphocytes and several accessory immune cells such as macrophages, natural killer cells or dendritic cells and triggers an immune reaction against the cancer cell) is active against epithelial tumours that express EpCAM,
  - ipilimumab (binds to cytotoxic T-lymphocyte antigen 4 and prevents inhibition of the cytotoxic action) used for metastatic melanoma.

CLINICAL USES OF ANTINEOPLASTIC DRUGS

Different forms of cancer vary in their sensitivity to chemotherapy. The most responsive include lymphomas, leukaemias, choriocarcinoma and testicular carcinoma, while solid tumours such as sarcomas, adrenocortical and squamous cell bronchial carcinomas generally have a poor response. An intermediate response is shown by other cancers, for example those of the bowel, bladder, head and neck, small cell bronchogenic tumours and hormone-related cancers (breast, ovary, endometrium and prostate). In addition, the sensitivity of an individual tumour can change during treatment with antineoplastic drugs, because of the development of resistance.

Chemotherapy can be used alone to treat cancer, or in combination with surgery or with radiation (chemoradiation). Chemotherapy may be given as a curative or a palliative treatment, or to reduce the risk of relapse after tumour removal. Adjuvant chemotherapy refers specifically to treatment following a surgical procedure that appears to have removed all tumour, with the intention of preventing relapse from occult disease. Neoadjuvant chemotherapy is given before surgery to reduce tumour size.

Chemotherapy is being supplemented in many cancers types by the use of orally effective small molecule inhibitors, which often require the presence of a particular gene mutation in the cancer for effect (see sections below). These are excellent examples of the increasing personalization of cancer treatments and such drugs have converted some solid cancers from rapidly fatal conditions to diseases that can remain well controlled or radiologically resolved for sometimes many years.

A major new development in systemic therapy over recent years is immunotherapy, which aims to target the cancer by immune attack. Examples for drugs that have become mainstream treatments are a vaccine in advanced prostate cancer and the immunostimulatory antibody ipilimumab in melanoma.

ANTI-CANCER DRUG THERAPY FOR SPECIFIC MALIGNANCIES

The following discussion selects some important cancers and outlines the role of chemotherapeutic drugs in their management. The choice of specific regimens is a complex process involving an assessment of prognosis, frailty, toxicity and the wishes of the individual. Clinical trials are producing a continuing flow of improved therapeutic options, and this is a field of medicine that changes rapidly.

OESOPHAGEAL CANCER

Oesophageal cancer usually presents with advanced disease, with 50% being unresectable or having radiological metastases at presentation. Two common forms are recognized: squamous cell carcinoma is more common in older smokers, and adenocarcinoma which is associated with gastro-oesophageal reflux, obesity and Barrett's metaplasia and accounts for 75% of cases in the UK. For squamous cell cancers, if the disease is localized chemoradiation followed by surgical resection or radical chemoradiation is used. For adenocarcinoma of the lower oesophagus tumours, combination chemotherapy with oxaliplatin, epirubicin and capecitabine is commonly given before and after surgery to improve cure rates.

GASTRIC CANCER

Surgery alone can be curative for early disease, but the majority present with more advanced disease. For those considered suitable for radical surgical resection, neoadjuvant and adjuvant chemotherapy using a combination of epirubicin, oxaliplatin and capecitabine improves survival. Fluorouracil or capecitabine combined with oxaliplatin and epirubicin can be palliative in advanced disease (response rate of 65%). Aproximately 15% of tumours are HER-2 positive, and cisplatin, fluoropyrimidine and trastuzumab can be considered for palliative treatment.

PANCREATIC CANCER

Most pancreatic cancers present late and 5-year survival is rare because of metastatic progression. For operable tumours, surgery followed by adjuvant chemotherapy with gemcitabine or fluorouracil is the treatment of choice. For inoperable locally advanced tumours, chemoradiation with capecitabine is used. Metastatic disease can be treated with gemcitabine alone or a combination of fluorouracil with oxaliplatin and irinotecan.

COLORECTAL CANCER

Surgery is the mainstay of treatment for people with colorectal cancer without metastatic disease. If there is a high risk of relapse (Duke's grade C or some grade B), a combination of oxaliplatin and fluoropyrimidine improves survival by 10–15%. Pre-operative chemoradiation reduces metastatic spread and for rectal cancer reduces local recurrence. Once a person has survived for 5 years, life expectancy is similar to that in the general population.

In advanced and metastatic colorectal cancer, fluorouracil or capecitabine, with or without oxapliplatin or irinotecan, improves survival and quality of life. The EGFR-targeted monoclonal antibodies cetuximab or panitumumab can be added to oxapliplatin or irinotecan-containing regimens in KRAS wild-type colorectal tumours, leading to increased response rates. Bevacizumab, a monoclonal antibody targetting VEGF, can also enhance the effect of standard chemotherapy.

LUNG CANCER

There are four principal types of lung cancer. Non-small-cell cancers (adenocarcinoma, squamous cell cancer and large-cell cancer) account for about three-quarters of cases, with small-cell cancer responsible for the remainder.

For non-small-cell lung cancer, superficial lesions are amenable to several treatments, including photodynamic therapy with porfimer sodium. Surgical resection can be curative in the early stages. Neoadjuvant or adjuvant chemotherapy with cisplatin combined with one of several other drugs improves survival if the tumour is resectable. Radiotherapy or chemoradiotherapy is used after surgery when the tumour is not fully resectable, or for palliation of metastases. Chemotherapy has a limited place for advanced or recurrent disease and is mainly palliative. The current gold standard is the combination of a platinum compound (carboplatin or cisplatin) with one of several newer generation drugs (pemetrexed, a taxane, vinorelbine, gemcitabine). More recently treatment has become stratified according to histological type: squamous cell carcinomas are best treated using a platinum compound with gemcitabine, and non-sqamous cell carcinomas using a platinum compound with pemetrexed.

About 15% of non-small cell lung cancers, mainly adenocarcinomas, carry an activating mutation in the epidermal growth factor receptor (EGFR) gene. These tumours are responsive to treatment with tyrosine kinase inibitors such as erlotinib and gefitinib, which have revolutionized the management of this subgroup of tumours and maintained remissions for years in some cases. Other treatment targets have been identified, such as the cMET/ALK translocation, which accounts for about 20% of non-squamous cell carcinomas and can be treated with crizotinib. A major area of progress has been immunotherapy with anti-PD1, with previously unheard-of disease control rates and survival in people with advanced lung cancer; it is expected that immunotherapy will play a major role in lung cancer management in the future.

Small-cell lung cancer is more sensitive to chemotherapy, and has an initial response rate of 60–70%, with complete remission in 20–30% of cases. Examples of regimens are cisplatin combined with etoposide or cyclophosphamide with doxorubicin and vincristine. Radiotherapy is also given for limited-stage disease.

MELANOMA

Survival in melanoma is related to tumour thickness, with 5-year survival falling from more than 95% with superficial tumours to less than 50% survival if the depth is greater than 4 mm. Wide surgical excision is the treatment of choice. Postsurgical adjuvant chemotherapy does not improve survival or disease-free outcome. Currently, interferon alfa is the only drug shown to increase disease-free survival, but it has only a small impact (3–5%) on overall survival.

The management of advanced (inoperable) disease is determined by the presence or absence of a mutation in the *BRAF* gene (mutation V600E). Tumours with this mutation (40–50%) can be treated with a B-Raf tyrosine kinase inhibitor, vemurafenib, with initial disease control in about 80% of cases. However the effect is sometimes short-lived with a median progression-free survival of 6 months. This appears to be mainly due to escape mutations in the *BRAF* gene. To overcome this, combinations with inhibitors of another intracellular signalling protein (MEK protein) appear promising. Tumours with *BRAF* wild-type gene or which progress after B-Raf inhibition can be treated with the immunotherapeutic antibody ipilimumab, which produces responses over 5 years in just over 20% of cases. Chemotherapy with dacarbazine, temozolamide or the vinca alkaloids (vincristine or vinblastine) produces tumour responses in 10–20% of people, but without any clear effect on survival. Combination chemotherapy increases toxicity with no improvement in response. Immunotherapy with interferon alfa has produced similar response rates to chemotherapy, but the addition of chemotherapy does not further increase survival.

RENAL CANCER

Nephrectomy is the treatment of choice for early stage renal cancer, but up to one-third of people have metastases at the time of diagnosis. Prior to the introduction of tyrosine kinase inhibitors for the treatment of advanced disease, interferon alfa was commonly used with response rates in the region of 10–15%. In people with significant primary tumours and modest volume metastatic disease, cytoreductive nephrectomy was generally offered and improves survival, with a small proportion of metastases spontaneously regressing after surgery. With the advent of more active systemic agents the role of nephrectomy in the presence of metastatic disease is less clear. The majority of people with renal cell cancer have the clear cell variant which is associated with high expression of VEGF. Agents that target this pathway are effective in the treatment of metastatic disease.

- Drugs that inibit multiple intracellular tyrosine kinases such as sorafenib, sunitinib or pazopanib are used as the first-line treatment for advanced disease. They produce high responses rates, with average duration of response of around 1 year.
- Both the mammalian target of rapamycin (mTOR) inhibitor everolimus and the VEGF-targeted kinase inhibitor axitinib are used after failure of tyrosine kinase inhibitors. By sequencing first-, second- and sometimes third-line treatment for those with advanced kidney cancer, the disease can now be controlled for several years.
- Immunotherapy with interferon alfa combined with bevacizumab or aldesleukin (interleukin-2) produces responses in about 15% of cases. The toxicity of treatment can be high, but for a small proportion of those treated extremely durable response can be achieved. More recently a peptide vaccine has shown encouraging effects on survival in those vaccinated at progression after first-line treatment with sunitinib or sorafenib.

BLADDER CANCER

Superficial bladder tumours are removed surgically, but recurrence rates are high. Intravesical immunotherapy with Bacillus Calmette–Guérin (BCG) vaccine is used to limit recurrence in superficial disease. For more advanced disease, neoadjuvant chemotherapy with gemcitabine and cisplatin improves survival. A bladder-sparing approach using transurethral resection followed by concurrent chemotherapy (cisplatin, methotrexate and vinblastine) and irradiation has given promising results for those who do not want cystectomy.

PROSTATE CANCER

Treatment is largely determined by the extent of spread of the cancer. There are several options:

- 'watchful waiting' for localised disease confined to the prostate. This is usually used for individuals with a life expectancy under 10 years, since many tumours do not progress in this time,
- radical prostatectomy for localised disease, usually in men under 70 years, in whom the risk of subsequent metastases is reduced from 25 to 15%. Impotence is a common sequel, occurring in 35–60% of cases,

- radiotherapy for localised disease or locally advanced disease in older men. Impotence follows therapy in 40–60% of cases,
- interstitial implantation of radioactive pellets for localised disease or locally advanced disease (brachytherapy),
- hormonal therapy for lymph node involvement or distant metastases. Prostate cancer is hormone-dependent for growth. Testosterone reduction can be achieved by bilateral orchidectomy or the use of GnRH analogues such as leuprolide or goserelin (Ch. 43). Tumour flare reactions are prevented by the use of anti-androgen therapy (e.g. with flutamide or cyproterone acetate; Ch. 46) for the first few weeks to block adrenal androgen activity,
- castration-resistant disease can be treated by chemotherapy with drugs such as docetaxel and cabazitaxel. Response rates of about 50% can be achieved. Painful metastatic deposits can be treated with radiotherapy or with strontium-89, which is taken up by sclerotic metastases,
- a new class of hormonal therapies has shown promising activity in advanced prostate cancer. Abiraterone is a 17-α hydroxylase inhibitor which prevents extratesticular synthesis of androgens. It has low toxicity and increases survival when used either before or after chemotherapy in those who have become resistant to castration levels of testosterone inhibition. New androgen receptor antagonists with enhanced potency such as enzalutamide also increase survival in people with castration-resistant disease.

TESTICULAR CANCER

Testicular tumours are either seminomas or non-seminomatous germ cell tumours, depending on the tissue of origin. Cure rates are now greater than 95%. For *seminomas*, treatment choice includes:

- orchidectomy then follow-up for recurrence or chemotherapy with carboplatin if the recurrence risk is high,
- for locally advanced disease, surgery is followed by radiotherapy, perhaps combined with carboplatin,
- for metastatic disease, chemotherapy with bleomycin, etoposide and cisplatin (BEP) is used.

For non-seminomatous germ cell tumours, treatment choice includes:

- orchidectomy for early disease, which may be followed by chemotherapy with a regimen containing cisplatin,
- for more advanced or recurrent disease, combination chemotherapy with BEP, which produces an 85% complete remission rate when combined with surgery.

OVARIAN CANCER

Initial surgery for ovarian cancer is followed by chemotherapy for all disease that is not localised to the ovary (which occurs in 80% of cases). About 70% of these women respond to chemotherapy, with complete remission in 10–20%. Carboplatin or cisplatin with paclitaxel is often used. Liposomal doxorubicin, radiotherapy and octreotide are among the options for more advanced disease.

CERVICAL CANCER

Surgery is the mainstay for local disease, but chemoradiation is used if there are poor prognostic predictors or advanced disease. Cisplatin is most frequently used and improves survival by 30%. For recurrent disease the combination of cisplatin and paclitaxel has a small advantage over cisplatin alone.

ENDOMETRIAL CANCER

Surgery is the usual initial treatment for endometrial cancer. Adjuvant radiotherapy is given to the pelvis, and radiotherapy is also used for extrauterine metastases. Disseminated disease can be treated by hormone therapy with progestogens, but responses are low (less than one-third of those treated) and depend on the presence of progesterone receptors on the tumour cells. Adjuvant chemotherapy with drugs such as carboplatin plus paclitaxel has a palliative role in advanced disease.

BREAST CANCER

Breast-conserving surgery is the treatment of choice for very early disease and for oestrogen receptor-positive tumours; it is usually followed by local radiotherapy. The risk of invasive recurrence is low; if this occurs, it is treated by mastectomy followed by chemotherapy. Chemotherapy or hormonal therapy is used for larger locally invasive tumours or distant spread, or as neoadjuvant treatment for recurrence.

Determination of the hormone receptor status of the tumour is an important guide to the most appropriate hormonal therapy or chemotherapy.

Oestrogen receptor-positive tumours

Options for adjuvant hormonal therapy for *postmenopausal* women with oestrogen receptor-positive tumours include the following.

- Non-steroidal aromatase inhibitors such as anastrazole or letrozole or the steroidal aromatase inhibitor exemestane are more effective than tamoxifen, which was long considered the treatment of choice. They can also be used as neoadjuvant therapy to reduce the extent of surgical resection.
- Anti-oestrogen therapy, e.g. with tamoxifen, is often considered second-line treatment for hormone-responsive cancer. If tamoxifen is used, then switching to an aromatase inhibitor after 2–3 years further improves disease-free survival.
- The selective oestrogen receptor downregulator (SERD) fulvestrant is an alternative second-line treatment for locally advanced or metastatic disease.
- Progestogens such as megestrol acetate are used as a third-line treatment.
- GnRH analogues such as goserelin (Ch. 43) are a fourth-line treatment.

For *premenopausal* women with oestrogen receptor-positive tumours:

- tamoxifen remains the cornerstone of treatment, with or without chemotherapy. Aromatase inhibitors are ineffective before the menopause,
- tamoxifen can be combined with ovarian ablation using a GnRH analogue such as goserelin.

Hormonal treatment for early disease is usually given for 5 years and reduces mortality by 30%, with continuing benefit after stopping treatment for 15 years. The benefit of extending treatment beyond 5 years is unproven. The 10–20% of women who become unresponsive to one hormonal treatment may still respond to the use of an alternative class of drug.

Oestrogen receptor-negative tumours

Chemotherapy (treatment which does not involve hormonal manipulation) is used for oestrogen receptor-negative tumours, HER2-positive tumours, and younger women (especially under 35 years but also up to 70 years of age) or for hormonally unresponsive disease. An example of a current regimen is doxorubicin or epirubicin with cyclophosphamide, combined with docetaxel for node-positive disease, which produces response rates of up to 40%. Trastuzumab can be added to chemotherapy for cancers that express HER2; it reduces early recurrence by 50% and improves survival by 25%. Trastuzumab can also be used as first-line therapy without cytotoxic drugs.

ACUTE MYELOID LEUKAEMIAS

The acute myeloid leukaemias are a heterogeneous group of disorders (Box 52.1) that are differentiated on morphological grounds. Acute myeloid leukaemia is responsible for up to 15% of childhood leukaemias and is the commonest leukaemia of adult life. Complications usually result from bone marrow failure, and management of serious infection or bleeding are important issues in supportive care. The risk of infection is amplified by chemotherapy. The initial aim of chemotherapy is to reduce 'blast' cells in the marrow to below 5% of the total cell population (remission) with induction therapy and then to eradicate the leukaemic cells with consolidation therapy, usually involving at least two or three cycles of additional treatment.

Intravenous chemotherapy with two or more drugs is used in the induction phase to reduce the development of resistance. A typical regimen consists of daunorubicin with

---

Box 52.1 Simplified classification of acute myeloid leukaemias

Acute myeloid leukaemia
Acute myeloblastic leukaemia
Acute promyelocytic leukaemia
Acute myelomonocytic leukaemia
Acute monocytic/monoblastic leukaemia
Acute erythroleukaemia
Acute megakaryoblastic leukaemia

cytarabine, which produces remission in 65–70% of individuals under 60 years old; older people have a less favourable response. Consolidation is achieved with further courses of similar therapy for three to four cycles. Haematopoietic stem cell transplantation may be considered after remission is achieved. In children, treatment for the central nervous system is also given with intrathecal methotrexate. Salvage treatment is used for failure to enter remission or for relapse, with high-dose cytarabine alone or combined with fludarabine.

For acute promyelocytic leukaemia, the best initial response is obtained with tretinoin (all-*trans* retinoic acid), a vitamin A derivative (see Ch. 49) and consolidation achieved by the addition of an anthracycline such as idarubicin or daunorubicin.

ACUTE LYMPHOBLASTIC LEUKAEMIA

Acute lymphoblastic leukaemia is most common in children under 10 years of age, with a few cases occurring after age 40 years. Supportive therapy is similar to that for acute myeloid leukaemia.

Remission induction (eradication of 99% of leukaemic cell burden) is achieved with combinations of three or more drugs. In children, vincristine and prednisolone or dexamethasone with crisantaspase, doxorubicin or daunorubicin is often used. Four or more drugs are used for children with high-risk disease and for most adults. Cyclophosphamide is often used for T-cell leukaemias, and imatinib or desatinib if the cells are Philadelphia chromosome-positive. Consolidation therapy is initially with at least two multidrug intensification modules, using various combinations of corticosteroid with vincristine, crisantaspase, methotrexate and mercaptopurine. Continuation therapy is used after the first 5 months with mercaptopurine and methotrexate for at least 2 years. Eradication of cranial disease is important, using intrathecal methotrexate, cytarabine and hydrocortisone; cranial irradiation is less commonly used. Selective use of haematopoietic stem cell transplantation can further improve outcome.

The results of treatment in childhood are excellent, with about 80% survival at 5 years, compared to 40% if the disease occurs in adult life.

CHRONIC MYELOID LEUKAEMIA

Chronic myeloid leukaemia occurs in all age groups but is rare in children. Most disease follows an initial chronic course, lasting 3–4 years, with subsequent transformation to an accelerated phase, when survival is just 3–6 months. Imatinib is standard treatment for the chronic phase, and achieves cytogenetic remission in up to 87% of people. Interferon alfa, usually given with cytarabine or hydroxycarbamide, is an alternative for those who do not tolerate imatinib. In younger people, allogeneic stem cell transplantation is the treatment of choice after failed chemotherapy.

For advanced disease with blast crisis, combination chemotherapy can be considered, such as the regimen used for acute myeloid leukaemia or acute lymphoblastic leukaemia depending on the type of transformation.

CHRONIC LYMPHOCYTIC LEUKAEMIA

Chronic lymphocytic leukaemia is predominantly a disease of the elderly. Cure is unusual and median survival is 5–8 years, but treatment is given to control symptoms due to the disease. Therefore, treatment may not be necessary if the disease is causing few problems, but oral chlorambucil, often combined with prednisolone, can be given for up to 6 months to regress the disease. Transformation of the disease to a more aggressive form can occur after several years, with increasing disease bulk, lymphoma-related symptoms or bone marrow failure. Standard therapy in these situations is either oral or intravenous fludarabine or oral chlorambucil, with the goal of reducing leukaemic cells in the marrow to below 30%. Rituximab and cyclophosphamide both enhance the efficacy of fludarabine.

MALIGNANT LYMPHOMAS

The malignant lymphomas are a diverse group of disorders comprising Hodgkin's disease and a variety of non-Hodgkin's lymphomas, which are classified by histopathological and cytochemical techniques. Low-grade non-Hodgkin's lymphomas are managed in a similar way to chronic lymphocytic leukaemia and have a similar prognosis. Non-Hodgkin's lymphomas of intermediate grade are curable in about 40% of cases, using courses of combination chemotherapy with cyclophosphamide, doxorubicin, vincristine and prednisolone ('CHOP' therapy, an acronym based on the generic and proprietary names of the drugs). Rituximab may improve survival when added to standard chemotherapy, and radiotherapy is sometimes used as adjunctive treatment, or for relapsed disease. More frequent, intensive therapy is required for high-grade, aggressive non-Hodgkin's lymphomas.

For Hodgkin's disease, radiotherapy is curative if the tumour is localised; combination chemotherapy is the usual approach for more extensive disease. The most frequently used regimen is doxorubicin, bleomycin, vinblastine and dacarbazine (ABVD).

MULTIPLE MYELOMA

Multiple myeloma is mainly a disorder of the elderly. Treatment is aimed at suppression of the monoclonal protein in the blood. Supportive therapy is often required to treat hypercalcaemia, renal impairment and infection. Rehydration and analgesia for bone pain are often required. Radiotherapy may be used to treat localized areas of disease for pain control, lytic bone lesions or fractures.

Autologous stem cell transplantation is increasingly used as primary therapy after intensive chemotherapy and can produce 30–50% complete remission. Induction chemotherapy is with either two or three drugs, using regimens such as dexamethasone in combination with cyclophosphamide, bortezomib, thalidomide or lenalidomide.

For those who are not eligible for transplantation, chemotherapy is usually with oral melphalan and prednisolone combined with either thalidomide or bortezomib. This reduces the myeloma protein in blood by more than 50% in half of those treated. Median survival with this treatment is 3 years.

SELF-ASSESSMENT

True/false questions

1. Cancer cells are not subject to the normal feedback mechanisms which restrict cell multiplication.
2. Resting cells in G_0 phase are most susceptible to anti-neoplastic drugs.
3. Adverse effects of some anti-cancer drugs include secondary carcinogenesis.
4. Alkylating agents interfere with normal DNA synthesis.
5. Methotrexate competitively inhibits deoxythymidylate kinase.
6. Folinic acid (leucovorin) reverses the action of methotrexate.
7. Fluorouracil is a purine antagonist.
8. The effects of cytotoxic antibiotics are due to their intercalation between DNA bases.
9. Most base analogue antimetabolites are prodrugs activated by dephosphorylation.
10. Vinca alkaloids and taxanes share a common mechanism of action.
11. Tyrosine kinase inhibitors block signalling by growth factors.
12. Tamoxifen blocks oestrogen receptors on bone cells, causing osteoporosis.

Case-based questions

1. What are the criteria for combination chemotherapy of cancer? How well do the following treatment regimens meet the criteria?
   A. Acute lymphoblastic leukaemia (initial phase for induction of remission): intravenous vincristine, subcutaneous crisantaspase (asparaginase) and oral prednisolone.
   B. Non-Hodgkin's lymphoma: cyclophosphamide, doxorubicin, vincristine and prednisolone (CHOP regimen).
   C. Testicular teratoma in an adult: intravenous etoposide, bleomycin and cisplatin.
2. Why are doses of anti-cancer drugs corrected to surface area rather than body weight? Does the use of surface area correction result in higher or lower doses for children compared with simple correction for body weight? Taking the example in Table 52.1 of an adult male (body weight 72.1 kg) given 100 mg of a drug, what doses would a 1-year-old child of body weight 9.9 kg be given if corrected for body weight or for surface area?

True/false answers

1. **True.** Dysfunction in the mechanisms that normally regulate cell multiplication is a characteristic of cancer cells.
2. **False.** Although some anti-cancer drugs affect the resting phase, cancer cells are typically most susceptible when they are actively dividing; the sensitivity of a tumour therefore depends on its growth fraction.

Table 52.1 Examples of body weights and surface areas in children and adults

Age (years)	Body weight (kg)	Height (m)	Body surface area (m²)
Children			
0.5	7.4	0.658	0.350
1.0	9.9	0.747	0.434
3	14.5	0.96	0.613
6	21.5	1.168	0.835
Adults			
Male	72.1	1.753	1.874
Female	60.3	1.676	1.681

3. **True.** Secondary cancers can occur such as bladder cancer with cyclophosphamide (due to urinary excretion of toxic metabolites) and lymphoma with alkylating agents.
4. **True.** The alkylated bases produce various effects on DNA function including misreading.
5. **False.** Methotrexate inhibits dihydrofolate reductase, a key enzyme in the folate pathway required for synthesis of purines and thymidine.
6. **True.** Leucovorin is used to rescue normal tissues when given after methotrexate; methotrexate has a preferential effect on cancer cells, and giving leucovorin 24 h afterwards overcomes its unwanted actions in normal tissues such as bone marrow and gut mucosa.
7. **False.** Fluorouracil is a pyrimidine analogue (fluorinated uracil).
8. **True.** As well as DNA intercalation, shown particularly by anthracyclines, cytotoxic antibiotics such as bleomycin also generate superoxide and hydrogen peroxide that cleave DNA.
9. **False.** Many base analogues such as cytarabine and gemcitabine are activated by intracellular phosphorylation to triphosphate derivatives, which are incorporated into DNA.
10. **False.** Vinca alkaloids prevent mitosis by inducing microtubule disassembly, whereas taxanes inhibit mitosis by promoting formation of stable but non-functional microtubules.
11. **True.** Drugs such as erlotinib, imatinib and pazopanib inhibit the receptor tyrosine kinase families associated with growth factors including epidermal growth factor (EGF), vascular endothelial growth factor (VEGF) and platelet-derived growth factor (PDGF); some also block kinases in downstream signalling pathways.
12. **False.** Tamoxifen is a selective oestrogen receptor modulator (SERM) that blocks oestrogen receptors on breast cancer cells but is an agonist at oestrogen receptors on bone cells, preventing osteoporosis.

Table 52.2 Effects of three treatment regimens

	Site of action	Principal toxicity
(A) Acute lymphoblastic leukaemia		
Vincristine	Binds to tubulin/metaphase arrest	BMS, peripheral neuropathy
Crisantaspase	Depletes asparagine in blood	Decreased clotting factors, albumin and insulin
Prednisolone	Reduces DNA transcription of cytokines	Glucocorticoid actions
(B) Non-Hodgkin's lymphoma (CHOP regimen)		
Cyclophosphamide	Alkylates DNA	BMS, nausea/vomiting
Doxorubicin	Intercalation into DNA, oxygen free radicals	BMS, cardiotoxicity
Vincristine	Binds to tubulin/metaphase arrest	BMS, peripheral neuropathy
Prednisolone	Reduces DNA transcription of cytokines	Glucocorticoid actions
(C) Testicular teratoma		
Etoposide	Increases DNA cleavage by topoisomerase II	BMS, nausea, alopecia
Bleomycin	Oxidative damage to DNA	Pulmonary fibrosis
Cisplatin	Crosslinks DNA	Nausea, BMS, nephrotoxicity, ototoxicity

BMS, bone marrow suppression.

Case-based answers

1. The criteria for combination therapy in cancer treatment are:

■ each drug should be active as a single agent; the ethics of clinical trials means that new drugs are not usually tested for this criterion in clinical studies,

■ each drug should have a different target within the cell; this increases cell kill and decreases drug resistance,

■ each drug should show different unwanted effects; ideally this will produce additive efficacy but not toxicity, and hence an increase in therapeutic index.

For each of the three drug regimens, the first criterion can be assumed to be met because all the agents are well-used drugs. The sites of action (second criterion) and side effects (third criterion) of the drugs in each regimen are shown in Table 52.2. All three regimens use drugs with different mechanisms of action, although regimen C is targeted only at DNA function. Regimen B contains three drugs that produce bone marrow toxicity and this will need careful monitoring during therapy.

2. Because many of the drugs used in cancer therapy are toxic at therapeutic doses, it is important to tailor the dosage to the individual. Children have a higher cardiac output and greater hepatic and renal blood flows than adults on a body weight basis. The clearance of drugs therefore tends to be faster in children than in adults and a proportionally higher dose is necessary to give the same blood levels. The liver and kidneys are essentially mature as the main organs of elimination by about 6–9 months of age. Hepatic and renal blood flows are related to body weight to the power of approximately 0.7. Since body surface area is also proportional to body weight$^{0.7}$, it is usual to correct the drug doses by surface area to take better account of clearance. Surface area is calculated from a nomogram, or estimated using the approximation that it correlates with weight$^{0.7}$, or by using the more accurate Du Bois equation:

$$\text{Surface area} = 71.84 \times \text{weight}^{0.425} \times \text{height}^{0.725}$$

where surface area is in metres squared, weight is in kilograms and height is in metres. In the example, the adult male (body weight 72.1 kg) is given 100 mg of a drug. Simple correction for body weight of the 1-year-old child (9.9 kg) would suggest 13.7 mg (100 mg × 9.9 kg/72.1 kg) is the appropriate dose. However, using the surface area values in Table 52.1 derived from the Du Bois formula, the dose would be 100 mg × 0.434 m^2/1.874 m^2 = 23.2 mg. An approximation using surface area estimated as weight$^{0.7}$ gives a calculated dose of 100 mg × 9.9$^{0.7}$/72.1$^{0.7}$ = 100 × 4.98/19.98 = 24.9 mg, close to that obtained using the Du Bois formula. These results appear counter-intuitive if children are assumed to be 'more sensitive' to drugs.

FURTHER READING

Drugs and drug action

Ambudkar SV, Dey S, Hrycyna CA, Ramachandra M, Pastan I, Gottesman MM (1999) Biochemical, cellular, and pharmacological aspects of the multidrug transporter. *Annu Rev Pharmacol Toxicol* 39, 361–398

Ciardiello F, Tortora G (2008) EGFR antagonists in cancer treatment. *N Engl J Med* 358, 1160–1174

Croce CM (2008) Oncogenes and cancer. *N Engl J Med* 358, 502–511

Dubowchik GM, Walker MA (1999) Receptor-mediated and enzyme-dependent targeting of cytotoxic anticancer drugs. *Pharmacol Ther* 83, 67–123

Eccles SA, Welch DR (2007) Metastasis: recent discoveries and novel treatment strategies. *Lancet* 369, 1742–1757

Efferth T, Volm M (2005) Pharmacogenetics for individualized cancer chemotherapy. *Pharmacol Ther* 107, 155–176

Gottesman MM (2002) Mechanisms of cancer drug resistance. *Annu Rev Med* 53, 615–627

Griffioen AW, Molema G (2000) Angiogenesis: potential for pharmacologic intervention in the treatment of cancer, cardiovascular diseases and chronic inflammation. *Pharmacol Rev* 52, 237–268

Links M, Lewis C (1999) Chemoprotectants: a review of their clinical pharmacology and therapeutic efficacy. *Drugs* 57, 293–308

Marsh S, McLeod HL (2004) Cancer pharmacogenetics. *Br J Cancer* 90, 8–11

Gastrointestinal cancer

Ballinger AB, Anggiansah C (2007) Colorectal cancer. *BMJ* 335, 715–718

Hartgrink HH, Jansen EPM, van Grieken NCT et al. (2009) Gastric cancer. *Lancet* 374, 477–490

Lagergren J, Lagergren P (2010) Oesophageal cancer. *BMJ* 341, c6280

Meyerhardt JA, Mayer RJ (2005) Systemic therapy for colorectal cancer. *N Engl J Med* 352, 476–487

Hidalgo M (2010) Pancreatic cancer. *New Engl J Med* 362, 1605–1617

Lung cancer

Booton R, Jones M, Thatcher N (2003) Lung cancer 7: management of lung cancer in elderly patients. *Thorax* 58, 711–720

Cullen M (2003) Lung cancer 4: chemotherapy for non-small cell lung cancer: the end of the beginning. *Thorax* 58, 352–356

Jackman DM, Johnson BE (2005) Small-cell lung cancer. *Lancet* 366, 1385–1396

Spira A, Ettinger DS (2004) Multidisciplinary management of lung cancer. *N Engl J Med* 350, 379–392

Urogenital cancer

Dahut N, Gulley JL, Dahut WL (2005) Androgen deprivation therapy for prostate cancer. *JAMA* 294, 238–244

Feldman DR, Bosl GJ, Sheinfeld J et al. (2008) Medical treatment of advanced testicular cancer. *JAMA* 299, 672–684

Hennessy BT, Coleman RL, Markman M (2009) Ovarian cancer. *Lancet* 374, 1371–1382

Hernandez J, Thompson IM (2004) Diagnosis and treatment of prostate cancer. *Med Clin North Am* 88, 267–279

Horwich A, Shipley J, Huddart R (2006) Testicular germ-cell cancer. *Lancet* 367, 754–765

Kaufman DS, Shipley WU, Feldman AS (2009) Bladder cancer. *Lancet* 374, 239–249

Petignat P, Roy M (2007) Diagnosis and management of cervical cancer. *BMJ* 335, 765–768

Rini BI, Campbell SC, Escudier B (2009) Renal cell carcinoma. *Lancet* 373, 1119–1132

Saso S, Chatterjee J, Georgiou E et al. (2011) Endometrial cancer. *BMJ*: d3954

Waggoner SE (2003) Cervical cancer. *Lancet* 361, 2217–2225

Walsh PC, DeWeese TL, Eisenberger MA (2007) Localized prostate cancer. *N Engl J Med* 357, 2696–2705

Wilt TJ, Thompson IM (2006) Clinically localized prostate cancer. *BMJ* 333, 1102–1106

Breast cancer

Benson JR, Jatoi I, Keisch M et al. (2009) Early breast cancer. *Lancet* 373, 1463–1479

Turner NC, Jones AL (2008) Management of breast cancer – Part 1. *BMJ* 337, 107–110

Turner NC, Jones AL (2008) Management of breast cancer – Part 2. *BMJ* 337, 164–169

Melanoma

Eggermont AMM (2002) European approach to the treatment of malignant melanoma. *Curr Opin Oncol* 14, 205–211

Acute leukaemias

Estey E, Döhner H (2006) Acute myeloid leukaemia. *Lancet* 368, 1894–1907

Pui C-H, Robinson LL, Look AT (2008) Acute lymphoblastic leukaemia. *Lancet* 371, 1030–1043

Ravandi F, Kantarajian H, Giles F et al. (2004) New drugs in acute leukemia and other myeloid disorders. *Cancer* 100, 441–454

Chronic leukaemias

Dighiero G, Hamblin TJ (2008) Chronic lymphocytic leukaemia. *Lancet* 371, 1017–1029

Hehlmann R, Hochhaus A, Baccarani M et al. (2007) Chronic myeloid leukaemia. *Lancet* 370, 342–350

Shanafelt TD, Byrd JC, Call TG et al. (2006) Narrative review: initial management of newly diagnosed, early-stage chronic lymphocytic leukaemia. *Ann Intern Med* 145, 435–447

Lymphomas

Evans LS, Hancock BW (2003) Non-Hodgkin lymphoma. *Lancet* 362, 139–146

Armitage JO (2010) Early-stage Hodgkin's lymphoma. *New Engl J Med* 363, 653–662

Multiple myeloma

Palumbo A, Anderson KA (2011) Multiple myeloma. *New Engl J Med* 364, 1046–1060

Raab MS, Podar K, Breitkreutz I (2009) Multiple myeloma. *Lancet* 374, 324–339

Compendium: drugs used in the treatment of cancer

Drug	Kinetics (half-life)	Comments	Atypical or dose-limiting toxicity[a]
Anti-cancer drugs			
Alkylating agents			
Widely used drugs; act by damaging DNA and thereby interfering with cell division.			
Bendamustine	Hepatic metabolism and conjugation (0.5 h)	Used for treatment of chronic lymphocytic leukaemia, non-Hodgkin's lymphoma and multiple myeloma; given intravenously	Risk of teratogenesis
Busulfan	Metabolism largely by interaction with thiol groups such as cysteine (2–3 h)	Mainly used for effects on the bone marrow (e.g. chronic myeloid leukaemia); given orally or by intravenous infusion	Myelosuppression and irreversible bone marrow aplasia; rare pulmonary fibrosis
Carmustine (BCNU)	Crosses blood–brain barrier; metabolites eliminated in urine (0.4–0.5 h)	Reactive molecule that crosslinks DNA, and nitroso function inactivates DNA repair; used for myeloma, lymphoma and brain tumours; given intravenously	Renal damage; progressive pulmonary fibrosis
Chlorambucil	Metabolism at alkylating groups and in the liver (1–2 h)	Used mainly in lymphocytic leukaemia, non-Hodgkin's lymphoma and Hodgkin's disease; given orally, usually after fasting	Vomiting
Cyclophosphamide	Good penetration of blood–brain barrier; hepatic metabolism, wide inter-subject variability (4–10 h)	Widely used for leukaemias, lymphomas and solid tumours; given orally or by intravenous injection	Haemorrhagic cystitis (see mesna antidote)
Estramustine	Dephosphorylated to the active drug, which is oxidised (20–24 h)	Oestrogen molecule linked to a nitrogen mustard group; acts as alkylating agent, especially on microtubule proteins, and increases circulating oestrogen levels; used for prostate cancer; given orally	
Ifosfamide	Metabolism similar to cyclophosphamide (4–15 h)	Uses similar to cyclophosphamide; given by intravenous injection	Cystitis (see mesna antidote)
Lomustine (CCNU)	Oxidised in gut wall and liver to product with half-life of 1–5 h	Mainly used for Hodgkin's disease and some solid tumours; similar to carmustine; given orally	Permanent bone marrow damage
Melphalan	Oral absorption incomplete and variable; metabolism not well defined (1.5 h)	Used mainly for multiple myeloma, ovarian adenocarcinoma, advanced breast cancer and neuroblastoma; given orally or by intravenous injection	
Thiotepa	Extensively absorbed from bladder lumen; converted to active metabolites (1.5–4 h)	Used for bladder cancer; given by intravesicular injection	
Treosulfan	High oral bioavailability; non-enzymatic degradation (1–2 h)	Used mainly for ovarian cancer; given orally or by intravenous injection	Allergic alveolitis; pulmonary fibrosis
Cytotoxic antibiotics			
Widely used drugs; many act as radiomimetics and should be avoided if overall treatment includes concomitant radiotherapy.			
Bleomycin	Slow uptake by tissues; inactivated by hydrolysis (2–4 h)	Used for testicular cancer, lymphomas and squamous cell carcinoma; given intravenously or intramuscularly	Dermatological effects; progressive pulmonary fibrosis
Dactinomycin (actinomycin D)	Negligible metabolism; eliminated in urine and bile (36 h)	Mainly used for paediatric solid tumours; given intravenously	Bone marrow toxicity; gastrointestinal toxicity
Daunorubicin	Metabolism to toxic superoxide radicals and H_2O_2 (24–48 h); liposomal formulation half-life 5 h	Used for acute leukaemias and AIDS-related Kaposi's sarcoma; given intravenously	Bone marrow toxicity

Compendium: drugs used in the treatment of cancer—cont'd

Drug	Kinetics (half-life)	Comments	Atypical or dose-limiting toxicity[a]
Doxorubicin	Reduced in liver to doxorubicinol; biliary excretion (2–10 h)	Widely used for leukaemias, lymphomas and a variety of solid tumours; given intravenously	Myelosuppression; cardiotoxicity
Epirubicin	Reduced to epirubicinol and also conjugated (11–69 h)	Uses are similar to doxorubicin; given intravenously	Myelosuppression; less cardiotoxic than doxorubicin
Idarubicin	Oral bioavailability 4–50%; metabolised (12–35 h) to active idarubicinol (half-life 50–70 h)	Used mainly for acute leukaemias and advanced breast cancer unresponsive to first-line treatments; given orally or intravenously	Myelosuppression
Mitomycin	Reduced to a hydroquinone then an unstable alkylating species that crosslinks DNA; metabolism gives toxic superoxide and hydroxyl radicals (0.5–1.5 h)	Mainly used for upper gastrointestinal and breast cancers and by bladder instillation for superficial bladder tumours; given intravenously	Myelosuppression; nephrotoxicity; lung fibrosis
Mitoxantrone	Highly variable hepatic metabolism (4–220 h)	Used to treat metastatic breast cancer, non-Hodgkin's lymphoma and non-lymphocytic leukaemia; given by intravenous infusion	Myelosuppression; cardiotoxicity

Antimetabolites

Incorporated into nucleic acids or combine irreversibly with cellular enzymes essential for normal cell division.

Drug	Kinetics (half-life)	Comments	Atypical or dose-limiting toxicity[a]
Azacitadine	Spontaneous hydrolysis and deamination (<1 h), urinary excretion	Pyrimidine analogue; used in treatment of myelodysplastic syndromes, chronic myelomonocytic leukaemia, and acute myeloid leukaemia in adults; given by subcutaneous injection	
Capecitabine	Prodrug hydrolysed to fluorouracil (0.5–1 h)	Used as monotherapy for metastatic colorectal cancer; given orally	
Cladribine	Intracellular phosphorylation by deoxycytidine kinase to the active triphosphate form (7 h)	Chlorine-substituted purine; the triphosphate is incorporated into DNA and blocks DNA polymerase and DNA ligase; used for hairy cell leukaemia; given by intravenous infusion	Myelosuppression; neurotoxicity
Clofarabine	Intracellular phosphorylation by deoxycytidine kinase; eliminated unchanged in urine (5 h)	Chlorine- and fluorine-substituted purine analogue; inhibits ribonucleotide reductase and terminates DNA chain elongation; used for acute lymphoblastic leukaemia in refractory or relapsed disease in people aged 1–21 years; given by intravenous infusion	
Cytarabine (cytosine arabinoside)	Intracellular phosphorylation to active triphosphate form (1–3 h)	The triphosphate is incorporated into DNA and blocks DNA polymerase and DNA ligase; mostly active in S phase; used for inducing remission in acute myeloblastic leukaemia; given intravenously, subcutaneously or intrathecally	Myelosuppression
Fludarabine phosphate	Rapidly hydrolysed to fludarabine then phosphorylated intracellularly by deoxycytidine kinase to active triphosphate (7–20 h)	Fluorine-substituted purine riboside; the triphosphate is incorporated into DNA and blocks DNA polymerase and DNA ligase; mostly active in S phase; used for B-cell chronic lymphocytic leukaemia; given orally or by intravenous injection or infusion	Myelosuppression

Compendium: drugs used in the treatment of cancer—cont'd

Drug	Kinetics (half-life)	Comments	Atypical or dose-limiting toxicity[a]
Fluorouracil	Converted intracellularly to fluorouridine monophosphate (FUMP) and the deoxy analogue (FdUMP); hepatic metabolism (0.25 h)	FUMP is converted to the triphosphate and incorporated into RNA; FdUMP inhibits thymidylate synthase, is converted to the triphosphate and incorporated into DNA; some selectivity for G_2 and S phases; used for cancers of the gastrointestinal tract and malignant and pre-malignant skin lesions; given topically or by intravenous injection or infusion or intra-arterial infusion	Relatively low toxicity
Gemcitabine	Intracellular conversion to active triphosphate; inactivated by deamination (0.2–0.5 h)	Deoxycytidine analogue with two fluorine atoms in the deoxyribose moiety; the triphosphate is incorporated into DNA and blocks elongation and promotes apoptosis; specific for S phase; used for palliative treatment of non-small-cell lung and pancreatic cancer; given intravenously	Limited toxicity
Mercaptopurine	Poor oral bioavailability (about 20%) due to first-pass metabolism; undergoes intracellular phosphorylation to mono- and triphosphates; inactivated mainly by xanthine oxidase, partly by thiopurine S-methyltransferase; renal excretion (1–1.5 h)	Sulphur-substituted purine; the monophosphate inhibits *de novo* purine synthesis; the triphosphate is incorporated into DNA and/or RNA, giving cytotoxicity; specific for S phase; used almost exclusively for maintenance therapy for acute leukaemias (also in inflammatory bowel disease); given orally	Limited toxicity
Methotrexate	Undergoes polyglutamate formation (like folate) and retained intracellularly for months; mainly renal elimination	Folate analogue, inhibits dihydrofolate reductase; used for maintenance therapy for childhood acute lymphoblastic leukaemia, choriocarcinoma, non-Hodgkin's lymphoma and some solid tumours (also for rheumatoid arthritis and psoriasis); given orally, intravenously, intramuscularly or intrathecally	Myelosuppression (folinic acid is an antidote; see below)
Nelarabine	Prodrug demethylated and converted intracellularly to active triphosphate, which inhibits DNA synthesis preferentially in T-cells (0.5 h)	Purine analogue; used for T-cell acute lymphoblastic leukaemia and T-cell lymphoblastic lymphoma in relapsing disease or those refractory to previous regimens; given by intravenous infusion	Neurotoxicity is common
Pemetrexed	Eliminated unchanged by glomerular filtration and tubular secretion (3.5 h)	Substituted purine compound; inhibits dihydrofolate reductase, thymidylate synthase and other folate-dependent enzymes; used with cisplatin for malignant pleural mesothelioma; given by intravenous infusion	
Raltitrexed	Retention within cells as polyglutamate gives prolonged inhibition of thymidylate synthase (10–12 days)	Folate analogue; used for palliation of metastatic colon cancer when fluorouracil cannot be used; given intravenously	Myelosuppression
Tegafur	A racemate that is metabolised to fluorouracil (8 h)	See fluorouracil; used with uracil folinic acid for management of metastatic colorectal cancer; also used with gimeracil, oteracil and cisplatin in advanced gastric cancer; given orally	

Compendium: drugs used in the treatment of cancer—cont'd

Drug	Kinetics (half-life)	Comments	Atypical or dose-limiting toxicity[a]
Tioguanine	Bioavailability 25–50%; rapidly converted intracellularly to thioguanylic acid; inactivated by methylation by thiopurine S-methyltransferase and by amination (3–6 h)	Tioguanine metabolites inhibit *de novo* purine synthesis and purine nucleotide interconversions; also incorporated into DNA; active in G_1 and S phases; used for acute leukaemia and chronic myeloid leukemia; given orally	Myelosuppression

Vinca alkaloids

Anti-microtubule and anti-mitotic agents used for a variety of cancers.

Drug	Kinetics (half-life)	Comments	Atypical or dose-limiting toxicity[a]
Vinblastine	Hepatic metabolism; biliary and renal elimination (20–80 h)	Used for acute leukaemias, lymphomas and non-solid tumours (e.g. breast and lung); given by intravenous injection	Myelosuppression
Vincristine	Hepatic metabolism; biliary excretion (85 h)	Used for acute leukaemias, lymphomas and non-solid tumours (e.g. breast and lung); given by intravenous injection	Neurotoxicity: peripheral and autonomic neuropathy (recovery slow but complete)
Vindesine	Hepatic metabolism; biliary and urinary excretion (25 h)	Used for acute leukaemias, lymphomas and non-solid tumours (e.g. breast and lung); given by intravenous injection	Myelosuppression
Vinflunine	Metabolised by plasma esterases to active metabolite; hepatic metabolism; biliary and urinary excretion (40 h),	Used for advanced or metastatic transitional cell carcinoma of the urothelial tract after failure of a platinum-containing regimen; given intravenously	Myelosuppression
Vinorelbine	Hepatic metabolism; biliary and urinary excretion (28–44 h)	Semi-synthetic vinca alkaloid made from vinblastine; used for advanced breast and non-small-cell lung cancer; given intravenously	Myelosuppression

Taxanes

Mitotic inhibitors.

Drug	Kinetics (half-life)	Comments	Atypical or dose-limiting toxicity[a]
Cabazitaxel	Hepatic metabolism, mainly faecal elimination (95 h)	Used with a corticosteroid for hormone-refractory metastatic prostate cancer in people previously treated with docetaxel; given by intravenous infusion	Hypersensitivity reactions are common
Docetaxel	Hepatic metabolism; mainly biliary excretion (11 h)	Used for advanced or metastatic anthracycline-resistant breast cancer; given by intravenous infusion	Hypersensitivity reactions; myelosuppression; peripheral neuropathy; fluid retention
Paclitaxel	Hepatic metabolism; biliary excretion (19 h)	Used for advanced ovarian cancer and as secondary treatment for breast and non-small-cell lung cancer; given by intravenous infusion	Hypersensitivity reactions; myelosuppression; peripheral neuropathy

Platinum compounds

Drug	Kinetics (half-life)	Comments	Atypical or dose-limiting toxicity[a]
Carboplatin	Parent compound eliminated by glomerular filtration (1.5 h);	Active form produced by interaction with water; used for ovarian cancer and some other solid tumours; given by intravenous injection	Myelosuppression; nausea and vomiting (less than with cisplatin)
Cisplatin	Parent compound eliminated by kidney (24–60 h)	Active form produced by interaction with water; used for solid tumours such as ovarian cancer and metastatic seminoma and testicular teratoma; given by intravenous injection	Nausea and vomiting; nephrotoxicity; myelosuppression; ototoxicity

Compendium: drugs used in the treatment of cancer—cont'd

Drug	Kinetics (half-life)	Comments	Atypical or dose-limiting toxicity[a]
Oxaliplatin	Parent drug undergoes rapid hydration; renal elimination of platinum (27 h)	Used for metastatic colorectal cancer; given intravenously	Neurotoxicity

Topoisomerase I inhibitors

Topoisomerase I is involved in maintaining the topographic structure of DNA during translation, transcription and mitosis.

Irinotecan	Metabolised to active and inactive metabolites; some renal excretion (6 h)	Used for metastatic colorectal cancer; given by intravenous infusion	Myelosuppression; gastrointestinal effects
Topotecan	Eliminated by hydrolysis and renal excretion (2–3 h)	Used for metastatic ovarian cancer when first-line treatment has failed; given by intravenous infusion	Myelosuppression; gastrointestinal effects

Topoisomerase II inhibitor

Topoisomerase II is involved in the breaking and religating of DNA strands during cell division.

Etoposide	Oral absorption 25–75%; metabolites eliminated in urine and bile (4–8 h)	Used for small-cell carcinoma of the bronchus, lymphomas and testicular cancer; given orally or by slow intravenous infusion	Myelosuppression; alopecia

Porfimer sodium and temoporfin

Used in photodynamic treatment of various tumours; the drugs accumulate in tumour tissue and are activated by laser light.

Porfimer sodium	Breakdown products eliminated in bile (40–50 h); photosensitised product has very long half-life (250 h)	Used in photodynamic treatment of small-cell lung cancer and for oesophageal cancer; given by intravenous injection	Photosensitivity
Temoporfin	Few data available; probably similar to porfimer	Used in photodynamic treatment of advanced refractory head and neck squamous cell carcinoma; given by intravenous injection	Photosensitivity

Tyrosine kinase receptor inhibitors

Bevacizumab	Peptide drug; clearance by proteolysis is higher in men than in women and is proportional to tumour burden (≈20 days)	VEGFR inhibitor antibody; used as part of first-line treatment of metastatic colorectal cancer; given by intravenous infusion	Mucocutaneous bleeding and arterial thromboembolism
Cetuximab	Peptide drug; largely restricted to the vascular space; proteolysis (≈100 h)	EGFR (HER1) inhibitor antibody; used for metastatic colorectal cancer expressing EGFR; given by intravenous infusion	Hypersensitivity reactions such as rash and airways obstruction; skin reactions
Panitumumab	Peptide drug (7.5 days)	EGFR (HER1) inhibitor antibody; used for metastatic colorectal cancer; given by intravenous infusion	Severe skin reactions
Trastuzumab	Probably cleared by the reticuloendothelial system (25 days)	HER2 receptor antibody, causes cell cycle arrest; used for metastatic breast cancer; given by intravenous infusion	Cardiotoxicity, especially if used with anthracyclines (see cytotoxic antibiotics above)

Tyrosine kinase inhibitors

Inhibit growth factor receptor-associated tyrosine kinase enzymes.

Dasatinib	Rapidly absorbed; hepatic metabolism, faecal elimination (3–5 h)	Multiple tyrosine kinase inhibitor; used for chronic myeloid leukaemia in those resistant to or intolerant of imatinib; given orally	Numerous, including gastrointestinal effects

Compendium: drugs used in the treatment of cancer—cont'd

Drug	Kinetics (half-life)	Comments	Atypical or dose-limiting toxicity[a]
Erlotinib	Bioavailability 60% (or 100% with food); hepatic metabolism, mainly faecal excretion (36 h)	Selective inhibitor of EGFR (HER1) tyrosine kinase; used for advanced or malignant small-cell lung cancer after failure of previous therapy; given orally	Numerous, including gastrointestinal effects
Everolimus	Hepatic metabolism; faecal elimination (30 h)	Protein kinase (mTOR) inhibitor; used for advanced renal cell carcinoma, neuroendocrine pancreatic tumours, giant cell astrocytoma, and HER2-negative advanced breast cancer; given orally	Hypersensitivity reactions; Q–T interval prolongation
Gefitinib	Oral bioavailability 59%; hepatic metabolism; faecal elimination (41 h)	EGFR tyrosine kinase inhibitor; used for advanced or metastatic non-small cell lung cancer with activating mutations of EGFR; given orally	Risk of interstitial lung disease; hepatotoxicity
Imatinib	Completely absorbed; hepatic metabolism (18 h) to active metabolite with half-life of 40 h	PDGFR inhibitor; used for newly diagnosed chronic myeloid leukaemia (under special circumstances); given orally	Numerous, including gastrointestinal effects
Lapatinib	Variable absorption; hepatic metabolism, mainly faecal elimination (24 h)	Dual EGFR (HER1) and HER2 tyrosine kinase inhibitor; ued for advanced or metastatic HER2-positive breast cancer; given orally	Pulmonary toxicity; hepatotoxicity
Nilotinib	Oral bioavailability 30%; hepatic metabolism, faecal elimination (17 h)	Multiple tyrosine kinase inhibitor; used for chronic myeloid leukaemia; given orally	Myelosuppression; Q–T interval prolongation
Pazopanib	Hepatic metabolism, faecal elimination (31 h)	Inhibitor of multiple tyrosine kinases, including VEGFR family and PDGFR; used for advanced renal cell carcinoma; given orally	Hepatotoxcity; hypertension; cardiac dysfunction
Sorafenib	Bioavailability 40%; hepatic metabolism; urinary and faecal elimination (25–48 h)	Inhibits VEGFR and PDGFR tyrosine kinases and other kinases; used for advanced renal cell carcinoma; given orally	Numerous, including gastrointestinal effects
Sunitinib	Hepatic metabolism (40–60 h) to an active product with half-life of 80–110 h; faecal elimination	Inhibits VEGFR and PDGFR tyrosine kinases; used for malignant gastrointestinal stromal tumours; given orally	Numerous, including gastrointestinal effects
Temsirolimus	Converted (17 h) to active sirolimus (73 h); mainly faecal elimination	Protein kinase (mTOR) inhibitor; used for advanced renal cell carcinoma, and for relapsed or refractory mantle cell lymphoma; given by intravenous infusion	Risk of life-threatening hypersensitivity reactions
Vandetanib	Hepatic metabolism and conjugation (19 days)	Tyrosine kinase inhibitor; used for aggressive and symptomatic medullary thyroid cancer; given orally	Significant Q–T prolongation; encephalopathy; skin reactions
Vemurafenib	Highly variable absorption; hepatic metabolism, faecal elimination (52 h)	B-Raf kinase inhibitor, causes apoptosis in melanoma cells; used for *BRAF* V600 mutation-positive unresectable or metastatic melanoma; given orally	Q–T prolongation; skin reactions; photosensitivity; risk of cutaneous squamous cell carcinoma
Proteasome inhibitors			
Bortezomib	Undergoes removal of boron and subsequent hepatic hydroxylation (9–15 h)	Boron-containing proteasome inhibitor; used for progressive multiple myeloma; given by intravenous injection	Nausea, vomiting and diarrhoea

Compendium: drugs used in the treatment of cancer—cont'd

Drug	Kinetics (half-life)	Comments	Atypical or dose-limiting toxicity[a]
Drugs for breast cancer			
See also Miscellaneous anti-cancer drugs, listed below.			
Anastrozole	Hepatic oxidation and glucuronidation; some is excreted unchanged (40–50 h)	Non-steroidal aromatase inhibitor; used as adjunct for oestrogen receptor-positive early breast cancer, and for advanced metastatic breast cancer in postmenopausal women; given orally	Hot flushes; vaginal dryness and bleeding; gastrointestinal effects
Exemestane	Bioavailability about 40%, increased by fatty meal; hepatic metabolism (24 h)	Irreversible steroid inhibitor of aromatase; used for advanced breast cancer in postmenopausal women in whom anti-oestrogen therapy has failed; given orally	Nausea and gastrointestinal effects; hot flushes
Fulvestrant	Slow uptake from injection; hepatic oxidation and conjugation (40 days)	Selective oestrogen receptor downregulator (SERD); used for oestrogen receptor-positive breast tumours; given by deep intramuscular depot injection	Hot flushes; nausea; gastrointestinal effects
Letrozole	High oral bioavailability; hepatic oxidation (2 days)	Non-steroidal aromatase inhibitor; used for advanced metastatic breast cancer unresponsive to other anti-oestrogens in postmenopausal women; given orally	Hot flushes; nausea; gastrointestinal effects
Tamoxifen	High bioavailability; hepatic oxidation (7 days); active metabolite has half-life of 14 days	Non-steroidal anti-oestrogen; used for oestrogen receptor-positive breast cancer; given orally	Exacerbation of pain from bone metastases
Toremifene	Well absorbed; hepatic metabolism by demethylation; undergoes enterohepatic circulation (5 days)	Non-steroidal oestrogen receptor antagonist; used for hormone-dependent metastatic breast cancer in postmenopausal women; given orally	Hot flushes; vaginal bleeding and discharge plus numerous other effects
Trastuzumab	See above	Used for metastatic breast cancer; see above	See above
Drugs for prostate cancer			
See also Miscellaneous anti-cancer drugs, listed below.			
Bicalutamide	Well absorbed; the active *R*-isomer undergoes hepatic oxidation and conjugation; urinary and biliary excretion (7–10 days)	Anti-androgen; used for advanced prostate cancer to cover the 'flare' associated with administration of gonadorelin analogues; given orally	Hot flushes; pruritus; gynaecomastia; rare serious hepatic and cardiovascular effects
Buserelin	Metabolism and some urinary excretion (1–1.5 h)	Gonadorelin analogue; used for advanced prostate cancer; given by subcutaneous injection for 7 days and then nasally	May cause tumour 'flare' leading to spinal cord compression; ureteric obstruction and bone pain
Cyproterone acetate	Hydrolysed and conjugated; metabolites eliminated in urine and bile (2 days)	Anti-oestrogen; used for prostate cancer and to cover 'flare' of gonadorelin analogues; given orally	See bicalutamide
Degarelix	Peptide hydrolysis (23–61 days)	Gonadotrophin-releasing hormone inhibitor used to treat advanced hormone-dependent prostate cancer; given by subcutaneous injection	Unlike gonaderelin analogues (see Ch. 43), does not induce a testosterone surge or tumour flare; susceptibility to Q–T interval prolongation

Compendium: drugs used in the treatment of cancer—cont'd

Drug	Kinetics (half-life)	Comments	Atypical or dose-limiting toxicity[a]
Flutamide	Complete bioavailability; rapid hepatic oxidation to an active hydroxy metabolite (8 h)	Anti-androgen; used for advanced prostate cancer and to cover 'flare' of gonadorelin analogues; given orally	See bicalutamide
Goserelin	Hepatic hydrolysis; about 20% excreted unchanged in urine (4 h)	Gonadorelin analogue; used for prostate cancer and advanced breast cancer; given by subcutaneous implant into anterior abdominal wall	See buserelin
Leuprorelin acetate (leuprolide)	Metabolised by proteases (3–4 h)	Gonadorelin analogue; used for advanced prostate cancer; given by subcutaneous or intramuscular injection	See buserelin; plus muscle weakness, hypertension, palpitations
Triptorelin	Metabolic routes not defined	Gonadorelin analogue; used for advanced prostate cancer (and endometriosis); given by intramuscular injection	See buserelin

Miscellaneous anti-cancer drugs

The drugs given below are those that affect the cancer *per se*; other drugs used in the management of people with cancer (e.g. anti-emetics) are described in the appropriate chapters.

Aldesleukin (interleukin-2)	Degraded by kidneys; half-life 0.5–6 h (intravenous), 3–12 h after subcutaneous dosage	Recombinant interleukin-2; use restricted to metastatic renal cell carcinoma; given by subcutaneous injection	Severe toxicity; pulmonary oedema; hypotension; bone marrow, hepatic, renal, thyroid and CNS toxicity
Alemtuzumab	Few data available; receptor-mediated uptake; probably eliminated by metabolism (1–14 days)	Antibody against CD52 antigen, causes lysis of B-lymphocytes; used for chronic lymphocytic leukaemia unresponsive to an alkylating agent; given by intravenous infusion	Cytokine release syndrome (characterised by severe dyspnoea)
Amsacrine	Hepatic metabolism, biliary elimination (4–7 h)	Planar fused ring system that intercalates into DNA; action and toxicity similar to doxorubicin; used for acute myeloid leukaemia; given as intravenous infusion	Myelosuppression; fatal arrhythmias when there is hypokalaemia
Arsenic trioxide	Kinetics not defined; metabolised by reduction and methylation	Mechanism of action not defined; used for acute promyelocytic leukaemia in disease that has relapsed or failed to respond to other treatment; given by intravenous infusion	Leucocyte activation syndrome (requires immediate treatment)
Bacillus Calmette–Guérin (BCG)	No kinetic data available	Immunostimulant that produces a non-specific, localised immune reaction with histocyte and leucocyte infiltration; used for primary or recurrent bladder carcinoma; given by bladder instillation	
Bexarotene	Hepatic metabolism (7 h)	Retinoid X receptor agonist; used for cutaneous T-cell lymphoma; given orally	Leucopenia
Crisantaspase (asparaginase)	Degraded by reticuloendothelial system (7–13 h)	Enzyme isolated from *Erwinia chrysanthemi* that depletes circulating L-asparagine; used for acute lymphoblastic leukaemia; given by intramuscular or subcutaneous injection	Anaphylaxis; CNS depression; nausea; hyperglycaemia
Catumaxomab	Low systemic exposure after intraperitoneal infusion (2 days)	Antibody to epithelial cell adhesion molecule (EpCAM) and CD3; used for malignant ascites associated with EpCAM-positive carcinomas; given by intraperitoneal infusion	Fever, vomiting

Compendium: drugs used in the treatment of cancer—cont'd

Drug	Kinetics (half-life)	Comments	Atypical or dose-limiting toxicity[a]
Dacarbazine	Activated by P450-mediated metabolism to cytotoxic and alkylating metabolite; about 50% excreted in urine unchanged (5 h)	Alkylating agent that interacts primarily with thiol groups; used for metastatic melanoma and soft tissue sarcomas; given intravenously	Myelosuppression; intense nausea and vomiting
Diethylstilbestrol	Eliminated by glucuronidation; undergoes enterohepatic cycling (2–3 days)	Oestrogen; inhibits hypothalamic–pituitary axis by negative feedback; used (very rarely) for prostate cancer, and occasionally for breast cancer; given orally	Nausea; fluid retention; thrombosis; impotence and gynaecomastia in men; hypercalcaemia and bone pain in women
Ethinylestradiol	See contraceptive hormones (Ch. 45)	Oestrogen; used for breast cancer (unlicensed indication in the UK); given orally	See contraceptive hormones (Ch. 45)
Hydroxycarbamide (hydroxyurea)	Eliminated unchanged by glomerular filtration (2–6 h)	Inhibits ribonucleotide reductase; used for chronic myeloid leukaemia; blocks; given orally	Myelosuppression
Interferon alfa	Catabolised by kidney (3–4 h)	Used for certain lymphomas and solid tumours; given by subcutaneous or intravenous injection	Nausea; lethargy; ocular effects; depression; myelosuppression; cerebrovascular, liver and kidney problems
Ipilimumab	Metabolic fate unknown (15 days)	Antibody that potentiates T-cells by blocking inhibitory signals from cytotoxic T-lymphocyte antigen 4 (CTLA-4); used for metastatic melanoma; given by intravenous infusion	Potentially fatal immune-mediated adverse reactions, particularly gastrointestinal, due to T cell activation
Lenalidomide	Bioavailability about 50%; mostly excreted unchanged in urine (3 h)	Immunomodulator with anti-angiogenic action; used in multiple myeloma unresponsive to other therapies; given orally	Thromboembolism, severe neutropenia; risk of teratogenesis
Medroxyprogesterone acetate	Complete oral bioavailability; eliminated as conjugated metabolites (30 days); half-life 50 days after intramuscular injection	Progestogen; used for endometrial and breast cancer, rarely for prostate and renal cancer; given orally or by deep intramuscular injection	Glucocorticoid effects at high doses
Megestrol acetate	Complete oral bioavailability; hepatic oxidation and conjugation (15–20 h)	Progestogen; used for endometrial and breast cancer; given orally	
Mitotane	Highly lipid-soluble compound; mostly eliminated unchanged in bile (0.5–6 months)	Selectively toxic to adrenal cortex, by unknown mechanism; used for advanced or inoperable adrenocortical carcinoma; given orally	Gastrointestinal effects; CNS disturbances
Norethisterone (norethindrone)	Complete oral bioavailability; hepatic metabolism (5–12 h)	Progestogen; used for endometrial cancer and also for renal and breast cancer; given orally	
Pentostatin	Eliminated unchanged by kidneys (3–15 h)	Adenosine deaminase inhibitor; used for hairy cell leukaemia; given intravenously	Myelosuppression; immunosuppression
Prednisolone	High oral bioavailability (70–80%); extensively metabolised (2–4 h)	Glucocorticoid; used for marked antitumour effect in acute lymphoblastic leukaemia, Hodgkin's disease and non-Hodgkin's lymphoma (also in palliative care); given orally, topically and by intramuscular injection	See corticosteroids (Ch. 44)

Compendium: drugs used in the treatment of cancer—cont'd

Drug	Kinetics (half-life)	Comments	Atypical or dose-limiting toxicity[a]
Procarbazine	Rapid hepatic metabolism, producing reactive methyl radicals; limited renal excretion (0.1 h)	Cytotoxic mechanism unclear; used in Hodgkin's disease; given orally	Nausea; myelosuppression; rash; ingestion with alcohol may give a disulfiram-like effect
Rituximab	Peptide hydrolysis (19–32 days)	Anti-CD20 antibody that lyses B-lymphocytes; used for chemotherapy-resistant advanced follicular lymphoma; given by intravenous infusion	Fever; chills; nausea; allergic reactions; cytokine release syndrome (characterised by severe dyspnoea)
Temozolomide	Non-enzymatic conversion to same active compound as dacarbazine (2 h)	Structural analogue of dacarbazine (see above); used as second-line treatment for malignant glioma; given orally	Myelosuppression
Thalidomide	Non-enzymatic hydrolysis; mainly urinary elimination (5–7 h)	Immunomodulator with anti-angiogenic action; used with an alkylating drug and a corticosteroid in multiple myeloma; given orally	Thromboembolism, peripheral neuropathy; risk of teratogenesis
Trabectedin	Highly protein bound; hepatic metabolism, mainly faecal elimination (180 h)	Used for advanced soft tissue sarcoma and with doxorubicin for ovarian cancer; given intravenously	Hepatotoxicity, myelosuppression
Tretinoin (all-*trans*-retinoic acid)	Hepatic oxidation, conjugation and isomerisation (1–2 h)	Retinoid RAR and RXR agonist; used for remission of acute promyelocytic leukaemia; given orally	Numerous symptoms (highly teratogenic)

Antidotes

Chemoprotectants: each agent is used reduce the toxicity of a specific anti-cancer drug or of a group of related anti-cancer drugs.

Drug	Kinetics (half-life)	Comments	Atypical or dose-limiting toxicity[a]
Amifostine	Rapid uptake by normal tissues, where it is dephosphorylated to active thiol form (<0.2 h)	Used before cytotoxic treatment to reduce risk of neutropenia-related infection in people treated with cisplatin or cyclophosphamide, and to reduce cisplatin nephrotoxicity; given by intravenous infusion	Hypotension
Dexrazoxane	Hepatic hydrolysis to EDTA-like compounds (2–4 h)	Chelating agent, protects against anthracycline-induced free radical damage; used for anthracycline-induced extravasation; given by intravenous infusion	–
Folinic acid (leucovorin) and levofolinate	Formyl group used in thymidate synthesis and folate enters body pool (0.75 h)	Given 24 h after methotrexate to speed recovery from myelosuppression; given orally or by intramuscular or intravenous injection	–
Mesna (mercaptoethane sulphonic acid)	Eliminated in the urine (1 h)	Highly polar molecule containing a thiol group; given orally before cyclophosphamide or ifosfamide treatment, or intravenously afterwards, to prevent urothelial toxicity	–
Palifermin	Peptide eliminated by proteolysis or by reticuloendothelial system (3–5 h)	Human keratinocyte growth factor, acts on epithelial cells to aid cellular defences; used for oral mucositis during treatment of haematological malignancies; given by intravenous injection	–

EGFR, epidermal growth factor receptor; mTOR, mammalian target of rapamycin; PDGFR, platelet-derived growth factor receptor; RAR, retinoic acid receptor; RXR, retinoid X receptors; VEGFR, vascular endothelial growth factor receptor.
[a]Typical toxicity for the class of drug is described in the general text; toxicity given in this column represents 'non-class' effects and/or severe dose-limiting toxicity.

12

General features: toxicity and prescribing

53 Drug toxicity and overdose

• •

Most therapeutic drugs produce their beneficial response by altering human homeostatic mechanisms; only antimicrobial agents and parasiticides have the theoretical possibility of a therapeutic response without some direct action on human metabolic or physiological processes. Some therapeutic agents, for example atropine (belladonna), tubocurarine (curare), ergot alkaloids (causing St. Anthony's fire), digoxin (digitalis) and dicoumarol (causing haemorrhagic disease in cattle), have pharmacological properties that were first recognised as a result of either accidental or intentional poisonings. It is hardly surprising that all drugs are capable of producing adverse effects if the dosage is high enough. The relationship between a potentially beneficial drug and a poison was recognised five centuries ago when Paracelsus stated: 'All things are toxic and it is only the dose which makes something a poison.'

Some of the medicines prescribed today were first used as relatively crude plant extracts, for example digitalis glycosides and opium extracts. It was the identification and isolation of the active chemical entities in plant extracts that allowed the dose and purity of the active ingredient to be controlled sufficiently to optimise the ratio between benefit and risk. In this respect, the current vogue for herbal remedies could be considered to represent a backward step in controlling the safety and efficacy of drugs.

Drug toxicity can develop at normal therapeutic doses of a drug or as a result of an acute overdose. In some cases, toxicity occurs in the majority of treated individuals because of the nature of the drug, for example cytotoxic agents used for cancer chemotherapy, but significant toxicity is rare with the majority of commonly prescribed drugs when used at recommended dosages. There is considerable inter-individual variability in both the nature and severity of adverse reactions, and toxicity can be reduced by taking into account factors that are known to increase susceptibility, such as age, concurrent disease or body weight, when selecting both the drug and the dosage. Usually, a reduction in dosage or a change of drug during chronic treatment will reduce the severity of adverse effects (but see immunological mechanisms discussed below).

Toxicity following an acute overdose usually produces predictable adverse reactions, which may be life-threatening and/or prejudice long-term health. Rapid treatment is then required and this may be aimed at preventing further drug absorption, increasing drug elimination/inactivation and managing the adverse effects produced.

This chapter is, therefore, divided into two main sections:

- **drug toxicity and adverse effects**, which discusses mechanisms for adverse effects produced both during normal drug therapy and after an overdose,
- **self-poisoning and drug overdose**, which is concerned with the management of drug overdose.

DRUG TOXICITY AND ADVERSE EFFECTS

There is no consistent use of terminology in describing effects of drugs that were not intended when the drug was prescribed. Adverse effects of a drug are those that can occur when the drug is used at therapeutic doses; these have also been referred to as collateral effects. Drug toxicity is more commonly applied to effects that occur at supra-therapeutic doses. This section provides a framework for classifying adverse and toxic effects of drugs which are referred to in the individual drug monographs as unwanted effects. The term side effect is a widely used alternative.

The beneficial effects of a drug in one situation (e.g. the antidiarrhoeal effect of opioids) may be an adverse effect in other circumstances (e.g. constipation, when an opioid is used for pain relief). Therefore, even classification of the nature of effect into beneficial or adverse may depend on the condition being treated. The adverse effects caused by different drugs are listed in the *British National Formulary* (BNF), and it is apparent that for most drugs' potential adverse effects are more numerous than beneficial properties. It is important to remember that such lists are not exhaustive, and prescribers should be alert to both predicted and unexpected reactions to medicines. The prescriber should consider the risk–benefit ratio for each individual and the suitability of alternative drugs and/or treatments and people who are prescribed drugs should be informed of the risk–benefit balance inherent in their treatment. The patient information leaflet (PIL) included with the dispensed medicine represents a useful way of providing such advice. Prescribers should also be aware of the risks of adverse and toxic effects arising from drug interactions.

It should be appreciated that all drugs are associated with some risk of adverse effects and toxicity, although both the severity and incidence differ widely among drugs. In general, the acceptability of a risk of an unwanted effect is related to the severity of the disease being treated; for example, serious idiosyncratic reactions with incidences of 1 in 10 000 have led to the withdrawal of some non-steroidal anti-inflammatory drugs (NSAIDs), whereas some cancer chemotherapeutic agents can cause significant toxicity in nearly all individuals.

A useful indication of the safety margin available for a drug is given by the therapeutic index (TI):

$$\text{Therapeutic index} = \frac{\text{Dose resulting in toxicity}}{\text{Dose giving therapeutic response}}$$

Drugs such as diazepam have a TI of about 50 and it is difficult for even the most inept doctor to cause serious toxicity with diazepam. In contrast, digoxin has a TI of only about 2, and for such drugs toxicity may be precipitated by relatively small changes in dosage regimen or the clearance of the drug from the body. The TI relates to serious toxicity and does not indicate the potential for minor adverse effects, which may inconvenience the person enough for him or her to stop treatment but are not considered to represent drug toxicity.

TYPES OF UNWANTED EFFECT

Adverse drug reactions are usually divided into two main types:

- **Type A (Augmented)**: these effects are usually dose-related and largely predictable from the known pharmacological and biochemical effects of the drug or its metabolites,
- **Type B (Bizarre)**: these effects are not obviously dose-related and are idiosyncratic and unpredictable; they are often immunological in nature.

This classification makes no allowance for time-dependency of some adverse events, or for the underlying susceptibility of the individual. Other types of adverse reactions have been defined as: continuing (type C), delayed (type D), end-of-use (type E), failure of therapy (type F) or genetic/genomic (type G). These types are not mutually exclusive, and classification of an adverse event along multiple axes, such as dose-relatedness, time-relatedness and susceptibility may be more meaningful.

PHARMACOLOGICAL TOXICITY

In 'pharmacological toxicity', the toxic reaction is a predictable extension of the known pharmacology of the drug at

Table 53.1 Examples of drugs with adverse effects related to their primary therapeutic properties

Drug	Adverse effect
Acetylcholinesterase inhibitors	Muscle weakness
Beta-adrenoceptor antagonists	Heart block when used as an antiarrhythmic
Insulin	Hypoglycaemia
General anaesthetics	Medullary depression
Loop diuretics	Hypokalaemia
Warfarin	Haemorrhage

its site(s) of action (Table 53.1), and should be recognised readily when monitoring the individual's response to treatment. There are numerous examples in this book where the adverse effect is really an excessive therapeutic action.

For many drug effects, the response increases with increase in dose, with low sub-therapeutic doses giving an inadequate response, therapeutic doses giving the desired response, but very high doses giving an excessive response that can be regarded as a form of toxicity (response 1 in Fig. 53.1). A good example is warfarin (Ch. 11), inadequate doses of which are associated with a lack of the desired anti-thrombotic effect, whereas at excessive doses there is a risk of haemorrhage. This has given rise to the concept of a 'therapeutic window', which is a range of doses or blood/plasma concentrations within which most individuals should show a beneficial response with minimal risk of adverse effects (illustrated by response 1 in Fig. 53.1). The concept is particularly valuable in the interpretation of measurements of drug concentrations in plasma, which can be used to monitor adherence to treatment and to assess likely response (Table 53.2).

In many other cases, the toxic reaction may be unrelated to the primary therapeutic effect (Table 53.3), and may be caused by a secondary effect that is not the primary aim of the treatment given (response 2 in Fig. 53.1). This toxicity will often be present to a limited extent at appropriate therapeutic doses.

The separation of therapeutic and toxic dose–response curves is a measure of the TI. If these are very close (e.g. responses 1 and 2 in Fig. 53.1), then there is a low safety margin (low TI) and most individuals will show some degree of toxicity at normal therapeutic doses, for example myelosuppression with cytotoxic anti-cancer drugs. For drugs with widely separated therapeutic and toxic dose–response curves (e.g. responses 1 and 3 in Fig. 53.1) – that is, those with high TIs – toxicity would not be seen at normal doses; for example a β-adrenoceptor antagonist would be very unlikely to cause myocardial depression and heart failure in people with normal left ventricular function. However, the toxic effect may occur in individuals who are unusually sensitive because of their genetics or their physical condition; for example, standard doses of a β-adrenoceptor antagonist can precipitate heart failure in people with pre-existing impaired left ventricular function.

Pharmacological toxicity is the most common cause of adverse effects. Such toxicity can be minimised by an assessment of the risk–benefit balance for the individual to

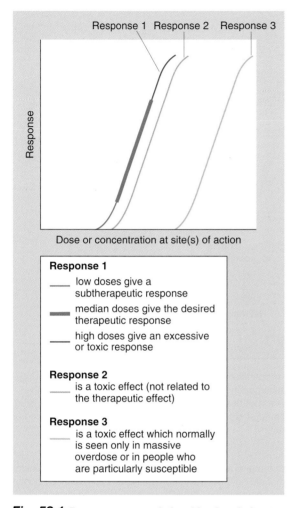

Response 1

— low doses give a subtherapeutic response

━ median doses give the desired therapeutic response

— high doses give an excessive or toxic response

Response 2

— is a toxic effect (not related to the therapeutic effect)

Response 3

— is a toxic effect which normally is seen only in massive overdose or in people who are particularly susceptible

Fig. 53.1 **Dose–response relationships in relation to toxicity.** Response 1 is the primary therapeutic effect, the magnitude of which increases with dose from sub-therapeutic, through therapeutic to potentially toxic. Response 2 is an undesired effect seen at a dose only slightly greater than those producing the therapeutic effect. Response 3 is an adverse effect normally seen only in overdose.

be treated. This should take into account factors that may influence both pharmacokinetics and target-organ sensitivity, including age, physiological status (e.g. renal function), concurrent medication, disease processes, environmental factors (e.g. smoking), etc.

Because of the predictable nature of pharmacological toxicity, it is usual for some treatments to be co-prescribed with drugs that will reduce the possibility of toxic effects; examples include anti-emetics given with cancer chemotherapy, vitamin B_6 given with isoniazid and leucovorin (folinic acid) given after high-dose methotrexate.

BIOCHEMICAL TOXICITY

In 'biochemical toxicity', the toxicity or tissue damage is caused by an interaction of the drug, or an active

Table 53.2 Examples of therapeutic windows based on plasma concentrations

Drug	Therapeutic concentration range (typical values)		Toxic response
	Minimum	*Maximum*[a]	
Aspirin (analgesia) ($\mu g \cdot mL^{-1}$)	20	300	Tinnitus, metabolic acidosis
Carbamazepine ($\mu g \cdot mL^{-1}$)	4	10	Drowsiness, visual disturbances
Digitoxin ($ng \cdot mL^{-1}$)	15	30	Bradycardia, nausea
Digoxin ($ng \cdot mL^{-1}$)	0.8	3	Bradycardia, nausea
Gentamicin ($\mu g \cdot mL^{-1}$)	2	12	Ototoxicity, renal toxicity
Kanamycin ($\mu g \cdot mL^{-1}$)	10	40	Ototoxicity, renal toxicity
Phenytoin ($\mu g \cdot mL^{-1}$)	10	20	Nystagmus, lethargy
Theophylline ($\mu g \cdot mL^{-1}$)	10	20	Tremor, nervousness

[a]The maximum concentration may be limited by toxicity related to the primary therapeutic response (e.g. carbamazepine) or to an unrelated effect (e.g. gentamicin).

Table 53.3 Examples of drugs with adverse effects unrelated to their primary therapeutic use

Drug	Adverse effects
Beta-adrenoceptor agonists	Increase in heart rate when used in asthma
Beta-adrenoceptor antagonists	Reduction in heart rate when used for hypertension
Aminoglycosides	Deafness
Anti-cancer drugs	Myelosuppression
Anticonvulsants	Sedation when used for epilepsy
Antipsychotics	Dystonias or parkinsonism
Corticosteroids	Glaucoma
Drugs for Parkinson's disease	Hallucinations and confusion
Opioid analgesics	Respiratory depression
Paracetamol	Liver failure
Statins	Rhabdomyolysis
Thalidomide	Birth defects
Thiazides	Glucose intolerance

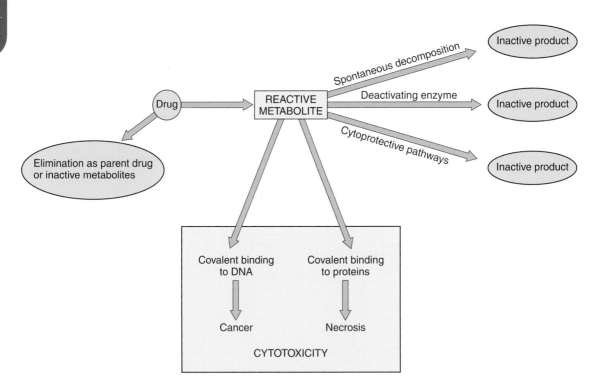

Fig. 53.2 **Metabolism and cytotoxicity.** In this scheme, the propensity of the reactive metabolite of a cytotoxic drug to cause adverse biochemical effects on cellular DNA and proteins depends on the balance between formation of the reactive metabolite from the parent drug, and the rate of elimination of both the reactive metabolite and the parent drug by alternative metabolic routes. Therapeutic interventions are aimed at either increasing elimination of the parent drug or enhancing cytoprotective pathways to reduce the cytotoxic effects.

metabolite, with cell components, especially macromolecules such as structural proteins and enzymes. A generalised scheme is given in Figure 53.2. For most licensed drugs this form of toxicity is identified and characterised during preclinical studies in animals and monitored in clinical trials (Ch. 3), for example by measuring changes in serum levels of liver or muscle enzymes.

In some situations, an understanding of the mechanism of toxicity has allowed the development of appropriate treatments or antidotes. An example is the key observation that the thiol (-SH) group of the endogenous tripeptide glutathione can prevent cell damage caused by highly reactive chemical species, such as the toxic metabolite of paracetamol (see below and Fig. 53.3). The nature of the cell damage is related to the stability of the toxic reactive chemical; extremely unstable metabolites may bind covalently to and inactivate the enzyme that forms them, whereas more stable species may be able to diffuse to a distant site, for example DNA, and initiate changes such as cancer. Important examples of biochemical toxicity are given below.

Paracetamol

Paracetamol-induced hepatotoxicity represents the result of an imbalance between metabolic detoxication of paracetamol, via conjugation with glucuronic acid and sulphate, and metabolic activation to an unstable toxic metabolite (*N*-acetyl-*p*-benzoquinone imine, NAPQI) via oxidation by cytochrome P450. This toxic metabolite can bind covalently

to proteins and cause cell necrosis. Low doses of paracetamol are safe because they are eliminated mainly by conjugation, and any NAPQI created by cytochrome P450 oxidation is inactivated by a cytoprotective pathway involving glutathione. However, in overdose, the sulphate conjugation reaction is saturated and there is increased cytochrome P450-mediated oxidation of paracetamol to NAPQI (Fig. 53.3). Once the hepatic glutathione is depleted this toxic metabolite binds covalently to proteins and causes oxidative stress and cell necrosis. This biochemical mechanism explains:

- the site of toxicity (centrilobular necrosis in the liver because of the large amounts of cytochrome P450 present),
- the increased toxicity seen in individuals treated with inducers of cytochrome P450 (especially alcohol-related induction of CYP2E1),
- the increased toxicity seen in individuals with low hepatic stores of glutathione due to poor nutrition,
- the successful treatment of paracetamol overdose with acetylcysteine, which provides an additional source of thiol groups for inactivation of NAPQI (see treatment of drug overdose, below).

Cyclophosphamide

Cyclophosphamide is an anti-cancer drug. Its highly toxic metabolites bind to DNA as part of their mechanism of

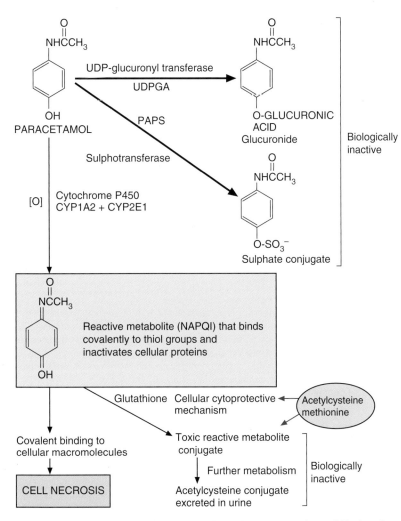

Fig. 53.3 Pathways of paracetamol metabolism. In overdose, the concentrations of 3′-phosphoadenosine 5′-phosphosulphate (PAPS) (for sulphation) and glutathione (for cytoprotection) are depleted, and extensive macromolecular binding leads to hepatocellular necrosis. *N*-Acetylcysteine and methionine replenish glutathione to conjugate the toxic metabolite. NAPQI, *N*-acetyl-*p*-benzoquinone imine; UDPGA, uridine diphosphate glucuronic acid.

action, but they are eliminated in the urine and cause haemorrhagic cystitis due to cell damage in the bladder (Ch. 52). This adverse effect can be prevented by prior treatment with mesna (mercaptoethane sulphonic acid), which possesses both a thiol group for cytoprotection and a highly polar sulphonic acid group, and results in high renal excretion and delivery of this cytoprotective molecule to the bladder epithelium. It is usually given either orally 2 h before the cyclophosphamide or intravenously at the same time to cover the period of maximum urinary excretion of toxic cyclophosphamide metabolites. It is not yet known whether mesna also protects against bladder cancer, which can arise about 10–20 years after initial treatment with cyclophosphamide.

Isoniazid

Isoniazid, which is used for the treatment of tuberculosis (Ch. 51), causes hepatitis in about 0.5% of treated

individuals. This is believed to result from the formation of a reactive metabolite, *N*-acetylhydrazine, which is produced by acetylation followed by oxidative metabolism. The biochemical basis for the susceptibility of some individuals to the hepatotoxic metabolite is not known. Fast acetylators (see Ch. 2) form more *N*-acetylhydrazine than do slow acetylators, but, unexpectedly, they are not more sensitive to isoniazid toxicity. Susceptibility may be related to the balance between further activation of *N*-acetylhydrazine (by oxidation) and its detoxification (by further acetylation); if this is so, then fast acetylators may produce more active metabolite but also inactivate it more rapidly.

Spironolactone

Spironolactone (Ch. 14) is oxidised by cytochrome P450. The metabolite formed in the testes binds to and destroys testicular cytochrome P450 and this causes a decrease in

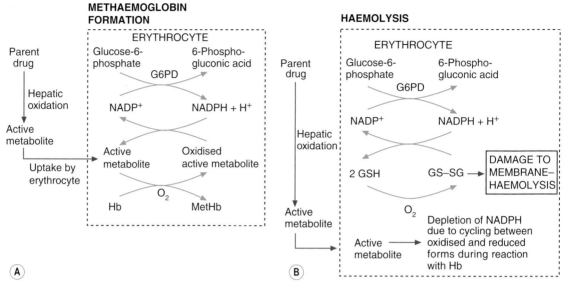

Fig. 53.4 **Mechanisms of methaemoglobinaemia and haemolysis.** In methaemoglobinamia (A), the active drug metabolite oxidises haemoglobin (Hb) to methaemoglobin (MetHb). The oxidised active metabolite is repeatedly recycled to the active metabolite by reduced nicotinamide adenine dinucleotide phosphate (NADPH) generated by glucose-6-phosphate dehydrogenase (G6PD). In (B), the depletion of NADPH as a result of methaemoglobinaemia depletes levels of the reduced glutathione (GSH) necessary for maintaining erythrocyte cell membrane integrity; the build-up of oxidised glutathione dimers (GS–SG) causes membrane damage and haemolysis. The active metabolite may also react directly with glutathione to lower GSH concentrations.

the metabolism of progesterone to testosterone (a step which is also catalysed by a cytochrome P450). This effect, combined with an anti-androgenic action at receptor sites (pharmacological toxicity), can result in gynaecomastia and decreased libido.

Aromatic amines and nitrites

Aromatic amines, such as the anti-leprosy drug dapsone and some antimalarials (e.g. primaquine), are oxidised in the liver to active metabolites, which are released into the circulation, where they can affect erythrocytes, causing methaemoglobinaemia and/or haemolysis.

Methaemoglobinaemia

In the erythrocyte, the active metabolite interacts with molecular oxygen (O_2), which then oxidises haemoglobin (Fe^{2+}) to methaemoglobin (Fe^{3+}) and also oxidises the active metabolite itself (Fig. 53.4A). Because of the large amounts of haemoglobin compared with the amount of drug given this would be inconsequential, were it not for the fact that the oxidised active metabolite can be recycled back to the active metabolite by reduction with NADPH (reduced nicotinamide adenine dinucleotide phosphate) in the erythrocyte. Consequently, each molecule of the metabolite undergoes repeated redox cycling and is able to oxidise many molecules of haemoglobin. NADPH is formed during the metabolism of glucose 6-phosphate by glucose-6-phosphate dehydrogenase (G6PD) (Fig. 53.4A). The activity of G6PD, and hence the amounts of NADPH, are determined genetically. There is a high incidence of G6PD deficiency in people of African ancestry and very high in those

of Mediterranean ancestry, such as Kurdish people. Such individuals have limited NADPH reserves and a low ability to reduce the oxidised active drug metabolite (Fig. 53.4A) back to the active metabolite. In consequence, there is limited redox cycling of the active drug metabolite and they are less susceptible to drug-induced methaemoglobinaemia, but they are more susceptible to haemolysis (see below).

Haemolysis

This arises from an increase in erythrocyte membrane permeability associated with accumulation of oxidised glutathione (GS–SG in Fig. 53.4B) in the erythrocyte. Oxidised glutathione accumulates because redox cycling of the drug metabolite linked to the formation of methaemoglobin (Fig. 53.4A) (see above) results in depletion of NADPH, which is the cofactor essential for maintaining glutathione in the reduced state. Individuals with G6PD deficiency are very susceptible to haemolysis caused by aromatic amines and nitrites because the low endogenous levels of NADPH are depleted rapidly and oxidised glutathione cannot then be reduced. Given the geographical distribution of G6PD deficiency, it is ironic that the amino groups associated with this form of toxicity are often present in drugs used to treat tropical infections (such as primaquine for the treatment of malaria; see Ch. 51 and Box 47.6).

IMMUNOLOGICAL TOXICITY

Immunological toxicity is frequently referred to as 'drug allergy' and is the form of toxicity with which people may be most familiar, for example penicillin allergy.

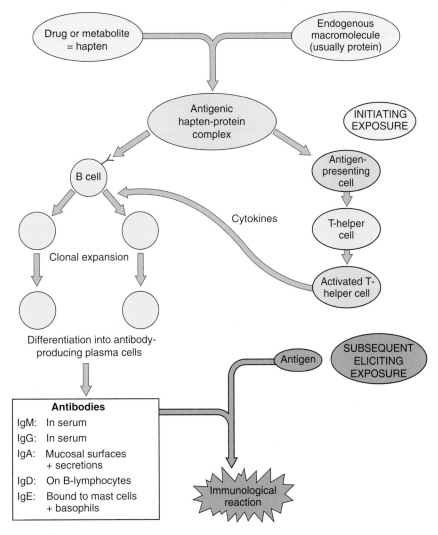

Fig. 53.5 **Mechanisms of drug allergy.** The drug or drug metabolite binds as a hapten to an endogenous macromolecule. The initial exposure produces an antigenic hapten–protein complex, which results in the production of antibodies via B-cell clonal expansion and differentiation, regulated by cytokines from activated T-helper cells. The eliciting exposure occurs later (usually at least 3 days later, during which time therapy may or may not be continuing); antigen–antibody interaction then exposes a complement-binding site, which triggers the reaction. The nature of the immunological reaction depends on the nature of the antibody and/or localisation of the antigen. Treatment is with immunosuppressant drugs (Ch. 38).

Immunological mechanisms are implicated in a number of common adverse effects, such as rashes and fever, but may also be involved in organ-directed toxicity. Although the term 'allergy' may not be strictly correct for all forms of immunologically mediated toxicity, it is probably better than 'hypersensitivity', which has also been used to describe an elevated sensitivity to any mechanism or effect.

Low-molecular-weight compounds (<1100 Da) are not able to elicit an allergic response directly but can do so after the compound, or a metabolite, has formed a stable or covalent bond with a macromolecule. Covalent binding to a normal protein produces a hapten–protein conjugate that is recognised as foreign by the immune system and can act as an antigen (Fig. 53.5).

Immunologically mediated toxicity can show a wide range of characteristics.

- Toxicity is unrelated to dose: once the antibody has been produced, even very small amounts of antigen can trigger a reaction.
- There is normally a lag of at least 3 days between initial exposure and the development of symptoms; however, the first dose of a subsequent treatment may give an immediate reaction.
- Cross-reactivity is possible among different compounds that share the same antigenic determinant or structural component involved in antibody recognition, such as the penicilloyl group of the penicillin family.

- The incidence varies widely between different drugs; for example, from about 1 in 10 000 people for phenylbutazone-induced agranulocytosis to 1 in 20 for ampicillin-related skin rashes.
- The response is idiosyncratic but genetically controlled. Individual responsiveness cannot be predicted, but individuals who have a history of atopic disease are more likely to develop a 'drug allergy'.

The effects produced may be subdivided into the classic four types of allergic reaction (see also Ch. 38).

- **Type 1: immediate or anaphylactic reactions**. These are mediated via IgE antibodies attached to the surface of basophils and mast cells; the release of numerous mediators, for example histamine, serotonin and leukotrienes, produces effects that include urticaria, bronchoconstriction, hypotension, oedema and shock. A skin-prick challenge test usually produces an acute inflammatory response. Examples of drugs having this type of effect are penicillins and peptide drugs, such as crisantaspase (asparaginase).
- **Type 2: cytotoxic reactions**. The antigen is formed by the drug binding to a cell membrane; subsequent interaction of this antigen with circulating IgG, IgM or IgA antibodies activates complement and initiates cell lysis. Depending on the carrier cell to which the drug is bound, cell lysis can result in thrombocytopenia (e.g. cephalosporins, quinine), neutropenia (e.g. metronidazole) or haemolytic anaemia (e.g. penicillins, rifampicin and possibly methyldopa).
- **Type 3: immune-complex reactions**. The antigen–antibody interaction occurs in serum and the complex formed is deposited on endothelial cells, basement membranes, etc., to initiate a more localised inflammatory reaction, such as arteritis or nephritis. Examples include serum sickness (urticaria, angioedema, fever) with penicillins, lupus erythematosus-like syndrome with hydralazine and procainamide (especially in slow acetylators) and possibly NSAID-related nephropathy.
- **Type 4: cell-mediated delayed-type reactions**. Reaction to the eliciting exposure is delayed. The reactions occur mostly in skin through the formation of an antigen between the drug (hapten) and skin proteins. This is followed by an infiltration of sensitised T-lymphocytes, which recognise the antigen and release cytokines to produce local inflammation, oedema and irritation; for example, contact dermatitis.

In addition to true immunologically mediated toxicity, as described above, there are examples of 'pseudoallergic' reactions, such as aspirin-intolerant asthma which shows many of the characteristics given above (e.g. induction of asthma only in susceptible individuals), but for which a true immunological basis has not been demonstrated. In aspirin intolerance, cross-reactivity with other NSAIDs in fact suggests a common pharmacological mechanism based on cyclo-oxygenase inhibition (Ch. 29).

It has been estimated that 'drug allergy' accounts for about 10% of adverse drug reactions but that severe reactions are rare. For example, only about 5 in 10 000 individuals develop an anaphylactic reaction to penicillins, but about a half of these are sufficiently serious to warrant hospital treatment (see Ch. 39). However, given the large numbers of people taking drugs such as penicillins, 'drug allergy' is an important source of iatrogenic morbidity.

SELF-POISONING AND DRUG OVERDOSE

Self-poisoning can be either accidental or deliberate. Approximately a quarter of a million episodes are believed to occur each year in England and Wales, although fewer than 40% of these reach hospital. Deaths from intentional self-poisoning and accidental overdose still average about 2500 each year in England and Wales, with about two-thirds being male. Accidental poisoning is common in children under 5 years of age, when it often involves household products as well as medicines. A second peak of self-poisoning occurs in the teens and early twenties, when it is more frequent in girls. The incidence then progressively falls with increasing age. Most deliberate self-poisoning represents 'parasuicide' or attention-seeking behaviour. True suicide attempts account for about 1000 deaths a year, occurring most frequently in those over 45 years. About 30% of the deaths from deliberate overdose are in those over 65 years of age: self-poisoning at this age occurs most often in response to depression or specific life events such as bereavement. It is important to recognise that at any age the severity of poisoning bears little relationship to suicidal intent.

Heroin and morphine overdoses are the most common single cause of death from drug overdose, accounting for almost 25% of the total. The drugs most frequently used for intentional self-poisoning are benzodiazepines, analgesics and antidepressants, often taken together with alcohol. It is important to attempt to identify the cause of the poisoning because it may determine the most suitable treatment. However, it should be remembered that information from the person, about which drug was taken, how much and the time of overdosing, is frequently unreliable. TICTAC (www.tictac.org.uk) is a computerised database which enables registered users to identify tablets and capsules.

MANAGEMENT PRINCIPLES

The emergency treatment of poisoning is described in the BNF. Additional sources of information include the UK National Poisons Information Service (www.npis.org) and its computer database TOXBASE (www.toxbase.co.uk), which has information on household products and industrial and agricultural chemicals as well as drugs, and is available to registered users.

The management of drug overdose outlined below has a number of principal aims (Fig. 53.6).

MANAGING ADVERSE EFFECTS

Immediate measures

There are certain immediate measures required when someone presents with a possible drug overdose or poisoning:

- remove the person from contact with the poison if appropriate; for example, gases, corrosives,

- assess vital signs, i.e. pulse, respiration and pupil size; inspect the person for injury,
- ensure a clear airway; if breathing but unconscious, place in the coma position,
- obtain a clear history if possible,
- preserve any evidence; for example, bottles, written notes, etc.

Supportive measures

Examples of unwanted effects seen in drug overdose are shown in Table 53.4. A number of the effects will require supportive measures (Fig. 53.7).

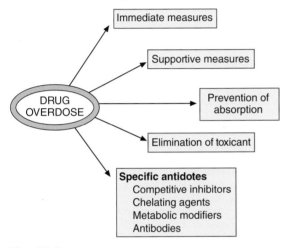

Fig. 53.6 Principles underlying the management of drug overdose.

Cardiac or respiratory arrest

This may result from a toxic effect of the drug on the heart, from depression of the respiratory centre or from metabolic disturbance. Assisted ventilation, ranging from mouth-to-mouth, or Ambu-bag inflation, to the use of a ventilator, may be required. In some circumstances, recovery is possible even after prolonged resuscitation.

Hypotension

A low blood pressure is common in severe poisoning with central nervous system depressants. A systolic blood pressure below 70 mmHg can cause irreversible brain damage, but any degree of low blood pressure should be treated if accompanied by poor tissue perfusion or low urine output. Depression of the vasomotor centre can cause arterial dilation and peripheral venous pooling, producing a low central venous pressure (CVP). The CVP should be raised

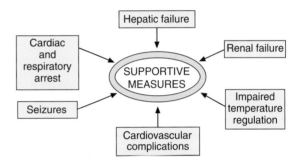

Fig. 53.7 Main effects of overdose requiring supportive measures.

Table 53.4 Complications of acute poisonings

Complication	Cause	Examples of poisons
Cardiac arrest	Direct cardiotoxicity	Many
	Hypoxia	Many
	Electrolyte/metabolic disturbance	Many
Central nervous system depression		Many
Seizures	Direct neurotoxicity	Tricyclic antidepressants, theophylline
	Hypoxia	Many
Hypotension	Myocardial depression	Beta-adrenoceptor antagonists, tricyclic antidepressants
	Peripheral vasodilation	Many
Arrhythmia	Direct cardiotoxicity	Beta-adrenoceptor antagonists, tricyclic antidepressants, verapamil, digoxin
	Hypoxia	Many
	Electrolyte/metabolic disturbance	Many
Renal failure	Hypotension	Many
	Rhabdomyolysis	Opioids, hypnotics, ethanol, carbon monoxide
	Direct nephrotoxicity	Paracetamol, heavy metals
Hepatic failure	Direct hepatotoxicity	Paracetamol, carbon tetrachloride
Respiratory depression	Direct neurotoxicity	Sedatives, hypnotics, opioids

to 10–15 cmH₂O (measured from the midaxillary line) by intravenous infusion of a crystalloid solution, such as 0.9% saline. A vasoconstrictor such as noradrenaline (norepinephrine; Ch. 4) is rarely required. If hypotension occurs in association with a normal or raised central venous pressure, this suggests myocardial depression. A positive inotropic drug such as the β_1-adrenoceptor agonist dobutamine (Ch. 7) should then be used.

Arrhythmias

Disturbances of cardiac rhythm should only be treated if they are severe. Ventricular arrhythmias causing hypotension often require intervention, but caution should be exercised if there is a long Q–T interval on the electrocardiogram, since the tachycardia often fails to respond to standard antiarrhythmic drugs. It is essential to correct metabolic derangements that predispose to arrhythmias, for example hypothermia, hypoxia, hypercapnia, hypokalaemia, hyperkalaemia and acidosis. If there is widening of the QRS complex after overdose of a tricyclic antidepressant, then intravenous sodium bicarbonate should be given to reduce the risk of serious arrhythmias.

Seizures

These may be caused by a treatable underlying cause such as hypoxia, hypoglycaemia or hypocalcaemia, or they may be a direct toxic effect of the drug on neuronal function. The treatment of choice is lorazepam or diazepam intravenously, or rectal diazepam if the intravenous route is unavailable (Ch. 20). Artificial ventilation with neuromuscular blockade (Ch. 27) is used if the seizures cannot be controlled.

Renal failure

Kidney damage is usually a consequence of prolonged hypotension. Other causes include a direct nephrotoxic effect of the drug and renal damage produced by the products of toxic muscle necrosis (rhabdomyolysis).

Hepatic failure

This usually results from the direct toxic effects of specific agents, such as paracetamol.

Impaired temperature regulation

Hypothermia is common, and can be caused by depression of the metabolic rate with reduced heat production and by increased heat loss from cutaneous vasodilation. It is common with phenothiazines and barbiturates, but is seen with any prolonged coma. Rewarming, preferably by wrapping in a 'space blanket', reduces the risk of serious ventricular arrhythmias. By contrast, CNS stimulants such as ecstasy can produce hyperthermia, as can aspirin, which uncouples cellular oxidative phosphorylation.

REDUCING TOXICITY

The adverse effects can be reduced by:

- minimising further drug absorption,
- maximising drug elimination,
- negating effects with antidotes, etc.

Prevention of absorption of poisons

There are two principal methods of preventing further absorption of the drug: gastric aspiration/lavage and activated charcoal. Inducing emesis with an irritant such as ipecacuanha is not recommended, since it has little effect on drug absorption and increases the risk of aspiration of gastric contents.

Gastric aspiration and lavage

Gastric lavage is rarely required, and should not be considered in unconscious or drowsy persons without protection of the airways by a cuffed endotracheal tube to prevent aspiration of gastric contents into the lungs. It should never be used after ingestion of corrosives or petroleum products. A large-bore orogastric tube is used to aspirate gastric contents initially and then to lavage with doses of water at body temperature. Its effectiveness is unproven. Gastric lavage can be considered for up to 1 h after ingestion of a drug that is not absorbed by activated charcoal, such as lithium or iron salts.

Activated charcoal

This formulation of charcoal has a large adsorbent area and is given as a suspension in water. Activated charcoal adsorbs or binds the drug and retains it in the gastrointestinal lumen. Not all drugs are adsorbed onto charcoal (see Table 53.5). About 10 g of charcoal is required for every 1 g of poison, which makes it impractical for poisons that are usually ingested in large quantities. For suitable drugs, an initial dose of 50 g of charcoal for adults can prevent absorption if given within 1 h of drug ingestion (later after poisoning with modified-release preparations, or drugs with antimuscarinic properties that delay gastric emptying). Charcoal should not be given to drowsy or comatose persons because of the risk of aspiration into the lungs. Constipation is the major unwanted effect of charcoal; charcoal should not be given in the absence of bowel sounds, because of the risk of bowel obstruction.

ELIMINATION OF POISONS

There are three principal methods of enhancing elimination of the drug: activated charcoal, renal elimination and haemodialysis/haemoperfusion.

Table 53.5 Drug adsorption onto activated charcoal

Drugs/compounds not adsorbed	Drugs/compounds adsorbed
Acids	Aspirin
Alkalis	Carbamazepine
Cyanide	Dapsone
DDT (insecticide)	Digoxin
Ethanol	Ecstasy
Ethylene glycol (antifreeze)	Paraquat (herbicide)
Ferrous salts	Phenobarbital
Lead	Quinine
Lithium	Sustained-release
Mercury	preparations
Methanol	Theophylline
Organic solvents	Tricyclic antidepressants

Activated charcoal

Repeated administration of 50 g of activated charcoal every 4 h for up to 24–36 h achieves further retention of adsorbed drug in the small intestine. Drug is continuously being transferred in both directions across the gut wall, with the concentration gradient normally favouring net absorption, owing to the high concentration free in solution within the gut lumen. If drug in the bowel is bound onto the charcoal, this lowers the free concentration and can result in net transfer from the body into the gut and thereby enhance elimination of the compound. Repeated-dose activated charcoal is useful for overdose with phenobarbital, carbamazepine, dapsone, quinine and theophylline.

Renal elimination

Altering urine pH, while maintaining normal urine flow, can be effective in increasing the renal elimination of drugs that are weak electrolytes. Modification of urine pH to increase the extent of ionisation of the drug will reduce reabsorption from the renal tubule (Ch. 2). Only a modest increase in urinary flow rate is required. Weak acids, such as salicylates, are excreted more readily when urine is alkalinised (alkaline diuresis, achieved by giving sodium bicarbonate),

Forced diuresis with intravenous infusion of large quantities of fluid was advocated in the past for drugs or toxic metabolites that are mostly eliminated unchanged by the kidney. However, serious disturbances of fluid or electrolyte balance can occur, and therefore it is no longer recommended.

Haemodialysis

This is reserved for the most severely poisoned individuals. The technique is only successful if a large proportion of the body burden of the drug is retained in the plasma and available for removal (i.e. the drug has a low apparent volume of distribution). Haemodialysis relies on diffusion of the drug from the blood across a semi-permeable membrane into the dialysis fluid; it is used for salicylates, phenobarbital, methanol, ethylene glycol, sodium valproate and lithium.

Specific antidotes

Antidotes are available for only a minority of the drugs commonly involved in poisoning cases. Some important examples are given below.

Competitive receptor antagonists

- Atropine acts at muscarinic receptors to block the parasympathetic effects of excess acetylcholine caused when organophosphate insecticides irreversibly inhibit acetylcholinesterase. It is given by intravenous or intramuscular injection.
- Naloxone acts at opioid receptors to reverse the effects of opioid analgesics. Its short half-life, compared with those of most opioids, means that repeated injections or preferably an infusion is usually needed. Naloxone can precipitate acute withdrawal in someone who is dependent on opioids.
- Flumazenil is an antagonist of benzodiazepine action on γ-aminobutyric acid type A (GABA$_A$) receptors. It is given intravenously, but is rarely needed for the treatment of intentional benzodiazepine overdose because fatalities are uncommon with this class of drug. Flumazenil can cause seizures in benzodiazepine-dependent individuals. It is used to reverse the effects of benzodiazepines when toxicity occurs in people with chronic liver disease.

Chelating agents

Chelating agents act by forming a complex with the drug or chemical, thereby reducing its free (active) concentration:

- desferrioxamine for iron salts; given by intravenous infusion,
- dicobalt edetate for cyanide; given by intravenous injection,
- sodium calcium edetate for lead; given by intravenous infusion,
- sodium nitrite, together with sodium thiosulphate, for cyanide; both given by intravenous injection.

Compounds that affect drug metabolism

- Fomepizole (available by special order) is a competitive inhibitor of alcohol dehydrogenase given by intravenous injection as the treatment of choice in methanol or ethylene glycol poisoning; it blocks the formation of their toxic metabolites formaldehyde and glycoaldehyde respectively. Alternatively, with caution, their formation can be slowed with oral or intravenous ethanol, which is a preferential substrate for alcohol dehydrogenase with less toxic metabolites.
- Acetylcysteine provides a substrate for conjugation of the cytotoxic metabolite of paracetamol (NAPQI) when the natural conjugating ligand, glutathione, is depleted (see below).

Antibodies

Digoxin can be neutralised in severe poisoning by specific antibody fragments. The antibodies are raised in sheep and cleaved to remove the antigenic crystalline (Fc) portion of the molecule while retaining the specific antigen-binding fragment (Fab).

SOME SPECIFIC COMMON POISONINGS

PARACETAMOL

Paracetamol overdose can be fatal, with about 150 deaths occurring each year in England and Wales. Metabolism of paracetamol takes place in the liver, mainly producing nontoxic conjugates (Fig. 53.3). A small amount is oxidised by the cytochrome P450 system to the reactive intermediate NAPQI, which is normally inactivated by conjugation with the thiol group of glutathione. When hepatic glutathione is depleted by paracetamol overdose, oxidative stress coupled with NAPQI-mediated denaturation of proteins produces hepatic necrosis. Similar processes in the kidney can cause renal tubular necrosis.

In the first 24 h there are few symptoms apart from nausea, vomiting, abdominal pain and sweating, which usually resolve. Liver damage begins within 24 h of a large overdose, producing right upper quadrant pain and tenderness. Jaundice is apparent by 36–48 h and liver damage is maximal by 3–4 days. Severe liver failure, requiring transplantation for survival, can ensue. The most sensitive measures of liver damage are the prothrombin time, or the international normalised ratio (INR), and the plasma unconjugated bilirubin. Renal failure is seen in about a quarter of cases with severe liver damage.

Activated charcoal in large doses is recommended within 1 h of a potentially serious paracetamol overdose. Because antidotes are most effective when given early, blood should be analysed for paracetamol if there is any suspicion of poisoning. Blood should be taken at 4 h or more after the suspected overdose. Earlier sampling is not informative because a low plasma level at that time could reflect incomplete absorption of a large overdose, rather than ingestion of a small overdose. Antidotes used in paracetamol poisoning, such as acetylcysteine and methionine, are used to replace glutathione as a thiol donor in the liver; glutathione itself is not used, because it cannot enter liver cells from the blood.

Intravenous acetylcysteine is the preferred treatment for potentially serious poisoning, and should be started prior to the analysis of a plasma paracetamol concentration. Methionine can be given orally if acetylcysteine is not available, but not with or after activated charcoal, because methionine can compete with paracetamol for adsorption. Methionine should not be used if there is vomiting, or started more than 10–12 h after ingestion of paracetamol, since the efficacy of methionine in late poisoning is unknown.

A graph is available (Fig. 53.8) to indicate the risk of liver damage for a given plasma paracetamol concentration related to the time after ingestion. Plasma concentrations after 15 h must be interpreted by extrapolation of the graph. Treatment is necessary if potentially toxic paracetamol concentrations are detected. However, after a staggered overdose or when the time of the overdose is unknown the plasma concentration is uninterpretable and treatment should always be given.

Treatment used to be confined to the first 15 h after overdose, but liver damage can be reduced even when the antidote is delayed for up to 36 h.

SALICYLATES

Salicylate poisoning is now uncommon in the UK. Aspirin is hydrolysed rapidly to salicylic acid after absorption, but further metabolism by conjugation with glycine is rate-limited. Symptoms of toxicity are nausea, vomiting, abdominal pain, tinnitus, deafness, hyperventilation and sweating. Agitation frequently occurs in adults, but children become comatose. The chain of metabolic events produced by aspirin is shown in Figure 53.9.

Activated charcoal is recommended for reducing absorption if given early. Correction of fluid, electrolyte and acid–base balance is fundamental to successful management; a fluid deficit of 3–4 L is not unusual in severe poisoning. Forced alkaline diuresis is no longer advocated to

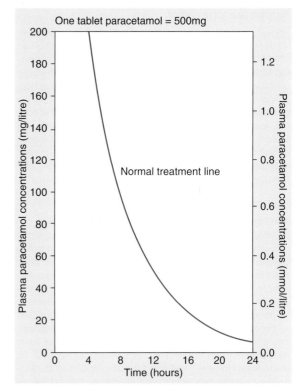

Fig. 53.8 Relationship between plasma paracetamol concentration and the risk of liver damage.

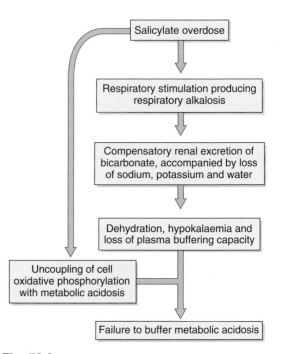

Fig. 53.9 The metabolic consequences of salicylate overdose.

enhance salicylate elimination (see above); simple alkalinisation of the urine with 1.26% oral sodium bicarbonate solution to raise the pH above 7.5 is effective and safer. Haemodialysis is the treatment of choice in severe poisoning, especially if there is severe metabolic acidosis.

TRICYCLIC ANTIDEPRESSANTS

Approximately 400 deaths per year occur in England and Wales from overdose with tricyclic antidepressants. The antimuscarinic effects of tricyclic antidepressants delay gastric emptying and oral activated charcoal is used routinely for up to 4 h after the overdose. Drowsiness and confusion are followed by seizures and coma in more severe poisoning. Cardiac depression can produce hypotension. Serious arrhythmias, such as ventricular tachycardia, can occur, and ECG monitoring is recommended for at least 24 h. If there is widening of the QRS complex on the ECG, then intravenous infusion of sodium bicarbonate can prevent or treat arrhythmias. Antiarrhythmic drugs should usually be avoided.

OPIOID ANALGESICS

The triad of signs characteristic of opioid overdose are:

- respiratory depression,
- pinpoint pupils,
- impaired consciousness.

They can be reversed rapidly by administration of naloxone (Ch. 19), which is a competitive antagonist at opioid μ-receptors. After an initial intravenous bolus dose of naloxone it is often necessary to give repeated boluses or a continuous infusion, because the half-life of naloxone is very short compared with those of most opioids. In poisoning with buprenorphine the effect of naloxone is often incomplete, and assisted ventilation may also be needed. Acute poisoning with organophosphorus insecticides can produce signs that are similar to those with opioids, but naloxone will have no effect.

BETA-ADRENOCEPTOR ANTAGONISTS

Poisoning by β-adrenoceptor antagonists usually presents with bradycardia and hypotension. More severe effects, including coma and convulsions, can occur with some drugs in this class. Treatment of the bradycardia is with intravenous atropine, which may increase the blood pressure. Cardiogenic shock that does not respond to atropine should initially be treated with intravenous glucagon, which has a positive inotropic effect. A temporary cardiac pacemaker may be necessary.

ECSTASY

Ecstasy (3,4-methylenedioxymetamfetamine, MDMA) toxicity is characterised by tachycardia, hyperreflexia, hyperpyrexia and initial hypertension followed by hypotension. In severe cases, delirium, seizures, coma and cardiac dysrhythmias may occur. MDMA is metabolised by CYP2D6 and genetic differences in this enzyme may result in wide inter-individual differences in susceptibility to the toxic effects of MDMA. Some people may present with hyponatraemia, possibly as a result of drinking excessive water as a precaution to prevent dehydration. Treatments include activated charcoal, but only for up to 2 h post-ingestion, since MDMA is absorbed rapidly, and diazepam for agitation or seizures.

SELF-ASSESSMENT

True/false questions

1. The therapeutic index (TI) is the ratio between the dose of a drug that results in significant toxicity and the dose that provides a therapeutic response.
2. Mesna reduces the cytotoxic effects of cyclophosphamide on the bladder.
3. Acidification of the urine (acid diuresis) enhances excretion of aspirin.
4. Flumazenil is a GABA$_A$ receptor antagonist.
5. Fomepizole accelerates the breakdown of methanol.

Case-based questions

A 70-year-old man with a history of depressive illness and alcohol abuse was prescribed a compound analgesic containing 30 mg codeine phosphate and 500 mg paracetamol (co-codamol 30/500) for back pain. Eight hours after collecting his prescription he was seen as an emergency by his GP, who considered the man had taken an overdose and admitted him to hospital.

A. What features might be seen soon after the overdosage and during the subsequent 24–48 h?
B. Outline suitable pharmacological treatments that should be undertaken.
C. Would co-dydramol have been a safer alternative to prescribe?

True/false answers

1. **True.** A high TI is a desirable property of a drug as it indicates that significant toxicity.
2. **True.** Mesna (mercaptoethane sulphonic acid) is a thiol donor which protects against haemorrhagic cystitis when administered with the cytotoxic drug cyclophosphamide.
3. **False.** Acidification of the urine would enhance excretion of weak bases. Weak acids such as aspirin are ionised by alkalinisation of the urine, so less is reabsorbed from the renal tubule.
4. **True.** Flumazenil is a competitive GABA$_A$ receptor antagonist that can be given intravenously in benzodiazepine overdose.
5. **False.** Fomepizole inhibits the metabolism of methanol by alcohol dehydrogenase, slowing the formation of its toxic metabolites formaldehyde and formic acid.

Case-based answers

A. Initial features would be those of opioid overdosage caused by the codeine, with possible symptoms of respiratory depression, pinpoint pupils, coma and cardiovascular collapse. Later symptoms of nausea, abdominal pain and sweating and, if untreated, jaundice, are due to liver damage caused by the toxic metabolite of paracetamol.

B. Naloxone is a rapid reversible antagonist of opioids at μ-, κ- and δ-receptors. It has a short half-life and may have to be given repeatedly. Acetylcysteine conjugates with the hepatotoxic metabolite of paracetamol (*N*-acetyl-*p*-benzoquinone imine, NAPQI) and is most effective when given early after an overdosage; the risk of liver damage is related to the time of ingestion before treatment and the plasma paracetamol concentrations. Chronic alcohol consumption would increase the toxic effects of codeine and paracetamol; alcohol enhances the central depressant actions of the opioid and also induces cytochrome P450 enzymes, increasing formation of NAPQI and causing toxicity at lower paracetamol doses. The toxicity of paracetamol would also be increased by other cytochrome P450-inducing drugs.

C. Codydramol contains paracetamol with the opioid dihydrocodeine and is likely to produce similar unwanted effects to co-codamol in overdose.

FURTHER READING

Adam J, Pichler WJ, Yerly D (2011) Delayed hypersensitivity: models of T-cell stimulation. *Br J Clin Pharmacol* 71, 701–707

Aronson JK (2009) Medication errors: definitions and classification. *Br J Clin Pharmacol* 67, 599–604

Ardern–Jones MR, Friedmann PS (2011) Skin manifestations of drug allergy. *Br J Clin Pharmacol* 71, 672–683

Buckley NA, Dawson AH, Whyte IM, O'Connell DL (1995) Relative toxicity of benzodiazepines in overdose. *BMJ* 310, 219–221

Dawson AH, Whyte IM (2001) Therapeutic drug monitoring in drug overdose. *Br J Clin Pharmacol* 52 (suppl 1), 97S–102S

Edwards IR, Aronson JK (2000) Adverse drug reactions: definitions, diagnosis and management. *Lancet* 356, 1255–1259

Ferner RE, Dear JW, Bateman DN (2011) Management of paracetamol poisoning. *BMJ* 342, d2218

Frew A (2011) General principles of investigating and managing drug allergy. *Br J Clin Pharmacol* 71, 642–646

Heard KJ (2008) Acetylcysteine for acetominophen poisoning. *N Engl J Med* 359, 285–292

Jick SS, Dean AD, Jick H (1995) Antidepressants and suicide. *BMJ* 310, 215–218

Lee WM (1995) Drug-induced hepatotoxicity. *N Engl J Med* 333, 1118–1127

Park BK, Kitteringham NR, Pirmohamed M, Tucker GT (1996) Relevance of induction of human drug-metabolising enzymes: pharmacological and toxicological implications. *Br J Clin Pharmacol* 41, 477–491

Park BK, Kitteringham NR, Powell H, Pirmohamed M (2000) Advances in molecular toxicology–towards understanding idiosyncratic drug toxicity. *Toxicology* 153, 39–60

Thong B Y-H, Tan T-C (2011) Epidemiology and risk factors for drug allergy. *Br J Clin Pharmacol* 71, 684–700

Vale JA, Proudfoot AT (1995) Paracetamol (acetaminophen) poisoning. *Lancet* 346, 547–552

Waring RH, Emery P (1995) The genetic origin of responses to drugs. *Br Med Bull* 51, 449–461

Compendium: drugs used to treat drug toxicity and drug overdose, and drugs used to treat toxicity due to environmental chemicals

Drug	Kinetics (half-life)	Comments
Drugs used to treat drug toxicity and drug overdose		
Acetylcysteine	Deacetylated to cysteine by the liver (5–6 h)	Used for paracetamol overdose; given by intravenous infusion
Charcoal activated	Not absorbed	Taken orally for a range of drug overdoses (see Table 53.5); adsorbs drug and reduces absorption
Methionine	Metabolised by normal pathways of amino acid metabolism	Used for paracetamol overdose; given orally
Naloxone	Half-life (1–1.5 h) shorter than that of morphine; eliminated by glucuronidation	Opioid antagonist used to treat opioid overdose; administered by injection; rapid onset of action (1–2 min)
Drugs used to treat toxicity due to environmental chemicals		
Iron poisoning/overload (see also Ch. 47)		
Desferrioxamine (deferoxamine) mesilate	Slowly eliminated in urine and by metabolism and chelation (6 h)	Given by continuous intravenous infusion
Cyanide poisoning		
Dicobalt edetate	Renal excretion	Chelating agent; given by intravenous injection
Hydroxocobalamin	Binds cyanide to form cyanocobolamin; urinary excretion (26 h)	Given by intravenous injection
Sodium nitrite	Oxidation to nitrate	Given by intravenous injection
Sodium thiosulphate	Acts as sulphur donor for conversion of cyanide to thiocyanate, which is excreted in urine	Given by intravenous injection
Heavy metals		
Dimercaprol	Drug–metal complexes are excreted in about 4 h	Largely superseded by other chelating agents; given by intramuscular injection
Sodium calcium edetate	Renal excretion	Chelating agent; used for various metals, especially lead; given by intravenous infusion
Organophosphate pesticides		
Pralidoxime	Hepatic metabolism and renal excretion (1 h)	Reactivates acetylcholinesterase (see Ch. 4); given by slow intravenous injection

54 Substance abuse and dependence

● ●

Substance abuse is characterised by compulsive drug-seeking and drug-taking behaviour and an inability to control intake (addiction); there may also be symptoms of withdrawal when the drug becomes unavailable (dependence).

Dependence-inducing drugs are mind modifying substances. They may be taken recreationally, initially because of the pleasurable effect they produce, but later to avoid unpleasant withdrawal symptoms. Dependence produces different degrees of need for the drug, from mild desire to an intense craving.

In other cases, the drug is initially prescribed to treat a medical problem.

THE BIOLOGICAL BASIS OF DEPENDENCE

The mechanisms of drug dependence are relatively poorly understood but involve complex dysfunctional adaptations of the neurocircuits in the brain that subserve physiological motivation and reward processes. The mesolimbic pathway is central to these processes and, depending upon the particular stimulus and the functional status of the individual, its activation can result in a spectrum of response from slight mood elevation to intense pleasure or euphoria. Stimulation can result from a plethora of factors that are very personal, for example food intake, sexual activity and the controlled and occasional use of lifestyle drugs such as alcohol and nicotine.

ACUTE ACTIVATION OF THE MESOLIMBIC DOPAMINE REWARD PATHWAYS

The mesolimbic pathway consists of several structures:

- the ventral tegmental area, which communicates with the nucleus accumbens via the medial forebrain bundle,
- the nucleus accumbens,
- the amygdala (associated with emotions, especially fear and anxiety),
- the hippocampus (associated with memory).

The reward pathway is activated by impulses arising in the ventral tegmental area of the brain. These impulses are relayed through the medial forebrain bundle, via the nucleus accumbens, to the prefrontal cortex (Fig. 54.1). Activation of the ventral tegmental area results in dopamine release in the nucleus accumbens and stimulation of postsynaptic D_2 receptors (acting via inhibitory G_i proteins to inhibit the generation of intracellular cAMP). This is thought to be central to the processes of motivation and reward.

Occasional and limited administration of most drugs of potential abuse directly or indirectly releases dopamine in the nucleus accumbens (Fig. 54.1). For example, morphine enhances dopaminergic input to the nucleus accumbens by stimulating opioid receptors in the ventral tegmental area. This effect may eventually drive the processes, resulting in drug dependence, because with repeated use, the drug-related dopamine release becomes essential to maintain a 'normal' level of pleasure.

CHRONIC STIMULATION OF THE MESOLIMBIC DOPAMINE REWARD PATHWAYS

The complexities of the changes involved are daunting and only a limited description of these events is given here. Chronic exposure of the mesolimbic system to drugs such as opioids, alcohol and cocaine eventually leads to neuro-adaptive changes and sensitisation of the mesolimbic system to further drug administration. Upregulation of neuronal cAMP in the nucleus accumbens results from chronic exposure to many drugs of abuse, with increased intraneuronal cAMP response element-binding protein (CREB). Increased CREB in the nucleus accumbens is probably important for the development of tolerance and dependence. CREB also activates dysphoria-inducing κ-opioid receptors that bind the opioid peptide dynorphin (Ch. 19) on dopamine- and glutamate-releasing neurons in the prefrontal cortex. The long-term actions of dependence-inducing drugs also affect plasticity in the neural circuits of the reward pathway. Upregulation of transcription factors such as CREB and ΔFosB leads to long-term changes in brain-derived neurotrophic factor (BDNF), which regulates the number of dendrites on various neurons in the pathway. Therefore, the changes in the reward and stress systems in the brain that arise with addiction may become 'imprinted' even if the causative drug is stopped for long periods. This would explain the vulnerability to relapse after detoxification. There are probably genetic influences on the neurochemical events involved in the reward pathways and stress systems that also increase susceptibility to addiction.

Nicotine stimulates transiently then
inhibits GABA release

Opioids and cannabis inhibit GABA release
Alcohol and benzodiazepines activate
presynaptic GABA autoreceptors,
and inhibit GABA release

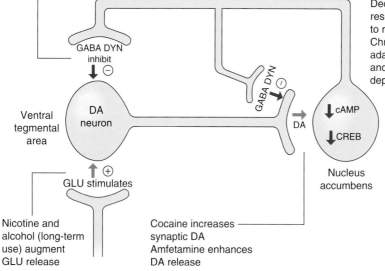

Decreased cAMP and CREB
results in pleasure and disposition
to repeat reward behaviours.
Chronic intake results in dysfunctional
adaptation with upregulation of cAMP
and CREB and DYN (a mechanism for
dependence and tolerance)

GABA DYN
inhibit

GABA DYN

Ventral
tegmental
area

DA
neuron

DA

cAMP

CREB

Nucleus
accumbens

GLU stimulates

Nicotine and
alcohol (long-term
use) augment
GLU release

Cocaine increases
synaptic DA
Amfetamine enhances
DA release

Fig. 54.1 **The role of dopamine and cAMP in reward pathways in the mesolimbic system and the relevance of these pathways to substance abuse.** This diagram illustrates only a small part of the complex mechanisms involved in the processes of reward and the ways that substances of abuse influence these pathways, leading to dependence and withdrawal effects. Dopaminergic neurons in the ventral tegmental area release dopamine (DA) at the nucleus accumbens, which decreases cAMP and its activation of the transcription factor, cAMP response element-binding protein (CREB). Many substances of abuse when administered acutely increase DA and consequently inhibit cAMP, providing the pleasurable and rewarding effects of the drug. However, chronic persistent intake eventually increases CREB and dynorphin (DYN), which will dampen reward mechanisms in the nucleus accumbens, providing a possible mechanism for drug dependence and tolerance (see further explanations in the text). GABA, γ-aminobutyric acid; GLU, glutamate.

Drug craving is also influenced by neural inputs to the 'reward' pathway from the amygdala, which are involved in emotion and conditioned responses. In particular, the amygdala is central to the reinforcing effects of drug binges and also the anxiety and negative effect involved in acute withdrawal. Conditioned responses provide powerful cues to drug-taking in specific social circumstances, and the conditioning is reinforced by aspects of the drug-taking process. Eventually, learning that a drug withdrawal can produce adverse effects that are relieved by the drug may lead to *any* source of stress or frustration becoming a cue for drug use. Dependence is associated with recruitment of stress systems in the brain on drug withdrawal, probably in an attempt to restore normal neuronal function. There is an elevation of corticotropin-releasing hormone (CRH) and noradrenaline, with suppression of the anti-stress neuropeptide Y.

In contrast, physical dependence on a drug is unrelated to activity in the mesolimbic system and arises from excessive noradrenergic output from the locus ceruleus, a structure in the base of the brain that is involved in arousal and vigilance.

This chapter covers drugs that are encountered in clinical practice primarily because of their abuse, such as ecstasy and cannabis, or because of their potential to cause dependence, such as nicotine and ethanol (Box 54.1).

Box 54.1	Common drugs of abuse

- Psychomotor stimulants
  - Cocaine
  - Amfetamine and derivatives
  - Nicotine
- Psychotomimetic agents
  - Hallucinogens, e.g. LSD, mescaline, psilocybin
  - Cannabis
  - Dissociative anaesthetics, e.g. ketamine, phencyclidine
- Central nervous system depressants
  - Alcohol (ethanol)
  - Benzodiazepines
  - Gamma-hydroxybutyric acid (GHB)
  - Inhaled solvents
- Opioids (see Ch. 19)

DRUGS OF ABUSE

PSYCHOMOTOR STIMULANTS

Several drugs that have central stimulant properties are abused and produce dependence. Those more commonly encountered are considered here.

Cocaine

Cocaine is an alkaloid obtained from the leaves of the coca plant. It is usually taken as the hydrochloride salt. 'Crack' cocaine is the free base form, named after the crackling sound produced when it is smoked.

Mechanism of action and effects

The psychomotor effects of cocaine are due to inhibition of reuptake transporters for monamines in presynaptic nerve terminals, particularly inhibiting the dopamine reuptake transporter (DAT), and to a lesser extent those for noradrenaline (NET) and serotonin (SERT). This in turn may activate opioid systems in the brain, with upregulation of μ-receptors (Ch. 19). Increased dopaminergic activity in the reward pathway promotes dependence. Changes in various pituitary neuroendocrine functions occur with more prolonged use; in particular, the release of corticotropin and luteinizing hormone (LH) are enhanced. Tolerance to the psychomotor effects of cocaine is limited. One of the metabolites of cocaine, norcocaine, has direct vasoconstrictor activity.

Effects of cocaine include:

- intense euphoria,
- alertness and wakefulness,
- increased confidence and strength,
- heightened sexual feelings,
- indifference to concerns and cares,
- anxiety, paranoia, restlessness and tactile hallucinations especially with habitual use,
- severe psychological, but not physical, dependence, brought about by the reinforcing effect of the rapid onset and brief duration of action; this develops particularly rapidly with 'crack' cocaine,
- despondency and despair rapidly follow withdrawal (the 'crash' or 'come down'). After chronic use, withdrawal can produce a dysphoric mood with fatigue, vivid dreams, insomnia, exhaustion, increased appetite and either psychomotor retardation or agitation, irritability and aggressive and stereotyped behaviour,
- toxic paranoid psychosis, with delusions of great stamina, occurs with chronic use,
- in overdose, excessive catecholamine concentrations produce convulsions, hypertension, cardiac rhythm disturbances and hyperthermia (due to excessive muscle activity and reduced heat loss); if severe, death can occur from respiratory depression and circulatory collapse. The cardiovascular toxicity can be treated with combined α- and β-adrenoceptor blockade, and seizures by intravenous diazepam,
- cocaine snuff produces necrosis of the nasal septum through its vasoconstrictor action,
- exposure in utero leads to impaired brain development and other teratogenic effects.

Pharmacokinetics

Cocaine, as the hydrochloride salt, is used orally, intranasally (cocaine snuff) or by intravenous injection; the intravenous route gives an intense and rapid onset of effect. 'Crack' cocaine is prepared by mixing cocaine hydrochloride with sodium bicarbonate or ammonia and water, then heating to volatilise the free base. The product is smoked and produces intense effects similar to intravenous use.

Cocaine is metabolised by plasma and liver esterases and its half-life is very short.

Management of cocaine dependence

There are no recognised drug treatments for cocaine dependence. Prolonged behavioural treatments remain the main approach. Tricyclic antidepressants (especially desipramine) are sometimes advocated for the severe depression that can occur on withdrawal.

Amfetamine and derivatives

Amfetamine, dexamfetamine, methamfetamine and 3,4-methylenedioxymetamfetamine (MDMA, 'ecstasy') have little medical value. Dexamfetamine is sometimes used as a treatment for attention deficit hyperactivity disorder (ADHD) (Ch. 22).

Mechanism of action and effects

Amfetamine and related drugs have indirect sympathomimetic effects, releasing monoamines from central nervous system (CNS) neurons (Ch. 4). They are taken up into presynaptic nerve terminals where they block vesicular uptake of dopamine, serotonin and noradrenaline by the vesicular monamine transporters (VMATs), increasing their concentrations in the cytoplasm. This induces release of the monoamines into the synapse by reversing the respective reuptake transporters for dopamine (DAT), serotonin (SERT) and noradrenaline (NET) in the neuronal membrane. CNS stimulation by amfetamine is most marked in the reticular formation although it also occurs in many other areas of the brain including the reward pathway. The D-isomer (dexamfetamine) is twice as potent as the L-isomer of amfetamine in its central stimulant activity. Effects of amfetamine include:

- euphoria, similar to that experienced with cocaine; this is particularly intense after intravenous use,
- increased self-confidence, reduced fatigue and increased alertness for repetitive tasks,
- anorexia,
- irritability, agitation,
- psychotic behaviour during repeated use over a few days or with acute intoxication, causing hallucinations, delusions of grandiosity, paranoia and aggressive behaviour and repetitive actions,
- acute intoxication can cause hyperthermia, cerebral haemorrhage. Other symptoms include panic, tremor, confusion, hallucinations and aggressiveness,
- peripheral sympathomimetic effects can lead to hypertension and cardiac arrhythmias,
- tolerance develops rapidly to some of the central effects of amfetamine, such as anorexia, presumably through central monoamine depletion; tolerance to the euphoric effects and motor stimulation is slower,
- withdrawal leads to prolonged sleep, followed by fatigue, depression and increased appetite. Other symptoms include anxiety, craving, headaches, restlessness and vivid dreams.

MDMA (ecstasy) is more selective than amfetamine for serotonin release, and produces euphoria similar to that of amfetamine but with less stimulant activity. Direct agonism of serotonin (5-hydroxytryptamine) $5\text{-}HT_1$ or $5\text{-}HT_2$ receptors may contribute to its effects, including release of oxytocin associated with the euphoric action. Disturbance of thermoregulatory homeostasis occurs, leading to a syndrome resembling heat stroke with hyperthermia and dehydration, usually after exertion in hot environments. Stimulation of antidiuretic hormone release can cause thirst and water retention with subsequent water intoxication and hyponatraemia. The toxic effects of MDMA include cardiac arrhythmias, seizures, muscle damage and severe metabolic acidosis, which may be fatal. The long-term toxicity may include memory impairment, anxiety or depression.

Pharmacokinetics

Although amfetamine is sometimes used intravenously or via nasal inhalation, absorption from the gut is rapid and complete. Amfetamine readily crosses the blood–brain barrier. About half is excreted unchanged in the urine and the rest is metabolised in the liver. Amfetamine is a basic drug and its half-life varies according to urine flow and pH; at low urine pH, greater ionisation of amfetamine increases its excretion, producing a shorter half-life, whereas at high urine pH the half-life is longer because of greater reabsorption of the non-ionised drug in the renal tubule. Metabolites of amfetamine are believed to contribute to the psychotic effects seen with long-term use.

Ecstasy is usually taken orally. It undergoes hepatic metabolism via CYP2D6, and polymorphism of this enzyme may explain some of the serious intoxication that occurs with the drug, although the half-life does not differ much between poor and extensive metabolisers (about 5 h in both).

Management of amfetamine dependence

There are no recognized treatments for amfetamine dependence, which relies on behavioural therapies.

Cathinone stimulants

Mechanism of action

Cathinone and cathine are derived from the khat plant, and there are several similar synthetic compounds such as mephedrone, methylone and flephedrone that are used recreationally. They probably stimulate release of monoamines from neuronal vesicles and inhibit their reuptake. Their psychoactive and physical effects resemble those of amfetamines. They are used intranasally or orally, although they can be injected, smoked or taken rectally.

Pharmacokinetics

They are metabolised in the liver, but there is little information about their pharmacokinetics. They have short half-lives in animal studies.

Nicotine and tobacco

Mechanism of action

Over 300 chemical compounds are present in tobacco smoke, but the actions of nicotine are central to the addictive pharmacological effects of smoking. Nicotine has dose-related peripheral actions. At low doses, stimulation of aortic and carotid chemoreceptors enhances sympathetic nervous system activity, and at higher doses there is direct stimulation of the nicotinic N_1 receptors in autonomic ganglia (Ch. 4). At even higher doses, nicotine acts as a ganglion-blocking agent. Initial stimulation of autonomic nervous tissue is therefore followed by depression. Effects on the CNS are mediated by presynaptic nicotinic receptors structurally distinct from those in the periphery. Stimulation of CNS nicotinic receptors increases neuronal permeability to Na^+ or Ca^{2+} and enhances the release of glutamate, which promotes dopamine release. With prolonged use nicotine inhibits the release of γ-aminobutyric acid (GABA). Nicotinic receptors are found in the mesocortical and mesolimbic dopaminergic systems, in projections from the ventral forebrain to the cortex that mediate arousal and in hippocampal projections where stimulation enhances learning and short-term memory. Tolerance to the CNS effects of nicotine is rapid due to receptor desensitisation.

Effects of nicotine and tobacco

Tobacco components, including nicotine, have effects on a number of organ systems.

Respiratory effects

The lungs are the first area to be in contact with the chemical components of tobacco smoke and are also exposed to particles and gases. Tars and other irritants, rather than nicotine, are responsible for the chronic damage to the lungs.

- An increase in blood carboxyhaemoglobin concentration (from carbon monoxide in tobacco smoke) decreases oxygen-carrying capacity. This may be important in ischaemic heart disease, increasing the chance of provoking angina.
- Increased mucus secretion, with reduced activity of bronchial cilia and consequent decreased clearance of lung secretions, leads to chronic bronchitis.
- Progressive destruction of the supporting tissue in the bronchioles produces emphysema and chronic obstructive pulmonary disease (COPD). Smoking is now the major cause of this condition.
- The risk of lung cancer is increased to about 20 times that of a non-smoker. Inhalation of tobacco smoke is a major contributory factor and explains the greater risk in cigarette smokers. Giving up smoking reduces the risk progressively over about 10 years of abstinence. The constituent of tobacco smoke responsible for altering DNA structure and initiating the cancer process remains controversial, but the relationship between smoking and lung cancer has been confirmed by numerous epidemiological studies. Compared with non-smokers, passive smokers also have a 20–25% increased risk of lung cancer.

Cardiovascular effects

- Stimulation of the autonomic nervous system and sensory receptors in the heart increases heart rate, blood pressure and cardiac output.
- The risk of cardiovascular disease is increased by smoking cigarettes, but not by pipe and cigar smoking,

and it occurs at a younger age. The overall risk of death from coronary artery disease is doubled in smokers compared with non-smokers, and the magnitude of the effect is related to the numbers of cigarettes smoked. Peripheral vascular disease and stroke are also increased. Even passive smokers have an excess risk of vascular disease of 25%. The major reason for the excess of events is accelerated formation of atheromatous plaques and enhanced platelet aggregability. The risk of vascular disease falls over the first 3–5 years after stopping smoking to a level close to that of non-smokers.

Psychological effects

The psychological effects of smoking are substantial, as indicated by the difficulties experienced by those attempting to quit.

- Decreased appetite, with weight gain on stopping smoking.
- Emotional dependence on nicotine and the physical act of smoking is powerful. Physical withdrawal is less marked than psychological withdrawal but includes restlessness, irritability, anxiety, depression, difficulty concentrating, sleep disturbance and increased appetite.

Other effects

Nicotine and smoking have a number of other effects.

- Peptic ulceration is twice as common in smokers.
- Smoking is a risk factor for osteoporosis.
- Smoking in pregnancy, especially during the second half, has several effects. The most important are an increased risk of a low-birth-weight child and increased perinatal mortality. The vasoconstrictor effects of nicotine are responsible. Physical and mental development is slowed in children born to mothers who smoked during pregnancy.
- Smoking induces several hepatic cytochrome P450 isoenzymes and increases the clearance of CYP1A2 substrates such as theophylline (Ch. 12) and imipramine (Ch. 22).

Pharmacokinetics of nicotine

Nicotine can be absorbed from the mouth in its non-ionised form, which is found in the less acidic environment of cigar and pipe tobacco smoke. Cigarette smoke, which is acidic, ionises nicotine, which can only be absorbed in significant amounts from the lungs. About 10% of the nicotine from a cigarette is absorbed, but at a faster rate than from cigars or a pipe owing to the larger surface area of the lungs, and results in a higher but less prolonged peak plasma concentration. Nicotine can also be absorbed transdermally. It is metabolised in the liver; the major metabolite, cotinine, has a much longer half-life (about 10–40 h) than nicotine (0.5–2 h) and its concentration in plasma, saliva or urine can be used as a monitor of smoking behaviour.

Dependence on and withdrawal from nicotine

Withdrawal is often difficult to achieve unless motivation is high. Smokers should be supported by counselling about the health benefits of quitting and advice on overcoming problems such as weight gain. Behavioural therapy as an aid to quitting has a success rate of 20% at 1 year. Pharmacotherapy is often used to reduce the intensity of withdrawal symptoms.

Nicotine-replacement therapy

Smokers usually adjust their smoking habit to maintain plasma nicotine concentrations just above a threshold that averts withdrawal symptoms. The plasma concentration falls rapidly within 1–2 h of the last cigarette, and rather more slowly after smoking a cigar or pipe. The resultant craving for nicotine can be reduced by nicotine replacement, delivered via transdermal patches, sublingual tablets, chewing gum, an inhaler (with most absorption occurring in the mouth) or a nasal spray. The delivery method determines the rate at which plasma nicotine concentrations increase, and is most rapid after the nasal spray. The individual can choose the most appropriate vehicle for his or her needs and preferences. Established cardiovascular disease is a caution for, but not a contraindication to, nicotine-replacement therapy. Behavioural therapy enhances the success rate achieved by nicotine-replacement therapy. Use of nicotine-replacement therapy doubles the chance of achieving abstinence.

Bupropion

This is an atypical antidepressant. Most antidepressants are ineffective for smoking cessation, but the use of bupropion gives smoking cessation rates equal to, or slightly greater than, nicotine-replacement therapy. Treatment should be started 1–2 weeks before a 'quit date'. Used together with nicotine-replacement therapy bupropion produces a modest increase in the chance of stopping. An additional benefit is that smokers who use bupropion as an aid to quitting are less likely to gain weight. Bupropion is a weak inhibitor of neuronal reuptake of noradrenaline and dopamine, and probably works by enhancing mesolimbic dopaminergic activity. It is given as a modified-release formulation and has a long half-life (24 h). Elimination is by hepatic metabolism, which also generates active metabolites. Unwanted effects include anxiety, headache, insomnia and dry mouth. There is an increased risk of epileptic seizures, and bupropion should be avoided if there is a past history of seizures. Nortriptyline is probably as effective as bupropion for smoking cessation.

Varenicline

This is a partial agonist at nicotine receptors, with high selectivity for the CNS receptor subtype involved in addiction. It produces about 30–45% of the response expected from nicotine, and blocks the effect of added nicotine. The modest release of dopamine reduces craving and nicotine withdrawal symptoms. Treatment should be started 1–2 weeks before a 'quit date', and combined with behavioural support. The oral bioavailability of varenicline has not been defined; it is excreted unchanged by the kidney and has a half-life of 24 h. Unwanted effects include gastrointestinal disturbances, dry mouth, headache, dizziness, drowsiness and sleep disturbance. Depression with suicidal thoughts has also been reported.

PSYCHOTOMIMETIC AGENTS

Hallucinogens

Lysergic acid diethylamide (LSD), psilocybin ('magic mushrooms'), mescaline (from peyote cactus) and the synthetic drug dimethyltryptamine (DMT) are adrenergic hallucinogens that have structural similarities to monoamine neurotransmitters. LSD is the most potent hallucinogen.

Mechanism of action and effects

The actions of hallucinogens on the brain are probably related to postsynaptic 5-HT$_2$ receptor stimulation in the cerebral cortex and locus coeruleus, a region of the midbrain that receives sensory signals. LSD also produces presynaptic 5-HT$_{1A}$ receptor blockade in the dorsal raphe neurons, inhibiting firing of neuronal projections to the forebrain. Tolerance to LSD occurs rapidly, and appears to be related to downregulation of these receptors. The actions of LSD, psilocybin and mescaline are similar, and they share several properties, including cross-tolerance.

- Visual hallucinations are frequent, especially with high doses, and auditory acuity is accentuated. There may be an overlap of sensory impressions such that music is 'seen' or colours 'heard', which can produce severe anxiety. Time appears to pass slowly. Emotions are altered, with either elation or depression, and rapid mood swings can occur. The overall experience can produce a good or a bad 'trip', and can vary in the same individual on different occasions.
- Serious psychotic reactions can occasionally occur, and long-term psychotic disorders can be precipitated. The other unpleasant persistent effect in some individuals is 'flashback', seeing bright flashes, or halos or trails attached to moving objects.
- Physical consequences of CNS stimulation include dizziness, weakness, drowsiness and paraesthesiae.
- Excessive sympathetic nervous system stimulation with large doses produces nausea, salivation, lacrimation, dizziness, mydriasis, tremor, hyperthermia, tachycardia and hypertension.
- Tolerance can occur within 5 days.
- Emotional dependence is frequent, but physical dependence is not seen.

Pharmacokinetics

Oral absorption of these drugs is good. Physical effects begin after about 20 min, but psychoactive effects are delayed for 2–4 h and then last up to 12 h. DMT has a rapid onset of hallucinogenic action, within 15–30 min, but the duration is only 1–2 h. Elimination is by hepatic metabolism and the half-lives are short.

Cannabis

Cannabis can be smoked as marijuana, which consists of dried leaves or flowers of the *Cannabis sativa* (hemp) plant, or as a resin extracted from the leaves of the plant and then dried, known as hashish. Solvent extraction of the resin produces cannabis oil, which can be added to tobacco. The hallucinogenic effects of cannabis are much less marked than those of the aminergic hallucinogens such as LSD.

Mechanism of action and effects

The constituent compounds (cannabinoids) interact with specific CB$_1$ receptors in the brain. These receptors are coupled to G$_i$ proteins that reduce intracellular cAMP production, and inhibit cell membrane Ca^{2+} and K$^+$ channels. The natural ligands are the arachidonic acid derivatives anandamide, 2-arachidonylglycerol and noladin ether. CB$_1$ receptors are found in greatest density in areas of the brain involved in cognition and pain recognition (cerebral cortex), memory (hippocampus), reward (mesolimbic system) and motor coordination (substantia nigra and cerebellum).

- The psychomotor effects result largely from tetrahydrocannabinol (THC) and one of its metabolites, 11-hydroxy-THC, which produce euphoria, heightened intensity of sensations, and relaxation. Occasionally panic reactions, hallucinations and depersonalisation can occur. Psychotic reactions are rare except in predisposed individuals, but the use of cannabis increases the risk of developing schizophrenia. Recent memory is markedly impaired and complex mental tests are executed less well, although the user may perceive that their performance is enhanced. Motor incoordination may affect driving ability.
- Effects on the cardiovascular system include tachycardia and increased systolic blood pressure with a postural fall.
- The tars inhaled during chronic use of cannabis predispose to heart disease, chronic bronchitis and lung cancer.
- THC has an anti-emetic action (Ch. 32), which may be useful during cancer chemotherapy (Ch. 52).
- Cannabinoids have analgesic effects that are used by some people with multiple sclerosis to control neuropathic pain.
- Tolerance to the psychomotor effects of cannabis occurs with regular use, and there is evidence of dependence.

Pharmacokinetics

Metabolism of THC is extensive, with some active metabolites being produced. The high lipid solubility of THC means that absorption from the lung or gut is high, and it has a large apparent volume of distribution; however, because of its very rapid metabolism its half-life is only 1.5 h. The psychomotor effects last for 2–3 h after inhalation.

Dissociative anaesthetics

Phencyclidine (PCP) and ketamine differ from adrenergic hallucinogens in their mode of action. Both drugs were developed as anaesthetics, but PCP was withdrawn because of severe adverse effects (hallucinations, mania, delirium and disorientation).

Mechanism of action and effects

Both drugs block the excitatory effects of glutamate at *N*-methyl-ᴅ-aspartate (NMDA) receptors. These receptors are abundant in the cortex, basal ganglia and sensory pathways of the CNS. PCP also releases dopamine from nerve terminals in a manner similar to amfetamine. The term dissociative anaesthetic refers to the feelings of detachment (dissociation) from the environment and self that are produced by the drugs. These are not true hallucinations.

- Acute effects include euphoria, decreased inhibition, a feeling of immense power, analgesia, altered perception of time and space, and depersonalisation. Ketamine creates a 'mellow, colourful wonderworld'.
- Catatonic rigidity can occur, followed by ataxia and slurring of speech.
- Adverse experiences include confusion, restlessness, disorientation and impaired judgement. Irritability, paranoia, depression and anxiety are also common. Psychotic reactions are precipitated in susceptible people.
- Ketamine can produce near-death experiences.
- Persistent abuse of PCP leads to memory loss, speech and thought difficulties, and depression that persist for months after the last use.
- Tolerance is unusual, but psychological dependence occurs.

Pharmacokinetics

PCP is rapidly absorbed from the gut, nose or lungs after smoking. Effects are seen within minutes of ingestion and usually last 4–6 h. It is a weak base that is excreted in the urine. It is also excreted into the stomach, and reabsorbed by the small intestine. The half-life is variable and can be up to 2 days. Ketamine is abused intravenously. It is metabolised in the liver and has a short half-life (see Ch. 17).

CNS DEPRESSANTS

Alcohol (ethyl alcohol, ethanol)

Mechanism of action and effects

Alcohol has multiple actions on the CNS. Non-specific actions such as increased fluidity of neuronal cell membranes (cf. general anaesthetics) may be important by reducing Ca^{2+} flux across the cell membrane, but several other actions have been described (Box 54.2). Overall, alcohol facilitates central inhibitory neurotransmission, particularly enhancing the effects of GABA, and therefore it is a general CNS depressant. With acute alcohol intake there is an initial depression of inhibitory neurons, particularly in

 Box 54.2 **Possible mechanisms of action of alcohol**

Activation of GABA$_A$ receptors
Inhibition of glutamate NMDA receptors
Activation of serotonin and opioid receptors
Inhibition of monoamine oxidase B in neurons
Inhibition of Na$^+$/K$^+$-ATPase in neuronal membranes
Increased neuronal adenylyl cyclase activity
Decreased intracellular phosphatidylinositol system
   activity, leading to reduced Ca^{2+} availability

Box 54.3 **Alcoholic content of alcoholic drinks**

1 unit of alcohol is about 10 g and is found in:
½ pint of normal-strength beer, lager, cider
⅓ pint of strong beer, lager, cider
⅕ pint of extra-strong beer, lager, cider
1 glass of wine (8 units per 75 cl bottle)
1 small measure of sherry (13 units per bottle)
1 standard measure of spirits (30 units per bottle)
⅔ bottle of 'alcopop'

the mesolimbic system, which produces a sense of relaxation, but this is followed by progressive depression of all CNS functions. Mental processes that are modified by education, training and previous experience are affected first, while relatively 'mechanical' tasks are less impaired. Despite subjective impressions, there is no increase in mental or physical capabilities, unless anxiety has previously reduced performance. All effects are closely related to blood alcohol concentration (Table 54.1).

In people who regularly use large amounts of alcohol, tolerance is seen to many of its psychological effects. Alcohol increases dopamine release in the nucleus accumbens indirectly by activating presynaptic GABA receptors that actually inhibit GABA release. This is explained by the different alpha subunits on the presynaptic receptors that are sensitive to alcohol, whereas the postsynaptic receptors are not. Long-term use of alcohol produces long-lasting adaptive changes in the NMDA receptor that enhance their function. Opioid and serotonin receptor stimulation is also involved in the reinforcing effects of alcohol on the brain.

Alcohol intake is usually measured in units (Box 54.3).

Other effects of alcohol

Alcohol has a range of effects.

Table 54.1 The effects of alcohol at various plasma concentrations

Plasma concentration (mg·100 mL^{-1})	Effects
30	Mild euphoria owing to suppression of social inhibitory pathways in the cortex; the individual is more talkative and emotionally labile with loss of self-control; the risk of accidental injury is increased
80	Delayed reactions and reduced comprehension; memory impairment; the risk of serious injury in a road accident is more than doubled (80 mg·100 mL^{-1} is the legal limit for driving in the UK)
100–200	Speech becomes slurred and motor coordination is impaired
>300	Often produces loss of consciousness
>400	Frequently fatal as a result of respiratory and vasomotor centre depression

Cardiovascular effects

- A modest alcohol intake may have protective effects on the circulation by inhibiting platelet aggregation and increasing high-density lipoprotein cholesterol. The form in which the alcohol is taken is probably not important. The extent of this beneficial effect is probably greatest at 1 unit per day and is lost when intake exceeds 3–4 units per day.
- Higher intake of alcohol has pressor effects that raise blood pressure, possibly through increased vascular sensitivity to catecholamines. This increases the risk of coronary artery disease and stroke.
- Cardiac arrhythmias can be provoked by high alcohol intake, particularly atrial fibrillation. This can occur after an alcoholic binge ('holiday heart' syndrome) or following more chronic abuse (Ch. 8).
- Alcoholic cardiomyopathy is a dilated cardiomyopathy that is only partially reversible with abstinence, and can lead to heart failure. An average intake of 10 units of alcohol daily for 8–10 years can produce this condition.

Liver

- Hypoglycaemia occurs as a consequence of the metabolism of alcohol in the liver. The metabolic process generates excess protons, which enhance the conversion of glucose, via pyruvate, to lactate and predisposes to lactic acidosis. Alcoholics often have a low-carbohydrate diet, which compounds the hypoglycaemia. Hypoglycaemia tends to occur several hours after heavy alcohol intake and can contribute to seizures on alcohol withdrawal.
- The lactic acidosis created by alcohol metabolism in the liver impairs the renal excretion of uric acid, which predisposes to gout.
- Lactic acidosis also facilitates the synthesis of saturated fatty acids, which accumulate in the liver, leading to a fatty liver, possibly with altered liver function. Plasma triglycerides are also increased.
- Alcoholic hepatitis is usually a consequence of short-term heavy alcohol abuse. It can be fatal.
- Cirrhosis occurs with prolonged alcohol abuse, but individual susceptibility varies widely. On average, consumption of more than 8 units per day for at least 10 years is required for cirrhosis to occur in men. About two-thirds of this amount creates the same risk for women. Established cirrhosis reduces the first-pass metabolism and clearance of drugs eliminated by the liver (Ch. 56).
- Chronic intake of alcohol induces hepatic drug-metabolising enzymes, especially CYP2E1, which decreases the effectiveness of some therapeutic drugs, for example warfarin, phenytoin and carbamazepine.

Other gastrointestinal consequences

- Erosive gastritis can occur as a result of stimulation of gastric secretions.
- Pancreatitis is probably caused by raised triglycerides or by pancreatic duct obstruction by proteinaceous secretions induced by alcohol.

Sexual function

- Sexual desire is often increased by alcohol, but the ability to sustain penile erection is reduced, possibly because of the vasodilator actions of alcohol.
- Direct damage to the Leydig cells of the testis reduces the circulating testosterone, leading to reduced libido, infertility and a loss of the male distribution of body hair. Altered steroid metabolism in the liver leads to an increase in circulating oestrone in males, which causes gynaecomastia.

Neuropsychiatric effects

- A combination of alcohol toxicity with deficiencies of vitamin B_6 and thiamine in the diet of alcoholics predisposes to peripheral neuropathy and dementia. Specific mid-brain damage can result and produces the syndromes of Wernicke's encephalopathy and Korsakoff's psychosis.
- Alcohol has anticonvulsant properties and withdrawal predisposes to seizures, even in individuals without a history of epilepsy.
- Alcohol can disturb sleep patterns, with decreased rapid eye movement (REM) sleep and increased stage 4 sleep during intoxication. Withdrawal increases REM sleep, with associated nightmares (Ch. 20).
- Dose-related memory impairment can be caused by suppressed hippocampal function.
- Subdural haematoma is more common after head injury in heavy drinkers, perhaps as a consequence of cerebral atrophy.
- Depression or anxiety states are more common in heavy drinkers.

Carcinogenesis and teratogenesis

- Cancer of the mouth, oesophagus and liver are more common with heavy alcohol use. Colon and breast cancer may also be increased.
- The fetal alcohol syndrome is believed to be caused by the effects of alcohol on neuronal adhesion molecules that regulate neuronal migration. Heavy maternal drinking during pregnancy leads to impaired learning and memory in the child. Genetic factors may be involved in the susceptibility of the fetus to these problems.

Pharmacokinetics

Although ethanol is absorbed from the stomach, the majority is absorbed from the small intestine, due to its larger surface area. High concentrations of alcohol (above 20%) and large volumes inhibit gastric emptying and delay absorption, as do foods high in fat or carbohydrate. Therefore, peak blood alcohol concentrations depend on the dose and strength of the alcohol and on whether or not it was taken with food. Following absorption, alcohol undergoes substantial first-pass metabolism in the liver. The extent of first-pass metabolism of alcohol is related to the speed of absorption; thus, with slower absorption, such as when alcohol is taken with food, less alcohol will reach the systemic circulation. Distribution of alcohol is fairly uniform and the ready passage across the blood–brain barrier and

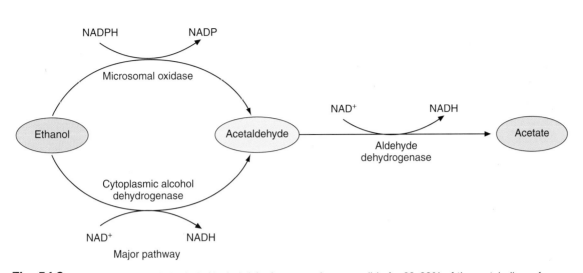

Fig. 54.2 **The metabolism of alcohol.** Alcohol dehydrogenase is responsible for 80–90% of the metabolism of ethanol. The microsomal oxidase is a minor pathway dependent on CYP2E1, the activity of which is increased by enzyme inducers such as alcohol itself.

high cerebral blood flow ensure rapid access to the CNS. The effects on the brain are more marked when the concentration is rising, indicating a degree of acute tolerance. Metabolism occurs mainly in the liver (Fig. 54.2), more than 90% being oxidised, mainly by alcohol dehydrogenase, while the rest is removed unchanged in expired air (in direct proportion to the blood concentration, which is the basis of the alcohol breath test) or in the urine. Alcohol metabolism shows saturation kinetics due to the limited supply of nicotine adenine nucleotide (NAD^+), which is the cofactor for the oxidative process. The maximum rate of alcohol metabolism averages 8 $g \cdot h^{-1}$. The initial metabolic reaction mediated by alcohol dehydrogenase produces acetaldehyde, which is subsequently metabolised by aldehyde dehydrogenase to acetic acid (Fig. 54.2). Genetic variability in alcohol and aldehyde dehydrogenases occurs among ethnic groups, leading to different capacities for alcohol or aldehyde metabolism. Accumulation of acetaldehyde in the circulation is responsible for many of the unpleasant effects of a hangover. Small amounts of alcohol are metabolised via the microsomal ethanol oxidising system (CYP2E1), the activity of which is increased by enzyme inducers such as alcohol itself (which does not affect the activity of alcohol dehydrogenase) (Ch. 36).

Some drugs, such as metronidazole (Ch. 51), inhibit aldehyde dehydrogenase, leading to acetaldehyde accumulation if alcohol is taken with them. Typical 'hangover' effects of flushing, sweating, headache and nausea then occur after even small amounts of alcohol.

Alcohol abuse and dependence

There are no reliable estimates of the number of people in the UK with alcohol-related problems, although it has been suggested that 1–2% of the population are affected. The distribution curve for alcohol consumption is continuous but skewed at higher alcohol intakes. The risk of alcohol-related problems rises with the average alcohol intake. Hazardous drinking is defined as a level or pattern of alcohol intake that will probably eventually cause harm. It applies to anyone drinking more than the recommended limits (21 units per week for men; 14 units per week for women). Harmful drinking is at a level that is already causing damage to physical or mental health. Dependent drinking is identified by features common to all drug dependence.

Up to 30% of hospital admissions are for alcohol-related problems, although the contribution of heavy drinking is often unrecognised. Screening for alcohol abuse can be carried out by obtaining a complete history of alcohol intake and using either the Alcohol Use Disorders Identification Test (AUDIT) or the Fast Alcohol Screening Test (FAST) (Box 54.4). Abnormal measurements of both the mean corpuscular volume (MCV) of red cells (which is raised with increasing alcohol intake because of an effect of alcohol on the cell membrane) and the liver enzyme γ-glutamyl transpeptidase (γGT) will identify about 75% of people with an alcohol problem.

Psychological dependence on alcohol is common, but physical dependence also occurs. Withdrawal symptoms occur 6–24 h after the last drink in dependent persons. If mild, these are related to autonomic hyperactivity and include anxiety, agitation, tremor, sweating, anorexia, nausea and retching. Convulsions can occur through neuronal excitation. Insomnia, tachycardia and hypertension are common with more severe withdrawal reactions. The most severe form of withdrawal is *delirium tremens*, with confusion, paranoia and visual and tactile hallucinations. Delirium tremens can cause death from respiratory and cardiovascular collapse.

If an individual is drinking excessively, controlled drinking may be an option. However, if there is alcohol dependence or alcohol-related problems, then abstinence is usually preferable.

Controlled detoxification is usually undertaken with a sedative agent, such as a benzodiazepine (Ch. 20), to attenuate withdrawal symptoms. Chlordiazepoxide or diazepam is usually used, decreasing the dose over 7–10 days. Clonidine (a presynaptic α_2-adrenoceptor agonist at the vasomotor centre in the brain; Ch. 6) can be useful, by reducing the excessive sympathetic stimulation that accompanies withdrawal. Beta-adrenoceptor antagonists (Ch. 5) may be helpful for the same reason. Multivitamin preparations containing an adequate amount of thiamine should be given for 1 month to prevent Wernicke's encephalopathy. Relapse is common after withdrawal from alcohol.

Two drugs are licensed in the UK to assist in the management of chronic alcoholism. *Disulfiram*, an inhibitor of acetaldehyde dehydrogenase, causes unpleasant hangover symptoms after small amounts of alcohol. Given alone, or with psychosocial rehabilitation, it can help to maintain abstinence. *Acamprosate* may activate GABA$_A$ receptors and block glutamate NMDA receptors, although several other contributory effects have been suggested. It has few unwanted effects, is non-addictive and can be used to reduce the craving for alcohol. *Naltrexone*, a long-acting opioid receptor antagonist, can reduce the craving associated with alcohol withdrawal. It is not licensed for this indication in the UK. Other potential agents to reduce the urge to drink include ondansetron (Ch. 32), topiramate and gabapentin (Ch. 23).

Gamma-hydroxybutyric acid

Mechanism of action and effects

Gamma-hydroxybutyric acid (GHB) was originally introduced as a general anaesthetic, but is now used illegally as an intoxicant, a 'date rape' drug or by athletes to improve performance. Its precursors γ-butyl-lactone (GBL) and 1,4-butanediol are also abused. GHB acts as an agonist at a specific inhibitory GHB receptor in the cortex and hippocampus of the brain, and also as an agonist at GABA$_B$ receptors, which mediate its sedative effects. GHB receptor activation stimulates dopamine release. GHB receptor stimulation also increases growth hormone release, which is the basis of its abuse by athletes and bodybuilders. In a similar manner to alcohol, GHB produces euphoria, increased libido and increased sociability. At high doses it produces nausea, dizziness, drowsiness, agitation, visual disturbances, amnesia and coma. Both psychological and physical dependence occur. Withdrawal can be treated with baclofen (Ch. 24).

Pharmacokinetics

GHB is usually taken orally, occasionally intravenously. It has low oral bioavailability, is metabolised in the liver and has a short half-life of 30 min. The clinical effect lasts for 1.5–3 h, and longer if taken with alcohol.

Inhaled solvents

Various organic solvents are abused as recreational drugs. Examples include butane, toluene and diethyl ether. Inhalation via a plastic bag held over the mouth or from an open container produces rapid intoxication resembling that produced by alcohol. These compounds probably act in a similar way to volatile general anaesthetics (Ch. 17). Death can occur from asphyxiation during inhalation, while long-term use produces brain damage by increasing neuronal apoptosis.

SELF-ASSESSMENT

True/false questions

1. Cocaine causes mydriasis by inhibiting the reuptake of noradrenaline into nerve terminals.
2. 'Crack' cocaine is the free-base form of cocaine.
3. Cocaine use has little damaging effect on the cardiovascular system.
4. Tolerance to the euphoric and anorexic effects of cocaine develops rapidly.
5. MDMA (ecstasy) blocks the release of serotonin from nerve endings.
6. In some individuals MDMA causes hyperthermia and dehydration.
7. MDMA suppresses appetite.
8. Amfetamines are used to treat attention deficit hyperactivity disorder (ADHD).
9. Cannabis impairs driving ability.
10. The euphoria caused by cannabis lasts for 24 h.

11. Tetrahydrocannabinol (THC), the main active ingredient of cannabis, causes nausea and vomiting.
12. Cannabis acts on specific receptors in the brain.
13. Nicotine causes tachycardia and reduced gut motility.
14. Tolerance to the effects of nicotine develops slowly.
15. Varenicline is a partial agonist of nicotine receptors in the central nervous system (CNS).
16. Cotinine has a long half-life and can be measured in serum to determine smoking habits.
17. Nicotine patches given alone are the optimum method for someone giving up smoking.
18. A physical withdrawal symptom does not occur when giving up smoking.
19. Alcohol is initially metabolised in the liver to acetaldehyde.
20. Chronic intake of alcohol induces hepatic drug-metabolising enzymes.
21. Even moderate alcohol intake increases the incidence of cardiovascular disease.
22. Some individuals have a genetically determined low ability to metabolise alcohol.
23. Disulfiram produces acute sensitivity to alcohol by blocking its conversion to acetaldehyde.
24. Acamprosate, which is used to encourage abstinence, acts on alcohol metabolism in a similar way to disulfiram.
25. The symptoms of alcohol withdrawal (detoxification) cannot be controlled by pharmacological means.
26. Alcohol can cause a macrocytosis.
27. Alcohol enhances antidiuretic hormone secretion.
28. Plasma levels of γ-glutamyl transpeptidase (γGT) are depressed with heavy alcohol intake.
29. Cathinone derivatives in the khat plant produce sedation.
30. Gamma-hydroxybutyric acid (GHB) may be abused by athletes.

True/false answers

1. **True.** Cocaine blocks monoamine reuptake; in the eye, the resulting increase in noradrenaline causes mydriasis by contraction of radial pupillary muscles.
2. **True.** Unlike the salt form of cocaine, the free base can be illicitly smoked.
3. **False.** Acute effects include cardiac arrhythmias and chronic use can lead to heart failure.
4. **True.** Tolerance develops to euphoria and appetite suppression in only a few days.
5. **False.** MDMA (ecstasy) increases release of serotonin and other monamines by preventing their uptake into synaptic vesicles and promoting their release from the cytoplasm into the synapse. It may also be an agonist at serotonin receptors.
6. **True.** Malignant hyperthermia resembling heat stroke and dehydration is observed in some individuals after ingesting MDMA.
7. **True.** Like other amfetamines, MDMA has a short-term effect to suppress appetite.
8. **True.** Amfetamines can be used to treat ADHD (but not an approved use in UK).

9. **True.** Cannabis impairs driving ability and the performance of complex mental tasks, and may give rise to psychotic reactions in predisposed individuals.
10. **False.** The euphoric effects last only 2–3 h.
11. **False.** The related cannabinoid, nabilone, is used to inhibit nausea and vomiting in patients taking cytotoxic drugs.
12. **True.** Cannabis acts on cannabinoid receptors CB_1 and CB_2 in the brain and periphery. The natural ligands for these receptors include anandamide.
13. **True.** These effects are caused by stimulation of nicotinic N_1 receptors in autonomic ganglia.
14. **False.** Tolerance to nicotine develops rapidly.
15. **True.** Varenicline reduces tobacco cravings by partial agonism at CNS nicotinic receptors, and it partially blocks the additional effect of nicotine if tobacco is smoked.
16. **True.** Cotinine is a stable and inactive nicotine metabolite; it can be measured in saliva, serum or urine.
17. **False.** Nicotine-replacement therapy should be supplemented with counselling.
18. **False.** Irritability, sleep disturbances and reduced psychomotor test performance occur on giving up smoking.
19. **True.** Alcohol is mainly metabolised to acetaldehyde (by alcohol dehydrogenase) and then to acetic acid (by aldehyde dehydrogenase).
20. **True.** The induction of CYP2E1 by alcohol can decrease the effectiveness of some drugs such as warfarin and phenytoin.
21. **False.** Moderate alcohol intake (below 3–4 units per day for men) has cardiovascular protective effects.
22. **True.** Some individuals have a genetically determined variant of alcohol dehydrogenase that has a reduced capacity to metabolise alcohol. Its incidence is low in white people but higher in people from some Far Eastern countries.
23. **False.** Disulfiram blocks conversion of acetaldehyde to acetic acid by aldehyde dehydrogenase; the accumulation of acetaldehyde causes sickness, headache and hangover symptoms following even a small amount of alcohol intake.
24. **False.** Acamprosate acts to reduce the craving for alcohol and not by affecting its metabolism.
25. **False.** Benzodiazepines can attenuate withdrawal symptoms but there is a risk of dependence to these agents.
26. **True.** Alcohol intake is a common cause of macrocytosis (increased red cell volume) in the absence of anaemia.
27. **False.** The diuresis resulting from alcohol intake is partly caused by inhibition of release of antidiuretic hormone.
28. **False.** Plasma γ-glutamyl transpeptidase (γGT) is elevated in heavy alcohol intake.
29. **False.** Cathinone and its derivatives have amfetamine-like properties and cause wakefulness and insomnia.
30. **True.** GHB has sedative activity but also increases growth hormone release, which is the basis of its abuse by athletes and bodybuilders.

FURTHER READING

Anton RF (2008) Naltrexone for the management of alcohol dependence. *N Engl J Med* 359, 715–721

Aveyard P, West R (2007) Managing smoking cessation. *BMJ* 335, 37–41

Barlecchi CE, MacKenzie TD, Schrier RW (1994) The human cost of tobacco. *N Engl J Med* 330, 907–912, 975–980

Benowitz NL (2010) Nicotine addiction. *N Engl J Med* 362, 2295–2303

Berke JD, Hyman SE (2000) Addiction, dopamine, and the molecular mechanisms of memory. *Neuron* 25, 515–532

Cami J, Farre M (2003) Drug addiction. *N Engl J Med* 349, 975–986

Farrell M, Wodak A, Gowing L (2012) Maintenance drugs to treat opioid dependence. *BMJ* 344, e2823

Gerdeman GL, Partridge JG, Lupica, CR et al. (2003) It could be habit forming: drugs of abuse and striatal synaptic plasticity. *Trends Neurosci* 26, 184–192

Hall W, Solowij N (1998) Adverse effects of cannabis. *Lancet* 352, 1611–1616

Hatsukami DK, Stead LF, Gupta PC (2008) Tobacco addiction. *Lancet* 371, 2027–2038

Hays JT, Ebbert JO (2008) Varenicline for tobacco dependence. *N Engl J Med* 359, 2018–2024

Hodgson RJ, Alwyn T, John B, Thom B, Smith, A (2002) The FAST Alcohol Screening Test. *Alcohol and Alcoholism* 37, 61–66

Johnson BA (2010) Medication treatment of different types of alcoholism. *Am J Psychiatry* 167, 630–639

Koob GF (2006) The neurobiology of addiction: a neuroadaptational view relevant for diagnosis. *Addiction* 101 (suppl 1), 23–30

Lancaster T, Hajek P, Stead LF et al. (2006) Prevention of relapse after quitting smoking. *Arch Intern Med* 166, 828–835

Mendelson JH, Mello NK (1996) Management of cocaine abuse and dependence. *N Engl J Med* 334, 965–972

Moore THM, Zammit S, Lingford-Hughes A et al. (2007) Cannabis use and risk of psychotic or affective mental health outcomes: a systematic review. *Lancet* 370, 319–328

Nides M (2008) Update on pharmacologic options for smoking cessation treatment. *Am J Med* 121 (suppl 4A), S20–S31

Parker AJ, Marshall EJ, Ball DM (2008) Diagnosis and management of alcohol use disorder. *BMJ* 336, 496–501

Rigotti A (2002) Treatment of tobacco use and dependence. *N Engl J Med* 346, 506–512

Saitz R (2005) Unhealthy alcohol use. *N Engl J Med* 352, 596–607

Schippenberg TS, Zapata A, Chefer VI (2007) Dynorphin and the pathophysiology of drug addiction. *Pharmacol Ther* 116, 306–321

Schuckit MA (2009) Alcohol-use disorders. *Lancet* 373, 492–501

Snead OC, Gibson KM (2005) γ-Hydroxybutyric acid. *N Engl J Med* 352, 2721–2732

Sullivan LE, Fiellin DA (2008) Narrative review: Buprenorphine for opioid-dependent patients in office practice. *Ann Intern Med* 148, 662–670

Winstock AR, Mitcheson L (2012) New recreational drugs and the primary care approach to patients who use them. *BMJ* 344, e288

Compendium: drugs of abuse and drugs used to treat drug dependence

Drug	Kinetics (half-life)	Comments
Drugs of abuse		
Alcohol (ethyl alcohol, ethanol)	Zero-order kinetics; oxidation by alcohol dehydrogenase is saturated at normal alcohol intakes	
Amfetamine	Rapidly absorbed; hepatic metabolism and renal excretion; half-life is dependent on urine pH (8–12 h)	Dexamfetamine is the active form and is sometimes used for treatment of hyperactivity in children (especially in the USA)
Benzodiazepines	–	See Ch. 20
Cannabis (Δ-9-tetrahydrocannabinol, THC)	Hepatic metabolism to numerous metabolites, including active 11-hydroxy-THC; eliminated in faeces and urine (1.5 h)	Delta-9-tetrahydrocannabinol is the main active constituent
Cathinone stimulants	Cathinine almost completely absorbed from chewing khat leaves; hepatic metabolism to norephedrine (1.5 h)	Main stimulant (with cathine) in khat plant; amfetamine-like actions
Cocaine	Oral bioavailability 30–40%; ester hydrolysed in the liver (1–1.5 h)	Limited use as a non-injection local anaesthetic; abuse involves non-oral routes (mostly nasal or inhalation)
Ecstasy (3,4-methylenedioxy-metamfetamine; MDMA)	Saturation of hepatic oxidation may contribute to risk of overdose; also excreted unchanged in urine (4–6 h)	The amfetamine analogue (MDA) and ethylamfetamine analogue (MDE or 'Eve') show similar properties
Gamma-hydroxybutyric acid (GHB)	Oral bioavailability 25%; eliminated by hepatic oxidation (0.5–1 h)	Sedative
Lysergic acid diethylamide (LSD)	Eliminated by hepatic metabolism (5 h); LSD is detectable in urine after oral dosage	Hallucinogen
Ketamine	–	Dissociative anaesthetic; see Ch. 17
Metamfetamine	Rapidly absorbed; hepatic oxidation; about 40% excreted in urine unchanged (pH-dependent) (10–12 h)	
Nicotine	Very rapidly absorbed after inhalation; rapid conversion to cotinine (0.5–2 h), which has longer half-life (10–40 h)	Exposure to nicotine can be assessed by measuring cotinine in saliva, blood or urine; for nicotine-replacement therapy see below
Opioids	–	See Ch. 19
Phencyclidine (PCP)	Oral bioavailability about 70%; mainly hepatic oxidation (7–57 h); about 10% excreted in urine unchanged	Dissociative anaesthetic
Psilocybin	Oxidised very rapidly (minutes) to psilocin and also in the intestine	Hallucinogen found in 'magic mushrooms'
Drugs used to treat drug dependence		
Cigarette smoking		
Bupropion	Oral bioavailability 5–20%; hepatic metabolism to three major active metabolites (24 h)	Atypical antidepressant; used as an adjunct to smoking cessation; given orally
Nicotine	See above; peak nicotine plasma concentrations occur at 4–15 min (nasal spray), 15–30 min (gum) or 2–12 h (patch), compared with 15 min after inhalation	Nicotine-replacement therapy; used as an adjunct to smoking cessation; given sublingually as chewing gum, transdermally as a patch or by inhaler or nasal spray
Varenicline	Eliminated by glomerular filtration and active tubular secretion (24 h)	Partial agonist of nicotine receptors in CNS; used as an adjunct to smoking cessation; given orally

Compendium: drugs of abuse and drugs used to treat drug dependence—cont'd

Drug	Kinetics (half-life)	Comments
Alcohol dependence		
Acamprosate calcium	Low oral bioavailability (11%); eliminated by renal excretion (20–33 h)	Used for the maintenance of abstinence; given orally
Disulfiram	Hepatic metabolism and renal excretion (60–120 h)	Acetaldehyde dehydrogenase inhibitor; used as an adjunct in the treatment of chronic alcohol dependence; given orally
Opioid dependence		
Opioid dependence is discussed in Ch. 19		
Buprenorphine	See Ch. 19	Used as an adjunct to treatment of dependence
Lofexidine	See Ch. 19	Used for management of symptoms of withdrawal
Methadone	See Ch. 19	Used as an adjunct to treatment of dependence
Naltrexone	See Ch. 19	Oral opioid receptor antagonist; longer duration of action than naloxone; used to prevent relapse in detoxified formerly opioid-dependent individuals

55

Prescribing, adherence and information about medicines

• •

About 80% of medicines are prescribed in general practice (primary medical care). On average, men visit their general practitioners three to four times each year and women visit five times. About two-thirds of consultations end with the issuing of a prescription. Prescribing is particularly frequent for elderly people, who are likely to continue treatment for long periods of time. For these reasons, regular review of prescribed treatment should take place to determine whether it is still appropriate or necessary, and to ensure that important drug interactions and unwanted effects are not overlooked. Some drugs also require regular monitoring of efficacy (e.g. warfarin, antihypertensive treatment), of blood concentrations (e.g. lithium) or for biochemical effects (e.g. amiodarone, thiazide diuretics).

DUTIES OF THE PRESCRIBER

There are certain legal requirements that must be met when a medicine is prescribed. The information to be recorded is:

- the name of the person for whom the drug is prescribed (surname and initial) and address; in the case of children up to 12 years, the person's age must be specified,
- drug name (without abbreviation),
- dose,
- route of administration (usually given on the manufacturer's product information rather than the prescription),
- frequency of administration (with minimum dose-interval for preparations to be taken 'as required'),
- either the quantity to be supplied or the duration of therapy,
- prescriber's name, address and signature,
- date.

GENERIC PRESCRIBING

In most situations the generic name (the officially accepted chemical name) of the drug is preferred to the proprietary trade name (a 'brand' name approved for use by a specific pharmaceutical company). One advantage of the generic name is that it is likely to indicate the nature of the drug. For example, all β-adrenoceptor antagonist drugs (β-blockers) end with -olol, such as atenolol, bisoprolol and metoprolol, but the trade names for these drugs, for example Tenormin®, Monocor® and Lopressor®, give little idea of the active ingredient. Another problem with trade names is that they rarely give any indication when there is more than one active ingredient; for example, Tenoret® contains both atenolol and chlortalidone. The generic names for many compound preparations have this indicated by the term 'co-'; for example, co-tenidone is the generic equivalent of Tenoret.

Another advantage of generic prescribing is that pharmacists can dispense any product that meets the necessary specifications, rather than having to buy in a specific brand. This helps to simplify stock holding and avoids unnecessary delays when dispensing. However, different generic preparations of the same drug may differ in the tablet size, colour or scoring as well as brand name. Therefore it is important to inform the person taking the drug if a different brand is dispensed.

Generic prescribing is sometimes cheaper than prescribing by trade name, although the difference depends on pack size and other commercial factors and is sometimes marginal. In recent years there has been an increasing tendency for doctors to prescribe by generic name. It is likely that economic arguments and the increasing use of electronic prescribing systems have been the chief factors leading to this change.

One potential hazard of generic prescribing involves drugs with a narrow therapeutic index. Stringent controls have eliminated the problem of variations in bioavailability from different brands, except for some modified-release formulations of drugs such as those for lithium or theophylline. Different release characteristics from the formulation can influence the plasma concentration profile of the drug and affect efficacy and toxicity, and in these situations prescribing by brand is recommended.

DOSAGE

The total exposure to a medicine during a course of treatment is related to the individual dose size, its frequency and the duration of therapy. The route of administration may also be important.

Dose

This is an essential item on all prescriptions and should be written in grams (g), milligrams (mg) or micrograms (which should not be abbreviated).

The route of administration

The route should be identified if there is any possibility of confusion. Confusion can arise with intravenous administration of drugs since there are numerous methods for delivery: drugs can be given by direct injection (either as a bolus or by slow injection) into a vein or can be infused, for example through the side-arm of a continuously running intravenous drip, via a motor-driven pump or added to the intravenous infusion fluid reservoir. It is particularly important when prescribing drugs for intravenous administration to make clear the precise intentions.

Frequency and times of administration

Sometimes, drugs are taken once only, while others must be given on a regular basis, in which case the frequency or times of administration should be specified, for example twice daily or at 12 h intervals.

The quantity to be supplied or the duration of therapy

Most general practice and outpatient prescriptions specify the amount to be dispensed, for example the total number of tablets or capsules. The duration of therapy will then be determined by the amount dispensed and the frequency of dosing. Duration can be specified in a number of ways. When the medicine is to be administered by a health professional or by a carer in a sheltered environment, the duration can be specified on the prescription sheet. Alternatively, it can be written on the prescription to be dispensed by a pharmacist. Medicines are now dispensed in original packs with tablets individually packed by the pharmaceutical company. Specifying the duration of therapy is essential in the case of controlled drugs (preparations that are subject to the prescription requirements of the UK Misuse of Drugs Regulations 2001 and subsequent amendments), such as opioids, for which there is a legal requirement that the total amount to be dispensed must be written in both figures and words.

OTHER ITEMS ON A PRESCRIPTION

Other essential items on prescriptions include the prescriber's signature and the address of his or her place of work. The latter is effectively waived for hospital prescriptions since it is assumed that the prescriber is based at the hospital in question. The prescription must be dated. Computer-issued prescriptions are now almost universal in primary care. The specific requirements for these are essentially similar to those outlined above. Use of computer-issued prescriptions avoids handwriting problems and assists in record keeping and in data collection and analysis.

ABBREVIATIONS

Directions for prescribing should preferably be in English (rather than Latin) without abbreviation. However, there are a number of abbreviations that are widely accepted. They include the following for route of administration: o or p.o., oral; i.v., intravenous; i.m., intramuscular; s.c., subcutaneous; and p.r., per rectum. Others, such as intrathecal, must not be abbreviated, because of the potential seriousness of inappropriate administration. Inappropriate intrathecal administration of vincristine, for example, has caused the death of several people. Besides the abbreviations already listed for quantities, ml or mL is acceptable. Quantities of less than 1 g should be written in milligrams (e.g. 400 mg, rather than 0.4 g), whereas quantities of less than 1 mg should be written in micrograms [e.g. 500 micrograms (in full), rather than 0.5 mg; when handwritten, μg is easily mistaken for mg]. Decimal points should be avoided wherever possible, but, if unavoidable, a zero should precede the decimal point when there is no figure (e.g. 0.5 mL, not .5 mL).

When indicating the timing of doses, od (*omni die*) is acceptable, but there is nothing wrong with saying once daily! The abbreviation om (*omni mane*) stands for in the morning and on (*omni nocte*) for at night; ac is short for ante cibum (before food) and pc for post cibum (after food). Twice daily can be abbreviated to bd (*bis die*), thrice daily to tds (*ter die sumendus*) and four times daily to qds (*quater die sumendus*).

ADHERENCE, CONCORDANCE AND COMPLIANCE

The term 'compliance' is used to describe the extent to which a person takes his or her medicine. However, other terms such as 'adherence' or 'concordance' are now preferred, because they emphasise the partnership between the person and health professions in the process of taking medicines, rather than simply following instructions. It is frequently assumed that once a prescription has been given, the recipient will automatically follow the prescriber's instructions. However, there is abundant evidence that this is often not the case. Indeed, many prescriptions are not even taken to the pharmacist for dispensing. Prescriptions are sometimes not presented to a pharmacist because of cost or because the prescriber failed to discuss the 'hidden agenda' for which the presenting complaint was an excuse to see the doctor. In addition, a very substantial proportion of medicines collected are not taken in the manner intended.

The degree of adherence is affected by many factors, which include the duration of treatment. Fewer than 50% of people adhere fully during long-term therapy, such as that for high blood pressure or psychotic illness. There is increasing evidence that adherence to prescribed therapy can determine the outcome of treatment. For example, in treating hypertension the control of blood pressure is substantially less good when adherence falls below 80% of prescribed doses.

The frequency of dosing has a major influence on adherence. Few people like taking their medicines with them to work. Therefore, adherence with twice-daily regimens tends to be much better than that for more frequent administration. There is a further improvement in the extent of adherence with once- rather than twice-daily dosing.

Unwanted effects can reduce the likelihood of a person complying with therapy, but at times this can be turned to an advantage. For example, giving the entire dose of a tricyclic antidepressant at night means that the sedation it produces can be used to aid sleep. Giving the person advanced warning of likely unwanted effects such as dry mouth with this compound may earn the person's trust and encourage continuation of the therapy.

A proportion of non-adherence is caused by people forgetting whether or not they have taken their medicine on a particular day. The use of calendar packs or prepacked dispensing boxes can be helpful in this situation.

The individual's health beliefs are also particularly important. Adherence can be improved by involving the person in monitoring his or her disease and its control by therapy, for example home monitoring of blood pressure, blood sugar in diabetes mellitus or peak flow measurements in people with asthma. Supplying accurate information about medicines can improve the level of satisfaction, and satisfied people are more likely to take their medicines.

INFORMING PEOPLE ABOUT THEIR MEDICINES

It is almost incredible to think that at one time doctors were reluctant to allow the name of a medicine to be shown on the container in which it was dispensed. However, paternalistic attitudes among the medical profession have been slow to disappear. Several surveys carried out in the early 1980s showed that most people felt that neither doctors nor pharmacists gave sufficient explanations about medicines. People are particularly keen to know:

- the name of the medicine,
- the purposes of treatment,
- when and how to take their medicine,
- how long to take it for and what to do if a dose is missed,
- unwanted effects and what to do about these,
- any necessary precautions to take, such as possible effects on driving,
- any problems with alcohol or with other drugs.

Manufacturers of pharmaceuticals now produce printed leaflets about medicines, which are included in original packs. However, leaflets are complementary to, and not a substitute for, discussion with the medical practitioner, pharmacist, practice nurse, etc. The internet provides an increasingly rich source of information for people about their medicines and the variety of treatments available for their condition(s). However, advertising and the lack of peer review of websites means that, in many cases, information the individual may have acquired before they first see their doctor may be incorrect and/or misunderstood.

RATIONAL PRESCRIBING

A definition of good prescribing has been proposed that encompasses four goals. These are to:

- maximise effectiveness,
- minimise harms,
- avoid wasting healthcare resources,
- respect the person's choice.

Irrational prescribing can take several forms, such as use of antibacterial drugs for viral infections, statin therapy for someone with late-stage malignancy, using expensive drugs when there are equally effective cheaper alternatives, using too high a drug dose in renal or hepatic impairment or under-dosage with an appropriate drug.

The standards against which rational prescribing can be judged will depend on locally or nationally agreed treatment protocols or an agreed list of therapeutic alternatives. Ideally, prescribing should follow evidence-based guidelines, but it is often necessary to extrapolate these guidelines to situations not covered by the evidence. In the absence of evidence from clinical trials it may be appropriate to use consensus guidelines produced by experts, and derived from a relevant evidence base.

There has been considerable debate about 'class effects' of drugs, and whether it is reasonable to extrapolate data from a clinical study with one drug to another in the same class. This is a complex area, and in part depends on the definition of a drug class (e.g. a group of drugs with similar chemical structure, similar mechanisms of action, or similar pharmacological effects). Class effect may be related to clinical outcome (such as death or risk of stroke), effects on surrogate end-points (such as reduction in blood pressure) or specific unwanted effects. Many consensus guidelines assume that drug efficacy is related to a class effect when there is a large body of information about several drugs in a class that suggests similar outcomes.

The sequence of events leading to a rational prescription involves initially making a diagnosis and determining prognosis. This may not always be possible, and it may be necessary to substitute differential diagnoses and rank these in order of probability and/or importance to treat. The goal of treatment must then be determined. This may be curative, symptom relief, prevention or occasionally an aid to the diagnostic process. The prescriber should then decide whether any treatment is necessary and, if so, then select an appropriate first choice. The process is completed by monitoring the outcome, and reaching a decision to stop, modify or continue treatment.

Assuming that the choice of drug is appropriate for the condition that the prescriber believes he or she is treating, there will be several further considerations involved in individualising drug treatment.

- Is this drug licensed for use in this condition? If it is not, prescribing may still be appropriate but the prescriber should be familiar with the evidence to support the use of the drug.
- How does the drug compare with available alternatives in relation to published evidence, efficacy, safety, convenience and cost?
- Does the individual have any coexisting conditions that will compromise the efficacy of the drug?
- Are there comorbidities that might benefit from the use of this or an alternative option?
- Are any other drugs being taken that might adversely interact with your choice?
- Are there any absolute contraindications to using the drug in this individual?

- Are there relative contraindications to use in this individual, including comorbidities or common unwanted effects?

- Has the individual suffered previous adverse drug events that should make you cautious about using this particular drug?

FURTHER READING

Aronson JK (2012) Balanced prescribing – principles and challenges. *Br J Clin Pharmacol* 74, 566–572

Bond C, Blenkinsopp A, Raynor DK (2012) Prescribing and partnership with patients. *Br J Clin Pharmacol* 74, 581–588

Burnier M (2006) Medication adherence and persistence as the cornerstone of effective antihypertensive therapy. *Am J Hypertens* 19, 1190–1196

Dans AL, Dans LF, Guyatt GH, Richardson S (1998) Users' guides to the medical literature: XIV. How to decide on the applicability of clinical trial results to your patient *JAMA* 279, 545–549

De Vries TPGM (1993) Presenting clinical pharmacology and therapeutics: a problem-based approach for choosing and prescribing drugs. *Br J Clin Pharmacol* 35, 581–586

Guyatt GH, Sinclair J, Cook DJ et al. (1999) Users' guides to the medical literature: XVI. How to use a treatment recommendation. *JAMA* 281, 1836–1843

Hogerzeil HV (1995) Promoting rational prescribing: an international perspective. *Br J Clin Pharmacol* 39, 1–6

McAlister FA, Laupacis A, Wells GA et al. (1999) Applying clinical trial results Part B. Guidelines for determining whether a drug is exerting (more than) a class effect. *JAMA* 282, 1371–1377

McAlister F, Strauss SE, Guyatt GH et al. (2000) Users' guides to the medical literature: XX. Integrating research evidence with the care of the individual patient. *JAMA* 283, 2829–2836

Osterberg L, Blaschke T (2005) Adherence to medication. *N Engl J Med* 353, 487–497

Rissman R, Dubois EA, Franson KL et al. (2012) Concept-based learning of personalized prescribing. *Br J Clin Pharmacol* 74, 589–596

Santaguida PL, Helfand M, Raina P (2005) Challenges in systematic reviews that evaluate drug efficacy. *Ann Intern Med* 142, 1066–1072

Shah RR, Shah DR (2012) Personalized medicine: is it a pharmacogenetic mirage? *Br J Clin Pharmacol* 74, 698–721

Spinewine A, Schmader KE, Barber N et al. (2007) Appropriate prescribing in elderly people: how well can it be measured and optimized? *Lancet* 370, 173–184

Thomas SHL, Yates LM (2012) Prescribing without evidence – pregnancy. *Br J Clin Pharmacol* 74, 691–697

56 Drug therapy in special situations

PRESCRIBING IN PREGNANCY

Guidelines for prescribing during pregnancy are set out in the *British National Formulary* (BNF). Pregnancy can be associated with medical problems that require treatment (Ch. 45), but exposure of the fetus to any unnecessary drugs is undesirable, particularly in the first trimester between the third and eleventh weeks of pregnancy, because of the risk of teratogenicity. In the second and third trimesters drugs may affect the growth or functional development of the fetus, whereas drugs given at full term may influence labour or affect the neonate after delivery. The magnitude of the potential problem is illustrated by the fact that about 50% of women take prescribed medication at some stage during pregnancy, and an unrecorded number will take over-the-counter medications, including herbal and homeopathic remedies, without guidance from a medical practitioner or a pharmacist.

Unequivocal teratogenic activity of drugs in humans is limited to a relatively small number of compounds, but the effects are irreversible and affect the whole life of the off-spring. The potential catastrophic consequences of the administration of a teratogenic drug were highlighted by the thalidomide tragedy in the 1960s. Thalidomide was introduced as a sedative and hypnotic and used for the treatment of pregnancy-associated morning sickness. Following its introduction there was a dramatic increase in the incidence of phocomelia (abnormal or absent development of limb buds). The drug was banned once the association had been recognised, and this resulted in the incidence of phocomelia decreasing to previous levels (Fig. 56.1). Thalidomide is not teratogenic in rodents, and teratogenic effects are seen in rabbits only at doses about 100 times higher than those in humans or other primates; this observation resulted in the requirement for two or more animal species in preclinical testing for teratogenicity. The thalidomide tragedy led to a significant reduction in the proportion of women taking any prescription drug during pregnancy, particularly in the first trimester. The recent use of thalidomide as an unlicensed treatment for leprosy raises the spectre of teratogenicity; the drug should never be given to women with child-bearing potential.

The list of drugs known to be teratogenic is relatively short but includes thalidomide, many anticonvulsants, some chemotherapeutic drugs (e.g. alkylating agents and antimetabolites), warfarin, androgens, danazol, diethylstilbestrol, lithium and retinoids (Table 56.1). Because of their long half-lives, some retinoids can result in teratogenesis even if treatment for the mother is stopped before pregnancy occurs. Although teratogenesis is commonly thought of in terms of structural abnormalities or dysfunctional growth *in utero*, it also refers to long-term functional defects. For example, maternal consumption of alcohol during pregnancy may cause behavioural and cognitive abnormalities in childhood, despite the birth of a seemingly unaffected infant. Some drugs may initially appear harmless yet exhibit a long latency period. Diethylstilbestrol, which was given during pregnancy between the 1940s and early 1970s in the mistaken belief that it reduced the risk of miscarriage, resulted in abnormalities in the offspring when they reached adulthood, including hypogonadism in males and vaginal adenocarcinoma in females.

Notwithstanding the limited list of drugs that are known to cause teratogenesis, there is a much larger number that should be avoided or used with caution in pregnancy because of their potential to produce detrimental effects in the fetus. Examples include warfarin-induced anticoagulation (Ch. 11), which may predispose to cerebral haemorrhage in the fetus during delivery; in contrast, heparin is an effective anticoagulant in the mother and does not cross the placenta. Non-steroidal anti-inflammatory drugs (NSAIDs; Ch. 29) can produce premature closure of the ductus arteriosus before delivery. Adverse effects produced

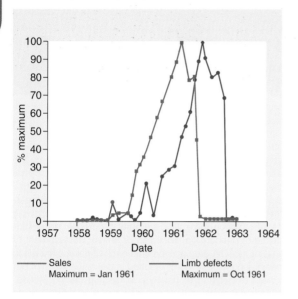

Fig. 56.1 Sales of thalidomide and the incidence of phocomelia. Thalidomide sales and phocomelia incidence are each expressed as a percentage of the reported maximum.

at therapeutic doses, such as tachycardia with tricyclic antidepressants and growth restriction with corticosteroids, may also affect the fetus or neonate.

Whenever a drug is given to a pregnant woman, or a woman who has child-bearing potential, an assessment should be made, taking into account any risk to the fetus balanced against the benefit to the mother and any risk associated with not treating the mother. For example, treatment with anticonvulsants or antimalarials may be essential for the mother, despite the possible risk to the fetus/neonate. The risk to the fetus/neonate should be minimised whenever possible by selecting the drug with the least potential for teratogenicity, by prescribing the lowest effective dose and minimizing the use of multiple drugs. Absence of evidence of teratogenicity does not imply that a risk does not exist. Drugs which have been used extensively in pregnancy and appear to be safe should nevertheless be preferred to new or untried drugs. The BNF provides detailed information on potential adverse drug effects on the fetus and neonate, and guidance is also available from the UK Teratology Information Service (www.uktis.org).

PHARMACOKINETICS IN PREGNANCY

The placenta provides a potential barrier to the transfer of macromolecules from the maternal circulation, but low-molecular-weight drugs will cross the placenta, particularly if they are lipid-soluble. Some metabolism of drugs can occur in the placenta, which may further restrict fetal exposure, although the placenta does not have a high drug-metabolising capacity. The fetal liver and kidneys have only modest abilities to eliminate drugs, so drugs in the fetal circulation are usually cleared by the maternal routes of elimination. The fetus therefore represents a slowly

equilibrating maternal kinetic compartment, with transfer across the placenta being determined by the concentration gradient between fetal and maternal circulations.

Maternal pharmacokinetics are affected by a number of physiological changes, especially in late pregnancy. Compared to non-pregnant women, these include:

- increased hepatic drug metabolism,
- increased renal perfusion and glomerular filtration rate,
- decreased plasma concentration of albumin.

These changes mean that maternal drug concentrations are often lower than those in a non-pregnant woman given the same dose, so drug doses may need to be increased in pregnancy to compensate.

DRUGS AND BREASTFEEDING

Almost any compound present in the maternal circulation will enter breast milk and be ingested by the suckling baby. However, with a few exceptions there is little evidence that drug intake via breastfeeding is of concern because most drugs enter breast milk in quantities too small to affect the baby. In general, drugs licensed for use in children can be safely given to the nursing mother, whereas drugs known to have serious toxic effects in adults, or known to affect lactation, such as bromocriptine, should be avoided.

The American Academy of Pediatrics (2001) divides drugs into:

i. cytotoxic drugs that may interfere with cellular metabolism of the nursing infant (e.g. cyclophosphamide, ciclosporin, doxorubicin, methotrexate),
ii. drugs of abuse for which adverse effects on the infant during breastfeeding have been reported (e.g. amfetamine, cocaine, heroin, marijuana),
iii. radioactive compounds that require temporary cessation of breastfeeding (e.g. radioiodine),
iv. drugs for which the effect on nursing infants is unknown but may be of concern (a list of about 40 miscellaneous drugs),
v. drugs that have been associated with significant effects on some nursing infants and should be given to nursing mothers with close monitoring (e.g. acebutolol, atenolol, bromocriptine, aspirin, ergotamine, lithium, phenindione, phenobarbital/primidone),
vi. maternal medication usually compatible with breastfeeding (the vast majority of drugs),
vii. food and environmental agents.

The reader should refer to the up-to-date information in the BNF for detailed advice. The absence of safety information for many drugs in lactation means that only essential drugs should be given to mothers during breastfeeding.

PHARMACOKINETICS IN LACTATION

Several factors influence drug transfer from the maternal circulation into breast milk, including the characteristics of the milk, the physicochemical properties of the drug and the amount of drug in the maternal circulation. The concentrations of drugs in breast milk are in equilibrium with those in the maternal circulation. At equilibrium, the free concentration in milk and plasma will be the same, but the total

Table 56.1 Examples of drug-induced teratogenicity and fetal/neonatal toxicity

Therapeutic drug	Teratogenic and adverse effects in fetus and neonate
ACE inhibitors	Affect fetal and neonatal blood pressure control and renal function; oligohydramnios
Alcohol	Fetal alcohol syndrome; growth restriction (Ch. 54)
Aminoglycosides	Auditory or vestibular nerve damage
Amiodarone	Neonatal goitre
Androgens	Virilisation of female fetus
Anti-cancer drugs	Carcinogenic and teratogenic effects (also avoid before pregnancy)
Barbiturates	Fetal abnormalities; withdrawal effects in neonates
Benzodiazepines	Withdrawal effects in neonates
Beta-adrenoceptor antagonists	Intra-uterine growth restriction, neonatal hypoglycaemia and bradycardia
Carbamazepine	Neural tube defects
Carbimazole	Neonatal goitre
Corticosteroids	Intra-uterine growth suppression (with prolonged treatment)
Dapsone	Neonatal haemolysis and methaemoglobinaemia
Diethylstilbestrol	Hypogonadism in male offspring and vaginal cancer in female offspring
Fibrinolytics	Premature separation of placenta in first 18 weeks
Lamotrigine	Teratogenicity
Leflunomide	Teratogenic in animals; effective contraception necessary for at least 2 years after end of treatment for women and 3 months for men
Lithium salts	Teratogenicity; cardiac abnormalities
NSAIDs	Premature closure of ductus arteriosus; pulmonary hypertension
Opioids	Neonatal respiratory depression and risk of withdrawal syndrome if the mother is habituated
Oral anticoagulants	Malformations; fetal or neonatal haemorrhage
Oxcarbazepine	Neural tube defects
Phenytoin	Congenital malformations; risk of neonatal haemorrhage due to vitamin K deficiency
Primaquine	Neonatal haemolysis and methaemoglobinaemia
Retinoids and retinoid-like drugs	Teratogenic, craniofacial malformations; some have long half-lives and effective contraception is essential for prolonged periods after stopping treatment and before pregnancy
Ribavirin	Teratogenic in animals; effective contraception necessary for at least 6 months after treatment for both women and men
Statins	Decreased cholesterol synthesis affects fetal development
Sulphonamides	Neonatal haemolysis and methaemoglobinaemia
Sulfonylureas	Neonatal hypoglycaemia
Thiazide diuretics	Growth retardation; electrolyte disturbance
Valproate	Congenital malformations and developmental delay in offspring

See BNF for detailed advice.
Manufacturers of most drugs advise that they should be taken in pregnancy only if the potential benefit outweighs the possible risk; also, many recommend that prescribing to women of childbearing age should be carried out with pregnancy in mind and contraception should be adequate before, during and after treatment. ACE, angiotensin-converting enzyme; NSAIDs, non-steroidal anti-inflammatory drugs.

concentration will be influenced by the extent of protein binding and uptake into the lipid phase (see Fig. 2.3). Water-soluble drugs diffuse from plasma into milk, and the concentration in breast milk is similar to the non-protein-bound fraction in the maternal plasma. Lipid-soluble compounds diffuse into breast milk and may concentrate because of the high fat content in milk.

The effects of drugs in breast milk depend not only on maternal pharmacokinetics but also on the extent of absorption, distribution and elimination of the drug in the neonate or infant (see below). Drugs may also have different pharmacodynamic properties in neonates or infants compared to older children and adults. If drugs are given during breast feeding, compounds with short half-lives are preferred because they are less likely to accumulate in neonates, who have lower drug clearance. Neonatal exposure can also be minimised if the feed is timed to coincide with the trough blood concentration in the mother, which is just before a dose is taken. The World Health Organization (WHO) nevertheless recommends that the health and developmental benefits of breastfeeding are usually greater than any likely risk from drugs in breast milk.

PRESCRIBING FOR CHILDREN

Both the pharmacokinetics and responses to drugs may differ in neonates, infants and children compared with adults. There are considerable differences among neonates (<1 month), infants (1–12 months) and children, because many metabolic and physiological processes are immature at birth and develop rapidly in the first months of life. These differences may affect the absorption and distribution of drugs and the rate of elimination of the drug from the body, and also the sensitivity of tissues to its actions or adverse effects. Particular care is needed in prescribing drugs that may affect growing or maturing organ systems such as the bones and teeth and the reproductive system. Box 56.1 shows some of the differences between the young and adults.

Although medicines should usually be used within the terms of the product license, many drugs given to children have not undergone formal clinical evaluation in this age group, and are not specifically licensed for paediatric use. It is recognised that 'off-label' prescribing may be necessary and the UK Medicines Act (1968) does not prohibit such unlicensed use. There is an increasing recognition of the need for formal clinical trials in the paediatric population, but such studies raise significant ethical issues. The BNF for Children (www.bnf.org/bnf/index.htm) gives specific guidance on prescribing for children in the UK and further information on the regulation of paediatric medicines is available at the following places.

UK: www.mhra.gov.uk/Howweregulate/Medicines/
Medicinesforchildren/index.htm

EU: http://ec.europa.eu/health/human-use/paediatric-
medicines/index_en.htm
USA: www.fda.gov/oc/opt/default.htm

PHARMACOKINETICS IN NEONATES AND CHILDREN

In neonates, inefficient metabolism and renal clearance mean that lower doses of some drugs are needed after allowing for body weight, and doses need to be calculated with special care. The processes of drug elimination are largely mature by a few weeks of age, after which drug clearance (adjusted to body weight) is similar to or higher than that in adults (see below). However, children may be more susceptible to effects on growing or maturing tissues and organs. Generalisations are difficult and each drug needs to be considered in its own right.

Absorption

Slow rates of gastric emptying and intestinal transit may reduce the rate of drug absorption in neonates, but total absorption of poorly absorbed drugs may eventually be more complete because of longer contact with the intestinal mucosa. In the neonate, gastric pH is neutral and this can reduce the absorption of weak acids but increase the absorption of weak bases.

Distribution

Neonates and young children have a lower body fat content and higher total body water than adults; this influences the distribution of both lipid- and water-soluble drugs. Neonates have a lower plasma albumin concentration, which also has a lower affinity for drug binding. In addition, the higher plasma concentrations of free fatty acids and bilirubin compete with drugs for plasma protein-binding sites. The overall effect is reduced plasma protein binding, which not only increases the apparent volume of distribution of the drug but also increases the proportion of drug able to cross the blood–brain barrier; it also increases the amounts diffusing into the liver and therefore available for metabolism. Drugs that are strongly bound to albumin should not be used during neonatal jaundice because the drugs may displace bilirubin (which is mostly in the unconjugated form) from protein-binding sites and increase the risk of kernicterus.

Metabolism

The drug-metabolising enzyme systems are immature in the neonatal liver, and first-pass metabolism and hepatic drug clearance are low, especially for substrates of CYP1A2, CYP3A4 and glucuronidation. The clearances for substrates for these enzymes are two to six times lower in neonates compared with adults. When the enzyme systems mature, drug metabolism processes become more extensive. Plasma drug clearance is often higher in young children than in adults, because of their higher relative liver mass and greater hepatic blood flow per kilogram of body weight; hepatic blood flow is the rate-limiting step in the elimination of high-clearance drugs.

Box 56.1 Developmental changes in the young that may alter drug handling compared with adults

Low production of gastric acid and erratic gastric emptying in first year of life
Smaller gut surface area/body mass ratio, but greater gut permeability to larger molecules
Greater proportion of body fat and larger extracellular volume may alter the volumes of distribution of some drugs
Maturation of drug metabolising enzyme pathways in the liver occurs at different rates over the first year
Glomerular filtration rate and tubular secretion are relatively low in the first year of life
Lower populations and reduced function of some gut flora

Renal elimination

Renal function in the neonate and infant is much less developed than in children or adults. The glomerular filtration rate in the newborn is about 40% of the adult level, and tubular secretory processes are poorly developed. Elimination of drugs such as digoxin, gentamicin and penicillin will therefore be slower until about 6–8 months of age.

In children, the larger volume of distribution and faster hepatic elimination mean that doses of metabolised drugs need to be higher than in adults after correcting for the difference in body weight. Prescribed doses are most accurately judged by considering both age and body surface area. In children, body surface area is a better guide to appropriate drug dosage than body weight. It can be estimated from a nomogram or by using the Du Bois formula:

$$\text{Body surface area} = 71.84 \times \text{weight}^{0.425} \times \text{height}^{0.725}$$

where body surface area is in square metres, weight in kilograms and height in metres. The drug dose for a child can be then approximated as:

$$\frac{\text{Adult dose} \times \text{surface area of child (in m}^2)}{1.8}$$

where 1.8 m^2 is the average body surface area of a 70 kg adult.

PRESCRIBING FOR THE ELDERLY

The elderly (usually taken to mean those over 70 years old) comprise a heterogeneous group who show considerable variation in 'biological' age. Changes occur in both the pharmacodynamics and pharmacokinetics of drugs with increasing age.

The density or numbers of receptors may be reduced with age; for example, β-adrenoceptors decrease in number, reducing the response to agonist drugs. The elderly are often more susceptible to sedatives, hypnotics and antipsychotic drugs, possibly because of changes in receptor numbers and/or reduced efficiency of the blood–brain barrier. They are also more susceptible to the adverse effects of NSAIDs on the gut.

Altered structure and function of target organs can also influence the effects of drugs. For example, baroreceptor function is impaired in the elderly and vasodilator drugs are more likely to provoke postural hypotension. The high peripheral resistance and less distensible arterial tree found with increasing age also respond less well to arterial vasodilators.

These changes reflect the ageing process itself, but they are often complicated by the presence of chronic disease (frequently involving multiple pathological processes) and variation due to both genetic and environmental influences. The risks of unwanted effects are higher in the elderly as a consequence of these changes. Significant numbers of hospital admissions in the elderly are due to adverse drug reactions, most of which are the more predictable type A effects (see Ch. 53). In addition, drug interactions are more common in the elderly because of the coexistence of different treatable conditions requiring the simultaneous use of several drugs (polypharmacy). For these reasons, it is usual to start drug treatment in the elderly with the smallest effective dose. Rational prescribers should also seek to minimise the numbers of drugs used, with clear explanations of usage instructions and regular review of drug regimens.

PHARMACOKINETICS IN THE ELDERLY

Absorption

Drug absorption across the gut wall is not greatly affected by ageing, although bioavailability may be increased due to reduced first-pass metabolism.

Distribution

Older people tend to have a lower lean body mass and a relative increase in body fat compared with young adults. The apparent volume of distribution (V_d) of water-soluble drugs such as digoxin may therefore be lower in the elderly and a smaller loading dose would be needed. Conversely, lipid-soluble drugs may be eliminated more slowly because of their increased V_d resulting from increased body fat and reduced hepatic metabolism.

Metabolism

The size of the liver and its blood flow decrease with age. Although enzyme activity per hepatocyte probably shows little change, the overall capacity for drug metabolism, particularly phase 1 metabolic reactions (Ch. 2), is reduced. This is particularly important for lipid-soluble drugs, such as nifedipine or propranolol, which undergo extensive first-pass metabolism, because lower hepatic metabolism increases bioavailability and reduces systemic clearance.

Renal elimination

Increasing age is also associated with a progressive reduction in glomerular filtration rate (GFR), so the elimination of polar drugs and metabolites is slower. This can produce toxicity when renally eliminated drugs with a low therapeutic index are prescribed in the elderly, for example lithium, digoxin or gentamicin. Creatinine clearance, which is an estimate of GFR, usually correlates well with the clearance of drugs that are eliminated in the urine unchanged as the parent drug. Reduced muscle mass in elderly people results in reduced creatinine production. Plasma creatinine in the elderly therefore frequently remains within the normal laboratory reference range even when renal function is substantially reduced, because the decreased creatinine production balances its reduced elimination. The Cockcroft and Gault equation, which relates plasma creatinine to creatinine clearance, contains elements reflecting sex- and age-dependent differences in muscle mass.

Creatinine clearance (mL·min^{-1}) for males equals:

$$\frac{1.23 \times (140 - \text{age in years}) \times \text{weight (in kg)}}{\text{plasma creatinine } (\mu \text{mol·L}^{-1})}$$

and for females it equals:

$$\frac{1.04 \times (140 - \text{age in years}) \times \text{weight (in kg)}}{\text{plasma creatinine } (\mu \text{ mol} \cdot \text{L}^{-1})}$$

As an alternative, the eGFR (see below) is used to approximate GFR.

PRESCRIBING IN RENAL FAILURE

Individuals with renal failure show increased responses to many drugs, especially when the drug, or its active metabolite, is eliminated in the urine. The extent to which dose adjustment is necessary depends on the extent of renal impairment and on the proportion of total plasma clearance that is due to renal clearance. The estimated glomerular filtration rate (eGFR) is often reported with laboratory estimations of serum creatinine. This is a useful guide to renal function, but does not consider weight as a variable that affects GFR. Nevertheless, for most drugs that are excreted by the kidney it is an adequate guide for dosage adjustment.

There are also pharmacodynamic changes in renal failure; for example, there are altered responses to drugs in people with uraemia, and drugs acting on the central nervous system (CNS) in particular produce enhanced responses, possibly because of increased permeability of the blood–brain barrier.

The BNF gives advice on drug prescribing to those with renal impairment. People with renal impairment may show an abnormal drug response due to one or more of the following factors:

- failure to excrete the drug or its metabolites may produce toxicity,
- there may be increased sensitivity, even if elimination is unaltered,
- many unwanted effects are poorly tolerated in such individuals,
- some drugs cease to be effective in such individuals.

PHARMACOKINETICS IN RENAL FAILURE

The activity of most drugs is not affected by impaired renal function, because most drugs are cleared by hepatic metabolism, but the kidneys provide the major route of elimination for water-soluble drugs and water-soluble metabolites (see Ch. 2). Renal elimination of drugs can be affected indirectly by abnormal renal perfusion, such as might occur in shock, or directly by changes in the kidney, for example renal tubular necrosis. Reduced renal function may increase the risk of toxicity from the parent drug or its metabolites due to their accumulation in the body, or toxicity may arise due to increased sensitivity in renal failure without an obvious impairment in drug elimination.

There are several other ways in which renal impairment may influence the handling of drugs.

- Metabolism in the liver can be impaired in people with uraemia, particularly metabolic reactions involving reduction, acetylation and ester hydrolysis.

- The kidney has important metabolic activities, such as the 1-α-hydroxylation of vitamin D and the degradation of insulin, both of which can be impaired in renal failure.
- The distribution of drugs can be affected by changes in fluid balance in renal failure, and more importantly by altered protein binding (see below). Circulating concentrations of albumin are decreased in severe renal failure with proteinuria. In addition, retained endogenous metabolites, such as the tryptophan metabolite indican, may compete for drug-binding sites on plasma proteins. The increased concentrations of free drug can lead to an enhanced response or to its increased elimination by glomerular filtration or metabolism.
- Tissue binding of digoxin is reduced in renal failure, so a lower loading dose should be given to compensate for the reduced volume of distribution.

The elimination of drugs by the kidney is significantly impaired only when the glomerular filtration rate is reduced below 50 mL·min^{-1}. For some drugs, clinically important accumulation does not occur until much lower filtration rates. Changes in renal tubular secretion of drugs in renal disease are less well understood.

A reduction in drug dosage in renal failure is usually necessary only if a high proportion of the drug is eliminated by the kidney and when the compound has a low therapeutic index. Maintenance dosage may be lowered by either reducing the dose or increasing the dose interval (see Ch. 2, equation 2.24). Loading doses do not usually require any modification. Large dose modifications are rarely needed for drugs that do not have dose-related unwanted effects. For the purposes of prescribing and dosage adjustment in renal impairment, the BNF uses the classification of Chronic Kidney Disease based on eGFR values (in mL/min/1.73 m^2):

- stage 1 (normal): eGFR >90 (with other evidence of kidney damage),
- stage 2 (mild): eGFR 60–89 (with other evidence of kidney damage),
- stage 3 (moderate): eGFR 30–59,
- stage 4 (severe): eGFR15–29,
- stage 5 (established renal failure): eGFR <15.

For some drugs, only established renal failure (stage 5) needs to be considered (for example, a reduction in dosage is recommended for ampicillin), while for other drugs even mild impairment (stage 2) may be important (for example, dosage reduction is recommended for carboplatin, whereas cisplatin should be avoided).

A further important consideration is the avoidance of drugs that have toxic effects on the kidney. Use of these in renal impairment can sometimes produce an irreversible decline in renal function.

PRESCRIBING IN LIVER DISEASE

Changes in both drug responses and pharmacokinetics can occur in liver disease. The BNF lists six main potential problems in prescribing for individuals with liver disease:

- impaired drug metabolism,
- hypoproteinaemia,
- reduced blood coagulation,

- hepatic encephalopathy,
- fluid overload,
- hepatotoxic drugs.

The severity of the liver disease is important, as is whether the disease is decompensated and includes jaundice, hypoproteinaemia or encephalopathy. Many of the pharmacodynamic and pharmacokinetic changes in liver failure arise from decreased hepatic synthesis of proteins that perform essential functions within the hepatocyte, or which are released into the blood, such as albumin and clotting factors.

CNS-depressant drugs such as morphine and chlorpromazine have an enhanced effect in people with liver failure. This is caused by increased sensitivity of neuronal tissue and can provoke encephalopathy in susceptible people. Decreased plasma protein binding may contribute to this greater sensitivity by increasing the percentage of free drug so that more drug crosses the blood–brain barrier. Benzodiazepines used during investigational procedures in individuals with liver failure can produce profound and long-lasting effects, which may require reversal by the administration of the benzodiazepine antagonist flumazenil.

Encephalopathy may be triggered by drugs that cause constipation (which increases the formation of potentially toxic metabolites, such as ammonia, by the intestinal bacteria). Diuretics that produce hypokalaemia can also precipitate hepatic encephalopathy in chronic liver disease. Therefore, potassium-sparing diuretics such as spironolactone are usually preferred to diuretics such as furosemide; an additional advantage of spironolactone is that it blocks the effects of circulating aldosterone, which is often increased in decompensated liver disease.

The reduced ability to synthesise vitamin K-dependent clotting factors makes people with chronic liver disease prone to clotting problems; they would be very sensitive to anticoagulant drugs, which are clearly contraindicated.

People with pre-existing liver disease are likely to be more susceptible to hepatotoxic drugs. This raises a problem for pain relief, since paracetamol is hepatotoxic at high doses, whereas NSAIDs can increase the risk of gastrointestinal bleeding and cause fluid retention, while opioids can precipitate encephalopathy. In practice, lower doses of paracetamol are usually given, taking care that the amounts do not exceed the reduced threshold for hepatotoxicity shown by such individuals (see Ch. 53).

PHARMACOKINETICS IN LIVER DISEASE

The rate of absorption of drugs from the gut lumen is not greatly affected in liver disease, but other aspects of drug handling may be altered. Distribution of drugs may be affected if synthesis of albumin is reduced, resulting in a higher percentage of free drug in plasma and possibly a greater risk of toxicity; examples of highly protein-bound drugs are phenytoin and prednisolone. Free drug concentrations may also be increased by elevated plasma bilirubin, which can displace drugs such as lidocaine and propranolol from their plasma protein-binding sites.

The liver has characteristics that facilitate the rapid and extensive uptake and metabolism of lipid-soluble drugs (Fig. 56.2). These include:

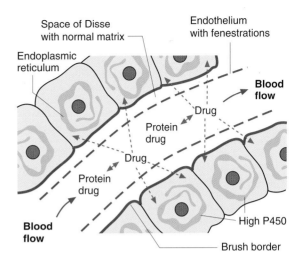

Fig. 56.2 Drug uptake from the sinusoid of a normal healthy liver.

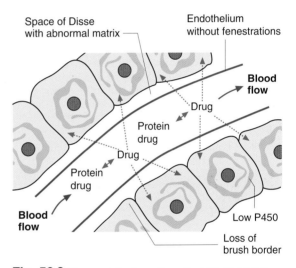

Fig. 56.3 Drug uptake from the sinusoid of a liver showing characteristic features of cirrhosis.

- fenestrations in the endothelium, allowing ready access to extracellular fluid,
- rapid diffusion across the space of Disse (which is a matrix consisting primarily of type 4 collagen),
- a brush border on hepatocytes, allowing rapid uptake,
- high intracellular enzyme activity for both phase 1 and phase 2 metabolism.

During chronic liver disease, a number of changes may occur that reduce the capacity of the liver to metabolise drugs (Fig. 56.3):

- fenestrations in the endothelium are lost,
- diffusion across the space of Disse may be reduced in fibrosis/cirrhosis as type 4 collagen is replaced by type 1 and type 3 collagen (which can form dense fibrils),
- the brush border on hepatocytes is lost,
- intracellular enzyme activity is reduced,
- intrahepatic vascular shunts may reduce the perfusion of hepatocytes.

Reduced hepatic uptake and metabolism or decreased biliary excretion of drugs may result in a greater proportion of the drug or its metabolites being eliminated by other routes, such as the urine.

First-pass metabolism may be considerably reduced in conditions such as liver cirrhosis; the consequences are most apparent with drugs that normally undergo extensive hepatic first-pass metabolism. In liver failure, their bioavailability may increase considerably from <20% to almost 100%.

Biliary excretion is impaired in conditions causing reduced formation of bile. A correlation between drug clearance and serum bilirubin would be expected for drugs eliminated unchanged in bile, such as rifampicin and fusidic acid. Reduced biliary elimination of drug metabolites could affect enterohepatic circulation (Ch. 2). Reduced bile production can affect the absorption of highly lipid-soluble molecules, such as the fat-soluble vitamins, that require micelle formation for effective absorption.

Systemic clearance may be reduced for drugs eliminated by hepatic metabolism. The changes that occur in liver disease affect both high-clearance drugs, where the elimination rate is dependent on effective liver blood flow, and low-clearance drugs, where it is dependent on hepatic extraction and enzyme activity.

Prescribing in liver disease should be undertaken with care, and drugs that are extensively metabolised by the liver should be given in smaller doses. The need for dose reduction arises primarily from an increase in bioavailability and a decrease in systemic clearance, both of which increase the average steady-state plasma concentration.

PRESCRIBING IN PALLIATIVE CARE

Symptom relief in palliative care often presents challenges to the prescriber, and the evidence to guide choice of treatments is often derived from experience rather than controlled trials. Palliative care services produce comprehensive guidelines for symptom control, often advising use of drugs for unlicensed indications. Awareness of psychological, emotional and social contributors to symptoms will help to guide strategies for management. The following synopsis is not comprehensive, but covers an approach to some key symptoms.

PAIN

Accurate diagnosis of the cause of pain is essential for a rational approach to therapy. The principles of the WHO analgesic ladder apply (Ch. 19). Analgesics should be given regularly, and preferably by mouth with additional methods of pain control considered in all cases. These may include co-analgesics for neuropathic pain (Ch. 19), surgery, radiotherapy, nerve blocks, TENS, acupuncture and addressing psychological problems.

If a strong opioid is needed, then immediate-release morphine every 4 h is preferred initially, increasing the dose by 30–50% every 2–3 days as required. When pain control is achieved, modified-release morphine every 12 h can be used (giving the same total daily dose), with immediate-release morphine for breakthrough pain. Continuing pain despite persisting unwanted effects such as drowsiness suggests that the pain is not fully opioid-responsive. A laxative should always be given with a strong opioid.

Alternative opioids for palliative care include oxycodone or hydromorphone (which have a slightly different unwanted effect profile), diamorphine for higher doses by subcutaneous infusion (can be given in a smaller volume of fluid), methadone (particularly for neuropathic pain) or fentanyl (for transcutaneous use or in severe chronic kidney disease). Transdermal delivery of an opioid can be helpful if there is vomiting, intractable constipation or other unwanted effects in the presence of opioid-responsive pain. Care must be taken to give equivalent doses when changing from one opioid to another.

NAUSEA AND VOMITING

It is important to identify the cause if possible, since this will guide treatment. Drug therapy should always be considered as a cause of vomiting, and the responsible drug stopped or the dose reduced if possible. Non-drug measures include psychotherapeutic techniques, acupuncture, acupressure and ginger.

If drug therapy is required, then the choice will depend on the predominant contributory causes (Ch. 32). Examples include dexamethasone for raised intracranial pressure, levomepromazine or benzodiazepines for anxiety, metoclopramide or prochlorperazine for drug-related vomiting, metoclopramide for gastric stasis, and metoclopramide, levomepromazine or cyclizine if the cause is not clear.

ANOREXIA/CACHEXIA/FATIGUE SYNDROME

This syndrome arises in terminal cancer, heart failure and with chronic infection or inflammation. There is usually profound loss of weight and muscle bulk. It is often not possible to deal with causative factors, and management may include dexamethasone to suppress inflammation, methylphenidate, or modafinil (Ch. 22) for fatigue and encouraging exercise.

Constipation

Constipation may arise from drug therapy (e.g. opioids, antidepressants, antispasmodics, ondansetron), inactivity, dehydration, hypercalcaemia or concurrent disease. Adequate fluid intake is important and if the underlying cause is not amenable to treatment then symptomatic treatment should be given (Ch. 35). Macrogols are usually used for opioid-induced constipation, although a stimulant such as senna may also be needed.

Breathlessness

Breathlessness is often multifactorial, and specific treatments may be successful. If there is no treatable cause then nebulised saline can help to loosen secretions. Morphine, sometimes together with a benzodiazepine such as diazepam, can reduce the subjective sensation of breathlessness.

Hiccups

Hiccups can have a peripheral cause such as gastric distention, diaphragmatic irritation, liver enlargement or intrathoracic tumour. A variety of treatments have been advocated, indicating that all have limited efficacy. Options include metoclopramide, domperidone, a proton pump inhibitor, dexamethasone, baclofen and nifedipine. Central causes include raised intracranial pressure and uraemia, and treatment options include dexamathasone, levomepromazine, haloperidol and diazepam.

Use of a syringe driver

Near the end of life drugs may need to be given by subcutaneous infusion via a small battery-powered pump. Maintaining steady plasma drug concentrations may aid symptom control or give relief in someone who cannot swallow. Examples of drugs given by this route are:

- cyclizine, haloperidol or metoclopramide for vomiting,
- dexamethasone for neuropathic pain, raised intracranial pressure or vomiting,
- morphine, oxycodone or diamorphine for pain control,
- glycopyrronium to reduce respiratory secretions,
- hyoscine to relieve intestinal colic and to reduce secretions,
- levomepromazine for vomiting or as a sedative,
- midazolam for vomiting or seizures.

DRUG INTERACTIONS

Many people take more than one drug during a course of treatment because:

- combination therapy is preferable or necessary for producing an adequate effect or response; important examples are the chemotherapy of malignant disease and the treatment of hypertension,
- a single condition or pathology may give rise to a variety of symptoms that are controlled by different drugs,
- the person may suffer from more than one condition or pathology requiring treatment with drugs that are unrelated pharmacologically.

The term 'interaction' implies that the response to the combination of drugs is different to that which could be predicted from a simple summation of the effects of each drug given singly.

The consequences of treatment with a combination of drugs can be divided into four different types:

- **dose-addition**, where each drug produces the same response and the magnitude of response to the combination of both drugs is given by simple addition of the doses, after allowing for any difference in potency; this is the usual situation when more than one drug is used to treat a single condition,
- **response-addition**, where each drug produces a different response and their combination gives each response as if the other drug were not present; this is the usual situation when two drugs are used to treat two different conditions,

- **synergism**, where the magnitude of response to a drug combination is greater than would be predicted by simple addition of the separate drug doses, after allowing for any difference in potency; synergism is often produced when the drugs have different mechanisms or act at different steps in the process leading to the overall response,
- **antagonism**, where the magnitude of response to a drug combination is lower than would be predicted by simple addition of the doses, after allowing for any difference in potency; this sort of interaction can occur if a partial receptor agonist is given with a full agonist at the same receptor and reduces the overall activity.

Interactions that result in antagonism or synergism may be beneficial, or potentially harmful because of a lack of clinical response or the risk of toxicity. Beneficial interactions are usually well characterised and have clear advantages – for example, combinations of different anti-cancer drugs – and are the basis of prescribing recommendations. This section therefore focuses on adverse interactions, which are of greatest importance for drugs that have a narrow therapeutic index and for groups of people at increased risk, such as the elderly.

Drug interactions may arise at the site of the mechanism of action (pharmacodynamic) or from altered delivery of the drug to its site of action (pharmacokinetic).

PHARMACODYNAMIC INTERACTIONS

Pharmacodynamic interactions are usually predictable based on the known mechanisms of action of the drugs. Interactions may relate to the principal site of action of the drug, or to secondary sites of action that are responsible for unwanted effects. In principle, drugs that are highly selective for a single site of action are less likely to produce pharmacodynamic interactions than drugs that show low selectivity. An example of a serious adverse synergistic interaction is between an angiotensin-converting enzyme (ACE) inhibitor, such as enalapril (Ch. 6) and spironolactone (Ch. 14); the ACE inhibitor reduces the production of aldosterone, thereby reducing the excretion of K^+, an effect which is exaggerated by the action of spironolactone, and the combination can cause potentially life-threatening hyperkalaemia.

PHARMACOKINETIC INTERACTIONS

Absorption

Co-administration of two drugs could give an interaction if one drug affects the rate or extent of absorption of the other drug. Changes in the rate of absorption, for example by increasing or decreasing gastric emptying or intestinal motility, will affect the peak concentration, but not usually the extent of absorption. Interactions affecting the extent of absorption are usually more important; examples include the retention of drugs in the gut lumen (e.g. tetracycline antibiotics bind to divalent or trivalent metals, such as Ca^{2+} or Fe^{3+}, to form complexes that are not absorbed) and the inhibition or induction of first-pass metabolism of drugs in the gut lumen, gut wall or liver.

Distribution

The main interactions affecting drug distribution arise from competition for the non-specific binding sites on plasma proteins, such as albumin (see Table 2.3). Interactions affecting plasma protein binding may be clinically relevant when:

- the displaced drug is highly protein bound; for example, if competition for protein-binding sites reduces binding from 98 to 96%, this will double the free drug concentration in plasma (from 2 to 4%); in contrast, a 2% change in the binding of a drug that is only 50% bound would not be clinically or biologically significant,
- the displaced drug has a narrow therapeutic index, so that a two- to three-fold change in free drug concentration greatly increases the risk of drug toxicity,
- the displaced drug has a low apparent volume of distribution, such that the plasma contains a significant proportion of the total body load,
- the displacing drug is of such low potency that large doses must be given and the number of protein-binding sites becomes limiting.

Metabolism

Perhaps surprisingly, the simultaneous administration of two drugs that share a common pathway of metabolism rarely causes an interaction. This is because therapeutic drug concentrations are usually far below the K_m values of the metabolising enzymes, such as cytochrome P450. The enzymes therefore do not become saturated and first-order kinetics (Ch. 2) still apply. An exception is the zero-order (saturated) metabolism of ethanol and methanol by alcohol dehydrogenase; this allows ethanol to be used to slow the metabolism of methanol to its toxic products and reduce the risk of blindness (Ch. 53).

Important interactions can occur, however, when one drug induces or inhibits the enzymes involved in the metabolism of another drug. This is well recognised for drugs affecting the cytochrome P450 enzyme system because of the large number of P450 isoenzymes and their importance for the elimination of most drugs (Table 2.7). Induction or inhibition of hepatic enzymes can affect both systemic clearance and first-pass metabolism after oral dosage.

Enzyme inhibition occurs as soon as the inhibiting drug concentration is sufficiently high, and can occur after a single dose (e.g. cimetidine). In contrast, enzyme induction requires a few days as it results from gene transcription and translation of additional enzyme; the increased enzyme activity then reduces the concentrations of the other drug. This may decrease the clinical response to the second compound, if it is an active drug, or it could increase the bioactivation of a prodrug to an active metabolite. When dosage with an enzyme-inducing drug is stopped, the enzyme activity usually declines over a period of 2–3 weeks. If the dosage of the second drug has been optimised for the drug combination, its plasma concentration may then increase markedly, giving a risk of toxicity.

Excretion

Each of the three processes involved in the renal elimination of drugs – that is, glomerular filtration, pH-dependent reabsorption and renal tubular secretion – can be a site for drug interactions.

- Glomerular filtration depends on renal perfusion and only removes free drug (not protein-bound). In consequence, drugs affecting renal perfusion or plasma protein binding can give rise to interactions.
- pH-dependent reabsorption could be altered by drugs that affect urine pH, either directly or via metabolic effects; for example, the pH changes associated with aspirin overdose can affect the excretion of drugs taken concurrently.
- Renal tubular secretion can give rise to interactions when there is competition for the transporter system. Aspirin can interfere with the transport of both endogenous compounds (e.g. uric acid) and drugs (e.g. methotrexate).

The biliary excretion of drugs is not an important site for drug interactions, but the enterohepatic cycling of drugs can be affected by the co-administration of poorly absorbed broad-spectrum antibacterials, which affect the hydrolysis of drug conjugates in the lower bowel (Fig. 2.13).

SELF-ASSESSMENT

True/false questions

1. The highest risk of teratogenicity is during the final trimester of pregnancy.
2. Drug doses may need to be increased in pregnancy.
3. After correction for body weight, drug doses in children are the same as for adults.
4. The bioavailability of lipid-soluble drugs is increased in the elderly.
5. Most drugs are not affected by impaired renal function.
6. Drugs that cause constipation can trigger encephalopathy in people with chronic liver disease.
7. Drugs that delay gastric emptying reduce the extent of absorption of other drugs.
8. Enzyme inducers can enhance clinical responses to prodrugs.

True/false answers

1. **False.** The greatest risk of teratogenicity is during organogenesis in the first trimester.
2. **True.** While only the lowest effective doses of essential drugs should be used in pregnancy, these may need to be higher than in non-pregnant women, due to increased volume of distribution and higher clearance.
3. **False.** Correction for body weight may underestimate drug doses in children due to their relatively high hepatic clearance; correction by body surface area is a better guide.
4. **True.** Lipid-soluble drugs are typically cleared by hepatic metabolism; lower hepatic blood flow in the elderly can reduce first-pass metabolism and increase oral bioavailability.

5. **True.** Most drugs are cleared by hepatic metabolism, so the plasma concentration of the parent drug is not affected by impaired renal function.

6. **True.** In chronic liver disease, constipation can increase the risk of encephalopathy from the generation of ammonia and other toxic products by the gut flora.

7. **False.** Delayed gastric emptying will slow the rate of absorption of most drugs and reduce their peak plasma concentrations, but the extent of absorption is not usually affected.

8. **True.** Bioconversion of a prodrug to its active derivative may be enhanced by an enzyme inducer.

FURTHER READING

American Academy of Pediatrics (2001) Committee on Drugs. The transfer of drugs and other chemicals into human milk. *Pediatrics* 108, 776–789

Bressler R, Bahl JJ (2003) Principles of drug therapy for the elderly patient. *Mayo Clin Proc* 78, 1564–1577

Briggs GG, Freeman RK, Yaffe SJ (1998) Drugs in Pregnancy and Lactation. A Reference Guide to Fetal and Neonatal Risk, 5th edn. Baltimore: Williams and Wilkins

Cresswell KM, Fernando B, McKinstry B, Sheikh A (2007) Adverse drug events in the elderly. *Br Med Bull* 83, 259–274

Dickinson BD, Altman RD, Nielsen NH, Sterling ML, Council on Scientific Affairs, American Medical Association (2001) Drug interactions between oral contraceptives and antibiotics. *Obstet Gynecol* 98, 853–860

Dorne JLCM, Walton K, Renwick AG (2005) Human variability in xenobiotic metabolism and pathway-related uncertainty factors for chemical risk assessment: a review. *Food Chem Toxicol* 43, 203–216

Ito S (2000) Drug therapy for breast-feeding women. *N Engl J Med* 343, 118–126

Johnson TN (2003) The development of drug metabolising enzymes and their influence on the susceptibility to adverse drug reactions in children. *Toxicology* 192, 37–48

Koren G, Pastuszak A, Ito S (2000) Drugs in pregnancy. *N Engl J Med* 338, 1128–1137

Mallet L, Spinewine A, Huang A (2007) Prescribing in elderly people 2. The challenge of managing drug interactions in elderly people. *Lancet* 370, 185–191

Nunn T, Williams J (2005) Formulation of medicines for children. *Br J Clin Pharmacol* 59, 674–676

O'Mahony D, Gallagher PF (2008) Inappropriate prescribing in the older population: need for new criteria. *Age Ageing* 37, 138–141

Patsalos PN, Perucca E (2003) Clinically important drug interactions in epilepsy: interactions between antiepileptic drugs and other drugs. *Lancet Neurol* 2, 473–481

Routledge PA, O'Mahony MS, Woodhouse KW (2004) Adverse drug reactions in elderly patients. *Br J Clin Pharmacol* 57, 121–126

Spina E, Scordo MG, D'Arrigo C (2003) Metabolic drug interactions with new psychotropic agents. *Fundam Clin Pharmacol* 17, 517–538

Spinewine A, Schmader KE, Barber N et al. (2007) Prescribing in elderly people 1. Appropriate prescribing in elderly people: how well can it be measured and optimised? *Lancet* 370, 173–184

Stephenson T (2006) The medicines for children agenda in the UK. *Br J Clin Pharmacol* 61, 716–719

Turnheim K (2003) When drug therapy gets old: pharmacokinetics and pharmacodynamics in the elderly. *Exp Gerontol* 38, 843–853

Index

Please note that page references relating to non-textual content such as boxes, figures or tables are in *italics*.